McGraw-Hill's NPTE

(NATIONAL PHYSICAL THERAPY EXAMINATION)

Notice

McGraw-Hill's
NPTE
(NATIONAL PHYSICAL THERAPY EXAMINATION)

Second Edition

Mark Dutton, PT
Allegheny General Hospital
West Penn Allegheny Health System (WPAHS)
Adjunct Clinical Instructor, Duquesne University
School of Health Sciences
Pittsburgh, Pennsylvania

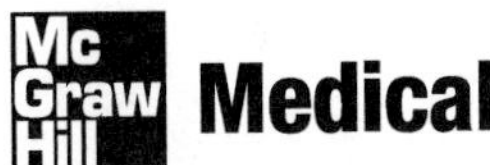

New York Chicago San Francisco Lisbon London
Madrid Mexico City Milan New Delhi
San Juan Seoul Singapore Sydney Toronto

The McGraw-Hill Companies

McGraw-Hill's NPTE (National Physical Therapy Examination), Second Edition

1 2 3 4 5 6 7 8 9 0 QDB/QDB 17 16 15 14 13 12

Set ISBN 978-0-07-177131-3
Set MHID 0-07-177131-X
Book ISBN 978-0-07-177129-0
Book MHID 0-07-177129-8
CD ISBN 978-0-07-177130-6
CD MHID 0-07-177130-1

The book was set in Garamond Light by Cenveo Publisher Services.
The editor was Brian Kearns.
The production supervisor was Sherri Souffrance.
Project management was provided by Kritika Kaul, Cenveo Publisher Services.
The cover designer was John Michael Graphics; main cover image © Michele Constantini/PhotoAlto/Corbis.
Quad/Graphics was printer and binder.

This book is printed on acid-free paper.

Library of Congress Cataloging-in-Publication Data

Dutton, Mark.
McGraw-Hill's NPTE (National Physical Therapy Exam) / Mark Dutton.—2nd ed.
p. ; cm.
NPTE (National Physical Therapy Examination)
National Physical Therapy Examination
Includes bibliographical references and index.
ISBN-13: 978-0-07-177131-3 (pbk. : alk. paper)
ISBN-10: 0-07-177131-X (pbk. : alk. paper)
I. Title. II. Title: NPTE (National Physical Therapy Examination).
III. Title: National Physical Therapy Examination.
[DNLM: 1. Physical Therapy Specialty—methods—Examination Questions.
2. Physical Therapy Modalities—Examination Questions. WB 18.2]
LC classification not assigned
615.8′2076—dc23 2011049555

Contents

Acknowledgments

- My family, especially my daughters Leah and Lauren. Time spent with my family is irreplaceable.
- My parents, Ron and Brenda.
- The exceptional team at McGraw-Hill—Joe Morita and Brian Kearns.
- To the production crew of Cenveo Publisher Services, especially the project manager Kritika Kaul.

Introduction

The purpose of this text is to help a physical therapist candidate prepare for the National Physical Therapy Examination (NPTE), and to equip the candidate with some excellent study tools. These study tools are designed to review the required level of didactic information, and to prepare for the NPTE by focusing on key topic areas.

The NPTE is a 5-hour, 250-question (200 scored, 50 pretest), multiple-choice examination. Preparing and sitting for such a comprehensive 5-hour examination can appear to be a daunting task. However, with the appropriate guidance about what to review from the pertinent subject areas, the student should be able to study with real direction and focus.

The information presented in this study guide is intended to be all-inclusive so that candidates do not have to use a number of texts to study for the examination. While it is hoped that the majority of information presented is familiar to candidates, some areas may require additional study prior to the examination. Special emphasis has been placed on subject areas that have traditionally been found to be weak. In addition to the chapters covering musculoskeletal, neuromuscular, cardiovascular, pulmonary, pediatric, geriatric, and integumentary physical therapy, there are also chapters on special topics such as administration, education, research, pharmacology, orthotics/prosthetics, adjuctive interventions, therapeutic exercise, and pathologic/psychological conditions. Given the importance that both the musculoskeletal and neurologic systems play in the field of physical therapy, greater emphasis is placed on these two systems, as is reflected in the relative size of their respective chapters. Illustrations and tables are provided throughout the text to help retain information. In addition, the layout of the book has been designed to allow candidates to add information in the margins.

The simulated examination questions on the CD-ROM are designed to help diagnose the strengths and vulnerabilities of the reader's academic and clinical backgrounds. After taking the simulated examination, the reader is provided with a performance analysis, which provides feedback about areas of vulnerability and strength, emphasizing those areas that require additional study. The examination that is provided on the CD-ROM is also available online, to provide the reader a true sense as to how it feels to sit in front of a computer and take the NPTE examination.

It is hoped that the contents of this book, the CD-ROM, and the online information will help the reader organize and focus his or her study in the most efficient and effective manner. This is a work in progress in the everchanging world of physical therapy. The author would welcome any suggestions for changes or additions. Please email your suggestions and comments to pt@mcgraw-hill.com.

Study Pearl

The Federation of State Boards of Physical Therapy (FSBPT) develops and administers the NPTE for both physical therapists and physical therapist assistants in 53 jurisdictions—the 50 states, the District of Columbia, Puerto Rico, and the Virgin Islands. Further information about the NPTE is available at http://www.fsbpt.org.

section I

The Profession

Who are Physical Therapists, and What Do They Do?

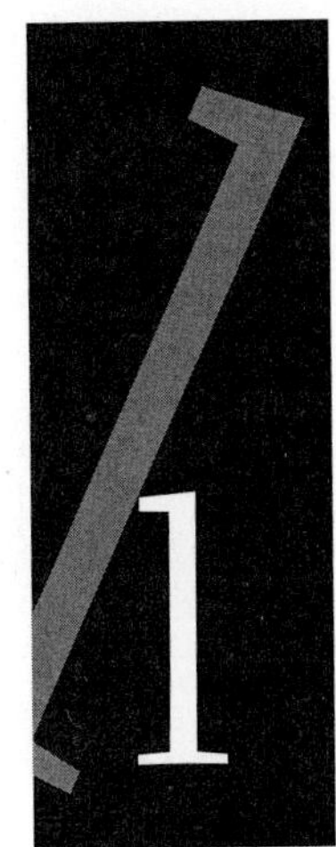

THE GUIDE

The *Guide to Physical Therapist Practice*, a detailed description of the practice of physical therapy, was first published in the November 1997 issue of *Physical Therapy*. A revision of the original *Guide* was published in 2001, and in 2003, the *Interactive Guide to Physical Therapist Practice* was released in the form of a CD-ROM. The purpose of the *Guide* was "to encourage a uniform approach to physical therapist practice and to explain to the world the nature of that practice."[1] The *Guide* is divided into two parts:

- Part 1: delineates the physical therapist's scope of practice and describes patient management by physical therapists (PTs).
- Part 2: describes each of the diagnostic preferred practice patterns of patients typically treated by PTs.

DEFINITION OF PHYSICAL THERAPY

The *Guide*[1] has defined physical therapy as follows:

> *Physical therapy includes diagnosis and management of movement dysfunction and enhancement of physical and functional abilities; restoration, maintenance, and promotion of optimal physical function, optimal fitness and wellness, and optimal quality of life as it relates to movement and health; and prevention of the onset, symptoms, and progression of impairments, functional limitations, and disabilities that may result from diseases, disorders, conditions, or injuries.*

SCOPE OF PRACTICE

Physical therapy is defined as the care and services provided by or under the direction and supervision of a PT.[1]

- PTs are the only professionals who provide physical therapy.
- Physical therapist assistants (PTAs)—under the direction and supervision of the PT—are the only paraprofessionals who assist in the provision of physical therapy interventions.

Study Pearl

- Patient—An individual who is receiving direct intervention for an impairment, functional limitation, disability, or changing physical function and health status resulting from injury, disease, or other causes; an individual receiving health care services.
- Client—A person who is not necessarily sick or injured but who can benefit from a PT's consultation, professional advice, or services. A client can also be a business, a school system, or other entity that may benefit from specific recommendations from a PT.

Education and Qualifications[1]

PTs are professionally educated at the college or university level and are required to be licensed in the state (or states) in which they practice. Education programs for the preparation of PTs have been recognized in some manner since 1928, when the American Physical Therapy Association (APTA) first published a list of approved programs.

> **Study Pearl**
>
> CAPTE only accredits entry-level PT and PTA education programs, not transitional Doctor of Physical Therapy (tDPT) programs, which are considered post-professional programs.

- Graduates from 1926 to 1959 who completed physical therapy curricula approved by appropriate accreditating bodies.
- Graduates from 1960 to the present who have successfully completed professional physical therapy education programs accredited by the Commission on Accreditation in Physical Therapy Education (CAPTE). CAPTE also makes autonomous decisions concerning the accreditation status of continuing education programs for the PTs and PTAs.

The APTA House of Delegates (HOD) first authorized the education of PTAs at the 1967 Annual Conference.

Practice Settings

PTs practice in a broad range of inpatient, outpatient, and community-based settings, including the following and those listed in Table 1-1.

Hospital. A hospital is an institution whose primary function is to provide inpatient diagnostic and therapeutic services for a wide variety of medical, surgical, and nonsurgical conditions. In addition, most hospitals provide some outpatient services, particularly emergency care. Hospitals may be classified in a number of ways, including:

- Length of stay (short-term or long-term).
  Acute-care (short-term hospital): an acute-care hospital can be defined as a facility that provides hospital care to patients who generally require a stay of up to 7 days, but less than 30 days, and whose focus is on a physical or mental condition requiring an immediate intervention and constant medical attention, equipment, and personnel. The goal of a hospital is for rapid discharge to the next level of care (home or to another health care facility) and the PT recommendation is very important in the discharge planning.
  Subacute: medical care provided to medically unstable patients who cannot return home. Required services (medical, nursing, rehabilitative) are provided within a hospital or skilled nursing facility.
- Teaching or nonteaching.
  Teaching: a hospital that serves as a teaching site for medicine, dentistry, allied health, nursing programs, or medical residency programs.
  Nonteaching: a hospital that has no teaching responsibilities, or one that serves as an elective site for health-related programs.

TABLE 1-1. PRACTICE SETTINGS

SETTING	CHARACTERISTICS	PHYSICAL THERAPIST ROLE
Primary care	▶ Basic or entry level of health care which includes diagnostic, therapeutic, or preventive services. ▶ Care is provided on an outpatient basis by primary-care physicians (PCP), including family practice physicians, internists, and pediatricians. These physicians often serve as *gatekeepers* to other subspecialists, such as physical therapy.	The physical therapist serves a supportive role for the primary care teams—provides examination, evaluation, diagnoses, prognosis, and intervention of musculoskeletal and neuromuscular dysfunctions.
Secondary (specialized) care	▶ Services provided by medical specialists, such as cardiologists, urologists, and dermatologists, who generally do not have first contact with the patients. ▶ This second level of care may require inpatient hospitalization or ambulatory same-day surgery.	Physical therapy involvement is minimal unless inpatient hospitalization is necessary.
Tertiary care (tertiary health care)	▶ Highly specialized care that is given to patients in a hospital setting who are in danger of disability or death (organ transplants, major surgical procedures). ▶ Services provided often require sophisticated technologies (eg, neurosurgeons or intensive care units). ▶ Specialized care usually provided because of a referral from primary or secondary medical care personnel.	Physical therapy may be consulted on an as-needed basis.
Transitional care unit	▶ Nonmedical-based facility, which may be in a group home or part of a continuum of a rehabilitation center. ▶ Typical stay is 4-8 months with discharge to home, assisted living facility, or skilled nursing facility (SNF). ▶ Greater focus placed on compensation versus restoration.	Physical therapy emphasis is on improving functional skills for maximum independence to prepare a patient for community reentry or for transfer to an assisted-living/skilled nursing facility.
Skilled nursing/ Extended care facility	▶ Freestanding facility or part of a hospital that is licensed and approved by the state (Medicare certified). ▶ Eligible individuals receive skilled nursing care and appropriate rehabilitative and restorative services. ▶ Accepts patients in need of rehabilitation and medical care that is of a lesser intensity than that received in the acute/subacute care setting of a hospital. ▶ Provides skilled services, including rehabilitation, and various other health services (nursing) on a daily basis (Medicare defines *daily* as 7 days a week of skilled nursing care and 5 days a week of skilled therapy). ▶ Physician orders must be rewritten every 60 days.	A SNF must be able to provide 24-hour nursing coverage, and the availability of physical, occupational, and speech therapy. Minimum data sets (MDS): federal data collection system for assessing nursing home patients. ▶ The MDS for nursing facility residents is a comprehensive resident assessment instrument (RAI) that measures functional status, mental health status, and behavioral status to identify chronic care patient needs and formalize a care plan in response to 18 resident assessment protocols (RAPs). ▶ Under federal regulation, assessments are conducted at a time of admission into a nursing facility, upon return from a 72-hour hospital admission, whenever there is a significant change in status, quarterly and annually.
Acute rehabilitation facility	▶ Usually based in a medical setting. ▶ Provides early rehabilitation, social, and vocational services once a patient is medically stable. ▶ Primary emphasis is to provide intensive physical and cognitive restorative services in the early months to disabled persons to facilitate their return to maximum functional capacity. ▶ Typical stay is 3-4 months (short-term).	Physical therapist involved in the coordinated services of medical, social, educational, vocational, and the other rehabilitative services (OT, speech).

(*Continued*)

TABLE 1-1. PRACTICE SETTINGS (*Continued*)

SETTING	CHARACTERISTICS	PHYSICAL THERAPIST ROLE
Chronic/Long-term care facility	▶ Long-term care facility that is facility- or community based. ▶ Sometimes referred to as *extended rehabilitation.* ▶ Designed for patients with permanent or residual disabilities caused by a nonreversible pathological health condition. Also used for patients who demonstrate slower than expected progress. ▶ Used as a placement facility—60 days or longer, but not for permanent stays.	The facility has a full range of rehabilitation services (physical, occupational, and speech therapy) available.
Comprehensive outpatient rehabilitation facility (CORF)	▶ A nonresidential facility established and operated exclusively for the purpose of providing outpatient diagnostic, therapeutic, and restorative services for the rehabilitation of injured, disabled, or sick persons, at a single fixed location, by or under the supervision of a physician. Services include: physician services, physical, occupational, and respiratory therapy; speech-language pathology services, prosthetic and orthotic devices, including testing, fitting, or training in the use of these devices, social and psychological services, nursing care provided by or under the supervision of a registered professional nurse, drugs and biologicals that cannot be self-administered, and supplies and durable medical equipment. ▶ CORFs are surveyed every 6 years at a minimum.	Physical therapy (and occupational therapy and speech-language pathology services) may be provided in an off-site location.
Custodial care facility	▶ Provides medical or nonmedical services, which do not seek to cure, but which are necessary for the patient who is unable to care for him/herself. ▶ Provided during periods when the medical condition of the patient is not changing. ▶ Patient does not require the continued administration of medical care by qualified medical personnel. ▶ This type of care is not usually covered under managed-care plans.	Physical therapy involvement is minimal.
Hospice care	▶ A facility or program that is licensed certified or otherwise authorized by law, which provides supportive care for the terminally ill. ▶ Focuses on the physical, spiritual, emotional, psychological, financial, and legal needs of the dying patient and the family. ▶ Services provided by an interdisciplinary team of professionals and perhaps volunteers in a variety of settings, including hospitals, freestanding facilities, and at home. ▶ Medicare and Medicaid require that at least 80% of hospice care is provided at home. Eligibility for reimbursement includes: • Medicare eligibility. • Certification of terminal illness (less than or equal to 6 months of life) by physician.	Physical therapy may be consulted on an as-needed basis.
Personal care	▶ Optional Medicaid benefit which allows a state to provide services to assist functionally impaired individuals in performing the activities of daily living (eg, bathing, dressing, feeding, grooming, etc.).	Physical therapy may be consulted on an as-needed basis.

(*Continued*)

TABLE 1-1. PRACTICE SETTINGS (*Continued*)

SETTING	CHARACTERISTICS	PHYSICAL THERAPIST ROLE
Ambulatory care (outpatient care)	▶ Includes outpatient preventative, diagnostic, and treatment services that are provided at medical offices, and surgery centers or outpatient clinics (including private practice physical therapy clinics, outpatient satellites of institutions, or hospitals). ▶ Designed for patients who do not require overnight hospitalization. ▶ More cost-effective than inpatient care, and therefore favored by managed-care plans.	Physical therapy may be consulted on an as-needed basis.

- Major types of services: psychiatric, tuberculosis, burn, general, and other specialties, such as maternity, pediatric, or ear, nose, and throat (ENT).
- Type of ownership or control: federal, state, or local government; for-profit and nonprofit.

Home Healthcare. Home healthcare involves the provision of medical or health care by a Home Health Agency (HHA), which may be governmental, voluntary, or private; nonprofit or for-profit. Home care services were introduced to reduce the need for hospitalization and its associated costs. A HHA provides part-time and intermittent skilled and non-skilled services and other therapeutic services on a visiting basis to persons of all ages in their homes. Patient eligibility includes:

- Any patient who is homebound or who has great difficulty leaving their home. A person may leave home for medical treatment or short infrequent nonmedical absences such as a religious service.
- Medicaid waiver clients. The Medicaid Waiver for the Elderly and Disabled (E&D Waiver) program is designed to provide services to seniors and the disabled whose needs would otherwise require them to live in a nursing home. The goal is for clients to retain their independence by providing services that allow them to live safely in their own homes and communities for as long as it is appropriate.
- A patient who requires skilled care from one of the following disciplines: nursing, physical therapy, occupational therapy, or speech therapy.
- Physician certification. In the case of an elderly patient, recertification by Medicare is required every 62 days. Medicare only pays for skilled home health services that are provided by a Medicare-certified agency. Medicare defines *intermittent* as skilled nursing care needed or given for less than 7 days each week, or less than 8 hours per day over a period of 21 days (or less) with some exceptions in special circumstances.
- Patients who continue to demonstrate the potential for progress.

The physical therapy focus includes:

- Environmental safety, including proper lighting, securing scatter rugs, handrails, wheelchair ramps, and raised toilet seats.
- Early intervention (refer to "School System")
- Addressing equipment needs:
  Equipment ordered in the hospital is reimbursable.
  Adaptive equipment ordered in the home is not reimbursable except for items such as wheelchairs, commodes, hospital beds, etc.
- Observing for any evidence of substance abuse, or physical abuse:
  Substance abuse should be reported immediately to the physician.
  Physical abuse should be immediately communicated to the proper authorities (varies from state to state).

School System. The major goal of physical therapy intervention in the school is to enhance the child's level of function in the school setting—the PT serves as a consultant to teachers working with children with disabilities in the classroom. Recommendations are made for adaptive equipment to facilitate improved posture, head control, and function.

- Early Intervention Program (EIP). National program designed for infants and toddlers with disabilities and for their families. The EIP was created by Congress in 1986 under the Individuals with Disabilities Education Act (IDEA)—refer to Chapter 16. To be eligible for services, children must be less than 3 years of age and have a confirmed disability, or established developmental delay, as defined by the State, in one or more of the following areas of development: physical, cognitive, communication, social-emotional, and/or adaptive.

Therapeutic and support services include:

- Family education and counseling, home visits, and parent support groups.
- Special instruction.
- Speech pathology and audiology.
- Occupational therapy.
- Physical therapy: PT can provide direct interventions within the classroom or other inclusion settings depending on the EIP.
- Psychological services.
- Service coordination.
- Nursing services.
- Nutrition services.
- Social work services.
- Vision services.
- Assistive technology devices and services.

Private Practice. Private practice settings are privately owned and freestanding independent physical therapy practices.

- Practice settings vary, from physical therapy and orthopedic clinics to rehabilitation agencies.
- Documentation is required for every visit. Reevaluations are required by Medicare every 30 days for reimbursement purposes.

CLINICAL EDUCATION OF STUDENTS

The term *clinical education* refers to the supervised practice of professional skills in a clinical setting. Clinical education is arranged by negotiation between the staff of the respective academic unit (Academic Coordinator of Clinical Education [ACCE]) and the director of the individual clinical setting (Center Coordinator of Clinical Education [CCCE]). In almost all cases, formal agreements are signed between the academic institution and the placement facility.

Instruction and supervision of a PT/PTA student are provided by a *clinical instructor* (CI) during scheduled clinical education experiences. The PT clinical instructor (CI) is responsible for all actions and duties of the affiliating student, and can supervise both physical therapy and PTA students (A PTA may only supervise a PTA student—not a PT student). The CI, in addition to carrying out their specific duties within the department, performs the role of teacher, facilitator, coordinator, and professional role model with the student, and evaluates the student on a regular basis.

The purpose of clinical education is to provide student clinicians with opportunities to:

- Observe and work with a variety of patients under professional supervision and in diverse settings and to integrate knowledge and skills at progressively higher levels of performance and responsibility.
- Work in situations where they can practice interpersonal skills and develop characteristics essential to productive working relationships.
- Develop clinical reasoning skills and management skills, as well as to master techniques that develop competence at the level of a beginning practitioner.

The nature of the student assessment varies across academic institutions but usually includes a student evaluation by both the CI and the student, the satisfactory completion of a specified number of hours, as well as a variety of assignments, including case studies, essays, and verbal presentations.

Students are expected to take an active responsibility for their own education by identifying their learning needs, assisting in the planning and implementation of the learning experiences, being familiar with and adhering to procedures and rules of the academic institution and the affiliating center, and in evaluating their own performance.

Study Pearl

In all clinical situations, the welfare of the patient/client is paramount. The patient's/client's dignity and rights to privacy and confidentiality must be respected at all times. Students who do not comply with the rules governing ethical practice may be removed from the clinical placement.

MODELS OF DISABLEMENT

A disablement model is designed to detail the functional consequences and relationships of disease, impairment, and functional limitations. *The Guide to Physical Therapist Practice*[2] employs

Study Pearl

Impairment—Loss or abnormality of anatomic, physiologic, or psychologic structure or function. Not all impairments are modified by physical therapy, and not all impairments cause activity limitations and participation restrictions.[1]
Primary Impairment—An impairment that can result from active pathology or disease. An example is a hip fracture with subsequent loss of ambulation and strength. Primary impairment can create secondary impairments and can lead to secondary pathology.
Secondary Impairment—An impairment that originates from primary impairment and pathology.[1] Using the hip fracture example, a secondary impairment could be the development of decubiti secondary to immobility.
Functional Limitation—A restriction of the ability to perform, at the level of the whole person, a physical action, activity, or task in an efficient, typically expected, or competent manner.[1]

terminology from the Nagi disablement model (Table 1-2),[3] but also uses components from other disablement models.[4] In 1980, the Executive Board of the World Health Organization published a document for trial purposes, the International Classification of Functioning, Disability and Health (ICFDH-I or ICF) (Table 1-2). In 2001, a revised edition was published (ICFDH-II) that emphasized "components of health" rather than "consequences of disease" (ie, participation rather than disability) and environmental and personal factors as important determinants of health (Table 1-2).[5]

THE FIVE ELEMENTS OF PATIENT/CLIENT MANAGEMENT

The PT integrates the following five elements of patient/client management:

1. Examination of the patient
2. Evaluation of the data and identification of problems
3. Determination of the diagnosis
4. Determination of the prognosis and plan of care (POC)
5. Implementation of the POC (intervention)[2]

EXAMINATION

The examination is an ongoing process that begins with the patient referral or initial entry and continues throughout the course of rehabilitation. The process of examination includes gathering information from the chart, other caregivers, the patient, the patient's family and friends, and caretakers in order to identify and define the patient's

TABLE 1-2. DISABLEMENT MODEL COMPARISONS

WHO (ICFDH-I)	WHO (ICFDH-II)	NAGI SCHEME
Disease The intrinsic pathology or disorder	**Health condition** Dysfunction of a body function and/or structure	**Pathology/Pathophysiology** Interruption or interference with normal processes and efforts of an organism to regain its normal state
Impairment Loss or abnormality of psychological, physiologic, or anatomic structure or function	**Impairment** Problems in body function or structure such as a significant deviation or loss	**Impairment** Anatomic, physiologic, mental, or emotional abnormalities or loss
Disability Restriction or lack of ability to perform an activity in a normal manner	**Activity limitation** Limitation in execution of a task or action by an individual	**Functional limitation** Limitation in performance at the level of the whole organism or person
Handicap Disadvantage or disability that limits or prevents fulfillment of a normal role (depends on age, sex, socoicultural factors for the person)	**Participation restriction** Prevents fulfillment of involvement in a life situation	**Disability** Limitation in performance of socially defined roles and tasks within a sociocultural and physical environment

Data from World Health Organization. International Classification of Impairments, Disabilities, and Handicaps. Geneva, Switzerland, 1993 (ICIDH).

problem(s).[6] The examination consists of three components of equal importance—patient history, systems review, and tests and measures.[2] These are closely related in that they often occur concurrently.

Patient History. The patient history (refer to Chapter 6) involves the information gathered from a review of the medical records and interviews with the patient, family members, caregiver, and other involved persons, about the patient's history and current functional and health status.[7] The medical record provides detailed reports from members of the health care team. The patient history usually precedes the systems review (see Chapter 6) and the tests and measures components of the examination, but it may also occur concurrently.

Observation. The observation includes but is not limited to, an analysis of posture, structural alignment or deformity, scars, crepitus, color changes, swelling, muscle atrophy, and the presence of any asymmetry.

The Systems Review. The systems review (see Chapter 6) is a brief or limited examination that provides additional information about the general health and the continuum of patient/client care throughout the lifespan. The patient history and systems review are used to generate diagnostic hypotheses.

Tests and Measures. The tests and measures portion of the examination involves the physical examination of the patient and is designed to provide objective data from which to accurately determine the degree of specific function and dysfunction.[7] The physical examination is modified based on the history and the systems review. For example, the examination of an acutely injured patient differs greatly from that of a patient in less discomfort or distress, and the examination of a child differs in some respects to that of an adult. Vital signs should be taken routinely, but are particularly warranted in those scenarios outlined in Table 1-3.

Anthropometrics. Anthropometrics are measurable physiological characteristics, and include height and weight.

> Height. Height is the anthropometric longitudinal growth of an individual. A stadiometer is the device used to measure height although often a height stick is more frequently used for adults or children older than 2 years of age (who are measured lying horizontally).
>
> Weight. Weight is the anthropometric mass of an individual. A scale is used to measure weight. Body mass index (BMI) is used to calculate the relationship between healthy height and weight and obesity or being overweight or underweight (see Chapter 5).

Pain. The assessment of pain is very important to the overall wellness of the patient. Clinically, pain can be measured using a wide variety of different scales. For example, the FACES scale which is a series of faces from "0" (no pain at all showing a normal happy face) to "5" (the worst pain ever experienced by the patient) can be used. There is also a visual analog scale using a straight line with a "0" at

Study Pearl

Reexamination allows the therapist to evaluate, progress, and modify interventions as appropriate.[2]

Study Pearl

It is estimated that at least 80% of the necessary information to explain the presenting patient problem can be provided by a thorough history.[8]

TABLE 1-3. CLINICAL INDICATORS THAT WARRANT DETERMINATION OF VITAL SIGN MEASURES

Dyspnea (shortness of breath, breathlessness)
Fatigue (weakness)
Syncope
Chest pain or discomfort
Irregular heartbeat
Cyanosis
Intermittent claudication
Pedal edema

Study Pearl

It is important, where possible, to allow patients to make their own choices on which pain scale to use.

one end and a "10" at the other end, with the 0 indicating no pain, and the 10 indicating "the worst pain imaginable."

EVALUATION

Following the history, systems review, and the tests and measures, an evaluation is made based on an analysis and organization of the collected data and information.[9] An evaluation is the level of judgment necessary to make sense of the findings in order to identify a relationship between the symptoms reported and the signs of disturbed function.[10] According to BOD P11-05-20-49 published by the APTA,[11] the evaluation includes the ability to:

- Synthesize available data on a patient/client expressed in terms of the disablement model to include impairment, functional limitation, and disability participation restrictions.
- Use available evidence in interpreting the examination findings.
- Verbalize possible alternatives when interpreting the examination findings.
- Cite the evidence (patient/client history, laboratory diagnostics, tests and measures, and scientific literature) to support a clinical decision.

The evaluation process may also identify possible problems that require consultation with, or referral to, another provider. A number of frameworks have been applied to clinical practice over the past 2 decades for guiding clinical decision making.[12-17] While the earliest frameworks were based on disablement models, the more recent models have focused on enablement perspectives.

DIAGNOSIS

A physical therapy diagnosis, which includes a prioritization of the identified impairments, functional limitations, and disabilities can only be made when all potential causes of the symptoms have been ruled out. In order to form a diagnosis, the clinician must be able to:[11]

- Integrate the examination findings to classify the patient/client problem in terms of a human movement dysfunction (ie, practice patterns).
- Identify and prioritize impairments to determine a specific dysfunction toward which the intervention will be directed.

The physical therapy diagnosis is a label ascribed to a cluster of signs and symptoms. The patient can be placed in a diagnostic category as well as in one or more of the practice patterns listed in the *Guide to Physical Therapist Practice*. Examples of the preferred practice patterns are outlined in (Table 1-4). Most of the time, these patterns do not occur in isolation, as a patient often presents with a mixture of signs and symptoms that indicate one or more possible problem areas. If more than one practice pattern is applicable, the therapist indicates which practice pattern is primary.

TABLE 1-4. EXAMPLES OF PREFERRED PRACTICE PATTERNS

CATEGORY/ PREFERRED PRACTICE PATTERN	IMPAIRMENT
Musculoskeletal	
Pattern 4A	Primary prevention/risk factor reduction for skeletal demineralization
Pattern 4B	Impaired posture
Pattern 4C	Impaired muscle performance
Pattern 4D	Impaired joint mobility, motor function, muscle performance, and range of motion associated with connective tissue dysfunction
Pattern 4E	Impaired joint mobility, motor function, muscle performance, and range of motion associated with localized inflammation
Pattern 4F	Impaired joint mobility, motor function, muscle performance, and range of motion, or reflex integrity secondary to spinal disorders
Pattern 4G	Impaired joint mobility, motor function, muscle performance, and range of motion associated with fracture
Pattern 4H	Impaired joint mobility, motor function, muscle performance, and range of motion associated with joint arthroplasty
Pattern 4I	Impaired joint mobility, motor function, muscle performance, and range of motion associated with bony or soft tissue surgical procedures
Pattern 4J	Impaired motor function, muscle performance, range of motion, gait, locomotion, and balance associated with amputation
Neuromuscular	
Pattern 5A	Primary prevention/risk reduction for loss of balance and falling
Pattern 5B	Impaired neuromotor development
Pattern 5C/D	Impaired motor function and sensory integrity associated with nonprogressive disorders of the central nervous system—congenital origin or acquired in infancy or childhood
Pattern 5D	Impaired motor function and sensory integrity associated with nonprogressive disorders of the central nervous system—acquired in adolescence or adulthood
Pattern 5E	Impaired motor function and sensory integrity associated with progressive disorders of the central nervous system
Pattern 5F	Impaired peripheral nerve integrity and muscle performance associated with peripheral nerve injury
Pattern 5G	Impaired motor function and sensory integrity associated with acute or chronic polyneuropathies
Pattern 5H	Impaired motor function, peripheral nerve integrity, and sensory integrity associated with nonprogressive disorders of the spinal cord
Pattern 5I	Impaired arousal, range of motion, and motor control associated with coma, near coma, and vegetative state
Cardiovascular/ Pulmonary	
Pattern 6B	Impaired aerobic capacity/endurance associated with deconditioning
Pattern 6C	Impaired ventilation, respiration/gas exchange, and aerobic capacity/endurance associated with airway clearance dysfunction
Pattern 6D	Impaired aerobic capacity endurance associated with cardiovascular pump dysfunction or failure
Pattern 6E	Impaired ventilation and respiration/gas exchange associated with ventilatory pump dysfunction or failure
Pattern 6F	Impaired ventilation and respiration/gas exchange associated with respiratory failure
Pattern 6H	Impaired circulation and anthropometric dimensions associated with lymphatic system disorders
Integumentary	
Pattern 7B	Impaired integumentary integrity associated with superficial skin involvement
Pattern 7C	Impaired integumentary integrity associated with partial-thickness skin involvement and scar formation
Pattern 7D	Impaired integumentary integrity associated with full-thickness skin involvement and scar formation

Data from *Guide to Physical Therapist Practice. Phys Ther.* 2001;81:S13-S95.

PROGNOSIS

The prognosis is the predicted level of function that the patient will attain and an identification of the barriers that may impact the achievement of optimal improvement (age, medication[s], socio-economic status, comorbidities, cognitive status, nutrition, social support, and environment) within a certain time frame.[10] This prediction helps guide the intensity, duration, frequency, and type of the intervention, in addition to providing justifications for the intervention. Knowledge of the severity of an injury, the age, physical and health status of a patient, and the healing processes of the various tissues involved are among the factors used in determining the prognosis.

PLAN OF CARE

The plan of care (POC), which outlines anticipated patient management, involves the setting of goals, coordination of care, progression of care, and discharge. The POC:[1]

- Is based on the examination, evaluation, diagnosis, and prognosis, including the predicted level of optimal improvement.
- Includes statements that identify anticipated goals and the expected outcomes
- Describes the specific interventions to be used, and the proposed frequency and duration of the interventions that is required to reach the anticipated goals and expected outcomes
- Includes documentation that is dated and appropriately authenticated by the PT who established the plan of care
- Includes plans for discharge of the patient/client taking into consideration achievement of anticipated goals and expected outcomes, and provides for appropriate follow-up or referral

To design a POC, the clinician must:[11]

- Write measurable functional goals (short-term and long-term) that are time-referenced with expected outcomes.
- Consult patient/client and/or caregivers to develop a mutually agreed to POC.
- Identify patient/client goals and expectations.
- Identify indications for consultation with other professionals.
- Make a referral to resources needed by the patient/client.
- Select and prioritize the essential interventions that are safe and meet the specified functional goals and outcomes in the plan of care: (a) identify precautions and contraindications, (b) provide evidence for patient-centered interventions that are identified and selected, (c) define the specificity of the intervention (time, intensity, duration, and frequency), and (d) set realistic priorities that consider relative time duration in conjunction with the family, caregivers, and other health care professionals.
- Establish criteria for discharge based on patient goals and functional status.

Study Pearl

Goals should be objective and quantifiable (measurable) and have anticipated dates.

- Short-term goals (STG) are used to indicate what progress is to be made in the near future.
- Long-term goals (LTG) are used to indicate how long it will take to restore function, or when the intervention is to be terminated.

Coordination of Care. The purpose of the coordination of care is to:[11]

1. Identify who needs to collaborate on the plan of care.
2. Identify additional patient/client needs that are beyond the scope of PT practice, level of experience and expertise, and warrant referral.
3. Refer and discuss coordination of care with other health care professionals.
4. Articulate a specific rationale for a referral.
5. Advocate for patient/client access to services.

Progression of Care. The purpose of the progression of care is to:[11]

1. Identify outcome measures of progress relative to when to progress the patient further.
2. Measure patient/client response to intervention.
3. Modify elements of the plan of care and goals in response to changing patient/client status, as needed.
4. Make ongoing adjustments to interventions according to outcomes including the physical and social environments, medical therapeutic interventions, and biological factors.
5. Make accurate decisions regarding intensity and frequency when adjusting interventions in the plan of care.

Discharge Plan. The purpose of the discharge plan is to:[11]

1. Reexamine the patient/client if not meeting the established criteria for discharge based on the plan of care.
2. Differentiate between the discharge of the patient/client, discontinuation of service, and transfer of care with reevaluation.
3. Prepare needed resources for the patient/client to ensure timely discharge, including follow-up care.
4. Include the patient/client and family/caregiver in the discharge planning.
5. Discontinue care when services are no longer indicated.
6. When services are still needed, seek resources and/or consult with others to identify alternative resources that may be available.
7. Determine the need for equipment and initiate requests to obtain the equipment.

INTERVENTION

The *Guide*[1] defines an intervention as "the purposeful and skilled interaction of the PT and the patient/client and, when appropriate, with other individuals involved in the patient/client care, using various physical therapy procedures and techniques to produce changes in the condition consistent with the diagnosis and prognosis." A physical therapy intervention is most effectively addressed from a problem-oriented approach, based on the evaluation, the patient's functional needs, and on mutually agreed-upon goals.[9]

The various intervention categories are listed in Table A-1 of the Appendix.

Study Pearl

Types of physical therapy interventions may include:

- Direct intervention (eg, manual therapy techniques, therapeutic exercise)
- Patient/client related instruction
- Coordination, communication, and documentation

COORDINATION, COMMUNICATION, AND DOCUMENTATION

Coordination, communication, and documentation may include:[11]

A. Addressing required functions:
   1. Establish and maintain an ongoing collaborative process of decision making with patients/clients, families, or caregivers prior to initiating care, and throughout the provision of services.
   2. Discern the need to perform mandatory communication and reporting (eg, incident reports, patient advocacy, and abuse reporting).
   3. Follow advance directives (see Chapter 2).

B. Admission and discharge planning.

C. Case management.

D. Collaboration and coordination with agencies, including:
   1. Home care agencies
   2. Equipment suppliers
   3. Schools
   4. Transportation agencies
   5. Payer groups

E. Communication across settings, including:
   1. Case conferences
   2. Documentation
   3. Education plans

F. Cost-effective resource utilization

G. Data collection, analysis, and reporting of:
   1. Outcome data
   2. Peer review findings
   3. Record reviews

H. Documentation across settings, following APTA's Guidelines for Physical Therapy Documentation, including:
   1. Elements of examination, evaluation, diagnosis, prognosis, and intervention
   2. Changes in impairments, functional limitations, and disabilities
   3. Changes in interventions
   4. Outcomes of intervention

I. Interdisciplinary teamwork:
   1. Patient/client family meetings
   2. Patient care rounds
   3. Case conferences

J. Referrals to other professionals or resources

DOCUMENTATION

Documentation in health care includes any entry into the patient/client record. The SOAP (Subjective, Objective, Assessment, Plan) note format has traditionally been used to document the examination and intervention process.

- Subjective: information about the condition from the patient or family member.
- Objective: measurement a clinician obtains during the physical examination.

- Assessment: analysis of problem including the long- and short-term goals.
- Plan: a specific intervention plan for the identified problem.

More recently, the Patient/Client Management Model is being used by those clinicians familiar with the *Guide to Physical Therapist Practice*.[6] The Patient/Client Management Model described in the *Guide to Physical Therapist Practice* has the following components:

- History: information gathered about the patient's history.
- Systems review: information gathered from performing a brief examination or screening of the patient's major systems addressed by physical therapy. Also includes information gathered about the patient's communication, affect, cognition, learning style, and education needs.
- Tests and measures: results from specific tests and measures performed by the therapist.
- Diagnosis: includes a discussion of the relationship of the patient's functional deficits to the patient's impairments and/or disability. The relevant practice pattern(s) may also be included, as well as a discussion on other health care professionals to which the therapist has referred the patient or believes the patient should be referred.
- Prognosis: includes the predicted level of improvement that the patient will be able to achieve and the predicted amount of time to achieve that level of improvement. The prognosis should also include the PT's professional opinion of the patient's rehabilitation potential.
- Plan of care: includes the expected outcomes (long-term goals), anticipated goals (short-term goals), and interventions, including an education plan for the patient or the patient's caregivers or significant others.

The purposes of documentation are as follows:[6]

- To document what the clinician does to manage the individual patient's case. This documentation, considered a legal document, becomes a part of the patient's medical record.
- To record examination findings, patient status, intervention provided, and the patient's response to treatment.
- To communicate with all other members of the health care team, including communication between the PT and the PTA; this helps provide consistency among the services provided.
- To provide information to third-party payers, such as Medicare and other insurance companies who make decisions about reimbursement based on the quality and completeness of the physical therapy note.
- To help the PT organize his/her thought processes involved in patient care.
- To be used for quality assurance and improvement purposes and for issues such as discharge planning.
- To serve as a source of data for peer and utilization review, and research.

APTA Guidelines for Documentation. The APTA Board of Directors has approved a number of guidelines for PT documentation to help develop and improve the art and science of PT, including practice, education, and research, although it is recognized that these guidelines do not reflect all of the unique documentation requirements associated with the many specialty areas within the PT profession. Applicable for both handwritten and electronic documentation systems, these guidelines are intended as a foundation for the development of more specific documentation guidelines in clinical areas, while at the same time providing guidance for the PT profession across all practice settings.[10]

The PTA or certified occupational therapy assistant (COTA) reads the initial documentation of the examination, evaluation, diagnosis, prognosis, anticipated outcomes and goals, and intervention plan, and is expected to follow the plan of care as outlined by the PT/OT in the initial patient note.[6] After the patient has been seen by the PTA or COTA for a time (the time varies according to the policies of each facility, health care system, and state law), the PTA or COTA must write a progress note documenting any changes in the patient's status that have occurred since the therapist's initial note was written.[6] Also, after discussion with the PT/OT about the diagnosis and prognosis, expected outcomes, anticipated goals, and interventions, the PTA/COTA rewrites or responds to the previously written expected outcomes, and then documents the revised POC accordingly.[6] In many facilities (according to the policies of each facility, health care system, and state law), the therapist then cosigns the PTA's/COTA's note, indicating agreement with what is documented.[7]

Study Pearl

Students in PT or PTA programs may document when the record is additionally authenticated by the PT or, when permissible by law, documentation by PTA students may be authenticated by a PTA.

Initial Examination/Evaluation. Documentation of the initial encounter is typically called the "initial examination," "initial evaluation," or "initial examination/evaluation." The examination/evaluation is typically completed by the end of the first visit, but may require several visits. Evaluation is a thought process that may not include formal documentation. However, the evaluation process may lead to documentation of impairments, functional limitations, and disabilities using formats such as:

- A problem list
- A statement of assessment of key factors (eg, cognitive factors, comorbidities, social support) influencing the patient/client status

Diagnosis. Documentation of a diagnosis determined by the PT may include impairment and functional limitations.

Visit/Encounter. Documentation of a visit or encounter, often called a progress note or daily note, describes the sequential implementation of the plan of care established by the PT. Documentation of each visit/encounter shall include the following elements:

- Patient/client self-reports (as appropriate)
- Identification of specific interventions provided, including frequency, intensity, and duration as appropriate. Examples include:
  - Knee extension, three sets, ten repetitions, 10 lb weight

  - Transfer training bed to chair with sliding board
  - Equipment provided
- Changes in patient/client impairment, functional limitation, and disability status as they relate to the plan of care
- Response to interventions, including adverse reactions, if any
- Factors that modify frequency or intensity of intervention and progression goals, including patient/client adherence to patient/client-related instructions
- Communication/consultation with providers/patient/client/family/significant other
- Documentation to plan for ongoing provision of services for the next visit(s), which is suggested to include, but not be limited to:
  - The interventions with objectives
  - Progression parameters
  - Precautions, if indicated

Reexamination. Documentation of a reexamination includes data from repeated or new examination elements, and is provided to evaluate progress and to modify or redirect the intervention. Specifically, the documentation shall include the following elements:

- Documentation of selected components of the examination to update the impairment, function, and/or disability status of a patient/client.
- Interpretation of findings and, when indicated, revision of goals.
- When indicated, revision of the plan of care, as directly correlated with the goals as documented.

Prognosis. Documentation of the prognosis is typically included in the POC.

Discharge or Discontinuation Summary. Documentation is required following conclusion of the current episode in the physical therapy intervention sequence to summarize progression toward goals and discharge plans. Documentation of discharge or discontinuation shall include the following elements:

- Current physical/functional status.
- Degree of goals achieved and reasons for goals not being achieved.
- Discharge/discontinuation plan related to the patient/client's continuing care. Examples include:
  - Home program
  - Referrals for additional services
  - Recommendations for follow-up physical therapy care
  - Family and caregiver training
  - Equipment provided

Basic Principles of Clinical Documentation[7]

- Never record falsely, exaggerate, guess at, or make up data. All documents must be legible and should be written in black or blue ink, typed, and/or transcribed.

- Keep the information objective and clear.
- Each episode of treatment must be documented and each entry must be dated and signed with first and last name and professional designation (PT, PTA). A professional license number may also be included, but is optional. The patient's name and ID number should be on each page.
- To avoid the potential for falsification, empty lines should not be left between one entry and another, nor should empty lines be left within a single entry.
- Avoid vague terminology.
- Information should be stated concisely. Abbreviations can help with brevity, however, only medically approved abbreviations or symbols can be used.
- Incorrect spelling, grammar, and punctuation can be misleading. Any mistake should be crossed out with a single line through the error, initialed, and dated by the clinician.

Study Pearl

Correction fluid/tape or similar products should never be used to correct text in the medical records.

PATIENT/CLIENT-RELATED INSTRUCTION

Patient/client-related instruction may include instruction, education, and training of patients/clients and caregivers regarding:

1. Current condition (pathology/pathophysiology [disease, disorder, or condition], impairments, functional limitations, or disabilities)
2. Enhancement of performance
3. Plan of care:
   a. Risk factors for pathology/pathophysiology (disease, disorder, or condition), impairments, functional limitations, or disabilities
   b. Preferred interventions, alternative interventions, and alternative modes of delivery
   c. Expected outcomes
4. Health, wellness, and fitness programs (management of risk factors)
5. Transitions across settings

Patient/client-related management forms the cornerstone of every patient visit. During the physical therapy visits, the clinician and the patient work to alter the patient's perception of their functional capabilities. Together, the patient and clinician discuss the parts of the patient's life that he or she can and cannot control and then consider how to improve those parts that can be changed. It is imperative that the clinician spend time educating patients as to their condition, so that they can fully understand the importance of their role in the rehabilitation process, and become educated consumers. The aim of patient education is to create independence, not dependence, and to foster an atmosphere of learning in the clinic. Patient/client education in its broadest sense involves informing, educating, or training patients/clients, families, significant others, and caregivers in order to promote and optimize physical therapy services.[9] Failure to identify the relevance of the presented material will promote disinterest and decreased compliance. Instruction should be provided across all settings for all patients/clients on promoting understanding of:

- Current condition, impairments, functional limitations, and disabilities.
- Anticipated goals and expected outcomes, the plan of care, specific intervention elements, and self-management strategies.
- The elements necessary for the smooth transition to home or an alternate setting, work, and community.
- Individualized family service plans or individualized education plans (IEPs).
- Safety awareness and risk factor reduction and prevention.

PROCEDURAL INTERVENTIONS

Procedural interventions can be broadly classified into three main groups:[7,16]

1. Restorative interventions: directed toward remediating or improving the patient's status in terms of impairments, functional limitations, and recovery of function. These strategies are particularly applicable for treating secondary impairments that may contribute to functional limitations and which are likely to improve with treatment. For example impaired lower extremity strength is associated with functional loss; strength training can improve gait.
2. Compensatory interventions: directed toward promoting optimal function using residual abilities. Examples include training patients with subtle left-sided neglect to consciously attend to the left side of space, using a cane for patients with impaired balance control that persists despite intervention, and functional training for patients with a complete spinal cord transection.
3. Preventative interventions: directed toward minimizing potential impairments, functional limitations, and disabilities and maintaining health. Examples include frequent changes in the seated position for a patient in a wheelchair to prevent decubiti.

CHOOSING AN INTERVENTION STRATEGY

Interventions are chosen on the basis of the data obtained, the diagnosis, prognosis, and anticipated goals and expected outcomes.[7] The goal of improving functional ability must be foremost in the clinician's reasoning when determining the intervention strategy. When deciding which intervention strategy to use, the clinician must weigh:

- The likelihood that the underlying impairments will improve (eg, through natural recovery from the injury, through neural plasticity) versus the requirements for immediate functional recovery despite the underlying impairments
- The contributions of risk factors:
  - Functional performance factors
  - Demographic, social lifestyle, behavioral, psychological, and environmental factors
  - Physiologic impairments

TABLE 1-5. QUESTIONS TO DETERMINE DESIRED OUTCOMES

1. If you were to concentrate your energies on one thing for yourself, what would it be?
2. What activities do you need help with that you would rather perform yourself?
3. What are your concerns about returning to work, home, school, or leisure activities?
4. What about your current situation would you like to be different in about 6 months? What would you like to be the same?

Data from Randall KE, McEwen IR: Writing patient-centered goals. *Phys Ther.* 2000;80:1197-1203 and Winton PJ, Bailey DB: Communicating with families: examining practices and facilitating change. In: Simeonsson JP, Simeonsson RJ, eds. *Children With Special Needs: Family, Culture, and Society.* Orlando, FL, Harcourt Brace Jovanovich. 1993.

- Comorbidities
- Anatomic impairments

The process of identifying meaningful, achievable functional goals should be a collaborative effort between the clinician and the patient, the patient's family, or the patient's significant other.[9] To identify functional goals, Randall and McEwen[18] recommend the following steps:

1. Determine the patient's desired outcome of the intervention.
2. Develop an understanding of the patient's self-care, work, and leisure activities and the environments in which these activities occur.
3. Establish goals with the patient that relate to the desired outcomes (Table 1-5).[18] Once the goals have been agreed upon, the clinician must write the goals so that they contain the following elements:[18,19]
   - Who (the patient)
   - Will do what (activities)
   - Under what conditions (the home or work environment)
   - How well (the amount of assistance, or number of attempts required for successful completion)
   - By when (target date)

OUTCOMES

The last step is ongoing and involves continuous reexamination of the patient and a determination of the efficacy of treatment.[7] The purpose of outcomes is to:[11]

- ▶ Summarize reexamination findings, and evaluation of the patient's abilities in terms of the anticipated goals and expected outcomes set forth in the POC.
- ▶ Make a determination as to whether the goals and outcomes are reasonable, given the patient's diagnosis and progress made.
  - If the patient attains the desired level of competence for the stated goals, revisions in the POC are indicated.
  - If the patient attains the desired level of competence for the expected outcomes, discharge is considered.
  - If the patient progresses more rapidly or more slowly than expected, revisions in the POC are indicated.
  - If the patient fails to achieve the stated goals or outcomes, the therapist must determine why (eg, were the goals and outcomes realistic; were the interventions selected at an appropriate level to challenge the patient; were any intervening and constraining factors identified?).

DISCHARGE/DISCONTINUATION OF INTERVENTION

Discharge planning, which is initiated during the data-collection phase, is the process of ending physical therapy services that have been provided during a single episode of care, when an analysis by the PT indicates that the anticipated goals and expected outcomes have been achieved.[1] Components of an effective discharge plan include:[7]

- Patient, family, or caregiver education
- Plans for appropriate follow-up care or referral to another agency

Instruction in a home exercise plan (HEP)

- Evaluation and modification of the home environment to assist the patient returning home

Discontinuation is the process of ending physical therapy services that have been provided during a single episode of care for any of the following reasons:[1]

- The patient/client, caregiver, or legal guardian declines to continue intervention.
- The patient/client is unable to continue to progress toward the anticipated goals and expected outcomes because of medical or psychosocial complications, or because financial/insurance resources have been expended (depending on the practice setting).
- The PT determines that the patient/client will no longer benefit from physical therapy.

PREVENTION AND PROMOTION OF HEALTH, WELLNESS, AND FITNESS

Three types of preventions are recognized:

1. Primary: prevention of disease in a susceptible or potentially susceptible population through the use of specific measures such as general health promotion offers.[1]
2. Secondary: efforts to decrease the duration of illness, severity of disease, and sequelae through early diagnosis and prompt intervention.[1]
3. Tertiary: efforts to decrease the degree of disability and promote rehabilitation and restoration of function in patients with chronic and irreversible diseases.[1]

Study Pearl

PTs can provide instructional and educational programs for other therapists, health care providers, staff, local, state, and federal agencies, and all patients/families in academic and/or clinical settings. These programs are provided to increase the awareness of health issues and the roles of the PT.

MEMBERS OF THE HEALTH CARE TEAM

Physical Therapy Director

The director of physical therapy is typically a PT who has demonstrated qualifications based on education and experience in the field of physical therapy and who has accepted the inherent responsibilities of a supervisory role.[9] The director of a physical therapy service must:

- Establish guidelines and procedures that will delineate the functions and responsibilities of all levels of physical therapy personnel in the service and the supervisory relationships inherent to the functions of the service and the organization (see Chapter 2).[9]

- Ensure that the objectives of the service are efficiently and effectively achieved within the framework of the stated purpose of the organization, and in accordance with safe PT practice.
- Interpret administrative policies.
- Act as a liaison between line staff and administration.
- Foster the professional growth of the staff.

Staff Physical Therapist

PTs engage in the examination, evaluation, diagnosis, prognosis, and intervention in an effort to maximize patient outcomes. The Commission on Accreditation in Physical Therapy Education (CAPTE) serves the public by establishing and applying standards that assure quality and continuous improvement in the entry-level preparation of PTs and PTAs. All states require PTs to obtain a license to practice.

Physical Therapist Assistant

A PTA must be supervised by a PT. Care provided by a PTA may include teaching patients/clients exercise for mobility, strength and coordination, training for activities such as walking with crutches, canes, or walkers, and the use of adjunctive interventions (see Chapter 18). A PTA may modify an intervention only in accordance with changes in patient status and within the established plan of care developed by the PT (see "Professional Standards"). Typically, a PTA has an associate's degree from an accredited PTA program and is licensed, certified, or registered in most states.

Physical Therapist/Occupational Therapist Aide

Physical therapist aides (PT aides), sometimes referred to as physical therapy aides, are considered support personnel who may be involved in support services directed by a PT. PT aides receive on-the-job training under the direction and supervision of a PT or PTA and are permitted to function only with continuous on-site supervision by a PT or in some cases a PTA. The duties of a PT aide are limited to those methods and techniques that do not require clinical decision making or clinical problem-solving by a PT or a PTA.

Study Pearl

Patients, parents, or legal guardians can refuse treatment by a student practitioner.

Physical Therapist and Physical Therapist Assistant Student

The PT or PTA student can perform duties commensurate with their level of education.

Physical Therapy Volunteer

A volunteer is usually a member of the community who has an interest in assisting PTs or PTAs with departmental activities. Responsibilities of a volunteer include:

- Taking phone messages.
- Basic nonclinical/secretarial duties.
- Volunteers may not provide or setup patient treatment, transfer patients, clean whirlpools, or maintain equipment.

HOME HEALTH AIDE

Home health aides provide health-related services to the elderly, disabled, and unwell in their homes. Their duties include performing housekeeping tasks, assisting with ambulation or transfers, and promoting personal hygiene. The registered nurse (RN), PT, or social worker caring for the patient may assign specific duties to, and supervise, the home health aide.

OCCUPATIONAL THERAPIST

An occupational therapist (OT) assesses patient function in activities of daily living (ADLs), including dressing, bathing, grooming, meal preparation, writing, and driving, which are essential for independent living. In making treatment recommendations, the OT addresses a number of factors including, but not limited to (1) fatigue management, (2) upper body strength, movement, and coordination, (3) adaptations to the home and work environment, including both structural changes and specialized equipment for particular activities, and (4) compensatory strategies for impairments in thinking, sensation, or vision. All states require an OT to obtain a license to practice.

CERTIFIED OCCUPATIONAL THERAPIST ASSISTANT

A certified occupational therapist assistant (COTA) works under the direction of an occupational therapist. COTAs perform a variety of rehabilitative activities and exercises as outlined in an established treatment plan. The minimum educational requirements for the COTA are described in the current *Essentials and Guidelines of an Accredited Educational Program for the Occupational Therapy Assistant.*[20]

SPEECH-LANGUAGE PATHOLOGIST (SPEECH THERAPIST)

A speech-language pathologist (SLP) evaluates speech, language, cognitive-communication, and swallowing skills of children and adults. SLPs are required to possess a master's degree or equivalent. The vast majority of states require a SLP to obtain a license to practice.

CERTIFIED ORTHOTIST

Certified orthotists (CO) design, fabricate, and fit orthoses (braces, splints, collars, corsets), prescribed by physicians, to patients with disabling conditions of the limbs and spine. A CO must have successfully completed the examination by the American Orthotist and Prosthetic Association.

Study Pearl

An individual may be certified in both orthotics and prosthetics (CPO).

CERTIFIED PROSTHETIST

A certified prosthetist (CP) designs, fabricates, and fits prostheses for patients with partial or total absence of a limb. A CP must have successfully completed the examination by the American Orthotist and Prosthetic Association.

Respiratory Therapists

Respiratory therapists evaluate, treat, and care for patients with breathing disorders. The vast majority of respiratory therapists are employed in hospitals. Patient care activities include performing bronchial drainage techniques, measuring lung capacities, administering oxygen and aerosols, and analyzing oxygen and carbon dioxide concentrations. Education programs for respiratory therapists are offered by hospitals, colleges, and universities, vocational-technical institutes, and the military. The vast majority of states require a respiratory therapist to obtain a license to practice.

Respiratory Therapy Technician Certified

A respiratory therapy technician certified (CRRT) is a skilled technician who:

- Holds an associates degree from a 2-year training program accredited by the Committee in Allied Health Education and Accreditation
- Has passed a national examination to become registered
- Administers respiratory therapy as prescribed and supervised by a physician, including:
  - Pulmonary function tests
  - Treatments consisting of oxygen delivery, aerosols, and nebulizers
  - Maintenance of all respiratory equipment

Primary Care Physician

A primary care physician (PCP) is a practitioner, usually an internist, general practitioner (GP), or family medicine physician, providing primary care services and managing routine health care needs. Most PCPs serve as gatekeepers for the managed-care health organizations and provide authorization for referrals to other specialty physicians or services, including physical therapy.

Physician's Assistant

A physician's assistant (PA) is a medically trained professional who can provide many of the health care services traditionally performed by a physician, such as taking medical histories and doing physical examinations, making a diagnosis, prescribing and administering therapies (see also "Registered Nurse").

Physiatrist

A physiatrist is a physician specializing in physical medicine and rehabilitation, who has been certified by the American Board of Physical Medicine and Rehabilitation. The primary role of the physiatrist is to diagnose and treat patients with disabilities involving musculoskeletal, neurological, cardiovascular, or other body systems.

CHIROPRACTOR

A chiropractor (DC) is an individual trained in the science, art, and philosophy of chiropractic. A chiropractic evaluation and treatment is directed at providing a structural analysis of the musculoskeletal and neurological systems of the body. According to chiropractic doctrine, abnormal function of these two systems may affect the function of other systems in the body. In order to practice, chiropractors are usually licensed by a state board. A patient may see a chiropractor and PT concurrently.

REGISTERED NURSE

A registered nurse (RN) is licensed by the state to provide nursing services after completing a course of study that results in a baccalaureate degree and who has been legally authorized or registered to practice as an RN and use the RN designation. A registered nurse may:

- Make referrals to other services under a physician's direction
- Supervise other levels of nursing care
- Administer medication, but cannot change drug dosages
- Communicate to the supervising physician any change in the patient's medical or social condition

NURSE PRACTITIONER

A nurse practitioner (NP) is a registered nurse with additional specialized graduate level training who can perform physical examinations and diagnostic tests, counsels patients, and develop treatment programs.

REHABILITATION (VOCATIONAL) COUNSELOR

Rehabilitation counselors help people deal with the personal, physical, mental, social, and vocational effects of disabilities resulting from congenital defects, illness or disease, accidents, or the stress of daily life. The role of the rehabilitation counselor includes:

- An evaluation of the strengths and limitations of individuals
- Providing personal and vocational counseling
- Arranging for medical care, vocational training, and job placement

AUDIOLOGIST

Audiologists evaluate and treat individuals of all ages with the symptoms of hearing loss and other auditory, balance, and related sensory and neural problems.

ATHLETIC TRAINER

The certified athletic trainer (ATC) is a professional specializing in athletic health care. In cooperation with the physician and other allied health personnel, the athletic trainer functions as an integral member of the athletic health care team in secondary schools, colleges, and universities, sports medicine clinics, professional sports programs, and other athletic health care settings.

Certified athletic trainers have, at minimum, a bachelor's degree, usually in athletic training, health, physical education, or exercise science.

Social Worker

Social workers help patients and their families to cope with chronic, acute, or terminal illnesses and attempt to resolve problems that stand in the way of recovery or rehabilitation. A bachelor's degree is often the minimum requirement to qualify for employment as a social worker, however, in the health field, the master's degree is often required. All states have licensing, certification, or registration requirements for social workers.

Massage Therapist

Massage therapy is a regulated health profession with a growing number of states and provinces now requiring a license. Registered massage therapists must uphold specific standards of practice and codes of ethics in order to hold a valid license. In order to become a licensed or registered massage therapist, most states and provinces require the applicant to pass specific government board examinations, which consist of a written and a practical portion. A registered massage therapist is covered under most health insurance plans.

Acupuncturist

An acupuncturist treats symptoms by inserting very fine needles, sometimes in conjunction with an electrical stimulus, into the body's surface to, theoretically, influence the body's physiological functioning. Typical sessions last between 30 minutes and an hour. At the end of the session, the acupuncturist may prescribe herbal therapies for the patient to use at home. At the time of writing, 32 states and the District of Columbia use National Certification Commission for Acupuncture and Oriental Medicine (NCCAOM) certification as the main examination criteria for licensure, which takes 3 to 4 years to achieve. Each state may also choose to set additional eligibility criteria (usually additional academic or clinical hours). A small number of states have additional jurisprudence or practical examination requirements such as passing the CNT (Clean Needle Technique) exam.

BUDGETS-FISCAL RESPONSIBILITIES

Budget

A budget is a financial document in which the costs associated with operating a business are estimated for a specific time period, usually for 1 year. Included in the budget is a projection of expected revenues and specific expenses. A number of budget plans or types are available:

Operating Budget. One of the most commonly used types of budgeting and one of the simplest and easiest ways to set up an effective, easy-to-follow plan of expenses and income.

It is composed of a plan for current costs of the day to day operation of a business and the future means of financing them. Categories include expenses associated with:

- Salaries, benefits (sick, vacation, short- and long-term disability etc.)
- Medical and office supplies
- Utilities (gas, electricity, phone)
- Housekeeping
- Continuing education
- Travel
- Postage

Capital Budget

- Details of expenditures for the purchase of more expensive equipment (ie, over $300-$500) with a life span of 3 to 5 years, repair needs, plans for purchasing buildings, and the means to finance each over lengthy time periods
- Similar to the operating budget except it is more highly detailed and focused on individual purchasing or business needs

Budget Calendar. The annual schedule of events needed to occur and a period of time in which the preparation, review, and adoption of a budget takes place—the amount of time in which a business needs to and can implement a successful plan of operation. Budget calendars can follow the normal calendar or a fiscal calendar, that is, July 1 to June 30, depending on the institution.

Zero-Base Budget

- An approach where the spending amount for each line item gets examined in its entirety annually, regardless of previous costs.
- Unjustifiable items often face eradication.
- Primarily used for essential cost planning.

Expenses/Costs

Business expenses/costs can be divided into such categories as direct, indirect, fixed, variable, contingency, and escalation costs.

- Direct: those that can be identified specifically with a particular project, an instructional activity, a specific service or any other institutional activity, or that can be directly assigned to such activities relatively easily with a high degree of accuracy. The basic principle is that direct costs must be allocable (have a direct benefit and be directly attributable to the activity), allowable, reasonable, and necessary. Examples include:
    - The salaries of professional staff

- Medical/surgical supplies (ultrasound gel, iontophoresis pads, etc.)
- Educational courses

▶ Indirect: those which are necessary for the general operation of a business and the conduct of activities, or those costs that are not deemed as direct costs. Examples include:
- Utilities (heating, phones, electricity)
- Housekeeping/cleaning/laundry
- Building maintenance

▶ Fixed: expenses that are not responsive to patient volume levels. Examples include property rental.

▶ Variable: expenses that increase and decrease in proportion to patient volume levels. By definition, a variable cost is one which will total out at zero if there is no patient volume. Examples include medical/surgical and office supplies.

▶ Contingency: the amount of additional money, above and beyond the base cost, that is required to ensure a project's success.

▶ Discretionary costs are not strictly necessary for the provision of the physical therapy service but correspond to strategic goals. Examples include advertising, community events, etc.

▶ Escalation: the expense/cost that may be added to proposal budgets in consideration of the effects of price/cost inflation on current year costs.

Accounts Payable

Accounts payable are the unpaid bills of the business; the money owed to the suppliers and other creditors of the business for goods or services received. The sum of the amounts owed is listed as a *current liability* on the business balance sheet.

Accounts Receivable

Accounts receivable are unpaid customer invoices, and any other money owed to the business by the customers/insurance companies/patients. The sum of all the customer accounts receivable is listed as a *current asset* on the business balance sheet.

QUALITY ASSURANCE/QUALITY IMPROVEMENT

Quality Assurance

Quality assurance (QA) is an interactive management process designed to objectively ensure the appropriateness and effectiveness of patient care. It includes identifying deficiencies, implementing corrective action(s) to improve the identified deficiencies, and the monitoring of corrective actions to ensure that the quality of care has been enhanced. In the broadest sense, this ongoing process should involve the medical and professional staff, the administration, and the governing body of the health care facility.

Continuous Quality Improvement

Continuous quality improvement (CQI) is a process that identifies problems in health care delivery, examines solutions to those problems, and regularly monitors the solutions for improvement.

Utilization Review

A utilization review (UR) is an evaluation of the correctness of the use of hospital services and resources, including the appropriateness of the admission, length of stay, and ancillary services. The review may be conducted prospectively, concurrently, retrospectively, or in combination. The utilization review:

- Uses objective clinical criteria to ensure that the services are/were medically necessary and provided at the appropriate level of care.
- Can be conducted by the hospital for its own QA and risk management system (peer review) using norms, criteria, and standards adopted by its medical staff. Reports summarizing the findings and actions taken as a result of the process are regularly provided to the hospital board.
- These types of reviews tend to be educational rather than punitive.

Hospitals conduct and comply with multiple delegated and nondelegated UR systems simultaneously:

- A delegated utilization review is an entity external to the hospital under contract with the payer to review services. The norms, criteria, and standards may be those adopted by the hospital medical staff, or the external agency may require that its own protocols be used. The hospital must report its patient-specific findings to the entity; it may also be required to summarize overall findings from its internal UR process.
- A nondelegated utilization review is an entity external to the hospital, which is under contract with the payer, and which reviews services using its own norms, criteria, and standards. This entity relies upon its own personnel to obtain clinical information from clinicians, the patient, family, medical records, or claims information submitted for payment after patient discharge. The review may be conducted concurrently or retrospectively, in person or on the hospital premises, by telephone or by review of documentation.

RISK MANAGEMENT

In general, risk management refers to the process of measuring or assessing risk and then developing strategies to manage that risk.

Measurement and Assessment

Traditional risk management focuses on risks stemming from physical or legal causes (eg, natural disasters or fires, accidents, death, and lawsuits). Ideally, risk management involves a process of prioritization that initially identifies those risks with the greatest potential for loss (patient or employee injury, property damage) and the greatest probability of occurring, followed by the identification of those risks with lower probability of occurrence and lower loss. Types of risk include:

- Knowledge risk: occurs when deficient knowledge is applied.
- Relationship risk: occurs when collaboration ineffectiveness occurs.
- Process-engagement risk: occurs when operational ineffectiveness occurs.

The level of risk can be significantly reduced by the following:

- Scheduling regular (biannual) equipment inspections and maintenance
- Safety training for staff in the use and care of equipment
- Creating and adhering to policies and procedures addressing the cleaning and maintenance of equipment, for example, whirlpools, exercise machines, treatment tables, and spill procedures
- Review of incident reports
- The prompt identification of risk factors in patient care
- Annual certification/recertification of staff in cardiopulmonary resuscitation (CPR)

STRATEGIES

In general, the strategies employed to address risk include:

- Transferring the risk to another party (insurance policies)
- Avoiding the risk
- Reducing the negative effect of the risk
- Accepting some or all of the consequences of a particular risk

PROGRAM DEVELOPMENT

Program development is a systematic process to plan, execute, and implement a program based on the needs of a specific population or group. Program development can be broken down into four phases:

1. Needs assessment: a needs assessment can be used to determine how well a department is currently meeting the needs of the community and the types of resources and services it can provide in the future. It can be in the form of a survey, community forum, or analysis of social indicators. To complete the needs assessment process, a determination must be made as to who will conduct the study, what kind of information needs to be collected (physical, social, cultural, and economic factors of the community), what is the target audience (demographics, perceived needs, real needs), how the information will be collected, and how the information will be used.

2. Program planning: in order to make use of the information collected, the results have to be interpreted. To interpret the data, some statistical analyses are often applied to identify what the majority of the community feels are the most important needs. An important feature of the results should be a reflection of whether the current goals of the department are meeting the needs of the community. When the data analysis is complete, it should be possible to produce a rank-ordered list of the most important changes identified by the community, which can be used to set budget priorities and to determine whether the program is viable.
3. Program implementation: at the end of the planning process, a timeframe should be set for implementation. At this stage, it is a good idea to share the plans with the community or target population.
4. Program evaluation: during this phase, a determination is made as to whether the program should be continued, modified, or discontinued.

PROFESSIONAL STANDARDS

Guide for Professional Conduct of the Physical Therapist[10]

The *Guide for Professional Conduct* was issued by the Ethics and Judicial Committee of the American Physical Therapy Association in 1981 (last amended in June 2009), and published in the *Guide to Professional Conduct*, APTA. The *Guide* is intended to serve the PT in interpreting the code of ethics of APTA the in matters of professional conduct. The code and the *Guide* apply to all PTs.

Interpreting Ethical Principles

The interpretations expressed in the *Guide* reflect the opinions, decisions, and advice of the Ethics and Judicial Committee. The interpretations are intended to assist a PT in applying general ethical principles to specific situations. They should not be considered inclusive of all situations that could evolve.

Principle 1. A physical therapist shall:

A. Respect the rights and dignity of all individuals and shall provide compassionate care.
B. Recognize individual differences and shall respect and be responsive to those differences.
C. Be guided by concern for the physical, psychological, and socioeconomic welfare of patients/clients.
D. Not harass, abuse, or discriminate against others.

Principle 2. A physical therapist shall act in a trustworthy manner toward patients/clients, and in all other aspects of physical therapy practice.

2.1 Patient–Physical Therapist Relationship

A. To act in a trustworthy manner the physical therapist shall act in the patient's/client's best interest. Working in the patient's/

client's best interest requires knowledge of the patient's/client's needs from the patient's/client's perspective. Patients/clients often come to the physical therapist in a vulnerable state and will only rely on the physical therapist's advice, which they perceive to be based on superior knowledge, skill, and experience. A trustworthy physical therapist acts to ameliorate the patient's/client's vulnerability, not to exploit it.

B. A physical therapist shall not exploit any aspect of the physical therapist–patient relationship.

C. A physical therapist shall not engage in any sexual relationship or activity, whether consensual or nonconsensual, with any patient while the physical therapist–patient relationship exists.

D. The physical therapist shall encourage an open and collaborative dialogue with the patient/client.

E. In the event the physical therapist or patient terminates the physical therapist–patient relationship while the patient continues to need physical therapy services, the physical therapist should take steps to transfer the care of the patient to another provider.

2.2 Truthfulness. A physical therapist shall not make statements that he/she knows or should know are false, deceptive, fraudulent, or unfair. See Sections 8.2 C and D.

2.3 Confidential Information

A. Information relating to the physical therapist–patient relationship is confidential and may not be communicated to a third party not involved in that patient's care without the prior consent of the patient, subject to applicable law.

B. Information derived from a peer-review shall be held confidential by the review unless the physical therapist who was reviewed consents to the release of the information.

C. A physical therapist may disclose information to appropriate authorities when it is necessary to protect the welfare of an individual or the community, or when required by law. Such disclosure shall be in accordance with applicable law.

2.4 Patient Autonomy and Consent

A. A physical therapist shall respect the patient's/client's right to make decisions regarding the recommended plan of care, including consent, modification, or refusal.

B. A physical therapist shall communicate to the patient/client the findings of his/her examination, evaluation, diagnosis, and prognosis.

C. A physical therapist shall collaborate with the patient/client to establish the goals of treatment and the plan of care.

D. A physical therapist shall use sound professional judgment in informing the patient/client of any substantial risks of the recommended examination and intervention.

E. A physical therapist shall not restrict patients' freedom to select their provider of physical therapy.

Principle 3. A physical therapist shall comply with rules and regulations governing physical therapy and shall strive to effect changes that benefit a patient/client.

3.1 Professional Practice. A physical therapist shall comply with laws governing the qualifications, functions, and duties of a physical therapist.

3.2 Just Laws and Regulations. A physical therapist shall abdicate the adoption of rules, regulations, and policies by providers, employers, third-party payers, legislatures, and regulatory agencies to provide and improve access to necessary health care services for all individuals.

3.3 Unjust Laws and Regulations. A physical therapist shall endeavor to change unjust laws, regulations, and policies that govern the practice of physical therapy. See Principle 10.2.

Principle 4. A physical therapist shall exercise sound professional judgment.

4.1 Professional Responsibility

A. A physical therapist shall make professional judgments that are in the patient's/client's best interests.

B. Regardless of practice setting, a physical therapist has primary responsibility for the physical therapy care of the patient and shall make independent judgments regarding that care consistent with accepted professional standards. See Section 2.4.

C. A physical therapist shall not provide physical therapy services to a patient/client while his/her ability to do so safely is impaired.

D. A physical therapist shall exercise sound professional judgment based upon his/her knowledge, skill, education, training, and experience.

E. Upon accepting a patient/client for physical therapy services, a physical therapist shall be responsible for: the examination, evaluation, and diagnosis of that individual; the prognosis and intervention; reexamination and modification of the plan of care; and the maintenance of adequate records, including progress reports. A physical therapist shall establish the plan of care and shall provide and/or supervise, and direct, the appropriate interventions. See Sections 2.4 and 6.1.

F. If the diagnostic process reveals findings that are outside the scope of the physical therapist's knowledge, experience, or expertise, the physical therapist shall so inform the patient/client and refer to an appropriate practitioner.

G. When the patient has been referred from another practitioner, the physical therapist shall communicate the findings and/or information to the referring practitioner.

H. A physical therapist shall determine when a patient/client will no longer benefit from physical therapy services. See Section 7.1D.

4.2 Direction and Supervision

A. The supervising physical therapist has primary responsibility for the physical therapy care rendered to a patient/client.

B. A physical therapist shall not delegate to a less qualified person any activity that requires the unique skill, knowledge, and judgment of the physical therapist.

4.3 Practice Arrangements

A. Participation in a business, partnership, corporation, or other entity does not exempt a physical therapist, whether an employer, partner, or stockholder, either individually or collectively, from the obligation to promote, maintain, and comply with the ethical principles of the Association.

B. A physical therapist shall advise his/her employer(s) of any employer practice that causes a physical therapist to be in conflict with the ethical principles of the Association. A physical therapist shall seek to eliminate aspects of his/her employment that are in conflict with the ethical principles of the Association.

4.4 Gifts and other Considerations

A. A physical therapist shall not invite or accept gifts, monetary incentives, or other considerations that affect, or give an appearance of affecting his/her professional judgment.

B. A physical therapist shall not offer or accept kickbacks in exchange for patient referrals. See Sections 7.1F and G and 9.1D.

Principle 5. A physical therapist shall achieve and maintain professional competence.

5.1 Scope of Competence. A physical therapist shall practice within the scope of his/her competence and commensurate with his/her level of education, training, and experience.

5.2 Self-Assessment. A physical therapist has a lifelong professional responsibility for maintaining competence through on-going self-assessment, education, and enhancement of knowledge and skills.

5.3 Professional Development. A physical therapist shall participate in educational activities to enhance his/her basic knowledge and skills. See Section 6.1.

Principle 6. A physical therapist shall maintain and promote high standards for physical therapy practice, education, and research.

6.1 Professional Standards. A physical therapist's practice shall be consistent with accepted professional standards. A physical therapist shall continuously engage in assessment activities to determine compliance with the standards.

6.2 Practice

A. A physical therapist shall achieve and maintain professional competence. See "Principle 5."

B. A physical therapist shall demonstrate his/her commitment to quality improvement by engaging in peer and utilization review and other self-assessment activities.

6.3 Professional Education

A. A physical therapist shall support high-quality education in academic and clinical settings.

B. A physical therapist participating in the educational process is responsible to the students, the academic institutions, and the clinical settings for promoting ethical conduct. A physical therapist shall model ethical behavior and provide the student with information about the Code of Ethics, opportunities to discuss ethical conflicts, and procedures for reporting unresolved ethical conflicts. See "Principle 9."

6.4 Continuing Education

A. A physical therapist providing continuing education must be competent in the content area.

B. When a physical therapist provides continuing education, he/she shall ensure that the course content, objectives, faculty credentials, and responsibilities of the instructional staff are accurately stated in the promotional and instructional course materials.

C. A physical therapist shall evaluate the efficacy and effectiveness of information and techniques presented in continuing education programs before integrating them into his or her practice.

6.5 Research

A. A physical therapist participating in research shall abide by ethical standards governing the protection of human subjects and dissemination of results.

B. A physical therapist shall support research activities that contribute knowledge for improved patient care.

C. A physical therapist shall report to appropriate authorities any acts in the conduct or presentation of research that appear unethical or illegal. See "Principle 9."

Principle 7. A physical therapist shall seek only such remuneration as is deserved and reasonable for physical therapy services.

7.1 Business and Employment Practices

A. A physical therapist's business/employment practices shall be consistent with the ethical principles of the Association.

B. A physical therapist shall never place his/her own financial interests above the welfare of individuals under his/her care.

C. A physical therapist shall recognize that third-party payer contracts may limit, in one form or another, the provision of physical therapy services. Third-party limitations do not absolve the physical therapist from making sound professional judgments that are in the patient's best interest. A physical therapist shall avoid underutilization of physical therapy services.

D. When a physical therapist's judgment is that the patient will receive negligible benefit from physical therapy services, the physical therapist shall not provide or continue to provide such services if the primary reason for doing so is to further the financial self-interest of the physical therapist or his/her employer.

E. Fees for physical therapy services should be reasonable for the service performed, considering the setting in which it is provided, practice costs in the geographic area, judgment of other organizations, and other relevant factors.

F. A physical therapist shall not directly or indirectly request, receive, or participate in the dividing, transferring, assigning, or rebating of an unearned fee. See Sections 4.4 A and B.

G. A physical therapist shall not profit by means of credit or other valuable consideration, such as an unearned commission, discount, or gratuity, in connection with the furnishing of physical therapy services. See Sections 4.4 A and B.
H. Unless laws impose restrictions to the contrary, physical therapists who provide physical therapy within a business entity may pool fees and monies received. Physical therapists may divide or apportion these fees and monies in accordance with the business agreement.
I. A physical therapist may enter into agreements with organizations to provide physical therapy services if such agreements do not violate the ethical principles of the Association or applicable laws.

7.2 Endorsement of Products or Services

A. A physical therapist should not exert influence on individuals under his/her care or their families to use products or services based on the direct or indirect financial interest of the physical therapist in such products or services. Realizing that these individuals will normally rely on the physical therapist's advice, their best interest must always be maintained, as must their right of free choice relating to the use of any product or service. Although it cannot be considered unethical for a physical therapist to own or to have a financial interest in the production, sale, or distribution of products/services, they must act in accordance with the law and make full disclosure of the interest whenever individuals under their care use such products/services.
B. A physical therapist may receive remuneration for endorsement or advertisement of products or services to the public, physical therapists, or other health professionals provided he/she discloses any financial interest in the production, sale, or distribution of said products or services.
C. When endorsing or advertising products or services, a physical therapist shall use sound professional judgment and shall not give the appearance of Association endorsement unless the Association has formally endorsed the products or services.

7.3 Disclosure. A physical therapist shall disclose to the patient if the referring practitioner derives compensation from the provision of physical therapy.

Principle 8. A physical therapist shall provide and make available accurate and relevant information to patients/clients about their care and to the public about physical therapy services.

8.1 Accurate and Relevant Information to the Patient

A. A physical therapist shall provide the patient/client information about his/her condition and plan of care. See Section 2.4.
B. Upon the request of the patient, the physical therapist shall provide, or make available, the medical records to the patient or a patient-designated third-party.
C. A physical therapist shall inform patients of any known financial limitations that may affect their care.

D. A physical therapist shall inform the patient when, in his/her judgment, the patient will receive negligible benefit from further care. See Section 7.1C.

8.2 Accurate and Relevant Information to the Public

A. A physical therapist shall inform the public about the societal benefits of the profession and who is qualified to provide physical therapy services.
B. Information given to the public shall emphasize that individual problems cannot be treated without individualized examination and plans/programs of care.
C. A physical therapist may advertise his/her services to the public. See Section 2.2.
D. A physical therapist shall not use, or participate in the use of, any form of communication containing a false, plagiarized, fraudulent, deceptive, unfair, or sensational statement or claim. See Section 2.2.
E. A physical therapist who places a paid advertisement shall identify it as such unless it is apparent from the context that it is a paid advertisement.

Principle 9. A physical therapist shall protect the public and the profession from unethical, incompetent, and illegal acts.

9.1 Consumer Protection

A. A physical therapist shall provide care that is within the scope of practice as defined by the state practice act.
B. A physical therapist shall not engage in any conduct that is unethical, incompetent, or illegal.
C. A physical therapist shall report any conduct that appears to be unethical, incompetent, or illegal.
D. A physical therapist may not participate in any arrangements in which patients are exploited due to the referring sources' enhancing their personal incomes as a result of referring for, describing, or recommending physical therapy. See Sections 2.1B, "Principle 4," and "Principle 7."

Principle 10. A physical therapist shall endeavor to address the health needs of society.

10.1 Pro Bono Services. A physical therapist shall render pro bono publico (reduced or no fee) services to patients lacking the ability to pay for services, as each physical therapist's practice permits.

10.2 Individual and Community Health

A. A physical therapist shall be aware of the patient's health-related needs and act in a manner that facilitates meeting those needs.
B. A physical therapist shall endeavor to support activities that benefit the health status of the community. See "Principle 3."

Principle 11. A physical therapist shall respect the rights, knowledge, and skills of colleagues and other health care professionals.

11.1 Consultation. A physical therapist shall seek consultation whenever the welfare of the patient will be safeguarded or advanced by consulting those who have special skills, knowledge, or experience.

11.2 Patient/Provider Relationships. A physical therapist shall not undermine the relationship(s) between his/her patient and other health care professionals.

11.3 Disparagement. A physical therapist shall not disparage colleagues and other health-care professionals. See "Principle 9" and Section 2.4A.

The guide for the conduct of the physical therapist assistant is provided in Table A-2 of the Appendix.

STANDARDS OF PRACTICE FOR PHYSICAL THERAPY AND THE CRITERIA[10]

Preamble

The physical therapy profession's commitment to society is to promote optimal health and function in individuals by pursuing excellence in practice. The American Physical Therapy Association (APTA) attests to this commitment by adopting and promoting the following Standards of Practice for Physical Therapy. These standards are the profession's statement of conditions and performances that are essential for the provision of high-quality professional service to society and provide a foundation for assessment of physical therapy practice.

Legal/Ethical Considerations

1. Legal considerations:
   a. A physical therapist complies with all the legal requirements of jurisdictions regulating the practice of physical therapy.
   b. The physical therapist assistant complies with all the legal requirements of jurisdictions regulating the work of the assistant.
2. Ethical considerations:
   a. The physical therapist practices according to the Code of Ethics of the APTA.
   b. The physical therapist assistant complies with the Standards of Ethical Conduct of the Physical Therapist Assistant of the APTA.

Administration of the Physical Therapy Service

1. Statement of mission, purposes, and goals
   a. The physical therapy service has a statement of mission, purposes, and goals that reflect the needs and interests of the patients and clients served, the physical therapy personnel affiliated with the service, and the community.
2. Organizational plan
   a. The physical therapy service has a written organizational plan.

3. Policies and procedures
   a. The physical therapy service has written policies and procedures that reflect the operation of the service and that are consistent with the Association's standards, mission, policies, positions, guidelines, and Code of Ethics.
4. Administration
   a. A physical therapist is responsible for the direction of the physical therapy service.
5. Fiscal management
   a. The director of the physical therapy service, in consultation with physical therapy staff and appropriate administrative personnel, participates in planning for, and allocation of, resources. Fiscal planning and management of the service is based on sound accounting principles.
6. Improvement of quality of care and performance
   a. The physical therapy service has a written plan for continuous improvement of quality of care and performance of services.
7. Staffing
   a. The physical therapy personnel affiliated with the physical therapy service have demonstrated competence and are sufficient to achieve the mission, purposes, and goals of the services.
   b. The physical therapy service has a written plan that provides for appropriate and ongoing staff development.
8. Physical setting
   a. The physical setting is designed to provide a safe and accessible environment that facilitates fulfillment of the mission, purposes, and goals of the physical therapy service. The equipment is safe and sufficient to achieve the purposes and goals of the service.
9. Collaboration
   a. The physical therapy service collaborates with all appropriate disciplines.

PATIENT/CLIENT MANAGEMENT

1. Patient client collaboration
   a. Within the patient/client management process, the physical therapist and patient/client establish and maintain an ongoing collaborative process of decision making that exists throughout the provision of services.
2. Initial examination/evaluation/diagnosis/prognosis
   a. A physical therapist performs an initial examination and evaluation to establish a diagnosis and prognosis prior to intervention.
3. Plan of care
   a. The physical therapist establishes a plan of care and manages the needs of the patient/client based on the examination, evaluation, diagnosis, prognosis, goals, and outcomes of the planned interventions for identified impairments, functional limitations, and disabilities.
   b. The physical therapist involves the patient/client and appropriate others in the planning, implementation, and assessment of the plan of care.

c. The physical therapist, in consultation with appropriate disciplines, plans the discharge of the patient/client taking into consideration the achievements of anticipated goals and expected outcomes, and provides for appropriate follow-up or referral.

4. Intervention
   a. The physical therapist provides, or directs and supervises, the physical therapy intervention consistent with the results of the examination, evaluation, diagnosis, prognosis, and plan of care.
5. Reexamination
   a. The physical therapist reexamines the patient/client as necessary during an episode of care to evaluate progress, or changes in the patient/client status, to modify the plan of care accordingly, or discontinue physical therapy services.
   b. The physical therapists reexamination
      (1) Identifies ongoing patient/client needs
      (2) May result in recommendations for additional services, discharge, or discontinuation of physical therapy needs
6. Discharge/discontinuation of intervention
   a. The physical therapist discharges the patient/client from physical therapy services when the anticipated goals or expected outcomes for the patient/client have been achieved.
   b. The physical therapist discontinues the intervention when the patient/client is unable to continue to progress toward goals or when the physical therapist determines that the patient/client will no longer benefit from physical therapy.
7. Communication/coordination/documentation
   a. The physical therapist communicates, coordinates, and documents all aspects of patient/client management including the results of the initial examination and evaluation, diagnosis, prognosis, plan of care, interventions, response to interventions, changes in patient/client status relative to the interventions, reexamination, and discharge/discontinuation of intervention and other patient/client management activities.
8. Education
   a. The physical therapist is responsible for individual professional development. The physical therapist assistant is responsible for individual career development.
   b. The physical therapist and the physical therapist assistant (under the direction and supervision of the physical therapist) participate in the education of students.
   c. The physical therapist educates and provides consultation to consumers and the general public regarding the purposes and benefits of physical therapy.
   d. The physical therapist educates and provides consultation to consumers and the general public regarding the roles of the physical therapist, the physical therapist assistant, and other support personnel.
9. Research
   a. The physical therapist applies research findings to practice and encourages, participates in, and promotes activities that establish the outcomes of patient/client management provided by the physical therapist.

10. Community responsibility
    a. The physical therapist demonstrates community responsibility by participating in community and community agency activities, educating the public, formulating public policy, or providing pro bono physical therapy services.

Questions for this chapter and the entire book appear on the included CD-ROM, with additional questions at www.DuttonNPTE.com.

REFERENCES

1. APTA: *Guide to Physical Therapist Practice, 2nd ed.* American Physical Therapy Association. *Phys Ther.* 2001;81:1-746.
2. APTA: *Guide to Physical Therapist Practice:* revisions. American Physical Therapy Association. *Phys Ther.* 2001;79:623-629.
3. Nagi S: Disability concepts revisited: implications for prevention. In: Pope A, Tartov A, eds. *Disability in America: Toward a National Agenda for Prevention.* Washington, DC: National Academy Press. 1991:309-327.
4. Brandt EN, Jr., Pope AM: *Enabling America: Assessing the Role of Rehabilitation Science and Engineering.* Washington, DC: Institute of Medicine, National Academy Press. 1997.
5. Palisano RJ, Campbell SK, Harris SR: Evidence-based decision-making in pediatric physical therapy. In: Campbell SK, Vander Linden DW, Palisano RJ, eds. *Physical Therapy for Children.* St. Louis, MO: Saunders. 2006:3-32.
6. Kettenbach G: Background information. In: Kettenbach G, ed. *Writing SOAP Notes with Patient/Client Management Formats, 3rd ed.* Philadelphia, PA: FA Davis. 2004:1-5.
7. O'Sullivan SB: Clinical decision-making. In: O'Sullivan SB, Schmitz TJ, eds. *Physical Rehabilitation, 5th ed.* Philadelphia, PA: FA Davis. 2007:3-24.
8. Goodman CC, Snyder TK: Introduction to the interviewing process. In: Goodman CC, Snyder TK, eds. *Differential Diagnosis in Physical Therapy.* Philadelphia, PA: Saunders. 1990:7-42.
9. APTA: *Guide to Physical Therapist Practice. Phys Ther.* 2001;81:S13-S95.
10. Grieve GP: *Common Vertebral Joint Problems.* New York, NY: Churchill Livingstone Inc. 1981.
11. APTA BOD: *Minimum Required Skills of Physical Therapist Graduates at Entry-Level,* BOD P11-05-20-49. Alexandria, VA: APTA. 2004.
12. Rothstein JM, Echternach JL, Riddle DL: The hypothesis-orientedalgorithm for clinicians II (HOAC II): a guide for patient management. *Phys Ther.* 2003;83:455-470.
13. Echternach JL, Rothstein JM: Hypothesis-oriented algorithms. *Phys Ther.* 1989;69:559-564.
14. Rothstein JM, Echternach JL: Hypothesis-oriented algorithm for clinicians. A method for evaluation and treatment planning. *Phys Ther.* 1986;66:1388-1394.
15. Schenkman M, Butler RB: A model for multisystem evaluation treatment of individuals with Parkinson's disease. *Phys Ther.* 1989; 69:932-943.

16. Schenkman M, Butler RB: A model for multisystem evaluation, interpretation, and treatment of individuals with neurologic dysfunction. *Phys Ther.* 1989;69:538-547.
17. Schenkman M, Donovan J, Tsubota J, et al.: Management of individuals with Parkinson's disease: rationale and case studies. *Phys Ther.* 1989;69:944-955.
18. Randall KE, McEwen IR: Writing patient-centered goals. *Phys Ther.* 2000;80:1197-1203.
19. O'Neill DL, Harris SR: Developing goals and objectives for handicapped children. *Phys Ther.* 1982;62:295-298.
20. American Occupational Therapy Association: Essentials and guidelines for an accredited educational program for the occupational therapy assistant. *Am J Occup Ther.* 1991;45:1085-1092.

Health Care Administration

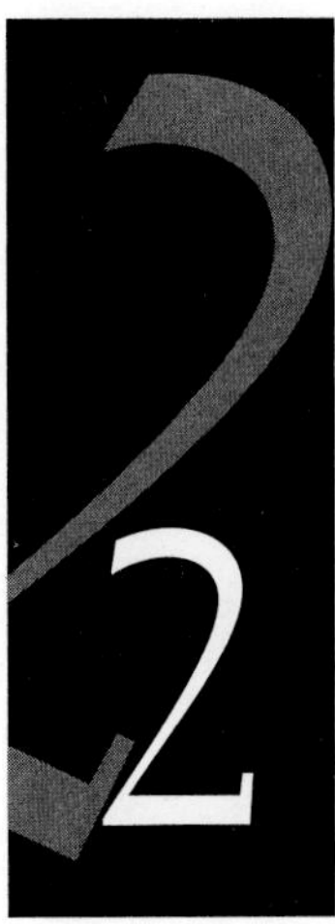

THE FUNDING OF HEALTH CARE

The traditional model provided health insurance in one of four ways:

1. Out-of-pocket payments.
2. Individual private insurance (generally for self-employed individuals). In return for paying a monthly sum, people receive assistance in case of illness.
3. Employment-based private insurance. Employers usually pay most of the premium that purchase health insurance for their employees as a benefit of employment. In most cases, employment-based plans now require employee contributions and co-payments. The government does not treat the health insurance fringe benefits as taxable income to the employee, so the government is in essence subsidizing employer-sponsored health insurance. A new form of employment-based private insurance is consumer-driven health care (CDH). Defined narrowly, consumer-driven health care refers to health plans in which individuals have a personal health account, such as a health savings account (HSA) or a health reimbursement arrangement (HRA), from which they pay medical expenses directly. The phrase is sometimes used more broadly to refer to defined contribution health plans, which allow employees to choose among various plans, often with a fixed dollar contribution from an employer. The characteristics of a CDH include:
   - High benefit level options involve significant employee contributions and deductibles in addition to an employer's contribution.
   - Lower benefit level options that involve less employee contributions and deductibles.
   - Greater choice and control over one's health plan.

- Economic incentives to better manage care—economic rewards for making good decisions and economic penalties for making ill-advised ones. These economic incentives make patients more likely to seek information about medical conditions and treatment options, including information about prices and quality.

4. Government financing through government funded programs, such as Medicare, Medicaid, and the Federal Employees Health Benefit Plans.
   - Medicare. Administered by the federal government—Center for Medicare and Medicaid Services (CMS)—an agency within the U.S. Department of Health and Human Services, through the extension of title XVIII of the Social Security Act, 1965 (law that created Medicare, Medicaid, and other federal programs). Two different varieties or parts are as follows:
     - Part A. On reaching the age of 65 years, people who are eligible for Social Security are automatically enrolled in Medicare part A whether or not they are retired. If a person has paid into the Social Security system for 10 years, his or her spouse is eligible for Social Security.[1] People who are not eligible for Social Security can enroll in Medicare part A by paying a monthly premium. People under the age of 65 who are totally and permanently disabled may enroll in Medicare part A after they have received Social Security disability benefits for 24 months. People with chronic renal disease requiring dialysis or transplant may also be eligible for Medicare part A without a 2-year waiting period. Part A helps pay for medically necessary inpatient hospital care (limits the number of hospital days), and, after a hospital stay, a limited inpatient care in a skilled nursing facility, or limited home health care or hospice care (Table 2-1).
     - Part B. The part B (Table 2-1) is for people who are eligible for Medicare part A and who elect to pay the Medicare part B premium of $96.40 a month (2008).[1] Some low income persons are not required to pay the premium.
   - Medicaid. A federal program mandated by title XIX of the Social Security Act, which is administered by the states, with the federal government paying between 50% and 76% of the total Medicaid costs. Benefits vary from state to state: The federal contribution is greater in states with lower per capita incomes. Medicaid pays for medical and other services on behalf of certain groups:
     - Low income families with children who meet certain eligibility requirements.
     - Most elderly, disabled, and blind individuals who receivecash assistance under the federal Supplemental Security Income (SSI) program.
     - Children younger than age 6 and pregnant women whose family income is at or below 133% of the federal poverty level. In 2008, the federal poverty level was $21,200 for a family of four.
     - School-age children (6-18 years) whose family income is at or below the federal poverty level.

Study Pearl

The Medicare Modernization Act of 2003 made two major changes in the Medicare program:

- Medicare advantage program: an expansion of the role of private health plans that rejuvenated the previous Medicare + Choice program by which Medicare beneficiaries could pay an additional premium to enroll in private Medicare HMO plans.
- Medicare part D: a prescription drug benefit. Has proved controversial as there are major gaps in coverage. Coverage has been farmed out to private insurance companies rather than administered by the federal Medicare program, and the government is not allowed to negotiate with pharmaceutical companies for lower drug prices.[1]

Study Pearl

Health Care Financing Administration (HCFA) was the previous name for Center for Medicare and Medicaid Services (CMS)

TABLE 2-1. MEDICARE PART A AND PART B (2008)

MEDICARE PART	METHOD OF FINANCING	BENEFIT	MEDICARE PAYS
A	Employers and employees each pay to Medicare 1.45% of wages and salaries into the Social Security system. Self-employed people pay 2.9%.	Hospitalization	
		First 60 days	All but a $1024 deductible per spell of illness
		61st-90th day	All but $256 per day
		91st-150th day	All but $512 per day
		Beyond 90 days if lifetime reserve days are used up	Nothing
		Skilled Nursing Facility (SNF)	
		First 20 days	All
		21st-100th day	All but $128 per day
		Beyond 100 days	Nothing
		Home health care	
		100 visits per spell of illness	100% for skilled care as defined by Medicare regulations
		Hospice care	
		Requires physician certification that individual has a terminal illness	100% form of services, co-pays for outpatient drugs and coinsurance for inpatient respite care
B	In part by general federal revenues (personal income and other federal taxes) and in part by part B monthly premium	Medical expenses	80% of approved amount after a $135 annual deductibles
		Physician services	
		Physical, occupational, and speech therapy	
		Medical equipment	
		Diagnostic tests	
		Preventative care (some Pap smears; some mammogram; hepatitis B, pneumococcal, and influenza vaccinations)	Included in medical expenses, with deductible and coinsurance waived for some services
		Outpatient medications. Partially covered under Medicare part D	All except for premium, deductible, coinsurance
		Eye refractions, hearing aids, dental services	Not covered

Data from Bodenheimer TS, Grumbach K: Paying for healthcare. In: Bodenheimer TS, Grumbach K, eds. *Understanding Health Policy: A Clinical Approach, 5th ed.* New York: McGraw-Hill. 2009:5-16.

Study Pearl

Medicaid Waivers are an exception to the usual requirements of Medicaid granted to a state by CMS. It allows states to:

- Waive provisions of the Medicaid law to test new concepts that are consistent with the goals of the Medicaid program. System-wide changes are possible under this provision. Frequently used to establish Medicaid-managed care programs.
- Waive freedom of choice. States may require that beneficiaries enroll in HMOs or other managed care programs, or select a physician to serve as their primary care case manager.
- Waive various Medicaid requirements to establish alternative, community-based services for (a) individuals who would otherwise require the level of care provided in a hospital or skilled nursing facility, and/or (b) persons already in such facilities who need assistance returning to the community. Target populations for 1915 (c) waivers include older adults, persons with disabilities, persons with mental retardation, persons with chronic mental illness, and persons with AIDS.
- Limit expenditures for nursing facility and home and community-based services for person 65 years and older so that they do not exceed a projected amount, determined by taking base year expenditure (last year before the waiver), and adjusting for inflation. Also eliminates requirements that programs are state-wide and be comparable for all target populations. Income rules for eligibility can also be waived.

Due to a large expenditure growth, the federal government ceded to states enhanced control of the Medicaid programs through Medicaid waivers, which allow states to reduce the number of people on Medicaid, to make alterations and scope of covered services, to require Medicaid recipients to pay part of their costs, and to obligate Medicaid recipients to enroll in managed care plans.[1]

In 1997, the federal government created the State Children's Health Insurance Program (SCHIP), a companion program for Medicaid designed to cover uninsured children in families with incomes at or below 200% of the federal poverty level, but above the Medicaid income eligibility level.[1]

> **Study Pearl**
>
> - Primary Care Case Management (PCCM). Medicaid managed care option allowed under Section 1915(b) of the Social Security Act in which each participant is assigned to a single primary care provider who must authorize most other services such as specialty physician care before they can be reimbursed by Medicaid.
> - Medicaid Prudent Pharmaceutical Purchasing Act (MPPPA). Enacted as part of the Omnibus Budget Reconciliation Act of 1990, MPPPA provides that Medicaid must receive the best-discounted price of any institutional purchaser of pharmaceuticals. In doing so, drug companies provide rebates to Medicaid equal to the difference between the discounted price and the price at which the drug was sold. This bill has resulted in cost shifting throughout the health industry.

MANAGED CARE PLANS

There are three major forms of managed care:

1. Fee-for-service reimbursement with utilization review. The third-party payer (whether private insurance company or government agency) has the authority to deny payment for expensive or unnecessary medical interventions.
2. Preferred provider organizations (PPOs). Insurers contract with a limited number of physicians and hospitals that agree to care for patients, usually on a discounted fee-for-service basis with utilization review.
3. Health maintenance organizations (HMOs). Organizations whose patients are required (except in emergencies) to receive their care from providers within that HMO. Several types of HMOs exist.

PERSONAL PAYMENT AND FREE CARE

An estimated 34 million Americans do not have health insurance: 56% are workers; 28% are children; and 16% are nonworking adults. About 83% of workers have private health insurance.

- Individuals who cannot pay for health care can receive pro bono or free care through philanthropic donations and services.
- Hill-Burton Act: Federal legislation enacted in 1947 to support the construction and modernization of health care institutions. Hospitals that receive Hill-Burton funds must provide specific levels of charity care.

> **Study Pearl**
>
> While the number of uninsured people is high, these people do have some recourse to emergency treatment. Hospital emergency rooms (those that receive tax-exemption, Federal Hill-Burton grants, or loans) are not allowed to turn away patients because of inability to pay. However, care is limited to emergency care only.
>
> The costs incurred by this population are covered by a surcharge on insurance payments.

BALANCED BUDGET ACT OF 1997

This law made sweeping changes in the Medicare and Medicaid programs. Several of the significant provisions of the Balanced Budget Act of 1997 (BBA) were payment reductions to health care providers, new prospective payment systems for health care providers, and reduction of coverage of health care services by the Medicare and Medicaid programs.

REIMBURSING HEALTH CARE PROVIDERS

Reimbursement to physicians, health care providers, and hospitals by insurance companies and government programs can occur in a number of ways:[2]

- Fee-for-service. The unit of payment is the visit or procedure.
- Payment by episode of illness. The entity is paid one sum for all services delivered during one illness.
- Per diem payments. Payments to hospitals for service delivered to a patient during 1 day.
- Capitation payment. One payment is made for each patient during a month or year.

ACCESS TO HEALTH CARE

The organizational task facing health care systems is one of assuring that the right patient receives the right service at the right time in the right place, and with the right caregiver.[3,4] The health care system is organized into three levels:[4]

1. Primary care: it involves common health problems and preventative measures that account for 80% to 90% of visits to a physician or other caregiver.
2. Secondary care: it involves problems that require more specialized clinical expertise such as hospital care for patients with a cardiac arrest.
3. Tertiary care: it involves the management of rare and complex disorders.

HEALTH INSURANCE AND PORTABILITY ACCOUNTABILITY ACT

The purpose of the Health Insurance and Portability Accountability Act (HIPAA) was to provide a mechanism to spread the risk of unforeseen medical expenditures across a broad base to protect the individual from personal expenditures. This 1996 federal legislation makes long-term care insurance premiums tax-deductible if non-reimbursable medical expenses, including part or all of long-term care premiums, exceed 7.5% of an individual's gross income. HIPAA also excludes long-term care insurance benefits from taxable income. Not all long-term care insurance coverage qualifies for this benefit.

Study Pearl

Regulatory controls within the U.S. healthcare system include the fraud and abuse provisions included in the HIPAA of 1996 and the 1997 BBA and those listed in Table 2-2.

EMERGENCY MEDICAL TREATMENT AND LABOR ACT

The Emergency Medical Treatment and Labor Act (EMTALA), also known as COBRA or the Patient Anti-Dumping Law, requires most hospitals to provide an examination and needed stabilizing treatment, without consideration of insurance coverage or ability to pay, when a patient presents to an emergency room for attention to an emergency medical condition.

TABLE 2-2. FISCAL REGULATIONS WITHIN THE U.S. HEALTH CARE

REGULATION	DESCRIPTION
False Claims Act of 1863	First signed into law in 1863. Underwent significant changes in 1986. Allows citizens to bring law suits against groups or other individuals who are defrauding the government through programs, agencies, or contracts (over-billing for services, "upcoding").
Medicare and Medicaid antifraud statutes	Stipulates that an individual who knowingly and willfully offers, pays, solicits, or receives any remuneration in exchange for referring an individual for the furnishing of any item or service (or for the purchasing, leasing, ordering, or recommending of any goods, facility, item, or service) paid for in whole or in part by Medicare or a state health care program (ie, Medicaid) shall be guilty of a felony. Often referred to as the "antikickback" statute.
The Civil Monetary Penalties Law (CMPL)	Authorizes the Secretary of Health and Human Services to impose civil money penalties, an assessment, and program exclusion for various forms of fraud and abuse involving the Medicare and Medicaid programs.
Federal self-referral prohibitions	Also known as Stark I and II. The first Self-Referral Prohibitions (Stark I) prohibited physicians from referring lab specimens obtained from Medicare patients to clinical laboratories with which the physician or an immediate family member of the physician had a financial relationship. In addition, any clinical laboratory that received a Medicare referral from a physician with which it had a financial relationship, could not bill Medicare for the performance of that procedure. A financial relationship is defined as either an ownership/investment interest or a compensation relationship. The expanded physician Self-Referral prohibitions (Stark II), introduced in 1995, prohibits self-referrals (Medicaid and Medicare) of not only lab services, but also many other designated health services, including physical therapy.
Pharmaceutical price regulation scheme	A scheme that ensures the national health system has access to good quality branded medicines at reasonable prices, and promotes a healthy, competitive pharmaceutical industry. Includes federal average wholesale price restrictions for Medicaid and state pharmaceutical regulations.
Certificate of Need (CON)	Intended to regulate major capital expenditures, which may adversely impact the cost of health care services, to prevent the unnecessary expansion of health care facilities, and encourage the appropriate allocation of resources for health care purposes. CON laws became part of almost every state by 1978 after the 1974 National Health Act was passed.

PATIENT SELF-DETERMINATION ACT OF 1990

The Patient Self-Determination Act (PSDA) requires many Medicare and Medicaid providers (hospitals, nursing homes, hospice programs, home health agencies, and HMOs) to give adult individuals, at the time of inpatient admission or enrollment, certain information about their rights under state laws including:

- the right to participate in and direct their own health care decisions
- the right to accept or refuse medical or surgical treatment
- the right to prepare an advance directive
- information on the provider's policies that govern the utilization of these rights

Study Pearl

An advance directive is a written instruction, such as a living will or a durable power of attorney for health care, that provides instructions for the provision of medical treatment *in anticipation* of those times when the individual executing the document no longer has decision-making capacity.

The act also prohibits institutions from discriminating against a patient who does not have an advance directive.

THE PATIENT PROTECTION AND AFFORDABLE CARE ACT

The Patient Protection and Affordable Care Act (PPACA) is a federal statute that was signed into U.S. law in March 2010, along with the Health Care and Education Reconciliation Act of 2010 (also signed into law in March, 2010). The law includes numerous health-related provisions to take effect over a 4-year period beginning in 2010:

- Guaranteed issue and community rating—insurers must offer the same premium to all applicants of the same age, sex, and geographical location regardless of whether the applicant has a preexisting condition.
- Medicaid eligibility is expanded to include individuals and families up to 133% of poverty level.
- New health insurance exchanges in each state will enhance competition by offering a marketplace where individuals and small businesses can compare policy premiums on a like for like basis, and buy insurance (with a government subsidy if eligible). Low income persons and families above the Medicaid level and up to 400% of poverty level will receive subsidies on a sliding scale if they choose to purchase insurance via a health insurance exchange.
- Introduction into the tax code of a "shared responsibility payment" which is a fine paid by any large employer (with 50 or more employees) if the government has had to subsidize an employee who bought insurance in the exchange because the employer did not offer a minimum coverage plan or better. Another form of shared responsibility payment or fine is imposed on certain persons who do not have minimum essential coverage for at least 1 month in the year (individual mandate), though being insured is not actually mandated by law.
- Improved benefits for Medicare prescription drug coverage.
- Establishment of national voluntary insurance program for purchasing community living assistance services and support.
- Very small businesses will be able to get subsidies if they purchase health insurance through the exchange.
- Additional support is provided for medical research and the National Institutes of Health.

HEALTH INSURANCE REGULATION

Health insurance regulation occurs at both the federal and state levels. Such regulations cover the gamut, regulating Blue Cross and Blue Shield carriers (which, if not for-profit, are often regulated somewhat differently than their commercial counterparts), commercial insurance companies, self-insured plans, and various flavors of managed care, including Health Maintenance Organizations (HMOs) and Preferred Provider Organizations (PPOs). These entities write group coverage for employers, associations, or similar groups, as well as individual coverage.

A number of regulations monitor the accessibility of health care. These include:

- Health Maintenance Organization Act of 1973.
- Anti-discriminatory restrictions (including the Rehabilitation Act of 1973, Pregnancy Discrimination Act of 1978, Americans with Disabilities Act of 1990, and Child Abuse Prevention and Treatment Act Amendments of 1984).
- Continuation of coverage requirements (including the Consolidated Omnibus Reconciliation Act of 1986 and state rules).
- Mandated health benefits (including mandated standards of care) such as bone marrow transplants. There are at present three federally mandated health insurance benefits:
  - The Mental Health Parity Act of 1996
  - Newborns' and Mothers' Protection Health Act of 1996
  - Women's Health and Cancer Rights Act of 1998

HEALTH CARE COMMON PROCEDURAL CODING SYSTEM

Health Care Common Procedural Coding System (HCPCS) is a federal coding system for medical procedures. It includes Current Procedural Terminology (CPT) codes, national alphanumeric codes, and local alphanumeric codes. The national codes are developed by the CMS to supplement CPT codes. They include physical services not included in CPT as well as nonphysician services such as ambulance, physical therapy, and durable medical equipment. The local codes are developed by local Medicare carriers to supplement the national codes. HCPCS codes are five-digit codes, the first digit is a letter followed by four numbers. HCPCS codes beginning with A through V are national; those beginning with W through Z are local. Also see physician's current procedural terminology.

CURRENT CONCERNS ABOUT QUALITY OF CARE

As health care costs have risen, efforts, both by government and private entities, to control costs have focused on a number of areas:

- Decreasing costs/expenses. Labor is the one of the biggest expenses to an organization. Decreasing or replacing manpower has the following disadvantages:
  - The use of lower cost paraprofessionals results in an increased share of the workload being performed by aides and technicians.
  - An increase in caseload size, resulting in less time spent with each patient.

Problems faced by health care providers include:

- Shortages in qualified personnel (physicians, pharmacists, nurses). Patients in rural areas face shortages of all types of health care personnel (about 20% of the U.S. population lives in areas that have a shortage of primary health care professionals).[5-7]

- An increasingly aging population.
- Lack of drug control. Although the drugs used in the United States must be approved for safety and efficacy, there are no constraints on either therapeutic duplication or price (see Chapter 19). Any drug that obtains approval from the Food & Drug Administration (FDA) may be marketed in the United States, and the distributor has full discretion over the price charged.

QUALITY OF CARE REGULATORS

A number of regulations exist within the U.S. health care that attempt to ensure quality of care. These include:

- Hospital accreditation and licensure, which includes Medicare Conditions of Participation (COP), and Joint Commission on Accreditation of Healthcare Organizations (JCAHO) (see "Voluntary Accreditation" section).
- State accreditation and licensure, including the Department of Health.
- Nursing home accreditation and licensure (including JCAHO, COP, the Nursing Home Reform Act, part of the Omnibus Budget Reconciliation Act of 1987, and state regulations).
- Licensure for all other health facilities (see "Voluntary Accreditation" section).
- Peer review, encompassing Quality Improvement Organizations and the Health Care Quality Improvement Act of 1986.
- The Clinical Laboratory Improvement Act of 1967 as amended.
- FDA regulation of blood banks.
- Blood-borne pathogen requirements imposed by the Occupational Safety and Health Administration (OSHA).
- Health outcomes reporting systems mandated by states.

Study Pearl

The goal of OSHA is to create a safe and healthy working environment for employees. Employers must provide a working environment that is free from recognized hazards and employees must adhere to health and safety standards. The National Institute for Safety and Health (NIOSH) is the research arm of OSHA. NIOSH has developed *Elements of Ergonomics Programs,* a primer based on workplace evaluations of musculoskeletal disorders that is useful in developing a program focusing on ergonomics (see Chapter 7).

VOLUNTARY ACCREDITING AGENCIES

Accreditation of health care institutions is a voluntary process by which an authorized agency or organization evaluates and recognizes health services according to a set of standards describing the structures and processes that contribute to desirable patient outcomes. Outpatient centers for comprehensive rehabilitation can be accredited by JCAHO, AC-MRDD, and/or CARF.

Joint Commission on Accreditation of Healthcare Organizations. Joint Commission on Accreditation of Healthcare Organizations (JCAHO) is a private organization created in 1951 to provide voluntary accreditation to hospitals. Many states rely on JCAHO accreditation as a substitute for their own inspection programs. In 1964, the JCAHO began charging hospitals for the surveys it performed. JCAHO has high standards of quality assurance and a rigorous process of evaluation, which makes it a much-esteemed agency for accreditation. Health services certified by JCAHO are given "deemed status" (in 1965, Congress passed amendments to the Social Security Act stating that hospitals accredited by JCAHO are "deemed" to be in compliance with most of Medicare's "Conditions of Participation for Hospitals" and therefore are able to participate in Medicare and Medicaid and are eligible for millions of federal health care dollars).

In the 1990s, JCAHO revised their standards to reflect the changing functions of hospitals, seeking to move away from departments and toward the patient experience of hospital systems. More recently, JCAHO has moved toward trying to find standards that reflect the integration of hospital services rather than examining them in isolation, and have begun to examine outcome measures instead of simple process standards for good practice.

Study Pearl

JCAHO accredits more than 80% of the nation's hospitals. It also accredits skilled nursing facilities, hospices, health plans, and other care organizations that provide home care, mental health care, laboratory, ambulatory care, and long-term services.

Disadvantages

- Hospitals pay for JCAHO surveys, and more than 70% of JCAHO's revenue comes directly from the organizations it is supposed to inspect.
- Hospitals and other health care providers are notified weeks or months in advance that a JCAHO survey team will be arriving—giving the provider plenty of time to make cosmetic changes, prepare staff to answer questions, update patient and personnel records, and increase staffing levels.
- Although JCAHO encourages workers to speak with survey-takers, most workers do not have legal protection from retaliation if they do so.

Study Pearl

The JCAHO surveys a hospital every 3 years.

Accreditation Council for Services for Mentally Retarded and Other Developmentally Disabled Persons. Accreditation Council for Services for Mentally Retarded and Other Developmentally Disabled Persons (AC-MRDD) is a voluntary agency that accredits programs or agencies that serve persons with developmental disabilities.

Commission on Accreditation of Rehabilitation Facilities. Commission on Accreditation of Rehabilitation Facilities (CARF) is a nonprofit organization designed to recognize standards of excellence in rehabilitation programs across the nation. CARF accreditation standards were developed with the input of consumers, rehabilitation professionals, state and national organizations, and third-party purchasers. It is designed to establish standards of quality for freestanding rehabilitation facilities and the rehabilitative programs of the largest hospital systems in the areas of behavioral health, employment (work hardening) and community support services and medical rehabilitation (spinal cord injury, chronic pain), and to determine how well an organization is serving its patients, consumers, and the community.

Programs accredited by CARF have demonstrated that they meet the national standards for rehabilitation programs.

Comprehensive Outpatient Rehabilitation Facility. The Comprehensive Outpatient Rehabilitation Facility (CORF) accreditation group conducts certification surveys for compliance with federal and state regulations and investigates any complaints filed against one of these providers. Certification is achieved by adherence to federal requirements including:

- Submission of a complete application.
- Required documentation.
- Successful completion of a survey. Each CORF must be surveyed for certification as directed by the Centers for Medicare/Medicaid Services (CMS). An application for certification includes submission of a completed application, required documentation, and successful completion of a survey. There are no fees and no renewal applications required for certification. There are no state licensing requirements imposed by the agency.

The Typical Accreditation Process

1. Organization submits an application for review.
2. A survey conducted by the accrediting agency.
3. The organization conducts a self-study or self-assessment to examine itself based on the accrediting agency standards.
4. An individual reviewer or surveyor, or a team visiting the organization conducts an on-site review.
5. The whole staff of the organization is involved in the accreditation and reaccreditation process. Tasks include document preparation, hosting the site visit team, and interviews with the accreditors.
6. Accreditation surveyor or team issues a report granting or denying accreditation.
   - If accredited, the organization undergoes periodic review, typically every 3 years.
   - Some accrediting bodies may perform unannounced or unscheduled site surveys to ensure ongoing compliance.

FEDERAL AND STATE HEALTH CARE REGULATIONS

In the United States, health care regulation is undertaken to improve performance and quality through an enormous variety of different governmental and nongovernmental agencies. These entities have varying statutory authority, scope and remit, approaches and outcomes resulting in a complex, overlapping, duplicative, and sometimes contradictory regulatory environment.

STATUTORY LAWS

Statutes are defined as laws that are passed by Congress and the various state legislatures. These statutes are the basis for statutory law. The legislature passes statutes that are later put into the federal code of laws or pertinent state code of laws. Statutory law consists of the acts of legislatures declaring, commanding, or prohibiting something; a particular law established by the will of the legislative department of government. A number of statutory laws impact physical therapy.

Licensure Laws

Under the U.S. federal system of government, each state regulates the practice of all health care professionals by establishing licensing or regulatory agencies or boards to generate regulations. State licensing statutes establish the minimum level of education and experience required to practice, define the functions of the profession, and limit the performance of these functions to licensed persons. These laws:

- Are designed to protect the consumer against professional incompetence and exploitation by opportunists.
- Make a determination as to the minimal standards of education. In the case of physical therapy, the minimal standards required include:
  - Graduation from an accredited program or its equivalent in physical therapy
  - Successful completion of a National Licensing Examination (NPTE)
- Licensure examination and related activities are the responsibility of the Federation of State Boards of Physical Therapy.
- All states belong to this association.
- Ethical and legal standards relating to the continuing practice of physical therapy.
- All physical therapists must have a license to practice.
- Each state determines the criteria to practice and issue a license.

Workers' Compensation Acts

The rules and regulations of individual state's workers' compensation systems are the primary factors influencing the provision of physical therapy services for patients with work-related injuries. Workers' compensation laws are designed to ensure that employees who are injured or disabled on the job are provided with fixed monetary awards, eliminating the need for litigation. The laws provide a no-fault system that pays all medical benefits and replaces salary (usually at 66%) until recovery occurs. In turn, employees forfeit the right to sue their employers for damages. These rules and regulations also provide benefits for dependents of those workers who are severely injured or killed because of work-related accidents or illnesses. Some of the rules and regulations also protect employers and fellow workers by limiting the amount an injured employee can recover from an employer and by eliminating the liability of coworkers in most accidents. State Workers Compensation statutes establish this framework for most employment. Federal statutes are limited to federal employees or those workers employed in some significant aspect of interstate commerce. The laws vary from state to state, but most states identify four types of disability:

- Temporary partial: the injured worker is able to do some work but is still recuperating from the effects of the injury, and is, thus, temporarily limited in the amount or type of work which can be performed compared to the pre-injury work.
- Temporary total: the injured worker is unable to work during a period when he/she is under active medical care and has not yet reached what is called "maximum medical improvement."

- Permanent partial: the injured worker is capable of employment, but is not able to return to the former job. Benefits are usually paid according to a prescribed schedule for a fixed number of weeks.
- Permanent total: the injured worker cannot return to any gainful employment, and lifetime benefits are provided to the employee.

Workers' Compensation Programs

- Are financed by covered employers insured or self-insured under property and casualty lines and are mandatory for employers in almost all states.
- Have a limit on the number of visits in some states based on the diagnosis, and/or require a preapproval process be followed for reimbursement. Other states require the total number of visits or total number of weeks (duration) and the number of treatments per week (frequency) to be usual, customary, and reasonable.
- Must be offered by all large employers (10 or more employees) or high-risk employers.

MALPRACTICE

Malpractice can be defined as a dereliction of professional duty or a failure to exercise an accepted degree of professional skill or learning by one rendering professional services which results in injury, loss, or damage. Malpractice also encompasses an injurious, negligent, or improper practice. Physical therapists are personally responsible for negligence and other acts that result in harm to a patient through professional/patient relationships. Negligence is defined as:

- Failure to do what reasonably competent practitioners would have done under similar circumstances.
- To find a practitioner negligent, harm must have occurred to the patient. Examples could include:
  - A burn caused by a hot pack.
  - Using defective equipment.
  - Failing to prevent a patient from falling.
  - Causing an injury to a patient through improper prescription of exercises.
  - Performing any action or inaction that is inconsistent with the code of ethics, or the standards of practice.

Study Pearl

- Every individual (PT, PTA, student PT, or student PTA) is liable for his or her own negligence.
- Supervisors or superiors may also be found "vicariously" negligent because of the actions of their workers if they provided faulty supervision or inappropriate delegation of responsibilities.
- Institutions can be found vicariously negligent if a patient is harmed as a result of an environmental problem such as a slippery floor, or a poorly lit area, or an employee is deemed to be incompetent or not properly licensed.

AMERICANS WITH DISABILITIES ACT

The Americans with Disabilities Act (ADA) of 1989[8] marked the first explicit national goal of achieving equal opportunity, independent living, and economic self-sufficiency for individuals with disabilities.[9] To qualify as a person with a disability, the individual must have a physical or mental impairment that substantially limits the performance of one of life's major activities (Table 2-3).

The ADA secures equal opportunity for individuals with disabilities in employment, public accommodations, transportation, state and

TABLE 2-3. MAJOR LIFE ACTIVITIES

Social/Emotional:

- Interaction with others (eg, speech difficulties such as pressured speech, lack of clarity, withdrawal, or responding with difficulty or too quickly; self-absorption; inability to relate to or listen to others, including inability to relate due to paranoia, delusions, hallucinations, obsessive-compulsive ideation, negativity; inability to regulate mood and anxiety; inability to maintain appropriate distance from others)
- Forming and maintaining relationships with others
- Communication with others (eg, answering questions, following directions, using intelligible speech, recognizing and expressing emotions appropriately, expressing needs, following a sequence)

Cognitive:

- Concentration (as a major life activity itself and also resulting in limitations on other major life activities, such as interaction with others, self-care)
- Making decisions
- Complex thinking (eg, planning, reconciling perceptions from different senses [seeing and hearing], sorting relevant from irrelevant details, problem solving, changing from one task to another)
- Abstract thinking (eg, difficulty generalizing or transferring learning from one setting to another, such as difficulty transferring the skill of cooking in one kitchen to another kitchen)
- Memory (long- or short-term)
- Attention
- Perception
- Distinguishing real from unreal events
- Initiating and completing actions
- Processing information

Physical:

- Taking care of personal needs, such as eating, dressing, toileting, bathing, hygiene, household chores, managing money, following medication or treatment regimens, following safety precautions
- Eating (eg, inability to regulate amounts appropriately, or to maintain appropriate diet; need for strict eating schedule)
- Sleeping (eg, inability to fall asleep, obtain restful sleep, or sleep without interruption; excessive sleeping)
- Reproduction
- Sexual activity
- Traveling

local government services, and telecommunications. Title III of the ADA applies to public entities that are open to the public (Table 2-4). Some examples of public accommodations are as follows:

- Restaurants
- Hotels
- Theaters
- Retail stores and shopping centers
- Grocery stores
- Parks that are not owned by the government
- Hospitals, doctor's offices, outpatient clinics
- Law offices

Public accommodations must make reasonable modifications to any policies, practices, and procedures that deny equal access to individuals with disabilities. However, a public accommodation does not have to modify a policy if it would greatly alter its goods, services, or operations. Other impacts of the ADA include:

- Employers may not ask job applicants about medical information, or require a physical examination prior to offering employment.

TABLE 2-4. ACCESSIBILITY REQUIREMENTS

Ramps	Grade: ≤ 8.3% Minimum width of 36 in Must-have hand rails on both sides 12 in of length for each inch of vertical rise Handrails required for a rise of 6 in or more or for horizontal runs of 72 in or more
Doorways	Minimum width of 32 in Maximum depth of 24 in
Thresholds	Less than ¾ in for sliding doors Less than ½ in for other doors
Carpet	Requires ½-in pile or less
Hallway clearance	36 in width
Wheelchair turning radius (U-turn)	60 in width 78 in length
Forward reach in wheelchair	Low reach 15 in High reach 48 in
Side reach in wheelchair	Reach over obstruction to 24 in
Bathroom sink	Not less than 29 in height Not greater than 40 in from floor to bottom of mirror or paper dispenser 17 in minimum depth under sink to back wall
Bathroom toilet	17-19 in from floor to top of toilet Grab bars should be 1¼-1½ in. in diameter 1½ in spacing between grab bars and wall Grab bar placement 33-36 in up from floor level
Hotels	Approximately 2% of total rooms must be accessible
Parking spaces	96 in wide. 240 in in length. Adjacent aisle must be 60 in × 240 in Approximately 2% of the total spaces must be accessible

1 in. = 2.54 cm

- After employment is offered, an employer can only ask for a medical examination if it is required of all employees holding similar jobs.
- If an individual is turned down for work based on the results of a medical examination, the employer must prove that it is physically impossible for that individual to do the work required.

UNIONS[10-14]

Over the last 200 years, trade unions have developed into a number of forms with differing political and economic climates influencing them. The immediate objectives and activities of trade unions vary, but may include:

- Provision of benefits to members: early trade unions often provided a range of benefits to insure members against unemployment, ill health, old age, and funeral expenses. In many developed countries, these functions have been assumed by the state; however, the provision of legal advice and representation for members remains an important benefit of trade union membership.

- Collective bargaining: where trade unions are able to operate openly and are recognized by employers, they may negotiate with employers over wages and working conditions.
- Industrial action: the inability of both parties to reach an agreement may lead to industrial action, culminating in either strike action or management lockout in furtherance of particular goals. In extreme cases, violent or illegal activities may develop around these events.
- Political activity: trade unions may promote legislation favorable to the interests of their members or workers as a whole. To this end they may pursue campaigns; undertake lobbying; financially support individual candidates or parties for public office.
- Sectional organization: unions may organize a particular section of skilled workers (craft unionism), a cross-section of workers from various trades (general unionism), or attempt to organize all workers within a particular industry (industrial unionism). These unions are often divided into "locals," and united in national federations.

MEDICAL RECORDS

Medical records contain sensitive information, and increasing computerization and other policy factors have increased threats to their privacy. Besides information about physical health, these records may include information about family relationships, sexual behavior, substance abuse, and even the private thoughts and feelings that come with psychotherapy.

Threats to Medical Record Privacy. Threats to medical record privacy include the following:

- Administrative actions: this includes errors that release, misclassify, or lose information. This includes compromised accuracy, misuse by legitimate users, and uncontrolled access.
- Computerization: while in some situations computerization increases privacy protection (eg, by adding passwords to sensitive areas), it may also decrease privacy protection for the following reasons:
    - Computerization enables storage of large amounts of data in small spaces. Thus when an intruder gains access, it is access not just to a certain discrete amount of data, but to larger collections, and perhaps keys to even further information.
    - Networked information is accessible from anywhere at any time, allowing a larger number of people access. This increases the possibility of mistakes or other problems such as misuse or leaks of data.
    - New databases and different types of data sets are more easily created. This both drives demand for new information and makes possible its creation.
    - Information is easily gathered, exchanged, and transmitted. Thus, potential for dissemination is theoretically limitless.
    - Access by unrelated parties.
- Insurance companies: they may either check records before approving treatment or may check records before extending coverage.

- Financial institutions: the federal Gramm-Leach-Bliley Act (GLB) allows financial companies such as banks, brokerage houses, and insurance companies to operate as a single entity.
- Drug companies: these companies may have deals with doctors and hospitals, and may use the list for marketing.
- Employers: employers could use sensitive information against employees.
- Court subpoenas: often a patient will be unaware when her or his records have been subpoenaed. Even worse, unnecessary information is often included when the records are not adequately screened.

Current Protections. Current protections for medical records privacy include:

- Medical ethics.
- The privacy portion of the Hippocratic Oath: "Whatsoever I shall see or hear in the course of my intercourse with men, if it be what should not be published abroad, I will never divulge, holding such things to be holy secrets."
- The 1992 AMA statement, which states that medical information must be kept confidential to the greatest possible degree.
- The Privacy Act of 1974, which states that no federal agency may disclose information without the consent of the person. Agencies must also meet certain requirements for protecting the information.
- Tort law. This may include defamation, breach of contract, and other privacy-related torts.
- HIPAA Privacy Rule, the U.S. Department of Health and Human Services ("HHS") issued the Privacy Rule to implement the requirement of the HIPAA Act of 1996. The Privacy Rule standards address the use and disclosure of individuals' health information—called "protected health information" by organizations subject to the Privacy Rule—called "covered entities," as well as standards for individuals' privacy rights to understand and control how their health information is used. A major goal of the Privacy Rule is to assure that individuals' health information is properly protected while allowing the flow of health information needed to provide and promote high-quality health care and to protect the public's health and well-being.
  - The Privacy Rule applies to those who transmit health information in electronic form in connection with transactions.
  - The Privacy Rule protects all "individually identifiable health information" (protected health information [PHI]) held or transmitted by a covered entity (health plans, health care clearinghouses, and to any health care provider) or its business associate (limited to legal, actuarial, accounting, consulting, data aggregation, management, administrative, accreditation, or financial services), in any form or media: electronic, paper, or oral.

HIPAA Terminology

- Protected health information (PHI): information, including demographic data, that relates to:

  - The individual's past, present, or future physical or mental health or condition.
  - The provision of health care to the individual.
  - The past, present, or future payment for the provision of health care to the individual, and that identifies the individual or for which there is a reasonable basis to believe that it can be used to identify the individual.
- Individually identifiable health information includes many common identifiers (eg, name, address, birth date, and Social Security Number).
- Required disclosures: a covered entity must disclose protected health information in only two situations:
  - To individuals (or their personal representatives) specifically when they request access to, or an accounting of disclosures of, their protected health information.
  - To Health and Human Services (HHS) when it is undertaking a compliance investigation, or review, or enforcement action.
- Permitted uses and disclosures: a covered entity is permitted, but not required, to use and disclose protected health information, without an individual's authorization, for the following purposes or situations:
  - To the individual (unless required for access or accounting of disclosures)
  - Treatment, payment, and health care operations
  - Opportunity to agree or object
  - Incident to an otherwise permitted use and disclosure
  - Public interest and benefit activities; and Office for Civil Rights (OCR)

Privacy Rule Summary

- Limited data set: for the purposes of research, public health, or health care operations.
- Covered entities may rely on professional ethics and best judgments in deciding which of these permitted uses and disclosures to make.
- Workforce training and management: workforce members include employees, volunteers, trainees, and may also include other persons whose conduct falls under the direct control of the entity (whether or not they are paid by the entity). A covered entity must train all workforce members on its privacy policies and procedures, as necessary and appropriate for them to carry out their functions. A covered entity must have and apply appropriate sanctions against workforce members who violate its privacy policies and procedures or the Privacy Rule.
- Data safeguards: a covered entity must maintain reasonable and appropriate administrative, technical, and physical safeguards to prevent intentional or unintentional use or disclosure of protected health information in violation of the Privacy Rule and to limit its incidental use and disclosure pursuant to otherwise permitted or required use or disclosure. For example, such safeguards might include shredding documents containing protected health information before discarding

them, securing medical records with lock and key or pass code and limiting access to keys or pass codes.

- Documentation and record retention: a covered entity must maintain, until 6 years after the later of the date of their creation or last effective date, its privacy policies and procedures, its privacy practices notices, disposition of complaints, and other actions, activities, and designations that the Privacy Rule requires to be documented.
- Criminal penalties: a person who knowingly obtains or discloses individually identifiable health information in violation of HIPAA faces a fine of $50,000 and up to 1-year imprisonment. The criminal penalties increase to $100,000 and up to 5-years imprisonment if the wrongful conduct involves false pretenses, and to $250,000 and up to 10-years imprisonment if the wrongful conduct involves the intent to sell, transfer, or use individually identifiable health information for commercial advantage, personal gain, or malicious harm.

INFORMED CONSENT

Informed consent is the process by which a fully informed individual can participate in choices about his or her health care. It originates from the legal and ethical right the patient has to direct what happens to his or her body and from the ethical duty of the physician to involve the patient in their health care.

The most important goal of informed consent is that the patient must have an opportunity to be an informed participant in his or her health care decisions. Basic consent entails letting the patient know what you would like to do and asking them if that will be all right. The more formal process should include a discussion of the following elements:

- The nature of the decision/procedure
- Reasonable alternatives to the proposed intervention
- The relevant risks, benefits, and uncertainties related to each alternative
- Assessment of patient understanding
- The acceptance of the intervention by the patient

Study Pearl

In order for the patient's consent to be valid, he/she must be considered competent to make the decision and his/her consent must be voluntary.

PERSONNEL SUPERVISION/MANAGEMENT OF THE DEPARTMENT

Administration, according to the *Guide to Physical Therapist Practice* is "the planning, directing, organizing, and managing of human, technical, environmental, and financial resources effectively and efficiently."[15] Examples of administrative activity in which the physical therapist may engage in during their career include:[15]

- Ensuring fiscally sound reimbursement for services rendered.
- Budgeting for physical therapy services.
- Managing staff resources, including the acquisition and development of clinical expertise and leadership abilities.
- Monitoring quality of care and clinical productivity.
- Negotiating and managing contracts.
- Supervising the physical therapist assistant, physical therapy aide, and other support personnel.

Direction and supervision are essential administrative responsibilities for the provision of high-quality physical therapy. The degree of direction and supervision necessary for ensuring high-quality physical therapy depends on many factors including the education, experience, and responsibilities of the parties involved; the organizational structure in which the physical therapy is provided; and applicable state law.[15]

MANAGEMENT AND LEADERSHIP THEORIES

Leadership is a process by which a person influences others to accomplish an objective and directs the organization in a way that makes it more cohesive and coherent. Leaders carry out this process by applying their leadership attributes, such as beliefs, values, ethics, character, knowledge, and skills. There are a number of leadership theories.[16-27]

Bass' Theory of Leadership

Bass' theory of leadership[28,29] states that there are three basic ways to explain how people become leaders:

1. Trait Theory: some personality traits may lead people naturally into leadership roles.
2. Great Events Theory: a crisis or important event may cause a person to rise to the occasion, which brings out extraordinary leadership qualities in an ordinary person.
3. Transformational Leadership Theory: people can choose to become leaders and can learn leadership skills.

Four Framework Approach[30]

The four framework approach suggests that leaders display leadership behaviors in one of four types of frameworks:

- Structural framework: structural leaders focus on structure, strategy, environment, implementation, experimentation, and adaptation.
  - In an effective leadership situation, the leader is a social architect whose leadership style involves analysis and design.
  - In an ineffective leadership situation, the leader is a petty autocrat whose leadership style is detail-oriented.
- Human resource framework: human resource leaders believe in people and communicate that belief; they are visible and accessible; they empower, increase participation, support, share information, and move decision-making down into the organization.
  - In an effective leadership situation, the leader is a catalyst and servant whose leadership style is support, advocate, and empowerment.
  - In an ineffective leadership situation, the leader is a pushover, whose leadership style is abdication and fraud.
- Political framework: political leaders clarify what they want and what they can get; they assess the distribution of power

and interests; they build linkages to other stakeholders, use persuasion first, then use negotiation and coercion only if necessary.

- In an effective leadership situation, the leader is an advocate, whose leadership style is coalition and building.
- In an ineffective leadership situation, the leader is a hustler, whose leadership style is manipulation.

▶ Symbolic framework: symbolic leaders view organizations as a stage or theater to play certain roles and give impressions; these leaders use symbols to capture attention; they try to frame experience by providing plausible interpretations of experiences; they discover and communicate a vision.

- In an effective leadership situation, the leader is a prophet, an inspirational leader.
- In an ineffective leadership situation, the leader is a fanatic or a fool, whose leadership style is smoke and mirrors.

MANAGERIAL GRID

The Blake and Mouton Managerial Grid[31] depicted in Figure 2-1 uses two axes:

1. "Concern for people" is plotted using the vertical axis.
2. "Concern for results" is plotted along the horizontal axis.

The managerial grid graphic is a very simple framework that elegantly defines the basic styles that characterize workplace behavior and the resulting relationships based on how two fundamental concerns (concern for people and concern for results) are manifested at

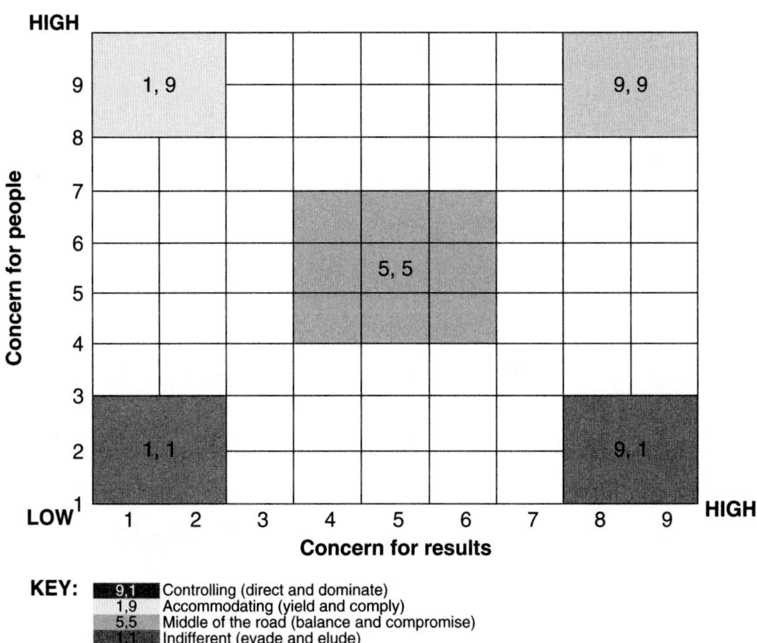

Figure 2-1. Managerial grid.

varying levels whenever people interact. Most people fall somewhere near the middle of the two axes, but people who score at the far end of the scales, can be categorized into five types of leaders:

1. **Controlling (produce or perish)** (9 on task [high task], 1 on people [low relationship]). People who get this rating are very much task-oriented and are hard on their workers (autocratic). There is little or no allowance for cooperation or collaboration. Heavily task-oriented people display these characteristics: They are very strong on schedules; they expect people to do what they are told without question or debate; when something goes wrong they tend to focus on who is to blame rather than concentrate on exactly what is wrong and how to prevent it; they are intolerant of what they see as dissent (it may just be someone's creativity), so it is difficult for their subordinates to contribute or develop.
2. **Team Leader** (9 on task [high task], 9 on people [high relationship]). This type of person leads by positive example and endeavors to foster a team environment in which all team members can reach their highest potential, both as team members and as people. They encourage the team to reach team goals as effectively as possible, while also working tirelessly to strengthen the bonds among the various members. They normally form and lead some of the most productive teams.
3. **Accommodating (Country Club)** (1 on task, 9 on people). This person uses predominantly reward power to maintain discipline and to encourage the team to accomplish its goals. Conversely, they are almost incapable of employing the more punitive coercive and legitimate powers. This inability results from fear that using such powers could jeopardize relationships with the other team members.
4. **Indifferent (Impoverished)** (1 on task, 1 on people). A leader who uses a "delegate and disappear" management style. Since they are not committed to either task accomplishment or maintenance; they essentially allow their team to do whatever it wishes and prefer to detach themselves from the team process by allowing the team to suffer from a series of power struggles.
5. **Middle of the Road** (5 on task, 5 on people). Managers using this style try to balance between company goals and workers' needs. By giving some concern to both people and production, managers who use this style hope to achieve acceptable performance.

Although it may appear that the most desirable place for a leader to be would be a 9 on task and a 9 on people (Team Leader), certain situations might call for one of the other four to be used at times.

MANAGEMENT AND LEADERSHIP STYLES

A number of management styles have been recognized (Table 2-5). A distinction is often made between being a manager versus being a leader (Table 2-6).

TABLE 2-5. MANAGEMENT STYLES

MANAGEMENT STYLE	DESCRIPTION
Management by coaching and development	Managers see themselves primarily as employee trainers.
Management by competitive edge	Individuals and groups within the organization compete against one another to see who can achieve the best results.
Management by consensus	Managers construct systems to allow for the individual input of the employees.
Management by decision models	Decisions are based on projections generated by artificially constructed situations.
Management by exception	Managers delegate as much responsibility and activity as possible to those below them, stepping in only when absolutely necessary.
Management by information systems	Managers depend on data generated within the company to help them increase efficiency and interrelatedness.
Management by interaction	Emphasizes communication and balance of male/female energy as well as integration of all human aspects (mental, emotional, physical, and spiritual), creating an empowered, high-energy, high-productive workforce.
Management by matrices	Managers study charted variables to discern their interrelatedness, probable cause and effect, and available options.
Management by objectives	The organization sets overall objectives, then managers set objectives for each employee.
Management by organizational development	Managers constantly seek to improve employee relations and communications.
Management by performance	Managers seek quality levels of performance through motivation and employee relations.
Management by styles	Managers adjust their approaches to meet situational needs.
Management by walking around	Managers walk around the company, getting a "feel" for people and operations; stopping to talk and to listen. Sometimes known as Management by Walking Around and Listening. This management style is based on the Hewlett-Packard (HP) Way developed by entrepreneur Dave Packard, cofounder of HP.
Management by work simplification	Managers constantly seek ways to simplify processes and reduce expenses.

MEETINGS

The most effective tool for accomplishing communication objectives within a department is the staff meeting (Table 2-7). Staff meetings can be used to:

- Chart progress
- Keep staff informed of all office activities
- Coordinate between offices and departments
- Determine how close the department is to meeting the goals of the strategic plan

JOB DESCRIPTIONS

- A job is a collection of tasks and responsibilities that an employee is responsible to conduct. Jobs have titles. Job descriptions (JDs) are lists of the general tasks, or functions, and responsibilities of a position.
  - A task is typically defined as a unit of work, that is, a set of activities needed to produce some result, for example, completing an examination and writing a memo. Complex positions in the organization may include a large number of tasks, which are sometimes referred to as functions.

TABLE 2-6. MANAGEMENT VERSUS LEADERSHIP TRAITS

MANAGEMENT TRAITS	LEADERSHIP TRAITS
Does not ensure imagination, inventiveness, or ethical behavior.	Uses personal power to affect the plans and endeavors of others.
Rationally analyzes, and builds a systematic selection of targets and objectives.	Intuitive, enigmatic understanding of what is essential.
Directs energy toward purposes, resources, organizational structure, and constructs a list of problems to resolve.	Directs energy toward guiding people to uncover practical solutions.
Can perpetuate group conflicts.	Works to develop compatible interpersonal relationships.
Becomes anxious when there is relative disorder.	Works best when circumstances are somewhat uncontrolled.
Uses an accumulation of concerted experience to effectively make decisions.	Often jumps to conclusions, without a logical progression of concepts or fact.
Innovates by modifying existing practices	Innovates through perception or intuition.
Sees the world as relatively impersonal and passive.	Sees the world as rich in color, constantly blending into new situations.
Influences people through reason, details, and rationale.	Influences people through altering moods, evoking images, and anticipation.
Views work as an enabling process, incorporating a merger of plans, skills, timing, and staff.	Views work as making new approaches to old problems, or discovering new options for old issues.
Has a low level of emotional involvement in their occupation.	Takes in emotional signals from others, making them mean something in the connection with an individual; often passionate about their career.
Relates to personnel by the role they play in the decision-making process.	Relates to people intuitively and empathically.
Focuses on how factors require completion.	Focuses on what needs to be done, leaving determinations to the personnel involved.
Focuses attention on the process.	Focuses on the determination to be made.
Forms moderate and widely distributed personal attachments with others.	Forms comprehensive one-on-one relationships, which may be of short duration; often has mentors.
Feels threatened by open challenges to their ideas, and are troubled by aggressiveness.	Able to tolerate aggressive interchanges, encouraging emotional involvement with others.

- A responsibility is the relationship between the value of a job outcome and the worker's input of effort; the employee's situation within, and their impact to the organization. A role is the set of responsibilities or expected results associated with a job. A job usually includes several roles.

▶ Typically, JDs also include to whom the position reports, specifications such as the qualifications (necessary skills and

TABLE 2-7. TIPS FOR EFFECTIVE STAFF MEETINGS

- ▶ Designate a meeting facilitator.
- ▶ Have a clear purpose and written agenda for the meeting.
- ▶ Establish a starting and ending time for the meeting.
- ▶ Inform staff ahead of time of their responsibilities for the meeting (bringing their calendars, briefing other staff on relevant issues, note-taking, etc).
- ▶ Encourage staff to participate but not to dominate.
- ▶ If certain issues or projects require extensive planning or discussion, schedule another meeting for the relevant staff rather than discussing it with the full group.
- ▶ Do not use staff meetings to discuss the performance of individuals, except for giving them a word of praise.
- ▶ Close the meeting with a bang—and a plan.

experience required) needed by the person in the job, salary range for the position, etc. To avoid age discrimination, experience should not include an upper limit.

- JDs are usually developed by conducting a job analysis, which includes examining the tasks and sequences of tasks necessary to perform the job. The analysis looks at the areas of knowledge and skills needed for the job.
- A JD should indicate the scope of the job, its responsibilities and duties and essential functions, and clearly indicate what contribution the position makes to the organization. The focus should be on major or critical activities with distinctions made between minor activities, which are done daily and major ones that might occur less frequently. The JD is usually not all-inclusive, and includes a statement at the end to indicate "...other duties as assigned."

PERFORMANCE APPRAISAL

The performance appraisal (performance review, performance evaluation, personal rating, merit rating, employee appraisal, or employee evaluation) is any personnel decision that affects the status of the employee regarding their retention, termination, promotion, transfer, salary increase or decrease, or admission into a training program.

The performance appraisal is a vehicle to:

- Validate and refine organizational actions and practices, or institute new ones.
- Provide feedback to employees with an eye on improving future performance. Although employees vary in their desire for improvement, generally workers want to know how well they are performing. People need positive feedback and validation on a regular basis. Once an employee has been selected, few management actions can have as positive an effect on worker performance as encouraging affirmation.

> **Study Pearl**
>
> Feedback may be qualitative or quantitative:
> - Qualitative: descriptive, such as expressing appreciation for the timeliness and quality of a clinician's documentation.
> - Quantitative: based on numerical figures, such as the number of patients seen by the clinician in a day.

RATING SYSTEMS

The various types of rating systems follow:

- Behavioral anchored rating scales: a performance rating that focuses on specific behaviors or sets as indicators of effective or ineffective performance, rather than on broadly stated adjectives such as "average, above average, or below average." Other variations are:
  - Behavioral observation scales
  - Behavioral expectation scales
  - Numerically anchored rating scales
- Checklists: a set of adjectives or descriptive statements.
  - If the rater believes the employee possesses a trait listed, the rater checks the item.
  - If the rater does not believe the employee possesses a trait listed, the rater leaves the item blank.
- Critical incident technique: a method of performance appraisal that makes lists of statements of very effective and very ineffective behaviors for employees. The lists are usually

combined into categories, which vary with each job. Once the categories have been developed and statements of effective and ineffective behavior have been provided, the evaluator prepares a log for each employee. During the evaluation period, the evaluator records examples of critical behaviors in each of the categories, and the log is used to evaluate the employee at the end of the evaluation period.

- Forced choice method: developed to prevent evaluators from rating employees too high. Using this method, the evaluator has to select from a set of descriptive statements that apply to the employee. The statements are weighted and summed to form an effectiveness index.
- Forced distribution: an appraisal system similar to grading on a curve. The evaluator is asked to rate employees in some fixed distribution of categories.
- Graphic rating scale: the oldest and most widely used performance appraisal method. The evaluators are given a graph and asked to rate the employees on a list of characteristics. The number of characteristics can vary from 1 to 100.
- Narrative or essay evaluation: the evaluator is asked to describe the strengths and weaknesses of an employee's behavior.
- Management by objectives: the supervisor and employee get together to set objectives in quantifiable terms. This method eliminates communication problems through the establishment of regular meetings, emphasizing results, and by being an ongoing process where new objectives are established and old objectives are modified as necessary according to changes in conditions.
- Paired comparison: an appraisal method for ranking employees. The names of the employees to be evaluated are first placed on separate sheets in a predetermined order, so that each person is compared with all other employees to be evaluated. The evaluator then checks the person he or she felt had been the better of the two on the criterion for each comparison. The number of times a person has been preferred is tallied, and the tally developed is an index of the number of preferences compared to the number being evaluated.

COMPLETING A PERFORMANCE APPRAISAL

- Translate organizational goals into individual job objectives.
- Communicate expectations regarding an employee performance.
- Provide feedback to the employee about job performance in light of departmental objectives.
- Coach the employee on how to achieve job objectives/ requirements.
- Diagnose the employee's strengths and weaknesses.
- Determine what kind of development activities might help the employee better utilize his or her skills to improve performance on the current job (development plan).
- Complete formal documentation of the performance appraisal and development plan (if necessary).

STAFF MOTIVATION

Some of the most effective ways for managers to motivate staff include giving praise; recognition; positive feedback; and the passing on of feedback from more senior managers. If staff feel that their decisions are generally supported, and when genuine mistakes are made they will be guided in the right direction; they will be more positive, confident, and prepared to take on responsibility and decision making.

Finally, when a staff is shown clear expectations and when they are valued, trusted, encouraged, and motivated; they will be more likely to give their best.

PROFESSIONAL GROWTH

It is the responsibility of the physical therapy director/manager/supervisor to provide ongoing educational program activities for the rehabilitation staff in order to enhance professional growth. Educational programs may occur during work time, in the evenings, or weekends. In addition, staff members should be encouraged to attend professional and educational development classes, including those outside of the organization, based on financial constraints.

POLICY AND PROCEDURE MANUALS

- Policy manual: the purpose of a policy manual is to familiarize employees with the specific mission, culture, expectations, and benefits of the department/organization.
- Procedure manual: procedure manuals differ from policy manuals in that they are used to assist employees in dealing with situations that may arise during the daily operations of the practice (eg, charge entry, patient scheduling and registration processes, answering the telephone, and appropriate handling of referrals to physicians, or other health care professionals).

While these manuals, which are often combined into one binder, are not a legal contract, they do help to provide a clear, common understanding of departmental/organizational goals, benefits, and policies, as well as what is expected with regard to performance and conduct. A typical policy and procedure manual has approximately eight sections, including the following:

- Introduction
- Employment
- Employment status and records
- Employee benefit programs
- Timekeeping/payroll
- Work conditions and hours
- Leaves of absence
- Employee conduct and disciplinary action

TABLE 2-8. VARIOUS STATE AND FEDERAL LEGISLATIONS

LEGISLATION	EXPLANATION
The Equal Employment Opportunity Act (EEO)	Prohibits discrimination on the basis of race or color, national origin, sex, and/or religion.
The Family and Medical Leave Act (FMLA)	Requires employers with 50 or more employees to allow up to 12 work-weeks of unpaid leave in any 12-month period for the birth, adoption, or foster care placement of a child, or serious health condition of the employee, spouse, parent, or child, provided the leave is taken within 12 months of such an event. Intermittent leave is allowed if there is a medical need for the leave. Intermittent leave is leave taken in separate blocks of time due to a single illness or injury, rather than in one continuous period.
Fair Labor Standards Act (FLSA)	The employers must pay overtime to their workers whenever they work more than 40 hours in any week. Varies from state to state. For example, under Pennsylvania's state wage and hour laws, individuals employed in a bona fide executive, administrative, or professional capacity (salaried) are exempt from the overtime provisions of the law.
Civil Rights Act of 1964	Prohibits employment discrimination based on race, color, sex, religion, and national origin.
The Age Discrimination and Employment Act of 1967	Prohibits employers from discriminating against persons from 40-70 years of age in any area of employment.
1973 Rehabilitation Act	Prohibits employment discrimination based on disability in federal executive agencies, and full institutions receiving Medicare, Medicaid, and other federal support.
The American with Disabilities Act (ADA)	Prohibits discrimination against "qualified individuals with disabilities." ▶ An individual is considered to have a "disability" if he or she has a physical or mental impairment that substantially limits one or more major life activities, has a record of such impairment, or is regarded as having such impairment. ▶ Persons discriminated against because they have a known association, or relationship with, an individual with a disability is also protected. ▶ Discrimination is prohibited in all employment practices, including job application procedures, hiring, firing, advancement, compensation, training, and other terms, conditions, and privileges of employment. ▶ Discrimination applies to recruitment, advertising, tenure, layoff, leave, fringe benefits, and all other employment-related activities. ▶ The ADA applies to employers with 15 or more employees.

The Policy and Procedure manual must be guided by various state and federal legislation, such as Equal Employment Opportunity (EEO)—protected classes, Americans with Disabilities Act (ADA), Family and Medical Leave Act (FMLA), and Fair Labor Standards Act (FLSA)—exempt versus nonexempt. Table 2-8 provides a brief description of each of these laws. A yearly review of the policies is recommended.

MATERIAL SAFETY DATA SHEET

The purpose of the Occupational Safety and Health Administration (OSHA) Hazard Communication Standard is to ensure the hazards of all chemical substances. Mixtures produced or imported are evaluated and any hazard information is communicated by means of a printed written document called the *Material Safety Data Sheet* (MSDS). The MSDS must be written in English and contain certain required information including the chemical identity or common name, health hazards, emergency and first aid procedures, and safety precautions.

Study Pearl

OSHA: A federal agency within the U.S. Department of Labor that is responsible for providing guidelines to promote employee safety in the workplace.

TABLE 2-9. EXAMPLES OF A SENTINEL EVENT

- Any patient death, paralysis, coma, or other major permanent loss of function associated with a medication error.
- Any suicide of a patient in a setting where the patient is housed around-the-clock, including suicides following elopement from such a setting.
- Any elopement, ie, unauthorized departure, of a patient from an around-the-clock care setting resulting in a temporally related death (suicide or homicide) or major permanent loss of function.
- Any procedure on the wrong patient, wrong side of the body, or wrong organ.
- Any intrapartum (related to the birth process) maternal death.
- Any perinatal death unrelated to a congenital condition in an infant having a birth weight greater than 2500 g.
- Assault, homicide, or other crime resulting in patient death or major permanent loss of function.
- A patient fall that results in death or major permanent loss of function as a direct result of the injuries sustained in the fall.
- Hemolytic transfusion reaction involving major blood group incompatibilities.

INCIDENT/OCCURRENCE REPORTING

The purpose of incident/occurrence reporting is to understand the underlying/contributing conditions that led to or contributed to the occurrence of a safety incident, identify appropriate corrective actions that must be taken to address these underlying/contributing conditions, and implement timely and effective corrective actions. An incident/occurrence report typically contains the following information:

- Name or description of the incident/occurrence. Attention should be placed on making the report simple, clear, and inclusive.
- Time and date of incident/occurrence.
- Brief description of the incident/occurrence location. A simple, chronological narrative works best.
- Brief description of incident.
- First and last names and titles of persons involved if appropriate.
- What's being done and/or will be done next.
- Other departments involved or to become involved in the incident (emergency services, physician etc).
- The name and title of the person submitting the report.

Sentinel Event Reporting

A sentinel event is an adverse health event that may have been avoided through appropriate care or alternative interventions. Examples of a sentinel event are provided in Table 2-9. Health care providers are required to alert JCAHO and often state licensing authorities of all sentinel events, including a review of risk factors, preventative measures, and case analysis.

Questions for this chapter and the entire book appear on the included CD-ROM, with additional questions at www.DuttonNPTE.com.

REFERENCES

1. Bodenheimer TS, Grumbach K: Paying for healthcare. In: Bodenheimer TS, Grumbach K, eds. *Understanding Health Policy: A Clinical Approach, 5th ed.* New York, NY: McGraw-Hill. 2009:5-16.
2. Bodenheimer TS, Grumbach K: Reimbursing healthcare providers. In: Bodenheimer TS, Grumbach K, eds. *Understanding Health Policy: A Clinical Approach, 5th ed.* New York, NY: McGraw-Hill. 2009:31-41.
3. Rodwin VG: *The Health Planning Predicament.* Berkeley, CA: University of California Press. 1984.
4. Bodenheimer TS, Grumbach K: How health care is organized. In: Bodenheimer TS, Grumbach K, eds. *Understanding Health Policy: A Clinical Approach, 5th ed.* New York, NY: McGraw-Hill. 2009:43-57.
5. Garrett N, Martini EM: The boomers are coming: a total cost of care model of the impact of population aging on the cost of chronic conditions in the United States. *Dis Manag.* 2007;10:51-60.
6. Hootman JM, Helmick CG: Projections of US prevalence of arthritis and associated activity limitations. *Arthritis Rheum.* 2006;54: 226-229.
7. Uphold CR, Rane D, Reid K, et al: Mental health differences between rural and urban men living with HIV infection in various age groups. *J Community Health.* 2005;30:355-375.
8. Americans with Disabilities Act of 1989: 104 Stat 327.101–336, 42 USC 12101 s2(a)(8). 1989.
9. Waddell G, Waddell H: A review of social influences on neck and back pain disability. In: Nachemson AL, Jonsson E, eds. *Neck and Back Pain: The Scientific Evidence of Causes, Diagnosis, and Treatment.* Philadelphia, PA: Lippincott Williams and Wilkins. 2000:13-55.
10. Trade unions and cleaner production: perspectives and proposals for action. *New Solut.* 1999;9:277-295.
11. Cohen P: Trade unions. United fronts? *Nurs Times.* 1993;89:40-41.
12. Johansson M, Partanen T: Role of trade unions in workplace health promotion. *Int J Health Serv.* 2002;32:179-193.
13. Myers ML: Professional trade unions. *Hospitals.* 1970;44:80-83.
14. O'Shea P: Nurses and trade unions: an uneasy relationship. *World Ir Nurs.* 1997;5:12-14.
15. Guide to physical therapist practice. *Phys Ther.* 2001;81:S13-S95.
16. Aaron L: Program director satisfaction with leadership skills. *Radiol Technol.* 2006;78:104-112.
17. Alimo-Metcalfe B: Leadership. Peak practice. *Health Serv J.* 2006;116:28-29.
18. Ausman JI: Leadership vs. consensus. *Surg Neurol.* 2006;66: 548-549.

19. Friedman PK: Mentoring: leadership, learning, legacy. *J Mass Dent Soc.* 2006;55:16-18.
20. Garman AN, Butler P, Brinkmeyer L: Leadership. *J Healthc Manag.* 2006;51:360-364.
21. Gifford WA, Davies B, Edwards N, et al: Leadership strategies to influence the use of clinical practice guidelines. *Can J Nurs Leadersh.* 2006;19:72-88.
22. Hohne K: The principles of leadership. *J Trauma Nurs.* 2006;13: 122-125.
23. Kerfoot K: Authentic leadership. *Medsurg Nurs.* 2006;15:319-320.
24. Naylor CD: Leadership in academic medicine: reflections from administrative exile. *Clin Med.* 2006;6:488-492.
25. Redman RW: Leadership strategies for uncertain times. *Res Theory Nurs Pract.* 2006;20:273-275.
26. Sternberg RJ: A systems model of leadership: WICS. *Am Psychol.* 2007;62:34-42; discussion 43-47.
27. Zaccaro SJ: Trait-based perspectives of leadership. *Am Psychol.* 2007;62:6-16; discussion 43-47.
28. Bass B: *Stogdill's Handbook of Leadership: A Survey of Theory and Research.* New York, NY: Free Press. 1989.
29. Bass B: From transactional to transformational leadership: learning to share the vision. *Organizational Dynamics.* 1990;18:19-31.
30. Bolman L, Deal T: *Reframing Organizations.* San Francisco: Jossey-Bass. 1991.
31. Blake RR, Mouton JS: *The Managerial Grid III: The Key to Leadership Excellence.* Houston: Gulf Publishing Co. 1985.

Research

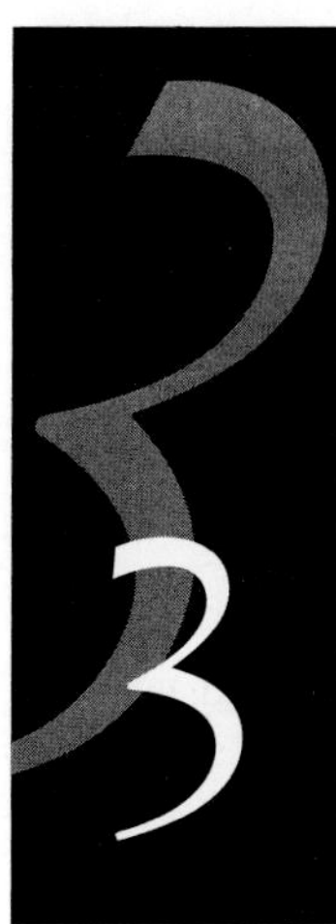

RESEARCH TYPES

Research involves a controlled, systematic approach to obtain an answer to a question.[1] A number of research types are recognized:

- Experimental research: involves the manipulation of a variable and then measuring the effects of this manipulation.[1] A variable is a measurement of phenomena that can assume more than one value or more than one category (see later).[1]
- Nonexperimental research: does not manipulate the environment but may describe the relationship between different variables, obtain information about opinions or policies, or describe current practice.[1]
- Basic research: generally thought of as laboratory-based research in which the researcher has control over nearly all aspects of the environment and subjects.[1]
- Clinical or applied research: refers to research that seeks to solve practical problems by finding solutions to everyday problems, cure illness, and develop innovative technologies.

> **Study Pearl**
>
> Much of the initial groundwork in statistics concerns making an accurate guess, or hypothesis.

STATISTICS

Statistics is a branch of applied mathematics concerned with finding patterns in data and inferring connections between events.[2] A number of statistical terms and definitions are outlined in Table 3-1.

POPULATIONS AND SAMPLES

A population consists of all subjects (human or otherwise) that are being studied.

- Prevalence: the proportion of a population who has a particular disorder or condition at a specific point in time.
- Incidence: a rate of development of new cases of a disorder in a particular at-risk population over a given period of time.

TABLE 3-1. STATISTICAL TERMS AND DEFINITIONS

TERM	DEFINITION
Abstract	A summary of the paper, usually between 100 and 500 words, that describes the most important aspects of the study, including: ▸ The problem investigated ▸ The subjects and instruments involved ▸ The design and procedures ▸ The major findings/conclusions
Conclusion	The conclusion responds to the original research question and hypothesis to describe what the study showed. It should bring coherence to the study.
Empirical methods	Research methods and data-gathering techniques supported by measurable evidence, not opinion or speculation.
Parameter	Numerical measurements describing some characteristic of the population.
Peer review	A process by which research studies are examined by an independent panel of researchers for review. The purpose of such a process is to open the study to examination, criticism, review, and replication by peer investigators and ultimately incorporate the new knowledge into the field.
Population	The population of a study refers to the group of people represented in a study. For example, if a researcher took a nationally representative sample of 1500 fourth-grade students, the sample is the 1500 fourth-grade students, but the population of the study would be fourth graders, in general.

- Parameter: a characteristic or measure obtained by using all the data values from a specific population.

A sample is a group of subjects selected from a population.

- Statistic: a characteristic or measure obtained by using all the data values from a sample.

VARIABLES

To gain knowledge about seemingly haphazard events, statisticians collect information called *variables*, which describe the event. Data are the values (measurements or observations) that the variables can assume.

Variables can be classified as qualitative or quantitative:

- Qualitative: a variable that can be placed into a distinct category according to some characteristic or attribute, eg, gender.
- Quantitative: a variable that is numeric and can be ordered or ranked, eg, age, height, and weight. Quantitative variables can be further classified into two groups: discrete and continuous.[2]
  - Discrete: a variable that can assume only certain values that are countable, eg, the number of children in a family
  - Continuous: a variable that can assume an infinite number of possible values in an interval between any two specific values, eg, temperature

In addition to being classified as qualitative and quantitative, variables can be classified by how they are categorized, counted, or measured. This type of classification uses measurement scales. The four classic scales (or levels) of measurement are[2]

Study Pearl

A valid informed consent for research purposes must include all of the following elements:

- An understandable explanation of the purpose and procedures to be used
- All reasonable and foreseeable risks and discomforts
- All potential benefits of participation

Study Pearl

The two traits of a variable that should always be achieved include:

- Each variable should be ***exhaustive***; it should include all possible answerable responses.
- Each variable should be ***mutually exclusive***; no respondent should be able to have two attributes simultaneously.

1. Nominal (Classificatory; Categorical): classifies data into mutually exclusive, exhausting categories in which no order or ranking can be imposed. Examples include arbitrary labels: zip codes, religion, and marital status.
2. Ordinal (Ranking): classifies data into categories that can be ranked, although precise differences between the ranks do not exist, eg, letter grades (A, B, C, etc) and body builds (small, medium, large).
3. Interval: ranks data where precise differences between units of measure do exist, although there is no meaningful zero. Examples include temperature (degrees centigrade, degrees Fahrenheit), IQ, and calendar dates.
4. Ratio: possesses all the characteristics of interval measurement, and a true zero exists. Examples include age and salary.

Types of Experiments

There are three basic types of statistical experiments: controlled, experimental, and field:

1. Controlled: a controlled experiment generally compares the results obtained from an experimental sample against a control sample, which is practically identical to the experimental sample except for the one aspect whose effect is being tested (the independent variable).
2. Natural: an observational study in which the assignment of treatments to subjects has been haphazard. The assignment of treatments to subjects has not been made by the researchers or by randomization.
3. Field: so named in order to highlight the contrast with laboratory experiments.

Study Pearl

Dependency refers to the "role" of the variable in the experiment or study.

- Independent variable: one that is manipulated by the researcher; independent variables are controlled or fixed in order to observe their effect on dependent variables. For example, a treatment or program or cause.
- Dependent variable: the variable that is measured by the researcher.

For example, if a study examines the effects of iontophoresis on pain levels, the iontophoresis is the independent variable and the measurement of pain levels is the dependent variable.

Other types of variables include:

- Random variable: one whose value is determined by chance.
- Controlled variable: a variable that the researcher wants to remain constant.
- Covariate: a phenomenon that affects the dependent variable and is not of interest to the researcher, but that the researcher is unable to control.[1]

RESEARCH DESIGN

There are a number of primary types of research designs (Table 3-2).

Control

Ideally, the researcher should attempt to remove the influence of any variable other than the independent variable in order to evaluate its effect on the dependent variable. An experimental design has the

TABLE 3-2. RESEARCH DESIGNS

Controlled trials	These require the experimental procedure to be compared with a placebo or another previously accepted procedure. Controlled studies are more likely than uncontrolled studies to determine whether differences are due to the experimental treatment or to some of the extraneous factor.
Uncontrolled trials	These involve the investigators describing their experience with an experimental procedure; however, the experimental procedure is not formerly compared with a placebo or another previously accepted procedure.
Single-blind study	A study in which the investigator does not know if the subject is in the treatment or the control group.
Double-blind study	A study in which neither the investigator nor the subject knows if the subject is in the treatment or the control group.

purpose of minimizing or controlling the effects on extraneous variables so that the relationship between the independent variable(s) and the dependent variable(s) can be ascertained.

Control Group

The control group is used as a standard for comparison with experimental groups in terms of age, abilities, race, etc. For example, a particular study may divide participants into two groups: an "experimental group" and a "control group." The experimental group is given the experimental treatment under study, while the control group may be given either the standard treatment for the illness or a placebo. At the end of the study, the results of the two groups are compared.

Experimental Group

Study participants in the experimental group receive the drug, device, treatment, or intervention under study. In some studies, all participants are in the experimental group. In "controlled studies," participants will be assigned either to an experimental group or to a control group.

Placebo Effect

The placebo effect is the measurable, observable, or felt improvement in health not attributable to treatment. Experimental research uses placebos (usually sugar or starch pills) to test the effect of a medication—an inactive substance that looks like medicine but contains no medicine and has no treatment value (placebo) is administered to the patient. While participants in the control group are given the placebo, the other members of the study are given the actual medication.

Random Assignment

Random assignment is assignment by chance, like flipping a coin or pulling numbers out of a hat. This method is sometimes used to determine who is in the experimental group and who is in the control group. For example, in a study with random assignment to one of two groups, participants have a 50% chance of being assigned to either group.

Study Pearl

Bias or systematic error refers to the tendency to consistently underestimate or overestimate a true value.

DATA COLLECTION AND SAMPLING TECHNIQUES

Researchers use samples to produce a representative sample of the target population. To avoid any biasing of the collected information, samples must be collected in a systematic fashion.

Four basic methods of sampling are employed:

1. Random sampling: all items have some chance of selection that can be calculated, thereby minimizing sampling bias.
2. Systematic sampling: sometimes referred to as interval sampling; means that there is a gap, or interval, between each selection (every 20th person).

3. Stratified sampling: sometimes called *proportional* or *quota* random sampling; involves dividing the population into homogeneous subgroups called strata and then taking a simple random sample from each subgroup. Stratified sampling assures that the overall population will be represented in addition to key subgroups of the population. For example, choosing only female patients.
4. Cluster sampling: involves dividing the population into groups or clusters (such as geographic boundaries) and then randomly selecting sample clusters and using all members of the selected clusters as subjects of the samples. For example, it may not be possible to list all of the patients of a chain of physical therapy clinics. However, it would be possible to randomly select a subset of clinics (stage 1 of cluster sampling) and then interview a random sample of patients who visit those clinics (stage 2 of cluster sampling).

GRAPHICAL REPRESENTATION OF ORGANIZED DATA

The most convenient method of organizing data is to construct a frequency distribution.[3] Two types of frequency distributions are[3]

1. Categorical frequency distribution: used for data that can be placed in specific categories, such as nominal- or ordinal-level data, eg, political affiliation.
2. Grouped frequency distribution: used when the range of data is large.

Data can be presented by constructing statistical charts and graphs. The choice of which chart/graph to use is determined by the type and breadth of the data, the audience it is directed to, and the questions being asked (Table 3-3). The three most commonly used graphs in research include the histogram, frequency polygon, and cumulative frequency graph (ogive) (Figure 3-1). In addition to these, the Pareto chart (Figure 3-1), the times series graph (Figure 3-1), and the pie graph (Figure 3-1) are also used. In those cases where the researchers are interested in determining if a relationship between two variables (independent and dependent) exists, a scatter plot or scatter diagram can be used (Figure 3-1).

SENSITIVITY AND SPECIFICITY

Sensitivity represents the proportion of a population with the target disorder, who has a positive result with the diagnostic test. A test that can correctly identify every person who has the target disorder has a sensitivity of 1.0. SnNout is an acronym for when Sensitivity of a symptom or sign is high, a Negative response rules out the target disorder. Thus, a "high" sensitive test helps rule out a disorder.

Specificity represents the proportion of the study population without the target disorder, in whom the test result is negative

TABLE 3-3. STATISTICAL GRAPHS

TYPE OF DISPLAY	ADVANTAGES	DISADVANTAGES
Pictograph A pictograph uses an icon to represent a quantity of data values in order to decrease the size of the graph. A key must be used to explain the icon.	Easy to read Visually appealing Handles large data sets easily using keyed icons	Hard to quantify partial icons Icons must be of consistent size Best for only 2-6 categories Very simplistic
Line plot A line plot can be used as an initial record of discrete data values. The range determines a number line which is then plotted with X's for each data value.	Quick analysis of data Shows range, minimum and maximum, gaps and clusters, and outliers easily Exact values retained	Not as visually appealing as pictograph Best for under 50 data values Needs small range of data
Pie chart A pie chart displays data as a percentage of the whole. Each pie section should have a label and percentage. A total data number should be included.	Visually appealing Shows percent of total for each category	No exact numerical data Hard to compare two data sets The "Other" category can be a problem Total unknown unless specified Best for 3-7 categories Used only with discrete data
Map chart A map chart displays data by shading sections of a map, and must include a key. A total data number should be included.	Good visual appeal Overall trends show well	Needs limited categories No exact numerical values Color key can skew visual interpretation
Histogram A histogram displays continuous data in ordered columns. Categories are of a continuous measure such as time, inches, temperature, etc.	Visually strong Can compare to normal curve The vertical axis is usually a frequency count of items falling into each category	Cannot read exact values because data is grouped into categories More difficult to compare two data sets Used only with continuous data
Bar graph A bar graph displays discrete data in separate columns. A double bar graph can be used to compare two data sets. Categories are considered unordered and can be rearranged alphabetically, by size, etc.	Visually strong Can easily compare two or three data sets	Graph categories can be reordered to emphasize certain effects Used only with discrete data
Line graph A line graph plots continuous data as points and then joins them with a line. Multiple data sets can be graphed together, but a key must be used.	Can compare multiple continuous data sets easily Interim data can be inferred from graph line	Used only with continuous data
Frequency polygon A frequency polygon can be made from a line graph by shading in the area beneath the graph. It can be made from a histogram by joining midpoints of each column.	Visually appealing	Anchors at both ends may imply zero as data points Used only with continuous data
Scatterplot A scatterplot displays the relationship between two factors of the experiment. A trend line is used to determine positive, negative, or no correlation.	Shows a trend in the data relationship Retains exact data values and sample size Shows minimum/maximum and outliers	Hard to visualize results in large data sets Flat trend line gives inconclusive results Data on both axes should be continuous

(Continued)

TABLE 3-3. STATISTICAL GRAPHS (*Continued*)

TYPE OF DISPLAY	ADVANTAGES	DISADVANTAGES
Stem and leaf plot Stem and leaf plots record data values in rows, and can easily be made into a histogram. Large data sets can be accommodated by splitting stems.	Concise representation of data Shows range, minimum and maximum, gaps and clusters, and outliers easily Can handle extremely large data sets	Not visually appealing Does not easily indicate measures of centrality for large data sets
Box plot A box plot is a concise graph showing the five point summary. Multiple box plots can be drawn side by side to compare more than one data set.	Shows five-point summary and outliers Easily compares two or more data sets Handles extremely large data sets easily	Not as visually appealing as other graphs Exact values not retained

Adapted with permission from Dr. Elaine Young at http://sci.tamucc.edu/~eyoung/1351/stat_graph_advantage.html.

(Table 3-4).[4] A test that can correctly identify every person who does not have the target disorder has a specificity of 1.0. SpPin is an acronym for when Specificity is extremely high, a Positive test result rules in the target disorder. Thus, a "high" specific test helps rule in a disorder or condition.

A test with a very high sensitivity, but low specificity, and vice versa, is of little value, and the acceptable levels are generally set at between 50% (unacceptable test) and 100% (perfect test), with an arbitrary cut off of about 80%.[4]

VALIDITY

Validity is defined as the degree to which a test measures what it purports to be measuring, and how well it correctly classifies individuals with or without a particular disease.[5-7] Validity is directly related to the

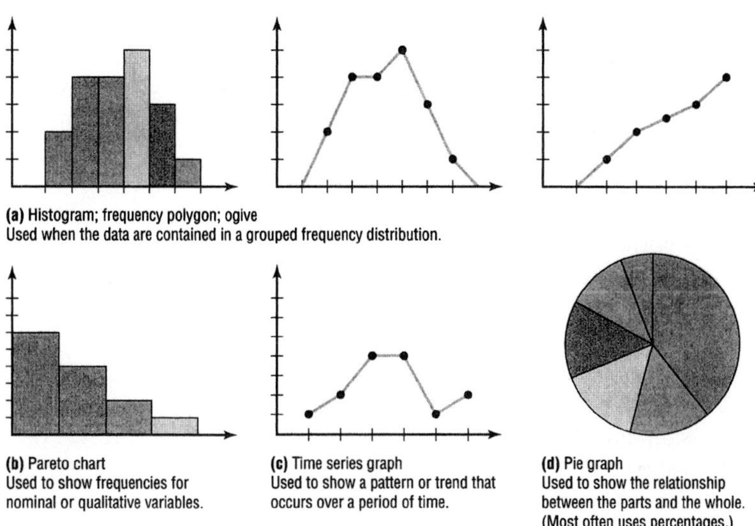

Figure 3-1. Summary of graphs and uses of each. (Reproduced, with permission, from Bluman A: *Elementary Statistics: A Step by Step Approach, 6th ed.* New York: McGraw-Hill. 2007:73.)

TABLE 3-4. CONCEPTS AND DEFINITIONS OF SENSITIVITY, SPECIFICITY, AND PREDICTIVE VALUES

CONCEPT	DEFINITION
Sensitivity	Proportion of patients with a disease who test positive.
Specificity	Proportion of patients without the disease who test negative.
Positive predictive value (PPV)	Proportion of patients who actually have the disease who test positive. If the target disease is uncommon, there are many more false positive results and the PPV goes down.
Negative predictive value	Proportion of patients who do not actually have the disease and who test negative.

notion of sensitivity and specificity. There are several types of validity, including construct validity, face validity, content validity, external validity, concurrent validity, criterion-referenced validity:

- Construct validity: refers to the ability of a test to represent the underlying construct (the theory developed to organize and explain some aspects of existing knowledge and observations). Construct validity refers to overall validity.
- Face validity: refers to the degree to which the questions or procedures incorporated within a test make sense to the users. The assessment of face validity is generally informal and non-quantitative and is the lowest standard of assessing validity. It is based on the notion that the finding is valid "on the face of it." For example, if a weighing scale indicates that a normal-sized person weighs 2000 lb, that scale does not have face validity.
- Content validity: refers to the assessment by experts that the content of the measure is consistent with what is to be measured. Content validity is concerned with sample-population representativeness, ie, the knowledge and skills covered by the test items should be representative of the larger domain of knowledge and skills. In many instances, it is difficult, if not impossible, to administer a test covering all aspects of knowledge or skills. Therefore, only several tasks are sampled from the population of knowledge or skills. In these circumstances, the proportion of the score attributed to a particular component should be proportional to the importance of that component to total performance. In content validity, evidence is obtained by looking for agreement in judgments by judges. In short, one person can determine face validity, but a panel should confirm content validity.
- External validity: deals with the degree to which study results can be generalized to different subjects, settings, and times.[8,9]
- Internal validity: can be defined as the degree to which the reported outcomes of the research study are a consequence of the relationship between the independent and dependent variables and not the result of extraneous factors.
- Criterion-referenced validity: determined by comparing the results of a test to those of a test that is accepted as a "gold standard" (a test which is accepted as being close to 100% valid).[4] There are three types of criterion-referenced validity: concurrent, predictive, and discriminant.
  - Concurrent: the degree to which the measurement being validated agrees with an established measurement standard administered at approximately the same time. Concurrent validity is a form of criterion validity.

- Predictive: the extent to which test scores are associated with future behavior or performance.
- Discriminant: the ability of a test to distinguish between two different constructs as is evidenced by a low correlation between the results of the test and those of tests of a different construct.

Diagnostic tests are used for the purpose of discovery, confirmation, and exclusion.[10] Tests for discovery and exclusion must have high sensitivity for detection, whereas confirmation tests require high specificity.[11] The sensitivity and specificity of any physical test to discriminate relevant dysfunction must be appreciated to make meaningful decisions.[12]

Prediction Value

The prediction value of a positive test indicates that those members of the study population who have a positive test outcome will have the condition under investigation (Table 3-4).[4] The diagnostic power of the negative test outcome relates to those of the study population with a negative test outcome who do not suffer from the condition under investigation.[4]

Likelihood Ratio

The likelihood ratio is the index measurement that is considered to combine the best characteristics of sensitivity, specificity, positive predictive value, and negative predictive value. Likelihood ratios are expressed as odds and are calculated from the values used to calculate sensitivity and specificity. The likelihood ratio indicates how much a given diagnostic test result will lower or raise the pretest probability of the target disorder.[4,13]

Reliability

Reliability is defined as the extent to which repeated measurements of a relatively stable phenomenon are close to each other.[14] Test-retest reliability is the consistency of repeated measurements that are separated in time when there is no change in what is being measured. Any difference between the two sets of scores represents measurement error, which can arise from a number of factors including intrarater variability, interrater reliability, or a lack of consistency of results. Reliability may be measured as repeatability between measurements performed by the same examiner (intrarater reliability), or between measurements by different examiners (interrater reliability). Instrument reliability deals with the tool used to obtain a measurement.

Reliability is quantitatively expressed by way of an index of agreement, with the simplest index being the percentage agreement value. The percentage agreement value is defined as the ratio of the number of agreements to the total number of ratings made.[15] However, because this value does not correct for chance agreement, it can provide a misleadingly high estimate of reliability.[6,15-17]

The results of an examination are of limited value if they are not consistently repeatable.[5,6] The kappa statistic (κ) is a chance-corrected index of agreement that overcomes the problem of chance agreement when used with nominal and ordinal data (Table 3-5).[18] However, with

TABLE 3-5. KAPPA (κ) BENCHMARK VALUES

VALUE (%)	DESCRIPTION
< 40	Poor to fair agreement
40-60	Moderate agreement
60-80	Substantial agreement
> 80	Excellent agreement
100	Perfect agreement

Data from Portney L, Watkins MP: *Foundations of Clinical Research: Applications to Practice.* Norwalk, CT: Appleton & Lange. 1993.

higher scale data such as ordinal and parametric, it tends to underestimate reliability, in which case a weight kappa (ranked) or intraclass correlation coefficient (ICC—see later) (parametric) should be used.[19] Theoretically κ can be negative if agreement is worse than chance. Practically, in clinical reliability studies, κ usually varies between 0.00 and 1.00.[19] The κ statistic does not differentiate among disagreements; it assumes that all disagreements are of equal significance.[19]

A number of calculations, including the Pearson product moment correlation coefficient and the ICC can be used to assess reliability.

THREATS TO VALIDITY AND RELIABILITY

The most common threats to validity and reliability are

- Ambiguity—when correlation is taken for causation
- Errors of measurement—random errors or systematic errors
- History—when some critical event occurs between pretest and posttest
- Instrumentation—when the researcher changes the measuring device
- Maturation—when people change or mature over the research period
- Mortality—when people die or drop out of the research
- Regression to the mean—a tendency toward middle scores
- The John Henry effect—when groups compete to score well
- Sampling bias—the tendency of a sample to exclude some members of the sampling population and overrepresent others
- Setting—something about the setting or context contaminates the study
- The Hawthorne effect—a tendency of research subjects to act atypically as a result of their awareness of being studied

DESCRIPTIVE STATISTICS

Descriptive statistics describe what is or what the data shows. Descriptive statistics include the collection, organization, summarization, and presentation of data to reduce lots of data into a simpler summary.[2] For example, the Grade Point Average (GPA) of a student describes the general performance of the student across a potentially wide range of course experiences.

Univariate analysis explores each variable in a data set, separately, focusing on the following:

- The central tendency: when populations are small, it is not necessary to use samples since the entire population can be used to gather information. Measures found by using all the data values in the population are called parameters. Measures of central tendency are measures of the location of the middle or the center of a distribution where data tends to cluster. Multiple metrics are used to describe this clustering, eg, mean, median, and mode:
  - Mean: the arithmetic mean is what is commonly called the average: When the word "mean" is used without a modifier, it can be assumed that it refers to the arithmetic mean.

The mean of a sample is typically denoted as $\bar{x}$. The mean is the sum of all the scores divided by the number of scores.
- Median: the median is the middle of a distribution. Half the scores are above the median and half are below the median. The median is less sensitive to extreme scores than the mean and this makes it a better measure than the mean for highly skewed distributions (see later).
- Mode: the mode is the most frequently occurring score in a distribution. The advantage of the mode as a measure of central tendency is that its meaning is obvious. Further, it is the only measure of central tendency that can be used with nominal data.

▶ Although measures of central tendency locate only the center of a distribution, other measures, such as a determination of the spread of a group of scores, are often needed to describe data. To examine the spread or variability of a data set, a number of measures are commonly used:[20]
- Range: the range is simply the highest value minus the lowest value.
- Variance: defined as the average of the squares of the distance that each value is from the mean.
- Standard deviation (σ): the standard deviation (SD) shows the relation that the set of scores has to the mean of the sample—it is a determination of the spread of a group of scores or the average deviation of values around the mean. The SD is based on the distance of sample values from the mean and provides information about how tightly all the various examples are clustered around the mean in a set of data. When the examples are pretty tightly bunched together, and the bell-shaped curve is steep, the standard deviation is small. When the examples are spread apart, and the bell curve is relatively flat, the standard deviation is relatively large. Mathematically, the standard deviation equals the square root of the mean of the square deviation, or the square root of the variance. The range can be used to approximate the standard deviation by dividing the range value by 4.

▶ A frequency distribution is a tabulation of the values that one or more variables take in a sample. These values can be graphed and frequency distributions can assume many shapes. Following are the most important shapes that are positively skewed, symmetric, and negatively skewed (Figure 3-2) (see "Measures of Position"):[20]
- Positively skewed: the majority of the data values fall to the left of the mean and cluster at the lower end of the distribution.
- Symmetric: the data values are evenly distributed on both sides of the mean.
- Negatively skewed: the majority of the data values fall to the right of the mean and cluster at the upper end of the distribution.

MEASURES OF POSITION

In addition to measures of central tendency and measures of variation, there are measures of position, which are used to locate the

Study Pearl

Normal distributions are a family of distributions that have a symmetrical and general shape with values that are more concentrated in the middle than in the tails (Figure 3-3). The standard normal distribution is a normal distribution with a mean of 0 and a standard deviation of 1.

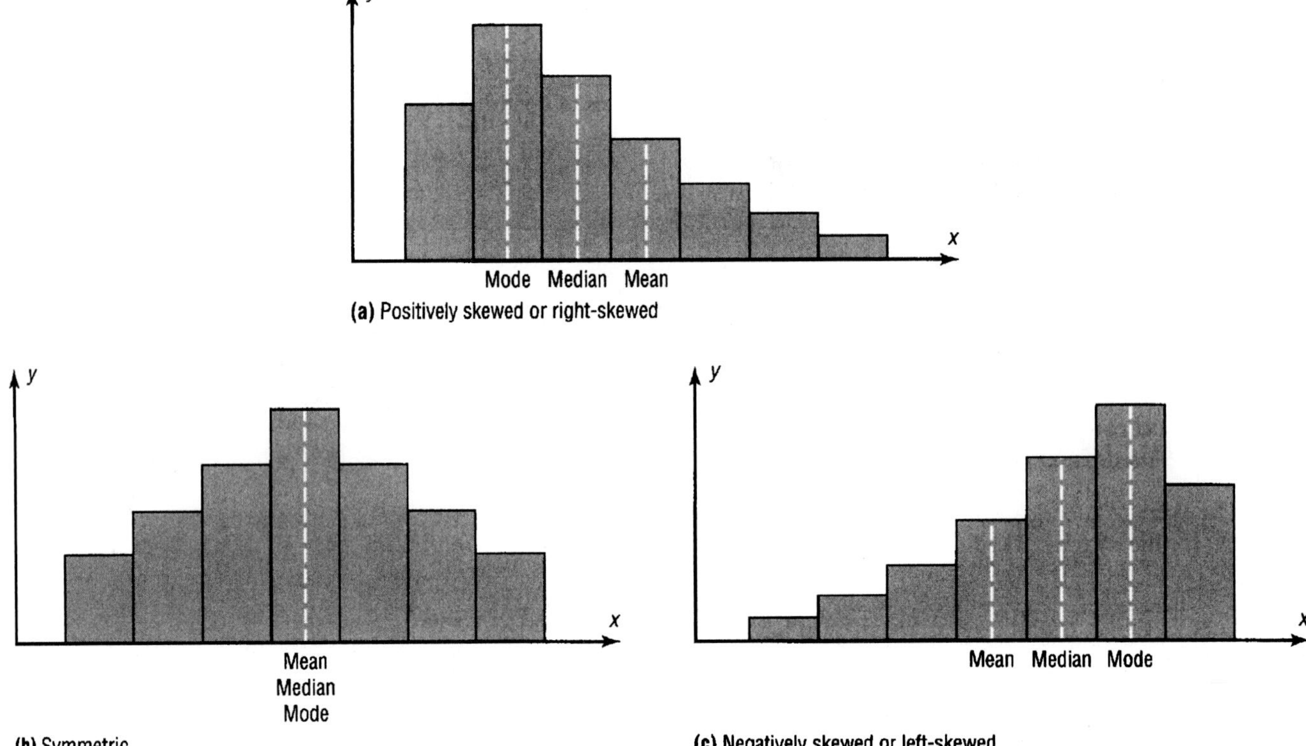

Figure 3-2. Types of distributions. (Reproduced, with permission, from Bluman A: *Elementary Statistics: A Step by Step Approach, 6th ed.* New York: McGraw-Hill. 2007:115.)

Study Pearl

Variances and standard deviations are used to determine the spread of data. If the variance or standard deviation is large, the data are more dispersed. The measures of variance and standard deviation are also used to determine the consistency of a variable, and the number of data values that fall within a specified interval in a distribution.

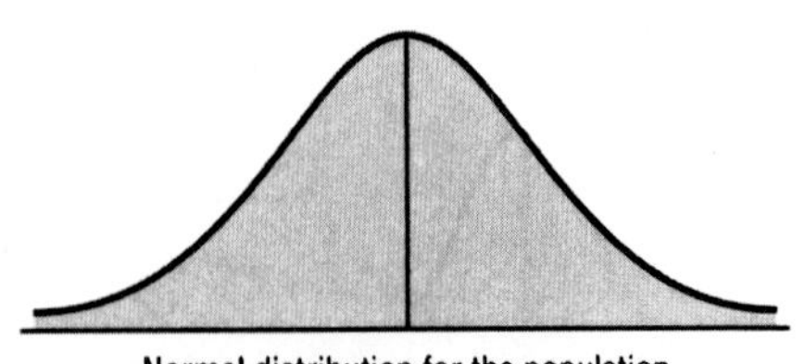

Figure 3-3. Histogram showing a normal distribution. (Reproduced, with permission, from Bluman A: *Elementary Statistics: A Step by Step Approach, 6th ed.* New York: McGraw-Hill. 2007:283.)

relative position of a data value in the data set.[20] One of the most common measures of position is the percentile. Percentiles divide the data set into 100 equal groups. The *N*th percentile is defined as the value such that *N* percent of the value lie below it. For example, a score in the 95th percentile represents the top 5% of scores.

- The lower quartile is defined as the 25th percentile—75% of the measures are above the lower quartile.
- The middle quartile is defined as the 50th percentile—the median of all the measures.
- The upper quartile is defined as the 75th percentile—25 percent of the measures are above the upper quartile.

No variable fits a normal distribution perfectly, since a normal distribution is a theoretical distribution.[21] The mean, median, and mode of a normal distribution have the same value due to the symmetry of the bell-shaped distribution (Figure 3-4). The curve has no boundaries and only a small fraction of the values fall outside of three standard deviations (a measure of how spread out a distribution is) above or below the mean:

- One standard deviation away from the mean in either direction on the horizontal axis accounts for approximately 68% of the people in the group (Figure 3-5).

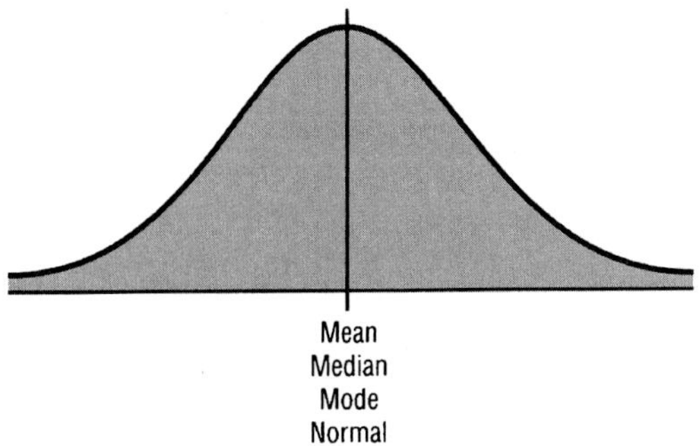

Figure 3-4. Normal distribution in relation to the mean, median, and mode. (Reproduced, with permission, from Bluman A: *Elementary Statistics: A Step by Step Approach, 6th ed.* New York: McGraw-Hill. 2007:283.)

Study Pearl

- Parametric statistical procedures, such as the ANOVA and *t*-test (see later), are performed on data that have a normal distribution, such as the distribution observed in a population.[1]
- Nonparametric procedures are performed on data that do not have a normal distribution, that is, a skewed distribution, as often is observed in a sample.[1]

- Two standard deviations away from the mean account for approximately 95% of the people (Figure 3-5).
- Three standard deviations account for about 99% of the people (Figure 3-5).
- The z value is actually the number of standard deviations that a particular x value is away from the mean.

Confidence Intervals

The sample mean will be, for the most part, somewhat different from the population mean due to sampling error.[22] An interval estimate of the parameter is an interval or a range of values used to estimate the parameter. This estimate may or may not contain the value of the parameter being estimated.[22] In interval estimates, the parameter is specified as being between two values.

The selection of a confidence level for an interval determines the probability that the CI produced will contain the true parameter value. Common choices for the CI are 0.90, 0.95, and 0.99. These levels correspond to percentages of the area of the normal density

Study Pearl

Skewness is a measure of the degree of asymmetry of a distribution. If the left tail (the tail at the small end of the distribution) is more pronounced that the right tail (the tail at the large end of the distribution), the function is said to have negative skewness (Figure 3-6). If the reverse is true, it has positive skewness (Figure 3-7). If the two halves of the curve are symmetrical (mirror images), the data distribution has zero skewness (Figure 3-4).

In a distribution displaying perfect symmetry, the mean, the median, and the mode are all at the same point, and skewness is zero.

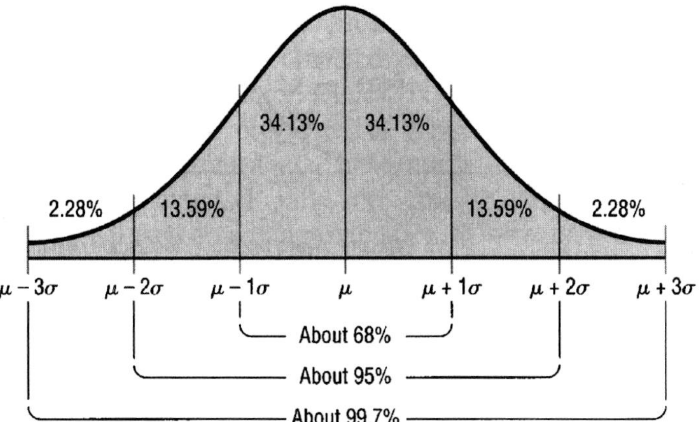

Figure 3-5. Areas under a normal distribution curve. (Reproduced, with permission, from Bluman A: *Elementary Statistics: A Step by Step Approach, 6th ed.* New York: McGraw-Hill. 2007:286.)

Study Pearl

A confidence interval (CI) is a statistical range with a specified probability that a given parameter lies within the range. The confidence level of an interval estimate of a parameter is the probability that the interval estimate will contain a parameter, assuming that a large number of samples are selected and that the estimation process on the same parameter is repeated.[22]

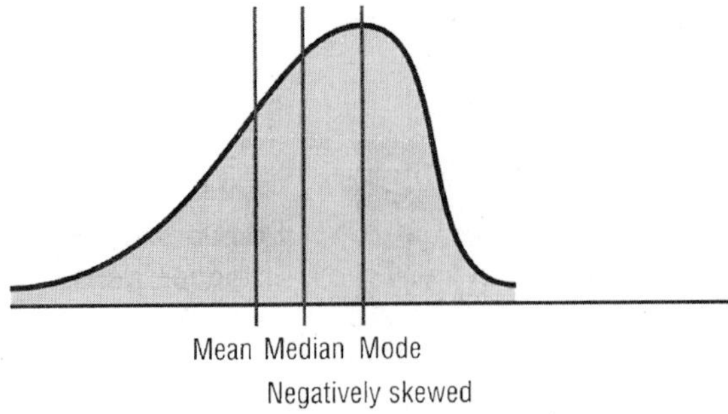

Figure 3-6. Negatively skewed distribution. (Reproduced, with permission, from Bluman A: *Elementary Statistics: A Step by Step Approach, 6th ed.* New York: McGraw-Hill. 2007:283.)

curve. For example, a 95% confidence interval covers 95% of the normal curve—the probability of observing a value outside of this area is less than 0.05.[4,13]

Confidence Intervals for the Mean. When the standard deviation is known and the variable is normally distributed, or when the standard deviation is unknown and the sample size is ≥30, the standard normal distribution is used to find confidence intervals for the mean.[22] However, in many situations, the population standard deviation is not known and the sample size is less than 30. In such situations, the standard deviation from the sample can be used in place of the population standard deviation for confidence intervals. A somewhat different distribution, called the *t distribution* (Figure 3-8), must be used when the sample size is less than 30, and the variable is normally or approximately normally distributed (Table 3-6).

Confidence Intervals for Variances and Standard Deviations. To calculate these confidence intervals, the chi-square distribution is used. The chi-square variable is similar to the *t* variable in that its distribution is a family of curves based on the number of degrees of freedom.[22] Several of the distributions are shown in Figure 3-9.

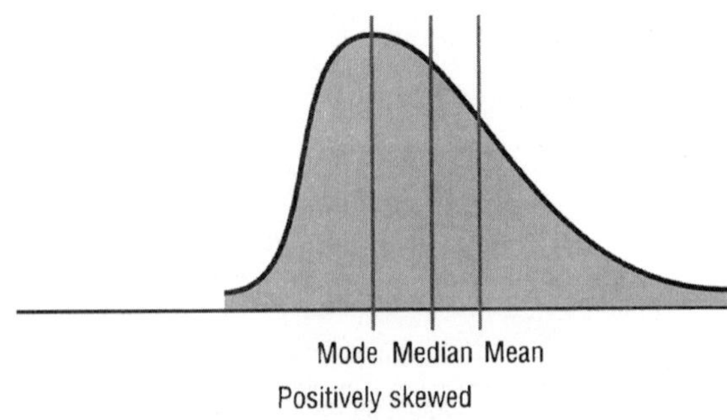

Figure 3-7. Positively skewed distribution. (Reproduced, with permission, from Bluman A: *Elementary Statistics: A Step by Step Approach, 6th ed.* New York: McGraw-Hill. 2007:283.)

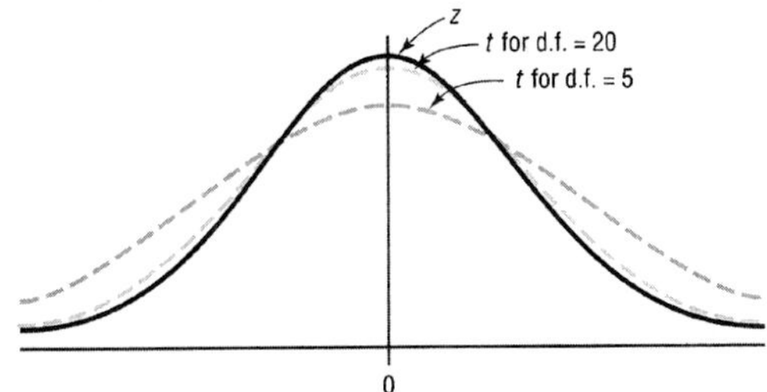

FIGURE 3-8. The *t* family of curves. (Reproduced, with permission, from Bluman A: *Elementary Statistics: A Step by Step Approach, 6th ed.* New York: McGraw-Hill. 2007:358.)

TABLE 3-6. SIMILARITIES AND DIFFERENCES BETWEEN THE *t* DISTRIBUTION AND THE STANDARD NORMAL DISTRIBUTION

SIMILARITIES	DIFFERENCES
Bell-shaped curve.	The variance is greater than one.
Symmetric about the mean: the mean, median, and node are equal to 0 and are located at the center of the distribution.	The key distribution is actually a family of curves based on the concept of degrees of freedom, which is related to sample size.[a]
The curve never touches the x-axis.	As the sample size increases, the *t* distribution approaches the standard normal distribution.

[a]The degrees of freedom are the number of values that are free to vary after a sample statistic has been computed, and they tell a researcher which specific code to use when a distribution consists of a family of curves. For example, if the mean of 5 values is 10, then 4 of the 5 values are free to vary. But once 4 values are selected, the fifth value must be a specific number to get a sum of 50, since 50 ÷ 5 = 10. Hence, the degrees of freedom are 5 − 1 = 4, and this value tells the researcher which *t* curve to use.

Reproduced, with permission, from Bluman AG: Confidence intervals and sample size. In: Bluman AG, ed. *Elementary Statistics: A Step by Step Approach, 4th ed.* New York: McGraw-Hill. 2008:343-385.

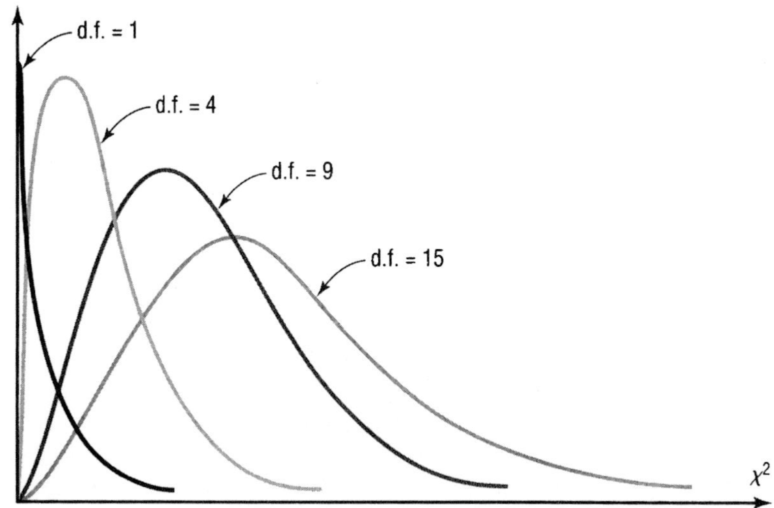

Figure 3-9. The chi-square family of curves. (Reproduced, with permission, from Bluman A: *Elementary Statistics: A Step by Step Approach, 6th ed.* New York: McGraw-Hill. 2007:374.)

INFERENTIAL STATISTICS

Inferential statistics are used to try to reach conclusions that extend beyond the immediate data alone. Inferential statistics include making inferences from samples to populations, estimations and hypothesis testing, determining relationships, and making predictions.[2] Inferential statistics are based on probability theory.[2] Probability deals with events that occur by chance. Probability can be defined as the chance of an event occurring. The classical theory of probability states that the chance of a particular outcome occurring is determined by the ratio of the number of favorable outcomes (or successes) to the total number of outcomes. An event consists of a set of outcomes of a probability experiment. Probabilities can be expressed as fractions, decimals, or percentages.

- Probability sampling: any method of sampling that utilizes some form of random selection, and uses a process or procedure that assures that the different units in the population have equal probabilities of being chosen.
- Non-probability sampling: does not require random selection or the parameters of the population to be identified. This type of sampling is often utilized in physical therapy due to the increased difficulty of meeting the more rigid requirements of probability sampling.
- Most of the major inferential statistics come from a general family of statistical models including the *t*-test, Analysis of Variance (ANOVA), and Analysis of Covariance (ANCOVA).
- *t*-Test: the *t-test* is the most commonly used method to evaluate the differences in means between two groups when the standard deviation is unknown, the sample size is less than 30, and the distribution of the variable is approximately normal. The groups can be independent (eg, blood pressure of patients who were given a drug vs a control group who received a placebo) or dependent (eg, blood pressure of patients "before" vs "after" they received a drug).
- Analysis of Variance (ANOVA): ANOVA is a useful tool that helps the user to identify sources of variability from one or more potential sources, sometimes referred to as "treatments" or "factors." ANOVA is used rather than performing multiple *t*-tests because it protects against an inflation of α that would otherwise result from multiple *t*-tests.

Study Pearl

The *t*-test and ANOVA determine whether the difference(s) between the means of two (*t*-test) or more samples (ANOVA) could be due to random sampling error alone.

- A *t*-test is used with one independent variable with two levels (ie, there are two groups, such as control vs experimental).
- ANOVA is used when there is one independent variable with three or more levels (conditions), or there are two or more independent variables.

By varying the factors in a predetermined pattern and analyzing the output, one can use statistical techniques to make an accurate assessment as to the cause of variation in a process. There are two common types of ANOVA:

- The one-way ANOVA: a method of analysis that requires multiple experiments or readings to be taken from a source that can take on two or more different inputs or settings. The one-way ANOVA performs a comparison of the means of a number of replications of experiments performed where a single input factor is varied at different settings or levels. The object of this comparison is to determine the proportion of the variability of the data that is due to the different treatment levels or factors as opposed to variability due to random error. Basically, rejection of the null hypothesis indicates that variation in the outcome is due to variation between the treatment levels and not due to random error. If the null hypothesis is rejected, there is a difference in the outcome of the different treatment levels at a significance α and it remains to be determined between which treatment levels the actual differences lie.

- The two-way Analysis of Variance: an extension to the one-way Analysis of Variance, in which comparisons can be made between two or more populations means with two or more independent variables (hence the name two-way) called factors.
- Analysis of Covariance (ANCOVA): ANCOVA is a test used to compare two or more treatment groups or conditions while also controlling for the effects of intervening variables (covariates), eg, two groups of subjects are compared on the basis of diet parameters using two different types of exercises; the subjects in one group are male and the subjects in the second group of female; sex then becomes the covariate that must be controlled during statistical analysis.

INTRACLASS CORRELATION COEFFICIENT

The intraclass correlation coefficient (ICC) is a reliability coefficient calculated with variance estimates obtained through an Analysis of Variance (ANOVA) (Table 3-7).[9] The ICC has been advocated as a statistic for assessing agreement or consistency between two methods of measurement, in conjunction with a significance test of the difference between means obtained by the two methods. The advantage of the ICC over correlation coefficients is that it does not require the same number of raters per subject, and it can be used for two or more raters or ratings.[9]

TABLE 3-7. INTRACLASS CORRELATION COEFFICIENT BENCHMARK VALUES

VALUE	DESCRIPTION
< 0.75	Poor to moderate agreement
> 0.75	Good agreement
> 90	Reasonable agreement for clinical measurements

Data from Portney L, Watkins MP: *Foundations of Clinical Research: Applications to Practice.* Norwalk, CT: Appleton & Lange. 1993.

Study Pearl

- Spearman's rank correlation coefficient or Spearman's rho (ρ): provides information as to the magnitude and direction of the association between two variables that are on an interval or ratio scale.
- The Pearson product-moment correlation coefficient (PPMCC, sometimes referred to as the Pearson correlation coefficient): measures the strength and direction of a *linear* relationship between the *X* and *Y* variables.[19] The PPMCC, which is denoted by the Greek letter "rho" (ρ), ranges from −1 to 1. A value of 1 implies a perfect relationship between *X* and *Y*:[19]
  - 0.00-0.25: Little or no relationship
  - 0.25-0.50: Fair relationship
  - 0.50-0.75: Moderate to good relationship
  - > 0.75: Good to excellent relationship

HYPOTHESIS TESTING

Statistical hypothesis testing is a decision-making process used for evaluating claims about a population.[23] Every hypothesis testing situation begins with a statement of a hypothesis.

There are two types of statistical hypothesis of each situation: the null hypothesis (H_0), and the alternative hypothesis (H_A).

1. Null hypothesis (H_0): a statistical hypothesis that states that there is no difference between a parameter and a specific value, or that there is no difference between two parameters.[23]
2. Alternative hypothesis (H_A): a statistical hypothesis that states the existence of a difference between a parameter and a specific value, or states that there is a difference between two parameters.[23]

Although the above definitions of null and alternative hypothesis use the word parameter, these definitions can be extended to include other terms such as distributions and randomness.[23]

In statistical hypothesis testing (Table 3-8), the null hypothesis (H_0) is initially believed to be true, and the researcher sees if the data provide enough evidence to abandon the belief in H_0 in favor of the

Study Pearl

A statistical hypothesis is a conjecture about a population parameter. This conjecture may or may not be true.[23]

TABLE 3-8. GUIDELINES FOR HYPOTHESIS TESTING

1. Make a claim—a hypothesis that is assumed to be/is correct—the research hypothesis. For example, the research hypothesis could be "I wonder whether sleep deprivation would have an effect on mental performance."
2. State the null hypothesis and the alternative hypothesis: The null hypothesis (denoted H_0) is a statement about the value of a population parameter that MUST contain equality (=, ≤, ≥). For example, in the sleep deprivation study, the null hypothesis could be that sleep deprivation will have no effect on mental performance. The alternative hypothesis (denoted H_1) is the opposite statement—the one that must be true if the null hypothesis is false. The alternative hypothesis is a statement of what a statistical hypothesis test is set up to establish. In this example, the alternative hypothesis would be that sleep deprivation would have a positive or negative effect, on mental performance. The goal is to ascertain a correct inference about the population that is being sampled with the experimental technique.
3. Decide on the appropriate test statistic. A test statistic is a quantity calculated from the sample of data and is determined by the assumed probability model and the hypotheses under question. Its value is used to decide whether or not the null hypothesis should be rejected in the hypothesis test.
4. Find the critical value for the test statistic and determine the critical region (see text).
5. Perform the calculations and state the conclusion.

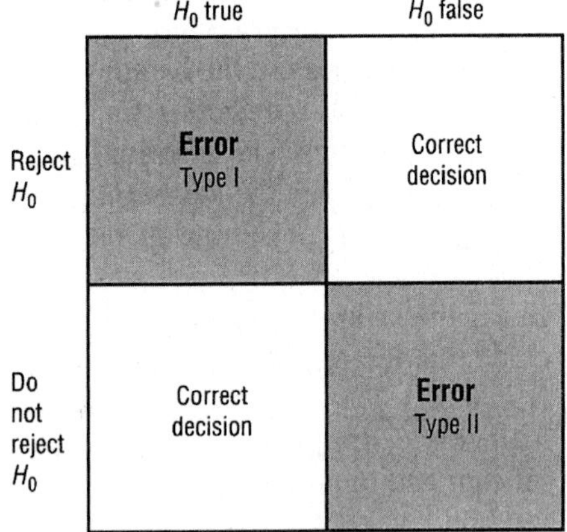

Figure 3-10. Possible outcomes of a hypothesis test. (Reproduced, with permission, from Bluman A: *Elementary Statistics: A Step by Step Approach, 6th ed.* New York: McGraw-Hill. 2007:392.)

alternative hypothesis H_A. For example, in a jury trial there is a presumption of innocence (eg, the population means of a control group and the experimental group are not different from each other). The null hypothesis is assumed to be true (the defendant is innocent) at the outset of inferential statistical analysis. The null hypothesis is only rejected in favor of the alternative hypothesis (eg, the two means differ) when the data provide the basis for "reasonable doubt about innocence," ie, based on the experimental data, it is more likely that the control and experimental groups are different from each other (Figure 3-10).

Type I Errors. In a hypothesis test, a type I error occurs when the null hypothesis is rejected when it is in fact true; that is, H_0 is wrongly rejected. For example, in a clinical trial of a new drug, the null hypothesis might be that the new drug is no better, on average, than the current drug; that is H_0: There is no difference between the two drugs on average. A type I error would occur if we concluded that the two drugs produced different effects when in fact there was no difference between them (Figure 3-11). A type I error is often considered to be more serious, and therefore more important to

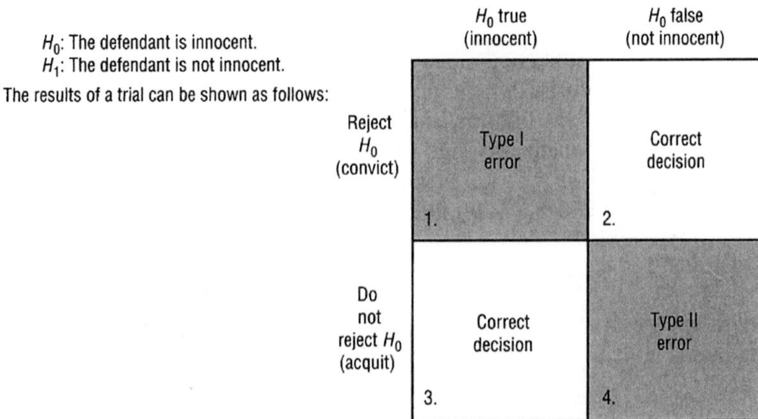

Figure 3-11. Hypothesis testing and a jury trial. (Reproduced, with permission, from Bluman A: *Elementary Statistics: A Step by Step Approach, 6th ed.* New York: McGraw-Hill. 2007:393.)

avoid, than a type II error (see next). The hypothesis test procedure is therefore adjusted so that there is a guaranteed "low" probability of rejecting the null hypothesis wrongly; this probability is never 0.

Type II Errors. In a hypothesis test, a type II error occurs when the null hypothesis H_0, is not rejected when it is in fact false. For example, in a clinical trial of a new drug, the null hypothesis might be that the new drug is no better, on average, than the current drug; that is H_0: There is no difference between the two drugs on average. A type II error would occur if it was concluded that the two drugs produced the same effect, that is, there is no difference between the two drugs on average, when in fact they produced different ones (Figure 3-11). A type II error is frequently due to sample sizes being too small.

Nothing can be proved absolutely. Likewise, the decision to reject or not reject the null hypothesis does not prove anything—the only way to prove anything statistically is to use the entire population.[23] The question as to how large the difference is necessary to reject the null hypothesis is answered somewhat using the level of significance.

Significance Level. The level of significance (denoted α) is the maximum probability of wrongly rejecting the null hypothesis H_0, when it is in fact true (committing a type I error). In simple terms, α is the preset risk one is willing to take in committing a type I error with an inferential statistical test. It is the bar over which the data needs to jump in order to reject the null hypothesis and be considered statistically significant. By convention, statisticians use three arbitrary significance levels (α): 0.10, 0.05, and 0.01 levels (although it can be any level, depending on the seriousness of the type I error).[23] That is, if the null hypothesis is rejected, the probability of a type I error will be 10%, 5%, or 1%, depending on which level of significance is used. For example, if the acceptable risk of committing a type I error is 5%, α is set to 0.05 (indicates that the expected difference due to chance is only 5 times out of every 100). While decreasing the α value reduces the risk of a type I error, decreasing it too much increases the chances of obtaining a type II error.

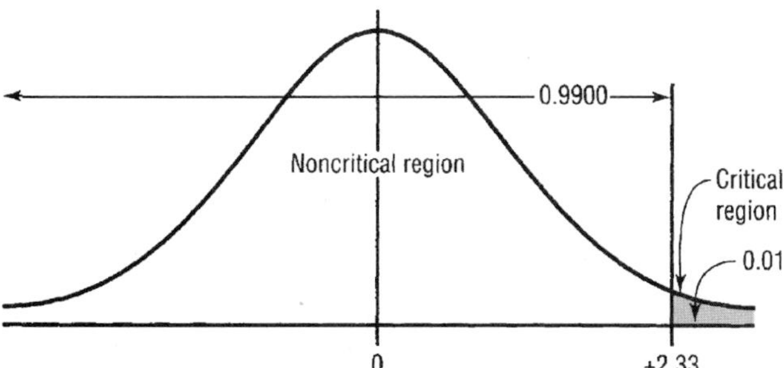

Figure 3-12. Critical and noncritical regions for $\alpha = 0.01$ (right-tailed test). (Reproduced, with permission, from Bluman A: *Elementary Statistics: A Step by Step Approach, 6th ed.* New York: McGraw-Hill. 2007:395.)

Study Pearl

- A type I error occurs if one rejects the null hypothesis when it is true.
- A type II error occurs if one does not reject the null hypothesis when it is false.

Study Pearl

- The critical or rejection region is the range of values of the test value that indicates that there is a significant difference and that the null hypothesis should be rejected (Figure 3-12); that is, the sample space for the test statistic is partitioned into two regions; one region (the critical region) will lead the researcher to reject the null hypothesis H_0,' the other not. So, if the observed value of the test statistic is a member of the critical region, the researcher concludes "reject H_0"; if it is not a member of the critical region then the researcher concludes "do not reject H_0."
- The noncritical or nonrejection region is the range of values of the test value that indicates that the difference was probably due to chance and that the null hypothesis should not be rejected.

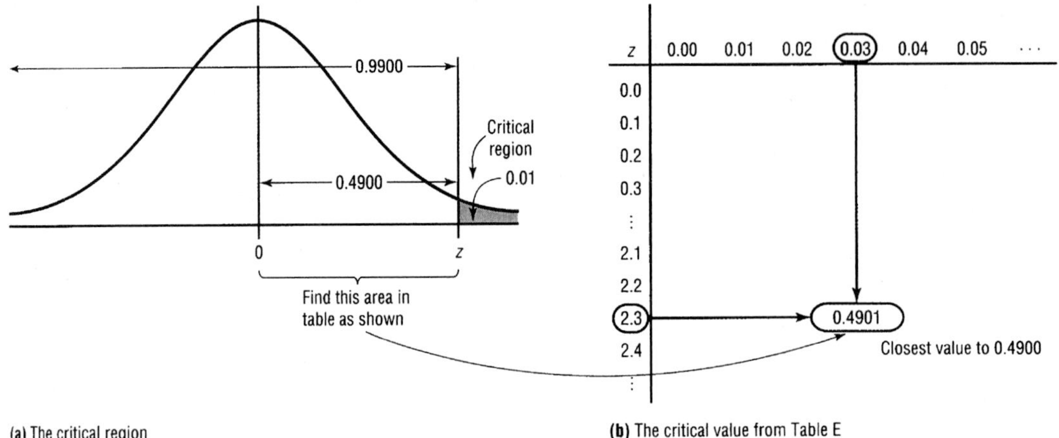

Figure 3-13. Finding the critical value for α = 0.01 (right-tailed test). (Reproduced, with permission, from Bluman A: *Elementary Statistics: A Step by Step Approach, 6th ed.* New York: McGraw-Hill. 2007:395.)

Study Pearl

A ***one-tailed*** (one-sided) test indicates that the null hypothesis should be rejected when the test value is in the critical region on one side of the mean; the region of rejection is entirely within one tail of the probability distribution. A one-tailed test is either a right-tailed test or a left-tailed test, depending on the direction of the inequality of the alternative hypothesis.

A ***two-tailed*** (two-sided) test indicates that the null hypothesis can be rejected when there is a significant difference in either direction, above or below the mean; the region of rejection is located in either of the two critical regions (Figure 3-14). An extreme test statistic in either tail of the distribution (positive or negative) will lead to the rejection of the null hypothesis of no difference.

The choice between a one-sided and a two-sided test is determined by the purpose of the investigation or prior reasons for using a one-sided test. In most scientific investigations a conservative approach is used where the problem is formulated with a two-sided alternative hypothesis, allowing the data to determine precisely how the null hypothesis might be false.

After a significance level is chosen, a critical value is selected from a table for the appropriate test. The critical value determines the critical and noncritical regions.

The critical value for any hypothesis test depends on the significance level at which the test is carried out, whether the test is one-tailed or two-tailed, and on the degrees of freedom (see next). The critical value can be on the right side of the mean or on the left side of the mean for one tail test—its location depends on the inequality sign of the alternative hypothesis. To obtain the critical value, the researcher must choose an alpha level (Figure 3-13).

Probability (*p*) Value. The probability value (*p*-value) is used in statistics to describe the probability of something happening. A study will generally give a value of *p* for any conclusions they draw. The *p*-value is the probability of getting a

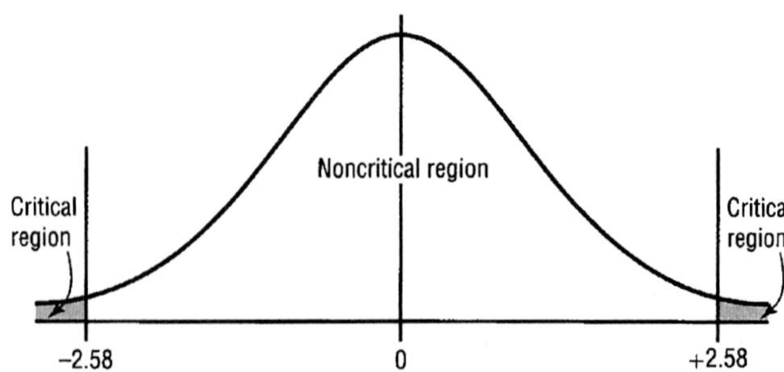

Figure 3-14. Critical and noncritical regions for α = 0.01 (two-tailed test). (Reproduced, with permission, from Bluman A: *Elementary Statistics: A Step by Step Approach, 6th ed.* New York: McGraw-Hill. 2007:395.)

sample statistic (such as the mean) or in more extreme sample statistic in the direction of the alternative hypothesis when the null hypothesis is true—the risk of committing a type 1 error if the null hypothesis is rejected.

Small *p*-values suggest a very unusual observation under H_0 indicating that the null hypothesis is unlikely to be true. The smaller the *p*-value, the more convincing is the rejection of the null hypothesis. H_0 is rejected when the *p*-value is less than α.

The *p*-value indicates the strength of evidence for rejecting the null hypothesis H_0, rather than simply concluding "reject H_0" or "do not reject H_0." For example, if a statistical test is run and yields $p = 0.25$, statistical significance is defined as a statistical test yielding a *p*-value that is less than α, ie, less than 0.05 (< 5% chance of committing a type 1 error).

Study Pearl

If the conclusion of a study finds that the intervention is better than the control with $p < 0.00001$, that is a very strong conclusion indeed. If, however, the conclusion is with $p < 0.25$, then there is a 25% chance of committing a type I error if the null hypothesis is rejected; this is considered too high a risk; too weak to rely on.

Study Pearl

It is important to remember that one does not know if a type I of type II error has been committed in a statistical inferential decision, rather, the α, and *p*-values provide information about the probability that such an error occurred, or the likelihood that such an error has occurred.

The Power of a Hypothesis Test. The power of a statistical hypothesis test measures the test's ability to reject the null hypothesis when it is actually false—that is, to make a correct inference.

- The power of a hypothesis test is the probability of not committing a type II error. It is calculated by subtracting the probability of a type II error from 1.
- The maximum power a test can have is 1, whereas the minimum is 0.
- Ideally a test should have a high power, close to 1.

z-Test. The z-test is a statistical test of the mean of a population. It can be used when the sample size is ≥ 30, of when the population is normally distributed and the standard deviation is known. For example, a z-test could be used if exam scores from a class of students is compared to a different class who took the same exam (when the population mean and standard deviation are known).

CHOOSING THE CORRECT STATISTICAL CALCULATION

The choice of how to analyze data depends on the question being asked:[1]

- If the design is to learn about the association between two variables (eg, what is the relationship between arm girth and elbow flexor strength), a correlation coefficient should be calculated.
- If the question deals with prediction (eg, if the patient has knee range of motion of 10-50 degrees on the second postoperative day, how many days will the patient likely remain in the hospital?), a regression analysis is appropriate.

Study Pearl

Sackett and colleagues[24] define best evidence as:

- Clinically relevant research, often from the basic sciences, but especially from patient-centered clinical research
- The accuracy and precision of diagnostic tests
- The power of prognostic markers
- The efficacy and safety of therapeutic, rehabilitative, and preventive regimens

- If the question is whether a treatment has an effect, or shows a difference (eg, does spinal traction reduce the signs and symptoms of a cervical root compression?), a chi-square, Analysis of Variance (ANOVA), or *t*-test is appropriate.
- For a correlation study to determine the degree of association, a Spearman rho is used for ordinal data, whereas a Pearson correlation coefficient is calculated for interval data.
- If the question is whether two groups differ on the dependent variable, and the data are normally distributed with equal variances, a *t*-test is appropriate.

USE OF EVIDENCE-BASED PRACTICE

Evidence-based practice (EBP), the integration of three key elements: best research evidence, clinical expertise, and patient values, is having an increasing impact on the profession of physical therapy.

When integrating evidence into clinical decision making, an understanding of how to appraise the quality of the evidence offered by clinical studies is important. Judging the strength of the evidence becomes an important part of the decision-making process.

Study Pearl

Clinical prediction rules (CPR) are tools designed to assist clinicians in decision making when caring for patients. However, although there is a growing trend to produce a number of CPRs in the field of physical therapy, few CPRs presently exist.

SCIENTIFIC RIGOR BY TYPE OF RESEARCH DESIGN

Unfortunately, many of the experimental studies that deal with physical therapy topics are not well-designed trials. Awareness of the distinction between efficacy and effectiveness is important for therapists attempting to translate evidence to practice.

- Efficacy: refers to outcomes of interventions provided in a controlled setting under experimental conditions. When attempting to apply the results of an efficacy study, a therapist must consider whether subject characteristics and the manner in which intervention was provided generalize to patients on their caseloads and how to adapt the intervention to constraints within their practice settings.[25]
- Effectiveness: refers to outcomes of interventions provided within the scope of clinical practice.

Study Pearl

Randomized controlled trials and systematic reviews provide the strongest, most relevant evidence to inform practice (Table 3-11).

Sackett[26] proposed a five-level system that relates the experimental design to levels of evidence and grades of recommendation (Table 3-9). A grade A recommendation (the randomized controlled trial) (Table 3-10) indicates that outcomes are supported by at least one level I study. A grade B recommendation indicates outcomes are supported by at least one level II study. A grade C recommendation indicates that outcomes are supported by level III, IV, or V studies.

TABLE 3-9. A HIERARCHY OF EVIDENCE GRADING

	LEVEL OF EVIDENCE GRADING = A	LEVEL OF EVIDENCE GRADING = B	LEVEL OF EVIDENCE GRADING = C	LEVEL OF EVIDENCE GRADING = D	LEVEL OF EVIDENCE GRADING = E
Type of Study	Randomized controlled trial	Cohort study	▶ Nonrandomized trial with concurrent or historical controls ▶ Case study ▶ Study of sensitivity and specificity of a diagnostic test ▶ Population-based descriptive study	▶ Cross-sectional study ▶ Case series ▶ Case report	▶ Expert consensus ▶ Clinical experience

Data from Sackett DL: Rules of evidence and clinical recommendations on the use of antithrombotic agents. *Chest.* 1986;89:2S-3S.

TABLE 3-10. THE RANDOMIZED CONTROLLED TRIAL

An experimental design in which subjects are randomly assigned to an experimental or control group permitting the strongest inferences about cause and effect. Typically volunteers agree to be randomly allocated to groups receiving one of the following:

- ▶ Treatment and no treatment
- ▶ Standard treatment and standard treatment plus a new treatment
- ▶ Two alternate treatments

The common feature is that the experimental group receives the treatment of interest, and the control group does not. At the end of the trial, outcomes of subjects in each group are determined—the difference in outcomes between groups provides an estimate of the size of the treatment effect.

- ▶ Less exposed to bias
- ▶ Ensures comparability of groups
- ▶ Provide evidence of efficacy

Data from Maher CG, Herbert RD, Moseley AM, et al: Critical appraisal of randomized trials, systematic reviews of radomized trials and clinical practice guidelines. In: Boyling JD, Jull GA, eds. *Grieve's Modern Manual Therapy: The Vertebral Column.* Philadelphia, PA: Churchill Livingstone. 2004:603-614; Petticrew M: Systematic reviews from astronomy to zoology: myths and misconceptions. *BMJ.* 2001;322:98-101; Palisano RJ, Campbell SK, Harris SR: Evidence-based decision-making in pediatric physical therapy. In: Campbell SK, Vander Linden DW, Palisano RJ, eds. *Physical Therapy for Children.* St. Louis: W.B. Saunders. 2006:3-32.

TABLE 3-11. SYSTEMATIC REVIEWS

Systematic review	Review of the literature conducted in a way that is designed to minimize bias—"a study of studies." Recently published reviews can be used to assess the effects of health interventions, the accuracy of diagnostic tests, or the prognosis for a particular condition. Usually involve criteria to determine which studies will be considered, the search strategy used to locate the studies, the methods for assessing the quality of the studies, and the process used to synthesize the findings of individual studies. Particularly useful for busy clinicians who may be unable to access all the relevant trials in an area and may otherwise need to rely upon their own incomplete surveys of relevant trials. NB: A systematic review is only as good as the quality of each study.
Meta-analysis	A mathematical synthesis of the results of two or more research reports. A meta-analysis can be performed on studies that used reliable and valid measures and report some type of inferential statistic (eg, *t*-test, ANOVA)—see "Parametric Statistics."

Data from Maher CG, Herbert RD, Moseley AM, et al: Critical appraisal of randomized trials, systematic reviews of radomized trials and clinical practice guidelines. In: Boyling JD, Jull GA, eds. *Grieve's Modern Manual Therapy: The vertebral Column.* Philadelphia, PA: Churchill Livingstone. 2004:603-614; Petticrew M: Systematic reviews from astronomy to zoology: myths and misconceptions. *BMJ.* 2001;322:98-101; Palisano RJ, Campbell SK, Harris SR: Evidence-based decision-making in pediatric physical therapy. In: Campbell SK, Vander Linden DW, Palisano RJ, eds. *Physical Therapy for Children.* St. Louis: W.B. Saunders. 2006:3-32.

TABLE 3-12. CLINICAL PRACTICE GUIDELINES

Recommendations for management of a particular clinical condition
Intended to provide current standards for quality practice in order to improve effectiveness and efficiency of health care
Involve compilation of evidence concerning needs and expectations of recipients of care, the accuracy of diagnostic tests, effects of therapy and prognosis
Usually necessitates the results from one, or sometimes several systematic reviews
May be presented as clinical decision algorithms
Can provide a useful framework upon which clinicians can build clinical practice

Data from Maher CG, Herbert RD, Moseley AM, et al: Critical appraisal of randomized trials, systematic reviews of radomized trials and clinical practice guidelines. In: Boyling JD, Jull GA, eds. *Grieve's Modern Manual Therapy: The Vertebral Column*. Philadelphia, PA: Churchill Livingstone. 2004:603-614.

Study Pearl

The critically appraised topic (CAT) provides a format for therapists to summarize the research evidence from a literature search conducted as part of clinical practice.[27] A critically appraised topic is a one- to two-page summary of research related to a focused clinical question that includes implications for practice.[25]

Evidence-based practice is a four-step process:

1. A clinical problem is identified and an answerable research question is formulated.
2. A systematic literature review is conducted and evidence is collected.
3. The research evidence is summarized and critically analyzed.
4. The research evidence is synthesized and applied to clinical practice.

Practice guidelines are systematically developed statements to assist patient and practitioner decisions about the management of a health condition (Table 3-12).[25] In general, practice guidelines include recommendations for the following:[25]

- Who should receive the intervention?
- Expected outcomes.
- Documentation including selection of reliable and valid tests and measures.
- Utilization of services (frequency and duration, number of visits).
- Procedural interventions.
- Coordination of care.
- Discharge planning.

In 1998, an international group of researchers and policymakers formed the AGREE (Appraisal of Guidelines for Research and Evaluation) collaboration in order to improve the quality and effectiveness of clinical practice guidelines.[25]

INSTRUMENTATION-GOLD STANDARD

The instrumentation-gold standard can be defined as an instrument with established validity that can be used as a standard for assessing or comparing other instruments.

Questions for this chapter and the entire book appear on the included CD-ROM, with additional questions at www.DuttonNPTE.com.

REFERENCES

1. Underwood FB: Clinical research and data analysis. In: Placzek JD, Boyce DA, eds. *Orthopaedic Physical Therapy Secrets.* Philadelphia, PA: Hanley & Belfus, Inc. 2001:130-139.
2. Bluman AG: The nature of probability and statistics. In: Bluman AG, ed. *Elementary Statistics: A Step by Step Approach, 4th ed.* New York, NY: McGraw-Hill. 2008:1-32.
3. Bluman AG: Organizing data. In: Bluman AG, ed. *Elementary Statistics: A Step by Step Approach, 4th ed.* New York, NY: McGraw-Hill. 2008:33-100.
4. Van der Wurff P, Meyne W, Hagmeijer RHM: Clinical tests of the sacroiliac joint, a systematic methodological review. part 2: validity. *Man Ther.* 2000;5:89-96.
5. Feinstein AR: *Clinimetrics.* Westford, MA: Murray Printing Company. 1987.
6. Marx RG, Bombardier C, Wright JG: What we know about the reliability and validity of physical examination tests used to examine the upper extremity. *J Hand Surg.* 1999;24A:185-193.
7. Roach KE, Brown MD, Albin RD, et al: The sensitivity and specificity of pain response to activity and position in categorizing patients with low back pain. *Phys Ther.* 1997;77:730-738.
8. Domholdt E: *Physical Therapy Research: Principles and Applications.* Philadelphia, PA: WB Saunders. 1993.
9. Huijbregts PA: Spinal motion palpation: a review of reliability studies. *J Man & Manip Ther.* 2002;10:24-39.
10. Feinstein AR: Clinical biostatistics XXXI: on the sensitivity, specificity & discrimination of diagnostic tests. *Clin Pharmacol Ther.* 1975;17:104-116.
11. Anderson MA, Foreman TL: Return to competition: functional rehabilitation. In: Zachazewski JE, Magee DJ, Quillen WS, eds. *Athletic Injuries and Rehabilitation.* Philadelphia, PA: WB Saunders; 1996:229-261.
12. Jull GA: Physiotherapy management of neck pain of mechanical origin. In: Giles LGF, Singer KP, eds. *Clinical Anatomy and Management of Cervical Spine Pain. The Clinical Anatomy of Back Pain.* London, England, Butterworth-Heinemann. 1998: 168-191.
13. Jaeschke R, Guyatt G, Sackett DL: Users guides to the medical literature. III. How to use an article about a diagnostic test. B. What are the results and will they help me in caring for my patients? *JAMA.* 1994;27:703-707.
14. Wright JG, Feinstein AR: Improving the reliability of orthopaedic measurements. *J Bone and Joint Surg.* 1992;74B:287-291.
15. Haas M: Statistical methodology for reliability studies. *J Manip Physiol Ther.* 1991;14:119-132.
16. Cooperman JM, Riddle DL, Rothstein JM: Reliability and validity of judgments of the integrity of the anterior cruciate ligament of the knee using the Lachman's test. *Phys Ther.* 1990;70:225-233.

17. Shields RK, Enloe LJ, Evans RE, et al: Reliability, validity, and responsiveness of functional tests in patients with total joint replacement. *Phys Ther.* 1995;75:169.
18. Laslett M, Williams M: The reliability of selected pain provocation tests for sacroiliac joint pathology. *Spine.* 1994;19:1243-1249.
19. Portney L, Watkins MP: *Foundations of Clinical Research: Applications to Practice.* Norwalk, CT. Appleton & Lange. 1993.
20. Bluman AG: Measures of central tendency. In: Bluman AG, ed. *Elementary Statistics: A Step by Step Approach, 4th ed.* New York, NY: McGraw-Hill. 2008:101-176.
21. Bluman AG: The normal distribution. In: Bluman AG, ed. *Elementary Statistics: A Step by Step Approach, 4th ed.* New York, NY: McGraw-Hill. 2008:281-341.
22. Bluman AG: Confidence intervals and sample size. In: Bluman AG, ed. *Elementary Statistics: A Step by Step Approach, 4th ed.* New York, NY: McGraw-Hill. 2008:343-385.
23. Bluman AG: Hypothesis testing. In: Bluman AG, ed. *Elementary Statistics: A Step by Step Approach, 4th ed.* New York, NY: McGraw-Hill. 2008:387-455.
24. Sackett DL, Strauss SE, Richardson WS, et al. *Evidence Based Medicine: How to Practice and Teach EBM, 2nd ed.* Edinburgh, Scotland, Churchill Livingstone. 2000.
25. Palisano RJ, Campbell SK, Harris SR: Evidence-based decision-making in pediatric physical therapy. In: Campbell SK, Vander Linden DW, Palisano RJ, eds: *Physical Therapy for Children.* St. Louis: Saunders. 2006:3-32.
26. Sackett DL: Rules of evidence and clinical recommendations on the use of antithrombotic agents. *Chest.* 1986;89:2S-3S.
27. Fetters L, Figueiredo EM, Keane-Miller D, et al: Critically appraised topics. *Pediatr Phys Ther.* 2004;16:19-21.

Education

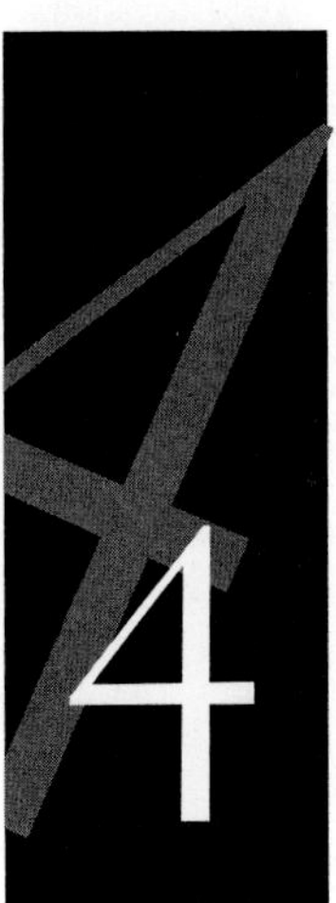

Education can be defined as any act or experience that has a formative effect on the mind, character, or physical ability of an individual.

Learning refers to the ways people acquire, process, store, and apply new information. Learning is most effective when an individual is ready to learn, that is, when one wants to know something.

MOTIVATION

Motivation plays a critical role in the learning process and success motivates more than failure (Table 4-1). Basic principles of motivation exist that are applicable to learning in any situation.

- The environment can be used to focus the patient's attention on what needs to be learned. For example, interesting visual aids, such as booklets, posters, or practice equipment, motivate learners by capturing their attention and curiosity.
- Incentives, including privileges and receiving praise from the educator, motivate learning. Both affiliation and approval are strong motivators.
- Internal motivation is longer lasting and more self-directive than is external motivation, which must be repeatedly reinforced by praise or concrete rewards.

MASLOW'S HIERARCHY OF NEEDS

Maslow's hierarchy of needs is based on the concept that there is a hierarchy of biogenic and psychogenic needs that humans must progress through. Maslow hypothesizes that the higher needs in this hierarchy only come into focus once all the needs that are lower

TABLE 4-1. LEARNING THEORIES

THEORY	PRINCIPLE ELEMENTS	STRATEGIES	PROMINENT THEORISTS	CLINICAL APPLICATION
Algo-Heuristic	Identifying the mental processes (conscious and subconscious) that underlie expert learning, thinking and performance in any area. All cognitive activities can be analyzed into operations of an algorithmic, semi-algorithmic, heuristic, or semi-heuristic nature. Teaching students how to discover processes is more valuable than providing them with already formulated processes.	Once discovered, the operations and their systems can serve as the basis for instructional strategies and methods.	L. Landa	Performing a task or solving a problem always requires a certain system of elementary knowledge units and operations.
Androgyny	Adults need to know why they need to learn something, and need to learn experientially as they approach learning as problem solving. Adults learn best when the topic is of immediate value.	There is a need to explain why specific things are being taught (eg, certain commands, functions, operations, etc). Learning activities should be in the context of common tasks to be performed instead of memorization. Instruction should take into account the wide range of different backgrounds of learners; learning materials and activities should allow for different levels/types of previous experience with computers. Since adults are self-directed, instruction should allow learners to discover things for themselves, providing guidance and help when mistakes are made.	M. Knowles	Can be applied to any form of adult learning. Has been used extensively in the design of organizational training programs.
Adult learning	Integrates other theoretical frameworks for adult learning such as andragogy (Knowles), experiential learning (Rogers), and lifespan psychology. Consists of two classes of variables: personal characteristics (aging, life phases, and developmental stages) and situational characteristics (part-time vs full-time learning, and voluntary vs compulsory learning).	The three personal characteristics must be taken into consideration. Aging results in the deterioration of certain sensory-motor abilities (eg, eyesight, hearing, reaction time) while intelligence abilities (eg, decision-making skills, reasoning, and vocabulary) tend to improve.	K. P. Cross	Adult learning programs should adapt to the aging limitations of the participants, while capitalizing on the experience of participants. Adults should be challenged to move to increasingly advanced stages of personal development.

Behaviorist (stimulus-response theory)-operant conditioning	Learning is a function of a change in overt behavior. Changes in behavior are the result of an individual's response to events (stimuli) and their consequences that occur in the environment. The response of one behavior becomes the stimulus for the next response. Learning occurs when an individual engages in specific behaviors in order to receive certain consequences (learned association). Behavior can be controlled or shaped by operant conditioning. Desired or correct behaviors are identified so that frequent and scheduled reinforcements (positive reinforcement) can be given to reinforce the desired behaviors. Negative behaviors are ignored (negative reinforcement) so that these behaviors become weakened to the point where they disappear (extinction).	Positive reinforcement is used through the use of rewards that are meaningful to the individual. **Timing of reinforcement** ▶ Continuous reinforcement: A behavior is reinforced every time it occurs. ▶ Partial reinforcement: A behavior is reinforced intermittently. ▶ Fixed interval: The period of time between the occurrences of each instance of reinforcement is fixed or set. ▶ Variable interval: The period of time between the occurrences of each instance of reinforcement varies around a constant average.	BF Skinner, G. Watson	Limited clinical use: behavior modification techniques may be used when working with adults with impaired or limited cognitive abilities or young children. Repetition is a necessary prerequisite for learning.
Classical conditioning	First model of learning to be studied in psychology. Demonstrate the environment's control over behavior. Type of associative learning—Relates the capacity of animals/humans to learn new stimuli and connect them to natural reflexes; allowing nonnatural cues to elicit a natural reflex. The conditioned stimulus, or conditional stimulus, is an initially neutral stimulus that elicits a response—known as a conditioned response—that is learned by the organism. Conditioned stimuli are associated psychologically with conditions such as anticipation, satisfaction (both immediate and prolonged), and fear. The relationship between the conditioned stimulus and conditioned response is known as the conditioned (or conditional) reflex. The process by which an individual learns to associate an unconditional stimulus with a conditional stimulus but receives no benefit from doing so.	Therapies associated with classical conditioning are aversion therapy, flooding, systematic desensitization, and implosion therapy. Much of what we like or dislike is a result of classical conditioning.	I. Pavlov J.B. Watson	These techniques have been criticized for being unethical since they have the potential to cause trauma. Perhaps the strongest application of classical conditioning involves emotion. Common experience and careful research both confirm that human emotion conditions vary rapidly and easily, particularly when the emotion is intensely felt or negative in direction, it will condition quickly.

(*Continued*)

TABLE 4-1. LEARNING THEORIES (*Continued*)

THEORY	PRINCIPLE ELEMENTS	STRATEGIES	PROMINENT THEORISTS	CLINICAL APPLICATION
Cognitive dissonance	There is a tendency for individuals to seek consistency among their cognitions (ie, beliefs, opinions). When there is an inconsistency between attitudes or behaviors (dissonance), something must change to eliminate the dissonance. In the case of a discrepancy between attitudes and behavior, it is most likely that the attitude will change to accommodate the behavior.	There are three ways to eliminate dissonance: 1. Reduce the importance of the dissonant beliefs. 2. Add more consonant beliefs that outweigh the dissonant beliefs. 3. Change the dissonant beliefs so that they are no longer inconsistent.	L. Festinger	Dissonance theory is especially relevant to decision making and problem solving.
Cognitive flexibility	Focuses on the nature of learning in complex and ill-structured domains. Emphasis is placed upon the presentation of information from multiple perspectives and use of many case studies that present diverse examples. Effective learning is context-dependent. Stresses the importance of constructed knowledge; learners must be given an opportunity to develop their own representations of information in order to properly learn.	Learning activities must provide multiple representations of content. Instructional materials should avoid oversimplifying the content domain and support context-dependent knowledge. Instruction should be case-based and emphasize knowledge construction, not transmission of information. Knowledge sources should be highly interconnected rather than compartmentalized.	R. Spiro, P. Feltovitch, and R. Coulson	Limited: Cognitive flexibility theory is especially formulated to support the use of interactive technology.
Cognitive load	Learning happens best under conditions that are aligned with human cognitive architecture. The contents of long-term memory are sophisticated structures (schema) that permit us to perceive, think, and solve problems, rather than a group of rote-learned facts. Schemas are acquired over a lifetime of learning, and may have other schemas contained within themselves. The difference between an expert and a novice is that a novice hasn't acquired the schemas of an expert.	Change problem-solving methods to use goal-free problems or worked examples. Eliminate the working memory load associated with having to mentally integrate several sources of information by physically integrating those sources of information. Eliminate the working memory load associated with unnecessarily processing repetitive information by reducing redundancy. Increase working memory capacity by using auditory as well as visual information under conditions where both sources of information are essential (ie, nonredundant) to understanding.	J. Sweller	Cognitive load theory has many implications in the design of learning materials such as handouts, and home exercise programs

Constructivist theory	Learning is an active process in which learners construct new ideas or concepts based upon their current/past knowledge. Cognitive structure (ie, schema, mental models) provides meaning and organization to experiences and allows the individual to "go beyond the information given."	Instruction must be concerned with the experiences and contexts that make the student willing and able to learn (readiness). Instruction must be structured so that it can be easily grasped by the student (spiral organization). Instruction should be designed to facilitate extrapolation and or fill in the gaps (going beyond the information given).	J. Bruner	Much of this theory is linked to child development
Experiential learning	Two types of learning: 1. Cognitive (meaningless)—academic knowledge such as learning vocabulary or multiplication tables. 2. Experiential (significant)—applied knowledge such as personal change and growth.	Significant learning takes place when the subject matter is relevant to the personal interests of the student. Learning which is threatening to the self (eg, new attitudes or perspectives) are more easily assimilated when external threats are at a minimum. Learning proceeds faster when the threat to the self is low. Self-initiated learning is the most lasting and pervasive.	C. Rogers	Applies primarily to adult learners and adult learning.
Genetic epistemology	Cognitive structures (ie, development stages) are patterns of physical or mental action that underlie specific acts of intelligence and correspond to stages of child development. There are four primary cognitive structures: 1. Sensorimotor stage (0-2 years)—intelligence takes the form of motor actions. 2. Preoperation period (3-7 years)—intelligence is intuitive in nature. 3. Concrete operational stage (8-11 years)—cognition is logical but depends upon concrete referents. 4. Formal operations (12-15 years)—thinking involves abstractions.	Children will provide different explanations of reality at different stages of cognitive development. Cognitive development is facilitated by providing activities or situations that engage learners and require adaptation (ie, assimilation and accommodation). Learning materials and activities should involve the appropriate level of motor or mental operations for a child of given age; avoid asking students to perform tasks that are beyond their current cognitive capabilities. Use teaching methods that actively involve students and present challenges	J. Piaget	The theory has been applied extensively to teaching practice and curriculum design in elementary education.

(Continued)

TABLE 4-1. LEARNING THEORIES (*Continued*)

THEORY	PRINCIPLE ELEMENTS	STRATEGIES	PROMINENT THEORISTS	CLINICAL APPLICATION
Modes of learning	Three modes of learning: 1. Accretion: the addition of new knowledge to existing memory, the most common form of learning 2. Structuring: involves the formation of new conceptual structures or schema. 3. Tuning: the adjustment of knowledge to a specific task usually through practice, the slowest form of learning and accounts for expert performance	Instruction must be designed to accommodate different modes of learning. Practice activities affect the refinement of skills but not necessarily the initial acquisition of knowledge.	D. Rumelhart and D. Norman	Multiple applications to physical therapy—general model for human learning.
Humanist	Emphasis placed on personal freedom and dignity of the individual and the learners' needs and feelings during the learning process The learner experiences unconditional positive regard, acceptance, and understanding Promotes active learning rather than passive	Teacher must function as a facilitator and resource finder. Learning must address relevant problems and issues.	AH Maslow	Used in clinical situations that emphasize self-discovery, self-appropriated learning, and experimental learning.
Social learning	The social learning theory emphasizes the importance of observing and modeling the behaviors, attitudes, and emotional reactions of others Social learning theory explains human behavior in terms of continuous reciprocal interaction between cognitive, behavioral, and environmental influences.	The highest level of observational learning is achieved by first organizing and rehearsing the modeled behavior symbolically and then enacting it overtly. Coding modeled behavior into words, labels, or images results in better retention than simply observing. Individuals are more likely to adopt a modeled behavior if it results in outcomes they value, or if the model is similar to the observer and has admired status and the behavior has functional value.	A. Bandura	Applied extensively to the understanding of aggression and psychological disorders, particularly in the context of behavior modification.

down in the pyramid are mainly or entirely satisfied. Maslow's hierarchy is often depicted as a pyramid consisting of five levels (Figure 4-1): The lower levels (physiological, and safety needs) are referred to as *deficiency needs*, while the top three levels (love/belonging, status, and self-actualization needs) are referred to as a *being needs*. According to Maslow, in order for an individual to progress up the hierarchy to the being needs, the deficiency needs must be met. Growth forces (eg, personal growth, integration, and fulfillment) create upward movement in the hierarchy, whereas regressive forces (eg, sickness, discomfort, lack of security) push predominant needs further down the hierarchy.

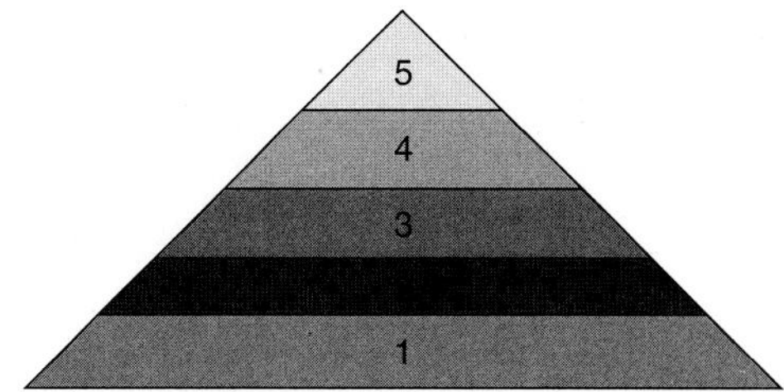

5. Actualization
4. Status (esteem)
3. Love/belonging
2. Safety
1. Physiological (biological needs)

Figure 4-1. Maslow's hierarchy of needs.

DOMAINS OF LEARNING

Bloom identified three domains of educational activities:[1]

- Cognitive: mental skills (knowledge)
  - Involves knowledge and the development of intellectual skills.
  - Includes the recall or recognition of specific facts, procedural patterns, and concepts that serve in the development of intellectual abilities and skills.
  - There are six major categories (degrees of difficulties) starting from the simplest behavior to the most complex, with the first one having to be mastered before the next one can take place (Table 4-2).

TABLE 4-2. COGNITIVE DOMAIN

CATEGORY	EXAMPLES AND KEY WORDS
Knowledge: Recall data or information.	Able to recite a poem; quote prices from memory. Key Words: defines, identifies, labels, lists, matches, names, outlines, recalls, recognizes, reproduces, selects.
Comprehension: Understand the meaning, translation, interpolation, and interpretation of instructions and problems.	Able to rewrite a policy and procedures manual; can explain the steps for performing a complex task. Key Words: comprehends, distinguishes, estimates, explains, interprets, paraphrases, predicts, summarizes.
Application: Use a concept in a new situation or unprompted use of an abstraction. Applies what was learned in the classroom into novel situations in the work place.	Can use a manual to set up a video recorder, can apply the laws of statistics to evaluate a research study Key Words: applies, computes, constructs, demonstrates, manipulates, modifies, operates, prepares, produces, relates, shows, solves.
Analysis: Separates material or concepts into component parts so that its organizational structure may be understood. Distinguishes between facts and inferences.	Can fix a piece of exercise equipment by using logical deduction, can gather information, and select the required tasks for staff training. Key Words: analyzes, breaks down, compares, contrasts, differentiates, distinguishes, identifies, illustrates, infers, outlines, separates.
Synthesis: Builds a structure or pattern from diverse elements. Put parts together to form a whole, with emphasis on creating a new meaning or structure.	Can design or revise a process to perform a specific task, is able to integrate training from several sources to solve a problem. Key Words: categorizes, combines, compiles, composes, creates, devises, designs, generates, modifies, rearranges, reconstructs, reorganizes, summarizes.
Evaluation: Make judgments about the value of ideas or materials.	Can select the most effective solution; hire the most qualified candidate; explain and justify a new budget. Key Words: appraises, compares, concludes, contrasts, critiques, discriminates, interprets, justifies, summarizes.

TABLE 4-3. AFFECTIVE DOMAIN: THE FIVE MAJOR CATEGORIES LISTED THE SIMPLEST BEHAVIOR TO THE MOST COMPLEX

CATEGORY	EXAMPLE AND KEYWORDS
Receiving phenomena: Awareness, willingness to hear, selected attention.	Able to listen to others with respect; listen for and remember the name of newly introduced people. Key words: chooses, describes, follows, identifies, locates, names, points to, selects.
Responding to phenomena: Active participation on the part of the learners. Attends and reacts to a particular phenomenon. Learning outcomes may emphasize compliance in responding, willingness to respond, or satisfaction in responding (motivation).	Is an active participant in staff discussions; able to present an in-service. Asks many questions about new ideas, concepts in order to fully understand them. Key words: answers, assists, complies, conforms, discusses, labels, performs, practices, reads, recites, reports, tells, writes.
Valuing: The worth or value a person attaches to a particular object, phenomenon, or behavior. This can range from simple acceptance to the more complex state of commitment.	Is sensitive toward individuals and the various cultural differences. Informs management on matters that one feels strongly about. Key words: completes, demonstrates, differentiates, initiates, invites, joins, justifies, proposes, reports, selects, shares.
Organization: Organizes values into priorities by contrasting different values, resolving conflicts between them, and creating an unique value system. The emphasis is on comparing, relating, and synthesizing values.	Able to recognize the need for balance between freedom and responsible behavior. Accepts professional ethical standards. Prioritizes time effectively to meet the needs of the organization, family, and self. Key words: adheres, alters, arranges, combines, compares, completes, defends, generalizes, identifies, integrates, modifies, organizes, relates, synthesizes.
Internalizing values (characterization): Has a value system that controls their behavior. The behavior is pervasive, consistent, predictable, and most importantly, characteristic of the learner. Instructional objectives are concerned with the patient's general patterns of adjustment (personal, social, emotional).	Demonstrates self-reliance and can work independently, but also cooperates in group activities as a team player. Uses an objective approach in problem solving. Values people for what they are, not how they look. Key words: discriminates, displays, influences, listens, modifies, performs, proposes, qualifies, questions, revises, solves, verifies.

- Affective: growth in feelings or emotional areas (attitude) (Table 4-3)
  - Includes the manner in which matters are dealt with from an emotional aspect
  - Includes feelings, values, appreciation, enthusiasms, motivations, and attitudes
- Psychomotor: manual or physical aspects (skills)
  - Includes physical movement, coordination, and use of the motor-skill areas.
  - Development of these skills requires practice and is measured in terms of speed, precision, distance, procedures, or techniques in execution.
  - Seven major categories are listed from the simplest behavior to the most complex (Table 4-4).

Decision Making. Most theories accept the idea that decision making consists of a number of steps or stages such as: recognition, formulation, the generation of alternatives, an information search, and then selection, and finally action. Furthermore, it is well-recognized that routine cognitive processes such as memory, reasoning, and concept formation play a primary role in decision making. In addition, decision-making behavior is affected (usually adversely) by anxiety and stress.

TABLE 4-4. PSYCHOMOTOR DOMAIN

CATEGORY	EXAMPLES AND KEY WORDS
Perception: The ability to use sensory cues to guide motor activity.	Able to detect nonverbal communication cues; can estimate where a moving ball will land and can move to the correct location to catch the ball. Key Words: chooses, detects, differentiates, distinguishes, identifies, isolates, relates, selects.
Set: Readiness to act: includes mental, physical, and emotional sets.	Knows and acts upon a sequence of steps in a construction process. Is able to recognize own abilities and limitations. Key Words: initiates, displays, explains, proceeds, reacts, states, volunteers.
Guided response: The early stages in learning a complex skill that includes imitation and trial and error.	Can perform an exercise as demonstrated; follows instructions well. Key Words: copies, traces, follows, reproduce.
Mechanism: This is the intermediate stage in learning a complex skill.	Can use a personal computer effectively; able to perform simple DIY projects at home; can drive a car. Key Words: assembles, calibrates, constructs, dismantles, fixes, manipulates, measures, mends, organizes.
Complex overt response: The skillful performance of motor acts that involve complex movement patterns in a quick, accurate, and highly coordinated manner and with a minimum expenditure of energy.	And parallel park a car into a tight spot. Displays skill and competence while playing sports. Key Words: the same as for Mechanism, except that the performance is quicker, better, more accurate, etc.
Adaptation: Skills are well developed and the individual can modify movement patterns to fit special requirements.	Responds effectively to unexpected experiences; able to modify instructions to meet the needs of the learners. Key Words: adapts, alters, changes, rearranges, reorganizes, revises, varies.
Origination: Can create new movement patterns to fit a particular situation or specific problem.	Able to independently develop a new and comprehensive training program, or exercise protocol. Key Words: arranges, builds, combines, composes, constructs, creates, designs, initiates.

Problem Solving. Problem-solving skills appear to be related to many other aspects of cognition such as schema (the ability to remember similar problems), pattern recognition (recognizing familiar problem elements), and creativity (developing new solutions). The issue of transfer is highly relevant to problem solving.

Sensory Motor Learning. Motor skills can be classified as continuous (eg, tracking), discrete (eg, skills that have a definite beginning and end), or procedural (eg, typing). Behavioral psychology emphasizes the use of practice variables in sensory-motor skills such as massed (concentrating the teaching or practice in a short period of time) versus spaced (distributing the teaching or practice over a longer period of time) practice, part versus whole task learning, and feedback/reinforcement schedules. Long-term retention of motor skills depends upon regular practice. Learning and retention of sensory-motor skills is improved by both the quantity and quality of feedback (knowledge of results) during training. Two ways in which learning/teaching of motor skills can be facilitated include:

1. Slowing down the rate at which the information is presented
2. Reducing the amount of information that needs to be processed

There is evidence that mental rehearsal, especially involving imagery, facilitates performance. This may be because it allows

Study Pearl

Some form of guided learning seems most appropriate when high proficiency on a new skill is involved. On the other hand, if the task is to be recalled and transferred to a new situation, then some type of problem-solving strategy may be better.

Study Pearl

Many forms of sensory-motor behavior are learned by imitation, especially complex movements such as dance, signing, crafts, or manual therapy techniques.

additional memory processing related to physical tasks (eg, the formation of schema) or because it maintains arousal or motivation for an activity.

LEARNING STYLES

There are several different theories regarding learning styles. However, it is not feasible to incorporate every learning theory into every session. One approach classifies learning styles as follows:[2]

- Accommodators. These type of learners look for the significance of the learning experience. These learners enjoy being active participants in their learning, and will ask many questions such as "What if?" and "Why not?"
- Divergers. These type of learners are motivated to discover the relevance of a given situation, and prefer to have information presented to them in a detailed, systematic, and reasoned manner.
- Assimilator. These type of learners are motivated to answer the question, "What is there to know?" They like accurate, organized delivery of information and they tend to respect the knowledge of the expert. These learners are perhaps less "instructor intensive" than some other learning styles. They will carefully follow prescribed exercises, provided a resource person is clearly available and able to answer questions.
- Convergers. These type of learners are motivated to discover the relevancy or "how" of a situation. The instructions given to this type of learner should be interactive, not passive.

Another series of learning styles that are used frequently were devised by Taylor,[3] who proposed that there are three common learning styles:

1. Visual. As the name suggests, the visual learner assimilates information by observation, using visual cues and information such as pictures, anatomical models, and physical demonstrations.
2. Auditory. Auditory learners prefer to learn by having things explained to them verbally.
3. Tactile. Tactile learners, who learn through touch and interaction, are the most difficult of the three groups to teach. Close supervision is required with this group until they have demonstrated to the clinician that they can perform the exercises correctly, and independently. Proprioceptive neuromuscular facilitation (PNF) techniques, with the emphasis on physical and tactile cues, often work well with this group.

Analytical Learner. The analytical/objective learner processes information in a step-by-step order, perceives information in an objective manner, and is able to use facts and easily understand the relationships between them. This type of learner perceives information in an abstract, conceptual manner; information does not need to be related to personal experience. As this type of learner may have difficulty comprehending the big picture, a step-by-step learning process with some form of structure is recommended.

Intuitive/Global Learner. The intuitive/global learner processes information all at once, and not in an ordered sequence. Global learners are spontaneous and intuitive, and tend to learn in layers, absorbing material almost randomly without seeing connections, and then suddenly "getting it." The learning of this type reflects personal life experiences and is thus subjective. As this type of learner tries to relate the subject matter to things they already know, information needs to be presented in an interesting manner using attractive materials.

Reasoning: Inductive Versus Deductive Reasoning. Inductive and deductive reasoning are two methods of logic used to arrive at a conclusion based on information assumed to be true. Both are used in research to establish hypotheses.

- Deductive reasoning: It involves a hierarchy of statements or truths and the arrival at a specific conclusion based on generalizations.
- Inductive reasoning: It is essentially the opposite of deductive reasoning. It involves trying to create general principles by starting with many specific instances.

Initiative: Active Versus Passive Learning

- Active/aggressive learner: exhibits initiative, actively seeks information; may reach conclusions quickly before all information is gathered.
- Passive learner: often exhibits little initiative; responds best to direct learning.

TEACHING STYLES

Bicknell-Holmes and Hoffman[4] describe a variety of teaching methods that correlate with most learning styles. These techniques involve active or discovery learning—the patient is able to actively participate in the learning process, which is in direct contrast with a teaching method like lecturing, where the patient is a passive observer. Discovery learning has certain attributes:

- Emphasizes learning over content
- Uses failure as an opportunity to learn
- More is learned by doing than by watching
- Involves patients in higher levels of cognitive processing

Some of the methods of discovery learning include:

- Case-based learning: a fairly common active learning strategy in which the patients are able to participate in the decision-making or problem-solving process.
- Incidental learning: learning is linked to game-like scenarios.
- Learning by exploring: a collection of questions and answers on a particular topic are organized into a system and patients can explore the various topics at their own pace.
- Learning by reflection: a type of active learning that involves higher level cognitive skills—patients are expected to model

certain skills or concepts which they have acquired through their instructor or through another system of learning.

- Simulation-based learning: the clinician creates an artificial environment in which patients can practice skills or apply concepts that they have learned, without the pressure of a real-world situation.
- Real-life examples: using real-life problems and examples in a variety of scenarios (buying a house/car; using a bus schedule etc).
- Relevant instruction: instruction should be practical and the examples and exercises should be important and meaningful to the patients, because patients often need to know why they need to learn a particular skill or concept, or how it will be useful to them in their everyday lives.
- Humor: to help keep the patients engaged and interested and to make their sessions more enjoyable.

Improving Compliance with Learning and Participation

A number of factors have been outlined to improve compliance, including:

- Involving the patient in the intervention planning and goal setting
- Realistic goal setting for both short- and long-term goals
- Promoting high expectations regarding final outcome
- Promoting perceived benefits
- Projecting a positive attitude
- Providing clear instructions and demonstrations with appropriate feedback
- Keeping the exercises pain-free or with a low level of pain
- Encouraging patient problem solving

Community and Staff Education

The strengths and weaknesses of various teaching methods when presenting community education programs, or when educating staff are outlined in Table 4-5.

Using Visual Aids. A number of guidelines when using visual aids are outlined in Table 4-6.

Cultural Influences

It is important that clinicians are sensitive to cultural issues in their interactions with patients. Cultural influences shape the framework within which people view the world, define and organize reality, and function in their everyday life.

In many cases individuals group themselves on the basis of cultural similarities, and, as a result, form cultural groups. Cultural groups share behavioral patterns, symbols, values, beliefs, and other characteristics that distinguish them from other groups.

At the group level, cultural differences are generally variations of differing emphasis or value placed on particular practices.

TABLE 4-5. TEACHING METHODS

TEACHING METHOD	STRENGTHS	WEAKNESSES	PREPARATION
Lecture	▶ Presents factual material in a direct, logical manner ▶ Contains experience which inspires ▶ Useful for large groups	▶ Experts are not always good teachers ▶ Audience is passive ▶ Learning is difficult to gauge ▶ Communication is one way	▶ Needs clear introduction and summary ▶ Needs time and content limit to be effective ▶ Should include examples, anecdotes
Lecture with discussion	▶ Involves audience at least after the lecture ▶ Audience can question, clarify, and challenge	▶ Time may limit discussion period ▶ Quality is limited to quality of questions and discussion	▶ Requires that questions be prepared prior to discussion
Panel of experts	▶ Allows experts to present different opinions ▶ Can provoke better discussion than a one-person discussion ▶ Frequent change of speaker keeps attention from lagging	▶ Experts may not be good speakers ▶ Personalities may overshadow content ▶ Subject may not be in logical order	▶ Facilitator coordinates focus of panel, introduces, and summarizes ▶ Briefs panel
Brainstorming	▶ Listening exercise that allows creative thinking for new ideas ▶ Encourages full participation because all ideas equally recorded ▶ Draws on group's knowledge and experience ▶ Spirit of congeniality is created ▶ One idea can spark off other ideas	▶ Can be unfocused ▶ Needs to be limited to 5-7 minutes ▶ People may have difficulty getting away from known reality ▶ If not facilitated well, criticism and evaluation may occur	▶ Facilitator selects issue ▶ Must have some ideas if group needs to be stimulated
Videotapes/slides	▶ Entertaining way of teaching content (colorful) and raising issues ▶ Keep group's attention ▶ Looks professional ▶ Stimulates discussion ▶ Demonstrates three-dimensional movement	▶ Can raise too many issues to have a focused discussion ▶ Discussion may not have full participation ▶ Only as effective as following discussion ▶ Can be expensive	▶ Need to set up equipment ▶ Effective only if facilitator prepares questions to discuss after the show
Discussion	▶ Pools ideas and experiences from group ▶ Effective after a presentation, film, or experience that needs to be analyzed ▶ Allows everyone to participate in an active process	▶ Not practical with more than 20 people ▶ Few people can dominate ▶ Others may not participate ▶ Is time consuming ▶ Can get off the track	▶ Requires careful planning by facilitator to guide discussion ▶ Requires question outline
Small group discussion	▶ Allows participation of everyone ▶ People often more comfortable in small groups ▶ Can reach group consensus	▶ Needs careful thought as to purpose of group ▶ Groups may get side tracked	▶ Need to prepare specific tasks or questions for group to answer

(*Continued*)

TABLE 4-5. TEACHING METHODS. (*Continued*)

TEACHING METHOD	STRENGTHS	WEAKNESSES	PREPARATION
Role-playing	▶ Introduces problem situation dramatically ▶ Provides opportunity for people to assume roles of others and thus appreciate another point of view ▶ Allows for exploration of solutions ▶ Provides opportunity to practice skills	▶ People may be too self-conscious ▶ Not appropriate for large groups ▶ People may feel threatened	▶ Trainer has to define problem situation and roles clearly ▶ Trainer must give very clear instructions
Case studies	▶ Develops analytic and problem-solving skills ▶ Allows for exploration of solutions for complex issues ▶ Allows patient to apply new knowledge and skills	▶ People may not see relevance to own situation ▶ Insufficient information can lead to inappropriate results	▶ Case must be clearly defined in some cases ▶ Case study must be prepared
Guest speaker	▶ Personalizes topic ▶ Breaks down audience's stereotypes	▶ May not be a good speaker	▶ Contact speakers and coordinate ▶ Introduce speaker appropriately

TABLE 4-6. GUIDELINES FOR THE USE OF VISUAL AIDS

OVERHEADS	FLIP CHARTS	SLIDES
▶ Use the most professional lettering available. ▶ Use transparencies of one color only and secure transparencies to cardboard frames (if available). ▶ Number each transparency. ▶ Prior to the session, check overheads for readability of type size by audience at far end of room. Printing should be no smaller than 1/4″ high. Information should be placed on the top two-thirds of the transparency ▶ Be familiar with the operation of the projector and make sure projector works. Have extra bulbs available. ▶ While presenting, be certain neither you nor the projector blocks anyone's view. ▶ Use a pencil rather than a finger to note a detail on the transparency. ▶ If you have a list of points, blackout all but the first point, then move the cover sheet at one point at a time.	▶ Choose a chart size that is appropriate for the design, your height, and the size of the audience. ▶ Draw the art to fit the vertical shape of the chart. ▶ Make the lettering dark enough and large enough to be read by everyone in the audience. ▶ During preparation, leave several blank pages between each one to allow for corrections and additions. For the final presentation, remove all but one blank page at the beginning so that you can turn to that blank page when there is no relevant visual. ▶ Securely attached the chart to the easel and adjust the easel height for the presentation. ▶ When writing on the flip chart, don't speak to the chart.	▶ Slides should be used instead of flip charts if the group is large. ▶ Design the visuals for continuous viewing and as notes. ▶ Maintain continuity—have all slides horizontal or vertical, not mixed. ▶ Allow sufficient production time. ▶ Place no more than 15 words per slide. ▶ Use black or blue background with bright colors. ▶ Check the position and order of the slide in the carousel or tray. ▶ Use a conventional pointer. ▶ Keep on as many lights as possible.

Questions for this chapter and the entire book appear on the included CD-ROM, with additional questions at www.DuttonNPTE.com.

REFERENCES

1. Bloom BS: *Taxonomy of Educational Objectives, Handbook I: The Cognitive Domain.* New York, NY: David McKay Co Inc. 1956.
2. Litzinger ME, Osif B: Accommodating diverse learning styles: designing instruction for electronic information sources. In: Shirato L, ed. *What is Good Instruction Now?* Library Instruction for the 90s. Ann Arbor, MI: Pierian Press. 1993.
3. Taylor JA: A practical tool for improved communications. *Supervision.* 1999;59:18-19.
4. Bicknell-Holmes T, Hoffman PS: Elicit, engage, experience explore: discovery learning in library instruction. *Reference Services Review.* Emerald, Simmons College Library. 2000:313-322.

Fundamentals and Core Concepts

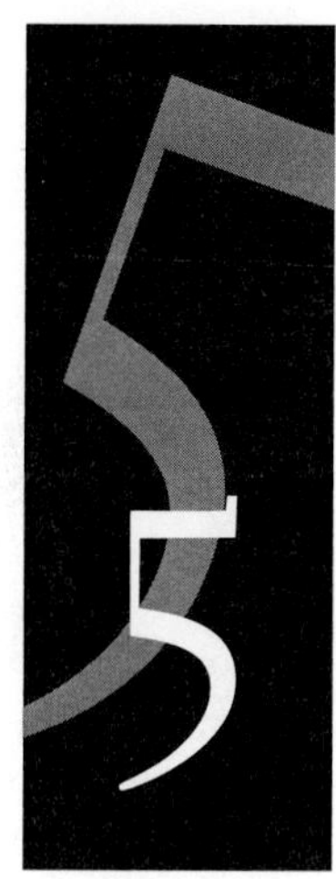

TISSUES OF THE BODY

Based on morphology and function, the tissues of the body are classified into four basic kinds: epithelial, nervous, connective, and muscle tissue:[1]

EPITHELIAL TISSUE

Epithelial tissue is found throughout the body in two forms: membranous and glandular.

- Membranous epithelium forms such structures as the outer layer of the skin, the inner lining of the body cavities and lumina, and the covering of visceral organs.
- Glandular epithelium is a specialized tissue that forms the secretory portion of glands.

NERVOUS TISSUE

Nervous tissue (see Chapter 9) helps coordinate body movements via a complex control system of prestructured motor programs and a distributed network of reflex pathways mediated throughout the CNS.[2]

> **Study Pearl**
>
> The primary types of CT cells are macrophages, which function to cleanup debris (phagocytes); mast cells, which release chemicals associated with inflammation; and the fibroblasts, which are the principal cells of CT.[3]

CONNECTIVE TISSUE

Connective tissue (CT) is found throughout the body. CT serves to provide structural and metabolic support for tissues and organs of the body. Connective tissue includes bone, cartilage, tendons, ligaments, and blood tissue.

The CT types are differentiated according to the extracellular matrix (ECM) that binds the cells:[1]

- Embryonic CT
- Connective tissue proper
  - Loose CT
  - Dense regular CT

Study Pearl

CT disorders include systemic lupus erythematosus (see Chapter 8), rheumatoid arthritis (see later), spondyloarthropathies (eg, ankylosing spondylitis—see Chapter 8, Reactive arthritis—see later), polymyalgia rheumatica, polymyositis, and dermatomyositis (see Chapter 13), scleroderma (see Chapter 13), Sjögren's syndrome (see later), crystal-induced arthropathies (eg, gout—see Chapter 8), and juvenile rheumatoid arthritis (see later).

Study Pearl

There are several protective mechanisms within CT that help it respond to stress or strain. These include:

- Crimp: the slack in collagen tissue, which serves as the tissue's first line of response to stress.
- Viscoelasticity: the principal mechanism used by ligaments, capsules, and muscle, to increase their length.
- Creep: the third line of response which increases the stiffness of the tissue in response to stress via a constant lengthening in the tissue.
- Stress or force relaxation: occurs in viscoelastic tissue when it is stretched to the end of its passive range.
- Stress reaction: the method by which the body responds to repeated stresses in an attempt to make itself stronger.

TABLE 5-1. MAJOR TYPES OF COLLAGEN

TYPE	LOCATION
I	Bone, skin, ligament, and tendon
II	Cartilage, nucleus pulposus
III	Blood vessels, gastrointestinal tract
IV	Basement membranes

  - Dense irregular CT
  - Elastic CT
- Reticular CT
- Adipose CT
- Cartilage and bone tissue
  - Hyaline cartilage
  - Fibrocartilage
  - Elastic cartilage
- Blood (vascular) tissue

Connective Tissue Proper. Connective tissue proper (CTP) has a loose, flexible matrix called ground substance. The most common cell within CTP is the fibroblast. Fibroblasts produce collagen, elastin, and reticulin fibers. Collagen and elastin are vital constituents of the musculoskeletal system.

Collagen. The collagens are a family of ECM proteins that play a dominant role in maintaining the structural integrity of various tissues and in providing tensile strength to tissues. The major forms of collagen are outlined in Table 5-1.[4]

Elastin. Elastic fibers are composed of a protein called elastin. Elastin provides the tissues in which it is situated with elastic properties. Elastin fibers can stretch, but they normally return to their original shape when the tension is released. The elastin determines the patterns of distension and recoil in most organs including the skin and lungs, blood vessels, and most CT.

Arrangement of Collagen and Elastin. Collagenous and elastic fibers are sparse and irregularly arranged in loose CT, but are tightly packed in dense CT.[5]

- Fascia is an example of loose CT. Fascia provides support and protection to the joint, and acts as an interconnection between tendons aponeurosis, ligaments, capsules, nerves, and the intrinsic components of muscle.[6,7]
- Tendons and ligaments are examples of dense regular CT.[8] At the microscopic level, tendons and ligaments are similar in composition—they are densely packed CT structures that consists largely of directionally oriented, high tensile strength collagen (mostly type I collagen).[9] Due to their function as support cables, ligaments and tendons must be relatively inextensible to minimize transmission loss of energy.
  - Tendons: cord-like structures that attach muscle to bone and transmit the forces generated by muscles to bone in order to achieve movement or stability.[10] The thickness of each tendon is proportional to the size of the muscle from which they originate. As the tendon joins the muscle, it fans out into a much wider and thinner structure called the myotendinous junction (MTJ). Despite its viscoelastic mechanical characteristics, the MTJ is very vulnerable to injury.[11,12] In particular, a tendency for a tear near the MTJ has been reported in the biceps and triceps brachii, the rotator cuff muscles, the fibularis (peroneus) longus, the

TABLE 5-2. MAJOR LIGAMENTS OF THE UPPER QUADRANT

JOINT	LIGAMENT	FUNCTION
Shoulder complex	Coracoclavicular	Fixes the clavicle to the coracoid process
	Costoclavicular	Fixes the clavicle to the costal cartilage of the first rib
Glenohumeral	Coracohumeral	Reinforces the upper portion of the joint capsule
	Glenohumeral ("Z")	Reinforces the anterior and inferior aspect of the joint capsule
	Coracoacromial	Protects the superior aspect of the joint
Elbow	Annular	Maintains the relationship between the head of the radius and the humerus and ulna
	Ulnar (medial) collateral	Provides stability against valgus (medial) stress, particularly in the range of 20-130 degrees of flexion and extension
	Radial (lateral) collateral	Provides stability against varus (lateral) stress and functions to maintain the ulnohumeral and radiohumeral joints in a reduced position when the elbow is loaded in supination
Wrist	Extrinsic palmar	Provides the majority of the wrist stability
	Intrinsic	Serves as rotational restraints, binding the proximal carpal row into a unit of rotational stability
	Interosseous	Binds the carpal bones together
Fingers	Volar and collateral interphalangeal	Prevent displacement of the interphalangeal joints

rectus femoris, the adductor longus, the iliopsoas, and the hamstrings group.[13-15] *Tendonitis* is an inflammatory condition characterized by pain at the point where tendons insert into bone.

- Skeletal ligaments, which contribute to the stability of joint function by preventing excessive motion, are fibrous bands of dense CT that connect bones across joints (Tables 5-2, 5-3, and 5-4). Ligaments[16] act as guides to direct motion, and provide proprioceptive information.[17]

Cartilage and Bone Tissue

Bone is a rigid, highly vascular, and dynamic form of CT, which undergoes constant metabolism and remodeling. A cell called the osteoblast produces the collagen of bone in the same manner as that of ligament and tendon.[5] At the microscopic level, each bone has a distinct morphology that consists of both cortical bone and cancellous bone (Table 5-5).

- Cortical bone is found in the outer shell of a bone.
- Cancellous bone is located within the epiphyseal and metaphyseal regions of long bones as well as throughout the interior of short bones.[11]

The function of bone is to provide support, store minerals (particularly calcium), enhance leverage by providing attachments for tendons, and to protect vital structures. The density of a bone determines its strength. A fracture is commonly defined as a loss of the continuity of a bone. A number of types of fractures exist (Table 5-6). The risk for a fracture depends largely on the nature of the applied force, the properties of the involved bone, patient age and health, and the presence of any comorbidities (eg, osteoporosis). Fractures may

Study Pearl

Complications following a fracture can include infection, embolism, and Volkmann's ischemic contracture (see Chapter 8), peripheral nerve damage, and hemorrhage.

TABLE 5-3. MAJOR LIGAMENTS OF THE SPINE AND LOWER QUADRANT

JOINT	LIGAMENT	FUNCTION
Spine	Anterior longitudinal ligament	Functions as a minor assistant in limiting anterior translation, and vertical separation of the vertebral body
	Posterior longitudinal ligament	Resists vertebral distraction of the vertebral body Resists posterior shearing of the vertebral body Acts to limit flexion over a number of segments Provides some protection against intervertebral disk protrusions
	Ligamentum flavum	Resists separation of the lamina during flexion
	Interspinous	Resists separation of the spinous processes during flexion
	Iliolumbar (lower lumbar)	Resists flexion, extension, axial rotation, and side bending of L5 on S1
Sacroiliac	Sacrospinous	Creates greater sciatic foramen Resists forward tilting of the sacrum on the hip bone during weight bearing of the vertebral column
	Sacrotuberous	Creates lesser sciatic foramen Resists forward tilting of the sacrum on the hip bone during weight bearing of the vertebral column
	Interosseous	Resists anterior and inferior movement of the sacrum
	Dorsal sacroiliac (long)	Resists backward tilting of the sacrum on the hip bone during weight bearing of the vertebral column
Hip	Ligamentum teres	Transports nutrient vessels to the femoral head
	Iliofemoral	Limits hip extension
	Ischiofemoral	Limits anterior displacement of the femoral head
	Pubofemoral	Limits hip extension
Knee	Medial collateral	Stabilizes medial aspect of tibiofemoral joint against valgus stress
	Lateral collateral	Stabilizes lateral aspect of tibiofemoral joint against varus stress
	Anterior cruciate	Resists anterior translation of the tibia and posterior translation of the femur
	Posterior cruciate	Resists posterior translation of the tibia and anterior translation of the femur
Ankle	Medial collaterals (Deltoid)	Provides stability between the medial malleolus, navicular, talus, and calcaneus against eversion
	Lateral collaterals	Static stabilizers of the lateral ankle especially against inversion
Foot	Long plantar	Provides indirect plantar support to the calcaneocuboid joint, by limiting the amount of flattening of the lateral longitudinal arch of the foot
	Bifurcate	Supports the medial and lateral aspects of the foot when weight bearing in a plantar flexed position
	Calcaneocuboid	Provides plantar support to the calcaneocuboid joint and possibly helps to limit flattening of the lateral longitudinal arch

TABLE 5-4. LIGAMENT INJURIES

GRADE	SIGNS	IMPLICATIONS
First degree (mild)	Minimal loss of structural integrity No abnormal motion Little or no swelling Localized tenderness Minimal bruising	Minimal functional loss Early return to training—some protection may be necessary
Second degree (moderate)	Significant structural weakening Some abnormal motion Solid end feel to stress More bruising and swelling Often associated with hemarthrosis and effusion	Tendency for recurrence Need protection from risk of further injury May need modified immobilization May stretch out further with time
Third degree (complete)	Loss of structural integrity Marked abnormal motion Significant bruising Hemarthrosis	Needs prolonged protection Surgery may be considered Often permanent functional instability

TABLE 5-5. GENERAL STRUCTURE OF BONE

SITE	COMMENT	CONDITIONS	RESULT
Epiphysis	Mainly develops under pressure	Epiphyseal dysplasias	Distorted joints
	Apophysis forms under traction	Joint surface trauma	Degenerative changes
	Forms bone ends	Overuse injury	Fragmented development
	Supports articular surface	Damaged blood supply	Avascular necrosis
Physis	Epiphyseal or growth plate	Physeal dysplasia	Short stature
	Responsive to growth and sex hormones	Trauma	Deformed or angulated growth or growth arrest
	Vulnerable prior to growth spurt	Slipped epiphysis	
	Mechanically weak		
Metaphysis	Remodeling expanded bone end	Osteomyelitis	Sequestrum formation
	Cancellous bone heals rapidly	Tumors	Altered bone shape
	Vulnerable to osteomyelitis	Metaphyseal dysplasia	Distorted growth
	Affords ligament attachment		
Diaphysis	Forms shaft of bone	Fractures	Able to remodel angulation
	Large surface for muscle origin	Diaphyseal dysplasias	Cannot remodel rotation
	Significant compact cortical bone	Healing slower than at metaphysis	Involucrum with infection
	Strong in compression		Dysplasia gives altered density and shape

Reproduced, with permission, from Reid DC: *Sports Injury Assessment and Rehabilitation*. New York: Churchill Livingstone. 1992. CopyrightElsevier.

be classified according to location, direction, mechanism, and whether the skin is broken or not (Table 5-7).

Cartilage Tissue. Cartilage tissue consists of cells called chondrocytes, which are specialized cells that are responsible for cartilage, and the maintenance of the ECM.[18] The ECM also contains proteoglycans, lipids, water, and dissolved electrolytes.[19]

Cartilage tissue exists in three forms: hyaline, elastic, and fibrocartilage.

1. Hyaline cartilage: Hyaline cartilage is the most common cartilage within the body. Most of the bones of the body form initially as hyaline cartilage, which later becomes bone through a process called endochondral ossification. Hyaline cartilage forms the articular surface of synovial joints as it covers the ends of long bones. Together with synovial fluid, hyaline cartilage provides a smoothly articulating surface while simultaneously protecting the underlying subchondral bone. Adult hyaline cartilage is an avascular and non-innervated structure.
2. Elastic cartilage is a very specialized CT primarily found in locations such as the outer ear.
3. Fibrocartilage, with its large and numerous collagen fiber content, functions as a shock absorber in all directions in both weight-bearing, and nonweight-bearing joints. Fibrocartilage is found in structures such as the intervertebral disc.

Pathology of Cartilage. The terms *arthritis*, *rheumatism*, and *rheumatoid disease* are generic references to an array of diseases that are divided into various categories.[20] Two major forms of arthritis

TABLE 5-6. TYPES OF FRACTURES

TYPES OF FRACTURE	DESCRIPTION
Avulsion	An avulsion fracture is an injury to the bone where a tendon or ligament pulls off a piece of the bone.
Closed	When there is a closed fracture there is no broken skin. The bones which brake do not penetrate the skin (but may be seen under the skin) and there is no contusion from external trauma.
Comminuted	A fracture that has more than two fragments of bone which have broken off. It is a highly unstable type of bone fracture with many bone fragments.
Complete	A fracture in which the bone has been completely fractured through its own width.
Complex	This type of fractured bone severely damages the soft tissue which surrounds the bone.
Compound (open)	When this occurs, the bone breaks and fragments of the bone penetrate through the internal soft tissue of the body and break through the skin from the inside. There is a high risk of infection if external pathogenic factors enter into the interior of the body.
Compression	This type of bone fracture occurs when the bone is compressed beyond its limits of tolerance. These fractures generally occur in the vertebral bodies as a result of a flexion injury or without trauma in patients with osteoporosis. Compression fractures of the calcaneus are also common when patients fall from a height and land on their feet.
Epiphyseal	A fracture of the epiphysis and physis—growth plate. These injuries are classified using the Salter-Harris Classification.
Greenstick	The pathology of this type of fracture includes an incomplete fracture in which only one side of the bone has been broken. The bone usually is "bent" and only broken on the outside of the bend. It is mostly seen in children and is considered a stable fracture because the whole bone has not been broken. As long as the bone is kept rigid healing is usually quick.
Hairline	This bone fracture has minimal trauma to the bone and surrounding soft tissues. It is an incomplete fracture with no significant bone displacement and is considered a stable fracture. In this type of fracture, the crack only extends into the outer layer of the bone but not completely through the entire bone. It is also known as a fissure fracture.
Impaction	Occurs when one fragment is driven into another. This type of fracture is common in tibial plateau fractures in adults.
Oblique	A fracture which goes at an angle from the axis to the bone.
Pathologic	A fracture that occurs when a bone breaks in an area that is weakened by another disease process. Causes of weakened bone include tumors, infection, and certain inherited bone disorders.
Spiral	In this pattern a bone has been broken due to a twisting type motion. It is highly unstable and may be diagnosed as an oblique fracture unless a proper x-ray has been taken. The spiral fracture will look like a corkscrew type which runs parallel with the axis of the broken bone.
Stress	These fractures may extend through all or only part of the way through the bone. These types of fractures are common in soldiers or runners and are far more common in women. They often occur in the spine, and lower extremity (most often in the fibula, tibia, or metatarsals). Stress fractures occur in a variety of age groups, ranging from young children to elderly persons. Stress fractures do not necessarily occur in association with a history of increased activity. Therefore, it is important to remember that the absence of a history of trauma or increased activity does not eliminate the possibility of stress or insufficiency fracture as a cause of musculoskeletal pain.

exist: osteoarthritis (OA), also referred to as degenerative joint disease (DJD), and rheumatoid arthritis (RA), also referred to as inflammatory arthritis.

BURSAE

Bursae are closed sacs that are lined by synovium that are located in areas of direct pressure, friction, or potential impingement. There are about 160 bursae throughout the body.

The synovial cells of the bursa secrete a fluid that acts as a lubricant that helps reduce friction between moving body parts, such as in the shoulder and elbow.

TABLE 5-7. SALTER-HARRIS CLASSIFICATION OF FRACTURES

Salter I	Epiphysis separate from shaft and metaphysis—through the physis Most common in newborns and young children Prognosis excellent
Salter II	Like Type I, through the physis with separation of physis from metaphysis, but with a small metaphysis triangle fracture Most common overall epiphyseal fracture Prognosis excellent although joint instability is possible
Salter III	Intra-articular fracture through epiphysis Uncommon Open reduction internal fixation (ORIF) is often necessary
Salter IV	Intra-articular: Through epiphysis, growth plate, and metaphysis Poor prognosis, lost blood supply Needs perfect reduction
Salter V	Crushing of physis Poor prognosis Early radiograph negative Rarely occurs
Salter VI (Rang)	Portion of growth plate sheared off Typically occurs with penetrating injuries Rare

Muscle Tissue

Muscle tissue is responsible for the movement of body parts, the movement of cellular materials throughout the body, and activities such as locomotion. Skeletal muscle consists of individual muscle cells or fibers called *muscle fibers* or *myofibers* (Figure 5-1). These individual myofibers are wrapped in a CT envelope called *endomysium.* Bundles of myofibers form a whole muscle (fasciculus). These bundles are encased in a structure called the perimysium, which is continuous with the deep fascia of the body. Groups of fasciculi are surrounded by epimysium. Each of the myofibers consists of thousands of *myofibrils,* which are composed of sarcomeres arranged in series.[21]

Each myofiber contains many fibers called *myofilaments* (Figure 5-1), which are made up of two protein filaments: actin (thin) and myosin (thick) that give myofibers a striped appearance.[22] The striped appearance is produced by alternating dark (A) and light (I) bands that appear to span the width of the myofiber. The myosin filaments form the A bands, whereas the I bands are composed of actin filaments. The actin filaments of the I band overlap into the A band, forming a central region (H band), which contains only myosin. At the center of each I band is a thin, dark Z line. The the distance between each Z line represents a *sarcomere.*

When a muscle contracts in a way in which the myofibers shorten, the distance between the Z lines decreases, the I band and H bands disappear, but the width of the A band remains unchanged.[22] This shortening of the sarcomeres is produced by a sliding of actin filaments over the myosin filaments, which pulls the Z lines together.

Structures called *cross-bridges* serve to connect the actin and myosin filaments. The myosin filaments contain two supple, hinge-like regions, which allow the cross-bridges to attach and detach from the actin filament. During contraction, the cross-bridges attach and undergo power strokes, which provide the contractile force, whereas

Study Pearl

The sarcomere is the contractile machinery of the muscle. The graded force of a muscle contraction can vary based on the number of fibers participating in the contraction. More force can be developed by recruiting more cells into cooperative action.

Study Pearl

Each myofiber is limited by a cell membrane called a *sarcolemma.* The protein *dystrophin,* which is lacking in patients with Duchenne muscular dystrophy, plays an essential role in the mechanical strength and stability of the sarcolemma.[23]

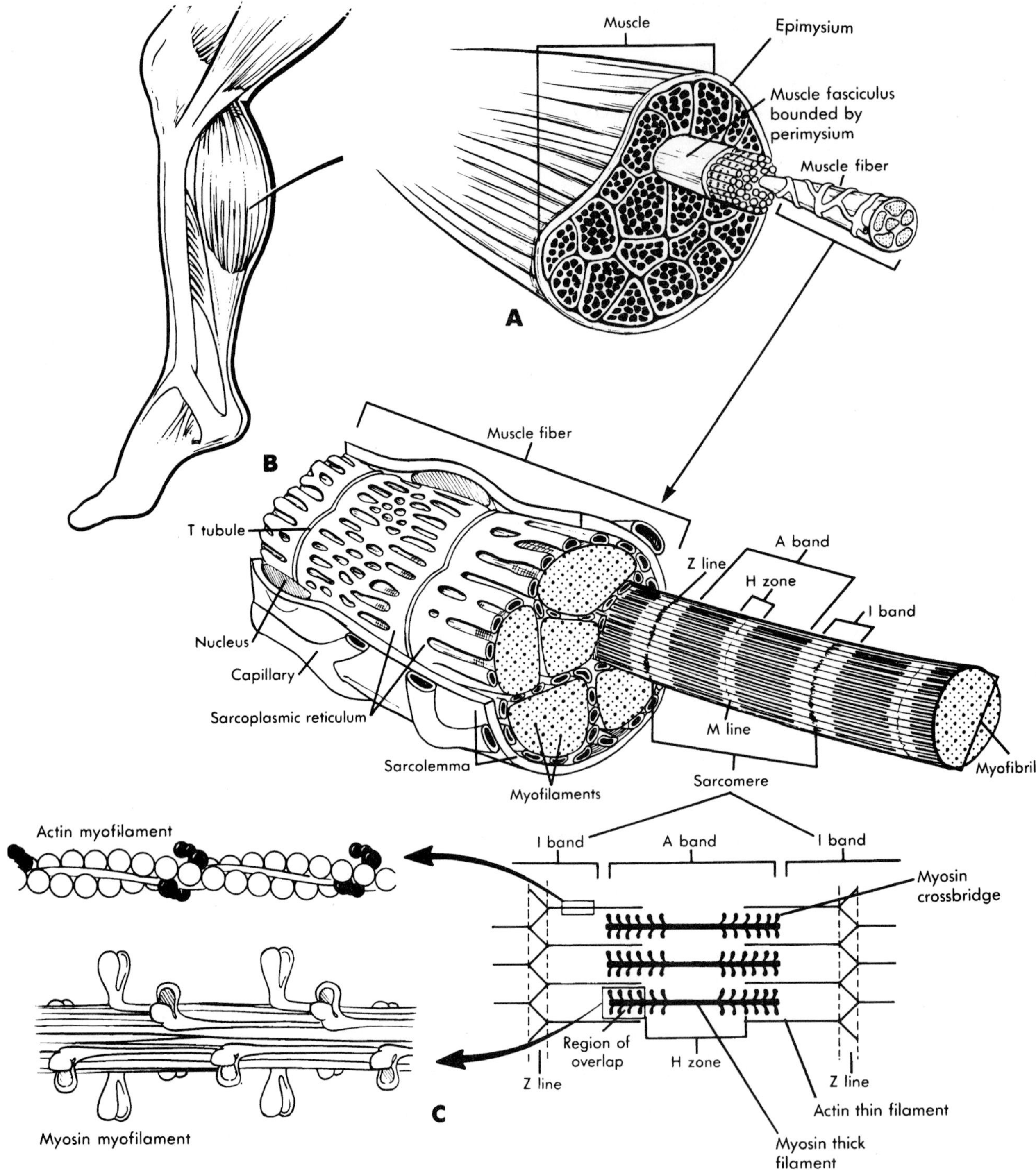

Figure 5-1. Parts of a muscle. (Reproduced, with permission, from Prentice WE, Voight MI: *Techniques in Musculoskeletal Rehabilitation.* New York: McGraw-Hill. 2001:31.)

during relaxation, the cross-bridges detach. This attaching and detaching occurs asynchronously, so that some are attaching while others are detaching.

The regulation of cross-bridge attachment and detachment is a function of two proteins located in the actin filaments: tropomyosin and troponin. Tropomyosin attaches directly to the actin filament. In contrast, troponin attaches to the tropomyosin rather than directly to the actin filament. Tropomyosin and troponin function as the toggle for muscle contraction and relaxation. In a relaxed state, the tropomyosin physically blocks the cross-bridges from binding to the actin. For contraction to take place, the tropomyosin must be moved.

Each myofiber is innervated by a somatic motor neuron. One neuron and the myofibers it innervates constitute a motor unit—the functional unit of the muscle. Each motor neuron branches as it enters the muscle to innervate a number of myofibers. The area of contact between a nerve and a myofiber is known as the motor end plate, or neuromuscular junction (NMJ). The release of acetylcholine from the axon terminals at the NMJs causes electrical activation of the myofibers. When an action potential propagates into the transverse tubule system (narrow membranous tunnels formed from and continuous with the sarcolemma), the voltage sensors on the transverse tubule membrane signal the release of Ca^{2+} from the terminal cisternae portion of the sarcoplasmic reticulum (SR)-(a series of interconnected sacs and tubes that surround each myofibril).[22] The released Ca^{2+} then diffuses into the sarcomeres and binds to troponin, displacing the tropomyosin, and allowing the actin to bind with the myosin cross-bridges. At the end of the contraction (the neural activity and action potentials cease), the SR actively accumulates Ca^{2+} and muscle relaxation occurs. The return of Ca^{2+} to the SR involves active transport, requiring the breakdown of adenosine triphosphate (ATP) to adenosine diphosphate (ADP)*.[22] Because SR function is closely associated with both contraction and relaxation, changes in its ability to release or sequester Ca^{2+} markedly affect both the time course and magnitude of force output by the myofiber.[24]

Activation of varying numbers of motor neurons results in gradations in the strength of muscle contraction. The stronger the electrical impulse, the stronger the muscle twitch. Whenever a somatic motor neuron is activated, all of the myofibers that it innervates are stimulated and contract with *all-or-none* twitches. Although the myofibers produce all-or-none contractions, muscles are capable of a wide variety of responses.

Based on contractile properties, four different types of skeletal myofibers have been recognized:

1. Type I (slow-twitch red oxidative)
2. Type IIa (fast-twitch red oxidative)
3. Type IIb (fast-twitch white glycolytic)
4. Type IIc (fast-twitch intermediate)

Human muscles contain a genetically determined mixture of both slow and fast fiber type. In humans, most limb muscles contain a relatively equal distribution of each myofiber type, while the back and trunk demonstrate a predominance of slow-twitch (ST) fibers. The use of specific myofibers is dependent on the required activity. Although, the two fiber types generally produce the same amount of force per contraction, the fast-twitch (FT) fibers produce that force at a faster

*The most readily available energy for skeletal muscle cells is stored in the form of ATP and phosphocreatine (see "Physiology of Exercise"). Through the activity of the enzyme ATPase, ATP promptly releases energy when required by the cell to perform any type of work, whether it is electrical, chemical, or mechanical.

Study Pearl

For the purpose of an orthopedic examination, Cyriax subdivided musculoskeletal tissues into those considered to be "contractile" and those considered as "inert" (noncontractile).[25]

- Contractile. Contractile tissue, as defined by Cyriax, is a bit of a misnomer, as the only true contractile tissue in the body is the myofiber. However, included under this term are the muscle belly, the tendon, the tenoperiosteal junction, the submuscular/tendinous bursa, and bone (teno-osseous junction), as all are stressed to some degree with a muscle contraction.
- Inert tissue. Inert tissue as defined by Cyriax includes the joint capsule, the ligaments, the bursa, the articular surfaces of the joint, and the synovium, the dura, bone and fascia. The teno-osseous junction and the bursae are placed in each of the subdivisions due to their close proximity to contractile tissue, and their capacity to be compressed or stretched during movement.

Study Pearl

Most muscles span only one joint. However, there are many muscles in the body that cross two or more joints. Examples of these include the erector spinae, the biceps brachii, the long head of the triceps brachii, the hamstrings, the rectus femoris, and a number of muscles crossing the wrist and finger joints.

TABLE 5-8. COMMON MUSCLE ATTACHMENTS OF THE UPPER EXTREMITY

ATTACHMENT SITE	MUSCLE
Greater tuberosity of the humerus	Supraspinatus, infraspinatus, teres minor
Lesser tuberosity of the humerus	Subscapularis
Medial epicondyle of humerus	Common flexor tendon origin
Lateral epicondyle of humerus	Common extensor tendon origin

rate (hence their name). Thus, activities that require a limited amount of time to generate maximal force use a predominance of FT fiber recruitment, whereas activities that involve repeated and extended muscle contractions entail more involvement of the ST fibers.

Muscle Function. There are approximately 430 muscles in the body, of which about 75 pairs, referred to as *agonists* and *antagonists*, provide the majority of body movements and postures.[26] An agonist muscle contracts to produce the desired movement, while the antagonist muscle opposes the desired movement by relaxing and lengthening in a gradual manner to ensure that the desired motion occurs in a coordinated and controlled fashion. Muscle groups that work together to produce a desired movement are called *synergists*.[27]

The effectiveness of a muscle to produce movement is dependent on a number of factors (see Chapter 17). These include the location and orientation of the muscle's attachment relative to the joint (Tables 5-8 and Table 5-9), the tightness or laxity present in the joint upon which it acts, and the actions and lengths of other muscles that cross the joint.[26]

Joint Classification. Joints may be classified as *diarthrosis*, which permit free bone movement and *synarthrosis*, in which very limited or no motion occurs (Table 5-10).

Diarthrosis (Synovial). Every synovial joint contains at least one "mating pair" of articular surfaces—one convex and one concave. If only one pair exists, the joint is called simple; more than one pair is called compound; and if an articular disk is present, the joint is termed complex. Synovial joints have five distinguishing characteristics: joint cavity, articular cartilage, synovial fluid, synovial membrane, and a fibrous capsule. Four types of synovial joint are recognized (Figure 5-2):

TABLE 5-9. COMMON MUSCLE ATTACHMENTS OF THE LOWER EXTREMITY

ATTACHMENT SITE	MUSCLE
Greater trochanter	Gluteus minimus, gluteus medius, piriformis, obturator internus, inferior and superior gemelli
Lesser trochanter	Psoas major
Ischial tuberosity	Semitendinosus, semimembranosus, biceps femoris, adductor magnus
Pubic ramus	Pectineus, adductor magnus, gracilis, adductor brevis

TABLE 5-10. JOINT TYPES

TYPE	CHARACTERISTICS	EXAMPLES
Diarthrosis	Generally unites long bones and has great mobility Fibroelastic joint capsule, which is filled with a lubricating substance called *synovial fluid*—referred to as a synovial joint.	Hip, knee, shoulder, and elbow joints
Synarthrosis		
Synostosis	United by bone tissue	Sutures of the skull and gomphoses (the teeth and their corresponding sockets in the mandible/maxilla)
Synchondrosis	Joined by either hyaline or fibrocartilage	The epiphyseal plates of growing bones and the articulations between the first rib and the sternum
Syndesmosis	Joined together by an interosseous membrane	The symphysis pubis Articulation between the tibia and fibula

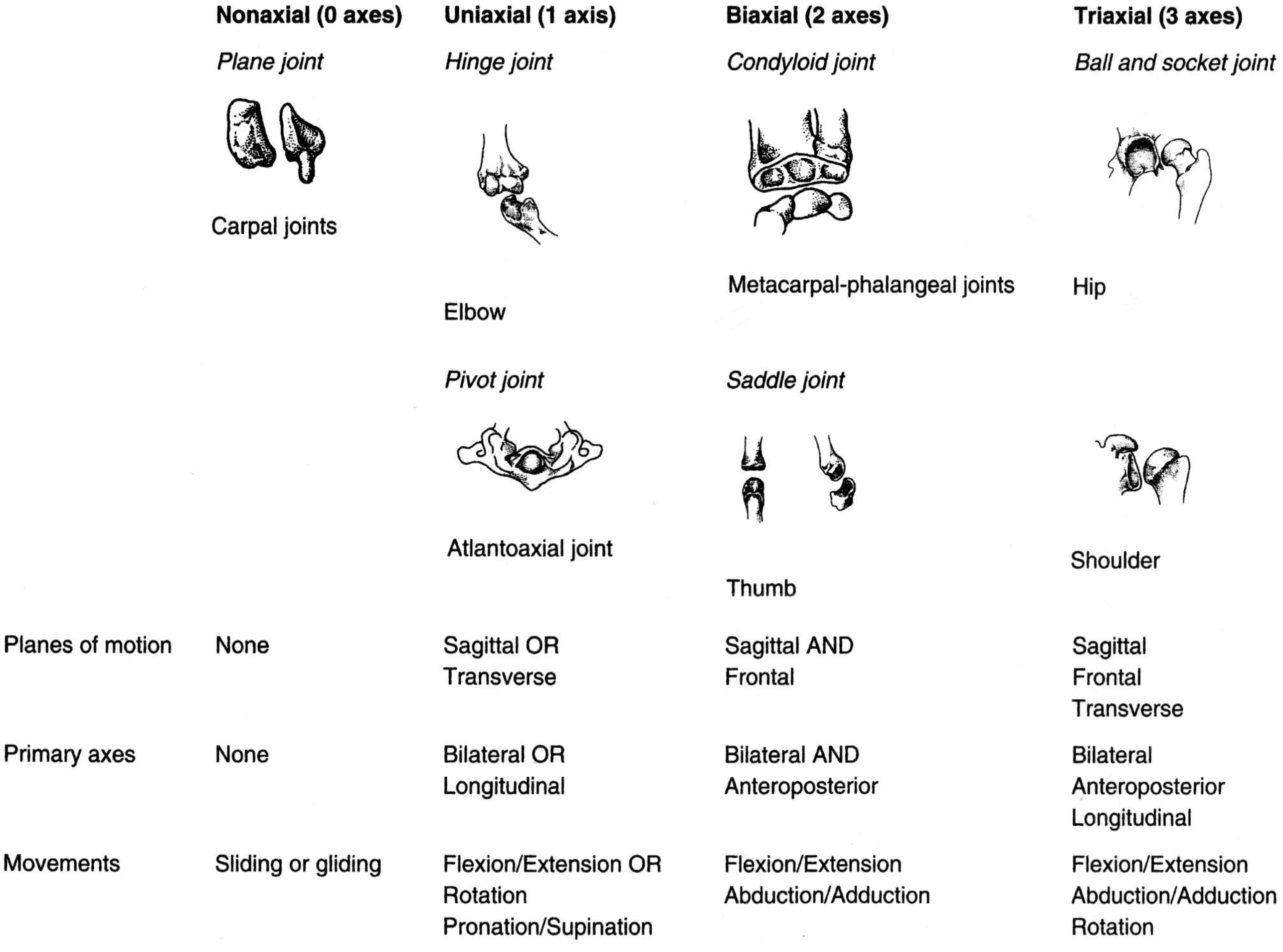

Figure 5-2. Joint classifications. (Reproduced, with permission, from Luttgens K, Hamilton N: *Kinesiology: Scientific Basis of Human Motion, 10th ed.* New York: McGraw-Hill. 2002:27.)

1. Nonaxial joint: these joints have no planes of motion or primary axes, and only permit sliding or gliding motions. Examples include the intercarpal joints.
2. Uniaxial joint: these joints allow one motion around a single axis and in one plane of the body. Two types are recognized:
   - Hinge (ginglymus): the elbow joint
   - Pivot joint (trochoid): atlantoaxial joint
3. Biaxial joint: these joints allow movement in two planes and around two axes based on their convex/concave surfaces. Two types are recognized:
   - Condyloid: one bone may articulate with another by one surface or by two, but never more than two. If two distinct surfaces are present, the joint is called condylar or bicondylar. Example: metacarpophalangeal joint of the finger.
   - Sellar (saddle): if a section is taken through a sellar surface in one plane, the joint surface can be seen to be convex, and the curvature of the joint in the opposite plane is concave. Example: carpometacarpal (CMC) joint of the thumb.
4. Multiaxial joint: these joints allow movement in and around three planes. An example includes the ball and socket joint of the hip.

Synarthrosis (Fibrous). There are three major types of synarthroses based on the type of tissue uniting the bone surfaces (Table 5-10).[28]

Mechanoreceptors. Articular mechanoreceptors, which are stimulated by mechanical forces (soft tissue elongation, relaxation, and compression), help mediate proprioception.[29-31] Wyke[31,32] categorized mechanoreceptors into four different types (Table 5-11).[30,31,33]

The mechanoreceptors translate mechanical deformation into electrical signals that provide information concerning joint motion and position.[34-38] Sensory information provided by the receptors travels through afferent pathways to the central nervous system (CNS), where it is integrated with information from other levels of the nervous system (see Chapter 9).[39]

Arthrokinematics. The small motion, which is available at musculoskeletal joint surfaces, is referred to as *accessory* or arthrokinematic motion. Normal arthrokinematic motions must occur for full-range physiological motion to take place. A restriction of arthrokinematic motion results in a decrease in osteokinematic (see "next section") motion—the motion of a bone in space. The three types of movement that occur at the articulating surfaces include:

1. Roll: a roll occurs when the points of contact on each joint surface are constantly changing (Figure 5-3). This type of movement is analogous to a tire on a car as the car rolls forward. The term rock is often used to describe small rolling motions.
2. Slide: a slide occurs if only one point on the moving surface makes contact with varying points on the opposing surface (Figure 5-3). This type of motion is also referred to

TABLE 5-11. MECHANORECEPTOR TYPES

TYPE	LOCATION	FUNCTION
I—Small Ruffini endings. Slow-adapting, low-threshold stretch receptors	The joint capsule, and in ligaments	▶ Important in signaling actual joint position or changes in joint positions. ▶ Contribute to reflex regulation of postural tone, to coordination of muscle activity, and to a perceptional awareness of joint position. ▶ An increase in joint capsule tension by active or passive motion, posture or by mobilization or manipulation, causes these receptors to discharge at a higher frequency.
II—Pacinian corpuscles. Rapidly adapting, low-threshold receptors	In adipose tissue, the cruciate ligaments, the anulus fibrosus, ligaments, and the fibrous capsule.	▶ Sense joint motion and regulate motor-unit activity of the prime movers of the joint. ▶ Type II receptors are entirely inactive in immobile joints and become active for brief periods at the onset of movement and during rapid changes in tension. ▶ The Type II receptors fire during active or passive motion of a joint, or with the application of traction.
III—Large Ruffini. Slowly adapting, high-threshold receptors	Ligaments and the fibrous capsule.	▶ Detect large amounts of tension. These receptors only become active in the extremes of motion or when strong manual techniques are applied to the joint.
IV—Nociceptors. Slowly adapting, high-threshold free nerve endings		▶ Inactive in normal circumstances but become active with marked mechanical deformation or tension. ▶ Also active in response to direct mechanical or chemical irritation.

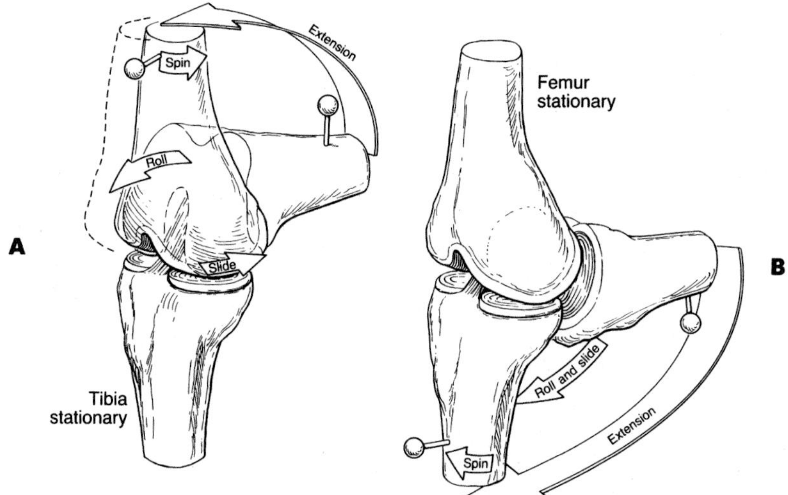

Figure 5-3. Joint movements. **A.** Roll and slide occurring with knee extension with a stationary tibia. **B.** Roll and slide occurring with knee extension with a staionary femur. (Reproduced, with permission, from Dutton M: *Manual Therapy of the Spine*. New York: McGraw-Hill. 2002:43.)

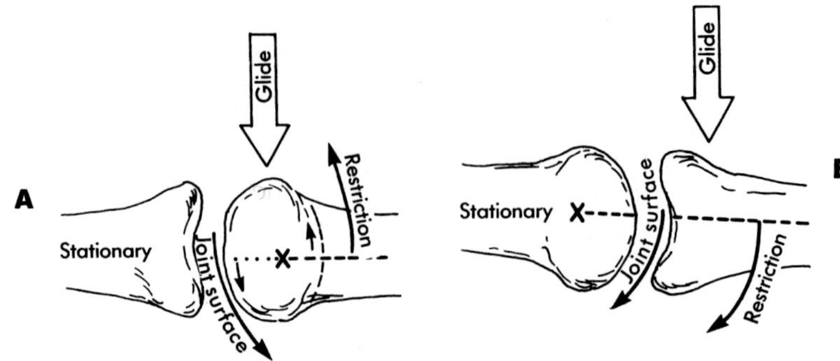

Figure 5-4. Gliding motions. **A.** Glides of the convex segment should be in the direction opposite to the restriction. **B.** Glides of the concave segment should be in the direction of the restriction. (Reproduced, with permission, from Dutton M: *Manual Therapy of the Spine.* New York: McGraw-Hill. 2002:44.)

as translatory or accessory motion and is analogous to a car tire skidding when the brakes are applied suddenly on a wet road. While the roll of a joint always occurs in the same direction as the swing of a bone, the direction of the slide is determined by the shape of the articulating surface (Figure 5-4). This rule is often referred to as the concave-convex rule: If the joint surface is convex relative to the other surface, the slide occurs in the opposite direction to the osteokinematic motion (Figure 5-4). If, on the other hand, the joint surface is concave, the slide occurs in the same direction as the osteokinematic motion (Table 5-12).

TABLE 5-12. CHARACTERISTICS OF CONVEX AND CONCAVE SURFACES

CONCAVE (FEMALE) SURFACES	CONVEX (MALE) SURFACES
Can both, spin and glide, on their convex partners. Spin and glides of the joint are combined in joints with 1 degree of freedom (DOF).[a] Spin and glides can occur independently in a joint with 2[b] or 3 degrees of freedom.[c] Can roll on the convex surface except when the joint is in the closed pack position. Rolling is accompanied by gliding except at the beginning and termination of a movement. Rolling and gliding occur in the same direction which is also the same direction as the swing of the bone. Rolling causes the leading edge of the concave surface to approximate the convex surface and the trailing edge to lift up from the convex surface. Rolling supplements gliding, the latter of which is the primary movement of the concave surface and makes for economy of articular cartilage.	Convex surfaces can both spin and glide on their concave partner. In addition convex surfaces can roll upon the concave surface and rolling is the primary movement of a convex surface. Rolling is always accompanied by gliding except at the beginning and termination of the movement. Rolling does not occur in the close pack position. Rolling always takes place in the same direction as the swing of the bone. Gliding always takes place in the opposite direction of the rolling movement. Since the convex surface is always larger than the concave surface, the gliding movement in the opposite direction prevents the convex surface from rolling off of the concave surface.

[a]1 DOF: a joint that can swing in one direction or can only spin. Examples include: the proximal interphalangeal joint.

[b]2 DOF: a joint that can swing in two directions or swing in one direction and spin. Examples include: the tibiofemoral joint, temporomandibular joint, proximal and distal radio-ulnar joints, subtalar joint, and talocalcaneal joint.

[c]3 DOF: a bone that can spin and also swing in two distinct directions. Examples include: ball and socket joints such as the shoulder and hip.

3. Spin: a spin is defined as any movement in which the bone moves but the mechanical axis remains stationary. A spin involves a rotation of one surface on an opposing surface around a longitudinal axis (Figure 5-3). This type of motion is analogous to the pirouette performed in ballet. Spin motions in the body include internal and external rotation of the glenohumeral joint when the humerus is abducted to 90 degrees.

Osteokinematics. Osteokinematics is defined as the study of bone motion. All human body segment motions involve osteokinematic motions. Actual bone movement is a combination of one or more basic movements:

- Spin: the motion of the chosen point is only rotation around the mechanical axis of the bone (pure spin). For example, internal and external rotation of the radius.
- Pure swing: also known as a cardinal swing. A pure swing involves no spin. The point moves from its initial position to the final position along the shortage path possible, with the path (chord) corresponding to a meridian of latitude or longitude, or a straight line on a flat surface.
- Swing: any motion of the point other than pure spin.
- Impure swing: also known as an arcuate swing. And impure swing is a combination of swing and spin. The point moves along a path (arc) that is other than the shortest-possible distance.

Degrees of Freedom. The number of independent modes of motion at a joint is called the *degrees of freedom* (DOF). When referring to degrees of freedom, the swings must be cardinal and the axis of swing must be at a 90 degrees angle to the other swing axes (Table 5-12).

Close-Packed and Open-Packed Positions of the Joint. Joint movements are usually accompanied by a relative compression (approximation) or distraction (separation) of the opposing joint surfaces. These relative compression or distractions affect the level of *congruity* of the opposing surfaces. The position of maximum congruity of the opposing joint surfaces is termed the *close-packed* position of the joint. The position of least congruity is termed the *open-packed* position. Thus, movements toward the close-packed position of a joint involve an element of compression and tension, whereas movements out of this position involve an element of distraction and slackening.

Close-Packed Position. The close-packed position of a joint is the joint position that results in:

- Maximal tautness of the major ligaments
- Maximal surface congruity
- The least trans-articular pressure
- The minimal joint volume
- The maximal stability of the joint

Study Pearl

The convex-concave rule describes the relationship between arthrokinematics and osteokinematics:

- Convex rule: If the moving joint surface is convex relative to the other surface, the slide occurs in the opposite direction to the movement of the bone shaft of the lever (angular motion).
- Concave rule: If the moving joint surface is concave, the slide occurs in the same direction to the movement of the bone shaft of the lever (angular motion).

This rule is very important to remember for joint mobility testing and for joint mobilizations. If during mobility testing, there is a limited glide:

- If the limitation occurs when the concave surface is moving, the restriction is likely due to a contracture of the trailing portion of the capsule.
- If the limitation occurs when the convex surface is moving, the restriction is likely due to an inability of the moving surface to move into the contracted portion of the capsule (may be due to adhesions between redundant folds of the capsule).

TABLE 5-13. CLOSE-PACKED POSITION OF THE JOINTS

JOINT	POSITION
Zygapophysial (spine)	Extension
Temporomandibular	Teeth clenched
Glenohumeral	Abduction and external rotation
Acromioclavicular	Arm abducted to 90 degrees
Sternoclavicular	Maximum shoulder elevation
Ulnohumeral	Extension
Radiohumeral	Elbow flexed 90 degrees; forearm supinated 5 degrees
Proximal radioulnar	5 degrees of supination
Distal radioulnar	5 degrees of supination
Radiocarpal (wrist)	Extension with radial deviation
Metacarpophalangeal	Full flexion
Carpometacarpal	Full opposition
Interphalangeal	Full extension
Hip	Full extension, internal rotation, and abduction
Tibiofemoral	Full extension and external rotation of tibia
Talocrural (ankle)	Maximum dorsiflexion
Subtalar	Supination
Midtarsal	Supination
Tarsometatarsal	Supination
Metatarsophalangeal	Full extension
Interphalangeal	Full extension

Once the close-packed position is achieved, no further motion in that direction is possible. This is the often-cited reason why most fractures and dislocations occur when an external force is applied to a joint that is in its close-packed position. The close-packed positions for the various joints are depicted in Table 5-13.

Open-Packed Position. In essence, any position of the joint, other than the close-packed position, could be considered as an open-packed position. The open-packed position, also referred to as the *loose-packed* position or resting position of a joint, is the joint position that results in:

- The slackening of the major ligaments of the joint
- Minimal surface congruity
- Minimal joint surface contact
- Maximal joint volume
- Minimal stability of the joint

The open-packed position permits maximal distraction of the joint surfaces. Because the open-packed position causes the brunt of any external force to be borne by the joint capsule or surrounding ligaments, most capsular or ligamentous sprains occur when a joint is in its open-packed position. The open-packed positions for the various joints are depicted in Table 5-14.

Study Pearl

The open-packed position is commonly used during joint mobilization techniques.

TABLE 5-14. OPEN-PACKED (RESTING) POSITION OF THE JOINTS

JOINT	POSITION
Zygapophysial (spine)	Midway between flexion and extension
Temporomandibular	Mouth slightly open (freeway space)
Glenohumeral	55 degrees of abduction, 30 degrees of horizontal adduction
Acromioclavicular	Arm resting by side
Sternoclavicular	Arm resting by side
Ulnohumeral	70 degrees of flexion, 10 degrees of supination
Radiohumeral	Full extension, full supination
Proximal radioulnar	70 degrees of flexion, 35 degrees of supination
Distal radioulnar	10 degrees of supination
Radiocarpal (wrist)	Neutral with slight ulnar deviation
Carpometacarpal	Midway between abduction-adduction and flexion-extension
Metacarpophalangeal	Slight flexion
Interphalangeal	Slight flexion
Hip	30 degrees of flexion, 30 degrees of abduction, slight lateral rotation
Tibiofemoral	25 degrees of flexion
Talocrural (ankle)	10 degrees of plantar flexion, midway between maximum inversion and eversion
Subtalar	Midway between extremes of range of movement
Midtarsal	Midway between extremes of range of movement
Tarsometatarsal	Midway between extremes of range of movement
Metatarsophalangeal	Neutral
Interphalangeal	Slight flexion

Capsular and Non-Capsular Patterns of Restriction

Broadly speaking, there are two patterns of range of motion used in the interpretation of joint motion:

1. A capsular pattern of restriction is a limitation of pain and movement in a joint-specific ratio, which is usually present with arthritis, or following prolonged immobilization (Table 5-15).
2. A non-capsular pattern of restriction is a limitation in a joint in any pattern other than a capsular one, and may indicate the presence of either a derangement, a restriction of one part of the joint capsule, or an extra-articular lesion that obstructs joint motion.

End Feels. End feels can be defined as the quality of resistance at end range. The end feel can indicate to the clinician the cause of the motion restriction (Tables 5-16 and 5-17).

Arc of Pain. The term "painful arc" is used to describe an occurrence of temporary pain during active or passive motion that disappears before the end of the movement. The presence of a painful arc indicates that some structure is being compressed.

Study Pearl

- A painful arc that occurs in association with a positive resistive test (for pain) usually indicates a contractile lesion.
- A painful arc that occurs in association with a negative resistive test (for pain) usually indicates an inert lesion.

Measuring Range of Motion

Overview. The term goniometry is derived from two Greek words, *gonia* meaning angle and *metron*, meaning measure. Thus, a goniometer is an instrument used to measure the total amount of available motion at a specific joint. Goniometry can be used to measure both active and passive range of motion.

TABLE 5-15. CAPSULAR PATTERNS OF RESTRICTION

JOINT	LIMITATION OF MOTION (PASSIVE ANGULAR MOTION)
Glenohumeral	External rotation > abduction > internal rotation (3:2:1)
Acromioclavicular	No true capsular pattern. Possible loss of horizontal adduction, pain (and sometimes slight loss of end range) with each motion
Sternoclavicular	See above: acromioclavicular joint
Humeroulnar	Flexion > extension (± 4:1)
Humeroradial	No true capsular pattern. Possible equal limitation of pronation and supination
Superior radioulnar	No true capsular pattern. Possible equal limitation of pronation and supination with pain at end ranges
Inferior radioulnar	No true capsular pattern. Possible equal limitation of pronation and supination with pain at end ranges
Wrist (carpus)	Flexion = extension
Radiocarpal	See above (carpus)
Carpometacarpal	
Mid carpal	
1st carpometacarpal	Retroposition
Carpometacarpal 2-5	Fan > fold
Metacarpophalangeal 2-5	Flexion > extension (±2:1)
Interphalangeal	
Proximal (PIP)	Flexion > extension (±2:1)
Distal (DIP)	
Hip	Internal rotation > flexion > abdduction = extension > other motions
Tibiofemoral	Flexion > extension (±5:1)
Superior tibiofibular	No capsular pattern: pain at end range of translatory movements
Talocrural	Plantar flexion > dorsiflexion
Talocalcaneal (subtalar)	Varus > valgus
Midtarsal	
Talonavicular calcaneocuboid	Inversion (plantar flexion, adduction, supination) > dorsiflexion
First metatarsophalangeal	Extension > flexion (±2:1)
Metatarsophalangeal 2-5	Flexion ≥ extension
Interphalangeal 2-5	
Proximal	Flexion ≥ extension
Distal	Flexion ≥ extension

Data from Cyriax J: *Textbook of Orthopaedic Medicine, Diagnosis of Soft Tissue Lesions, 8th ed.* London: Bailliere Tindall. 1982.

Goniometers are produced in a variety of sizes and shapes and are usually constructed of either plastic or metal. The two most common types of instruments used to measure joint angles are the bubble inclinometer and the traditional goniometer.

- Bubble goniometer: the bubble goniometer, which has a 360 degrees rotating dial and scale with fluid indicator can be used for flexion and extension; abduction and adduction; and rotation in the neck, shoulder, elbow, wrist, hip, knee, ankle, and the spine.
- Traditional goniometer: the traditional goniometer, which can be used for flexion and extension; abduction and adduction; and rotation of the shoulder, elbow, wrist, hip, knee, and ankle, consists of three parts:
  - A body: the body of the goniometer is designed like a protractor and may form a full or half circle. A measuring scale is located around the body. The scale can extend either from 0 to 180 degrees and 180 to 0 degrees for the half circle models, or from 0 to 360 degrees and from 360 to 0 degrees

TABLE 5-16. NORMAL END FEELS

TYPE	CAUSE	CHARACTERISTICS AND EXAMPLES
Bony	Produced by bone to bone approximation	Abrupt and unyielding with the impression that further forcing will break something **Examples** Normal: elbow extension Abnormal: cervical rotation (may indicate osteophyte)
Muscular	1. Insufficiency: produced by the muscle-tendon unit; may occur with adaptive shortening 2. Slow guarding: resistance that is felt, slowly releases with sustained force	Stretch with elastic recoil exhibits constant-length phenomenon, similar to Capsular (see below), further forcing feels as if it will snap something **Examples** Normal: wrist flexion with finger flexion, the straight leg raise, and ankle dorsiflexion with the knee extended Abnormal: decreased dorsiflexion of the ankle with the knee flexed
Soft tissue approximation	Produced by the contact of two muscle bulks on either side of a flexing joint where the joint range exceeds other restraints	A very forgiving end-feel that gives the impression that further normal motion is possible if enough force could be applied **Examples** Normal: knee flexion, elbow flexion in extremely muscular subjects Abnormal: elbow flexion with the obese subject
Capsular	Produced by capsule or ligaments	Various degrees of stretch without elasticity, stretch ability is dependent on thickness of the tissue ▶ Strong capsular or extra-capsular ligaments produce a hard capsular end-feel while a thin capsule produces a softer one ▶ The impression given to the clinician is, if further force is applied something will tear **Examples** Normal: wrist flexion (soft), elbow flexion in supination (medium) and knee extension (hard) Abnormal: inappropriate stretch ability for a specific joint, if too hard, may indicate a hypomobility due to arthrosis; if too soft, a hypermobility

on the full circle models. The intervals on the scales can vary from 1 to 10 degrees.

- A stationary arm: the stationary arm is structurally a part of the body and therefore cannot move independently of the body.
- A moving arm: the moving arm is attached to the fulcrum in the center of the body by a rivet or screw-like device that allows the moving arm to move freely on the body of the device. In some instruments, the screw-like device can be tightened to fix the moving arm in a certain position or loosened to permit free movement.

The correct selection of which goniometer device to use depends on the joint angle to be measured. The length of arms varies. Extendable goniometers allow varying ranges from 9½ in to 26 in. The longer armed goniometers, or the bubble inclinometer are recommended when the landmarks are further apart, such as when measuring hip, knee, elbow, and shoulder movements. In the smaller joints such as the wrist and hand and foot and ankle, a traditional goniometer with a shorter arm is used.

Grading Accessory Movements. The range of motion at a joint is defined as the available range, not the full range, and is usually in one direction only (Figure 5-5). Each joint has an anatomical limit (AL), which is determined by the configuration of the joint

TABLE 5-17. ABNORMAL END FEELS

TYPE	CAUSES	CHARACTERISTICS AND EXAMPLES
Springy	Produced by the articular surface rebounding from an intra-articular meniscus or disc. The impression is that if forced further, something will collapse.	A rebound sensation as if pushing off from a Sorbo rubber pad. **Examples** Normal: axial compression of the cervical spine Abnormal: knee flexion or extension with a displaced meniscus.
Boggy	Produced by viscous fluid (blood) within a joint.	A "squishy" sensation as the joint is moved towards its end range further forcing feels as if it will burst the joint **Examples** Normal: none Abnormal: hemarthrosis at the knee
Fast guarding (spasm)	Produced by reflex and reactive muscle contraction in response to irritation of the nociceptor predominantly in articular structures and muscle. Forcing it further feels as if nothing will give.	An abrupt and "twangy" end to movement that is unyielding while the structure is being threatened, but disappears when the threat is removed (kicks back) With joint inflammation, it occurs early in the range especially toward the close pack position to prevent further stress With an irritable joint hypermobility it occurs at the end of what should be normal range as it prevents excessive motion from further stimulating the nociceptor Spasm in grade II muscle tears becomes apparent as the muscle is passively lengthened and is accompanied by a painful weakness of that muscle Note: Muscle guarding is not a true end feel as it involves a co-contraction **Examples** Normal: none Abnormal: significant traumatic arthritis, recent traumatic hypermobility, grade II muscle tears
Empty	Produced solely by pain. Frequently caused by serious and severe pathological changes that do not affect the joint or muscle and so do not produce spasm. Demonstration of this end-feel is, with the exception of acute sub-deltoid bursitis, de facto evidence of serious pathology. Further forcing simply increases the pain to unacceptable levels.	The limitation of motion has no tissue resistance component and the resistance is from the patient being unable to tolerate further motion due to severe pain. It is not the same feeling as voluntary guarding but rather it feels as if the patient is both resisting and trying to allow the movement simultaneously **Examples** Normal: none Abnormal: acute sub-deltoid bursitis, sign of the buttock
Facilitation	Not truly an end-feel as facilitated hypertonicity does not restrict motion. It can, however, be perceived near the end range.	A light resistance as from a constant light muscle contraction throughout the latter half of the range that does not prevent the end of range being reached. The resistance is unaffected by the rate of movement **Examples** Normal: none Abnormal: spinal facilitation at any level

Study Pearl

Caution must be used when basing clinical judgments on the results of accessory motion testing because few studies have examined the validity and reliability of accessory motion testing of the spine or extremities and little is known about the validity of these tests for most inferences.[40]

surfaces and the surrounding soft tissues. The point of limitation (PL) is that point in the range which is short of the anatomical limit and which is reduced by either pain or tissue resistance.

Maitland advocated five grades of accessory movements at a joint, each of which falls within the available range of motion that exists at the joint—a point somewhere between the beginning point and the anatomic limit (Figure 5-5). These grades can be used to assess arthrokinematic motion (see "Hypomobility, Hypermobility, and Instability") of the joint.

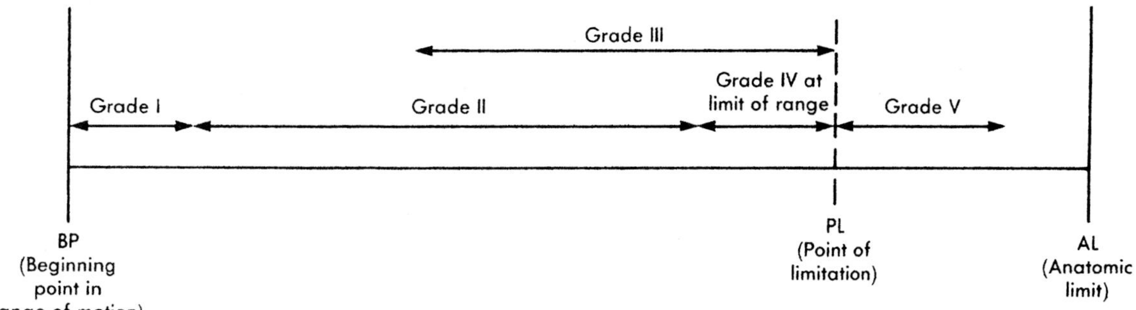

Figure 5-5. Maitland's five grades of motion. PL = point of limitation; AL = anatomic limit. (Reproduced, with permission, from Dutton M: *Manual Therapy of the Spine*. New York: McGraw-Hill. 2002:44.)

Hypomobility, Hypermobility, and Instability. If a joint moves less than what is considered normal, or when compared to the same joint on the opposite extremity, it may be deemed *hypomobile*. Hypomobility may be caused by a contracture of connective tissue (CT). A joint that moves more than considered normal when compared to the same joint on the opposite extremity may be deemed *hypermobile*. Hypermobility may occur as a generalized phenomenon or be localized to just one direction of movement—the result of damaged CT.

The term *stability*, specifically related to the joint, has been the subject of much research.[41-56] In contrast to a hypermobile joint, an unstable joint involves a disruption of the osseous and ligamentous structures of that joint, and results in a loss of function. Joint stability may be viewed as a factor of joint integrity, elastic energy, passive stiffness, and muscle activation:

- Joint integrity: joint integrity is enhanced in those ball and socket joints with deeper sockets, or steeper sides as opposed to those with planar sockets and shallower sides. Joint integrity is also dependent on the attributes of the supporting structures around the joint, and the extent of joint disease.
- Elastic energy: connective tissues are elastic structures and as such are capable of storing elastic energy when stretched. This stored elastic energy may then be used to help return the joint to its original position when the stresses are removed.
- Passive stiffness: individual joints have passive stiffness that increases toward the joint end range. An injury to these passive structures causing inherent loss in the passive stiffness, results in joint laxity.[57]
- Muscle activation: muscle activation increases stiffness, both within the muscle and within the joint(s) it crosses.[58] However, the synergists and antagonist muscles that cross the joint must be activated with the correct and appropriate activation in terms of magnitude or timing. A faulty motor control system can lead to inappropriate magnitudes of muscle force and stiffness, allowing for a joint to buckle or undergo shear translation.[58]

Study Pearl

- The presence of hypomobility in the absence of contraindications is an indication for joint mobilizations as the intervention of choice.
- The presence of hypermobility is a contraindication to joint mobilizations.

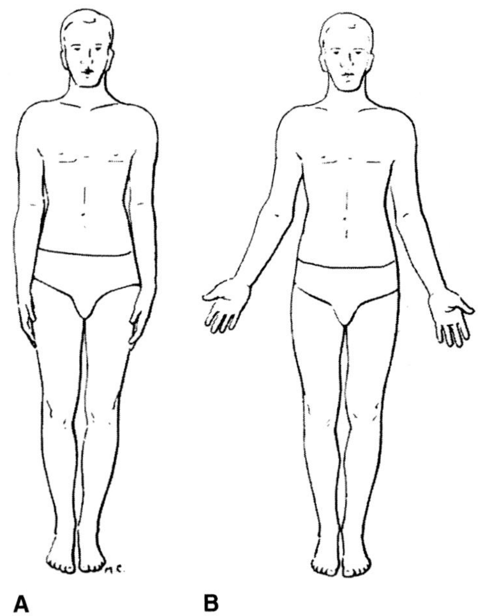

Figure 5-6. Standing positions: **A.** fundamental standing position; **B.** anatomical standing position. (Reproduced, with permission, from Luttgens K, Hamilton N: *Kinesiology: Scientific Basis of Human Motion, 10th ed.* New York: McGraw-Hill. 2002:38.)

Pathological breakdown of the above factors may result in *instability*. Two types of instability are recognized: articular and ligamentous.

1. Articular instability can lead to abnormal patterns of coupled and translational movements.[59]
2. Ligamentous instability may lead to multiple planes of aberrant joint motion.[60]

KINESIOLOGY

GENERAL PRINCIPLES OF BIOMECHANICS

The science of biomechanics involves the application of mechanical principles in the study of the structure and function of movement. When describing joint movements, it is necessary to have a starting position as the reference position. This starting position is referred to as the *anatomical reference position*. The anatomical reference position for the human body is described as the erect standing position with the feet just slightly separated and the arms hanging by the side, the elbows straight and with the palms of the hand facing forward (Figure 5-6).

DIRECTIONAL TERMS

Directional terms are used to describe the relationship of body parts or the location of an external object with respect to the body.[61] The following are commonly used directional terms:

- Superior or cranial—closer to the head
- Inferior or caudal—closer to the feet
- Anterior or ventral or volar—toward the front of the body
- Posterior or dorsal—toward the back of the body
- Medial—toward the midline of the body
- Lateral—away from the midline of the body
- Proximal—closer to the trunk
- Distal—away from the trunk
- Superficial—toward the surface of the body
- Deep—away from the surface of the body in the direction of the inside of the body

MOVEMENTS OF THE BODY SEGMENTS

Movements of the body segments occur in three dimensions along imaginary planes and around various axes of the body.

Planes of the Body. There are three traditional planes of the body corresponding to the three dimensions of space: sagittal, frontal, and transverse (Figure 5-7).[61]

- Sagittal: the sagittal plane, also known as the anterior-posterior or median plane, divides the body vertically into left and right halves.
- Frontal: the frontal plane, also known as the lateral or coronal plane, divides the body into front and back halves.

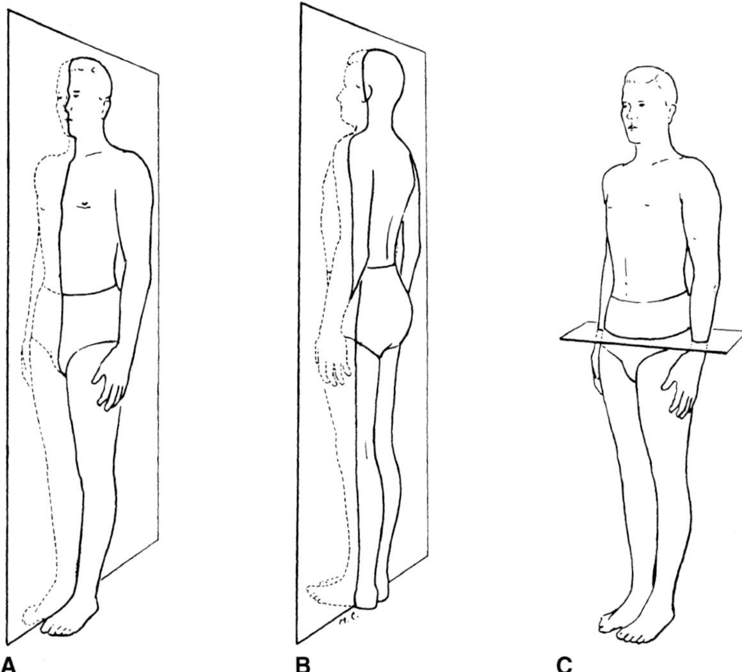

Figure 5-7. The planes of the body: **A.** sagittal, or anteroposterior, plane; **B.** frontal or lateral, plane; **C.** horizontal, or transverse, plane. (Reproduced, with permission, from Luttgens K, Hamilton N: *Kinesiology: Scientific Basis of Human Motion, 10th ed.* New York: McGraw-Hill. 2002:36.)

- Transverse: the transverse plane, also known as the horizontal plane, divides the body into top and bottom halves.

Axes of the Body. Three reference axes are used to describe human motion: frontal, sagittal, and longitudinal. The axis around which the movement takes place is always perpendicular to the plane in which it occurs.

- Frontal: the frontal axis, also known as the transverse axis, is perpendicular to the sagittal plane.
- Sagittal: the sagittal axis is perpendicular to the frontal plane.
- Longitudinal: the longitudinal axis, also known as the vertical axis, is perpendicular to the transverse plane.

The planes and axes for the more common planar movements are described below:

- Flexion, extension, hyperextension, dorsiflexion, and plantar flexion occur in the sagittal plane around a frontal-horizontal axis.
- Abduction, adduction; side flexion of the trunk; elevation and depression of the shoulder girdle; radial and ulnar deviation of the wrist; eversion and inversion of the foot occur in the frontal plane around a sagittal-horizontal axis.

- Rotation of the head, neck and trunk; internal rotation and external rotation of the arm or leg; horizontal adduction and abduction of the arm or thigh; pronation and supination of the forearm occur in the transverse plane around the longitudinal axis.
- Arm circling and trunk circling are examples of circumduction. Circumduction involves an orderly sequence of circular movements that occur in the sagittal, frontal, and intermediate oblique planes, so that segment as a whole incorporates a combination of flexion, extension, abduction, and adduction. Circumduction movements can occur at biaxial and triaxial joints. Examples of these joints include the tibiofemoral, radiohumeral, hip, glenohumeral, and the spinal joints.

LEVERS

Biomechanical levers can be defined as rotations of a rigid surface about an axis. For simplicity's sake, levers are usually described using a straight bar which is the lever, and the fulcrum, which is the point on which the bar is resting. The effort force attempts to cause movement of the load. That part of the lever between the fulcrum and the load is load arm. There are three types of levers:

1. First-class: occurs when two forces are applied on either side of an axis and the fulcrum lies between the effort and the load (Figure 5-8), like a seesaw. Examples in the human body include the contraction of the triceps at the elbow joint, or tipping of the head forward and backward.
2. Second-class: occurs when the load (resistance) is applied between the fulcrum and the point where the effort is exerted (Figure 5-8). This has the advantage of magnifying the effects of the effort so that it takes less force to move the resistance. Examples of second-class levers in everyday life include the nutcracker, and the wheelbarrow—with the wheel acting as the fulcrum. An example of a second class lever in the human body is weight-bearing plantarflexion (rising up on the toes).

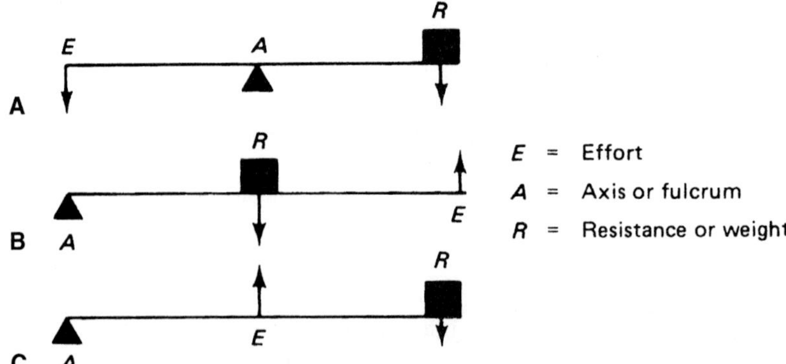

Figure 5-8. Levers: **A.** a lever of the first class; **B.** a lever of the second class; **C.** a lever of the third class. (Reproduced, with permission, from Luttgens K, Hamilton N: *Kinesiology: Scientific Basis of Human Motion, 10th ed.* New York: McGraw-Hill. 2002:350.)

Another would be an isolated contraction of the brachioradialis to flex the elbow, which could not occur without the other elbow flexors being paralyzed.

3. Third class: occurs when the load is located at the end of the lever (Figure 5-8) and the effort lies between the fulcrum and the load (resistance), like a drawbridge or a crane. The effort is exerted between the load and the fulcrum. The effort expended is greater than the load, but the load is moved a greater distance. Most movable joints in the human body function as third-class levers—flexion at the elbow.

Study Pearl

When considering both concentric and eccentric contractions, all peripheral joint muscles act as both a third- and a second-class lever—as a third class in concentric contractions and as a second class in eccentric contractions.

PHYSIOLOGY

THERMOREGULATION

The purpose of the thermoregulatory system is to maintain a relatively constant internal body temperature. The thermoregulatory system consists of three primary components:[62]

- Thermoreceptors: provide input to the temperature-regulating center located in the hypothalamus. Peripheral and central thermoreceptors provide afferent temperature input to the regulating center.
- Peripheral receptors: composed primarily of free nerve endings, and have a high distribution in the skin. Also located in the abdominal organs and nervous system.
- Central receptors: located in the hypothalamus and are sensitive to temperature changes in blood perfusing the hypothalamus.
- Regulating center: dependent on information from thermoreceptors to achieve constant temperatures. Once this information reaches the regulatory center, it is compared with a *set point* standard or optimal temperature value and, depending on the contrast between *set* value and incoming information, mechanisms may be activated either to conserve or dissipate heat.
- Effector organs: respond to both increases and decreases in temperature. The primary effector systems include vascular, metabolic, skeletal muscle responses (shivering), and sweating.

CONSERVATION AND PRODUCTION OF BODY HEAT[62]

When body temperature is lowered, the following mechanisms are activated to conserve heat and increase heat production:

- Vasoconstriction of blood vessels: the hypothalamus activates sympathetic nerves, resulting in vasoconstriction of cutaneous vessels throughout the body, thereby reducing the amount of heat loss to the environment.
- Decrease (or abolition) of sweat gland activity: reduces or prevents heat loss by evaporation.
- Piloerection: although less significant in humans, this mechanism functions to trap a layer of insulating air near the skin and decrease heat loss.

Study Pearl

For the purposes of establishing baseline data in determining response to treatment, physical therapists generally measure body temperature using a thermometer (refer to Chapter 11). A variety of thermometer designs exist:[62]

- Glass mercury
- Electronic
- Disposable single use
- Temperature-sensitive strips
- Tympanic membrane (infrared)

- Shivering: the primary motor center for shivering is located in the posterior hypothalamus.
- Hormonal regulation: serves to increase cellular metabolism, which subsequently increases body heat.

Excess heat is dissipated from the body through four primary methods:

1. Radiation: the transfer of heat by electromagnetic waves from one object to another.
2. Conduction: the transfer of heat from one object to another through a liquid, solid, or gas.
3. Convection: the transfer of heat by movement of air or liquid (water).
4. Evaporation: dissipation of body heat by the conversion of a liquid to a vapor.

THE HEALING PROCESS

Fortunately, the majority of soft tissue injuries heal without complication in a predictable series of events. This chain of events can be conveniently divided into stages or phases:

- Coagulation and inflammation: this stage is initiated almost immediately following injury and represents the normal immune system reaction to injury—a series of defensive events that involves the recognition of a pathogen and the mounting of a reaction against it.
- Coagulation involves temporary repair: apart from an initial period of vasoconstriction lasting for 5 to 10 minutes, tissue injury causes vasodilation, the disruption of blood vessels and extravasation of blood constituents.[63] Extravasated blood contains platelets, which secrete substances that attract and activate macrophages and fibroblasts.[64] Coagulation and platelet release results in the excretion of platelet-derived growth factor (PDGF),[65] platelet factor 4,[66] transforming growth factor-[alpha] (TGF-[alpha]),[67] and transforming growth factor-[beta] (TGF-[beta]).[68] The main functions of a cell-rich tissue exudate are to provide cells capable of producing the components and biologic mediators necessary for the directed reconstruction of damaged tissue while diluting microbial toxins and removing contaminants present in the wound.[69]
- Inflammation: inflammation is mediated by chemotactic substances, including anaphylatoxins. Anaphylatoxins serve to attract neutrophils and monocytes:
  - Neutrophils: neutrophils are white blood cells of the polymorphonuclear (PMN) leukocyte subgroup (the others being eosinophils, and basophils) that are filled with granules of toxic chemicals (phagocytes) that enable them to bind to microorganisms, internalize them, and kill them.
  - Monocytes: monocytes are white blood cells of the mononuclear leukocyte subgroup (the other being lymphocytes). The monocytes migrate into tissues and develop into macrophages, and provide immunological defences against

many infectious organisms. Macrophages serve to orchestrate a "long-term" response to injured cells subsequent to the acute response.[70]

The white blood cells of the inflammatory stage serve to clean the wound of foreign substances, increase vascular permeability, and promote fibroblast activity.[70] The extent and severity of the inflammatory response depends on the size and the type of the injury, the tissue involved, and the vascularity of that tissue.[71-75] Local vasodilation is promoted by biologically active products of the complement and kinin cascades:[69]

- The complement cascade involves 20 or more proteins that circulate throughout the blood in an inactive form.[69]After tissue injury, activation of the complement cascade produces a variety of proteins with activities essential to healing.
- The kinin cascade is responsible for the transformation of the inactive enzyme kallikrein, which is present in both blood and tissue, to its active form, bradykinin. Bradykinin also contributes to the production of tissue exudate through the promotion of vasodilation and increased vessel wall permeability[76]
- Migratory and proliferative stage: this stage, which begins within days and includes the major processes of healing, is responsible for the development of wound tensile strength. A collagenous matrix facilitates angiogenesis by providing protection to new and friable vessels. The process of neovascularization during this phase provides a granular appearance to the wound due to the formation of loops of capillaries and migration of macrophages, fibroblasts, and endothelial cells into the wound matrix.
- Remodelling: the remodeling phase of wound healing involves a conversion of the initial healing tissue to scar tissue. This lengthy phase of contraction, tissue remodeling, and increasing the tensile strength of the wound lasts for up to a year.[63,73,80-83] The application of controlled stresses to the new scar tissue must occur during this stage to help prevent it from shortening.[63,75] If the healing tissues are kept immobile, the fibrous repair is weak, and there are no forces influencing the collagen. Scarring that occurs parallel to the line of force of a structure is less vulnerable to reinjury than a scar, which is perpendicular to those lines of force.[84]

IMAGING STUDIES

The role of diagnostic imaging in physical therapy is rapidly evolving, although the availability or access to diagnostic images varies greatly depending on the practice setting. Diagnostic imaging should not be used as a substitute for the normal procedures of patient management, but instead serve as an adjunct and in context with the results from the tests and measures.

Although the ordering of imaging studies is not within the scope of physical therapy practice (with the exception of PTs in the US Army who have primary care physical therapy provider credentials),

Study Pearl

This stage of healing is characterized by swelling, redness, heat, and impairment or loss of function. The edema is due to an increase in the permeability of the venules, plasma proteins, and leukocytes, which leak into the site of injury.[77,78] Usually there is pain at rest or with active motion, or when specific stress is applied to the injured structure. The pain, if severe enough, can result in muscle guarding, and a loss of function. If this phase is interrupted or delayed, chronic inflammation can result, lasting from months to years.

Study Pearl

Upon progressing to this stage, the "active" effusion and local erythema of the inflammatory stage are usually no longer present. However, residual effusion may still be present at this time and resist resorption.[16,79]

Study Pearl

Despite the presence of an intact epithelium at 3 to 4 weeks after the injury, the tensile strength of the wound has been measured at approximately 25% of its normal value. Several months later, only 70% to 80% of the strength may be restored.[85] This would appear to demonstrate that the remodeling process may last many months or even years, making it extremely important to continue applying controlled stresses to the tissue long after healing appears to have occurred.[85]

TABLE 5-18. STRENGTHS AND WEAKNESSES OF VARIOUS IMAGING STUDIES

IMAGING STUDY	ADVANTAGES	DISADVANTAGES
Plain-film or conventional radiograph	Helpful in detecting fractures and subluxations in patients with a history of trauma Highlight the presence of degenerative joint disease	Do not provide an image of soft tissue structures such as muscles, tendons, ligaments, and intervertebral disks
Stress radiograph	Helpful in assessing spinal mobility and stability in the spine	Patient may not tolerate stress position
Arthrogram	Outlines the soft tissue structures of a joint that would otherwise not be visible with a plain-film radiograph Good for detecting internal derangements	Mildly invasive May require imaging guidance to place the needle
Myelography	Provides image of the spinal cord, nerve roots, dura mater, and the spinal canal	Potential for a post-myelogram headache Potential for seizure (rare)
Computed tomography (CT)	Provides good visualization of the shape, symmetry, and position of structures by delineating specific areas Quicker scan than MRI Better detail of bone than MRI	Generally limited to axial plane Soft tissue contrast not as good as MRI
Magnetic resonance imaging (MRI)	Excellent tissue contrast No streak artifacts Ability to provide cross-sectional images Noninvasive nature Complete lack of ionizing radiation Can take images of any plane	Expensive Time consuming Poor visualization of cortical bone detail or calcifications Limited spatial resolution compared with CT
Diagnostic ultrasound	Readily available Noninvasive Much less expensive than CT or MRI Can be used in any plane (sagittal, coronal, axial, and at any obliquity) Can detect soft tissue injuries, tumors, bone infections, bone mineral density, and arthropathy	Not a sharp, clear image compared to images produced by other radiologic modalities Because of the degrees of obliquity, one cannot easily tell what one is looking at without knowledge of cross-sectional anatomy; sonographer identifies anatomic segment Visualization of structures limited by bone and gas (lung, bowel)

clinicians frequently receive imaging study reports (Table 5-18). Thus, it is important for the clinician to know what relevance to attach to these reports, and the strengths and weaknesses of the various imaging techniques. In general, imaging tests have a high sensitivity (few false negatives), but low specificity (high false-positive rate).

MISCELLANEOUS INFORMATION

Standard and Transmission-Based Precautions

See Tables 5-19 and 5-20.

The Intensive Care Unit Environment

A working knowledge of ICU equipment is important for the clinician so that interventions may be performed with the least disruption to the patient's care.

TABLE 5-19. STANDARD PRECAUTIONS

Hand Washing
1. Wash hands after touching blood, body fluids, secretions, excretions, and contaminated items, whether or not gloves are worn.
2. Wash hands immediately after removing gloves, between patient contacts, and when otherwise indicated to reduce transmission of microorganisms.
3. Wash hands between tasks and procedures on the same patient to prevent cross-contamination of different body sites.
4. Use plain (non-antimicrobial) agent for routine handwashing.
5. An antimicrobial agent or a waterless antiseptic agent may be used for specific circumstances (hyperendemic infections) as defined by infection control.

Gloves
1. Wear gloves (clean, unsterile gloves are adequate) when touching blood, body fluids, secretions, excretions, and contaminated items; put on clean gloves just before touching mucous membranes and nonintact skin.
2. Change gloves between tasks and procedures on the same patient after contact with materials that may contain high concentrations of microorganisms.
3. Remove gloves promptly after use, before touching uncontaminated items and environmental surfaces, and before going on to another patient; wash hands immediately after glove removal to avoid transfer of microorganisms to other patients or environments.

Mask and Eye Protection or Face Shield
1. Wear a mask and eye protection or a face shield to protect mucous membranes of the eyes, nose, and mouth during procedures and patient care activities that are likely to generate splashes or sprays of blood, body fluids, secretions, and excretions.

Gown
1. Wear a gown (a clean, unsterile gown is adequate) to protect skin and prevent soiling of clothing during procedures and patient care activities that are likely to generate splashes or sprays of blood, body fluids, secretions, and excretions.
2. Select a gown that is appropriate for the activity and the amount of fluid likely to be encountered.
3. Remove a soiled gown as soon as possible and wash hands to avoid transfer of microorganisms to other patients or environments.

Patient Care Equipment
1. Handle used patient care equipment soiled with blood, body fluids, secretions, and excretion in a manner that prevents skin and mucous membrane exposures, contamination of clothing, and transfer of microorganisms to other patients or environments.
2. Ensure that reusable equipment is not used for the care of another patient until it has been cleaned and reprocessed appropriately.
3. Ensure that single-use items are discarded properly.

Environmental Control
1. Follow hospital procedures for the routine care, cleaning and disinfection of environmental surfaces, beds, bed rails, bedside equipment, and other frequently touch surfaces.

Linen
1. Handle, transport, and process used linen soiled with blood, body fluids, secretions, and excretion in a manner that prevents skin and mucous membrane exposures and contamination of clothing, and avoids transfer of microorganisms to other patients or environments.

Occupational Health and Blood-Borne Pathogens
1. Prevent injuries when using needles, scalpels, and other sharp instruments or devices; when handling sharp instruments and procedures; when cleaning used instruments; and when disposing of used needles.
2. Never recap used needles, or otherwise manipulate them using both hands, or use any other technique that involves directing the point of the needle toward any part of the body; rather, use either a one-handed "scoop" technique or mechanical device designed for holding the needle sheath.
3. Do not remove used needles from disposable syringes by hand, and do not bend, break, or otherwise manipulate used needles by hand.
4. Place used disposable syringes and needles, scalpel blades, or other sharp items in appropriate puncture-resistant container for transport to the reprocessing area.
5. Use mouthpieces, resuscitation bags, or other ventilation devices as an alternative to mouth-to-mouth resuscitation.

Patient Placement
1. Use a private room for a patient who contaminates the environment or who does not (or cannot be expected to) assist in maintaining appropriate hygiene or environmental control.
2. Consult Infection Control if private room is not available.

From WHO Guidelines on Hand Hygiene in Health Care (Advanced draft), at: http://www.who.int/patientsafety/information_centre/ghhad_download/en/index.html (2007).

Airways

- Endotracheal tube: artificial airway inserted into a patient who is unable to oxygenate/ventilate on their own. The tube may be placed in the mouth or the nose. Verification of correct placement is done by x-ray, and once correctly placed must not be moved unless there is a written order from the physician.

TABLE 5-20. AIRBORNE, DROPLET, AND CONTACT PRECAUTIONS

Airborne Precautions

In addition to standard precautions, use airborne precautions, or the equivalent with all patients known or suspected to be infected with serious illness transmitted by airborne droplet nuclei (small-particle residue) that remain suspended in the air and that can be dispersed widely by air currents within a room or over long-distance (eg, *Mycobacterium tuberculosis*, measles virus, chickenpox virus).

1. Respiratory isolation room.
2. Wear respiratory protection (mask) when entering room.
3. Limit movement and transport of patient to essential purposes only. Mask patient when transporting out of area.

Droplet Precautions

In addition to standard precautions, use droplet precautions, or the equivalent, for patients known or suspected to be infected with serious illness microorganisms transmitted by large particle droplets that can be generated by the patient during coughing, sneezing, talking, or the performance of procedures (eg, mumps, rubella, pertussis, influenza).

1. Use isolation room.
2. Wear respiratory protection (mask) when entering room.
3. Limit movement and transport of patient to essential purposes only. Mask patient when transporting out of area.

Contact Precautions

In addition to standard precautions, use contact precautions, or the equivalent, for specified patients known or suspected to be infected or colonized with serious illness transmitted by direct patient contact (and or skin to skin contact) or contact with items in patient environment.

1. Use isolation room.
2. Wear gloves when entering room, change gloves after having contact with infective material, remove gloves before leaving patient's room, wash hands immediately with an antimicrobial agent or waterless antiseptic agent. After glove removal and hand washing, ensure that hands do not touch contaminated environmental items.
3. Wear a gown when entering room if you anticipate your clothing will have substantial contact with the patient, environmental surfaces, or items in the patient's room, or if the patient is incontinent or has diarrhea, ileostomy, colostomy, or wound drainage not contained by dressing. Remove gown before leaving patient's room; after gown removal, ensure that clothing does not contact potentially contaminated environmental surfaces.
4. Use single patient use equipment.
5. Limit movement and transport of patient to essential purposes only. Use precautions when transporting patient to minimize risk of transmission of microorganisms to other patients and contamination of environmental surfaces or equipment.

Data from Siegel JD, Rhinehart E, Jackson M, Chiarello L, and the Healthcare Infection Control Practices Advisory Committee, 2007: *Guideline for Isolation Precautions: Preventing Transmission of Infectious Agents in Healthcare Settings*, June 2007. www.cdc.gov/ncidod/dhqp/pdf/isolation2007.pdf.

- Tracheostomy tube: artificial airway inserted into a patient who is unable to oxygenate/ventilate on their own. This type of tube is usually not placed unless the patient has had an endotracheal tube in for an extended period of time and is unable to be weaned from the ventilator. Other instances in which the tracheostomy tube may be inserted include facial trauma, or difficulty placing the standard endotracheal tube.

Lines

- Arterial line: a catheter inserted to monitor arterial pressure at all times. Also used for drawing arterial blood gases. May be inserted into one of four arteries—radial, femoral, pedal, axillary. Arterial lines are usually changed every 4 to 5 days to decrease the risk of infection.
- Triple lumen: a venous catheter that is placed in the femoral vein, internal jugular vein, or subclavian vein to monitor central venous pressure (CVP). The tip of the catheter is usually placed in the superior vena cava.
- PA catheter (Swan-Ganz): very large venous catheter placed in the subclavian vein, the internal jugular vein, or the femoral vein (rarely). The catheter is inserted into the pulmonary artery via the heart.

- Uldall catheter: not strictly an IV—venous catheter used for dialysis, and continuous renal replacement therapy. Can be placed in the same areas as a triple lumen and a PA catheter.

Miscellaneous Equipment

- Chest tube: placed by a physician into the pleural space for drainage of fluid or air. The chest tube is connected to a large bottle, which is responsible for collecting air/fluid without permitting the lung to collapse. If the tube is accidentally dislodged or disconnected from the bottle, the patient's lung will collapse completely.
- Pigtail catheter: small catheter inserted into the pleural space for drainage of fluid only. The catheter may also be inserted into the peritoneum to drain ascites in a patient with liver disease. The catheter is connected to a drainage bag for collection of fluid.
- T-tube: placed into the common bile duct in order to drain bile after liver transplantation to assess if the liver is producing bile adequately.
- Jackson-Pratt: placed in a patient after liver transplantation to drain fluid and blood.
- ICP drain: inserted to remove excess fluid from the ventricles of the brain. Extreme care must be taken with patients who have an ICP inserted, as raising (increases the drainage, thereby lowering the ICP) or lowering (increases the ICP) the head of the bed can significantly change the ICP.

Study Pearl

The clinician should be very careful when doing range of motion exercises in an extremity in which a catheter has been placed, because if the catheter becomes disconnected or accidentally removed, it can result in hemorrhage, air emboli, arrhythmia, and/or catheter contamination.

Questions for this chapter and the entire book appear on the included CD-ROM, with additional questions at www.DuttonNPTE.com.

REFERENCES

1. Van de Graaff KM, Fox SI: Histology. In: Van de Graaff KM, Fox SI eds. *Concepts of Human Anatomy and Physiology.* New York: WCB/McGraw-Hill. 1999; 130-158.
2. Williams GR, Chmielewski T, Rudolph KS, et al: Dynamic knee stability: current theory and implications for clinicians and scientists. *J Orthop Sports Phys Ther.* 2001;31:546-566.
3. Prentice WE: Understanding and managing the healing process. In: Prentice WE, Voight ML, eds. *Techniques in Musculoskeletal Rehabilitation.* New York: McGraw-Hill. 2001;17-41.
4. Burgeson RE: New collagens new concepts. *Ann Rev Cell Biol.* 1988;4:551-577.
5. Engles M: Tissue response. In: Donatelli R, Wooden MJ, eds. *Orthopaedic Physical Therapy, 3rd ed.* Philadelphia, PA: Churchill Livingstone. 2001:1-24.
6. Barnes J: Myofascial Release: A Comprehensive Evaluatory and Treatment Approach. Paoli, PA: MFR Seminars. 1990.
7. Smolders JJ: Myofascial pain and dysfunction syndromes. In: Hammer WI, ed. *Functional Soft Tissue Examination and Treatment by Manual Methods—The Extremities.* Gaithersburg, MD: Aspen. 1991:215-234.

8. Ham AW, Cormack DH: *Histology, 8th ed.* Philadelphia, PA: Lippincott. 1979.
9. Clancy WG, Jr: Tendon trauma and overuse injuries. In: Leadbetter WB, Buckwalter JA, Gordon SL, eds. *Sports-Induced Inflammation.* Park Ridge, Illinois, IL: The American Academy of Orthopaedic Surgeons. 1990:609-618.
10. Teitz CC, Garrett WE, Jr., Miniaci A, et al: Tendon problems in athletic individuals. *J Bone and Joint Surg.* 1997;79-A:138-152.
11. Reid DC: *Sports Injury Assessment and Rehabilitation.* New York: Churchill Livingstone. 1992.
12. Garrett W, Tidball J: Myotendinous junction: structure, function, and failure. In: Woo SL-Y, Buckwalter JA, eds. *Injury and Repair of the Musculoskeletal Soft Tissues.* Rosemont, IL: AAOS. 1988.
13. Garrett WE: Muscle strain injuries. *Am J Sports Med.* 1996;24: S2-S8.
14. Safran MR, Seaber AV, Garrett WE: Warm-up and muscular injury prevention: an update. *Sports Med.* 1989;8:239-249.
15. Huijbregts PA: Muscle injury, regeneration, and repair. *J Man & Manip Ther.* 2001;9:9-16.
16. Safran MR, Benedetti RS, Bartolozzi AR, III., et al: Lateral ankle sprains: a comprehensive review: part 1: etiology, pathoanatomy, histopathogenesis, and diagnosis. *Medicine & Science in Sports & Exercise.* 1999;31:S429-S437.
17. Smith RL, Brunolli J: Shoulder kinesthesia after anterior glenohumeral dislocation. *Phys Ther.* 1989;69:106-112.
18. Mankin HJ, Mow VC, Buckwalter JA, et al: Form and function of articular cartilage. In: Simon SR, ed. *Orthopaedic Basic Science.* Rosemont, IL: American Academy of Orthopaedic Surgeons; 1994:1-44.
19. Woo SL-Y, Buckwalter JA: *Injury and Repair of the Musculoskeletal Tissue.* Park Ridge, IL: American Academy of Orthopaedic Surgeons. 1988.
20. Guccione AA, Minor MA: Arthritis. In: O'Sullivan SB, Schmitz TJ, eds. *Physical Rehabilitation, 5th ed.* Philadelphia, PA: FA Davis. 2007:1057-1085.
21. Jones D, Round D: Skeletal muscle in health and disease. *A Textbook of Muscle Physiology. Manchester: Manchester University Press.* 1990.
22. Van de Graaff KM, Fox SI: Muscle tissue and muscle physiology. In: Van de Graaff KM, Fox SI, eds. *Concepts of Human Anatomy and Physiology.* New York: WCB/McGraw-Hill. 1999:280-305.
23. Armstrong RB, Warren GL, Warren JA: Mechanisms of exercise-induced muscle fibre injury. *Med Sci Sports Exerc.* 1990;24: 436-443.
24. Williams JH, Klug GA: Calcium exchange hypothesis of skeletal muscle fatigue. A brief review. *Muscle & Nerve.* 1995;18:421.
25. Cyriax J: *Textbook of Orthopaedic Medicine, Diagnosis of Soft Tissue Lesions, 8th ed.* London: Bailliere Tindall. 1982.
26. Hall SJ: The biomechanics of human skeletal muscle. In: Hall SJ, ed. *Basic Biomechanics.* New York: McGraw-Hill. 1999:146-185.
27. MacConnail MA, Basmajian JV: *Muscles and Movements: A Basis for Human Kinesiology.* New York: Robert Krieger Pub Co. 1977.
28. Junqueira LC, Carneciro J: Bone. In: Junqueira LC, Carneciro J, eds. *Basic Histology, 10th ed.* New York: McGraw-Hill. 2003:141-159.

29. Chusid JG: *Correlative Neuroanatomy & Functional Neurology, 19th ed.* Norwalk: Conn, Appleton-Century-Crofts. 1985:144-148.
30. Freeman MAR, Wyke BD: An experimental study of articular neurology. *J Bone Joint Surg.* 1967;49B:185.
31. Wyke BD: The neurology of joints: a review of general principles. *Clinics in Rheumatic Diseases.* 1981;7:223-239.
32. Wyke BD: Articular neurology and manipulative therapy. In: Glasgow EF, Twomey LT, Scull ER, et al, eds. *Aspects of Manipulative Therapy, 2nd ed.* New York: Churchill Livingstone; 1985:72-77.
33. Wyke BD: The neurology of joints. *Ann R Coll Surg Engl.* 1967;41:25-50.
34. Grigg P: Peripheral neural mechanisms in proprioception. *J Sport Rehabil.* 1994;3:1-17.
35. Grigg P, Hoffmann AH: Properties of Ruffini afferents revealed by stress analysis of isolated sections of cat knee capsule. *J Neurophysiol.* 1982;47:41-54.
36. Borsa PA, Lephart SM, Kocher MS, et al: Functional assessment and rehabilitation of shoulder proprioception for glenohumeral instability. *J Sport Rehabil.* 1994;3:84-104.
37. Clark R, Wyke BD: Contributions of temporomandibular articular mechanoreceptors to the control of mandibular posture: an experimental study. *J Dent Assoc S Africa.*1974;2:121-129.
38. Skaggs CD: Diagnosis and treatment of temporomandibular disorders. In: Murphy DR, ed. *Cervical Spine Syndromes.* New York: McGraw-Hill. 2000:579-592.
39. Lephart SM, Pincivero DM, Giraldo JL, et al: The role of proprioception in the management of and rehabilitation of athletic injuries. *Am J Sports Med.* 1997;25:130-137.
40. Riddle DL: Measurement of accessory motion: critical issues and related concepts. *Phys Ther.* 1992;72:865-874.
41. Answorth AA, Warner JJP: Shoulder instability in the athlete. *Orthop Clin North Am.* 1995;26:487-504.
42. Bergmark A: Stability of the lumbar spine. *Acta Orthop Scand.* 1989;60:1-54.
43. Boden BP, Pearsall AW, Garrett WE, Jr., et al: Patellofemoral instability: evaluation and management. *J Am Acad Orthop Surgeons.* 1997;5:47-57.
44. Callanan M, Tzannes A, Hayes KC, et al: Shoulder instability. Diagnosis and management. *Austr Fam Phy.* 2001;30: 655-661.
45. Cass JR, Morrey BF: Ankle instability: current concepts, diagnosis, and treatment. *Mayo Clinic Proceedings.* 1984;59:165-170.
46. Clanton TO: Instability of the subtalar joint. *Orthop Clin N Am.* 1989;20:583-592.
47. Cox JS, Cooper PS: Patellofemoral instability. In: Fu FH, Harner CD, Vince KG, eds. *Knee Surgery.* Baltimore: Williams & Wilkins. 1994:959-962.
48. Freeman MAR, Dean MRE, Hanham IWF: The etiology and prevention of functional instability of the foot. *J. Bone Joint Surg.* 1965;47B:678-685.
49. Friberg O: Lumbar instability: a dynamic approach by traction-compression radiography. *Spine.* 1987;12:119-129.
50. Grieve GP: Lumbar instability. *Physiotherapy.* 1982;68:2.

51. Hotchkiss RN, Weiland AJ: Valgus stability of the elbow. *J Orthop Res.* 1987;5:372-377.
52. Kaigle A, Holm S, Hansson T: Experimental instability in the lumbar spine. *Spine.* 1995;20:421-430.
53. Kuhlmann JN, Fahrer M, Kapandji AI, et al: Stability of the normal wrist. In: Tubiana R, ed. *The Hand.* Philadelphia, PA: WB Saunders. 1985:934-944.
54. Landeros O, Frost HM, Higgins CC: Post traumatic anterior ankle instability. *Clin Orthop.* 1968;56:169-178.
55. Luttgens K, Hamilton N: The center of gravity and stability. In: Luttgens K, Hamilton N, eds. *Kinesiology: Scientific Basis of Human Motion, 9th ed.* Dubuque, IA: McGraw-Hill. 1997: 415-442.
56. Wilke H, Wolf S, Claes L, et al: of the lumbar spine with different muscle groups: a biomechanical in vitro study. *Spine.* 1995;20: 192-198.
57. Panjabi MM: The stabilizing system of the spine. Part 1. Function, dysfunction adaption and enhancement. *J Spinal Disord.* 1992;5:383-389.
58. McGill SM, Cholewicki J: Biomechanical basis for stability: an explanation to enhance clinical utility. *J Orthop Sports Phys Ther.* 2001;31:96-100.
59. Gertzbein SD, Seligman J, Holtby R, et al: Centrode patterns and segmental instability in degenerative disc disease. *Spine.* 1985;10:257-261.
60. Cholewicki J, McGill S: Mechanical stability of the in vivo lumbar spine: implications for injury and chronic low back pain. *Clin Biomech.* 1996;11:1-15.
61. Hall SJ: Kinematic concepts for analyzing human motion. In: Hall SJ, ed. *Basic Biomechanics.* New York: McGraw-Hill. 1999:28-89.
62. Schmitz TJ: Vital signs. In: O'Sullivan SB, Schmitz TJ, eds. *Physical Rehabilitation, 5th ed.* Philadelphia, PA: FA Davis. 2007:81-120.
63. Singer AJ, Clark RAF. Cutaneous wound healing. *N Engl J Med.* 1999;341:738-746.
64. Heldin C-H, Westermark B: Role of platelet-derived growth factor in vivo. In: Clark RAF, ed. *The Molecular and Cellular Biology of Wound Repai, 2nd ed.* New York: Plenum Press. 1996:249-273.
65. Katz MH, Kirsner RS, Eaglstein WH, et al: Human wound fluid from acute wounds stimulates fibroblast and endothelial cell growth. *J Am Acad Dermatol.* 1991;25:1054-1058.
66. Deuel TF, Senior RM, Chang D, et al: Platelet factor 4 is a chemotaxtic factor for neutrophils and monocytes. *Proc Natl Acad Sci.* 1981;74:4584-4587.
67. Schultz G, Rotatari DS, Clark W: EGF and TGF[alpha] in wound healing and repair. *J Cell Biochem.* 1991;45:346-352.
68. Sporn MB, Roberts AB: Transforming growth factor beta: recent progress and new challenges. *J Cell Biol.* 1992;119:1017-1021.
69. Wong MEK, Hollinger JO, Pinero GJ: Integrated processes responsible for soft tissue healing. *Oral Surg Oral Med Oral Pathol Oral Radiol Endod.* 1996;82:475-492.
70. Sen CK, Khanna S, Gordillo G, et al: Oxygen, oxidants, and antioxidants in wound healing: an emerging paradigm. *Ann N Y Acad Sci.* 2002;957:239-249.
71. Kellett J: Acute soft tissue injuries: a review of the literature. *Med Sci Sports Exerc.* 1986;18:5.

72. Amadio PC: Tendon and ligament. In: Cohen IK, Diegelman RF, Lindblad WJ, eds. *Wound Healing: Biomechanical and Clinical Aspects.* Philadelphia, PA: WB Saunders. 1992:384-395.
73. Hunt TK: *Wound Healing and Wound Infection: Theory and Surgical Practice.* New York: Appleton-Century-Crofts. 1980.
74. Peacock EE: *Wound Repair, 3rd ed.* Philadelphia, PA: WB Saunders. 1984.
75. Ross R: The fibroblast and wound repair. *Biol Rev.* 1969; 43:51-96.
76. McAllister BS, Leeb-Lunberg LM, Javors MA, et al: Bradykinin receptors and signal transduction pathways in human fibroblasts: integral role for extracellular calcium. *Arch Biochem Biophys.* 1993;304:294-301.
77. Evans RB: Clinical application of controlled stress to the healing extensor tendon: a review of 112 cases. *Phys Ther.* 1989; 69:1041-1049.
78. Emwemeka CS: Inflammation, cellularity, and fibrillogenesis in regenerating tendon: implications for tendon rehabilitation. *Phys Ther.* 1989;69:816-825.
79. Safran MR, Zachazewski JE, Benedetti RS, et al: Lateral ankle sprains: a comprehensive review part 2: treatment and rehabilitation with an emphasis on the athlete. *Med & Sci Sports Exerc.* 1999;31:S438-S447.
80. Oakes BW: Acute soft tissue injuries: nature and management. *Austr Family Physician.* 1982;10:3-16.
81. Van der Mueulin JHC: Present state of knowledge on processes of healing in collagen structures. *Int J Sports Med.* 1982;3:4-8.
82. Clayton ML, Wier GJ: Experimental investigations of ligamentous healing. *Am J Surg.* 1959;98:373-378.
83. Mason ML, Allen HS: The rate of healing of tendons. An experimental study of tensile strength. *Ann. Surg.* 1941;113:424-459.
84. Farfan HF: The scientific basis of manipulative procedures. *Clin Rheumat Dis.* 1980;6:159-177.
85. Orgill D, Demling RH: Current concepts and approaches to wound healing. *Crit Care Med.* 1988;16:899.

section II

Tests and Measures

Musculoskeletal Disorders and Diseases

Fractures

Neurologic Disorders and Diseases

Cerebrovascular Accident (Stroke)

Degenerative Diseases

Cognitive Disorders

Delirium, Dementia

Cardiovascular Disorders and Diseases

Hypertension

Coronary Artery Disease

Pulmonary Disorders and Diseases

Chronic Bronchitis/Chronic Obstructive Pulmonary Disease (COPD)

Asthma

Pneumonia

Lung Cancer

Integumentary Disorders and Diseases

Decubitus Ulcers

Metabolic Pathologies

Diabetes Mellitus

Ethical and Legal Issues

The Living Will (Advanced Care and Medical Directive)

Refusal of Treatment/Informed Consent

Do Not Resuscitate (DNR) Orders

Health-Care Proxy

Common Functional Problem Areas in the Geriatric Population

Immobility-Disability

Physical Therapy Intervention

Falls and Instability

Evaluation of the Elderly Patient Who Falls

Physical Therapy Intervention

Nutritional Deficiency

Physical Therapy Role

General Principles of Geriatric Rehabilitation

Chapter 15
Prosthetics, Orthotics, and Assistive Devices

Amputation

Levels of Amputation

Postoperative Period

Postoperative Dressings

Postoperative Physical Therapy

Postoperative Intervention

Lower Limb Prosthetic Designs

Partial Foot Amputations

Transphalangeal (Toe Disarticulation)

Transtibial (Below the Knee)

Transfemoral (Above the Knee)

Hip Disarticulation

Hemipelvectomy

Hemicorporectomy

Prosthetic Components

Shanks

Foot Socket Designs

Knee Socket Designs

Hip Joints

Hip Flexion Bias System

Littig Hip Strut

Lower Limb Prosthetic Training

Proprioceptive training

Gait Examination and Training

Abnormal Transtibial Gait

Abnormal Transfemoral Gait

Upper Limb Prosthetic Devices

Levels of Upper Limb Amputation

Terminal Devices

Hooks

Wrist Units

Transradial Sockets

Hinges

Transradial Harness and Controls

Elbow Units

Use of the Prosthesis

Orthotics

General Concepts

Lower Limb Orthoses: Components/ Terminology

Shoe Components

Foot Orthoses

Shoe Modifications

Ankle–Foot Orthoses (AFO)

Knee–Ankle–Foot Orthoses

Knee Orthotics

Hip–Knee–Ankle–Foot Orthoses

Reciprocal Gait Orthosis

Standing Frame and Swivel Walker

Parapodium

Thoracic and Lumbosacral Orthoses

Cervical Orthoses

Upper Limb Orthoses

Hand and Wrist Orthoses

Elbow Orthoses

Athletic Taping

Skin Preparation

Patent Ductus Arteriosus (PDA)
Tetralogy of Fallot

Musculoskeletal System

Congenital Muscular Torticollis
Talipes Equinovarus (Club Foot)
Developmental (Congenital)
Dysplasia of the Hip
Osteogenesis Imperfecta
Physical Therapy Role

Neurologic System

Hydrocephalus
Arthrogryposis
Brachial Plexus Injury
Spina Bifida
Prader-Willi Syndrome

The Role of the Physical Therapist in the Special Care Nursery

Developmental Interventions
Discharge Planning

Physical Therapy Roles for Specific Pediatric Pathologies

Asthma (Hyperreactive Airway Disease)

Physical Therapy Role

Cystic Fibrosis

Physical Therapy Role

Nursemaid's Elbow

Torsional Conditions

Slipped Capital Femoral Epiphysis

Physical Therapy Role

Legg-Calvé Perthes Disease

Physical therapy Role

Osgood Schlatter

Physical Therapy Role

Idiopathic Scoliosis

Physical Therapy Role

Cerebral Palsy

Physical Therapy Role

Myelodysplasia

Physical Therapy Role

Down Syndrome (Trisomy 21)

Physical Therapy Role

Brain Injury

Traumatic Brain Injury
Near-Drowning
Brain Tumors
Physical Therapy Role

Seizure Disorders

Duchenne Muscular Dystrophy

Physical Therapy Role

Spinal Muscular Atrophy

Physical Therapy Role

Oncology

Leukemia
Neuroblastoma
Lymphomas
Wilms Tumor
Bone Tumors
Physical Therapy Role in Oncology Cases

Rheumatology: Juvenile Rheumatoid Arthritis

Physical Therapy Role

Hematopoietic System: Hemophilia

Physical Therapy Role

The History and Systems Review

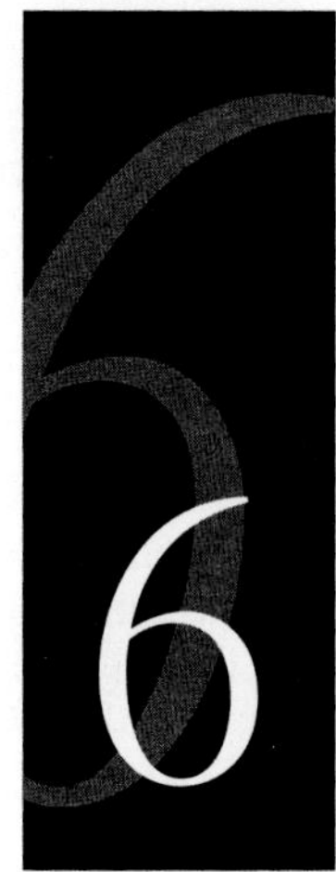

THE HISTORY

The purpose of the history (Table 6-1) is to:

1. Develop a working relationship and establish lines of communication with the patient.
2. Elicit reports of potentially dangerous symptoms, or *red flags,* that require an immediate medical referral (Table 6-2).[1]
3. Determine the chief complaint, its mechanism of injury, its severity, and its impact on the patient's function.
4. Ascertain the specific location and nature of the symptoms.
5. Determine the irritability of the symptoms.
6. Establish a baseline of measurements.
7. Elicit information on the history and past history of the current condition.
8. Gather information about the patient's past general medical and surgical history, which can afford the clinician some insight as to the impact the information may have on the patient's tolerance or response to the planned intervention.
9. Determine the goals and expectations of the patient from the physical therapy intervention, and the functional demands of a specific vocational or avocational activity to which the patient is planning to return.

HISTORY OF CURRENT CONDITION

This portion of the history taking involves the gathering of both positive and negative findings, followed by the dissemination of the information into a working hypothesis. An understanding of the patient's history of the current condition can often help determine the prognosis and guide the intervention.

Onset. The mode of onset, or mechanism of injury, can be either traumatic (macrotraumatic) or atraumatic (microtraumatic), and can give clues as to the extent and nature of the damage caused.

Study Pearl

Constant pain following an injury continues until the healing process has sufficiently reduced the concentration of noxious irritants.

TABLE 6-1. CONTENTS OF THE HISTORY

HISTORY OF CURRENT CONDITION
Did the symptoms begin slowly or was trauma involved?
How long has the patient had the presenting symptoms?
Where are the symptoms located?
How does the patient describe the symptoms?

PAST HISTORY OF CURRENT CONDITION
Has the patient had a similar injury in the past?
Was it treated or did it resolve on its own? If it was treated, how was it treated and did intervention help?
How long did the most recent episode last?

PAST MEDICAL/SURGERY HISTORY
How is the patient's general health?
What pertinent surgeries has the patient had?
Does the patient have any allergies?

MEDICATIONS PATIENT IS PRESENTLY TAKING, OTHER TESTS AND MEASURES
Has the patient had any imaging studies?
Has the patient had an EMG test, or a nerve conduction velocity test, which would suggest compromise to muscle tissue and/or neurologic system?

SOCIAL HABITS (PAST AND PRESENT)
Does the patient smoke? If so, how many packs per day?
Does the patient drink alcohol? If so, how often and how much?
Is the patient active or sedentary?

SOCIAL HISTORY
Is the patient married, living with a partner, single, divorced, widowed?
Is the patient a parent or single parent?

FAMILY HISTORY
Is there a family history of the present condition?

GROWTH AND DEVELOPMENT
Is the patient right- or left-handed?
Were there any congenital problems?

LIVING ENVIRONMENT
What type of home does the patient live in with reference to accessibility?
Is there any support at home?
Does the patient use any extra pillows or special chairs to sleep?

OCCUPATIONAL/EMPLOYMENT/SCHOOL
What does the patient do for work?
How long has he or she worked there?
What does the job entail in terms of physical requirements?
How does the present condition affect the patient at work?
What level of education did the patient achieve?

FUNCTIONAL STATUS/ACTIVITY LEVEL
How does the present condition affect the patient's ability to perform activities of daily living?
How does the patient's condition affect sleep?
Is the patient able to drive? If so, for how long?

CT, computed tomography; EMG, electromyogram; MRI, magnetic resonance imaging.
Data from Clarnette RG, Miniaci A: Clinical exam of the shoulder. *Med & Sci Sports Exercise.* 1998;30:1-6.

TABLE 6-2. SIGNS AND SYMPTOMS OF SERIOUS PATHOLOGY

SIGN OR SYMPTOM	POSSIBLE CAUSE
Fevers, chills, or night sweats	Systemic problem (infection, cancer, disease). Increased sweating can have a myriad of causes ranging from increased body temperature due to exertion, fever, apprehension, and compromise to the autonomic system. Night sweats are of particular concern as they can often indicate the presence of a systemic problem.[1]
Recent unexplained weight changes	An unexplained weight gain could be due to congestive heart failure, hypothyroidism, or cancer.[2] An unexplained weight loss could be due to a gastrointestinal disorder, hyperthyroidism, cancer, or diabetes.[2]
Malaise or fatigue	Systemic disease. Thyroid disease. Iron deficiency.
Unexplained nausea or vomiting	Never a good sign.
Dizziness	Although most causes of dizziness can be relatively benign, dizziness may signal a more serious problem, especially if the dizziness is associated with trauma to the neck or head, or with motions of cervical rotation and extension (vertebral artery compromise). The clinician must ascertain whether the symptoms result from vertigo, nausea, giddiness, unsteadiness, fainting, etc. Vertigo requires that the patient's physician be informed, for further investigation. However, in of itself, it is not usually a contraindication to the continuation of the examination.
Unilateral, bilateral, or quadrilateral paresthesias.	The seriousness of the paresthesia depends upon its distribution. Quadrilateral paresthesia always indicates the presence of central nervous system involvement.
Shortness of breath	Systemic problem.
Bowel or bladder dysfunction	Bowel and bladder dysfunction may indicate involvement of the cauda equina.
Night pain	Malignancy, if not related to movement.
Pain following eating	Gastrointestinal problems.
Weakness	Any weakness should be investigated by the clinician to determine whether it is the result of spinal nerve root compression, a peripheral nerve lesion, disuse, inhibition due to pain or swelling, an injury to the contractile or inert tissues (muscle, tendon, bursa etc), or a more serious pathology such as a fracture.
A gradual increase in the intensity of the pain	Radiating pain refers to an increase in pain intensity and distribution. Radiating pain typically travels distal from the site of the injury.
Radicular pain	Nerve root irritation.
Numbness	Numbness that is a dermatomal pattern indicates spinal nerve root compression.

Data from D'Ambrosia R: *Musculoskeletal Disorders: Regional Examination and Differential Diagnosis, 2nd ed.* Philadelphia, PA: Lippincott; 1986; and Goodman CC, Snyder TEK. *Differential Diagnosis in Physical Therapy.* Philadelphia, PA: W.B. Saunders. 1990.

Intensity. One of the simplest methods to quantify the intensity of pain is to use a 10-point visual analogue scale (VAS). The VAS is a numerically continuous scale that requires the pain level be identified by making a mark on a 100-mm line.[2] The patient is asked to rate their present pain compared with the worst pain they have ever experienced, with zero representing no pain, 1 representing minimally perceived pain, and 10 representing pain that requires immediate attention.[3]

Pain Perception. It is important to remember that pain perception is highly subjective. Pain is a broad and significant symptom that can be described using many descriptors.

Study Pearl

The aching type of pain, associated with degenerative arthritis and muscle disorders is often accentuated by activity and lessened by rest. Pain that is not alleviated by rest, that is not associated with acute trauma, may indicate the presence of a serious disorder such as a tumor or aneurysm. This pain is often described as deep, constant, and boring, and is apt to be more noticeable and more intense at night.[4]

Study Pearl

Patients with chronic pain may be more prone to depression and disrupted interpersonal relationships.[5-8]

Study Pearl

Because motor and sensory axons run in the same nerves, disorders of the peripheral nerves (neuropathies) usually affect both motor and sensory functions.

The symptoms of chronic pain typically behave in a mechanical fashion, in that they are provoked by activity or repeated movements, and reduced with rest, or a movement in the opposite direction.

Quality of Symptoms. The quality of the symptoms depends on the type of receptor being stimulated.

- Stimulation of the cutaneous A-delta nociceptors leads to pricking pain.[9]
- Stimulation of the cutaneous C nociceptors results in burning or dull pain.[10]
- Activation of the nociceptors in muscle by electrical stimulation produces aching pain.[11]
- Electrical stimulation of visceral nerves at low intensities results in vague sensations of fullness and nausea, but higher intensities cause a sensation of pain.[12]

Peripheral neuropathies can manifest as abnormal, frequently unpleasant sensations, which are variously described by the patient as numbness, pins and needles, and tingling.[13] When these sensations occur spontaneously without an external sensory stimulus, they are called *paresthesias* (Table 6-3).[13] Patients with paresthesias typically demonstrate a reduction in the perception of cutaneous and proprioceptive sensations.

Motivational-affective circuits can also mimic pain states, most notably in patients with anxiety, neurotic depression, or hysteria.[7] The MADISON mnemonic outlines the behavioral indicators that suggest motivational-affective pain.[14,15]

Multiple complaints, including complaints about unrelated body parts

Authenticity claims in an attempt to convince the clinician the symptoms exist

Denial of the negative effect the pain is having on function

Interpersonal variability, manifested by different complaints to different clinicians or support staff

Singularity of symptoms, where the patient requests special consideration due to their type and level of pain

Only you, where the clinician is placed at a special level of expertise

Nothing works, where every attempt and approach provides no relief

TABLE 6-3. CAUSES OF PARESTHESIA

PARESTHESIA LOCATION	PROBABLE CAUSE
Lip (perioral)	Vertebral artery occlusion
Bilateral lower or bilateral upper extremities	Central protrusion of intervertebral disk impinging on spine
All extremities simultaneously	Spinal cord compression
One half of body	Cerebral hemisphere
Segmental (in dermatomal pattern)	Disk or nerve root
Glove-and-stocking distribution	Diabetes mellitus neuropathy, lead or mercury poisoning
Half of face and opposite half of body	Brain stem impairment

Frequency and Duration. The frequency and duration of the patient's symptoms can help the clinician to classify the injury according to its stage of healing: acute (inflammatory), subacute (migratory and proliferative), and chronic (remodeling) (Table 5-31).

Study Pearl

The persistence of symptoms usually indicates a poorer prognosis, as it may indicate the presence of a chronic pain syndrome. Chronic pain syndromes have the potential to complicate the intervention process.[16]

Aggravating and Easing Factors. Of particular importance are the patient's chief complaint and the relationship of that complaint to specific aggravating activities or postures. Musculoskeletal conditions are typically aggravated with movement and alleviated with rest (Table 6-4). If no activities or postures are reported to aggravate the symptoms, the clinician needs to probe for more information. Nonmechanical events that provoke the symptoms could indicate a non-musculoskeletal source for the pain:[17]

- Night pain: pain at night, unrelated to movement, that disturbs or prevents sleep may indicate a malignancy.
- Eating: pain that increases with eating may suggest gastrointestinal involvement.
- Stress: an increase in overall muscle tension prevents muscles from resting.
- Cyclical pain: cyclical pain can often be related to systemic events, eg, menstrual pain.

If aggravating movements or positions have been reported, they should be tested at the end of the tests and measures, to avoid any overflow of symptoms, which could confuse the clinician.

Study Pearl

Any relieving factors reported by the patient can often provide sufficient information to assist the clinician in the intervention plan.

Location. The clinician should determine the location of the symptoms, as this can indicate which areas need to be included in the physical examination. Information about how the location of the symptoms has changed since the onset can indicate whether a condition is worsening or improving. In general, as a condition worsens, the symptom distribution becomes more widespread and distal (peripheralizes). As the condition improves, the symptoms tend to become more localized (centralized). A body chart may be used to record the location of symptoms.

It must be remembered that the location of symptoms for many conditions is quite separate from the source. The term *referred pain* is used to describe those symptoms that have their origin at a site other than where the patient feels the pain. If the extremity appears to be the source of the symptoms, the clinician should attempt to reproduce the symptoms by loading the peripheral tissues. If this proves unsuccessful, a full investigation of the spinal structures must ensue.

Study Pearl

Symptoms that are distal and superficial are easier for the patient to specifically localize than those that are proximal and deep.

TABLE 6-4. DIFFERENTIATION BETWEEN MUSCULOSKELETAL AND SYSTEMIC PAIN

MUSCULOSKELETAL PAIN	SYSTEMIC PAIN
Usually decreases with cessation of activity	Reduced by pressure
Generally lessens at night	Disturbs sleep
Aggravated with mechanical stress	Not aggravated by mechanical stress
Usually continuous or intermittent	Usually constant or in waves

Reproduced, with permission, from Meadows J: *Orthopedic Differential Diagnosis in Physical Therapy*. New York: McGraw-Hill. 1999.

Behavior of Symptoms. The behavior of the symptoms aids the clinician in determining the stage of healing and the impact it has on the patient's function. Whether the pain is worsening, improving, or unchanging provides information on the effectiveness of an intervention. In addition, a gradual increase in the intensity of the symptoms over time may indicate to the clinician that the condition is worsening, or that the condition is nonmusculoskeletal in nature.[17,18]

Maitland[19] introduced the concept of the *degree of irritability*. An irritable structure has the following characteristics:

- A progressive increase in the severity of the symptoms with movement or a specific posture. An ability to reproduce constant symptoms with a specific motion or posture indicates an irritable structure.
- Symptoms increased with minimal activity. An irritable structure is one which requires very little to increase the symptoms.
- Increased latent response of symptoms. Symptoms do not usually resolve within a few minutes following a movement or posture.

According to McKenzie,[16] the intervention for the patient whose symptoms have a low degree of irritability, and are gradually resolving, should focus on only education initially. However, if the improvement ceases, a mechanical intervention may then be necessary.[16]

The Nature of the Symptoms. The clinician must determine whether pain is the only symptom, or whether there are other symptoms that accompany the pain, such as dizziness, bowel and bladder changes, tingling (paresthesia), radicular pain/numbness, weakness, and increased sweating.

- Dizziness. Dizziness (vertigo) is a nonspecific neurologic symptom that requires a careful diagnostic workup. A report of vertigo, although potentially problematic, is not a contraindication to the continuation of the examination. Differential diagnosis includes primary central nervous system diseases, vestibular and ocular involvement, and, more rarely, metabolic disorders (see Systems Review).
- Bowel or bladder dysfunction usually indicates a compromise (compression) of the cauda equina.
- Paresthesia. The seriousness of the paresthesia depends upon its distribution. While complaints of paresthesia can be the result of a relatively benign impingement of a peripheral nerve, the reasons for its presence can vary in severity and seriousness (Table 6-3).
- Radicular pain is produced by nerve root irritation. This type of pain is typically sharp or shooting. Numbness that is a dermatomal pattern indicates spinal nerve root compression. Radiating pain refers to an increase in pain intensity and distribution. Radiating pain typically travels distally from the site of the injury.

- Weakness. Any weakness should be investigated by the clinician to determine whether it is the result of spinal nerve root compression, a peripheral nerve lesion, disuse, inhibition due to pain or swelling, an injury to the contractile or inert tissues (muscle, tendon, bursa etc), or a more serious pathology such as a fracture.

Past History of Current Condition. It is important for the clinician to determine whether the patient has had successive onsets of similar symptoms in the past, as recurrent injury tends to have a detrimental effect on the potential for recovery. If it is a recurrent injury, the clinician should note how often, and how easily, the injury has recurred, and the success or failure of previous interventions.

PAST MEDICAL AND SURGICAL HISTORY

The patient's past medical history (PMH) can be obtained through a questionnaire (Table 6-5). The PMH can provide information with regard to allergies, childhood illnesses, and previous trauma. In addition, information on any health conditions such as cardiac problems, high-blood pressure, or diabetes should be elicited as these may impact exercise tolerance (cardiac problems, high-blood pressure) and speed of healing (diabetes).

If the surgical history (Table 6-5) is related to the current problem, the clinician should obtain as much detail about the surgery as possible from the surgical report, including any complications, precautions, or postsurgical protocols.

FAMILY HISTORY AND GENERAL HEALTH STATUS

Certain diseases, such as rheumatoid arthritis, diabetes, cardiovascular disease, and cancer have familial tendencies.

The general health status refers to a review of the patient's health perception, physical and psychological function, as well as any specific questions related to a particular body region or complaint.[20]

MEDICATIONS

Although the dispensing of medications is out of the scope of practice for a physical therapist, questioning the patient about their prescribed medications can reveal medical conditions that the patient might not consider related to his or her present problem.[1] Medications can also have an impact on clinical findings and the success of an intervention (see Chapter 19).[21]

SYSTEMS REVIEW

The purpose of the systems review is to:

- Help determine the anatomical and physiological status of all systems (ie, musculoskeletal, neurological, cardiovascular, pulmonary, integumentary, gastrointestinal [GI], urinary, and genital reproductive).[22]

> **Study Pearl**
>
> Symptom magnification, an exaggerated subjective response to symptoms in the absence of adequate objective findings, is an increasingly common occurrence in the clinic.

TABLE 6-5. SAMPLE MEDICAL HISTORY QUESTIONNAIRE

GENERAL INFORMATION

____Date: ________________

Last Name First Name

The information requested may be needed if you have a medical emergency.

____________________________ ____________________________ ______________________________________

Person to be notified in emergency Phone Relationship

Are you currently working? (Y) or (N) Type of work: If not, why?

GENERAL MEDICAL HISTORY:

Please check (√) if you have been treated for:

( ) Heart problems
( ) Fainting or dizziness
( ) Shortness of breath
( ) Calf pain with exercise
( ) Severe headaches
( ) Recent accident
( ) Head trauma/concussion
( ) Muscular weakness
( ) Cancer
( ) Joint dislocation(s)
( ) Broken bone
( ) Difficulty sleeping
( ) Frequent falls
( ) Unexplained weight loss
( ) Tremors
( ) High blood pressure (hypertension)
( ) Kidney disease
( ) Liver disease
( ) Weakness or fatigue
( ) Hernias
( ) Blurred vision
( ) Bowel/bladder problems
( ) Difficulty swallowing
( ) A wound that does not heal
( ) Unusual skin coloration
( ) Lung disease/problems
( ) Arthritis
( ) Swollen and painful joints
( ) Irregular heart beat
( ) Stomach pains or ulcers
( ) Pain with cough or sneeze
( ) Back or neck injuries
( ) Diabetes
( ) Stroke(s)
( ) Balance problems
( ) Muscular pain with activity
( ) Swollen ankles or legs
( ) Jaw problems
( ) Circulatory problems
( ) Epilepsy/seizures/convulsions
( ) Chest pain or pressure at rest
( ) Allergies (latex, medication, food)
( ) Constant pain unrelieved by rest
( ) Pregnancy
( ) Night pain (while sleeping)
( ) Nervous or emotional problems
( ) Any infectious disease (TB, AIDS, hepatitis)
( ) Tingling, numbness, or loss of feeling? If yes, where?
( ) Constant pain or pressure during activity

Do you use tobacco? (Y) or (N) If yes, how much?

Are you presently taking any medications or drugs? (Y) or (N)

If yes, what are you taking them for?

1. Pain

On the line provided, mark where your "pain status" is today.

|———————————————————|

No pain Most severe pain

2. Function. On a scale of 0 to 10 with 0 being able to perform all of your normal daily activities, and 10 being unable to perform any of your normal daily activities, give yourself a score for your *current ability* to perform your activities of daily living.

Please list any major surgery or hospitalization:

Hospital:_____________________ Approx. Date:__________________

Reasons:

Hospital:_____________________ Approx. Date:__________________

Reasons:

Have you recently had an x-ray, MRI, or CT scan for your condition? (Y) or (N)

Facility:______________________ Approx. date:__________________

Findings:

Please mention any additional problems or symptoms you feel are important:

Have you been evaluated and/or treated by another physician, physical therapist, chiropractor, osteopath, or health care practitioner for this condition? (Y) or (N) If yes, please circle which one.

- Provide information about communication skills, affect, cognition, language abilities, education needs, and learning style of the patient.[22]
- Narrow the focus of subsequent tests and measures.
- Define areas that may cause complications or indicate a need for precautions during the examination and intervention processes.
- Screen for physical, sexual, and psychological abuse.
- Make a determination of the need for further physical therapy services based on an evaluation of the information obtained.
- Identify problems that require consultation with, or referral to, another health care provider.

With the majority of states now permitting direct access to physical therapists, many physical therapists now have the primary responsibility for being the gatekeepers of health care and for making medical referrals. In light of the American Physical Therapy Association's (APTA's) movement toward realizing "Vision 2020," an operational definition of autonomous practice and the related term autonomous physical therapist practitioner is defined by the APTA's Board as follows:

- Autonomous physical therapist practice is practice characterized by independent, self-determined professional judgment and action.
- An autonomous physical therapist practitioner within the scope of practice defined by the *Guide to Physical Therapist Practice* provides physical therapy services to patients who have direct and unrestricted access to their services, and may refer as appropriate to other health care providers and other professionals and for diagnostic tests.[22]

The systems review, in addition to the scanning examination (Table 6-6) is the critical part of the examination that identifies possible health problems that require consultation with, or referral to, another health care provider.[20] All patients should be questioned about their general health. This is usually obtained using a patient self-report questionnaire (Table 6-5). The self-report questionnaire should be designed to address such issues as:[23]

- Fatigue: complaints of feeling tired or run down are extremely common and therefore often only become significant if the

TABLE 6-6. COMPONENTS OF THE SCANNING EXAMINATION AND THE STRUCTURES TESTED

ACTIVE ROM	Willingness to move, ROM, integrity of contractile and inert tissues, pattern of restriction (capsular, or non-capsular), quality of motion, and symptom reproduction
PASSIVE ROM	Integrity of inert and contractile tissues, ROM, end feel, sensitivity/irritability
RESISTED	Integrity of contractile tissues (strength, sensitivity)
STRESS	Integrity of inert tissues (ligamentous/disc stability)
DURAL	Dural mobility
NEUROLOGICAL	Nerve conduction
DERMATOME	Afferent (sensation) pathway
MYOTOME	Efferent (strength, fatigability) pathway
REFLEXES	Afferent-efferent pathways and central nervous systems

TABLE 6-7. CONDITIONS PRESENTING AS CHRONIC FATIGUE

Psychological	Depression
	Anxiety
	Somatization disorder
Endocrine/metabolic	Hypothyroidism
	Diabetes mellitus
	Pituitary insufficiency
	Addison disease
	Chronic renal failure
	Hyperparathyroidism
Infectious	Endocarditis
	Tuberculosis
	Mononucleosis
	Hepatitis
	HIV infection
Neoplasms	Occult malignancy
Cardiopulmonary	Congestive heart failure
	Chronic obstructive pulmonary disease
Connective tissue disease	Rheumatic disorders
Sleep disturbances	Sleep apnea
	Esophageal reflux
Allergic rhinitis	Lethargy

Reproduced, with permission, from Boissonnault WG: Review of systems. In: Boissonnault WG, ed. *Primary Care for the Physical Therapist: Examination and Triage* St. Louis: Elsevier W.B. Saunders. 2005:87-104. Copyright © Elsevier.

patient reports that tiredness interferes with the ability to carry out typical daily activities and when the fatigue has lasted for 2 to 4 weeks or longer. Many serious and benign illnesses can cause fatigue (Table 6-7).

- Malaise: a sense of uneasiness or general discomfort that is often associated with conditions that generate fever.
- Fever/chills/sweats: these are signs and symptoms that are most often associated with systemic illnesses such as cancer, infections, and connective tissue disorders such as rheumatoid arthritis. To qualify as a red flag, the fever should have some longevity (2 weeks or longer).
- Unexpected weight change: a sensitive but non-specific finding that can be a normal physiologic response, but may also be associated with depression, cancer, or gastrointestinal disease.
- Nausea/vomiting: persistent vomiting is an uncommon complaint reported to a physical therapist, as the physician will have already been contacted. However, a low-grade nausea, which can be caused by systemic illness or an adverse drug reaction, may be reported.
- Dizziness/lightheadedness: [24] careful questioning can help in the differentiation of central and peripheral causes of vertigo. Dizziness provoked by head movements or head positions could indicate an inner ear dysfunction. Dizziness provoked by certain cervical motions, particularly extension or rotation, also may indicate vertebral artery compromise.
- Paresthesia/numbness/weakness (Table 6-3).

- Change in mentation/cognition: this can be a manifestation of multiple disorders including delirium, dementia, head injury, stroke, infection, fever, and adverse drug reactions. The clinician notes whether the patient's communication level is age appropriate, whether the patient is oriented to person, place, and time, and whether her emotional and behavioral responses appear to be appropriate to his or her circumstances.

The systems review includes an assessment of the anatomical and physiological status of all systems including:[22]

- The cardiopulmonary system, the assessment of heart rate, respiratory rate, blood pressure, and edema. The four so-called *vital signs* which are standard in most medical settings include: temperature, heart rate, blood pressure, and respiratory rate. Pain is considered by many to be the fifth vital sign.[25-36] The clinician should monitor at least heart rate and blood pressure in any person with a history of cardiovascular disease or pulmonary disease, or those at risk for heart disease.[37] The equipment needed to assess these vital signs is a thermometer, a blood pressure (BP) cuff with a stethoscope (or an automatic BP machine), and a watch or clock.
  - ***Temperature.*** Body temperature is one indication of the metabolic state of an individual; measurements provide information concerning basal metabolic state, possible presence or absence of infection, and metabolic response to exercise.[38] "Normal" body temperature of the adult is 98.4°F (37°C). However, a temperature in the range of 96.5°F (35.8°C) and 99.4°F (37.4°C) are not at all uncommon. Fever or pyrexia is a temperature exceeding 100°F (37.7°C).[39] Hyperpyrexia refers to extreme elevation of temperature above 106°F (41.1°C).[36] Hypothermia refers to an abnormally low temperature (below 95°F [35°C]). The temperature is generally taken by placing the bulb of a thermometer under the patient's tongue for 1 to 3 minutes depending on the device. In most individuals, there is a diurnal (occurring everyday) variation in body temperature of 0.5° F to 2° F. The lowest ebb is reached during sleep. Menstruating women have a well-known temperature pattern that reflects the effects of ovulation, with the temperature dropping slightly before menstruation, and then dropping further 24 to 36 hours prior to ovulation.[37] Coincident with ovulation, the temperature rises and remains at a somewhat higher level until just before the next menses. It is also worth noting that in adults over 75 years of age and in those who are immunocompromised (eg, transplant recipients, corticosteroid users, persons with chronic renal insufficiency, or anyone taking excessive antipyretic medications) fever response may be blunted or absent.[36]
  - ***Heart rate.*** In most people, the pulse is an accurate measure of heart rate. The heart rate or pulse is taken to a contain information about the resting state of the cardiovascular system and the system's response to activity or exercise and recovery.[36] It is also used to assess patency of the specific arteries palpated, and the presence of any irregularities in the rhythm[36] (see Chapter 11).

- ***Respiratory rate.*** The normal chest expansion difference between the resting position and the fully inhaled position is 2 to 4 cm (females > males). The clinician should compare measurements of both the anterior-posterior diameter and the transverse diameter during rest and at full inhalation. Normal respiratory rate is between 8 and 14 breaths per minute in adults, and slightly quicker in children. The examination of breathing patterns is described in Chapter 10.
- ***Blood pressure.*** Blood pressure is a measure of vascular resistance to blood flow (see Chapter 12).[36]
- ***Edema.*** Edema is an observable swelling from fluid accumulation in certain body tissues. Edema most commonly occurs in the feet and legs, where it also is referred to as peripheral edema. Swelling or edema may be localized at the site of an injury or diffused over a larger area due to a systemic disorder (eg, congestive heart failure or renal disease). In general, the amount of swelling is related to the severity of the condition. The swelling occurs as a result of changes in the local circulation and an inability of the lymphatic system to maintain equilibrium, which causes an accumulation of excess fluid under the skin in the interstitial spaces or compartments within the tissues that are outside of the blood vessels.

The more serious reasons for swelling include fracture, tumor, and deep vein thrombosis. See Chapters 11 and 12 for more details regarding the lymphatic system and the various types of edema.

- ▶ For the integumentary system, the assessment of skin integrity, skin color, and presence of scar formation (see Chapter 13).
- ▶ For the musculoskeletal system, the assessment of gross symmetry, gross range of motion, gross strength, weight, and height (see Chapter 8).
- ▶ For the neuromuscular system, a general assessment of gross coordinated movement (eg, balance, locomotion, transfers, and transitions). In addition, the clinician observes for peripheral and cranial nerve integrity (see Chapter 9) and notes any indication of neurological compromise. For communication ability, affect, cognition, language, and learning style, it is important to verify that the patient can communicate his or her needs. The clinician should determine whether the patient has a good understanding about his or her condition, the planned intervention, and the prognosis. The clinician should also determine the learning style that best suits the patient.

Finally, it is well worth investigating the possibility that the presenting signs and symptoms are because of an adverse drug reaction (Table 6-8).

THE SCANNING EXAMINATION FOR NEUROMUSCULOSKELETAL CONDITIONS

Designed by Cyriax,[38] the scanning (screening) examination traditionally follows the history and is often incorporated as part of the systems review. Although two studies[39,40] questioned the validity of some

TABLE 6-8. MEDICATION SIDE EFFECTS AND SUBJECTIVE SYMPTOMS

SIDE EFFECTS AND SUBJECTIVE SYMPTOMS	MEDICATIONS (IN ORDER OF MOST COMMON OCCURRENCE)
Gastrointestinal distress (dyspepsia, heartburn, nausea, vomiting, abdominal pain, constipation, diarrhea, bleeding)	Salicylates Nonsteroidal anti-inflammatory drugs (NSAIDs) Opioids Corticosteroids Beta-blockers Calcium channel blockers Skeletal muscle relaxants Diuretics Angiotensin-converting enzyme (ACE) inhibitors Digoxin Nitrates Cholesterol-lowering agents Antiarrhythmic agents Antidepressants (tricyclic antidepressants, monoamine oxidase inhibitors, lithium) Neuroleptics Antiepileptic agents Oral contraceptives Estrogens and progestins Theophylline
Pulmonary (bronchospasm, shortness of breath, respiratory depression)	Salicylates NSAIDs Opioids Beta blockers ACE inhibitors
Central nervous system (dizziness, drowsiness, insomnia, headaches, hallucinations, confusion, anxiety, depression, muscle weakness)	NSAIDs Skeletal muscle relaxants Opioids Corticosteroids Beta-blockers Calcium channel blockers Nitrates ACE inhibitors Digoxin Antianxiety agents Antidepressants (tricyclic antidepressants, monoamine oxidase inhibitors) Neuroleptics Antiepileptic agents Oral contraceptives Estrogens and progestins
Dermatologic (skin rash, itching, flushing of face)	NSAIDs Corticosteroids Beta-blockers Opioids Calcium channel blockers ACE inhibitors Nitrates Cholesterol-lowering agents Antiarrhythmic agents Antidepressants (monoamine oxidase inhibitors, lithium) Oral contraceptives Estrogens and progestins Antiepileptics

(*Continued*)

TABLE 6-8. MEDICATION SIDE EFFECTS AND SUBJECTIVE SYMPTOMS (*Continued*)

SIDE EFFECTS AND SUBJECTIVE SYMPTOMS	MEDICATIONS (IN ORDER OF MOST COMMON OCCURRENCE)
Musculoskeletal (weakness, fatigue, cramps, arthritis, reduced exercise tolerance, osteoporosis)	Corticosteroids Beta-blockers Calcium channel blockers ACE inhibitors Diuretics Digoxin Anti-anxiety agents Anti-epileptic agents Antidepressants Neuroleptic agents
Cardiac (bradycardia, ventricular irritability, AV block, congestive heart failure, PVCs, ventricular tachycardia)	Opioids Diuretics Beta-blockers Calcium channel blockers Digoxin Antiarrhythmic agents Tricyclic antidepressants Neuroleptics Oral antiasthmatic agents
Vascular (claudication, hypotension, peripheral edema, cold extremities)	NSAIDs Corticosteroids Diuretics Beta-blockers Calcium channel blockers ACE inhibitors Nitrates Antidepressants (tricyclic antidepressants, monoamine oxidase inhibitors) Neuroleptics Oral contraceptives Estrogens and progestins
Genitourinary (sexual dysfunction, urinary retention, urinary incontinence)	Opioids Diuretics Beta-blockers Antiarrhythmic agents Antidepressants (tricyclic antidepressants, monoamine oxidase inhibitors) Neuroleptics Oral contraceptives Estrogens and progestins
Head, eyes, ears, nose, and throat (tinnitus, loss of taste, headache, lightheadedness, dizziness)	Salicylates NSAIDs Opioids Skeletal muscle relaxants Beta-blockers Nitrates Calcium channel blockers ACE inhibitors Digoxin Antiarrhythmic agents Antianxiety agents Antidepressants (tricyclic antidepressants, monoamine oxidase inhibitors) Antiepileptic agents

Reproduced, with permission, from Boissonnault WG: Review of systems. In: Boissonnault WG, ed. *Primary Care for the Physical Therapist: Examination and Triage.* St. Louis: Elsevier W.B. Saunders. 2005:87-104; and Data from Cain SD, Janos SC: Clinical pharmacology for the physical therapist. In: Boissonnault W, ed. *Examination in Physical Therapy Practice: Screening for Medical Disease, 2nd ed.* New York: Churchill Livingstone. 1995:350-351.

aspects of the selective tissue tension examination, no definitive conclusions were drawn from these studies. The scarcity of research to refute the work of Cyriax would suggest that its principles are sound, and that its use should be continued.

The purpose of the scanning examination is to help rule out the possibility of symptom referral from other areas, and to ensure that all possible causes of the symptoms are examined. In addition, the scanning examination helps narrow the search for the source(s) of symptoms to a specific body region and to identify any red flags that were alluded to during the history or physical examination. It was Grieve[41] who coined the term *masqueraders* to indicate those conditions which may not be musculoskeletal in origin, and which may require skilled intervention elsewhere (Table 6-9).

The scanning examination is divided into two examinations: one for the lower quarter/quadrant (Table 6-10) and the other for the upper quarter/quadrant (Table 6-11). The tests that comprise the scanning examination are designed to detect neurological weakness, the patient's ability to perceive sensations, and the inhibition of the muscle stretch (deep tendon reflexes, DTR) and other reflexes by the central nervous system.

TABLE 6-9. EXAMINATION FINDINGS AND THE POSSIBLE CONDITIONS CAUSING THEM

FINDINGS	POSSIBLE CONDITION
Dizziness	Upper cervical impairment, vertebrobasilar ischemia, craniovertebral ligament tear; may also be relatively benign
Quadrilateral paresthesia	Cord compression, vertebrobasilar ischemia
Bilateral upper limb paresthesia	Cord compression, vertebrobasilar ischemia
Hyper-reflexia	Cord compression, vertebrobasilar ischemia
Babinski or clonus sign	Cord compression, vertebrobasilar ischemia
Consistent swallow on transverse ligament stress tests	Instability, retropharyngeal hematoma, rheumatoid arthritis
Nontraumatic capsular pattern	Rheumatoid arthritis, ankylosing spondylitis, neoplasm
Arm pain lasting > 6-9 mo	Neoplasm
Persistent root pain < 30 y	Neoplasm
Radicular pain with coughing	Neoplasm
Pain worsening after 1 mo	Neoplasm
> 1 level involved (cervical region)	Neoplasm
Paralysis	Neoplasm or neurologic disease
Trunk and limb paresthesia	Neoplasm
Bilateral root signs and symptoms	Neoplasm
Nontraumatic strong spasm	Neoplasm
Nontraumatic strong pain in elderly patient	Neoplasm
Signs worse than symptoms	Neoplasm
Radial deviator weakness	Neoplasm
Thumb flexor weakness	Neoplasm
Hand intrinsic weakness and/or atrophy	Neoplasm, thoracic outlet syndrome, carpal tunnel syndrome
Horner syndrome	Superior sulcus tumor, breast cancer, cervical ganglion damage, brain stem damage
Empty end-feel	Neoplasm
Severe posttraumatic capsular pattern	Fracture
Severe posttraumatic spasm	Fracture
Loss of range of motion posttrauma	Fracture
Posttraumatic painful weakness	Fracture

Reproduced, with permission, from Meadows J: *Orthopedic Differential Diagnosis in Physical Therapy*. New York: McGraw-Hill. 1999.

TABLE 6-10. THE LOWER QUARTER SCANNING MOTOR EXAMINATION

MUSCLE ACTION	MUSCLE TESTED	ROOT LEVEL	PERIPHERAL NERVE
Hip flexion	Iliopsoas	L1-L2	Femoral to iliacus and lumbar plexus to psoas
Knee extension	Quadriceps	L2-L4	Femoral
Hamstrings	Biceps femoris, semimembranosus, and semitendinosus	L4-S3	Sciatic
Dorsiflexion with inversion	Tibialis anterior	Primarily L4	Deep peroneal
Great toe extension	Extensor hallicus longus	Primarily L5	Deep fibular (peroneal) nerve
Ankle eversion	Fibularis (peroneus) longus and brevis	Primarily S1	Superficial fibular (peroneal) nerve
Ankle plantarflexion	Gastrocnemius and soleus	Primarily S1	Tibial
Hip extension	Gluteus maximus	L5-S2	Inferior gluteal nerve

The tests used in the scanning examination (Table 6-6) produce a medical diagnosis, rather than a physical therapy one.[42] Those diagnoses can include:

- Neurological pathology, which can either be treated (mechanical nerve root compression from a disc protrusion, or inflammation), or is out of the scope of a physical therapist (tumor, upper motor neuron impairment, and cauda equina impairment) (Table 6-2)
- Fracture
- Tendinitis, bursitis, muscle tear
- Tendon avulsion

If a diagnosis is rendered from the scan, an intervention may be initiated using the guidelines outlined in Table 6-12.

Often though, the scanning examination does not generate enough signs and symptoms to formulate a working hypothesis or a diagnosis. In which case, further testing with the tests and measures is required in order to proceed.

TABLE 6-11. THE UPPER QUARTER SCANNING MOTOR EXAMINATION

RESISTED ACTION	MUSCLE TESTED	ROOT LEVEL	PERIPHERAL NERVE
Shoulder abduction	Deltoid	Primarily C5	Axillary
Elbow flexion	Biceps brachii	Primarily C6	Musculocutaneous
Elbow extension	Triceps brachii	Primarily C7	Radial
Wrist extension	Extensor carpi radialis longus, brevis, and extensor carpi ulnaris	Primarily C6	Radial
Wrist flexion	Flexor carpi radialis and flexor carpi ulnaris	Primarily C7	Median nerve for radialis and ulnar nerve for ulnaris
Finger flexion	Flexor digitorum superficialis, flexor digitorum profundus, and lumbricales	Primarily C8	Median nerve superficialis, both median and ulnar nerve for profundus and lumbricales
Finger abduction	Dorsal interossei	Primarily T1	Ulnar

TABLE 6-12. SCAN FINDINGS AND INTERVENTIONS

CONDITIONS	FINDINGS	PROTOCOL
Disk protrusion, prolapse, and extrusion	Severe pain. All movements reduced	Gentle manual traction in progressive extension
Anterior-posterior instability	Flexion and extension reduction greater than rotation	Traction and/or traction manipulation in extension
Arthritis	Hot capsular pattern	PRICEMEM (Protection, Rest, Ice, Compression, Elevation, Medication Electrotherapeutics, Manual therapy)
Subluxation of segment	One direction restricted	Exercises in pain-free direction
Arthrosis of segment	All directions restricted	Exercises in the most painless direction

Questions for this chapter and the entire book appear on the included CD-ROM, with additional questions at www.DuttonNPTE.com.

REFERENCES

1. Boissonnault WG: *Examination in Physical Therapy Practice: Screening for Medical Disease.* New York, NY: Churchill Livingstone. 1991.
2. Huskisson EC: Measurement of pain. *Lancet.* 1974;2:127.
3. Halle JS: Neuromusculoskeletal scan examination with selected related topics. In: Flynn TW, ed. *The Thoracic Spine and Rib Cage: Musculoskeletal Evaluation and Treatment.* Boston: Butterworth-Heinemann. 1996:121-146.
4. Judge RD, Zuidema GD, Fitzgerald FT: Musculoskeletal system. In: Judge RD, Zuidema GD, Fitzgerald FT, eds. *Clinical Diagnosis.* 4th ed. Boston: Little, Brown and Company. 1982:365-403.
5. Bonica JJ: Neurophysiological and pathological aspects of acute and chronic pain. *Arch Surg.* 1977;112:750-761.
6. Burkhardt CS: The use of the McGill Pain Questionnaire in assessing arthritis pain. *Pain.* 1984;19:305.
7. Chaturvedi SK: Prevalence of chronic pain in psychiatric patients. *Pain.* 1987;29:231-237.
8. Dunn D: Chronic regional pain syndrome, type 1: part I. *AORN J.* 2000;72:421-424,426,428-432,435,437-442,444-449,452-458.
9. Konietzny F, Perl ER, Trevino D, et al: Sensory experiences in man evoked by intraneural electrical stimulation of intact cutaneous afferent fibers. *Exp Brain Res.* 1981;42:219-222.
10. Ochoa J, Torebjörk E: Sensations evoked by intraneural microstimulation of C nociceptor fibres in human skin nerves. *J Physiol.* 1989;415:583-599.
11. Torebjörk HE, Ochoa JL, Schady W: Referred pain from intraneural stimulation of muscle fascicles in the median nerve. *Pain.* 1984;18:145-156.
12. Ness TJ, Gebhart GF: Visceral pain: a review of experimental studies. *Pain.* 1990;41:167-234.
13. Rowland LP: Diseases of the motor unit. In: Kandel ER, Schwartz JH, Jessell TM eds. *Principles of Neural Science.* 4th ed. New York, NY: McGraw-Hill. 2000:695-712.
14. Goldstein R: Psychological evaluation of low back pain. *Spine: State of the Art Rev.* 1986;1:103.

15. Norris TR: History and physical examination of the shoulder. In: Nicholas JA, Hershman EB, Posner MA, eds. *The Upper Extremity in Sports Medicine, 2d ed.* St Louis, MO: Mosby Year-Book. 1995;39-83.
16. McKenzie R, May S: History. In: McKenzie R, May S, eds. *The Human Extremities: Mechanical Diagnosis and Therapy.* Waikanae, New Zealand: Spinal Publications. 2000;89-103.
17. Goodman CC, Snyder TEK: *Differential Diagnosis in Physical Therapy.* Philadelphia, PA: WB Saunders Company. 1990.
18. Maitland G: *Vertebral Manipulation.* Sydney: Butterworth; 1986.
19. Maitland G: *Peripheral Manipulation, 3rd ed.* London: Butterworth. 1991.
20. American Physical Therapy Association: Guide to physical therapist practice. *Phys Ther.* 2001;81:S13-S95.
21. Magarey ME: Examination of the cervical and thoracic spine. In: Grant R, ed. *Physical Therapy of the Cervical and Thoracic Spine.* 2nd ed. New York, NY: Churchill Livingstone. 1994;109-144.
22. American Physical Therapy Association: *Guide to Physical Therapist Practice, 2nd ed. Phys Ther.* 2001;81:1-746.
23. Boissonnault WG: Review of systems. In: Boissonnault WG, ed. *Primary Care for the Physical Therapist: Examination and Triage.* St Louis, MO: Elsevier Saunders. 2005;87-104.
24. Mohn A, di Ricco L, Magnelli A, et al: Celiac disease—associated vertigo and nystagmus. *J Pediatr Gastroenterol Nutr.* 2002;34:317-318.
25. Davis MP, Walsh D: Cancer pain: how to measure the fifth vital sign. *Cleve Clin J Med.* 2004;71:625-632.
26. Salcido RS: Is pain a vital sign? *Adv Skin Wound Care.* 2003;16:214.
27. Sousa FA: Pain: the fifth vital sign. *Rev Lat Am Enfermagem.* 2002;10:446-447.
28. Lynch M: Pain: the fifth vital sign. Comprehensive assessment leads to proper treatment. *Adv Nurse Pract.* 2001;9:28-36.
29. Lynch M: Pain as the fifth vital sign. *J Intraven Nurs.* 2001;24:85-94.
30. Merboth MK, Barnason S: Managing pain: the fifth vital sign. *Nurs Clin North Am.* 2000;35:375-383.
31. Torma L: Pain: the fifth vital sign. *Pulse.* 1999;36:16.
32. Newman BY: Pain as the fifth vital sign. *J Am Optom Assoc.* 1999;70:619-620.
33. Joel LA: The fifth vital sign: pain. *Am J Nurs.* 1999;99:9.
34. McCaffery M, Pasero CL: Pain ratings: the fifth vital sign. *Am J Nurs.* 1997;97:15-16.
35. Frese EM, Richter RR, Burlis TV: Self-reported measurement of heart rate and blood pressure in patients by physical therapy clinical instructors. *Phys Ther.* 2002;82:1192-1200.
36. Bailey MK: Physical examination procedures to screen for serious disorders of the low back and lower quarter. In: Wilmarth MA, ed. *Medical Screening for the Physical Therapist.* Orthopaedic Section Independent Study Course 14.1.1 La Crosse, WI: Orthopaedic Section, APTA. 2003:1-35.
37. Judge RD, Zuidema GD, Fitzgerald FT: Vital signs. In: Judge RD, Zuidema GD, Fitzgerald FT, eds. *Clinical Diagnosis.* 4th ed. Boston: Little, Brown and Company. 1982:49-58.

38. Cyriax J: *Textbook of Orthopaedic Medicine, Diagnosis of Soft Tissue Lesions, 8th ed.* London, Bailliere Tindall; 1982.
39. Hayes KW: An examination of Cyriax's passive motion tests with patients having osteoarthritis of the knee. *Phys Ther.* 1994; 74:697.
40. Franklin ME: Assessment of exercise induced minor lesions: the accuracy of Cyriax's diagnosis by selective tissue tension paradigm. *J Orthop Sports Phys Ther.* 1996;24:122.
41. Grieve GP: The masqueraders. In: Boyling JD, Palastanga N, eds. *Grieve's Modern Manual Therapy, 2nd ed.* Edinburgh: Churchill Livingstone. 1994:841-856.
42. Meadows JTS: *Manual Therapy: Biomechanical Assessment and Treatment, Advanced Technique.* Calgary: Swodeam Consulting. 1995.

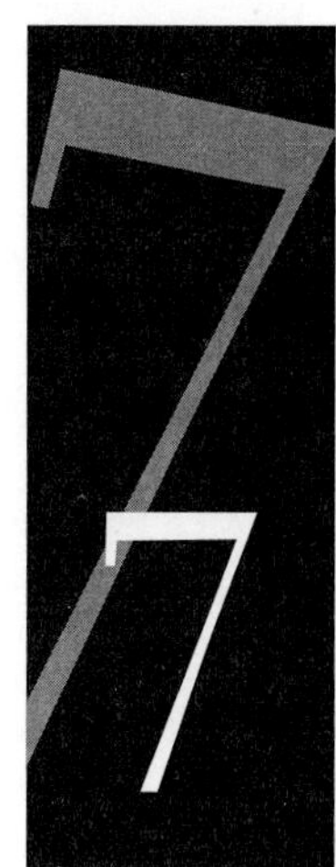

Gait, Posture, Ergonomics, and Occupational Health

GAIT

The major requirements for successful walking include:[1]

- Support of body mass by the lower extremities.
- Production of a locomotor rhythm—the stretch reflex and the extensor thrust.[2] The stretch reflex is involved in the extremes of joint motion, while the extensor thrust may facilitate the extensor muscles of the lower extremity during weight bearing.[3]
- Dynamic balance control of the moving body.
- Propulsion of the body in the intended direction.
- Adaptability of locomotor responses to changing task and environmental demands.

A number of parameters are used to describe gait (Table 7–1).

THE GAIT CYCLE

The *gait cycle* is defined as the interval of time between any of the repetitive events of walking.[4] During the gait cycle:

- The swing of the arms is out of phase with the legs. Unless they are restrained, the arms tend to swing in opposition to the legs, the left arm swinging forward as the right leg swings forward and vice versa.[3]
- As the upper body moves forward, the trunk twists about a vertical axis. The shoulders and trunk rotate out of phase with each other during the gait cycle.[5] Although the majority of the arm swing results from momentum, the pendular actions of the arms are also produced by gravity and muscle action.[3,6]
- The thoracic spine and the pelvis rotate in opposite directions to each other to enhance stability and balance. In contrast, the lumbar spine tends to rotate with the pelvis.

TABLE 7-1. GAIT PARAMETERS

Step length: measured as the distance between the same point of one foot on successive footprints (ipsilateral to the contralateral foot fall).

Stride length: the distance between successive points of foot-to-floor contact of the same foot. A stride is one full lower extremity cycle. The average stride length for normal individuals is 1.41 m.[a]

- Two step lengths added together make the stride length.
- Men typically have longer stride lengths than women.

Typically, the stride length does not vary more than a couple of inches between tall and short individuals. Stride length decreases with age, pain, disease, and fatigue.[b] It also decreases as the speed of gait increases.[c] A decrease in stride length may also result from a forward-head posture, a stiff hip, or a decrease in the availability of motion at the lumbar spine.

Cadence: the number of steps taken per unit of time (steps/min) = velocity (m/s) × 120/stride length (m). Normal cadence is between 90 and 120 steps/min, with an average of 113 steps/min.[d,e] The cadence of women is usually 6-9 steps/min slower than that of men.[f] Cadence is also affected by age, with cadence decreasing from the age of 4 to the age of 7, and then again in advancing years.

Velocity (m/s) = cadence (steps/min) × stride length (m)/120. Normal free gait velocity on a smooth and level surface averages about 82 m/min for adults, with men being about 5% faster than women. Walking velocity declines with age at a rate of 3%-11% in healthy adults > 60 years old.[a]

Data from:
[a]Perry J: Stride Analysis. In: Perry J, ed. *Gait Analysis: Normal and Pathological Function. Thorofare,* NJ: Slack Inc. 1992:431-441.
[b]Ostrosky KM, Van Sweringen JM, Burdett RG, et al: A comparison of gait characteristics in young and old subjects. *Phys Ther.* 1994;74:637-646.
[c]Adelaar RS: The practical biomechanics of running. *Am J Sports Med.* 1986;14:497-500.
[d]Perry J: *Gait Analysis: Normal and Pathological Function.* Thorofare, NJ: Slack Inc. 1992.
[e]Rogers MM: Dynamic foot mechanics. *J Orthop Sports Phys Ther.* 1995;21:306-316.
[f]Gage JR, Deluca PA, Renshaw TS: Gait analysis: principles and applications with emphasis on its use with cerebral palsy. *Inst Course Lect.* 1996;45:491-507.

Study Pearl

Two types of terminology are commonly used to describe gait:
- Traditional: refers to points in time in the gait cycle
- Rancho Los Amigos (RLA): refers to the length of time in the gait cycle

- Maximum flexion of both the elbow and shoulder joints occurs when the opposite foot initially makes contact with the ground, while maximum extension occurs when the foot on the same side initially makes contact with the ground.[7]

According to the RLA terminology, the gait cycle consists of two periods: stance and swing (Figure 7-1):

- The stance period: This period constitutes approximately 60% of the gait cycle[8,9] and describes the entire time that the foot is in contact with the ground and the limb is bearing weight.

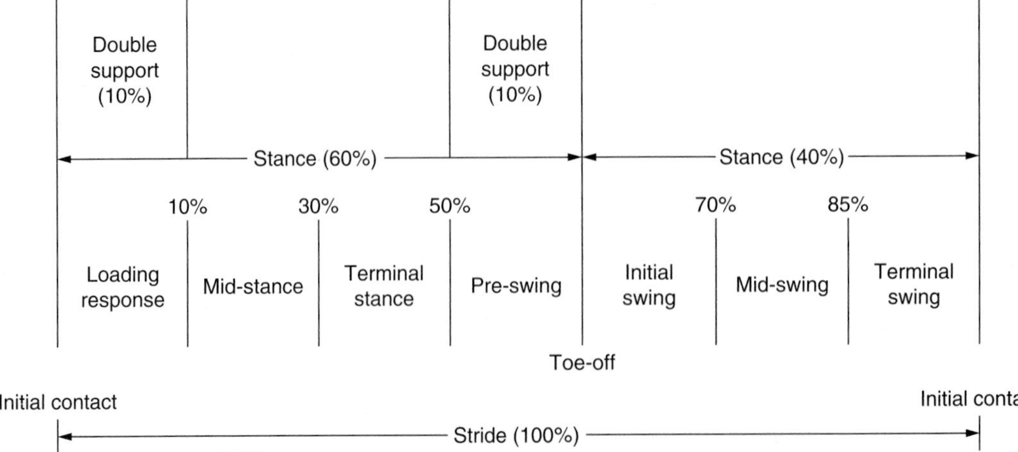

Figure 7-1. Approximate values for the two phases of gait. (Reproduced, with permission, from Dutton M: *Orthopaedic Examination, Evaluation, and Intervention.* New York: McGraw-Hill. 2004:374.)

The stance period begins with the initial contact of the foot on the ground (heel strike), and concludes when the ipsilateral foot leaves the ground (initial swing or toe-off).

- The swing period: The swing period constitutes approximately 40% of the gait cycle[8,9] and describes the period when the foot is not in contact with the ground. The swing period begins as the foot is lifted from the ground (initial swing or toe-off) and ends with initial contact (heel strike) with the ipsilateral foot.[4]

Stance Period. Initial contact (heel strike) and initial swing (toe-off) are instantaneous events. The initial contact, which occurs when one foot makes contact with the ground, takes place at the beginning of the stance period. As the initial contact of one foot is occurring, the contralateral foot is preparing to come off the floor. The traditional terminology includes the following during the stance period:

- Heel strike: the instant that the heel touches the ground to begin the stance phase
- Foot flat: the point in which the entire foot makes contact with the ground, which normally occurs immediately after heel strike
- Mid stance: the point during the stance phase when the entire body weight is taken through the stance limb
- Heel off: the point in which the heel of the stance limb leaves the ground
- Toe-off: the point in which only the toe of the stance limb remains on the ground

The RLA terminology describes:

- Initial contact: the beginning of the stance phase—when the foot first touches the ground.
- Loading response: begins as one limb bears weight while the other leg begins to go through its swing period. This interval may be referred to as the *initial double stance* period and consists of the first 0% to 10% of the gait cycle.[10]
- Mid stance: begins as one foot is lifted, and continues until the body weight is aligned over the forefoot.[10] The mid-stance interval comprises the 10% to 30% phase of the gait cycle.[10]
- Terminal stance: begins when the heel of the weight-bearing foot lifts off the ground and continues until the contralateral foot strikes the ground. Terminal stance comprises the 30% to 50% phase of the gait cycle.[10]
- Pre-swing: begins with initial contact of the contralateral limb and ends with ipsilateral toe-off. As both feet are on the floor at the same time during this interval, double support occurs for the second time in the gait cycle. This last portion of the stance period is therefore referred to as the *terminal double stance.*

Timing for the phases of stance is 10% for each double stance interval, and 40% for single limb support, so that the period of single limb support of one limb equals the period of swing for the other.[10]

Study Pearl

During the stance period, three *ankle rocker periods* are recognized.

1. The first rocker occurs between the initial contact and when the foot is flat on the floor. This rocker involves the ankle dorsiflexors working eccentrically to gradually permit the foot to come into full contact with the ground.
2. During the second rocker, the foot remains flat on the ground while the tibia advances. This motion is due to the plantar flexors working eccentrically to control the ankle dorsiflexion that occurs.
3. The third rocker is the push-off required for advancement of the limb. This is the period of power generation.

Thus, the first two rockers are deceleration rockers, where the perspective muscles are working eccentrically by undergoing a lengthening contraction with energy absorption. The third rocker is an acceleration rocker and aids in propulsion.

Swing Period. Gravity and momentum are the primary sources of motion for the swing period.[3] Three terms are used in traditional terminology:

1. Acceleration: begins when toe-off is complete and ends when the reference limb swings until positioned directly under the body.
2. Mid swing: the point at which the reference extremity moves directly below the body.
3. Deceleration: begins directly after mid swing when the reference extremity is slowing down in preparation for heel strike

The RLA terminology also uses three terms:

1. Initial swing: begins with the lifting of the foot from the floor and ends when the swinging foot is opposite the stance foot. It represents the 60% to 73% phase of the gait cycle.[10] Knee flexion to 60 degrees (owing to passive and active factors) assists in clearing the limb.[11] Hip flexion to 25 degrees, in combination with ankle dorsiflexion to neutral, is necessary to achieve foot clearance.[11]
2. Mid swing: begins as the swinging limb is opposite the stance limb, and ends when the swinging limb is forward and the tibia is vertical. It represents the 73% to 87% phase of the gait cycle.[10]
3. Terminal swing: begins with a vertical tibia of the swing leg with respect to the floor, and ends the moment the foot strikes the floor. It represents the last 87% to 100% of the gait cycle.

Study Pearl

A number of factors contribute to shock absorption during the stance period. These include:[11]

- Eccentric control of knee flexion to 15 degrees allows the dissipation of forces generated by the abrupt transfer of body weight onto the limb.
- Movement of the foot into 4 degrees to 6 degrees of eversion functions to unlock the midtarsal joints (talonavicular and calcaneocuboid), creating a more flexible foot that is able to adapt to uneven surfaces.

Study Pearl

Three functional tasks are achieved during the eight phases of the gait cycle:

1. Weight acceptance, which includes the initial contact and the loading response phases
2. Single limb support, which includes the midstance and terminal stance phases
3. Limb advancement, which includes the pre-swing, initial swing, mid swing, and terminal swing phases

CHARACTERISTICS OF NORMAL GAIT

Perry lists five *priorities* of normal gait:[13,14]

1. Stability of the weight-bearing-foot throughout the stance period
2. Clearance of the non-weight-bearing foot during the swing period
3. Appropriate prepositioning (during terminal swing) of the foot for the next gait cycle
4. Adequate step length
5. Energy conservation

In order for gait to be efficient and to conserve energy, the center of gravity (COG) must undergo minimal displacement. During the gait cycle, the COG is displaced both vertically and laterally, described below.

- Vertical displacement: Vertical displacement of the whole trunk occurs twice during each cycle—the lowest in double support, and the highest around mid stance and mid swing.[4] This vertical displacement of the COG is minimized through pelvic rotation, flexion and extension movements at the hip and knee, and rotation of the tibia and subtalar joint.[5]

Study Pearl

As gait speed increases, it develops into jogging and then running with changes occurring with each of the intervals. For example, as speed increases, the stance period decreases and the terminal double stance phase disappears altogether. This produces a double unsupported phase.[12]

- Lateral displacement: The lateral displacement of the COG occurs during the left and right stance periods.[4] Under normal conditions, the lateral displacement of the COG occurs in a sinusoidal manner. The amount of lateral tilting of the pelvis may be accentuated in the presence of a leg length discrepancy, or hip abductor weakness, the latter of which results in a Trendelenburg sign. The Trendelenburg sign is said to be positive if, when standing on one leg, the pelvis drops on the side opposite to the stance leg. The weakness is present on the side of the stance leg—the gluteus medius is not able to maintain the center of gravity on the side of the stance leg.

When considering the energy costs of walking, two factors are important

1. Any displacement that elevates, depresses, or moves the COG beyond normal maximum excursion limits wastes energy.
2. Any abrupt or irregular movement will waste energy even when that movement does not exceed the normal maximum displacement limits of the COG.

The three-dimensional excursion of the center of gravity/body mass is minimized through the intricate interactions of the segments of the lower extremity, especially at the knee and pelvis.[14] It has been proposed that six kinematic features, the so-called Six Determinants, are employed to reduce the energy cost of human walking:[16,17]

1. Pelvic rotation: the rotation of the pelvis normally occurs about a vertical axis in the transverse plane toward the weight-bearing limb. The total pelvic rotation is approximately 4 degrees to each side.[14] Forward rotation of the pelvis on the swing side prevents an excessive drop in the body's center of gravity. The pelvic rotation also results in a relative lengthening of the femur, and thus step length, during the termination of the swing period.[10] If the pelvis does not rotate, the COG's position is somewhat lower during periods of double limb support, and the COG's total vertical displacement.
2. Pelvic tilt: lateral pelvic tilting (dropping on the unsupported side) during midstance prevents an excessive rise in the body's center of gravity. If the pelvis does not drop, the COG's position is somewhat higher during midstance, and the COG's total vertical displacement is greater.
3. Displacement of the pelvis: to avoid significant muscular and balancing demands, the pelvis shifts over the support point of the stance limb. If the lower extremities dropped directly vertical from the hip joint, the center of mass would be required to shift 3 to 4 in to each side to be positioned effectively over the supporting foot. The combination of femoral varus and anatomical valgum at the knee permits a vertical tibial posture with both tibias in close proximity to each other. This narrows the walking base to 5 to 10 cm (2-4 in) from heel center to heel center, thereby reducing the lateral shift required of the COG to 2.5 cm (1 in) toward either side.

Study Pearl

The COG of the body is located approximately midline in the frontal plane and slightly anterior to the second sacral vertebra in the sagittal plane. The COG in men is at a point that corresponds to 56.18% of their height. In women, the COG is at a point that corresponds to 55.44% of their height.[15]

4. Knee flexion during stance: in normal walking, about 60 degrees of knee motion are required for adequate clearance of the foot in the swing period. A loss of knee extension, which can occur with a flexion deformity, results in the hip being unable to extend fully, which can alter the gait mechanics. Knee motion is intrinsically associated with foot and ankle motion. At initial contact, before the ankle moves into a plantarflexed position and thus is relatively more elevated, the knee is in relative extension. Responding to a plantarflexed posture at loading response, the knee flexes. Midstance knee flexion prevents an excessive rise in the body's COG during that period of the gait cycle. If not for the midstance knee flexion, the COG's rise during midstance would be larger, as would its total vertical displacement. Passing through midstance as the ankle remains stationary with the foot flat on the floor, the knee again reverses its direction to one of extension. As the heel comes off the floor in terminal stance, the heel begins to rise as the ankle plantar flexes, and the knee flexes. In pre-swing, as the forefoot rolls over the metatarsal heads, the heel elevates even more as further plantarflexion occurs and flexion of the knee increases.
5. Ankle mechanism: for normal foot function and human ambulation the amount of ankle joint motion required is approximately 10 degrees of dorsiflexion (to complete midstance and begin terminal stance) and 20 degrees of plantarflexion (for full push-off in pre-swing). At initial contact, the foot is in relative dorsiflexion due to the muscle action of the pretibial muscles and the triceps surae. This muscle action produces a relative lengthening of the leg, resulting in a smoothing of the pathway of the COG during stance phase. An adaptively shortened gastrocnemius muscle may produce movement impairment by restricting normal dorsiflexion of the ankle from occurring during the midstance to heel raise portion of the gait cycle. This motion is compensated for by increased pronation of the subtalar joint, increased internal rotation of the tibia, and the resultant stresses to the knee joint complex.
6. Foot mechanism: the controlled lever arm of the forefoot at pre-swing is particularly helpful as it rounds out the sharp downward reversal of the COG. Thus it does not reduce a peak displacement period of the COG as the earlier determinants did but rather smoothes the pathway.

Joint Motions and Muscle Actions During Gait

The joint motions and muscle actions that occur during gait are depicted in Table 7-2.

Abnormal Gait Syndromes

Each of the attributes of normal gait described under characteristics of normal gait are subject to compromise by disease states particularly neuromuscular conditions (Table 7-3).[18] In general, gait deviations

TABLE 7-2. JOINT MOTIONS AND MUSCLE ACTIVITY DURING GAIT

PHASE	HIP	KNEE	TIBIA	ANKLE	FOOT
Initial contact/ heel strike	▶ Gluteus maximus and hamstrings work eccentrically to resist flexion moment at the hip ▶ Erector spinae working eccentrically to control trunk flexion ▶ Reaction force anterior to the hip joint creating a flexion moment ▶ Hip positioned in slight adduction and external rotation	▶ Positioned in full extension before initial contact, but flexing as initial makes contact ▶ Reaction force behind knee causing flexion moment ▶ Quadriceps contracting eccentrically to control knee flexion	▶ Slight external rotation	▶ Moving into plantarflexion	▶ Supination
Loading response/ foot flat	▶ Gluteus maximus and hamstrings shift from eccentric to slight concentric activation, guiding the hip toward extension ▶ The hip begins to extend from a position of 20 degrees to 40 degrees of flexion ▶ Hip moving into extension, adduction, and internal rotation	▶ In 20 degrees of knee flexion, moving toward extension ▶ Flexion moment ▶ The quadriceps begin working eccentrically but, once the foot is flat, work concentrically to bring the femur over tibia	▶ Internal rotation	▶ Plantarflexion to dorsiflexion over a fixed foot	▶ Pronation, adapting to support surface
Midstance	▶ The hip approaches 0 degrees of extension at which point the hip extensors are only slightly active (to help stabilize the hip as the body is propelled forward). This activation is minimal during slow walking on level surfaces, but increases significantly with increasing speed and slope of the walking surface. During midstance, the stance leg is in single limb support as the other leg is freely swinging toward the next step. The hip abductor muscles (eg, gluteus medius) of the stance leg therefore are active to stabilize the hip in the frontal plane, preventing the opposite side of the pelvis from dropping excessively ▶ Pelvis rotates posteriorly ▶ Iliopsoas contracting eccentrically to resist hip extension ▶ Gluteus medius creating reverse action to stabilize opposite pelvis	▶ Quadriceps activity decreasing as the knee reaches near full extension. Because the line of gravity falls just anterior to the medial-lateral axis of rotation of the knee, the knee is mechanically locked into extension, requiring little activation from the quadriceps at this time	▶ Neutral rotation	▶ 3 degrees of dorsiflexion	▶ Neutral
Terminal stance/heel off	▶ Hip positioned in 10 degrees to 15 degrees of hip extension, abduction, and external rotation ▶ Iliopsoas activity continuing ▶ Extension moment decreases after double-limb support begins	▶ In slight flexion, moving toward extension ▶ Maximum flexion moment ▶ Quadriceps activity decreasing	▶ External rotation	▶ 15 degrees dorsiflexion toward plantarflexion ▶ Maximum dorsiflexion moment	▶ Supination as foot becomes rigid for push-off
Pre-swing/toe off	▶ The hip continues to extend to about 10 degrees of extension with eccentric activation of the hip flexors, in particular the iliopsoas, helping to control the rate and amount of extension ▶ Adductor magnus working eccentrically to control pelvis	▶ Moving from near full extension to 40 degrees of flexion ▶ Reaction forces moving posterior to knee as knee flexes ▶ Flexion moment ▶ Quadriceps contracting eccentrically	▶ External rotation	▶ 20 degrees of plantarflexion ▶ Dorsiflexion moment	▶ Supination

TABLE 7-3 GAIT DEVIATIONS RELATED TO DISEASE

DEVIATION	CHARACTERISTICS
Sensory ataxic	Characterized by staggering and unsteadiness. With this type of ataxia, because the patient is unaware of the position of the limbs, the gait is broad-based, and the patient tends to lift the feet too high and slap on the floor in an uncoordinated and abrupt manner. The patient tends to watch the floor and the feet to maximize attempts at visual correction, and may have difficulty walking in the dark.
Cerebellar ataxic	The nature of the gait abnormality with a cerebellar lesion is determined by the site of the lesion. In *vermal* lesions, the gait is broad-based, unsteady, and staggering with an irregular sway. The patient is unable to walk in tandem or in a straight line. The ataxia of gait worsens when the patient attempts to stop suddenly or to turn sharply, with a tendency to fall. In *hemispheral* lesions, the ataxia tends to be less severe, but there is persistent lurching or deviation toward the involved side.
Double step	Characterized by alternate steps which are of a different length or at a different rate.
Equinus	Equinus gait (toe-walking) is one of the more common abnormal patterns of gait of patients with spastic diplegia. Spastic diplegia is the most common pattern of motor impairment in patients with cerebral palsy (CP).[19] In these patients, motor impairment is due to a number of deficits, including poor muscle control, weakness, impaired balance, hypertonicity, and spasticity.[20] Equinus gait is characterized by forefoot strike to initiate the cycle and premature plantar flexion in early stance to midstance.[21] Toe-walking may be a primary gait deviation, which is the consequence of excessive myostatic contracture of the triceps surae, excessive dynamic contraction of the ankle plantarflexors, or a combination of both factors. Additionally, toe-walking may be a compensatory deviation for myostatic deformity or dynamic overactivity of the ipsilateral hamstring muscles, which directly limit knee alignment and secondarily compromise foot and ankle position during stance phase. Associated gait deviations are frequently seen at the knees, hips, and pelvis in children with CP who are walking on their toes:[22] ▶ Deviations seen at the knees include increased flexion in stance phase at initial contact and in midstance, and delayed and diminished peak knee flexion in swing phase. ▶ The hips often show diminished extension in the sagittal plane at terminal stance. ▶ A common deviation seen at the pelvis in children with CP who are toe-walking is increased anterior tilt.
Gluteus maximus	The gluteus maximus gait, which results from weakness of the gluteus maximus, is characterized by a posterior thrusting of the trunk at initial contact in an attempt to maintain hip extension of the stance leg. The hip extensor weakness also results in a forward tilt of the pelvis, which eventually translates into a hyperlordosis of the spine to maintain posture.
Trendelenburg	This type of gait is due to weakness of the hip abductors (gluteus medius and minimus). The normal stabilizing affect of these muscles is lost and the patient demonstrates an excessive lateral list in which the trunk is thrust laterally in an attempt to keep the center of gravity over the stance leg. A positive Trendelenburg sign is also present.
Quadriceps	Quadriceps weakness can result from a peripheral nerve lesion (femoral), a spinal nerve root lesion, from trauma, or from disease (muscular dystrophy). Quadriceps weakness requires that forward motion be propagated by circumducting each leg. The patient leans the body toward the other side to balance the center of gravity, and the motion is repeated with each step.
Parkinsonian	The parkinsonian gait is characterized by a flexed and stooped posture with flexion of the neck, elbows, metacarpophalangeal joints, trunk, hips, and knees. The patient has difficulty initiating movements and walks with short steps with the feet barely clearing the ground. This results in a shuffling type of gait with rapid steps. As the patient gets going, he/she may lean forward and walk progressively faster as though chasing his or her center of gravity (propulsive or festinating gait). Less commonly, deviation of the center of gravity backward may cause retropulsion. There is also a lack of associated arm movement during the gait as the arms are held stiffly.
Hysterical	The hysterical gait is nonspecific and bizarre. It does not conform to any specific organic pattern with the abnormality varying from moment to moment and from one examination to another. There may be ataxia, spasticity, inability to move, or other types of abnormality. The abnormality is often minimal or absent when the patient is unaware of being watched or when distracted. However, while all hysterical gaits are bizarre, all bizarre gaits are not hysterical.
Hemiplegic	Abduction and circumduction of the paralyzed limb in order to move the foot forward.
Scissor	Crossing of the legs in midline upon advancement.

(*Continued*)

TABLE 7-3 GAIT DEVIATIONS RELATED TO DISEASE (*Continued*)

DEVIATION	CHARACTERISTICS
Spastic	Characterized by stiff movements, toes seeming to catch and drag, hips and knees joints slightly flexed, and legs held together.
Steppage	Gait in which elevation of the feet and toes appears exaggerated. This type of gait occurs in patients with a foot drop. A foot drop is the result of weakness or paralysis of the dorsiflexor muscles due to an injury to the muscles, their peripheral nerve supply, or the nerve roots supplying the muscles.[23] The patient lifts the leg high enough to clear the flail foot off the floor by flexing excessively at the hip and knee, and then slaps the foot on the floor.
Tabetic	Slapping of the feet on the ground associated with high-stepping.
Waddling	Characterized by feet that are wide apart. Associated with coax vara.

(Table 7-4) fall under four headings: those caused by weakness, those caused by abnormal joint position or range of motion, those caused by muscle contracture, and those caused by pain.[14] These have been described below:

- Weakness implies that there is an inadequate internal joint moment or loss of the natural force couple relationship. Neuromuscular conditions may be associated with abnormalities of muscle tone, the timing of muscle contractions, and proprioceptive and sensory disturbances, the latter of which can profoundly affect reflex postural balance.
- Abnormal joint position can be caused by an imbalance of flexibility and strength around a joint or by contracture.
- Contractures, changes in the connective tissue of muscles, ligaments, and the joint capsule, may produce changes in gait. If the contracture is elastic, the gait changes are apparent in the swing period only. If the contractures are rigid, the gait changes are apparent during the swing and the stance periods.
- Pain can alter gait as the patient attempts to use the position of minimal articular pressure. Pain may also produce muscle inhibition and eventual atrophy. The antalgic gait is characterized by a decrease in the stance period on the involved side in an attempt to eliminate the weight from the involved leg and use of the injured body part as much as possible. In the case of joint inflammation, attempts may be made to avoid positions of maximal intra-articular pressure and to seek the position of minimum articular pressure:[24]
- Minimum articular pressure occurs at the ankle at 15 degrees plantar flexion.
- Minimum articular pressure occurs at the knee at 30 degrees of flexion. With a painful knee, the gait is characterized by a decrease in knee flexion at initial contact and the loading response interval, and an increase in knee extension during the remainder of the stance period.
- Minimum articular pressure occurs at the hip at 30 degrees flexion.

Spastic Gait. A spastic gait may result from either unilateral or bilateral upper motor neuron lesions.

TABLE 7-4. SOME GAIT DEVIATIONS AND THEIR CAUSES

GAIT DEVIATIONS	REASONS
Slower cadence than expected for person's age	Generalized weakness Pain Joint motion restrictions Poor voluntary motor control
Shorter stance phase on the involved side and a decreased swing phase on the uninvolved side -Shorter stride length on the uninvolved side -Decrease lateral sway over the involved stance limb -Decrease in cadence -Decrease in velocity -Use of an assistive device	Antalgic gait, resulting from a painful injury to the lower limb and pelvic region
Stance phase longer on one side	Pain Lack of trunk and pelvic rotation Weakness of lower limb muscles Restrictions in lower limb joints Poor muscle control Increased muscle tone
Lateral trunk lean The purpose is to bring the center of gravity of the trunk nearer to the hip joint.	Ipsilateral lean—hip abductor weakness (gluteus medius/ Trendelenburg gait) Contralateral lean—decreased hip flexion in swing limb Painful hip Abnormal hip joint (congenital dysplasia, coxa vara, etc) Wide walking base Unequal leg length
Anterior trunk leaning Occurs at initial contact to move the line of gravity in front of the axis of the knee	Weak or paralyzed knee extensors, or gluteus maximus Decreased ankle dorsiflexion Hip flexion contracture
Posterior trunk leaning Occurs at initial contact to bring the line of the external force behind the axis of the hip	Weak or paralyzed hip extensors, especially the gluteus maximus (gluteus maximus gait) Hip pain Hip flexion contracture Inadequate hip flexion in swing Decreased knee range of motion
Increased lumbar lordosis Occurs at the end of the stance period	Inability to extend the hip, usually due to a flexion contracture or ankylosis
Pelvic drop during stance	Contralateral gluteus medius weakness Adaptive shortening of quadratus lumborum on the swing side Contralateral hip adductor spasticity
Excessive pelvic rotation	Adaptively shortened/spasticity of hip flexors on same side Limited hip joint flexion
Circumducted hip Ground contact by the swinging leg can be avoided if it is swung outward (in order for natural walking to occur, the leg which is in its stance phase needs to be longer than the leg which is in its swing phase in order to allow toe clearance of the swing foot)	Functional leg length discrepancy Arthrogenic stiff hip or knee
Hip hiking The pelvis is lifted on the side of the swinging leg, by contraction of the spinal muscles and the lateral abdominal wall	Functional leg length discrepancy Inadequate hip flexion, knee flexion, or ankle dorsiflexion Hamstring weakness Quadratus lumborum shortening

TABLE 7-4. SOME GAIT DEVIATIONS AND THEIR CAUSES (*Continued*)

GAIT DEVIATIONS	REASONS
Vaulting The ground clearance of the swinging leg will be increased if the subject goes up on the toes of the stance period leg	Functional leg length discrepancy Vaulting occurs on the shorter limb side
Abnormal internal hip rotation Produces a "toe in" gait	Adaptive shortening of the iliotibial band Weakness of the hip external rotators Femoral anteversion Adaptive shortening of the hip internal rotators
Abnormal external hip rotation Produces a "toe out" gait	Adaptive shortening of the hip external rotators Femoral retroversion Weakness of the hip internal rotators
Increased hip adduction (scissor gait) Results in excessive hip adduction during swing (scissoring), decreased base of support, and decreased progression of opposite foot	Spasticity or contracture of ipsilateral hip adductors Ipsilateral hip adductor weakness Coxa vara
Inadequate hip extension/excessive hip flexion Results in loss of hip extension in midstance (forward leaning of trunk, increased lordosis, and increased knee flexion and ankle dorsiflexion) and late stance (anterior pelvic tilt), and increased hip flexion in swing	Hip flexion contracture Iliotibial band contracture Hip flexor spasticity Pain Arthrodesis (surgical or spontaneous ankylosis) Loss of ankle dorsiflexion
Inadequate hip flexion Results in decreased limb advancement in swing, posterior pelvic tilt, circumduction, and excessive knee flexion to clear foot	Hip flexor weakness Hip joint arthrodesis
Decreased hip swing through (psoatic limp) Manifested by exaggerated movements at the pelvis and trunk to assist the hip to move into flexion	Legg-Calve-Perthes disease Weakness or reflex inhibition of the psoas major muscle
Excessive knee extension/inadequate knee flexion Results in decreased knee flexion at initial contact and loading response, increased knee extension during stance, and decreased knee flexion during swing	Pain Anterior trunk deviation/bending Weakness of the quadriceps. The hyperextension is a compensation and places the body weight vector anterior to the knee Spasticity of the quadriceps. This is noted more during the loading response and during the initial swing intervals Joint deformity
Excessive knee flexion/inadequate knee extension At initial contact or around midstance. Results in increased knee flexion in early stance, decreased knee extension in midstance and terminal stance, and decreased knee extension during swing	Knee flexion contracture resulting in decreased step length, and decreased knee extension in stance Increased tone/spasticity of hamstrings or hip flexors Decreased range of motion of ankle dorsiflexion in swing period Weakness of plantar flexors resulting in increased dorsiflexion in stance Lengthened limb
Inadequate dorsiflexion control ("foot slap") during initial contact to midstance	Weak or paralyzed dorsiflexors Lack of lower limb proprioception
Steppage gait during the acceleration through deceleration of the swing phase Exaggerated knee and hip flexion are used to lift the foot higher than usual, for increased ground clearance resulting from a foot drop	Weak or paralyzed dorsiflexor muscles Functional leg length discrepancy

(*Continued*)

TABLE 7-4. SOME GAIT DEVIATIONS AND THEIR CAUSES (*Continued*)

GAIT DEVIATIONS	REASONS
Increased walking base (> 20 cm)	Deformity such as hip abductor muscle contracture Genu valgus Fear of losing balance Leg length discrepancy
Decreased walking base (< 10 cm)	Hip adductor muscle contracture Genu varum
Excessive eversion of calcaneus during initial contact through midstance	Excessive tibia vara (refers to the frontal plane position of the distal 1/3 of the leg as it relates to the supporting surface) Forefoot varus Weakness of tibialis posterior Excessive lower extremity internal rotation (due to muscle imbalances, femoral anteversion)
Excessive pronation during midstance through terminal stance	Insufficient ankle dorsiflexion (< 10 degrees) Increased tibial varum Compensated forefoot or rearfoot varus deformity Uncompensated forefoot valgus deformity Pes planus Long limb Uncompensated medial rotation of tibia or femur Weak tibialis anterior
Excessive supination during initial contact through midstance	Limited calcaneal eversion Rigid forefoot valgus Pes cavus Uncompensated lateral rotation of the tibia or femur Short limb Plantar flexed first ray Upper motor neuron muscle imbalance
Excessive dorsiflexion	Compensation for knee flexion contracture Inadequate plantar flexor strength Adaptive shortening of dorsiflexors Increased muscle tone of dorsiflexors Pes calcaneus deformity
Excessive plantarflexion	Increased plantar flexor activity Plantar flexor contracture
Excessive varus	Contracture Overactivity of the muscles on the medial aspect of the foot
Excessive valgus	Weak invertors Foot hypermobility
Decreased or absence of propulsion (plantar flexor gait)	Inability of plantar flexors to perform function resulting in a shorter step length on the involved side

Data from Giallonardo LM: Clinical evaluation of foot and ankle dysfunction. *Phys Ther.* 1988;68:1850-1856; Epler M: Gait. In: Richardson JK, Iglarsh ZA, eds. *Clinical Orthopaedic Physical Therapy.* Philadelphia, PA: Saunders. 1994:602-625; Hunt GC, Brocato RS: Gait and foot pathomechanics. In: Hunt GC, ed. *Physical Therapy of the Foot and Ankle.* Edinburgh: Churchill Livingstone. 1988; Krebs DE, Robbins CE, Lavine L, et al: Hip biomechanics during gait. *J Orthop Sports Phys Ther.* 1998;28:51-59; Larish DD, Martin PE, Mungiole M: Characteristic patterns of gait in the healthy old. *Ann NY Acad Sci.* 1987;515:18-32; Levine D, Whittle M: *Gait Analysis: The Lower Extremities.* La Crosse, WI, Orthopaedic Section, APTA, Inc. 1992; Perry J: *Gait Analysis: Normal and Pathological Function.* Thorofare, NJ: Slack. 1992; and Song KM, Halliday SE, Little DG: The effect of limb-length discrepancy on gait. *J Bone Joint Surg.* 1977;79A:1690-1698.

Spastic Hemiplegic (Hemiparetic) Gait. This type of gait results from a unilateral upper motor neuron lesion (see Chapter 9). This type is frequently seen following a complete stroke. There is spasticity of all muscles on the involved side, but is more marked in some muscle groups. During gait, the leg tends to circumduct in a semicircle, rotating outward, or is pushed ahead and the foot drags and scrapes the floor. The upper limb is held adducted at the shoulder and flexed at the elbow and wrist, with the fist closed, and is typically carried across the trunk for balance.

Spastic Paraparetic Gait. This type of gait results from bilateral upper motor neuron lesions (eg, cervical myelopathy in adults and cerebral palsy in children). The gait is characterized by slow, stiff, and jerky movements. There is spastic extension at the knees with adduction at the hips (scissors gait).

Clinical Examination of Gait

The clinical examination of gait can be performed using a number of methods ranging from observation to computerized analysis. The most commonly used gait analysis chart is the one designed by the Rancho Los Amigos Medical Center (Figure 7-2), which involves a systematic examination of the movement patterns of the following body segments at each point in the gait cycle: ankle, foot, knee, hip, pelvis, and trunk.

A paper walkway, approximately 25-ft long, on which the patient's footprints can be recorded, is very useful for gait analysis.[26,27] The patient should be asked to walk on their toes, and then on their heels. An inability to perform either of these could be the result of pain, weakness, or a motion restriction.

The patient's footwear is examined for patterns of wear. The greatest amount of wear on the sole of the shoe should occur beneath the ball of the foot, and in the area corresponding to the first, second, and third MTP joints, and slight wear to the lateral side of the heel. The upper portion of the shoe should demonstrate a transverse crease at the level of the MTP joints. A stiff first MTP joint can produce a crease line that runs obliquely, from forward and medial to backward and lateral.[28] Scuffing of the shoe might indicate tibialis anterior weakness or adaptively shortened heel cords.[25]

The patient's foot is also examined for callus formation, blisters, corns, and bunions. Callus formation on the sole of the foot is an indicator of dysfunction and provides the clinician with an index to the degree of shear stresses applied to the foot, and clearly outlines abnormal weight-bearing areas.[29] Adequate amounts of calluses may provide protection, but in excess amounts they may cause pain. Callus formation under the second and third metatarsal heads could indicate excessive pronation in a flexible foot, or Morton's neuroma if just under the former. A callus under the fifth, and sometimes the fourth metatarsal head may indicate an abnormally rigid foot.

The clinician begins the gait assessment with an overall look at the patient while they walk and notes the cadence, stride length, step length, and velocity. The arm swing during gait should also be observed. If an individual has a problem with the foot and/or ankle on one side, the opposite arm swing is often decreased.[29,30]

Study Pearl

Barefoot walking provides information regarding foot function without support, and can highlight compensations such as excessive pronation, and foot deformities such as claw toes.[25] Having the patient walk with footwear can provide information about the effectiveness of the footwear to counteract the compensations.

Study Pearl

Metatarsalgia is indicated if the metatarsal heads are made more painful with barefoot walking. Pain at initial contact may indicate a heel spur, bone contusion, calcaneal fat pad injury, or bursitis.

GAIT ANALYSIS: FULL BODY

RANCHO LOS AMIGOS MEDICAL CENTER
PHYSICAL THERAPY DEPARTMENT

Reference Limb:

L ☐ R ☐

☐ Major Deviation
▒ Minor Deviation

	Weight Accept		Single Limb Support		Swing Limb Advancement			
	IC	LR	MSt	TSt	PSw	ISw	MSw	TSw
Trunk: Lean: B/F								
Lateral Lean: R/L								
Rotates: B/F								
Pelvis: Hikes								
Tilt: P/A								
Lacks Forward Rotation								
Lacks Backward Rotation								
Excess Forward Rotation								
Excess Backward Rotation								
Ipsilateral Drop								
Contralateral Drop								
Hip: Flexion: Limited								
Excess								
Inadequate Extension								
Past Retract								
Rotation: IR/ER								
Ad/Abduction: Ad/Ab								
Knee: Flexion: Limited								
Excess								
Inadequate Extension								
Wobbles								
Hyperextend								
Extension Thrust								
Varus/Valgus: Vr/Vl								
Excess Contralateral Flex								
Ankle: Forefoot Contact								
Foot-Flat Contact								
Foot Slap								
Excess Plantar Flexion								
Excess Dorsiflexion								
Inversion/Everson: Iv/Ev								
Heel Off								
No Heel Off								
Drag								
Contralateral Vaulting								
Toes: Up								
Inadequate Extension								
Clawed								

Major Problems

Weight Acceptance

Single Limb Support

Swing Limb Advancement

Excessive UE Weight Bearing ☐

Name ______

Diagnosis ______

Figure 7-2. Rancho Los Amigos gait analysis chart. (Reproduced, with permission, from Dutton M: *Orthopaedic Examination, Evaluation, and Intervention.* New York: McGraw-Hill. 2004:388.)

The patient is observed from head to toe and then back again, from the side, from the front, and then from the back.

In addition to observing the patient walking at their normal pace, the clinician should observe the patient walking at varying speeds. This can be achieved on a treadmill by adjusting speed, or by asking the patient to change their walking speed.

Once an overall assessment has been made of the patient's gait, the clinician can focus their attention on the various segments of the kinetic chain of gait, including the trunk, the pelvis, the lumbar spine, the hip, the knee, and the ankle and foot (Table 7-2). Attempts are made to determine the primary cause of any gait deviations or compensations (Table 7-4).

Anterior View. When observing the patient from the front, the clinician can note the following:

- The subject's head should not move too much during gait in a lateral or vertical direction, and should remain fairly stationary during the gait cycle.
- The amount of lateral tilt of the pelvis.
- The amount of lateral displacement of the trunk and pelvis.
- Whether there is excessive swaying of the trunk or pelvis.
- The amount of vertical displacement. Vertical displacement can be assessed by observing the patient's head. A "bouncing" gait is characteristic of adaptively shortened gastrocnemii, or increased tone of the gastrocnemius and soleus.
- The reciprocal arm swing. Movements of the upper trunk and limbs usually occur in the opposite directions to the pelvis and the lower limbs.
- Whether the shoulders are depressed, retracted, or elevated.
- Whether the elbows are flexed or extended.
- The amount of hip adduction/abduction that occurs. Causes of excessive adduction include an excessive coxa vara angle, hip abductor weakness, hip adductor contracture or spasticity, or contralateral hip abduction contracture. Excessive hip abduction may be caused by an abduction contracture, a short leg, obesity, impaired balance, or hip flexor weakness.[31]
- The amount of valgus or varus at the knee. During gait, there may be an obvious varus-extension thrust. According to Noyes et al, this gait pattern is characteristic of chronic injuries to the posterolateral structures of the knee.[32]
- The width of the base of support. A wider base of support suggests poor balance.
- The degree of toe-out. The term toe-out refers to the angle formed by the intersection of the foot's line of progression and the line extending from the center of the heel through the second metatarsal. The normal toe-out angle is approximately 7 degrees, which decreases as the speed of gait increases.[33]
- Whether any circumduction occurs. Hip circumduction can indicate a leg length discrepancy, decreased ability of the knee to flex, or hip abductor shortening or overuse.
- Whether any hip hiking occurs. Hip hiking can indicate a leg length discrepancy, hamstring weakness, or quadratus lumborum shortening.
- Evidence of thigh atrophy.
- The degree of rotation of the whole lower extremity. Because positioning the lower extremity in external rotation decreases the stress on the subtalar joint complex, an individual with a foot/ankle problem will often adopt this position during gait.[29] Excessive internal or external rotation of the femur can indicate adaptive shortening of the medial or lateral hamstrings respectively, anteversion or retroversion respectively.

Lateral View. When observing the patient from the side, the clinician can note the following:

- The amount of thoracic and shoulder motion during the arm swing. Each shoulder and arm should swing reciprocally with equal motion.
- Orientation of trunk: The trunk should remain erect and level during the gait cycle as it moves in the opposite direction to the pelvis. Compensation can occur in the lumbar spine for a loss of motion at the hip. A backward lean of the trunk may result from weak hip extensors or inadequate hip flexion. A forward lean of the trunk may result from pathology of the hip, knee or ankle, abdominal muscle weakness, decreased spinal mobility, hip flexion contracture. Forward leaning during the loading response and early midstance intervals may indicate hip extensor weakness.[34]
- Orientation of the pelvic tilt: An anterior pelvic tilt of 10 degrees is considered normal. Excessive anterior tilting can be due to weak hip extensors, a hip flexion contracture, or hip flexor spasticity. Excessive posterior pelvic tilting during gait usually occurs in the presence of hip flexor weakness.
- Degree of hip extension: Causes of inadequate hip extension and excessive hip flexion include a hip flexion contracture, iliotibial band contracture, hip flexor spasticity, or pain.[31] Causes of inadequate hip flexion may include hip flexor weakness, or a hip joint arthrodesis.[31]
- Knee flexion and extension: The knee should be extended during the initial contact interval, followed by slight flexion during the loading response interval. During the swing period there must be sufficient knee flexion. Causes of excessive knee flexion and inadequate knee extension include inappropriate hamstring activity, knee flexion contracture, soleus weakness, or excessive ankle plantar flexion. Causes of inadequate flexion and excessive extension at the knee include quadriceps weakness, pain, quadriceps spasticity, excessive ankle plantar flexion, hip flexor weakness, or knee extension contractures.[35] Individuals with genu recurvatum may have a functional strength deficit in the quadriceps muscle or gastrocnemius that allows knee hyperextension.[36]
- Ankle dorsiflexion and plantar flexion: During the midstance, the ankle dorsiflexors, and the body pivot over the stationary foot. At the end of the stance period, the ankle should be seen to plantarflex to raise the heel. At the beginning of the swing period, the ankle is plantarflexed, moving into dorsiflexion as the swing period progresses, reaching a neutral position at the time of heel contact at the termination of the swing. Excessive plantar flexion in mid swing, initial contact, and loading response may be due to pretibial (especially the anterior tibialis) weakness. Excessive plantar flexion may also be due to a plantar flexion contracture, soleus and gastrocnemius spasticity, or weak quadriceps.[37] Excessive dorsiflexion may be due to soleus weakness, ankle fusion, or persistent knee flexion during the midstance period.[34]
- The stride length of each limb.
- Cadence: The cadence should be normal for the patient's age.

- Heel rise: An early heel rise indicates an adaptively shortened Achilles tendon.[30] Delayed heel rise may indicate a weak gastrocnemius-soleus complex.
- Heel contact: A low heel contact during initial contact may be due to a plantar flexion contracture, tibialis anterior weakness, or premature action by the calf muscles.[37]
- Pre-swing: An exaggerated pre-swing is manifested by the patient walking on their toes. The causes for this include pes equines deformity, adaptive shortening or increased tone of the triceps surae, weakness of the dorsiflexors, and knee flexion occurring at midstance. A decreased pre-swing is often characterized by a lack of plantarflexion at terminal stance and pre-swing. The causes for this can be ankle or foot pain or weakness of the plantar flexor muscles.

Posterior View. When observing the patient from the back, the clinician can note the following:

- The amount of subtalar inversion (varus)/eversion (valgus). Excessive inversion and eversion usually relate to abnormal muscular control. Generally speaking, varus tends to be the dominant dysfunction in spastic patients, while valgus tends to be more common with flaccid paralysis.[37]
- Base of support.
- Pelvic list.
- Degree of hip rotation: As in standing, excessive femoral internal rotation past the midstance of gait will accentuate genu recurvatum. Causes of excessive external hip rotation may include gluteus maximus overactivity and excessive ankle plantar flexion.[31] Cause of excessive internal hip rotation include medial hamstring overactivity, hip adductor overactivity, anterior abductor overactivity, or quadriceps weakness.[31]
- The amount of hip adduction/abduction.
- The amount of knee rotation.

QUANTITATIVE GAIT ANALYSIS

Quantitative gait analysis (Table 7-5) is used to obtain information on spatial and temporal gait variables, as well as motion patterns.[38,39] Imaging-based systems are the most sophisticated and expensive methods of obtaining quantitative data.

TABLE 7-5. GAIT VARIABLES FOR QUANTITATIVE GAIT ANALYSIS

VARIABLE	DESCRIPTION
Speed	A scalar quantity that has magnitude but not direction.
Acceleration	The rate of change of velocity with respect to time.
Stride time	The amount of time that elapses during one stride. Both stride times should be measured.
Step time	The amount of time that elapses between consecutive right and left foot contacts (heel strikes). Both right and left step times should be measured.
Swing time	The amount of time during the gait cycle that one foot is off the ground.
Step width	The width of the walking base (base of support) is the linear distance between one foot and the opposite foot.
Foot angle	The angle of foot placement with respect to the line of progression (degree of toe-out or toe-in).

GAIT ANALYSIS PROFILES AND/OR SCALES[39]

- Functional ambulation profile (FAP): designed to examine gait skills on a continuum from standing balance in the parallel bars to independent ambulation.[40] A more recent version of the FAP, which incorporates five environmental challenges which the individual may negotiate with or without use of orthotics or assistive devices, is called the Emory Functional Ambulation Profile (EFAP).
- Functional independence measure (FIM):[41-45] a multidimensional scale that assesses locomotion as one dimension of overall functional status. The FIM has two domains of function: motor (self-care, sphincter control, ability to transfer, and locomotion) and cognitive (communication and social cognition). The scoring criteria for the ambulation component of the locomotion subscale are summarized in Table 7-6.
- Iowa Level of Assistance Scale: examines four functional tasks (one of which involves gait): getting out of bed, standing from the bed, ambulating 15 ft (4.57 m), and walking up and down three steps.
- Gait Abnormality Rating Scale (GARS):[46] designed to identify patients living in nursing homes who are at risk for falling. The Modified GARS (GARS-M) is a modified seven-item version.
- Fast Evaluation of Mobility Balance and Fear (FEMBAF): an instrument designed to identify risk factors, functional performance, and factors that hinder mobility.
- Functional ambulation classification (FAC):[47,48] Six functional categories are defined.
  1. Nonfunctional ambulation.
  2. The assistance of another for support and balance is required.
  3. Light touch assistance is required.
  4. The patient needs verbal queuing for occasional safety assistance.

TABLE 7-6. SCORING CRITERIA FOR THE LOCOMOTION COMPONENT OF THE FIM

SCORE	CRITERIA
7	Able to walk at least 150 ft (50 m) completely independently, without any type of assistive device or wheelchair, safely, and within a reasonable (functional) period of time
6	Able to walk at least 150 ft (50 m) independently but requires an assistive device (orthosis, prosthesis, wheelchair, special shoes, cane, crutches, walker), or takes more than reasonable time, or has safety concerns
5	Required standby supervision, cueing, or coaxing to walk or propel wheelchair at least 150 ft (50 m)
4	Requires minimum contact assistance (patient contributes 75% effort) to walk or propel wheelchair at least 150 ft (50 m)
3	Requires moderate assistance (patient contributes 50%-74% effort) to walk or propel wheelchair a minimum of 150 ft (50 m)
2	Requires maximal assistance of one person (patient contributes 25%-49% effort) to walk or propel wheelchair 50 ft (17 m)
1	Requires total assistance (patient contributes less than 25% effort) or requires assistance of more than one helper, or is unable to walk or propel wheelchair at least 50 ft (17 m)

Data from Dickson HG, Kohler F: Functional independence measure (FIM). *Scand J Rehabil Med.* 1999;31:63-64; Grey N, Kennedy P: The Functional Independence Measure: a comparative study of clinician and self ratings. *Paraplegia.* 1993;31:457-461; Hamilton BB, Laughlin JA, Fiedler RC, et al: Interrater reliability of the 7-level functional independence measure (FIM). *Scand J Rehabil Med.* 1994;26:115-119. Keith RA, Granger CV, Hamilton BB, et al: The functional independence measure: a new tool for rehabilitation. *Adv Clin Rehabil.* 1987;1:6-18.

5. Patient is independent in ambulation on level surfaces.
6. Patient is independent in ambulation on all surfaces, including stairs and inclines.

- Timed up and go:[49-54] Patients are asked to rise from a seated position in a standard high chair, walk 3 m on a level surface, turn, walk back to the chair, and return to a seated position, moving as quickly and safely as they are able to. Performance is based on total time to complete the task.

Specific Interventions for Gait

The interventions for gait deviations are based on the findings of the clinical examination. Ideally, each deviation is broken down into its functional components and addressed accordingly before combining the various components to produce normal gait. A series of therapeutic progressions for gait are listed in Table 7-7.

TABLE 7-7. THE MAJOR ELEMENTS OF PHYSICAL THERAPY INTERVENTION THAT COMPRISE LOCOMOTOR TRAINING

MAJOR ELEMENT	INTERVENTION–INSTRUCTION AND TRAINING IN
Preparation for locomotor training	Bridging exercises Quadruped exercises Sitting balance and perturbations Sit to stand activities Kneeling and half kneeling activities Modified plantigrade exercises Standing balance and perturbations
Parallel bar progression	Moving from sitting to standing and reverse Standing balance and stability training Stepping, sidestepping, cross-stepping Use of appropriate gait pattern, forward progression, and turning Moving from sitting to standing position with assistive device, then from standing to sitting position Standing balance and weight shifting activities with assistive device Use of assistive device (with appropriate gait pattern) for forward progression and turning
Indoor overground progression	Walking forward and backward with resistance Sidestepping and cross-stepping Braiding Stair climbing Falling techniques (as appropriate)
Outdoor overground progression	Opening doors and passing through thresholds Curb climbing; negotiating ramps, stairs, and sloped surfaces Walking on even and uneven surfaces Walking with imposed timing requirements Use of open community environments; outside doors and thresholds Entering/exiting transportation vehicles Use of elevators, revolving doors
Locomotor training using body weight support and a motorized treadmill	Walking on treadmill using body weight support progressing to no body weight support Production of locomotor rhythm: initiating with slow speed and then progressing to faster speeds Dynamic balance control of the moving body Reciprocal stepping patterns: assisted movements to unassisted Strategies to improve speed, symmetry, and endurance
Indoor overground progression using body weight support	Indoor walking on level surfaces with body weight support progressing to no body weight support Use of assistive devices (as indicated) for ambulation on level surfaces

Data from Schmitz TJ: Locomotive training. In: O'Sullivan SB, Schmitz TJ, eds. *Physical Rehabilitation, 5th ed.* Philadelphia, PA: FA Davis. 2007: 523-560.

Study Pearl

Good posture may be defined as "the optimal alignment of the patient's body that allows the neuromuscular system to perform actions requiring the least amount of energy to achieve the desired effect."[54]

POSTURE

Posture describes the relative positions of different joints at any given moment.[55] Like "good movement," "good posture" is a subjective term based on what the clinician believes to be correct based on ideal models. Over the course of time, various definitions have been put forward to describe the attributes of good posture.[18,56-60]

Postural control is fundamental to movement allowing an individual to:[61]

- Maintain a position
- Move into and out of positions
- Recover from instability
- Anticipate and prepare for instability

Postural control is described under three conditions:[62]

1. Steady-state adjustments: require movement strategies that control a stable, quiet position in which the center of body mass is kept within the base of support.
2. Anticipatory adjustments: require movement strategies that recover stability in response to a planned, voluntary movement.
3. Reactive adjustments: require strategies that recover stability in response to an unexpected, external disturbance

Study Pearl

- In the lateral view, normal postural alignment is defined as balance about a coronal line of reference or gravity line that passes through the external auditory meatus, acromioclavicular joints, greater trochanters, and lateral malleoli.
- In the anteroposterior view, approximate skeletal symmetry allows division of the body into symmetrical halves with bisection of the following points: glabella; frenulum; episternal notch; xiphoid process; symphysis pubis; and a point midway between the medial malleoli of the ankle joints.

The postural examination may be assessed statically, when the body is at rest, or dynamically with the body in motion. The clinician observes the patient from the front, the back, and the sides, ideally with a patient standing near a plumbline for vertical reference for each view and with the clinician positioned to be able to see the patient's entire body:

- Standing: when observing from the anterior or posterior view, the plumbline should be aligned with a point midway between the feet and should divide the patient equally into the left and right halves. When observing the patient from the side, the plumbline should be aligned slightly anterior to the lateral malleolus.
- Dynamic: refer to "Clinical Examination of Gait."

The postural assessment gives an overall view of the patient's muscle function in both chronic and acute pain states. The examination enables the clinician to differentiate between possible provocative causes, such as structural variations, altered joint mechanics, muscle imbalances, and/or the residual effects of pathology.

Skeletal malalignment may be defined as either abnormal joint alignment or deformity within a bone. Abnormal, or *nonneutral* alignment, is defined as "positioning that deviates from the midrange position of function."[63] To be classified as abnormal, nonneutral alignment must produce physical functional limitations. Nonneutral alignment may produce neuromusculoskeletal pathology at adjacent or distal joints through compensatory motions or postures. Nonneutral alignment, whether maintained statically, or performed repetitively, appears to be a key precipitating factor in soft tissue and neurological pain.[64] This may be due to an alteration in joint load distribution, or the force transmission of the muscles.

Nonneutral alignment can occur in the frontal (scoliosis, a leg length discrepancy) and sagittal plane (forward head, anteriorly rotated pelvis, a decrease in the lumbar lordosis, knee recurvatum, shoulder protraction), and can progress to a somatic dysfunction.[65-69]

Sustained postures can also produce muscle imbalances and pain, especially if the joint is held at the end of its range.[70]

It is theorized that, if a muscle lengthens as part of a compensation, muscle spindle activity increases within that muscle, producing reciprocal inhibition of that muscle's functional antagonist, and resulting in an alteration in the normal force-couple and arthrokinematic relationship, thereby effecting the efficient and ideal operation of the movement system.[71-74]

The pain from sustained positions is thought to result from ischemia of the isometrically contracting muscles, localized fatigue, or an excessive mechanical strain on the structures. Intramuscular pressure can compress the blood vessels and prevent the removal of metabolites, and the supply of oxygen, either of which can cause temporary pain.[75]

It is quite normal for muscles to frequently change their lengths during movements. However, this change in resting length becomes pathological when it is sustained through incorrect habituation, or as a response to pain.

Muscles maintained in a shortened or lengthened position will eventually adapt to their new positions. Although these muscles are initially incapable of producing a maximal contraction in the newly acquired positions,[76] changes at the sarcomere level allow the muscle to eventually produce maximal tension at this new length.[77] While this may appear to be a satisfactory adaptation, the changes in length produce changes in tension development, as well as changes in the angle of pull.[78] For example, a passively insufficient muscle is activated earlier in a movement than a normal muscle, and has a tendency to be more hypertonic, thereby producing a reflex inhibition of the antagonists.[79-82]

Common lower limb skeletal malalignments and possible correlated and compensatory motions or postures are compiled in Table 7-8. Common postural deformities of the thoracic region include:[83]

- *Dowager's hump:* This deformity is characterized by a severely kyphotic upper dorsal region, which results from multiple anterior wedge compression fractures in several vertebrae of the middle to upper thoracic spine, usually caused by postmenopausal osteoporosis or long-term corticosteroid therapy (specificity, 0.99).[84]
- *Hump back:* This deformity is a localized, sharp, posterior angulation, called *gibbus,* produced by an anterior wedging of one of two thoracic vertebra as a result of infection (tuberculosis), fracture, or congenital bony anomaly of the spine.[85]
- *Round back:* This deformity is characterized by decreased pelvic inclination and excessive kyphosis.
- *Flat back:* This deformity is characterized by decreased pelvic inclination, increased kyphosis, and a mobile thoracic spine.

Study Pearl

A muscle imbalance occurs when the resting length of the agonist and the antagonist changes, with one adopting a shorter resting length than normal, and the other adopting a longer resting length than normal. The inert tissues, such as the ligaments and joint capsules react in a similar fashion, thereby altering joint play, which in turn alters arthrokinematic function, and force transmission as the muscles around that joint alter their length in an attempt to minimize the stresses at that joint.[61,66,67]

Study Pearl

While most clinicians can appreciate that repeated movement patterns performed in a therapeutic manner can be beneficial, it must also be remembered that repeated motions performed erroneously can produce negative changes in muscle tension, muscle strength, length, and stiffness.[72]

Study Pearl

A sustained change in muscle length is postulated to influence the information sent by the proprioceptors, which can cause alterations in recruitment patterns, and the dominance of one synergist over another.[145,147]

Study Pearl

Postural imbalances involve the entire body, as should any corrections. It is important to remember that, prior to any intervention, an appropriate examination must take place.

TABLE 7-8. SKELETAL MALALIGNMENT OF THE LOWER QUARTER AND CORRELATED AND COMPENSATORY MOTIONS OR POSTURES

MALALIGNMENT	POSSIBLE CORRELATED MOTIONS OR POSTURES	POSSIBLE COMPENSATORY MOTIONS OR POSTURES
Ankle and Foot		
Ankle equinus		Hypermobile first ray Excessive pronation at subtalar or midtarsal joints Hip or knee flexion compensation Genu recurvatum
Rearfoot (subtalar) varus (calcaneal valgus) Excessive subtalar supination	Tibial; tibial and femoral; or tibial, femoral, and pelvic external rotation	Excessive internal rotation along the lower quarter chain Hallux valgus Plantar flexed first ray Functional forefoot valgus Excessive or prolonged midtarsal pronation
Rearfoot (subtalar) valgus (calcaneal varus)	Tibial; tibial and femoral; or tibial, femoral, and pelvic internal rotation	Excessive external rotation along the lower quarter chain
Excessive subtalar pronation	Hallux valgus	Functional forefoot varus
Forefoot varus	Subtalar supination and related rotation along lower quarter	Plantar flexed first ray Hallux valgus Excessive midtarsal or subtalar pronation or prolonged pronation Excessive tibial; tibial and femoral; or tibial, femoral, and pelvic internal rotation, or all with contralateral lumbar spine rotation
Forefoot valgus	Hallux valgus Subtalar pronation and related rotation along lower quarter	Excessive midtarsal or subtalar supination Excessive tibial; tibial and femoral; or tibial, femoral, and pelvic external rotation, or all with ipsilateral lumbar spine rotation
Metatarsus adductus	Hallux valgus Internal tibial torsion Flat foot In-toeing	
Hallux valgus	Forefoot valgus Subtalar pronation and related rotation along the lower quarter	Excessive tibial; tibial and femoral; or tibial, femoral, and pelvic external rotation, or all with ipsilateral lumbar spine rotation
Knee and Tibia		
Genu valgus	Pes planus Excessive subtalar pronation External tibial torsion Lateral patellar subluxation Excessive hip adduction Ipsilateral hip excessive internal rotation Lumbar spine contralateral rotation	Forefoot varus Excessive subtalar supination to allow lateral heel to contact ground In-toeing to decrease lateral pelvic sway during gait Ipsilateral pelvic external rotation
Genu varus	Excessive lateral angulation of tibia in frontal plane (tibial varum, tibia vara) Internal tibial torsion Ipsilateral hip external rotation Excessive hip abduction	Forefoot valgus Excessive subtalar pronation to allow medial heel to contact ground Ipsilateral pelvic internal rotation

(*Continued*)

TABLE 7-8. SKELETAL MALALIGNMENT OF THE LOWER QUARTER AND CORRELATED AND COMPENSATORY MOTIONS OR POSTURES (*Continued*)

MALALIGNMENT	POSSIBLE CORRELATED MOTIONS OR POSTURES	POSSIBLE COMPENSATORY MOTIONS OR POSTURES
Genu recurvatum	Ankle plantar flexion Excessive anterior pelvic tilt	Posterior pelvic tilt Flexed trunk posture Excessive thoracic kyphosis
External tibial torsion	Out-toeing Excessive subtalar supination with related rotation along lower quarter	Functional forefoot varus Excessive subtalar pronation with related rotation along lower quarter
Internal tibial torsion	In-toeing Metatarsus adductus Excessive subtalar pronation with related rotation along lower quarter	Functional forefoot valgus Excessive subtalar supination with related rotation along lower quarter
Excessive tibial retroversion (posterior slant of tibial plateaus)	Genu recurvatum	
Inadequate tibial retrotorsion (posterior deflection of proximal tibia due to hamstrings pull)	Flexed knee posture	
Inadequate tibial retroflexion (bowing of the tibia)	Altered alignment of Achilles tendon causing altered associated joint motion	
Bowleg deformity of tibia (tibia vara, tibial varum)	Internal tibial torsion	Forefoot valgus Excessive subtalar pronation
Hip and Femur		
Excessive femoral anteversion (anteversion)	In-toeing Excessive subtalar pronation Lateral patellar subluxation	Excessive external tibial torsion Excessive knee external rotation Excessive tibial; tibial and femoral; or tibial, femoral, and pelvic external rotation; or all with ipsilateral lumbar spine rotation
Femoral retrotorsion (retroversion)	Out-toeing Excessive subtalar supination	Excessive knee internal rotation Excessive tibial; tibial and femoral; or tibial, femoral, and pelvic internal rotation; or all with contralateral lumbar spine rotation
Excessive femoral neck to shaft angle (coxa valga)	Long ipsilateral lower limb and correlated motions or postures of a long limb Posterior pelvic rotation Supinated subtalar joint and related external rotation along the lower quarter	Excessive ipsilateral subtalar pronation Excessive contralateral subtalar supination Contralateral plantar flexion Ipsilateral genu recurvatum Ipsilateral hip or knee flexion Ipsilateral forward pelvis with contralateral lumbar spine rotation
Decreased femoral neck to shaft angle (coxa vara)	Pronated subtalar joint and related internal rotation along lower quarter Short ipsilateral lower limb and correlated motions or postures along lower quarter: anterior pelvic rotation	Excessive ipsilateral subtalar supination Excessive contralateral subtalar pronation Ipsilateral plantar flexion Contralateral genu recurvatum Contralateral hip or knee flexion Ipsilateral backward pelvic rotation with ipsilateral lumbar spine rotation

Reproduced, with permission, from Riegger-Krugh C, Keysor JJ: Skeletal malalignments of the lower quarter: correlated and compensatory motions and postures. *J Orthop Sports Phys Ther.* 1996;23:164-170. With permission of the Orthopaedic and Sports Physical Therapy Section of the American Physical Therapy Association.

Other deformities associated with this region include:

- *Barrel chest:* In this deformity, a forward and upward projecting sternum increases the anteroposterior diameter. The barrel chest results in respiratory difficulty, stretching of the intercostal and anterior chest muscles, and adaptive shortening of the scapular adductor muscles.
- *Pigeon chest:* In this deformity, a forward and downward projecting sternum increases the anteroposterior diameter. The pigeon chest results in a lengthening of the upper abdominal muscles and an adaptive shortening of the upper intercostal muscles.
- *Funnel chest:* In this deformity, a posterior-projecting sternum occurs secondary to an outgrowth of the ribs.[86] The funnel chest results in adaptive shortening of the upper abdominals, shoulder adductors, pectoralis minor, and intercostal muscles, and in lengthening of the thoracic extensors and middle and upper trapezius.

LATERAL CURVATURE OF THE SPINE

Two terms, *scoliosis* and *rotoscoliosis,* are used to describe a lateral curvature of the spine. Scoliosis is the older term and refers to an abnormal side bending of the spine, but gives no reference to the coupled rotation that also occurs. Rotoscoliosis is a more detailed definition, used to describe the curve of the spine by detailing how each vertebra is rotated and side flexed in relation to the vertebra below. For example, with a left lumbar convexity, the L5 vertebra would be found to be side flexed to the right and rotated to the left in relation to the sacrum. The same would be true with regard to the relation between L4 and L5. This rotation, toward the convexity, continues in small increments until the apex at L3. L2, which is above the apex, is right rotated and right side-flexed in relation to L3. The small increments of right rotation continue up until the thoracic spine, where the side bending and rotation return to the neutral position. Lateral curvature of the spine can be described as being structural or functional:[87,88]

Study Pearl

The curve patterns are named according to the level of the apex of the curve. For example, a right thoracic curve has a convexity toward the right, and the apex of the curve is in the thoracic spine.

- Functional: This type of scoliosis is classified as postural, which disappears on forward bending, and is compensatory; most commonly due to a short leg.
- Structural: may be genetic, congenital, or idiopathic, producing a structural change to the bone and a loss of spinal flexibility. With a structural scoliosis, the vertebral bodies rotate toward the convexity of the curve (the spinous processes deviate toward the concave side), producing a distortion, called a *rib hump.*[89] The rib hump occurs on the convex side of the curve. Persistent scoliosis during forward bending (Adam sign) is indicative of a structural curve.

The curvature results in an adaptive shortening of the intrinsic trunk muscles on the concave side, and lengthening of the intrinsic muscles on the convex side. A number of radiographic classification systems exist to describe the types of scoliotic curves including:

- Ponseti-Friedman classification.[90-91] There are five types:
  - I—a single major lumbar curve at T11-L3 with an apex at L1-2
  - II—a single major dorsolumbar curve at T6-7 to L1-2 with an apex at T11-12
  - III—combined thoracic and lumbar with a dorsal curve on the right side at T5-6 or T10-11 and an apex at T7-8 and a lumbar curve on the left side at T10-11 to L3-4 with an apex at L1-2
  - IV—a single major thoracic curve at T5-6 to T11-12 with an apex at T8-9
  - V—cervicothoracic at C7-T1 or T4-5 with an apex at T3
- King-Moe classification.[86] There are four types:
  - I—lumbar dominant and *S* shaped
  - II—thoracic dominant and *S* shaped
  - III—thoracic where the thoracic and lumbar curves do not cross the midline
  - IV—long thoracic or double thoracic with T1 tilted into the upper curve
- Lenke classification.[92,93] There are three components:
  - Type of curves:
    - I—primary thoracic
    - II—double thoracic scoliosis
    - III—double major scoliosis
    - IV—triple major scoliosis
    - V—dorsolumbar-lumbar scoliosis
- Lumbar modifier: based on the relationship of the central sacral vertical line to the apex of the lumbar curve and is classified into A, B, and C categories.
- Sagittal thoracic modifier: the sagittal curve measurement from T5-12; designations are for less than 10 degrees, N for 10 degrees to 40 degrees, and + for greater than 40 degrees.

> **Study Pearl**
>
> The significant incidence of scoliosis in the adolescent population has prompted the creation of school screening programs in all 50 states. From the fifth grade onward, children should be screened approximately every 6 to 9 months.

A number of techniques, measures, and indices are used to assess scoliosis: the Cobb-Webb technique, the Ferguson technique, the Greenspan method, the Nash-Moe technique of measuring vertebral rotation, the Cobb method of assessing vertebral rotation, the Risser index, the observation for ossification of the vertebral ring apophysis, the difference in the rib-vertebral angle, the Perdriolle method, and the Lytilt method.

There is no literature that examines why patients and/or their surgeons choose surgical *versus* nonsurgical treatment. Parameters to consider include preoperative risks, radiographic measures, clinical symptoms, functional limitations and appearance, or social issues. The conservative approach for scoliosis runs the gamut from bracing to monitoring. Electrical stimulation of muscles for the correction of scoliosis has not been found to be effective in preventing scoliosis progression.[94]

Posture at Work

Posture for Standing, Sitting in Office Chairs, or Driving

Standing Posture. It is important to maintain the natural curve of the spine when standing. The patient should be advised to:

- Keep the head directly over the shoulders and the shoulders over the pelvis.

- Tighten the abdominal muscles and tuck in their buttocks.
- Place the feet slightly apart with one foot in front of the other and knees slightly flexed. Use a railing or box to prop one foot up while standing.
- Wear shoes with good support and cushioning. A rubber mat can ease the pressure and enhance favorable ergonomic conditions.
- Change feet positions every 20 minutes.

Sitting Posture. Many of the problems associated with sitting may be avoided by a combination of the following techniques:

- Provide support for the lumbar spine. Maintaining a similar lumbar lordosis in sitting as one maintains in standing is generally thought to be better than either a reduced lordosis or a kyphotic lumbar spine posture.[95,96]
- Modifying the sitting position. As with standing, there are many potential sitting postures, although three are commonly described:
  - Anterior (forward) sitting: involves either an anterior rotation of the pelvis or increased kyphosis of the spine so that more than 25% of the body's weight is transmitted through the feet to the floor and the center of gravity is anterior to the ischial tuberosities.
  - Middle (erect) sitting: involves sitting with the center of gravity directly over the ischial tuberosities with approximately 25% of the body's weight transmitted through the feet to the floor.
  - Posterior sitting: involves sitting so that less than 25% of the body's weight is transmitted through the feet to the floor and the center of gravity is posterior to the ischial tuberosities.
- Taking stretch breaks from sitting in office chairs or standing for long periods of time.
- Make the workstation as consistent and comfortable as possible.
  - *Choose the surface height for the desk* (standing, sitting, or semi-seated) best for the task to be performed. Architects and drafters may want a higher surface for drawing while computer entry work could be seated or standing, depending on the need to use other tools or references. The workstation top should be big enough to allow space not only for all computer-related necessary equipment, but also for paperwork, books, and other materials needed while working at the computer. Working with materials on chairs and at odd angles has the potential for neck and other body strain. Frequently used items should be kept close to avoid long reaches. A general recommendation is that the work area top should be at least as big as the standard office desk—30 in by 60 in. A depth of at least 30 in allows flexibility in use/reuse of the work area. Usable space may be maximized by good wire/cable management. The thickness of the work surface should be 1 in.

Study Pearl

Nachemson found that intervertebral disk pressure was higher in anterior sitting than in middle sitting, and that disk pressure in middle sitting, in turn, was greater than in posterior sitting.[169]

TABLE 7-9. CHAIR DIMENSIONS

Seat height	Seat height should be pneumatically adjusted while seated. A range of 16-20.5 in off the floor should accommodate most users. Thighs should be horizontal, lower legs vertical, feet flat on the floor or on a footrest. The seat height should be 1-2 in below the knee fold when the lower leg is vertical. Seat height should also allow a 90 degrees angle at the elbows for typing.
Seat width and depth	A seat width of 17-20 in suffices for most people and should be deep enough to permit the back to contact the lumbar backrest without cutting into the backs of knees (there should be approximately 4 in between the back of the lower leg in the seat). The front edge should be rounded and padded. Avoid bucket-type seats. The seat should swivel easily.
Seat slope	The seat slope should be adjustable (0 degrees to 5 degrees is ideal). A forward slope is required for raised seats and semi-sitting. A backward slope of 5 degrees is suggested for normal sitting
Backrest	The backrest should offer firm support, especially in the lumbar region. Should be convex top to bottom; concave side to side. Should be 12-19 in wide, and should be easily adjustable both in angle and height, while sitting. The optimum angle between seat and back should permit a working posture of at least 90 degrees between the spine and thighs. Seat pan angle and backrest height and angle should be coordinated to allow for the most comfortable weight load on the spinal column.
Seat material	A chair seat and back should be padded enough to allow comfortable circulation. If a seat is too soft, the muscles must always adjust to maintain a steady posture, causing strain and fatigue. The seat fabric should "breathe" to allow air circulation through clothes to the skin.
Armrests	Armrests are optional, depending on user preference and task performed. They should not restrict movement or impede the worker's ability to get close enough to the work surface. If the width between the armrests is too wide, the user must raise their shoulders and abduct their arms. The worker should not rest his or her forearms while keying. When using the arm rests, shoulder abduction angle should be 15 degrees to 20 degrees or less and shoulder flexion angle should be 25 degrees or less.

1 in = 2.54 cm

- *Adjust the seat of the office chair* (Tables 7-9 and 7-10) so that the work surface is "elbow high." The individual's fist should be able to pass easily behind his or her calf and in front of the seat edge to provide enough space for the legs. Two fingers should slip easily under the thighs. If not, use a couple of telephone books or a footrest to raise the knees level with the hips. The backrest of the office chair should push the low back forward slightly.
- *Fit the height of the computer screen.* Ask the individual to sit comfortably in their office chair, and to close their eyes and relax. Ask the individual to slowly reopen their eyes and see whether the center of the screen is level with their gaze.
- *Adjust the workstation accessories* (Table 7-11).

TABLE 7-10. ERGONOMIC CHAIR CHECKLIST

1. Chair has wheels or castors suitable for the floor surface.	Yes	No
2. Chair swivels.	Yes	No
3. Backrest is adjustable for both height and angle.	Yes	No
4. Backrest supports the inward curve of the lower back.	Yes	No
5. Chair height is appropriate for the individual and the work surface height.	Yes	No
6. Chair is adjusted so there is no pressure on the backs of the legs, and feet are flat on the floor or on a foot rest.	Yes	No
7. Chair is adjustable from the sitting position.	Yes	No
8. Chair upholstery is a breathable fabric.	Yes	No
9. Footrests are used if feet do not rest flat on the floor.	Yes	No

TABLE 7-11. WORK STATION ACCESSORIES

Footrest:	Situations will arise in which a user is perfectly adjusted for keyboard use and with the monitor at a correct angle, but his/her feet do not rest flat on the floor. A footrest may be used to correct this problem.
Document holder:	Use a document holder instead of resting copy on the table top. This helps to eliminate strain and discomfort by keeping the copy close to the monitor and at the same height and distance from the users face as the screen.
Wrist rests:	Wrists should only be used to support the wrist in pauses between typing if this is comfortable for the individual. Placing the wrists on a wrist rest while typing can create a bend in the wrists and pressure on the carpal tunnel. Wrist rests should have rounded, not sharp, edges and should provide a firm but soft cushion.

Driving Posture. The individual should be advised to:

- Sit with the knees level with the hips. A rolled up towel or a commercial back support can be placed at the back of the seat for added support.
- Sit as close to the steering wheel as possible as reaching increases the pressure on the lumbar and cervical spines, shoulder, and wrist.

THE EXAMINATION OF THE ENVIRONMENT

The *Guide to Physical Therapist Practice* includes examination of environmental, home, and work (job/school/play) barriers among the list of categories of test and measures that may be used by physical therapists.[97] Treating the injured worker requires that the physical therapist must be knowledgeable regarding the following:[98]

- An understanding of all aspects of the patient's community, home, and work. This includes the physical environment in which an individual functions, including both built and natural objects. This aspect of the examination may entail the clinician visiting the patient's home or worksite. Detailed information about the patient's work history and available resources at the worksite may also be obtained from the company representative responsible for implementing change on the worker's behalf.
- The psychosocial issues and cultures of the patient's environment.
- The most appropriate avenues for minimizing loss of function while maximizing recovery for a specific patient and workplace.
- Accessibility: the degree to which an environment affords use of its resources with respect to an individual's level of function.
- Universal design (lifespan design): this design concept emphasizes social inclusion by creating environments that are usable by a wide range of individuals of different ages, stature, sizes, and abilities as well as addresses the changing needs of human beings across the lifespan.[99]
- Environmental barriers: defined as physical impediments to prevent individuals from functioning optimally in their surroundings. Environmental barriers can be external or internal.[100]

EXTERIOR BARRIERS

- Exterior access routes: includes consideration of the frequency and mode of transportation typically used to reach the destination, parking, lighting in the parking area, and safely traveling to the entrance.
- Stairs: steps should have a maximum height of 7 in and depth of at least 11 in and should not have tread lip projections.[99]
- Ramps: if the patient has to use a ramp for home or work, the clinician should ensure that they can safely ascend and descend it, and that it is soundly built. For safety and ease of use, a ramp should ideally have an inclined of at least 1-ft length for each inch of rise (1:12 ratio). For example a 6-in-step leading into the home/building requires a 6-ft ramp.[100]
- Handrails: particularly important for those who ambulate with difficulty, and for those with impaired balance, especially on stairs and ramps.

INTERIOR BARRIERS

- Interior access routes: should be checked to ensure that there is enough space for basic mobility in and out of rooms with any assistive device the patient requires.
- Floor surface: type and resistance of floor covering.
- Doorways: a door must be at least 32 in wide for a standard wheelchair to pass and ideally 1 to 2 in wider than this to account for inaccurate maneuvering and the usual oblique approach to doors.[100]
- Lighting: check that lighting in all areas is bright enough for safe task performance and that light switches can be reached by the patient or the lights come on automatically as the patient enters the environment.[101]
- Seating: examine the height, width, depth, and stability of all seating.

TEST AND MEASURES

Environmental Impact. A variety of instruments have been developed that address the impact of environmental determinants on function. These include:[99]

- The Physical Activity Resource Assessment (PARA):[102] designed to examine and document the available resources that promote activity within the neighborhood or community environment.
- Home and Community Environment (HACE):[103] a self-report instrument used to identify features of the patient's home or community that may impact level of function.
- Safety Assessment of Function and the Environment for Rehabilitation (SAFER) tool:[104] a comprehensive functional and environmental examination tool designed for use with the elderly.
- Environmental Analysis of Mobility Questionnaire (EAMQ):[105] a self-report instrument that examines the impact of the environment on community mobility.

Study Pearl

Most products are designed to work well for people within the 5th to 95th percentile of the general population of nondisabled individuals.[105-108] The clinician should measure the patient's height, reach, depth, hip, shoulder, and hand width to identify individuals who do not fit within the typical range.

Study Pearl

The multidirectional reach test, an expanded version of the functional reach test is an effective test of functional range of motion.[109,110] Another measure of functional ROM is a map of the patient's reach zones, which look like semicircles extending in front of and to the side of the patient.[100] These items can be classified as primary, secondary, or tertiary. Objects are then placed in the zones according to frequency of use.

- Primary zone: Frequently used objects, which can be used while keeping elbows at the side of the body.
- Secondary zone: all objects that are used 4 to 10 times an hour and which can be reached without the elbow moving further forward than the anterior portion of the rib cage.
- Tertiary zone: infrequently used objects, which can be reached without exceeding full elbow extension or 90 degrees of shoulder flexion.

Study Pearl

Repetitive, forceful, or prolonged exertions of the hands; frequent or heavy lifting, pushing, pulling, or carrying of heavy objects; prolonged awkward postures; and vibration contribute to WMSDs.

TABLE 7-12. COMMON UPPER EXTREMITY WORK-RELATED NEUROMUSCULOSKELETAL DISORDERS

Carpal tunnel syndrome
Tendinitis
Tenosynovitis
Ganglion cysts
Bursitis
Myositis
Synovitis
Fibromyalgia
Osteoarthritis
Raynaud syndrome
Complex regional pain syndrome

Range of Motion. Functional range of motion rather than individual joint motion is generally most relevant to the examination of environmental barriers.

Muscle Performance. Functional muscle testing, such as whether the individual has the strength to handle the required tools, operate levers and lifts, carry, push, and pull objects as required by the expected roles, can be more useful than an examination of strength by measurement of individual muscle performance with manual muscle test or other approaches.[100]

Gait, Locomotion, and Balance. The patient's movement patterns and balance should be observed throughout the environmental assessment, including how the patient moves in and out of the vehicle or other equipment, climb steps, traverses uneven surfaces, anticipates and maneuvers trip hazards, stand and sits while talking, and balances when sitting and standing, as well as how fatigue impacts these motions.[100]

WORK-RELATED MUSCULOSKELETAL DISORDERS

Work-related musculoskeletal disorders (WMSDs) represent a wide range of disorders involving dysfunction of the neuromusculoskeletal system caused or made worse by the work environment, which can differ in severity from mild periodic symptoms to severe chronic and debilitating conditions.

Examples of WMSDs include carpal tunnel syndrome, tenosynovitis, tension neck syndrome, and low back pain (Table 7-12).

WMSDs can cause symptoms such as pain, numbness, and tingling; reduced worker productivity; lost time from work; temporary or permanent disability; inability to perform job tasks; and an increase in workers' compensation costs. The Occupational Safety and Health Administration (OSHA) has issued directives to minimize risk for WMSDs in the form of the Ergonomic Programs Rule.[111-113]

The following is adapted from Physical Therapist Management of the Acutely Injured Worker, BOD G03-01-17-56 (Program 32), retitled Occupational Health Guidelines: Physical Therapist Management of the Acutely Injured Worker, amended BOD 03-00-25-61; BOD 03-99-16-51; BOD 03-98-11-32; initial BOD 03-97-26-68.

PRINCIPLE: MANAGEMENT OF LOST TIME AND MINIMIZATION OF DISABILITY

The global outcomes of effective physical therapist management of the injured worker are to optimize work performance and minimize the development of work-related occupational disability. Effective and timely management of the injured worker is enhanced by participation in some form of productive duty, and access to on-site or convenient off-site services. The physical therapist may recommend making accommodations to normal duty or providing alternative or transitional duty work. The physical therapist needs to have a working knowledge of the critical work demands obtained through a job-site analysis, video analysis, or written physical job demands analysis, or through communication with the employer.

Principle: Management of Neuromusculoskeletal Injury

The physical therapist has unique qualifications to facilitate optimal functional outcomes through:

- Diagnosis of the neuromusculoskeletal condition and application of interventions to specific systems and tissues affected by the injury.
- Determination of safe work activity that will not compromise medical stability.
- The design of safe, progressive rehabilitation programs that aggressively recondition the injured worker. These programs are specific to the workers' job demands and are within their functional and medical limitations.
- Minimization of lost work time, through aggressive clinical management and promotion of productive work.

Principle: Facilitation of Timely and Appropriate Referrals

The physical therapist facilitates timely and appropriate referrals for other necessary intervention, that is, physician specialists or other providers, through the constant monitoring of neuromusculoskeletal signs, symptoms, medical stability, and progress. Injured workers are directed through the employer's health system working interdependently with physicians and other health care providers.

Principle: Minimization of Injury/Reinjury Incident Rate

The physical therapist's role in minimizing injury recurrence is in making sound and practical ergonomic recommendations for work station design, work performance, and worker training to improve knowledge of personal responsibilities for fatigue control. For the injured worker these recommendations may be specific to the worker's neuromusculoskeletal condition.

Ideally, physical therapy services are provided on-site or in close proximity to the workplace. Workers with potentially disabling neuromusculoskeletal signs or symptoms are directed early to the physical therapist service. Supervisors are trained to detect signs of cumulative trauma disorders, thus facilitating early referral.

The physical therapist should be knowledgeable of workplace duties, physical job requirements, equipment, and pertinent company policies and procedures.

If the neuromusculoskeletal problem is not satisfactorily resolved within a limited number of visits, a referral for further examination and evaluation by another health professional may be indicated. As soon as medically prudent, the injured worker is referred again to the physical therapist. The injured worker is then progressed, as above, to a self-paced program with the worker assuming, as possible via appropriate education and training, the responsibility for continued improvement.

Clear, concise, functionally relevant information about the injured worker's physical therapist management and recovery progress must be documented and conveyed in a timely manner to all team members. A comprehensive "team" may include: the physician, the physical therapist, employer representative (such as human resources, safety management, and department contact person), the injured worker, the worker's supervisor, insurance carrier, and the occupational health nurse.

The management of neuromusculoskeletal problems can be divided into four phases. The admission of an injured worker to a particular phase of care is based upon the physical therapist's examination/evaluation/diagnosis/prognosis of the worker's functional and neuromusculoskeletal status. Progression from one phase to the next is based on objective functional tests and measures. The level of physical activity required by the job, if a reasonable alternative job placement is not available, influences the duration of a treatment phase.

- Acute phase (immediate post-trauma): Patient management focused on the control and reduction of localized inflammatory response, joint and soft tissue swelling or restriction, and the stabilization and containment of the injury.
- Post-acute phase: Involvement of the injured worker in more active/functional activities. Graduated therapeutic exercises to increase muscle performance, improve joint integrity and mobility, and improve motor function (motor control and motor learning). Functional training to increase ability to perform physical tasks related to community and work reintegration.
- Reconditioning phase: More vigorous therapeutic exercises emphasizing daily functional and work activities and improved endurance. The injured worker's neuromusculoskeletal status is in the end phase of physiologic healing and ready for restoration of objectively measured functional capacities.
- Return-to-work phase: This phase is indicated for worker's who have progressed satisfactorily through the reconditioning phase but are not yet ready to return to work because of identifiable physical, functional, behavioral, or vocational deficits. An objective Functional Capacity Evaluation may be used as a basis for entry into this phase. This examination and evaluation serve, with a review of previous treatment progression, to form the entry into an appropriate work conditioning or work hardening program. The ultimate anticipated goal is the restoration of the injured worker's physical and functional capacity for a safe and expeditious return-to-work.

Inherent in the management of all of the phases is frequent and open communication between the physical therapist and the injured worker, his/her supervisor, and the other members of the employee health team. The ongoing emphasis on injury prevention education, including proper body mechanics, self-responsibility, worker compliance with their physician and the physical therapist's instructions, safe workplace practices, and workstation modifications is essential.

PERSONAL PROTECTIVE EQUIPMENT

The Occupational Safety and Health Administration (OSHA) requires the use of personal protective equipment (PPE) to reduce employee exposure to hazards when engineering and administrative controls are not feasible or effective in reducing this exposure to acceptable levels. Employers are required to determine if PPE should be used to protect their workers. Personal protective equipment may include gloves, mask, protective guards, protective clothing, or goggles.

If PPE is to be used, a PPE program should be implemented. This program should address the hazards present; the selection, maintenance, and the use of the PPE; the training of employees; and monitoring of the program to ensure its ongoing effectiveness.

Study Pearl

An FCE measures the ability of an individual to perform functional or work-related tasks and predicts the potential to sustain these tasks over a defined time frame. A job-specific FCE is one that is required to evaluate a client's ability to perform the physical demands of a specific, identified job.

FUNCTIONAL CAPACITY EVALUATION

The purpose of a Functional Capacity Evaluation (FCE) is to provide performance-based measures of a worker's safe functional abilities compared to the physical demands of work.

In an effort to provide more objectivity to the diagnoses and prognoses or work-related injuries, occupational therapists and then physical therapists have developed a battery of tasks that involve the testing and measurement of physical work functions (lifting, carrying, pushing and pulling, activities or positions required). These measurements of function are used to make return-to-work/activity decisions, disability determinations, or to generate a rehabilitation plan.

Definitions Specific to FCE

- Capacity: The ability of the client to work safely at maximal or submaximal levels over a selected period of time.
- Functional activity: Any physical activity that generically or specifically simulates a work or practical task. Functional activities as defined by the Department of Labor may include, but are not limited to, balancing, carrying, climbing, crawling, kneeling, lifting, pulling, pushing, reaching, sitting, standing, stooping, and walking.
- Job modification: Change in a task to allow the demands of the job to match the abilities of the patient/client.
- Medically stable: Medical stability is defined as that state in which primary healing is complete, or the progression of primary healing is not compromised.
  - Clinically, medical stability refers to the consistent presence of a set of signs and symptoms. Consistent means that the location of the symptoms and the presence of the signs have reached a plateau.
  - The intensity of the symptoms may vary with activity or intervention/treatment, but the location or pattern of change of symptoms remains consistent.
- Categories of work demands include: sedentary, light, medium, heavy, and very heavy.
- The frequency of work demands is classified as never, occasional, frequent, and constant.
- Functional capacity evaluation provider: A provider is someone licensed in the jurisdiction in which the services are performed, who is able to demonstrate evidence of education, training, and competencies specific to the delivery of FCEs.
- Physical demands of the workplace: Those physical abilities required to perform work tasks successfully. Physical demands

include work postures (positions), body movements, forces applied to the worker, repetition of the work tasks, and other work stressors and hazards as defined by OSHA. For safe FCE administration and useful interpretation, the FCE provider should have adequate knowledge in the following areas:

- Administration of FCEs and interpretation of tests results.
- Evaluation of physical demands of the workplace.
- Identification of patient/client behaviors that interfere with physical performance.
- Biomechanical components of safe work practices.
- Relevant laws and regulations, including, but not limited to:
  - Americans with Disabilities Act (ADA)
  - Code of Federal Regulations
  - Occupational Safety and Health Administration (OSHA)
  - Social Security Disability Administration
  - Workers' Compensation
  - Admission criteria.

FCE Protocols. A standard protocol includes tests and measures consistently applied to all patients/clients undergoing a functional capacity evaluation. Some clinics use their own approach, whereas others purchase a commercially available FCE system.

A job-specific protocol includes tests and measures consistently applied to a patient/client undergoing a functional capacity evaluation with reference to a specific, identified job. The test length can range from 1 hour to multiple weeks.

The five recommended test components to the FCE are

1. Intake interview
2. Subjective test
3. Neuromusculoskeletal evaluation
4. Baseline functional test
5. Work specific test

It is important to remember that injury can occur during an FCE as a result of exceeding the patient's musculoskeletal, cardiovascular, or neurologic system tolerances. Specific decision-making criteria help to standardize the process and protect the patient from overexertion. Controversy exists surrounding the safety of isometric lift testing due to the potential of generating significant amounts of force.

Applications and indications for an FCE in work injury management include:

- Determination of work function or work level with nonwork-related illnesses and injuries.
- Determination of work function or work level with work-related illnesses and injuries.
- Return to work and job placement decisions and programs.
- Disability evaluation and rating.
- Determination of function in nonoccupational settings.
- Medical and rehabilitation treatment intervention and planning.
- Case management and case closure.

Reporting Process and Format. The primary elements of the report should include:[171]

1. The patient's overall level of work, ranging from sedentary to very heavy.
2. Abilities on specific tasks within that overall level.
3. Tolerance for an 8-hour day. During an FCE, each physical demand of work is typically assessed for a brief period, usually no more than 5 to 10 minutes. Based on his brief assessment, the clinician must determine the duration of day that this level of demand could be performed by the worker.
4. Level of cooperation with the testing or sincerity of effort. This is one of the most challenging and controversial aspects of the FCE. Patients who perceive secondary financial gain to the worker's compensation system may exaggerate their symptoms and limitations.
5. Comparison of the patient's abilities with the job demands or former occupation.
6. Conclusion/summary/recommendation.

For FCE tests to be reliable and valid, the following FCE criteria must be met:

- Objectivity: objectivity refers to the indication that the test and measurement are relatively unbiased by either the participant or the evaluator. Objectivity in testing can be increased when the testing procedures and practices for observation and scoring are clearly defined and documented.
- Reliability: reliability refers to consistency in measurement and scoring. The test measures and scores must be consistent across evaluators, participants, and the date or time of test administration. Interrater and intra-rater reliability have been noted to be the most two important forms of reliability in FCE test administration and evaluation.
- Practicality: refers to the reasonableness of the testing procedure. The test must be practical to administer. The direct and indirect costs of the evaluation procedure must be reasonable and appropriate.
- Safety: refers to the level of risk in performing the test. The test must be safe to administer and must not be expected to lead to injury.
- Utility: refers to the test being useful. The evaluation procedure must meet the needs of, and provide useful information to, the participant, the evaluator, the referral source, and the payor.
- Validity: a measurement of how real the test results are. Without validity testing, there is no way of knowing whether or not the results are truly accurate and meaningful.

WORK CONDITIONING AND WORK HARDENING PROGRAMS

The following is adapted from Guidelines: Occupational Health Physical Therapy: Work Conditioning and Work Hardening Programs,

BOD G03-01-17-58 (Program 32), retitled Occupational Health Guidelines: Work Conditioning and Work Hardening Programs, amended BOD 03-00-25-62; BOD 03-99-16-49; BOD 11-94-33-109; initial BOD 11-92-29-134.

Introduction. Injured workers benefit from physical therapist services from the onset of injury through their return to work. Early physical therapy intervention consists of treatment for acute neuromusculoskeletal problems and other injuries. Many patients/clients who receive appropriate early care return to their job without additional rehabilitation services.

For those who are not able to return to work because of unresolved physical problems following acute care, the treatment focus changes to restoration of work-related function. Defined as *Work Conditioning*, these programs address the physical issues of flexibility, strength, endurance, coordination, and work-related function for the global outcome of return to work.

For the limited number of patients/clients with behavioral and vocational dysfunction, *Work Hardening* may be indicated. Work hardening programs are interdisciplinary and address the physical, functional, behavioral and vocational needs of the injured worker, with the global outcome of return to work. Physical therapists provide the physical and functional components within both of these programs.

The following guidelines identify *Work Conditioning* and *Work Hardening* as separate and distinct programs for injured workers. These guidelines describe program elements that should be used to develop and guide practice.

The guidelines serve the following purposes:

- For physical therapists—to design, implement, and evaluate structured programs for injured workers.
- For medical referral sources—to facilitate appropriate referral to structured programs.
- For insurance companies and managed care organizations—to develop appropriate methods of program authorization, monitoring, and payment.
- For Departments of Labor and Industry—to utilize as definitions and guidelines for worker compensation patients.
- For managed care organizations, regulators, and providers—to serve as resource documents.

Operational Definitions

Work Conditioning. An intensive, work-related, goal-oriented conditioning program designed specifically to restore systemic neuromusculoskeletal functions (eg, joint integrity and mobility), muscle performance (including strength, power, and endurance), motor function (motor control and motor learning), range of motion (including muscle length), and cardiovascular/pulmonary functions (eg, aerobic capacity/endurance, circulation, and ventilation and respiration/gas exchange). The objective of the work conditioning program is to restore physical capacity and function to enable the patient/client to return to work.

Work Conditioning Examination and Evaluation. Examination by history, systems review, and selected tests and measures required to identify the patient's/client's individual work-related, systemic, neuromusculoskeletal restoration needs. Evaluation of examination data shall be used to identify eligibility, design a plan of care, monitor progress, plan for discharge, and return to work.

A work conditioning provider is a licensed physical therapist, although the APTA recognizes that other professionals may be work conditioning providers.

Work Hardening. A highly structured, goal-oriented, individualized intervention program designed to return the patient/client to work. Work hardening programs, which are multidisciplinary in nature, use real or simulated work activities designed to restore physical, behavioral, and vocational functions. Work hardening addresses the issues of productivity, safety, physical tolerances, and worker behaviors.

Work Hardening Examination and Evaluation. Multidisciplinary examination including history, systems review, and selected tests and measures required to identify the patient's/client's individual restoration needs related to physical, functional, behavioral, and vocational status. The initial multidisciplinary evaluation of examination data is used to identify patient/client eligibility, design a plan of care, monitor progress, plan for discharge, and return to work.

Work Hardening Providers. Work hardening providers include the following professionals: physical therapists, occupational therapists, psychologists, and vocational specialists (Table 7-13).

Work Conditioning Guidelines

Patient/Client Eligibility. To be eligible for Work Conditioning, a patient/client must:

- Have a job goal.
- Have stated or demonstrated willingness to participate.
- Have identified systemic neuromusculoskeletal physical and functional deficits that interfere with work.

Work conditioning generally follows acute medical care or may begin when the patient/client meets the eligibility criteria. Work

TABLE 7-13 PROGRAM COMPARISON

WORK CONDITIONING	WORK HARDENING
Addresses physical and functional needs; which may be provided by one discipline (single discipline model)	Addresses physical, functional, behavioral, vocational needs within a multidisciplinary model
Requires work conditioning examination and evaluation	Requires work hardening examination and evaluation
Utilizes physical conditioning and functional activities related to work	Utilizes real or simulated work activities
Provided in multi-hour sessions up to:	Provided in multi-hour sessions up to:
4 h/d	8 h/d
5 d/wk	5 d/wk
8 wk	8 wk

conditioning should not begin after 365 days have elapsed following the injury without a comprehensive multidisciplinary examination and evaluation.

Provider Responsibility

- The employer and/or carrier should be notified prior to initiation of the program.
- The need for a program shall be established by a work conditioning provider based on the results of a work conditioning examination and evaluation.
- The program shall be provided by or under the direction and supervision of a work conditioning provider.
- The work conditioning provider shall document all examinations, evaluations, and services provided, patient/client progress, and discharge plans. Information shall be available with appropriate authorization to the patient/client, employer, other providers, insurance carriers, and any referral source.
- The work conditioning provider shall develop and utilize an outcome assessment system designed to evaluate, at a minimum, achievement of goals and outcomes, and program effectiveness and efficiency.
- The work conditioning providers should be appropriately familiar with job expectations, work environments, and skills required of the patient/client through means such as site visitation, videotapes, and functional job descriptions.

Program Content

- Development of program goals in relation to job skills and job requirements.
- Interventions to improve strength, endurance, movement, flexibility, motor control, and cardiovascular/pulmonary capacity related to the performance of work tasks.
- Practice, modification, and instruction in work-related activities.
- Education related to safe job performance and injury prevention.
- Promotion of patient/client responsibility and self-management.

Program Termination. The patient/client shall be discharged from the work conditioning program when the goals and outcomes for the patient/client have been met.

Work conditioning may be discontinued when any of the following occur:

- The patient/client is unable to continue to progress toward goals and outcomes because of medical or psychosocial complications or because financial/insurance resources have been expended.
- The patient/client declines to continue intervention.
- The patient/client fails to comply with the requirements of participation.
- The physical therapist determines that the patient/client will no longer benefit from physical therapy.

When the patient/client is discharged or discontinued from the work conditioning program, the work conditioning provider shall notify the employer, insurance carrier and/or any referral source, and include the following information:

- Reasons for program termination
- Clinical and functional status
- Recommendations regarding return to work
- Recommendations for follow-up services

MANAGEMENT MODEL

The following is adapted from *Guidelines: Occupational Health Physical Therapy: Work-Related Injury/Illness Prevention and Ergonomics*, BOD G03-01-17-57 (Program 32), retitled *Occupational Health Physical Therapy Guidelines: Prevention of Work-Related Injury/Illness*; initial BOD 11-99-25-71.

Physical therapists, in their management of individual patients/clients, integrate five elements in the management scheme; examination, evaluation, diagnosis, prognosis, and intervention(s). These elements are incorporated in a manner designed to maximize anticipated outcomes. This approach is also successfully employed by physical therapists in the development, implementation, and management of workplace injury/illness prevention programs.

EXAMINATION

When investigating the potential for injury/illness prevention and ergonomics programs, the first step is to take a complete history of the client company's injury/illness experience. The first tests and measures to be performed relate to individual work sites and work stations.

- Ergonomic tests and measures examine the environment, site, tools, equipment, materials and machinery, individual work flow, general production processes, rate, quality, and production demands, physical demands, physical stressors, and task rotation.
- Environmental factors of noise, ambient temperature, humidity, light, and air quality all may contribute to potential injury/illness during performance of occupational tasks.
- Physical characteristics of the work site and workstation (Table 7-14), including surfaces, work station area size and configuration, and seating also may contribute to potential injury/illness during performance of occupational tasks.
- Individual aspects of occupational tasks that may contribute to potential injury/illness may include tools, equipment, materials, machinery, individual work sequencing and pacing, general production processes, and rate, quality, and production demands.
- Specific physical demands placed on individuals during occupational tasks may include force, repetition, postures and motions, vibration, and surface temperature of materials.

TABLE 7-14. VDT CHECKLIST

Keyboard height (home row above floor): 71-87 cm (28-34 in).	Yes	No
Top surface of the keyboard space bar is no higher than 6 cm (2.5 in) about the work surface.	Yes	No
During keyboard use, the forearm and upper arm form an angle of 90-100 degrees with the upper arm almost vertical, the wrist is relaxed and not bent, wrist rests are available.	Yes	No
If used primarily for text entry, keyboard is directly in front of the operator.	Yes	No
If used primarily for data entry, keyboard is directly in front of the keying hand.	Yes	No
Top of screen is at eye level or slightly lower, with the center above the floor at 92-116 cm (36-45.5 in).	Yes	No
Viewing distance (eye to screen): 61-93 cm (24-36.5 in).	Yes	No
Viewing angles (eye to screen center): +2 to −26 degrees.		
Screen is free of glare or shadows.	Yes	No
Images on the screen are sharp, easy to read, and do not flicker.	Yes	No

The second tests and measures to be performed relate to individuals who will perform occupational tasks.

- Examination of each worker and the work force includes anthropometrics, including age and gender, examination of the individual worker, evaluation of the physical capacities of the worker, and assessment of work and health habits, risk behaviors, and worker/work force characteristics.
- Health habits should include nutrition, exercise, and smoking history.

Evaluation, Diagnosis, and Prognosis. Reports relating to the evaluation and diagnosis of work sites or work stations, with respect to preventing injury or illness, should include data analysis; work analysis; evaluation of worker/work force, safety, behavior, and compliance; identification of at-risk employees; identification of at-risk work processes/work stations; and identification of solutions. Reports relating to prognosis of work sites or work stations, with respect to preventing injury/illness, should include an estimate of goals and outcomes for all interventions.

INTERVENTIONS

Successful injury/illness prevention and ergonomics programs address the needs of both individual workers and employers. The dynamic nature of these programs mandates careful analysis and balancing of relevant components of the intervention.

There are two major areas of intervention. The first area of intervention includes those aspects of prevention programs where physical therapists take primary leadership roles. Procedural intervention components include monitoring at-risk employees and work processes, ergonomics, education and training, health promotion, return-to-work case management, and occupational health committee/team development.

The second area of intervention includes those aspects of injury/illness prevention and ergonomics programs in which physical therapists most often participate as team members. Participatory intervention components include involvement as a team member in work assignment, human resources management, compensation and benefits, labor relations, corporate values and work culture, and design and production standards.

A comprehensive occupational health injury/illness prevention and ergonomics program developed, implemented, and managed by a physical therapist will explicitly define the; (1) scope of the program, program plan, relevant policies and procedures, (2) authorities, responsibilities, accountabilities of those participating in the program, (3) surveillance strategy, benchmark, baseline, and triggering indicators, and intervention protocols, (4) content and process of report generation, report distribution, (5) maintenance of the program, and (6) methods of program evaluation and improvement through measures that determine actual outcomes.

OUTCOMES

Generating, analyzing, and interpreting data related to injury/illness prevention and ergonomics is performed by physical therapists using the full range of statistical and epidemiological methods, and appropriate application of such methods.

Questions for this chapter and the entire book appear on the included CD-ROM, with additional questions at www.DuttonNPTE.com.

REFERENCES

1. Schmitz TJ: Locomotor training. In: O'Sullivan SB, Schmitz TJ, eds. *Physical Rehabilitation, 5th ed.* Philadelphia, PA: FA Davis; 2007:523-560.
2. Burnett CN, Johnson EW: Development of gait in children: I. Method; II. Results. *Dev Med Child Neurol.* 1971;13:196.
3. Luttgens K, Hamilton N: Locomotion: solid surface. In: Luttgens K, Hamilton N, eds. *Kinesiology: Scientific Basis of Human Motion, 9th ed.* Dubuque, IA: McGraw-Hill. 1997:519-549.
4. Levine D, Whittle M: *Gait Analysis: The Lower Extremities.* La Crosse, WI: Orthopaedic Section, APTA Inc; 1992.
5. Richardson JK, Iglarsh ZA: Gait. In: Richardson JK, Iglarsh ZA, eds. *Clinical Orthopaedic Physical Therapy.* Philadelphia, PA: Saunders. 1994:602-625.
6. Hogue RE: Upper extremity muscular activity at different cadences and inclines during normal gait. *Phys Ther.* 1969;49:963-972.
7. Murray MP, Sepic SB, Barnard EJ: Patterns of sagittal rotation of the upper limbs in walking. *Phys Ther.* 1967;47:272-284.
8. Mann RA, Hagy J: Biomechanics of walking, running, and sprinting. *Am J Sports Med.* 1980;8:345-350.
9. Murray MP: Gait as a total pattern of movement. *Am J Phys Med.* 1967;46:290.
10. Perry J: Gait cycle. In: Perry J, ed. *Gait Analysis: Normal and Pathological Function.* Thorofare, NJ: Slack Inc. 1992:3-7.
11. Powers CM, Burnfield JM: Normal and pathologic gait. In: Placzek JD, Boyce DA, eds. *Orthopaedic Physical Therapy Secrets.* Philadelphia, PA: Hanley & Belfus Inc. 2001:98-103.
12. Mann RA, Moran GT, Dougherty SE: Comparative electromyography of the lower extremity in jogging, running and sprinting. *Am J Sports Med.* 1986;14:501-510.

13. Perry J: *Gait Analysis: Normal and Pathological Function.* Thorofare, NJ: Slack Inc. 1992.
14. Gage JR, Deluca PA, Renshaw TS: Gait analysis: principles and applications with emphasis on its use with cerebral palsy. *Inst Course Lect.* 1996;45:491-507.
15. Croskey MI, Dawson PM, Luessen AC, et al: The height of the center of gravity in man. *Am J Physiol.* 1922;61:171-185.
16. Saunders JBD, Inman VT, Eberhart HD: The major determinants in normal and pathological gait. *J Bone Joint Surg Am.* 1953; 35:543-558.
17. Whitehouse PA, Knight LA, Di Nicolantonio F, et al: Heterogeneity of chemosensitivity of colorectal adenocarcinoma determined by a modified ex vivo ATP-tumor chemosensitivity assay (ATP-TCA). *Anticancer Drugs.* 2003;14:369-375.
18. Dee R: Normal and abnormal gait in the pediatric patient. In: Dee R, Hurst LC, Gruber MA, et al, eds. *Principles of Orthopaedic Practice, 2nd ed.* New York: McGraw-Hill. 1997:685-692.
19. Blair E, Stanley F: Issues in the classification and epidemiology of cerebral palsy. *Mental Retard Devel Disab Res Rev.* 1997;3:184-193.
20. Baddar A, Granata K, Damiano DL, et al: Ankle and knee coupling in patients with spastic diplegia: effects of gastrocnemius-soleus lengthening. *J Bone and Joint Surg.* 2002;84A:736-744.
21. Abel MH, Damiano DL, Pannunzio M, et al: Muscle-tendon surgery in diplegic cerebral palsy: functional and mechanical changes. *J Pediatr Orthop.* 1999;19:366-375.
22. Davids JR, Foti T, Dabelstein J, et al: Voluntary (normal) versus obligatory (cerebral palsy) toe-walking in children: a kinematic, kinetic, and electromyographic analysis. *J Pediatr Orthop.* 1999;19: 461-469.
23. Morag E, Hurwitz DE, Andriacchi TP, et al: Abnormalities in muscle function during gait in relation to the level of lumbar disc herniation. *Spine.* 2000;25:829-833.
24. Eyring EJ, Murray W: The effect of joint position on the pressure of intra-articular effusion. *J Bone and Joint Surg.* 1965;47A:313-322.
25. Appling SA, Kasser RJ: Foot and ankle. In: Wadsworth C, ed. *Current Concepts of Orthopedic Physical Therapy—Home Study Course.* La Crosse, WI: Orthopaedic Section, APTA; 2001.
26. Boeing DD: Evaluation of a clinical method of gait analysis. *Phys Ther.* 1977;57:795-798.
27. McPoil TG, Schuit D, Knecht HG: A comparison of three positions used to evaluate tibial varum. *J Am Podiat Med Assn.* 1988; 78:22-28.
28. Hertling D, Kessler RM: *Management of Common Musculoskeletal Disorders: Physical Therapy Principles and Methods, 3rd ed.* Philadelphia, PA: Lippincott Williams & Wilkins; 1996.
29. Reid DC: *Sports Injury Assessment and Rehabilitation.* New York: Churchill Livingstone. 1992.
30. Mann RA: Biomechanical approach to the treatment of foot problems. *Foot & Ankle.* 1982;2:205-212.
31. Perry J: Hip Gait Deviations. In: Perry J, ed. *Gait Analysis: Normal and Pathological Function.* Thorofare, NJ: Slack, Inc. 1992:245-263.
32. Noyes FR, Dunworth LA, Andriacchi TP, et al: Knee hyperextension gait abnormalities in unstable knees. *Am J Sports Med.* 1996; 24:35-45.

33. Murray MP, Drought AB, Kory RC: Walking patterns of normal men. *J Bone Joint Surg Am.* 1964;46A:335-360.
34. Perry J: Pelvis and trunk pathological gait. In: Perry J, ed. *Gait Analysis: Normal and Pathological Function.* Thorofare, NJ: Slack, Inc; 1992:265-279.
35. Perry J: Knee abnormal gait. In: Perry J, ed. *Gait Analysis: Normal and Pathological Function.* Thorofare, NJ: Slack Inc. 1992:223-243.
36. Stauffer RN, Chao EYS, Gyory AN: Biomechanical gait analysis of the diseased knee joint. *Clin Orthop.* 1977;126:246-255
37. Perry J: Ankle and foot gait deviations. In: Perry J, ed. *Gait Analysis: Normal and Pathological Function.* Thorofare, NJ: Slack Inc. 1992:185-220
38. Oatis CA: Role of the hip in posture and gait. In: Echternach J, ed. *Clinics in Physical Therapy: Physical Therapy of the Hip.* New York: Churchill Livingstone. 1983:165-179.
39. Norkin CC: Examination of gait. In: O'Sullivan SB, Schmitz TJ, eds. *Physical Rehabilitation, 5th ed.* Philadelphia: FA Davis; 2007:317-363.
40. Nelson AJ: Functional ambulation profile. *Phys Ther.* 1974; 54:1059-1065.
41. Dickson HG, Kohler F: Functional independence measure (FIM). *Scand J Rehabil Med.* 1999;31:63-64.
42. Grey N, Kennedy P: The Functional Independence Measure: a comparative study of clinician and self ratings. *Paraplegia.* 1993; 31:457-461.
43. Hamilton BB, Laughlin JA, Fiedler RC, et al: Interrater reliability of the 7-level functional independence measure (FIM). *Scand J Rehabil Med.* 1994;26:115-119.
44. Keith RA, Granger CV, Hamilton BB, et al: The functional independence measure: a new tool for rehabilitation. *Adv Clin Rehabil.* 1987;1:6-18.
45. Wolfson L, Whipple R, Amerman P, et al: Gait assessment in the elderly: a gait abnormality rating scale and its relation to falls. *J Gerontol.* 1990;45:M12-M19.
46. Holden MK, Gill KM, Magliozzi MR: Gait assessment for neurologically impaired patients. Standards for outcome assessment. *Phys Ther.* 1986;66:1530-1539.
47. Holden MK, Gill KM, Magliozzi MR, et al: Clinical gait assessment in the neurologically impaired. Reliability and meaningfulness. *Phys Ther.* 1984;64:35-40.
48. Mathias S, Nayak US, Isaacs B: Balance in elderly patients: the "get-up and go" test. *Arch Phys Med Rehabil.* 1986;67:387-389.
49. Kristensen MT, Foss NB, Kehlet H: Timed "up & go" test as a predictor of falls within 6 months after hip fracture surgery. *Phys Ther.* 2007;87:24-30. Epub 2006 Dec 1.
50. Large J, Gan N, Basic D, et al: Using the timed up and go test to stratify elderly inpatients at risk of falls. *Clin Rehabil.* 2006; 20:421-428.
51. Ng SS, Hui-Chan CW: The timed up & go test: its reliability and association with lower-limb impairments and locomotor capacities in people with chronic stroke. *Arch Phys Med Rehabil.* 2005; 86:1641-1647.
52. Podsiadlo D, Richardson S: The timed "Up & Go": a test of basic functional mobility for frail elderly persons. *J Am Geriatr Soc.* 1991;39:142-148.

53. Goodman CC, Snyder TEK: *Differential Diagnosis in Physical Therapy.* Philadelphia, PA: WB Saunders Company. 1990.
54. Ayub E: Posture and the upper quarter. In: Donatelli RA, ed. *Physical Therapy of the Shoulder, 2nd ed.* New York: Churchill Livingstone. 1991:81-90.
55. Janda V: On the concept of postural muscles and posture in man. *Aust J Physiother.* 1983;29:83-84.
56. Turner M: Posture and pain. *Phys Ther.* 1957;37:294.
57. Kendall FP, McCreary EK, Provance PG: *Muscles: Testing and Function.* Baltimore, MD: Williams & Wilkins. 1993.
58. Greenfield B, Catlin P, Coats P, et al: Posture in patients with shoulder overuse injuries and healthy individuals. *J Orthop Sports Phys Ther.* 1995;21:287-295.
59. Clayton-Krasinski D, Klepper S: Impaired neuromotor development. In: Cameron MH, Monroe LG, eds. *Physical Rehabilitation: Evidence-Based Examination, Evaluation, and Intervention.* St Louis, MO: Saunders/Elsevier. 2007:333-366.
60. Putz-Anderson V: *Cumulative Trauma Disorders: A Manual for Musculoskeletal Diseases of the Upper Limbs.* Bristol, PA: Taylor & Francis. 1988.
61. Keller K, Corbett J, Nichols D: Repetitive strain injury in computer keyboard users: pathomechanics and treatment principles in individual and group intervention. *J Hand Ther.* 1998; 11:9-26.
62. Korr IM, Wright HM, Thomas PE: Effects of experimental myofascial insults on cutaneous patterns of sympathetic activity in man. *J Neural Transm.* 1962;23:330-355.
63. Travell JG, Simons DGL: *Myofascial Pain and Dysfunction—The Trigger Point Manual.* Baltimore, MD: Williams & Wilkins; 1983.
64. Beal MC: The short leg problem. *JAOA.* 1977;76:745-751.
65. Wilder DG, Pope MH, Frymoyer JW: The biomechanics of lumbar disc herniation and the effect of overload and instability. *J Spinal Disord.* 1988;1:16.
66. Kiser DM: Physiological and biomechanical factors for understanding repetitive motion injuries. *Semin Occup Med.* 1987; 2:11-17.
67. Greenfield B: Upper quarter evaluation: structural relationships and interindependence. In: Donatelli R, Wooden M, eds. *Orthopedic Physical Therapy.* New York: Churchill Livingstone. 1989:43-58.
68. Janda V: Muscle strength in relation to muscle length, pain and muscle imbalance. In: Harms-Ringdahl K, ed. *Muscle Strength.* New York: Churchill Livingstone. 1993:83-91.
69. Janda V: *Muscle Function Testing.* London: Butterworths; 1983.
70. Lewit K: *Manipulative Therapy in Rehabilitation of the Motor System, 3rd ed.* London: Butterworths. 1999.
71. Lewit K: Simons DG. Myofascial pain: relief by post-isometric relaxation. *Archives of Physical Medicine & Rehabilitation.* 1984; 65:452-426.
72. Sahrmann SA: *Diagnosis and Treatment of Movement Impairment Syndromes.* St Louis: Mosby. 2001.
73. Smith A: Upper limb disorders—time to relax? *Physiotherapy.* 1996;82:31-38.
74. Babyar SR: Excessive scapular motion in individuals recovering from painful and stiff shoulders: causes and treatment strategies. *Phys Ther.* 1996;76:226-247.

75. Tardieu C, Tabary JC, Tardieu G, et al: Adaptation of sarcomere numbers to the length imposed on muscle. In: Guba F, Marechal G, Takacs O, eds. *Mechanism of Muscle Adaptation to Functional Requirements.* Elmsford, NY: Pergamon Press. 1981:99-114.
76. Seidel-Cobb D, Cantu R: Myofascial treatment. In: Donatelli RA, ed. *Physical Therapy of the Shoulder, 3rd ed.* New York: Churchill Livingstone. 1997:383-401.
77. Janda V: Muscles, motor regulation and back problems. In: Korr IM, ed. *The Neurological Mechanisms in Manipulative Therapy.* New York: Plenum. 1978:27-41.
78. Jull GA, Janda V: Muscle and motor control in low back pain. In:Twomey LT, Taylor JR, eds. *Physical Therapy of the Low Back: Clinics in Physical Therapy.* New York: Churchill Livingstone. 1987:258-278.
79. Janda V: Muscles and motor control in cervicogenic disorders: assessment and management. In: Grant R, ed. *Physical Therapy of the Cervical and Thoracic Spine.* New York: Churchill Livingstone. 1994:195-216.
80. Wiles P, Sweetnam R: *Essentials of Orthopedics.* London: J.A. Churchill; 1965.
81. Deyo RA, Rainville J, Kent DL: What can the history and physical examination tell us about low back pain? *JAMA.* 1992;268: 760-765.
82. Bland JH: Diagnosis of thoracic pain syndromes. In: Giles LGF, Singer KP, eds. *Clinical Anatomy and Management of the Thoracic Spine.* Oxford: Butterworth-Heinemann; 2000:145-156.
83. Sutherland ID: Funnel chest. *J Bone Joint Surg.* 1958;40B:244-251.
84. Bradford S: Juvenile kyphosis. In: Bradford DS, Lonstein JE, Moe JH, et al, eds. *Moe's Textbook of Scoliosis and Other Spinal Deformities.* Philadelphia, PA: W.B. Saunders; 1987:347-368.
85. McKenzie RA: Manual correction of sciatic scoliosis. *N Z Med J.* 1972;76:194-199.
86. Keim HA: *The Adolescent Spine.* New York: Springer-Verlag; 1982.
87. Ponseti IV, Friedman B: Prognosis in idiopathic scoliosis. *J Bone Joint Surg Am.* 1950;32A:381-395.
88. Ponseti IV, Pedrini V, Wynne-Davies R, et al: Pathogenesis of scoliosis. *Clin Orthop Relat Res.* 1976;120:268-280.
89. Weinstein SL, Ponseti IV: Curve progression in idiopathic scoliosis. *J Bone Joint Surg Am.* 1983;65:447-455.
90. Lowe T, Berven SH, Schwab FJ, et al: The SRS classification for adult spinal deformity: building on the King/Moe and Lenke classification systems. *Spine.* 2006;31:S119-125.
91. Lenke LG: Lenke classification system of adolescent idiopathic scoliosis: treatment recommendations. *Instr Course Lect.* 2005; 54:537-542.
92. Lenke LG, Edwards CC, 2nd, Bridwell KH: The Lenke classification of adolescent idiopathic scoliosis: how it organizes curve patterns as a template to perform selective fusions of the spine. *Spine.* 2003;28:S199-S207.
93. Durham JW, Moskowitz K, Whitney J: Surface elcetrical stimulation versus brace in treatment of idiopathic scoliosis. *Spine.* 1990;15:888-892.
94. Andersson BJ, Ortengren R, Nachemson AL, et al: The sitting posture: an electromyographic and discometric study. *Orthop Clin North Am.* 1975;6:105-120.

95 Williams MM, Hawley JA, McKenzie RA, et al: A comparison of the effects of two sitting postures on back and referred pain. *Spine.* 1991;16:1185-1191.
96. Nachemson A: Towards a better understanding of low-back pain: a review of the mechanics of the lumbar disc. *Rheumatol Rehabil.* 1975;14:129-143.
97. American Physical Therapy Association. *Guide to Physical Therapist Practice, 2nd ed. Phys Ther.* 2001;81:1-746.
98. Lechner D, Daly J, Maltchev K, et al: The work-injured population. In: Boissonnault WG, ed. *Primary Care for the Physical Therapist: Examination and Triage.* St Louis: Elsevier Saunders; 2005:271-287.
99. Schmitz TJ: Examination of the environment. In: O'Sullivan SB, Schmitz TJ, eds. *Physical Rehabilitation, 5th ed.* Philadelphia, PA: FA Davis; 2007:401-467.
100. Paterson M, Mets T: Environmental assessment: home, community, and work. In: Cameron MH, Monroe LG, eds. *Physical Rehabilitation: Evidence-Based Examination, Evaluation, and Intervention.* St Louis, MO: Saunders/Elsevier; 2007:918-936.
101. Lee RE, Booth KM, Reese-Smith JY, et al. The Physical Activity Resource Assessment (PARA) instrument: evaluating features, amenities and incivilities of physical activity resources in urban neighborhoods. *Int J Behav Nutr Phys Act.* 2005;2:13.
102. Keysor J, Jette A, Haley S: Development of the home and community environment (HACE) instrument. *J Rehabil Med.* 2005; 37:37-44.
103. Oliver R, Blathwayt J, Brackley C, et al: Development of the Safety Assessment of Function and the Environment for Rehabilitation (SAFER) tool. *Can J Occup Ther.* 1993;60:78-82.
104. Gerr F, Marcus M, Monteilh C, et al: A randomised controlled trial of postural interventions for prevention of musculoskeletal symptoms among computer users. *Occup Environ Med.* 2005; 62:478-487.
105. Dainoff MJ, Cohen BG, Dainoff MH: The effect of an ergonomic intervention on musculoskeletal, psychosocial, and visual strain of VDT data entry work: the United States part of the international study. 2005;11:49-63.
106. Moise A, Atkins MS: Design requirements for radiology workstations. *J Digit Imaging.* 17:92-99. Epub 2004 Apr 19, 2004.
107. Ong CN, Chia SE, Jeyaratnam J, et al: Musculoskeletal disorders among operators of visual display terminals. *Scand J Work Environ Health.* 1995;21:60-64.
108. Horii SC: Electronic imaging workstations: ergonomic issues and the user interface. *Radiographics.* 1992;12:773-787.
109. Mackenzie M: A simplified measure of balance by functional reach. *Physiother Res Int.* 1999;4:233-236.
110. Duncan PW, Weiner DK, Chandler J, et al: Functional reach: a new clinical measure of balance. *J Gerontol.* 1990; 45:M192-M197.
111. Nelson A, Matz M, Chen F, et al: Development and evaluation of a multifaceted ergonomics program to prevent injuries associated with patient handling tasks. *Int J Nurs Stud.* 2005;43: 717-733. Epub 2005 Oct 25, 2006.

112. Punnett L: Commentary on the scientific basis of the proposed Occupational Safety and Health Administration Ergonomics Program Standard. *J Occup Environ Med.* 2000;42:970-981.
113. Hadler NM: Comments on the "Ergonomics Program Standard" proposed by the Occupational Safety and Health Administration. *J Occup Environ Med.* 2000; 42:951-969.

Musculoskeletal Physical Therapy

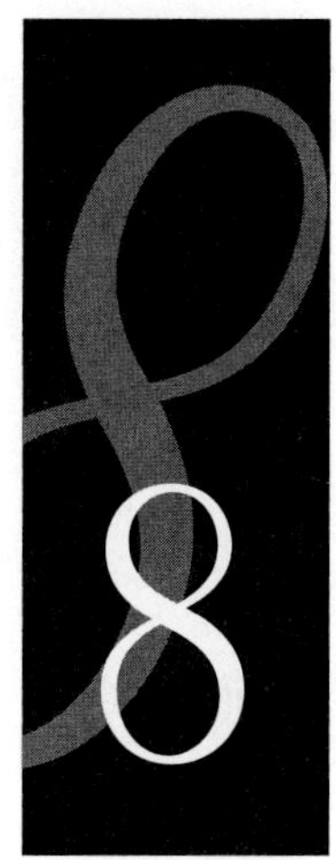

The musculoskeletal system includes bones; muscles with their related tendons and synovial sheaths; bursae; and joint structures such as cartilage, menisci, capsules, and ligaments.

FUNCTIONAL ANATOMY AND BIOMECHANICS OF SPECIFIC JOINTS

Shoulder Complex

The shoulder complex (Figure 8-1) is composed of four separate articulations:

1. The glenohumeral (GH) joint
2. The acromioclavicular (AC) joint
3. The sternoclavicular (SC) joint
4. The scapulothoracic pseudoarticulation

The subacromial junction between the coracoacromial arch (a rigid structure above the humeral head and rotator cuff tendons) and the rotator cuff tendons—is considered by some as a fifth "articulation".[1]

Bursae. Approximately eight bursae are distributed throughout the shoulder complex. The subdeltoid-subacromial bursae, collectively referred to as the subacromial bursa, are the most significant with relation to pathology. As the humerus elevates, the bursae permit the rotator cuff to slide easily beneath the deltoid muscle.

Biomechanics. Complete movement at the shoulder girdle involves a complex interaction between the glenohumeral; AC and SC complex; scapulothoracic, upper thoracic, costal, and sternomanubrial joints; and the lower cervical spine.

Study Pearl

An important bony landmark in the shoulder is the coracoid process, medial to which run the major blood vessels and the brachial plexus complex. The coracoid serves as a muscular attachment for the pectoralis minor, the short head of the biceps, and the coracobrachialis. The acromion and the acromioclavicular joint are also important bony landmarks that can be easily palpated.

Study Pearl

Injury to the long thoracic nerve leads to paralysis of the serratus anterior muscle, resulting in medial scapular winging.

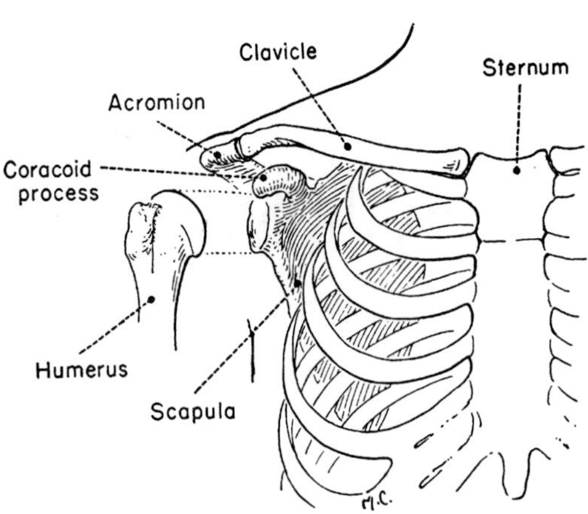

Figure 8-1. Anterior view of right shoulder joints. (Reproduced, with permission, from Luttgens K, Hamilton N: *Kinesiology: Scientific Basis of Human Motion, 10th ed.* New York, NY: McGraw-Hill. 2002:104.)

Study Pearl

Sprengel's deformity, a failure of the scapula to descend during normal musculoskeletal development, is characterized as a prominent lump in the web of the neck. This condition may be associated with scoliosis and rib abnormalities.

GH Joint

- The convex humeral head articulates with the concave glenoid fossa of the scapula (Table 8-1). The humeral head is retroverted 20 to 30 degrees. The longitudinal axis of the head is 135 degrees from the axis of the neck.
- The glenoid is retroverted approximately 7 degrees. It faces anteriorly at an angle of approximately 45 degrees to the coronal plane, as it sits on the chest wall. The depth of the glenoid fossa is enhanced by the glenoid labrum, which can contribute up to 50% of the fossa's depth.
- The scapula is a flat triangular bone, situated over the second to seventh ribs. The glenoid fossa is located on the lateral angle of the scapula and faces anteriorly, laterally and superiorly. This orientation places true abduction at 30 degrees anterior to the frontal plane.

Study Pearl

Snapping scapula is a condition resulting from friction between the scapula and its attached soft tissues and the thoracic wall. Causes for snapping scapula include thickened bursa and bone spurs on the scapula or a rib.

The GH joint is relatively unstable:

- Static stability for the joint is provided by the previously mentioned labrum, and a variety of ligaments (Table 8-2). The joint capsule is reinforced by the GH ligaments, which are distinct capsular thickenings that limit excessive rotation and translation of the humeral head by reinforcing the connection between the glenoid fossa and the humerus. The GH ligaments have a number of subdivisions:

Study Pearl

The term "scaption" refers to the forward elevation of an internally rotated arm in the scapular plane (30-45 degrees from the coronal plane) with the thumb pointed to the floor.

TABLE 8-1. GLENOHUMERAL JOINT MOTIONS AND THEIR APPROPRIATE AXIS AND ACCESSORY MOTIONS

PLANE/AXIS OF MOTION	PHYSIOLOGICAL MOTION	ACCESSORY MOTION
Sagittal/medial-lateral	Flexion/extension	Spin
Coronal/anterior–posterior	Abduction	Inferior glide of humeral head
	Adduction	Superior glide of humeral head
Transverse/longitudinal	Internal rotation	Posterior glide of humeral head
	External rotation	Anterior glide of humeral head

TABLE 8-2. LIGAMENTS OF THE SHOULDER

LIGAMENT	DESCRIPTION	FUNCTION
Coracohumeral Ligament	Runs from the lateral end of the coracoid process and inserts either side of the greater and lesser tuberosities	Provides anterior support by tightening with flexion
Transverse Humeral Ligament	Traverses the bicipital groove	Maintains the long head of the biceps muscle in the intertubercular groove
Coracoclavicular Ligament	Comprised of the conoid and trapezoid ligaments	Reinforces the connection between the coracoid process and the clavicle
Acromioclavicular Ligament	Runs between the acromion process and the clavicle	Stabilizes the acromioclavicular joint
		Reinforces the connection between the acromion and the clavicle
Sternoclavicular Ligaments	Comprised of anterior and posterior ligaments	Reinforces the connection between the sternum and the clavicle
Interclavicular Ligament	Connects the superior-medial sternal ends of each clavicle with the capsular ligaments and the upper sternum	Strengthens the articular capsule
Costoclavicular Ligament	The strongest of the sternoclavicular ligaments	Reinforces the connection between the first rib and the clavicle and stabilizes the joint
Intrinsic Ligaments of the Scapula	Attached by one end to the base of the coracoid process, and by the other to the medial end of the scapular notch	Reinforces the connection between the coracoid process and the medial border of the scapular notch
Inferior Transverse Scapular Ligament	An inconstant fibrous band that passes from the lateral border of the spine of the scapula to the posterior margin of the glenoid cavity	Reinforces the connection between the lateral aspect of the root of the spine of the scapula and the margin of the glenoid fossa
Coracoacromial Ligament	Runs from the coracoid process to the anteriorñinferior aspect of the acromion, with some of its fibers extending to the AC joint	Reinforces the connection between the coracoid process and the acromion, stabilizing the joint

- Inferior glenohumeral ligament (IGHL): A ligamentous complex—parts include the anterior band, axillary pouch, and the posterior band. The IGHL provides anterior stabilization, especially during abduction of the arm.
- Middle glenohumeral ligament: Strongest of the glenohumeral ligaments and provides anterior stabilization during the combined motion of external rotation and 45 degrees of abduction.

▶ Superior glenohumeral ligament: Runs from the glenoid rim to the anatomical neck and works in conjunction with the coracohumeral ligament to provide inferior stabilization during adduction.

▶ Dynamic stability for the joint is afforded by the muscular dynamic stabilizers, in particular the rotator cuff, the biceps tendon, and the muscles of scapular motion (Tables 8-3 and Table 8-4). The normal strength ratios of the shoulder are outlined in Table 8-5.

Available ranges of motion of the shoulder complex, end feels, and potential causes of pain are listed in Table 8-6.

Study Pearl

Superior labrum anterior and posterior (SLAP) lesions most often result from a sudden downward force on a supinated outstretched upper extremity or from a fall on the lateral aspect of the shoulder.

Study Pearl

- ▶ The capsular pattern of the shoulder is a motion restriction of external rotation > abduction > internal rotation, often noted in frozen shoulders.
- ▶ The reverse capsular pattern of the shoulder is internal rotation > elevation (abduction/flexion), often noted in impingement syndrome.

TABLE 8-3 MUSCLES OF THE SHOULDER COMPLEX ACCORDING TO THEIR ACTIONS ON THE SCAPULAR AND AT THE GLENOHUMERAL JOINT

ACTION	MUSCLES	NERVE SUPPLY
Glenohumeral Flexors	Coracobrachialis	Musculocutaneous
	Short and long head of the biceps brachii	Musculocutaneous
	Pectoralis major (clavicular head)	Lateral and medial pectoral
	Anterior deltoid	Axillary
Glenohumeral Extensors	Triceps (long head)	Radial
	Posterior deltoid	Axillary
	Pectoralis major	Lateral and medial pectoral
	Teres major	Thoracodorsal
	Latissimus dorsi	Thoracodorsal
Glenohumeral Abductors	Supraspinatus	Suprascapular
	Anterior and middle deltoid	Axillary
Glenohumeral Adductors	Pectoralis major	Lateral and medial pectoral
	Latissimus dorsi	Thoracodorsal
	Teres major	Thoracodorsal
	Coracobrachialis	Musculocutaneous
Glenohumeral Internal Rotators	Pectoralis major	Lateral and medial pectoral
	Subscapularis	Subscapular
	Latissimus dorsi	Thoracodorsal
	Teres major	Thoracodorsal
Glenohumeral External Rotators	Infraspinatus	Suprascapular
	Posterior deltoid	Axillary
	Teres minor	Axillary
Scapular Abductors/Protractors	Pectoralis minor	Lateral and medial pectoral
	Serratus anterior (upper fibers)	Long thoracic
Scapular Adductors/Retractors	Levator scapulae	Dorsal scapular
	Rhomboids	Dorsal scapular
	Middle trapezius (upper and lower trapezius assist)	Spinal accessory
Scapular Elevators	Upper trapezius	Spinal accessory
	Levator scapula	Dorsal scapular
	Rhomboids	Dorsal scapular
Scapular Depressors	Lower trapezius	Spinal accessory
	Latissimus dorsi	Thoracodorsal
	Pectoralis minor	Medial pectoral
	Subclavius	Nerve to subclavius
Scapular Upward Rotators	Serratus anterior	Long thoracic
	Upper trapezius	Spinal accessory
	Lower trapezius	Spinal accessory
Scapular Downward Rotators	Rhomboids	Dorsal scapular
	Pectoralis minor	Medial pectoral
	Levator scapula	Dorsal scapular
Scapular Retractors/Abductors	Rhomboids	Dorsal scapular
	Middle trapezius	Spinal accessory

The Scapulohumeral Rhythm. The scapula provides a mobile base for humeral motions in all directions. Scapular motion occurs in all three cardinal planes:

- Rotation of the scapula occurs in the transverse plane.
- The scapula externally rotates from a starting point of approximately 33 degrees internal rotation to 20 degrees internal rotation as the arm is elevated from 0 to 140 degrees in the scapular plane.
- Tilting of the scapula involves rotation in the sagittal plane.

TABLE 8-4. DYNAMIC RESTRAINTS ABOUT THE GLENOHUMERAL JOINT

Humeral stabilizers	Supraspinatus Infraspinatus Subscapularis Teres minor
Movers of glenohumeral joint	Pectoralis major Latissimus dorsi Biceps (long head) Triceps Deltoid Teres major
Movers of scapula	Serratus anterior Latissimus dorsi Trapezius Rhomboids Levator scapulae Pectoralis minor

TABLE 8-5. NORMAL STRENGTH RATIOS OF THE SHOULDER

Internal to external rotation: 3 to 2
Adduction to abduction: 2 to 1
Extension to flexion: 5 to 4

TABLE 8-6. MOVEMENTS OF THE SHOULDER COMPLEX, NORMAL RANGES, END FEELS, AND POTENTIAL CAUSES OF PAIN

MOTION	RANGE NORMS (DEGREES)	END FEEL	POTENTIAL SOURCE OF PAIN
Elevation—flexion	0-180	Tissue stretch Motion limited by: posterior band of the coracohumeral ligament, inferoposterior joint capsule	-Suprahumeral impingement -Stretching of glenohumeral, acromioclavicular, sternoclavicular joint capsule -Triceps tendon if elbow flexed
Extension	0-60	Tissue stretch Motion limited by: coracohumeral ligament, anterior joint capsule	-Stretching of glenohumeral joint capsule -Severe suprahumeral impingement -Biceps tendon if elbow extended
Elevation—abduction	0-180	Tissue stretch Motion limited by: inferior joint capsule, glenohumeral ligament, approximation of greater tuberosity and glenoid labrum	-Suprahumeral impingement -Acromioclavicular arthritis at terminal abduction
External rotation	0-85	Tissue stretch Motion limited by: anterior capsule, glenohumeral ligament	-Anterior glenohumeral instability
Internal rotation	0-95	Tissue stretch Motion limited by: posterior capsule	-Suprahumeral impingement -Posterior glenohumeral instability

Study Pearl

Scapular dyskinesia (also referred to as abnormal scapulohumeral rhythm, scapular winging, and scapular dysrhythmia) refers to an abnormal or atypical movement of the scapula during normal active motion. Scapular dyskinesia is common in patients with an unstable glenohumeral joint or patients with impingement syndrome.

Study Pearl

- Shoulder dislocation: a true separation between the head of the humerus and the glenoid. Can occur posteriorly or, more commonly, anteriorly. The most commonly injured nerve with an anterior shoulder dislocation is the axillary nerve.
- Hill-Sachs lesion: a compression fracture of the poster lateral aspect of the humeral head, which results from impact on the anteroinferior rim of the glenoid during an anterior dislocation of the shoulder.
- Reverse Hill-Sachs lesion: a compression fracture of the anteromedial humeral head as result of a posterior dislocation.
- Bankart lesion: an avulsion or detachment of the anterior portion of the inferior glenohumeral ligament complex and glenoid labrum of the anterior rim of the glenoid. Bankart lesions can contribute to recurrent instability.
- Shoulder subluxation: excessive movement of the humeral head with respect to the glenoid, but not a true separation.
- Shoulder separation: disruption of the acromioclavicular joint.

During elevation of the arm in the scapular plane, the scapula rotates upwardly, externally rotates, and tilts posteriorly. The combination and synchronization of the motions that occur between the scapula and the humerus during elevation is termed "scapulohumeral rhythm." With 180 degrees of abduction there is an approximate 2:1 ratio of movement between the two structures—120 degrees of movement occurs at the GH joint, with 60 degrees of motion occurring at the scapulothoracic joint. The scapulohumeral rhythm (Figure 8-2) decreases the potential for shear and translatory forces at the GH joint by actively positioning the scapula in relation to the moving humerus, thereby providing a stable base of muscle origin for the rotator cuff muscles.

By allowing the glenoid to stay centered under the humeral head, the strong tendency for a downward dislocation of the humerus is resisted and the glenoid is maintained within a physiologically tolerable range. At full abduction, the glenoid completely supports the humerus.

Sternoclavicular and Acromioclavicular Joints

- SC joint: The clavicle, which is convex in a superior/inferior direction and concave in an anterior/posterior direction articulates with the reciprocal shape of the sternum in a fibrocartilaginous joint (Table 8-7). The SC joint is the only joint that

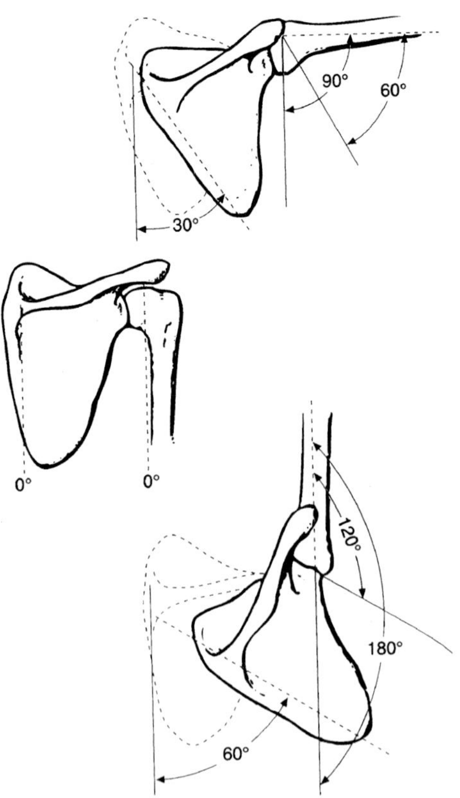

Figure 8-2. Normal scapulohumeral rhythm. (Reproduced, with permission, from Brukner P, Khan K: *Clinical Sports Medicine, 3rd ed.* Sydney, Australia: McGraw-Hill. 2007:64.)

TABLE 8-7. MOVEMENTS OF THE ACROMIOCLAVICULAR AND STERNOCLAVICULAR COMPLEX

MOTION	RANGE OF MOTION	MOTION LIMITED BY
Protraction (sagittal plane: clavicle glides posteriorly, acromion glides anteriorly)	The distal clavicle moves approximately 10 cm	Anterior SC ligament, costoclavicular ligament (posterior portion), anterior capsule of the SC joint
Retraction (transverse plane: clavicle glides anteriorly, acromion glides posteriorly)	Distal clavicle moves approximately 3 cm	Posterior SC ligament, costoclavicular ligament (anterior portion), posterior capsule of the SC joint
Elevation (frontal plane: clavicle glides superiorly, only slight angular motion occurs at AC joint)	The distal clavicle moves approximately 10 cm	Costoclavicular ligament, inferior capsule of the SC joint
Depression (frontal plane: clavicle glides inferiorly, only slight angular motion occurs at AC joint)	Distal clavicle moves approximately 3 cm	Interclavicular ligament, SC ligament, articular disk of SC joint, superior capsule of SC joint
Rotation (transverse plane)	30 degrees at AC joint then 30 degrees at SC joint	SC: anterior and posterior sternoclavicular ligament, interclavicular ligament, costoclavicular ligament AC: acromioclavicular ligament, coracoclavicular ligament (conoid [limits backward rotation], trapezoid [limits forward rotation])

directly attaches the upper extremity to the thorax. The allowed movements are elevation and depression, protraction and retraction, and rotation.

- AC joint: A plane joint, but also described as diarthrodial, with fibrocartilage surfaces—a convex clavicle and a concave acromion. The joint contains an intra-articular fibrocartilaginous disk, which degenerates during the third and fourth decades of life.

Study Pearl

Sternoclavicular joint injuries are relatively rare but can result from indirect or direct trauma. Posterior dislocations can have serious implications.

Nerve Supply. The shoulder complex is embryologically derived from C5 to C8, except the AC joint, which is derived from C4.[2-4] The sympathetic nerve supply to the shoulder originates primarily in the thoracic region from T2 down as far as T8.[5]

Blood Supply. The vascular supply to the shoulder girdle is primarily provided by branches of the axillary artery (including the thoracoacromial artery, subscapular artery, and the anterior and posterior circumflex humeral arteries), which begins at the outer border of the first rib as a continuation of the subclavian artery.

ELBOW COMPLEX

The elbow is composed of three articulations (Figure 8-3 and Table 8-8). The elbow is a very congruous joint, and, hence, inherently very stable.

Muscles. Details about the muscles of the elbow and forearm are provided in Table 8-9

Ligaments

Medial (Ulnar) Collateral Ligament. There are three distinct components of the ulnar collateral ligament (UCL): anterior bundle, transverse

Study Pearl

There are two anatomic intervals of note in the region[1]:

1. The quadrangular space is formed by the shaft of the humerus laterally, the long head of the triceps medially, the teres minor muscle superiorly, and teres major muscle inferiorly. Through it passes the axillary nerve and the posterior humeral circumflex artery.
2. The triangular space is formed by the long head of the triceps laterally, the teres minor superiorly, and the teres major inferiorly. Through it passes the circumflex scapular artery, a branch of the scapular artery.

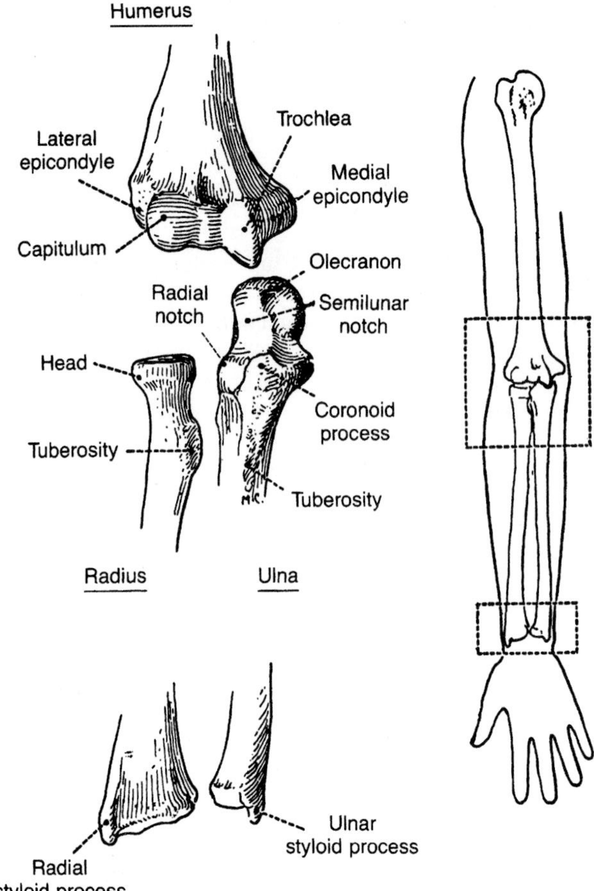

Figure 8-3. The lateral aspect of the elbow joint showing ligaments. (Reproduced, with permission, from Luttgens K, Hamilton N: *Kinesiology: Scientific Basis of Human Motion, 10th ed.* New York, NY: McGraw-Hill. 2002:129.)

bundle, and posterior bundle. The fan-shaped UCL is functionally the most important ligament in the elbow for providing stability against valgus stress.[6,7]

Lateral Collateral Ligament. The lateral collateral ligament (Figure 8-3) consists of the annular ligament, the fan-like radial collateral ligament (RCL) that originates from the lateral humerus

TABLE 8-8. MUSCLES OF THE ELBOW AND FOREARM

ACTION	MUSCLES	NERVE	NERVE ROOT
Elbow flexion	Brachialis (workhorse of elbow flexion)	Musculocutaneous	C5-C6, (C7)
	Biceps brachii	Musculocutaneous	C5-C6
	Brachioradialis	Radial	C5-C6, (C7)
		Median	C6-C7
Elbow extension	Triceps	Radial	C7-C8
	Anconeus	Radial	C7-C8, (T1)
Forearm supination	Supinator	Posterior interosseous (radial)	C5-C6
	Biceps brachii	Musculocutaneous	C5-C6
Forearm pronation	Pronator quadratus	Anterior interosseous (median)	C8, T1
	Pronator teres	Median	C6-C7

TABLE 8-9. ARTICULATIONS OF THE ELBOW

JOINT	DESCRIPTION	FUNCTION
Humeroulnar	The concave ulna articulates with the convex distal humerus (trochlea)	A hinged articulation that permits motion in a single plane, allowing for flexion and extension of the elbow.
Humeroradial (radiocapitellar)	The concave head of the radius articulates with the capitellum, which is the convex lateral articular surface of the distal humerus.	The joint permits the radius to rotate to any degree of flexion or extension of the humeroulnar joint, and this rotation allows supination and pronation of the forearm (in association with the proximal radioulnar joint [the third articulation of the elbow]).
Proximal radioulnar	Formed between the periphery of the convex radial head, and the fibrous osseous ring formed by the concave radial notch of the ulna	This is an uniaxial pivot joint, which lies distal to the trochlear notch, and the annular ligament. The proximal and distal radioulnar joints together form a bicondylar joint. An interosseous membrane located between the radius and ulna serves to help distribute forces throughout the forearm, and provide muscle attachment.

at the center of the trochlea and capitellum, the accessory collateral ligament, and the lateral aspect of the UCL. As the axis for rotation passes through the origin of the RCL, the anterior, middle, and posterior fibers of this ligament maintain consistent patterns of tension whether varus, valgus, or no force is applied to the elbow throughout the arc of flexion.[8,9] The RCL functions to maintain the ulnohumeral and radiohumeral joints in a reduced position when the elbow is loaded in supination. Secondary restraints of the lateral elbow consist of the bony articulations, the joint capsule, and the extensor muscles with their fascial bands and intermuscular septa.

Annular Ligament. The annular ligament functions to maintain the relationship between the head of the radius and the humerus and ulna.

Bursae. There are numerous bursae in the elbow region:

- Olecranon bursa: the main bursa of the elbow complex. It lies posteriorly between the skin and the olecranon process.
- Deep intratendinous bursa and deep subtendinous bursa: present between the triceps tendon and olecranon.
- Bicipitoradial bursa: separates the biceps tendon from the radial tuberosity.
- Subcutaneous medial epicondylar bursa.
- Subcutaneous lateral epicondylar bursa.

Nerve Supply. The elbow has a complex innervation (Table 8-10).

Blood Supply. The elbow complex receives its blood supply from the brachial artery, anterior ulnar recurrent artery, posterior ulnar recurrent artery, radial recurrent artery, and middle collateral branch of the arteria profunda brachii.

Study Pearl

The cubital tunnel is a fibro-osseous canal, through which the ulnar nerve passes.

The volume of the cubital tunnel is greatest with the elbow held in extension and the least in full elbow flexion. A number of factors have been associated with a decrease in the size of the cubital tunnel:

- Space-occupying lesions
- Bulging of the UCL
- Osteoarthritis
- Rheumatoid arthritis
- Heterotopic bone formation
- Trauma to the nerve

Patients with systemic conditions such as diabetes mellitus, hypothyroidism, alcoholism, and renal failure also may have a predisposition.

TABLE 8-10 NERVE INNERVATION OF THE ELBOW COMPLEX AND INJURY CONSEQUENCES

NERVE	PERTINENT ANATOMY	MOTOR LOSS	SENSORY LOSS	FUNCTIONAL LOSS
Median nerve (C6-C8, T1)	Passes through the two heads of the pronator teres, which is a potential site of entrapment	Pronator teres Flexor carpi radialis Palmaris longus Flexor digitorum superficialis Flexor pollicis longus Lateral half of flexor digitorum profundus Pronator quadratus Thenar eminence Lateral two lumbricals	Palmar aspect of hand with thumb, index, middle, and lateral half of ring finger. Dorsal aspect of distal third of index, middle, and lateral half of ring finger.	Pronation weakness Wrist flexion and abduction weakness Loss of radial deviation at wrist Inability to oppose or flex thumb Thumb abduction weakness Weak grip Weak or no pinch (ape hand deformity)
Anterior interosseous nerve (branch of median nerve)		Flexor pollicis longus Lateral half of flexor digitorum profundus Pronator quadratus Thenar eminence muscles Lateral two lumbricals	None	Pronation weakness especially at 90 degrees elbow flexion Weakness of opposition and thumb flexion Weak finger flexion Weak pinch (no tip-to-tip)
Ulnar nerve (C7-C8, T1)	Passes along the medial arm and posterior to the medial epicondyle through the cubital tunnel, a likely site of compression	Flexor carpi ulnaris Medial half of flexor digitorum profundus Palmaris brevis Hypothenar eminence Adductor pollicis Medial two lumbricals All interossei	Dorsal and palmar aspect of little and medial half of ring finger	Weak wrist flexion Loss of ulnar deviation at wrist Loss of distal flexion of little finger Loss of abduction and adduction of fingers Inability to extend second and third phalanges of little and ring fingers (benediction hand deformity) Loss of thumb adduction
Redial nerve (C5-C8, T1)	Divides into the superficial (sensory) branch and the deep (motor, or posterior interosseous) branch. The deep branch must then pass through the arcade of Fröhse, a fibrous arch formed by the proximal margin of the superficial head of the supinator muscle, where it is most susceptible to injury	Anconeus Brachioradialis Extensor carpi radialis longus and brevis Extensor digitorum Extensor pollicis longus and brevis Abductor pollicis longus Extensor carpi ulnaris Extensor indices Extensor digiti minimi	Dorsum of hand (lateral two-thirds) Dorsum and lateral aspect of thumb Proximal two-thirds of dorsum of index, middle, and half of ring finger	Loss of supination Loss of wrist extension (wrist drop) Inability to grasp Inability to stabilize wrist Loss of finger extension Inability to abduct thumb
Posterior interosseous nerve		Extensor carpi radialis brevis Extensor digitorum Extensor pollicis longus and brevis Abductor pollicis longus Extensor carpi ulnaris Extensor indices Extensor digiti minimi	None	Weak wrist extension Weak finger extension Difficulty stabilizing wrist Difficulty with grasp Inability to abduct thumb

Reproduced, with permission, from Magee DJ: *Orthopedic Physical Assessment.* Philadelphia, PA: WB. Saunders; 2002.

Biomechanics. A number of articular and ligamentous structures contribute to elbow stability. In flexion, the coronoid process locks into the coronoid fossa, while the medial rim of the radial head engages in the trochleocapitellar groove. In extension, the apex of the olecranon is held in the olecranon fossa. Elbow stability is enhanced by the perfect congruency between the radial head and the radial notch of the ulna. As a rough estimation, the bony surfaces contribute 50% of the mediolateral stability of the elbow, while the other 50% comes from the ligaments, although the role of each of these structures varies with the degree of flexion or extension of the elbow.

Humeroulnar Joint. The motions that occur at the humeroulnar joint involve impure flexion and extension, which are primarily the result of rotation of the ulna about the trochlea. The range of flexion-extension is from 0 to 150 degrees, with about 10 degrees of hyperextension being available. Full active extension in the normal elbow is some 5 to 10 degrees short of that obtainable by forced extension, due to passive muscular restraints (biceps, brachialis, and supinator).[10,11]

- Passive extension is limited by the impact of the olecranon process on the olecranon fossa, and tension on the UCL and anterior capsule.[12]
- Passive flexion is limited by bony structures (the head of the radius against the radial fossa, and the coronoid process against the coronoid fossa), tension of the posterior capsular ligament, and passive tension in the triceps (Figure 8-4).[12]

Activities of daily living usually can be accomplished with an elbow range of motion of 30 to 130 degrees of flexion, 50 degrees of supination, and 50 degrees of pronation.

Humeroradial Joint. The motions occurring at this joint include flexion and extension of the elbow. Some supination and pronation also occurs at this joint due to a spinning of the radial head.

Study Pearl

The cubital fossa represents the triangular space, or depression, which is located over the anterior surface of the elbow joint, and which serves as an "entrance" to the forearm or antebrachium. The boundaries of the fossa are

- Lateral: brachioradialis and extensor carpi radialis longus muscles
- Medial: pronator teres muscle
- Proximal: an imaginary line that passes through the humeral condyles
- Floor: brachialis muscle

The contents of the fossa include:

- The tendon of the biceps brachii, which lies as the central structure in the fossa
- The median nerve, which runs along the lateral edge of the pronator teres muscle
- The brachial artery, which enters the fossa just lateral to the median nerve and just medial to the biceps brachii tendon
- The radial nerve, which runs along the medial edge of the brachioradialis and ECRL muscles, and is vulnerable to injury here
- The median cubital or intermediate cubital cutaneous vein, which crosses the surface of the fossa

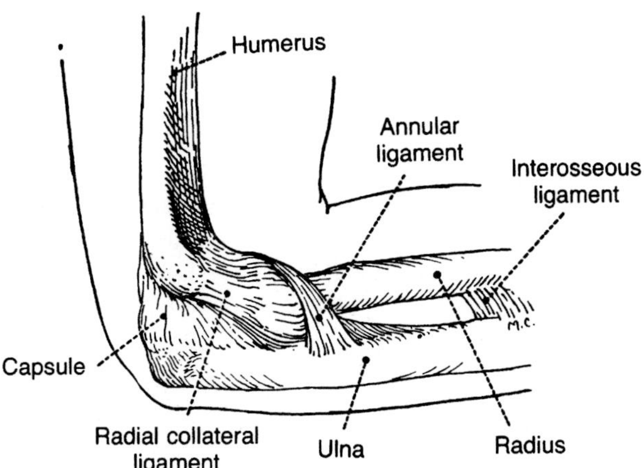

Figure 8-4. The bony structures of the elbow and radioulnar joints. (Reproduced, with permission, from Luttgens K, Hamilton N: *Kinesiology: Scientific Basis of Human Motion, 10th ed.* New York, NY: McGraw-Hill. 2002:128.)

Study Pearl

- The normal carrying angle of the elbow varies with flexion and extension, ranging from 6 degrees of varus with full flexion to 11 degrees of valgus in full extension. In men, the mean value is between 11 and 14 degrees (full extension). Women tend to have a larger carrying angle, with an average value between 13 and 16 degrees.
- The resting, or open pack, position for the humeroulnar joint is 70 degrees of flexion with 10 degrees of forearm supination.
- The closed pack position is full extension and maximum forearm supination.
- The capsular pattern is much more limited in flexion than extension.

Study Pearl

- The resting, or open pack, position of the humeroradial joint is extension and forearm supination.
- The closed pack position is approximately 90 degrees of elbow flexion and 5 degrees of supination.
- There is no true capsular pattern at this joint, although clinically an equal limitation of pronation and supination is observed.

Study Pearl

Wrist instability can be classified in the following manner:

- Dorsal intercalated segment instability (DISI): results from disruption between the scaphoid and lunate, allowing the scaphoid to rotate into volar flexion. The remaining components of the proximal row rotate into dorsiflexion because of loss of connection to the scaphoid.
- Volar intercalated segment instability (VISI): results from disruption of the ligamentous support to the triquetrum and lunate and leads to volar rotation of the lunate and extension of the triquetrum.

Proximal Radioulnar Joint. At the proximal radioulnar joint (PRUJ), 1 degree of freedom exists, permitting pronation and supination. Pronation and supination involve the articulations at the elbow as well as the distal radioulnar joint (DRUJ) and the radiocarpal articulation.

Motion at the elbow is primarily gliding for both flexion and extension. Rolling occurs in the final 5 to 10 degrees of range of motion for both flexion and extension.

WRIST AND HAND

Distal Radioulnar Joint. The DRUJ is a double pivot joint that unites the distal radius and ulna and an articular disc. The articular disc, known as the triangular fibrocartilaginous complex (TFCC), assists in binding the distal radius, and is the main stabilizer of the DRUJ as it improves joint congruency and cushions against compressive forces. A number of ligaments originate from the TFCC and provide support to it.

The articular capsule, which attaches to the articular margins of the radius and ulna, and to the disc, enclosing the inferior radioulnar joint is lax. Palmar and dorsal radioulnar ligaments strengthen the capsule anteriorly and posteriorly. Supination tightens the anterior capsule while pronation tightens the posterior part, adding to the overall stability of the wrist.

The Wrist. The wrist joint is comprised of the distal aspects of the radius and ulna, eight carpal bones, and the bases of five metacarpals (Figure 8-5).

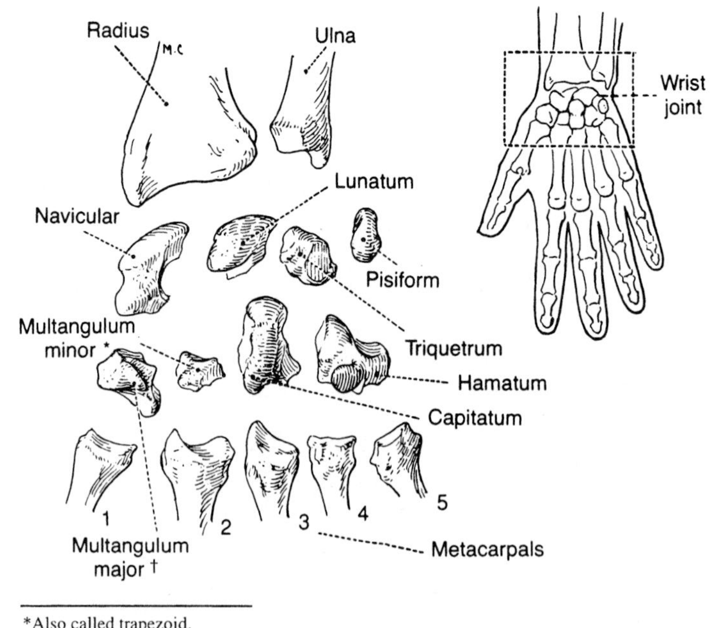

*Also called trapezoid.

†Also called trapezium.

Figure 8-5. Bones of the wrist, anterior view. (Reproduced, with permission, from Luttgens K, Hamilton N: *Kinesiology: Scientific Basis of Human Motion, 10th ed.* New York, NY: McGraw-Hill. 2002:137.)

The Carpals. The carpal bones lie in two transverse rows. The proximal row contains (radial to ulnar) the scaphoid (navicular), lunate, triquetrum, and pisiform. The distal row holds (radial to ulnar) the trapezium, trapezoid, capitate, and hamate.

Midcarpal Joints. The midcarpal joint lies between the two rows of carpals. It is referred to as a "compound" articulation because each row has both concave and convex segments. Wrist flexion, extension, and radial deviation are mainly midcarpal joint motions. Approximately, 50% of the total arc of wrist flexion and extension occur at the midcarpal level with more flexion (66%) occurring than extension (34%).[13,14]

The proximal row of the carpals is convex laterally and concave medially.

- The scaphoid, lunate, trapezium trapezoid, and triquetrum present with a concave surface to the distal row of carpals.
- The scaphoid, capitate, and hamate present a convex surface to a reciprocally arranged distal row.

Carpal Ligaments. Migration of the carpal bones is prevented by strong ligaments, and by the ulnar support provided by the TFCC. The major ligaments of the wrist include the palmar (volar) intrinsic ligaments, the palmar (volar) extrinsic, and the posterior (dorsal) extrinsic, and intrinsic ligaments.

Radiocarpal Joint. The radiocarpal joint is formed by the large articular concave surface of the distal end of the radius, the scaphoid and lunate of the proximal carpal row, and the TFCC.

Antebrachial Fascia. The antebrachial fascia is a dense connective tissue "bracelet" that encases the forearm and maintains the relationships of the tendons that cross the wrist.

The Extensor Retinaculum. Where the tendons cross the wrist, a retinaculum serves to prevent the tendons from "bow-stringing" when the tendons turn a corner at the wrist.[15] The tunnel-like structures formed by the retinaculum and the underlying bones are called fibro-osseous compartments. There are six fibro-osseous compartments on the posterior aspect (dorsum) of the wrist. The compartments, from lateral to medial, contain the tendons of:

1. Abductor pollicis longus (APL) and extensor pollicis brevis (EPB)
2. Extensor carpi radialis longus (ECRL) and brevis (ECRB)
3. Extensor pollicis longus (EPL)
4. Extensor digitorum (ED) and indicis (EI)
5. Extensor digiti minimi (EDM)
6. Extensor carpi ulnaris (ECU)

The Flexor Retinaculum. The flexor retinaculum (transverse carpal ligament) spans the area between the pisiform, hamate, scaphoid, and trapezium. It transforms the carpal arch into a tunnel, through which pass the median nerve and some of the tendons of the hand. Proximally, the retinaculum attaches to the tubercle of the scaphoid

Study Pearl

A scapholunate dissociation is a complete tear of the scapholunate ligaments which may result from a hyperextension injury. The lunate and triquetrum extend abnormally, supinate, and deviate radially, while the scaphoid tilts into flexion, pronation, and ulnar deviation (see "Watson Test").

Study Pearl

The mnemonic 2 2 1 2 1 1 can be used to remember the number of tendons in each compartment.

and the pisiform. Distally it attaches to the hook of the hamate, and the tubercle of the trapezium. The tendons that pass deep to the flexor retinaculum include:

- Flexor digitorum superficialis (FDS)
- Flexor digitorum profundus (FDP)
- Flexor pollicis longus (FPL)
- Flexor carpi radialis (FCR)

Study Pearl

Some surgeons refer to the area where the sheaths contain two tendons as "no man's land."

Structures that pass *superficial* to the flexor retinaculum include the:

- Ulnar nerve and artery
- The tendon of the palmaris longus
- The sensory branch (palmar branch) of the median nerve

Carpal Tunnel. The carpal tunnel serves as a conduit for the median nerve and nine flexor tendons (the eight tendons of the FDS and FDP, and the FPL).

- The palmar radiocarpal ligament and the palmar ligament complex form the floor of the canal.
- The roof of the tunnel is formed by the flexor retinaculum (transverse carpal ligament).
- The ulnar and radial borders are formed by carpal bones (trapezium and hook of hamate, respectively).

Within the tunnel, the median nerve divides into a motor branch and distal sensory branches.

Tunnel of Guyon. The tunnel of Guyon is a depression superficial to the flexor retinaculum, located between the hook of the hamate and the pisiform bones. From radial to ulnar, the ulnar artery and ulnar nerve pass through the canal. The flexor carpi ulnaris (FCU) tendon is most ulnar but lies outside the tunnel.

PHALANGES

The fourteen phalanges each consist of a base, shaft, and head. Two shallow depressions, which correspond to the pulley-shaped heads of the adjacent phalanges, mark the concave proximal bases.

Metacarpophalangeal Joints of the Second Through Fifth Fingers. The second through fifth metacarpals articulate with the respective proximal phalanges in biaxial joints. The metacarpophalangeal (MCP) joints allow flexion-extension and medial-lateral deviation associated with a slight degree of axial rotation.

- Approximately 90 degrees of flexion is available at the second MCP. The amount of available flexion progressively increases toward the fifth MCP.
- Active extension at these joints is 25 to 30 degrees, while 90 degrees is obtainable passively.

- Approximately 20 degrees of abduction/adduction can occur in either direction, with more being available in extension than in flexion.
- Abduction-adduction movements of the MCP joints are restricted in flexion and freer in extension.[16]

The joint capsule of these joints is relatively lax and redundant, endowed with collateral ligaments, which pass posterior to the joint axis for flexion/extension of the MCP joints. Although lax in extension, these collateral ligaments become taut in approximately 70 to 90 degrees of flexion of the MCP joint.

Carpometacarpal Joints. The distal borders of the distal carpal row bones articulate with the bases of the metacarpals, thereby forming the carpometacarpal (CMC) joints. The CMC joints progress in mobility from the second to the fifth.

The anterior (palmar) and posterior (dorsal) carpometacarpal and intermetacarpal ligaments provide stability for the CMC joints. While the trapezoid articulates with only one metacarpal, all of the other members of the distal carpal row combine one carpal bone with two or more metacarpals.

First Carpometacarpal Joint. The thumb is the most important digit of the hand and the sellar (saddle-shaped) carpometacarpal (CMC) joint is the most important joint of the thumb. Motions that can occur at this joint include flexion/extension, adduction/abduction, and opposition, the latter of which includes varying amounts of flexion, internal rotation, and palmar adduction.

Metacarpophalangeal Joint of the Thumb. The metacarpophalangeal (MCP) joint of the thumb is a hinge joint. Its bony configuration, which resembles the interphalangeal joints, provides it with some inherent stability. In addition, palmar and collateral ligaments provide support for the joint. Approximately 75 to 80 degrees of flexion is available at this joint. The extension movements as well as the abduction and adduction motions are negligible. Traction, gliding, and rotatory accessory movement are also present.

Interphalangeal Joints. Adjacent phalanges articulate in hinge joints that allow motion in only one plane. The congruency of the interphalangeal (IP) joint surfaces contributes greatly to finger joint stability.

Proximal Interphalangeal Joint (PIP). The PIP joint is a hinged joint capable of flexion and extension and is stable in all positions. The supporting ligaments and tendons provide the bulk of the static and dynamic stability of this joint. The motions available at these joints consist of approximately 110 degrees of flexion at the PIP joints and 90 degrees at the thumb interphalangeal (IP) joint. Extension reaches 0 degree at the PIP joints, and 25 degrees at the thumb IP joint. Traction, gliding, and accessory movement also occur at the IP joints.

Distal Interphalangeal Joints. The distal interphalangeal joint (DIP) has similar structures but less stability and allows some hyperextension. The motions available at these joints consist of

Study Pearl

Although sellar surfaces follow the same rules as ovid surfaces, because of the nature of the curvature of their joint surfaces, a swing in one direction involves movement of the male surface and a swing in a direction at 90 degrees to the first swing involves movement of the female surface. For example, at the first carpometacarpal joint, the following biomechanics are involved:

- Flexion/extension of metacarpal: the moving surface is concave
  - The swing of the bone occurs in an anteromedial/posterolateral direction
  - The base glides and rolls in an anteromedial/posterolateral direction.
- Abduction/adduction of metacarpal: the moving surface is convex
  - The swing of the bone occurs in an anterolateral/postermedial direction.
  - The base glides in the opposite direction to the swing, and rolls in the same direction as the swing.

Study Pearl

Dupuytren's contracture is a fibrotic condition of the palmar aponeurosis that results in nodule formation or scarring of the aponeurosis, and which may ultimately cause finger flexion contractures (see "Common Orthopedic Conditions").

approximately 90 degrees of flexion, and 25 degrees of extension. Traction, gliding, and accessory movement also occur at the DIP joints.

Palmar Aponeurosis. The palmar aponeurosis is located just deep to the subcutaneous tissue. It is a dense fibrous structure continuous with the palmaris longus tendon and fascia covering the thenar and hypothenar muscles.

Extensor Hood. At the level of the MCP joint, the tendon of the extensor digitorum (ED) fans out to cover or shroud the dorsal aspect of the joint in a hood-like structure. A complex tendon, which covers the posterior (dorsal) aspect of each digit is formed from a combination of the tendons of insertion from the extensor digitorum, EI, and EDM. The distal portion of the hood receives the tendons of the lumbricales and interossei over the proximal phalanx. The tendons of the intrinsic muscles pass palmar to the MCP joint axes, but dorsal to the PIP and DIP joint axes. Between the MCP and PIP joints, the complete, complex ED tendon (after all contributions have been received) splits into three parts—a central band, and two lateral bands:

- Central band. This band inserts into the proximal posterior (dorsal) edge of the middle phalanx.
- Lateral bands. These lateral bands rejoin over the middle phalanx into a terminal tendon, which inserts into the proximal posterior (dorsal) edge of the distal phalanx. Rupture of the tendon insertion into the distal phalanx produces a "mallet" finger.

The arrangement of the muscles and tendons in this expansion hood, creates a "cable" system that provides a mechanism for *extending* the MCP and IP joints, and allows the lumbrical, and possibly interosseous muscles, to assist in the *flexion* of the MCP joints.

Synovial Sheaths. Synovial sheaths can be thought of as long narrow balloons filled with synovial fluid, which wrap around a tendon so that one part of the balloon wall (visceral layer) is directly on the tendon, while the other part of the balloon wall (parietal layer) is separate.[15] During wrist motions, the sheaths move longitudinally, reducing friction.

At the wrist, the tendons of both the FDS and FDP are essentially covered by a synovial sheath and pass posterior (dorsal) and deep to the flexor retinaculum. The FDP tendons are dorsal to those of the FDS.

In the palm, the FDS and FDP tendons are covered for a variable distance by a synovial sheath.

At the base of the digits, both sets of tendons enter a "fibro-osseous tunnel" formed by the bones of the digit (head of the metatarsals and phalanges) and a fibrous digital tendon sheath on the palmar surface of the digits.

Flexor Pulleys. Annular (A) and cruciate (C) pulleys restrain the flexor tendons to the metacarpals and phalanges and contribute to fibro-osseous tunnels through which the tendons travel.

MUSCLES OF THE WRIST AND FOREARM

The muscles of the forearm, wrist, and hand (Table 8-11 and Table 8-12) can be subdivided into the 19 intrinsic muscles that arise and insert within the hand, and the 24 extrinsic muscles that originate in the forearm and insert within the hand.

Anatomic Snuff Box. The anatomic snuffbox is represented by a depression on the posterior (dorsal) surface of the hand at the base of the thumb, slightly distal to the radius. The tendons of the APL and EPB form the lateral (radial) border of the snuffbox, while the tendon of the EPL forms the medial (ulnar) border. The deep branch of the radial artery and the tendinous insertion of the ECRL are located along the floor of the snuffbox. Underneath these structures, the scaphoid and trapezium bones are found.

Neurology. The three peripheral nerves that supply the skin and muscles of the wrist and hand include the median, ulnar, and radial nerve (refer to Chapter 9).

Vasculature of the Wrist and Hand. The brachial artery bifurcates at the elbow into radial and ulnar branches, which are the main arterial branches to the hand.

Biomechanics. The open pack and close pack positions, and capsular patterns for the articulations of the wrist and hand are listed in Table 8-13. Table 8-14 outlines the active range of motion norms for the forearm. Table 8-15 outlines the functional range of motion of the hand and wrist.

Movement of the Hand on the Forearm. The proximal and distal radioulnar joints are intimately related biomechanically, with the function and stability of both joints dependent on the configuration of,

TABLE 8-11. MUSCLE COMPARTMENTS OF THE FOREARM

COMPARTMENT	PRINCIPAL MUSCLES
Anterior	Pronator teres
	Flexor carpi radialis
	Palmaris longus
	Flexor digitorum superficialis
	Flexor digitorum profundus
	Flexor pollicis longus
	Flexor carpi ulnaris
	Pronator quadratus
Posterior	Abductor pollicis longus
	Extensor pollicis brevis
	Extensor pollicis longus
	Extensor digitorum communis
	Extensor digitorum proprius
	Extensor digiti quinti
	Extensor carpi ulnaris
Mobile wad	Brachioradialis
	Extensor carpi radialis longus
	Extensor carpi radialis brevis

Study Pearl

The following areas of the hand typically have autonomous innervation:

- The dorsal thumb-index webspace (radial nerve)
- The distal tip of the little finger (ulnar nerve)
- The anterior (volar) tip of the index finger

Study Pearl

Tenderness with palpation in the anatomic snuffbox is indicative of a scaphoid fracture, but also can be present in minor wrist injuries or other conditions.

Study Pearl

Kienböck's disease, an avascular necrosis of the lunate, usually results from trauma to the hand, but has also been associated with relative shortening of the ulnar compared with the radius bone. The four stages of the disease are sclerosis, fragmentation, collapse, and arthritis.

TABLE 8-12. MUSCLES OF THE WRIST AND HAND: THEIR ACTIONS AND NERVE SUPPLY

ACTION	MUSCLES	NERVE SUPPLY
Wrist extension	Extensor carpi radialis longus	Radial
	Extensor carpi radialis brevis	Posterior interosseous
	Extensor carpi ulnaris	Posterior interosseous
Wrist flexion	Flexor carpi radialis	Median
	Flexor carpi ulnaris	Ulnar
Ulnar deviation of wrist	Flexor carpi ulnaris	Ulnar
	Extensor carpi ulnaris	Posterior interosseous
Radial deviation of wrist	Flexor carpi radialis	Median
	Extensor carpi radialis longus	Radial
	Abductor pollicis longus	Posterior interosseous
	Extensor pollicis brevis	Posterior interosseous
Finger extension	Extensor digitorum communis	Posterior interosseous
	Extensor indicis	Posterior interosseous
	Extensor digiti minimi	Posterior interosseous
Finger flexion	Flexor digitorum profundus	Anterior interosseous, lateral two digits Ulnar, medial two digits
	Flexor digitorum superficialis	Median
	First and second: median	
	Lumbricals	Third and fourth: ulnar
	Interossei	Ulnar
	Flexor digiti minimi	Ulnar
Abduction of fingers	Dorsal interossei	Ulnar
	Abductor digiti minimi	Ulnar
Adduction of fingers	Palmar interossei	Ulnar
Thumb extension	Extensor pollicis longus	Posterior interosseous
	Extensor pollicis brevis	Posterior interosseous
	Abductor pollicis longus	Posterior interosseous
Thumb flexion	Flexor pollicis brevis	Superficial head: median Deep head: ulnar
	Flexor pollicis longus	Anterior interosseous
	Opponens pollicis	Median
Abduction of thumb	Abductor pollicis longus	Posterior interosseous
	Abductor pollicis brevis	Median
Adduction of thumb	Adductor pollicis	Ulnar
Opposition of thumb and little finger	Opponens pollicis	Median
	Flexor pollicis brevis	Superficial head: median
	Abductor pollicis brevis	Median
	Opponens digiti minimi	Ulnar

TABLE 8-13. THE OPEN PACK AND CLOSE PACK POSITIONS, AND CAPSULAR PATTERNS FOR THE ARTICULATIONS OF THE WRIST AND HAND

JOINT	OPEN PACK	CLOSE PACK	CAPSULAR PATTERN
Distal radioulnar	10 degrees of supination	5 degrees of supination	Minimal to no limitation with pain at the end ranges of pronation and supination
Radiocarpal (wrist)	Neutral with slight ulnar deviation	Extension	Equal limitation of flexion and extension
Intercarpal	Neutral or slight flexion	Extension	None
Midcarpal	Neutral or slight flexion with ulnar deviation	Extension with ulnar deviation	Equal limitation of flexion and extension
Carpometacarpal	Thumb: midway between abduction and adduction and midway between flexion and extension	Thumb: full opposition	Thumb: abduction then extension
	Fingers: midway between flexion and extension	Fingers: full flexion	Fingers: equal limitation in all directions
Metacarpophalangeal	Slight flexion	Thumb: full opposition Fingers: full flexion	Flexion then extension
Interphalangeal	Slight flexion	Full extension	Flexion, extension

TABLE 8-14. ACTIVE RANGE OF MOTION NORMS FOR THE FOREARM, WRIST, AND HAND

MOTION	DEGREES
Forearm pronation	85-90
Forearm supination	85-90
Radial deviation	15
Ulnar deviation	30-45
Wrist flexion	80-90
Wrist extension	70-90
Finger flexion	MCP: 85-90; PIP: 100-115; DIP: 80-90
Finger extension	MCP: 30-45; PIP: 0; DIP: 20
Finger abduction	20-30
Finger adduction	0
Thumb flexion	CMC: 45-50; MCP: 50-55; IP: 85-90
Thumb extension	MCP: 0; IP: 0-5
Thumb adduction	30
Thumb abduction	60-70

CMC, carpometacarpal; DIP, distal interphalangeal; IP, interphalangeal; MCP, metacarpophalangeal; PIP, proximal interphalangeal.

and distance between, the two bones. Wrist movements occur around a combination of three functional axes: longitudinal, transverse, and anterior–posterior. In a neutral wrist position, the scaphoid contacts the radius, and the lunate contacts the radius and disc. Due to the morphology of the wrist, movement at this joint complex involves a coordinated interaction between a number of articulations including the radiocarpal joint, the proximal row of carpals, and the distal row of the carpals.[16] The movements of flexion and extension of the wrist are shared among the radiocarpal articulation and the intercarpal articulation, in varying proportions.

TABLE 8-15. FUNCTIONAL RANGE OF MOTION OF THE HAND AND WRIST

JOINT MOTION	FUNCTIONAL RANGE OF MOTION (DEGREES)
Wrist flexion	5-40
Wrist extension	30-40
Radial deviation	10-20
Ulnar deviation	15-20
MCP flexion	60
PIP flexion	60
DIP flexion	40
Thumb MCP flexion	20

DIP, distal interphalangeal; MCP, metacarpophalangeal; PIP, proximal interphalangeal.

Data from Blair SJ, McCormick E, Bear-Lehman J, et al: Evaluation of impairment of the upper extremity. *Clin Orthop.* 1987;221:42-58; Brumfield RH, Champoux JA: A biomechanical study of normal functional wrist motion. *Clin Orthop Rel Res.* 1984;187:23-25; Lamereaux L, Hoffer MM: The effect of wrist deviation on grip and pinch strength. *Clin Orthop.* 1995;314:152-155; Kapandji IA: *The Physiology of the Joints, Upper Limb.* New York: Churchill Livingstone. 1991; Tubiana R, Thomine J-M, Mackin E: *Examination of the Hand and Wrist.* London: Mosby. 1996; Palmer AK, Werner FW, Murphy D, et al: Functional wrist motion: a biomechanical study. *J Hand Surg.* 1985;10A:39-46; and Ryu J, Cooney WP, Askew LJ, et al: Functional ranges of motion of the wrist joint. *J Hand Surg.* 1991;16A:409-420.

- Wrist extension is accompanied by a slight radial deviation, and pronation of the forearm. During wrist extension, most of the motion occurs at the radiocarpal joint (66.5% or 40 degrees versus 33.5% or 20 degrees at the midcarpal joint), and is associated with slight radial deviation and pronation of the forearm.[17]
- Wrist flexion is accompanied by a slight ulnar deviation, and supination, of the forearm. During wrist flexion, most of the motion occurs in the midcarpal joint (60% or 40 degrees versus 40% or 30 degrees at the radiocarpal joint), and is associated with slight ulnar deviation and supination of the forearm.[17]

The wrist also allows relatively extensive traction and gliding accessory movements. There is a physiological ulnar deviation at rest. The amount of deviation is approximately 40 degrees of ulnar deviation, and 15 degrees of radial deviation.

The position of the wrist in flexion or extension influences the tension of the long or "extrinsic" muscles of the digits. Neither the flexors nor the extensors of the fingers are long enough to allow maximal range of motion at the wrist and the fingers simultaneously.

Thumb Movements

- Thumb flexion and extension occur around an anterior–posterior axis in the frontal plane (Figure 8-6) that is perpendicular to the sagittal plane of finger flexion and extension. In this plane, the metacarpal surface is concave, and the trapezium surface is convex. Flexion occurs with a conjunct rotation of internal rotation of the metacarpal. Extension occurs with a conjunct rotation of external rotation of the metacarpal. A total range of 50 to 70 degrees is available.
- Thumb abduction and adduction occur around a medial-lateral axis in the sagittal plane (Figure 8-6), which is perpendicular to the frontal plane of finger abduction and adduction. During thumb abduction and adduction, the convex metacarpal surface moves on the concave trapezium. Abduction occurs with a conjunct rotation of internal rotation. Adduction occurs with a conjunct rotation of external rotation. A total range of 40 to 60 degrees is available.
- Opposition of the thumb involves a wide arc motion comprised of sequential palmar abduction, and flexion from the anatomic position, accompanied by internal rotation of the thumb. Retroposition of the thumb returns the thumb to the anatomic position, a motion that incorporates elements of adduction with extension and external rotation of the metacarpal.

HIP

Anatomy. The hip joint is classified as an unmodified ovoid (ball and socket) joint. The acetabulum is made up of three bones: the ilium, ischium, and pubis (Figure 8-7). The acetabulum is deepened by the acetabular labrum, which increases articular congruence. A number of muscles act across the hip (Table 8-16). The femur is held in the acetabulum by five separate ligaments.

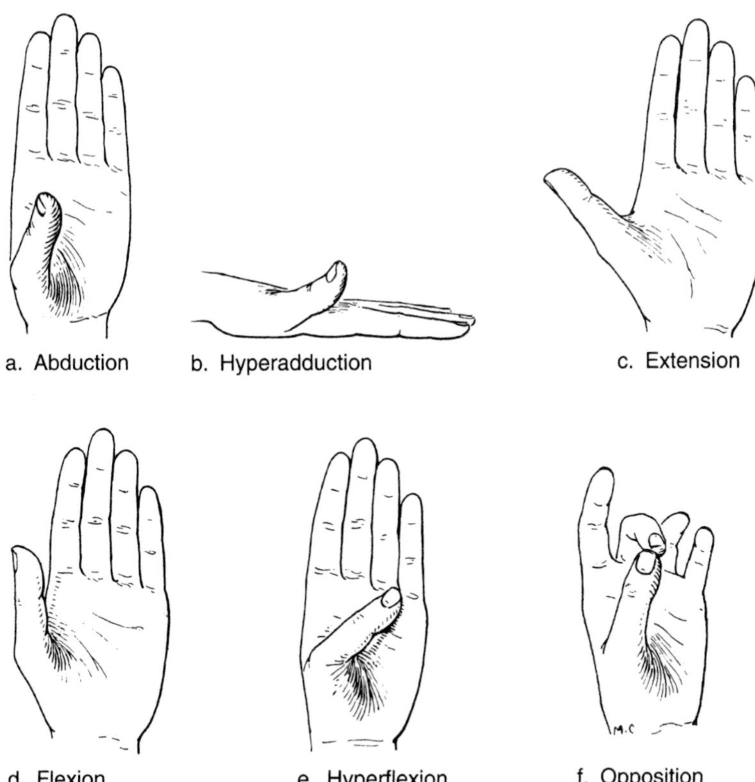

Figure 8-6. Movements of the thumb at the carpometacarpal joint. (Reproduced, with permission, from Luttgens K, Hamilton N: *Kinesiology: Scientific Basis of Human Motion, 10th ed.* New York, NY: McGraw-Hill. 2002:141.)

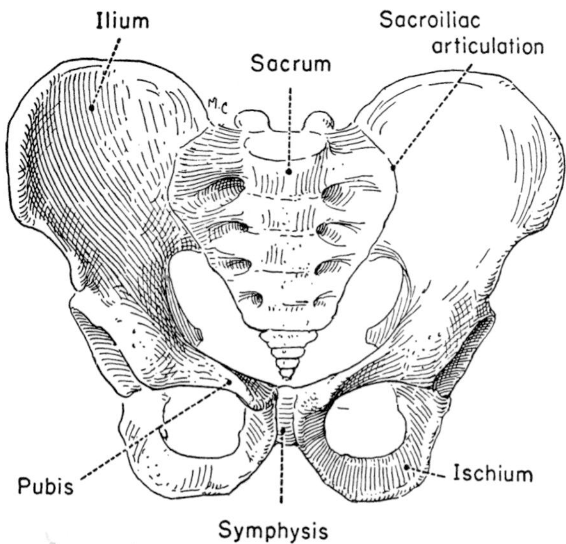

Figure 8-7. Anterior view of the sacroiliac joint showing bones and ligaments. (Reproduced, with permission, from Luttgens K, Hamilton N: *Kinesiology: Scientific Basis of Human Motion, 10th ed.* New York, NY: McGraw-Hill. 2002:160.)

TABLE 8-16. MUSCLES ACTING ACROSS THE HIP JOINT

MUSCLE	ORIGIN	INSERTION	INNERVATION
Adductor Brevis	External aspect of the body and inferior ramus of the pubis	By an aponeurosis to the line from the greater trochanter of the linea aspera of the femur	Obturator nerve, L3
Adductor Longus	Pubic crest and symphysis	By an aponeurosis to the middle third of the linea aspera of the femur	Obturator nerve, L3
Adductor Magnus	Inferior ramus of pubis, ramus of ischium, and the inferolateral aspect of the ischial tuberosity	By an aponeurosis to the linea aspera and adductor tubercle of the femur	Obturator nerve and tibial portion of the sciatic nerve, L2-L4
Biceps Femoris (Long Head)	Arises from the sacrotuberous ligament and posterior aspect of the ischial tuberosity	By way of a tendon, on the lateral aspect of the head of the fibula, the lateral condyle of the tibial tuberosity, the lateral collateral ligament, and the deep fascia of the leg	Tibial portion of the sciatic nerve, S1
Gemelli (Superior and Inferior)	Superior-dorsal surface of the spine of the ischium, inferior-upper part of the tuberosity of the ischium	Superior and inferior-medial surface of the greater trochanter	Sacral plexus, L5-S1
Gluteus Maximus	Posterior gluteal line of the ilium, iliac crest, aponeurosis of the erector spinae, dorsal surface of the lower part of the sacrum, side of the coccyx, sacrotuberous ligament, and intermuscular fascia	Iliotibial tract of the fascia lata, gluteal tuberosity of the femur	Inferior gluteal nerve, S1-S2
Gluteus Medius	Outer surface of the ilium between the iliac crest and the posterior gluteal line, anterior gluteal line, and fascia	Lateral surface of the greater trochanter	Superior gluteal nerve, L5
Gluteus Minimus	Outer surface of the ilium between the anterior and inferior gluteal lines, and the margin of the greater sciatic notch	A ridge laterally situated on the anterior surface of the greater trochanter	Superior gluteal nerve, L5
Gracilis	The body and inferior ramus of the pubis	The anterior-medial aspect of the shaft of the proximal tibia, just proximal to the tendon of the semitendinosus	Obturator nerve, L2
Iliacus	Superior two-thirds of the iliac fossa, upper surface of the lateral part of the sacrum	Fibers converge with the tendon of the psoas major to lesser trochanter	Femoral nerve, L2
Obturator Externus	Rami of the pubis, ramus of the ischium, medial two-thirds of the outer surface of the obturator membrane	Trochanteric fossa of the femur	Obturator nerve, L4
Obturator Internus	Internal surface of the anterolateral wall of the pelvis, and obturator membrane	Medial surface of the greater trochanter	Sacral plexus, S1
Pectineus	Pecten pubis	Along a line leading from the lesser trochanter to the linea aspera	Femoral or obturator or accessory obturator nerves, L2

Piriformis	Front of the sacrum, gluteal surface of the ilium, capsule of the sacroiliac joint, and sacrotuberous ligament	Upper border of the greater trochanter of femur	Sacral plexus, S1
Psoas Major	Transverse processes of all the lumbar vertebrae, bodies, and intervertebral discs of the lumbar vertebrae	Lesser trochanter of the femur	Lumbar plexus, L2-L3
Quadratus Femoris	Ischial body next to the ischial tuberosity	Quadrate tubercle on femur	Nerve to quadratus femoris
Rectus Femoris	By two heads, from the anterior inferior iliac spine, and a reflected head from the groove above the acetabulum	Base of the patella	Femoral nerve, L3-L4
Sartorius	Anterior superior iliac spine and notch below it	Upper part of the medial surface of the tibia in front of the gracilis	Femoral nerve, L2-L3
Semimembranosus	Ischial tuberosity	The posterior-medial aspect of the medial condyle of the tibia	Tibial nerve, L5-S1
Semitendinosus	Ischial tuberosity	Upper part of the medial surface of the tibia behind the attachment of the sartorius and below that of the gracilis	Tibial nerve, L5-S1
Tensor Fasciae Latae	Outer lip of the iliac crest and the lateral surface of the anterior superior iliac spine	Iliotibial tract	Superior gluteal nerve, L4-L5

Study Pearl

The hip region is a common site of symptom referral from other regions and, therefore, its examination rarely occurs in isolation. Typically, an examination of the hip, almost always involves an assessment of the lumbar spine, pelvis, and knee joint complex.

Study Pearl

Motions about the hip joint can occur independently; however the extremes of motion require motion at the pelvis.[19] For example, end-range hip flexion is associated with a posterior rotation of the ilium bone; end range of hip extension is associated with an anterior rotation of the ilium. Hip abduction and adduction are associated with a medial and lateral tilt of the pelvis respectively.

Study Pearl

The angle between the femoral shaft and the neck is called the collum/inclination angle. This angle is approximately 125 to 130 degrees,[22] but can vary with body types. In a tall person the collum *angle* is larger (valga). The opposite is true with a shorter individual.

- The iliofemoral ligament is thought to limit hip extension and external rotation, while the superior portion tightens with hip adduction.
- The pubofemoral ligament limits extension and abduction, and reinforces the joint capsule along its medial surface.
- The ischiofemoral ligament limits extension and internal rotation of the hip, and when the hip is flexed, the ligament serves to limit hip adduction.
- The transverse acetabular ligament, which covers the acetabular notch, contributes little to joint stability.
- The femoral head ligament connects the femoral head to the transverse ligament and acetabular notch.

Vascular Supply. The proximal shaft of the femur and the femoral neck has a plentiful blood supply from the medial circumflex femoral artery and its branches. The femoral head, on the other hand, has an extremely tenuous blood supply from a small branch of the obturator artery that passes together with the femoral ligament.

Biomechanics. Loads of up to eight times body weight have been demonstrated in the hip joint during jogging, with potentially greater loads present during vigorous athletic competition.[18] Motion at the hip occurs in three planes: sagittal (flexion and extension around a transverse axis), frontal (abduction and adduction around an anterior–posterior axis), and transverse (internal and external rotation around a vertical axis). All three of these axes pass through the center of the femoral head.

In the anatomic position, the orientation of the femoral head causes the contact force between the femur and acetabulum to be high in the anterior-superior region of the joint.[20] Because the anterior aspect of the femoral head is somewhat exposed in this position, the joint has more flexibility in flexion than extension.[21]

An increase in the collum angle causes the femoral head to be directed more superiorly in the acetabulum, and is known as coxa valga. Coxa valga has the following effects at the hip joint:

- It changes the orientation of the joint reaction force from the normal vertical direction, to one that is almost parallel to the femoral shaft.[23,24] This lateral displacement of the joint reaction force reduces the weight-bearing surface, resulting in an increase in stress applied across joint surfaces not specialized to sustain such loads.
- It shortens the moment arm of the hip abductors, placing them in a position of mechanical disadvantage.[24] This causes the abductors to contract more vigorously to stabilize the pelvis, producing an increase in the joint reaction force.[21]
- It increases the overall length of the lower extremity, affecting other components in the kinetic chain. Coxa valga has the effect of decreasing the normal physiological valgus angle at the knee. This places an increased mechanical stress on the medial aspect of the knee joint and more tensile stress on the lateral aspect of the joint.

If the collum angle is reduced, it is known as coxa vara. The mechanical effects of coxa vara are, for the most part, the opposite of those found in coxa valga, although they appear to be less deleterious than those of coxa valga.[25]

Femoral alignment in the transverse plane also influences the mechanics of the hip joint.

Anteversion is defined as the anterior position of the axis through the femoral condyles.[26,27] Retroversion is defined as a femoral neck axis that is parallel or posterior to the condylar axis.[21] The normal range for femoral alignment in the transverse plane in adults is 12 to 15 degrees of anteversion.[27,28]

Excessive anteversion directs the femoral head toward the anterior aspect of the acetabulum when the femoral condyles are aligned in their normal orientation. Some studies have supported the hypothesis that a persistent increase in femoral anteversion predisposes to osteoarthritis of the hip, although other studies have refuted this.

Hip flexion averages 110 to 120 degrees, extension 10 to 15 degrees, abduction 30 to 50 degrees, and adduction 25 to 30 degrees. Hip external rotation averages 40 to 60 degrees and internal rotation averages 30 to 40 degrees (Table 8-17).

The degree of pelvic tilt, which is measured as the angle between the horizontal plane and a line connecting the ASIS with the posterior superior iliac spine, varies from 5 to 12 degrees in normal individuals.[29] Both a low ASIS in women, and a structurally flat back in men, can cause structural variations in pelvic alignment, which can be misinterpreted as acquired postural impairments.

The most stable position of the hip is the normal standing position: hip extension, slight abduction, and slight internal rotation.[30-32]

TABLE 8-17. HIP MOTIONS AND THEIR ASSOCIATED INNOMINATE MOTIONS

Flexion (posterior rotation)
Extension (anterior rotation)
Abduction (upward)
Adduction (downward)
Internal rotation (internal rotation)
External rotation (external rotation)

Study Pearl

Version is the normal angular difference between the transverse axis of each end of a long bone. The terms of femoral anteversion (FA) and femoral retroversion (FR) refer to the relationship between the neck of the femur and the femoral shaft/condyles, that dictates the position of the femoral head when the knee is pointing straight ahead.

Study Pearl

Subjects with excessive anteversion usually have more hip internal rotation range of motion than external rotation, and gravitate to the typical "frog-sitting" posture as a position of comfort. There is also associated intoeing while weight bearing.[21]

Study Pearl

The commonly cited open packed (resting) positions of the hip are between 10 to 30 degrees flexion, 10 to 30 degrees abduction, and 0 to 5 degrees of external rotation. According to Cyriax,[33,34] the capsular pattern of the hip is a marked limitation of flexion, abduction, and internal rotation. Kaltenborn[30] considers the capsular pattern at the hip to be extension more limited than flexion, internal rotation more limited than external rotation, and abduction more limited than adduction.

KNEE JOINT COMPLEX

The knee is the largest and most complex joint in the body. It is considered a "physiological" joint because it requires the normal functioning of all its parts (ie, bony, ligamentous, and muscular) to simultaneously provide smooth motion, stability in stance, and protection against deterioration over time.[35,36] The knee joint complex includes three articulating surfaces, which form two distinct joints contained within a single joint capsule: the patellofemoral and tibiofemoral joint. Despite its proximity to the tibiofemoral joint, the patellofemoral joint can be considered as its own entity, in much the same way as the craniovertebral joints are when compared to the rest of the cervical spine.

Tibiofemoral Joint. The tibiofemoral joint, or knee joint, is a modified hinge joint, which has 6 degrees of freedom. The bony configuration of this joint is geometrically incongruous and lends little inherent stability to the joint. Joint stability is therefore dependent upon the static restraints of the joint capsule, ligaments, and menisci (Figure 8-8 and Table 8-18), and the dynamic restraints of the quadriceps, hamstrings, and gastrocnemius.

Patellofemoral Joint. The quadriceps tendon, which represents the confluence of four muscle tendon units (rectus femoris, vastus lateralis, vastus intermedius, and the vastus medialis), inserts on the superior pole of the patella.

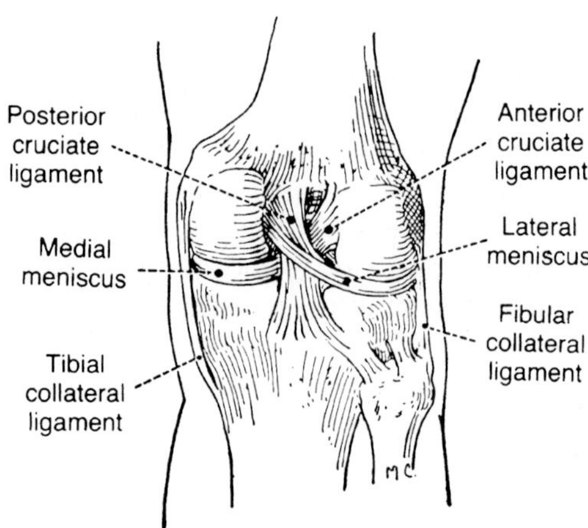

Figure 8-8. Posterior view of the knee joint showing menisci and ligaments. (Reproduced, with permission, from Luttgens K, Hamilton N: *Kinesiology: Scientific Basis of Human Motion, 10th ed.* New York, NY: McGraw-Hill. 2002:185.)

Laterally, the iliotibial band, which originates above the hip joint as a wide fascial band, supports the extensor mechanism, and is an important lateral stabilizer of the patellofemoral joint. Distally, the iliotibial band inserts on the Gerdy tubercle of the lateral tibial plateau.

The patellar retinaculum is an important soft tissue stabilizer of the patellofemoral joint. The thicker lateral retinaculum comprises a distinct, thick deep layer and a thin superficial layer.

The patella, the largest sesamoid bone in the body, possesses the thickest articular cartilage. The articular surface, which can have a variable contour, articulates with the trochlear groove of the femur.

The patellar tendon, occasionally termed the patellar ligament, originates at the inferior pole of the patella and inserts onto the tibial tuberosity.

TABLE 8-18. COMMON LIGAMENTOUS AND MENISCAL INJURIES

STRUCTURE	MECHANISM OF INJURY	SUBJECTIVE COMPLAINTS
MCL	Most commonly involves valgus (contact) stress or external rotational force with the leg firmly planted. Often associated with ACL injury	Reports of swelling developing within 12 hours of injury; localized swelling and tenderness over injured area
ACL	Most commonly injured with noncontact pivoting/twisting mechanism while the foot is planted; noncontact hyperextension; sudden deceleration; forced internal rotation; sudden valgus impact	Reports of being immediately disabled/unable to continue activity; extreme pain at time of injury; hearing "pop" in the knee; experiencing tearing sensation; acute knee swelling (within 1-2 hours of injury); episodes of "giving way"
Meniscus	Usually caused by noncontact injury; rotational force applied to partly or completely flexed knee, as occurs with squatting then rapidly rotating while coming to a standing position	Reports being able to continue/complete with activity. Reports of swelling developing within 12 hours of injury; localized swelling and tenderness over injured area. History of popping or clicking with knee motions

Data from Austermuehle PD: Common knee injuries in primary care. *Nurse Practit.* 2001;26:32-45; quiz 46-47.

Biomechanics

Tibiofemoral Joint. The motions that occur about the tibiofemoral joint consist of flexion and extension, coupled with other motions such as varus and valgus motions, and external and internal rotation. All of the motions about the tibiofemoral joint consist of a rolling, gliding, and rotation between the femoral condyles and the tibial plateaus. This rolling, gliding, and rotation occurs almost simultaneously, albeit in different directions.

During flexion of the knee, the femur rolls posteriorly and glides anteriorly, with the opposite occurring with extension of the knee. This arrangement resembles a twin wheel, rolling on a central rail. 120 to 160 degrees of knee flexion are available, depending on the position of the hip and the girth of the soft tissues around the leg and the thigh.

In the last 30 to 35 degrees of weight bearing knee extension, the lateral condyle of the femur, together with the lateral meniscus, become congruent, moving the axis of movement more laterally. The tibial glide now becomes much greater on the medial side, which produces internal rotation of the femur, and the ligaments, both extrinsic and intrinsic, start to tighten near terminal extension. At this point, the cruciates become crossed and are tightened.

In the last 5 degrees of extension, rotation is the only movement accompanying the extension. This rotation is referred to as the *screw home mechanism*, and is a characteristic motion in the normal knee, in which the tibia externally rotates, and the femur internally rotates, as the knee approaches extension. Knee hyperextension ranging from 0 to 15 degrees is usually available.[37] During knee hyperextension, the femur does not continue to roll anteriorly but instead tilts forward. This creates anterior compression between the femur and tibia.[38] In the normal knee, hyperextension is checked by the soft tissue structures. When the knee hyperextends, the axis of the thigh runs obliquely inferiorly and posteriorly, which tends to place the ground reaction force anterior to the knee. In this position, the posterior structures are placed on tension, which helps to stabilize the knee joint, negating the need for quadriceps muscle activity.[39]

Patellofemoral Joint. The static and dynamic relationships of the underlying tibia and femur determine the patellar-tracking pattern. To assist in the control of the forces around the patellofemoral joint, there are a number of static and dynamic restraints. The static restraints include:

- The medial retinaculum: This is the primary static restraint to lateral patellar displacement at 20 degrees of knee flexion, contributing 60% of the total restraining force.[40]
- Bony configuration of the trochlea: The patellofemoral joint is intrinsically unstable because the tibial tubercle lies lateral to the long axis of the femur and the quadriceps muscle, and the patella is therefore subject to a laterally directed force.
- The medial patellomeniscal ligament and the lateral retinaculum contribute 13% and 10% of the restraint to lateral translation of the patella, respectively.

The passive restraints to medial translation of the patella are provided by the structures that form the superficial and deep lateral retinaculum.

Study Pearl

For flexion to be initiated from a position of full extension, the knee joint must first be "unlocked." The service of locksmith is provided by the popliteus muscle, which acts to internally rotate the tibia with respect to the femur, enabling the flexion to occur.

Study Pearl

The normal capsular pattern of the tibiofemoral joint is gross limitation of flexion and slight limitation of extension. The ratio of flexion to extension is roughly 1:10, thus 5 degrees of limited extension corresponds to a 45 to 60 degree limitation of flexion.

The primary dynamic restraints to patellar motions are the quadriceps muscles, particularly the VMO. However, the muscle vector of the VMO is more vertical than normal when a patella malalignment is present, making it less effective as a dynamic stabilizer.[41,42] The timing of the VMO contractions relative to those of other muscles, especially the vastus lateralis, also appears to be critical, and has been found to be abnormal with patellar malalignment.

Patellar Tracking. In the normal knee, the patella glides in a sinuous path inferiorly and superiorly during flexion and extension respectively, covering a distance of 5 to 7 cm with respect to the femur.[45] The patella produces a concave lateral C-shaped curve as it moves from a knee flexion of approximately 120 degrees toward approximately 30 degrees of knee extension. Further extension of the knee (between 30 and 0 degree) produces a lateral glide of the patella in the frontal plane and a lateral tilt in the sagittal plane.

Study Pearl

Various normal values have been reported in the literature. The most common ranges cited for the Q-angle are 8 to 14 degrees for males and 15 to 17 degrees for females.[43,44]

The Quadriceps Angle. The quadriceps angle (Q-angle) is the angle formed by the bisection of two lines, one line drawn from the anterior superior iliac spine (ASIS) to the center of the patella, and the other line drawn from the center of the patella to the tibial tubercle.

The Q-angle can vary significantly with the degree of foot pronation and supination, and when compared with measurements made in the supine position.[43,44]

Patella-Femur Contact and Loading. The amount of contact between the patella and the femur appears to vary according to a number of factors including (1) the angle of knee flexion, (2) the location of contact, (3) the surface area of contact, (4) the patellofemoral joint reaction force.[46] Each of these factors is discussed separately.

The Angle of Knee Flexion. As knee flexion proceeds, the stress on the patella increases significantly.[47]

The Location of Contact. In the normal knee, as the knee flexes from 10 to 90 degrees, the contact area shifts gradually from the distal to the proximal pole of the patella.

- At full extension, the patella is not in contact with the femur, but rests on the supratrochlear fat pad.[48]
- From full extension to 10 degrees of flexion, the tibia internally rotates, allowing the patella to move into the trochlea.[46] This brings the inferior third of the patellar into contact with the femur.
- From 10 to 20 degrees of flexion, the patella contacts the lateral surface of the femur on the inferior patellar surface.[49,50]
- The middle surfaces of the inferior aspect of the patellar come into contact with the femur at around 30 to 60 degrees of flexion, at which point the patella is well-seated in the groove.[49,50]
- As the knee continues to flex to 90 degrees the patella moves laterally, and the area of patella contact moves proximally.[46] At 90 degrees of knee flexion, the entire articular surface of the patella (except the odd facet) is in contact with the femur.[49,50]

- Beyond 90 degrees, the patella rides down into the intercondylar notch. At this point, the medial and lateral surfaces of the patella are in contact with the femur, and the quadriceps tendon articulates with the trochlear groove of the femur.[46]
- At approximately 120 degrees of knee flexion, there is no contact between the patella and the medial femoral condyle. At 135 degrees of knee flexion, the odd facet of the patella makes contact with the medial femoral condyle.

The Surface Area of Contact.[51] From 0 to 60 degrees of flexion, the magnitude of the patellofemoral contact area increases as flexion proceeds. Between 30 and 60 degrees of flexion, the patella moves medially to become centered in the trochlear groove. Contact between the quadriceps tendon and the femur begins at more than 70 degrees of flexion.[51] When the knee is flexed beyond 90 degrees, the patella tilts so that its medial facet articulates with the medial femoral condyle.[46] As knee flexion approaches 120 degrees, the contact area moves back toward the center of the patella. This is the point of maximum contact area between the patella and the femur.[52]

The Patellofemoral Joint Reaction Force. The patellofemoral joint reaction force (PJRF) causes compression of the patellofemoral joint. The PJRF is due to the increase in patellar and quadriceps tendon tension and the increase in the acuity of the Q-angle that occurs during knee flexion. Maximum force in the quadriceps muscle and patellar tendon is generated at 60 degrees of flexion.

Open- and Closed-Kinetic Chain Activities. A closed chain motion at the knee joint complex occurs when the knee bends or straightens while the lower extremity is weight bearing, or when the foot is in contact with any firm surface. An open chain motion occurs when the knee bends or straightens when the foot is not in contact with any surface.

Whether the motion occurring at the knee joint complex occurs as a closed or open kinetic chain, it has implications on the biomechanics and the joint compressive forces induced.

Closed-Chain Motion

Tibiofemoral Joint. During closed-chain knee flexion, the femoral condyles roll backward and glide forward on the tibia. During closed-chain knee extension, the femoral condyles roll forward and slide backward. During closed-chain knee flexion, as the femur rolls posteriorly, the distance between the tibial and femoral insertions of the ACL increases. Since the ACL cannot lengthen, it guides the femoral condyles anteriorly.[37] In contrast, during closed chain extension of the knee, the distance between the femoral and tibial insertions of the PCL increases. Since the PCL cannot lengthen, the ligament pulls the femoral condyles posteriorly as the knee extends.[37]

Patellofemoral Joint. During closed-kinetic exercises, the flexion moment of the arm increases as the angle of knee flexion increases. In addition, the joint-reaction force increases proportionately more during knee flexion than the magnitude of the contact area.[42] Thus, the articular pressure gradually increases as the knee flexes from 0 to

90 degrees,[42] with maximum values occurring at 90 degrees of flexion.[52] However, because this increasing force is distributed over a larger patellofemoral contact area, the contact stress per unit area is minimized. Some studies have demonstrated that CKC exercises at greater than 30 degrees of knee flexion can exacerbate patellofemoral problems.[53,54]

From 90 to 120 degrees of flexion, the articular pressure remains essentially unchanged because the quadriceps tendon is in contact with the trochlea, which effectively increases the contact area.[55]

Study Pearl

Due to the effect of joint reaction forces, CKC exercises involving the patellofemoral joint are performed in the 0 to 45 degrees range of flexion, with caution used when exercising between 90 and 50 degrees of knee flexion, where the patellofemoral joint reaction forces can be significantly greater.[55]

Open-Chain Motion

Tibiofemoral Joint. During open-chain flexion the tibia rolls and glides posteriorly on the femur, while during extension the opposite occurs. Open-chain knee extension involves a conjunct external rotation of the tibia, while open-chain knee flexion involves a conjunct internal rotation of the tibia.

Open-chain activities produce shear forces at the tibiofemoral joint in the direction of tibial movement.

Open-chain knee flexion, resulting from an isolated contraction of the hamstrings reduces ACL strain throughout the ROM,[56] but increases the strain on the PCL as flexion increases from 30 to 90 degrees.[57]

Study Pearl

Due to the effect of joint reaction forces, OKC exercises for the patellofemoral joint should be performed from 25 to 90 degrees of flexion (60 to 90 degrees if there are distal patellar lesions), or at 0 degree of extension (or hyperextension) from a point of view of cartilage stress.[55] OKC exercises are not recommended for the patellofemoral joint between 0 to 45 degrees of knee flexion, especially if there are proximal patellar lesions, as the PJRF are significantly greater.[55]

Patellofemoral Joint. In an open-chain activity, the forces across the patella are their lowest at 90 degrees of flexion. As the knee extends from this position, the flexion moment arm (contact stress/unit) for the knee increases, peaking between 35 and 40 degrees of flexion, while the patella contact area decreases.[53,58] This produces an increase in the PJRF at a point when the contact area is very small. At 0 degrees of flexion (full knee extension), the quadriceps force is high, but the contact stress/unit is low.

ANKLE AND FOOT JOINT COMPLEX

The majority of the support provided to the ankle and foot joints (Table 8-19) is provided through the anatomical arrangement of the ankle mortise and by the numerous ligaments (Table 8-20). Further

TABLE 8-19. THE JOINTS OF THE FOOT AND ANKLE: THEIR OPEN PACK, CLOSE PACK POSITIONS, AND CAPSULAR PATTERNS

JOINTS OF THE HIND FOOT	OPEN PACK POSITION	CLOSE PACK POSITION	CAPSULAR PATTERN
Tibiofibular joint	Plantar flexion	Maximum dorsiflexion	Pain on stress
Talocrural joint	10 degrees plantar flexion and midway between inversion and eversion	Maximum dorsiflexion	Plantar flexion, dorsiflexion
Subtalar joint	Midway between extremes of range of motion	Supination	Varus, valgus
Joints of the midfoot			
Midtarsal joints	Midway between extremes of range of motion	Supination	Dorsiflexion, plantar flexion, adduction, medial rotation
Joints of the forefoot			
Tarsometatarsal joints	Midway between extremes of range of motion	Supination	None
Metatarsophalangeal joints	10 degrees extension	Full extension	Great toe: extension, flexion 2nd-5th toes: variable
Interphalangeal joints	Slight flexion	Full extension	Flexion, extension

TABLE 8-20. ANKLE AND FOOT JOINTS AND ASSOCIATED LIGAMENTS

JOINT	ASSOCIATED LIGAMENT	FIBER DIRECTION	MOTIONS LIMITED
Distal tibiofibular	Anterior tibiofibular	Distolateral	Distal glide of fibula
	Posterior tibiofibular	Distolateral	Plantar flexion
	Interosseous		Distal glide of fibular Plantar flexion Separation of tibia and fibula
Ankle	Deltoid (medial collateral)		
	Superficial		
	Tibionavicular	Plantar-anterior	Plantar flexion, abduction
	Tibiocalcaneal	Plantar, plantar-posterior	Eversion, abduction
	Posterior tibiotalar	Plantar-posterior	Dorsiflexion, abduction
	Deep		
	Anterior tibiotalar	Anterior	Eversion, abduction, plantar flexion
	Lateral or fibular collateral		
	Anterior talofibular	Anterior-medial	Plantar flexion Inversion
	Calcaneofibular	Posterior-medial	Anterior displacement of foot Posterior displacement of foot Inversion Dorsiflexion
	Posterior talofibular	Horizontal (lateral)	Dorsiflexion Posterior displacement of foot
	Lateral and cervical talocalcaneal	Posterior-medial	Inversion Dorsiflexion
	Anterior capsule		Plantar flexion
	Posterior capsule		Dorsiflexion
Subtalar	Interosseous talocalcaneal		
	Anterior band	Proximal-anterior-lateral	Inversion Joint separation
	Posterior band	Proximal-posterior-lateral	Inversion Joint separation
	Lateral talocalcaneal	(See ankle)	
	Deltoid	(See ankle)	
	Lateral collateral	(See ankle)	
	Posterior talocalcaneal	Vertical	Dorsiflexion
	Medial talocalcaneal	Plantar-anterior	Eversion
	Anterior talocalcaneal (cervical ligaments)	Plantar-posterior-lateral	Inversion
Main ligamentous support of longitudinal arches	Long plantar	Anterior, slightly medial	Eversion
	Short plantar	Anterior	Eversion
	Plantar calcaneonavicular	Dorsal-anterior-medial	Eversion
	Plantar aponeurosis	Anterior	Eversion
Midtarsal or transverse	Bifurcated		Joint separation
	Medial band	Longitudinal	Plantar flexion
	Lateral band	Horizontal	Inversion
	Dorsal talonavicular	Longitudinal	Plantar flexion of talus on navicular
	Dorsal calcaneocuboid	Longitudinal	
	Ligaments supporting the arches		Inversion, plantar flexion

(Continued)

TABLE 8-20. ANKLE AND FOOT JOINTS AND ASSOCIATED LIGAMENTS (*Continued*)

JOINT	ASSOCIATED LIGAMENT	FIBER DIRECTION	MOTIONS LIMITED
Intertarsal	Numerous ligaments named by two interconnected bones (dorsal and plantar ligaments)		Joint motion in direction causing ligament tightness
	Interosseous ligaments connecting cuneiforms, cuboid, and navicular		Flattening of transverse arch
	Ligaments supporting arches		
Tarsometatarsal	Dorsal, plantar, and interosseous		Joint separation
Intermetatarsal	Dorsal, plantar, and interosseous		Joint separation
	Deep transverse metatarsal		Joint separation Flattening of transverse arch
Metatarsophalangeal	Fibrous capsule		
	Dorsally, thin—separated from extensor tendons by bursae		Flexion
	Inseparable from deep surface of plantar and collateral ligaments		Extension
	Collateral	Plantar-anterior	Flexion, abduction, or adduction in flexion
	Plantar, grooved for flexor tendons		Extension
Interphalangeal	Collateral		Flexion, abduction, or adduction in flexion
	Plantar		Extension
	Extensor hood replaces dorsal ligaments		Flexion

stabilization is provided by a host of tendons that cross this joint complex (Table 8-21), which are also involved in producing foot and ankle movements.

Even with this level of protection, the foot and ankle complex is at the mercy of truly impressive forces that act upon it during normal and athletic activities. As elsewhere, injuries to this area can be either microtraumatic or macrotraumatic.

Biomechanics

Terminology. Motions of the leg foot and ankle consist of single plane and multi-plane movements (Table 8-22). The single plane motions include:

- The motions of inversion and eversion that occur in the frontal plane.
- The motions of dorsiflexion and plantar flexion that occur in the sagittal plane.
- The motions of adduction and abduction that occur in the horizontal plane.

Triplanar motions occur at the talocrural, subtalar, and midtarsal joints, and at the first and fifth rays. Pronation and supination are considered triplanar motions.

TABLE 8-21. EXTRINSIC MUSCLE ATTACHMENTS AND INNERVATION

MUSCLE	PROXIMAL	DISTAL	INNERVATION
Gastrocnemius	Medial and lateral condyle of femur	Posterior surface of calcaneus through Achilles tendon	Tibial S2 (S1)
Plantaris	Lateral supracondylar line of femur	Posterior surface of calcaneus through Achilles tendon	Tibial S2 (S1)
Soleus	Head of fibula, proximal third of shaft, soleal line and midshaft of posterior tibia	Posterior surface of calcaneus through Achilles tendon	Tibial S2 (S1)
Tibialis anterior	Distal to lateral tibial condyle, proximal half of lateral tibial shaft, and interosseous membrane	First cuneiform bone, medial and plantar surfaces, and base of first metatarsal	Deep fibular (peroneal) L4 (L5)
Tibialis posterior	Posterior surface of tibia, proximal two-thirds posterior of fibula, and interosseous membrane	Tuberosity of navicular bone, tendinous expansion to other tarsals and metatarsals	Tibial L4 and L5
Fibularis longus	Lateral condyle of tibia, head and proximal two-thirds of fibula	Base of first metatarsal and first cuneiform, lateral side	Superficial fibular (peroneal) L5 and S1 (S2)
Fibularis brevis	Distal two-thirds of lateral fibular shaft	Tuberosity of fifth metatarsal	Superficial fibular (peroneal) L5 and S1 (S2)
Fibularis tertius	Lateral slip from extensor digitorum longus	Tuberosity of fifth metatarsal	Deep fibular (peroneal) L5 and S1
Flexor hallucis brevis	Plantar surface of cuboid and third cuneiform bones	Base of proximal phalanx of great toe	Medial plantar S3 (S2)
Flexor hallucis longus	Posterior distal two-thirds fibula	Base of distal phalanx of great toe	Tibial S2 (S3)
Flexor digitorum brevis	Tuberosity of calcaneus	One tendon slip into base of middle phalanx of each of the lateral four toes	Medial and lateral plantar S3 (S2)
Flexor digitorum longus	Middle three-fifths of posterior tibia	Base of distal phalanx of lateral four toes	Tibial S2 (S3)
Extensor hallucis longus	Middle half of anterior shaft of fibula	Base of distal phalanx of great toe	Deep fibular (peroneal) L5 and S1
Extensor hallucis brevis	Distal superior and lateral surfaces of calcaneus	Dorsal surface of proximal phalanx	Deep fibular (peroneal) S1 and S2
Extensor digitorum longus	Lateral condyle of tibia proximal anterior surface of shaft of fibula	One tendon to each lateral four toes, to middle phalanx, and extending to distal phalanges	Deep fibular (peroneal) L5 and S1

TABLE 8-22. NORMAL RANGES OF MOTION, AND END FEELS, FOR THE LOWER LEG, ANKLE, AND FOOT

MOTION	NORMAL RANGE (DEGREES)	END FEEL
Plantar flexion	30-50	Tissue stretch
Dorsiflexion	20	Tissue stretch
Hind foot inversion (supination)	20	Tissue stretch
Hind foot eversion (pronation)	10	Tissue stretch
Toe flexion	Great toe: MTP, 45; IP, 90 Lateral four toes: MTP, 40; PIP, 35; DIP, 60	Tissue stretch
Toe extension	Great toe: MTP, 70; IP, 0 Lateral four toes: MTP, 40; PIP, 0; DIP, 30	Tissue stretch

Data from Rasmussen O: Stability of the ankle joint. *Acta Orthop Scand.* 1985; 211(suppl):56-78; and Seto JL, Brewster CE. Treatment approaches following foot and ankle injury. *Clin Sports Med.* 1985;13:295.

Study Pearl

In pronation, the forefoot is rotated inward and downward, whereas in supination, the reverse occurs.

- The three body plane motions in pronation are abduction in the transverse plane, dorsiflexion in the sagittal plane, and eversion in the frontal plane.
- The three body plane motions in supination are a combined movement of adduction, plantar flexion, and inversion.

Distal Tibiofibular Joint. Although the two tibiofibular joints (proximal and distal) are described as individual articulations, they function as a pair. The movements that occur at these joints are primarily a result of the ankle's influence.

The ligaments of the distal tibiofibular joint are more commonly injured than any other ligament. Injuries to the ankle syndesmosis most often occur as a result of forced external rotation of the foot or during internal rotation of the tibia on a planted foot. Hyperdorsiflexion may also be a contributing mechanism.

Talocrural Joint. The primary motions at this joint are dorsiflexion and plantar flexion, with a total range of 70 to 80 degrees. The orientation of the talocrural joint axis is oriented, on average, 20 to 30 degrees posterior to the frontal plane as it passes posteriorly from the medial malleolus to the lateral malleolus. Although talocrural motion occurs primarily in the sagittal plane, an appreciable amount of horizontal motion appears to occur in the horizontal plane, especially during internal rotation of the tibia, or pronation of the foot.

The tibia follows the talus during weight bearing so that the talocrural joint externally rotates with supination, and internally rotates with pronation.[59] Therefore the tibia internally rotates during pronation and externally rotates during supination.[60]

Stability for this joint in weight bearing is provided by the articular surfaces, while in non-weight bearing, the ligaments appear to provide the majority of stability.

Subtalar Joint. The subtalar joint is responsible for inversion and eversion of the hindfoot—approximately 50% of apparent ankle inversion observed actually comes from the subtalar joint. In normal individuals, there is an inversion to eversion ratio of 2:3 to 1:3, which amounts to approximately 20 degrees of inversion and 10 degrees of eversion. For normal gait, a minimum of 4 to 6 degrees of eversion, and 8 to 12 degrees of inversion are required.[61] The axis of motion for the subtalar joint is approximately 45 degrees from horizontal and 20 degrees medial to the midsagittal plane. This axis, which moves during subtalar joint motion, allows the subtalar joint to produce a triplanar (pronation/supination), and varies according to whether the joint is weight bearing (close chain), or non-weight bearing (open chain).[62]

- During weight-bearing activities, pronation involves a combination of calcaneal eversion, adduction and plantar flexion of the talus, and internal rotation of the tibia, whereas supination involves a combination of calcaneal inversion, abduction and dorsiflexion of the talus, and external rotation of the tibia.
- During non-weight-bearing activities, pronation involves a combination of calcaneal eversion, abduction and dorsiflexion of the talus, whereas supination involves a combination of calcaneal inversion, adduction and plantar flexion of the talus.

The subtalar joint controls supination and pronation in close conjunction with the transverse tarsal joints of the mid foot.

Stability for the subtalar joint is provided by the calcaneofibular ligament, the cervical ligament, the interosseous ligament, the lateral talocalcaneal ligament, the fibulotalocalcaneal ligament (ligament of Rouviere), and the extensor retinaculum.

Midtarsal (Transverse Tarsal) Joint Complex. The function of the midtarsal joint complex is to provide the foot with an additional mechanism for raising and lowering the arch, and to absorb some of the horizontal plane tibial motion that is transmitted to the foot during stance.[59,63] The talocalcaneal joint has two degrees of freedom: plantar flexion/dorsiflexion and inversion/eversion, with motion occurring around a longitudinal and oblique axis, both of which are independent of each other.[63]

Cuneonavicular Joint. The cuneonavicular joint has 1 to 2 degrees of freedom: plantar/dorsiflexion, inversion/eversion.

Intercuneiform and Cuneocuboid Joints. Due to their very plane curvature, these joints have only 1 degree of freedom: inversion/eversion.

Metatarsophalangeal Joints. The metatarsophalangeal (MTP) joints have 2 degrees of freedom: flexion/extension and abduction/adduction. Range of motion of these joints is variable (Table 8-22).

First Metatarsophalangeal Joint. The function of the great toe is to provide stability to the medial aspect of the foot, and to provide for normal propulsion during gait. Normal alignment of the first MTP joint varies between 5 degree varus and 15 degrees valgus.

The great toe is characterized by having a remarkable discrepancy between active and passive motion. Approximately 30 degrees of active plantar flexion is present, and at least 50 degrees of active extension, which can be frequently increased passively to between 70 and 90 degrees.

Interphalangeal Joints. Each of the interphalangeal (IP) joints has 1 degree of freedom: flexion/extension.

CRANIOVERTEBRAL JOINTS

The term craniovertebral (CV) junction refers to the region of the cervical spine where the skull and vertebral column articulate and which is comprised of the bony structures of the foramen magnum, occiput, atlas, axis, and their supporting ligaments. The brainstem-spinal cord junction is housed in the posterior portion of the foramen magnum.

Occipito-Atlantal (OA) Joint. The OA joint is formed between the two occipital condyles, which are ovoid structures with their long axis situated in a posterolateral to anteromedial orientation, and the superior articular facets of the atlas (C1).

Atlanto-Axial Joint. This complex articulation consists of:

- Two zygapophysial joints between the articular surfaces of the inferior articular processes of the atlas and the superior processes of the axis.
- Two medial joints: one between the anterior surface of the atlas and the anterior surface of the dens of the axis, and the other between the anterior surface of the transverse ligament and the posterior surface of the dens.

Craniovertebral Ligaments

- Capsule and accessory capsular ligaments: By necessity, these ligaments are quite lax, to permit maximal motion, so they provide only moderate support to the joints during contralateral head rotation.
- Apical: The apical ligament of the dens extends from the apex of the dens to the anterior rim of the foramen magnum. The apical ligament appears to be only a moderate stabilizer against posterior translation of the dens relative to both the atlas and the occipital bone.
- Vertical and transverse bands of the cruciform ligament: The transverse portion stretches between tubercles on the medial aspects of the lateral masses of the atlas. The major responsibility of the transverse portion is to counteract anterior translation of the atlas relative to the axis, thereby maintaining the position of the dens relative to the anterior arch of the atlas. The transverse ligament also limits the amount of flexion between the atlas and axis.[64] These limiting functions are of extreme importance because excessive movement of either type could result in the dens compressing the spinal cord, epipharynx, vertebral artery, or superior cervical ganglion.
- Alar and accessory alar: The alar ligaments connect the superior part of the dens to fossae on the medial aspect of the occipital condyles, although they can also attach to the lateral masses of the atlas. The function of the ligament is to resist flexion, contralateral side bending, and rotation.[65] Due to the connections of the ligament, side bending of the head produces a contralateral rotation of the C2 vertebra.[66]

- Anterior occipito-atlantal membrane: The anterior occipito-atlantal membrane is thought to be the superior continuation of the anterior longitudinal ligament. It extends from the anterior arch of vertebra C1 to the anterior aspect of the foramen magnum.
- Posterior occipito-atlantal membrane: The posterior occipito-atlantal membrane is a continuation of the ligamentum flavum. This ligament interconnects the posterior arch of the atlas and the posterior aspect of the foramen magnum.
- Tectorial membrane: The tectorial membrane is the most posterior of the three ligaments and interconnects the occipital bone and the axis. This ligament is the superior continuation of the posterior longitudinal ligament, and connects the body of vertebra C2 to the anterior rim of the foramen magnum. This bridging ligament is an important limiter of upper cervical flexion.

Craniovertebral Muscles

Anterior Suboccipital Muscles

- Rectus Capitis Anterior
- Rectus Capitis Lateralis

Posterior Suboccipital Muscles. These muscles function in the control of segmental sliding between C1 and C2,[67] and may have an important role in proprioception, having more muscle spindles than any other muscle for their size.[67] All of the posterior suboccipital muscles are innervated by the posterior ramus of C1, and are also strongly linked with the trigeminal nerve.[68,69] The suboccipitals receive their blood supply from the vertebral artery.

Nerve Supply. The dorsal ramus of spinal nerve C1 is larger than the ventral ramus and supplies most of the muscles that form that triangle. It usually has no cutaneous distribution.

The dorsal ramus of spinal nerve C2, also known as the greater occipital nerve, supplies most of the posterior aspect of the scalp, extending anteriorly to a line across the scalp that extends from one external auditory meatus to the other.

Blood Supply. The cervical cord is supplied by two arterial systems, central and peripheral, which overlap but are discrete. The first is dependent entirely on the single anterior spinal artery (ASA). The second, without clear-cut boundaries, receives supplies from the ASA and both posterior spinal arteries.[70]

Biomechanics. The upper cervical spine is responsible for approximately 50% of the motion that occurs in the entire cervical spine. Motion at the A-A joint occurs relatively independently, while below C2, normal motion is a combination of motion occurring at other levels.

Occipito-Atlantal Joint. The primary motion that occurs at this joint is flexion and extension, although side bending and rotation also occur. It is generally agreed that rotation and side bending at this joint occur to opposite sides when they are combined.

Occipital rotation and, to some degree, anterior–posterior translation of the occiput on C1 is thought to be limited by the alar ligaments.

Atlanto-Axial Joint. The major motion that occurs at all three of the A-A articulations is axial rotation, totaling approximately 40 to 47 degrees to each side. This large amount of rotation has the potential to cause compression of the vertebral artery if it becomes excessive. As the atlas rotates, the ipsilateral facet moves posteriorly and inferiorly while the contralateral facet moves anteriorly and inferiorly, so that each facet of the atlas slides along the convex surface of the axial facet, telescoping the head downward.

Flexion and extension movements of the A-A joint amount to a combined range of 10 to 15 degrees: 10 degrees of flexion and 5 degrees of extension.

Cervical Spine

There are seven vertebrae in the entire cervical spine. As previously mentioned, C1 articulates with the occiput of the skull above and with C2 below. Vertebrae C3 through C7, which are considered the cervical spine proper, collectively allow for varying degrees of flexion, extension, side bending, and rotation. Each cervical spinal nerve, which exit bilaterally through the intervertebral foramina is named for the vertebra above which it exits; for example, the C5 nerve exits above the C5 vertebra.

Due to the high degree of mobility but low degree of stability, the cervical spine is vulnerable to both direct and indirect trauma.

Biomechanics. At the zygapophyseal joints there is a combined sagittal range of 30 to 60 degrees.[71] Significant flexion occurs at C5 to C6, and extension around C6 to C7.

The only significant arthrokinematic available to the zygapophyseal joint is an inferior, medial glide of the inferior articular process of the superior facet during extension, and a superior, lateral glide during flexion. Segmental side bending is, therefore, extension of the ipsilateral joint and flexion of the contralateral joint. Rotation, coupled with ipsilateral side bending, involves extension of the ipsilateral joint and flexion of the contralateral.

Muscle Control. The muscle groups of the cervical region may be divided into those that produce movement and those that sustain postures or attempt to stabilize the segments.[72-74]

- The global muscles of the neck are thought to be the sternocleidomastoid (anteriorly), the semispinalis capitis and splenius capitis (posteriorly).
- The local system is thought to comprise the longus capitis and longus colli[75] and semispinalis cervicis and multifidus.[76]

Temporomandibular Joint

Three bony components make up the masticatory system: the maxilla and the mandible, which support the teeth, and the temporal bone, which supports the mandible at its articulation with the skull. The temporomandibular joint (TMJ) is formed between the articular eminence of the temporal bone, the intra-articular disc, and the head of the mandible. The TMJ differs from other joints in that the articulating surfaces of the bones are covered, not by hyaline cartilage, but by fibrocartilage. The development of fibrocartilage provides a greater capacity for self-repair than would hyaline cartilage.

A fibrocartilaginous disc (sometimes inappropriately referred to as "meniscus") is located between the articulating surface of the temporal bone, and the mandibular condyle. The shape of the condyle and the articulating fossa determines the biconcave shape of the disc.

The disc is usually located on top of the condyle in the 12 o'clock to 1 o'clock position on the mandibular head when the jaw is closed. Because the only firm attachment of the disc to the condyle occurs medially and laterally, the disc can move somewhat independently of the condyle.

The disc effectively divides the TMJ into a lower and upper joint cavity.

Supporting Structures. The supporting structures of the TMJ consist of periarticular connective tissue (ligament, tendon, capsule, and fascia). As its name implies, the periarticular connective tissue serves to keep the joints together and to limit the ranges of motion at the joint.

The intercapsular structures are located posteriorly to the condyle. Anterior to the joint are the muscles of the medial and lateral pterygoid. Two strong ligaments help to provide joint stability:

- The joint capsule or capsular ligament: This structure, which surrounds the entire joint, is thought to provide proprioceptive feedback regarding joint position and movement.
- The temporomandibular (or lateral) ligament: The capsule of the TMJ is reinforced laterally by an outer oblique portion, and an inner horizontal portion of the temporomandibular ligament, which function as a suspensory mechanism for the mandible during moderate opening movements. The ligament also functions to resist rotation, and posterior displacement of the mandible.

Two other ligaments assist with joint stability:

1. Stylomandibular ligament. This ligament acts as a guiding mechanism for the mandible, keeping the condyle, disc, and temporal bone firmly opposed.
2. Sphenomandibular ligament. This ligament acts to check the angle of the mandible from sliding, as far forward as the condyles during the translatory cycle, and serves as a suspensory ligament of the mandible during wide opening.

Muscles. The muscles of the face and mouth and pharynx are described in Table 8-23.

The Infrahyoid or "Strap" Muscles

- The infrahyoid muscles comprise the sternohyoid, omohyoid, sternothyroid, and thyrohyoid muscles.
- The sternohyoid muscle is a strap-like muscle, which functions to depress the hyoid as well as assist in speech and mastication.

TABLE 8-23. MUSCLES OF THE FACE, MOUTH, AND PHARYNX

	ANATOMY	ACTION	INNERVATION
Muscles of the face			
Levator anguli oris	Arises from the canine fossa of the maxilla and inserts into the upper and lower lips	Contraction results in drawing the corner of the mouth up and medially	Superior buccal branches of CN VII
Zygomatic major (zygomaticus)	Arises lateral to the zygomatic minor on the zygomatic bone. Courses obliquely and inserts into the corner of the orbicularis oris	Elevates and retracts the angle of the mouth (smiling)	
Depressor labii inferioris	Originates from the mandible and courses up and in to insert into the lower lip	Dilation of the orifice of the mouth; pulls the lips down and out; counterpart to the levator triad	Mandibular marginal branches of VII
Depressor anguli oris (triangularis)	Originates along the lateral margins of the mandible. Fanlike fibers converge on the orbicularis oris and upper lip at the corner	Depresses the corners of the mouth and compresses the upper lip against the lower lip	
Mentalis	Arises from the region of the incisive fossa of the mandible, and inserts into the skin of the chin	Contraction elevates and wrinkles the chin and pulls the lower lip out	Innervated by the mandibular marginal branch of the facial nerve
Platysma (also considered a neck muscle)	Arises from the fascia overlying the pectoralis major and deltoid. Courses up and inserts into the corner of the mouth below the symphysis mente, the lower margin of the mandible, and then into the skin near the masseter	Appears to assist in depression of the mandible	The cervical branch of CN VII
Muscles of the mouth			
Orbicularis oris	Considered a single muscle encircling the mouth opening as well as paired upper and lower muscles (obicularis oris superior, obicularis oris inferior)	Serves as a point of insertion for other muscles	Branches of the VII facial nerve
Risorius	Superficial to the buccinators, originates from the posterior region of the face along the fascia of the masseter muscle; courses forward and inserts into the corners of the mouth	Retracts the lips at the corners (smiling)	Cranial nerve VII (facial nerve)
Buccinator	Deep to the risorius; originates on the pterygomandibular ligament and the posterior alveolar portion of the mandible and maxillae; courses forward to insert into the upper and lower orbicularis oris	Involved in mastication; also constricts the oropharynx	Cranial nerve VII (facial nerve)
Levator triad—A group of three muscles	1. Levator labii superioris alaeque nasi (most medial)—courses vertically along the lateral margin of the nose, arising from the frontal process of maxilla; inserts into the wing of the nostril and UL (flares the nares) 2. Levator labii superioris (intermediate)—originates from the infraorbital margin of the maxilla; courses down and into the upper lip 3. Zygomatic minor (lateral)—originates at the facial surface of the zygomatic bone and courses downward into the upper lip	Dominant muscles for lip elevation and also dilate oral opening	Buccal branches of CN VII

Intrinsic muscles of the tongue		
Median fibrous septum	Divides right and left halves of the tongue—originates on the body of the hyoid bone via the hyoglossal membrane; courses the length of the tongue	Serves as the point of origin for transverse muscle of the tongue, Forms tongue attachment with the hyoid
Longitudinal muscle (superior lingualis)	Thin layer of oblique and longitudinal muscle fibers lying just deep to the mucous membrane of the dorsum tongue Fibers arise from the submucous fibrous tissue near the epiglottis, hyoid, and the median fibrous septum Fibers fan forward and outward then insert into the lateral margins of the tongue	Bilateral contraction will elevate the tongue tip Unilateral contraction will pull the tongue toward the side of contraction
Inferior longitudinal muscle (inferior lingualis)	A bundle of muscle fibers located on the undersurface of the tongue (absent in the medial tongue base) Originates at the root of the tongue and corpus hyoid Courses between the genioglossus and hyoglossus muscles and to the apex of the tongue Longitudinal muscle fibers interdigitate with them	Bilateral contraction will pull the tip of the tongue downward and assist in retraction of the tongue if co-contracted with the superior longitudinal Unilateral contraction will cause the tongue to turn toward the contracted side and downward
Transverse muscle (transverse lingualis)	Fibers originate at the median fibrous septum Course laterally to insert into the submucous tissue at the lateral margins of the tongue Some fibers continue as the palatopharyngeus muscle	Contraction pulls the edges of the tongue toward midline, narrowing and elongating the tongue
Vertical muscles (vertical lingualis)	Originate from the mucous membrane of the dorsum Course vertically downward and somewhat laterally Fibers of the transverse and vertical muscles interweave Insert into the sides and inferior surface of the tongue	Contraction flattens the tongue
Extrinsic tongue muscles		
Genioglossus	Flat, triangular muscle located close to the median plane Arises from the inner mandibular surface at the symphysis Lower fibers course to the hyoid bone and attach by a thin aponeurosis to the upper part of the body Remainder of fibers radiate fanlike to the dorsum of the tongue inserting into the submucous fibrous	The prime mover of the tongue (strongest and largest of the extrinsic muscles) Contraction of the anterior fibers results in retraction of the tongue Contraction of the posterior fibers draws the tongue forward to aid protrusion of the apex Contraction of both anterior and posterior fibers will draw the middle portion of the tongue down into the floor of the mouth (cupping the tongue)

(Continued)

TABLE 8-23. MUSCLES OF THE FACE, MOUTH, AND PHARYNX (*Continued*)

	ANATOMY	ACTION	INNERVATION
Hyoglossus	Arises from the length of the greater cornu and lateral body of the hyoid Courses upward and inserts into the lateral portions of the tongue	Contraction pulls the sides of the tongue down Antagonist to the palatoglossus	
Styloglossus	Originates from the anterolateral margin of styolid process Courses forward and down to insert into the inferior sides of the tongue Divides into two portions: One interdigitates with the inferior longitudinal muscle and the other with the hyoglossus	Bilateral contraction draws the tongue back and up	
Chondroglossus	Also considered to be a part of the hyoglossus Arises from the lesser cornu of the hyoid Courses up to interdigitate with the intrinsic muscles of the tongue medial to the point of insertion of the hyoglossus	Contraction depresses the tongue	
Palatoglossus	Can be considered a muscle of the tongue or the velum	Serves a dual purpose—depresses the soft palate and elevates the back of the tongue	
Mandibular elevators			
Masseter	Most superficial of the mastication muscles Originates on the lateral, inferior, and medial surfaces of the zygomatic arch External fibers insert into the ramus Internal (deep) fibers terminate on the coronoid process	Places maximum force on the molars Contraction elevates the mandible, closing the jaw Clenching the teeth will make the muscular belly visible	Innervated by CN V- trigeminal nerve
Temporalis	Deep to the masseter Arises from the temporal fossa (a region of the temporal and parietal bones) The broad, thin, fan-shaped muscle converges as it courses down and forward Terminal tendon passes through the zygomatic arch and inserts in the coronoid process and ramus	Contraction elevates the mandible and draws it back if protruded	Innervated by CN V-trigeminal
Medial pterygoid (internal pterygoid muscle, internal masseter)	Originates primarily in the vertically directed pterygoid fossa and from the medial surface of the lateral pterygoid plate Fibers course down and back inserting into the ramus	Contraction elevates the mandible in conjunction with the masseter	Innervated by CN V

Mandibular protrusors		
Lateral pterygoid	Arises from the sphenoid bone Two heads—lateral pterygoid plate; greater wing of the sphenoid bone Fibers course back to insert into the pterygoid fossa (fovea) of the mandible (a depression on the anterior neck of the condyle of the mandible) and to the anterior margin of the articular disc of the temporomandibular articulation	Contraction protrudes the mandible, causing the condyle to slide down and forward on the articular eminence Unilateral contraction moves the jaw in a grinding motion
Mandibular depressors		
Digastricus	Anterior and posterior	When infrahyoid musculature is fixed, contraction of anterior digastricus will depress the mandible. Bilaterally, the digastrics assist in forced mouth opening by stabilizing the hyoid. The posterior bellies are especially active during coughing and swallowing
Mylohyoid	Forms floor of the mouth	When hyoid is in fixed position, contraction will depress the mandible. Stabilizes or elevates the tongue during swallowing, and elevates the floor of the mouth in the first stage of deglutition
Geniohyoid	A narrow muscle situated under the mylohyoid muscle	Contraction depresses the mandible if the hyoid is fixed; elevates the hyoid bone if mandible fixed
Platysma	Also considered a muscle of the face	Contraction depresses the mandible
Pharyngeal constrictors		
	Superior pharyngeal constrictor Middle pharyngeal constrictor Inferior pharyngeal constrictor Cricopharyngeal muscle Thyropharyngeus muscle	

Study Pearl

Working in combinations, the muscles of the TMJ are involved as follows:

- Mouth opening: bilateral action of the lateral pterygoid and digastric muscles
- Mouth closing: bilateral action of the temporalis, masseter and medial pterygoid muscles
- Lateral deviation: action of the ipsilateral masseter, and contralateral medial pterygoid muscles
- Protrusion: bilateral action of the lateral pterygoid, medial pterygoid, and anterior fibers of the temporalis muscles
- Retrusion: bilateral action of the posterior fibers of the temporalis muscle, the digastric, stylohyoid, geniohyoid, and mylohyoid muscles

- The omohyoid muscle, situated lateral to the sternohyoid, consists of two bellies, and functions to depress the hyoid.
- The sternothyroid and thyrohyoid muscles are located deep to the sternohyoid muscle. The sternothyroid muscle is involved in drawing the larynx downward, while the thyrohyoid depresses the hyoid and elevates the larynx.

These infrahyoid muscles are innervated by fibers from the upper cervical nerves. The nerves to the lower part of these muscles are given off from a loop, the ansa cervicalis (cervical loop).

The Stylohyoid. The stylohyoid muscle elevates the hyoid and base of the tongue and has an undetermined role in speech, mastication, and swallowing. Although these muscles work most efficiently in groups, an understanding of the specific anatomy and action(s) of the individual muscles is necessary for an appreciation of their coordinated function during masticatory activity.

Nerve Supply. The TMJ is primarily supplied from three nerves that are part of the mandibular division of the fifth cranial (trigeminal) nerve.

Biomechanics. The movements that occur at the TMJ are extremely complex. The TMJ has 3 degrees of freedom, with each of the degrees of freedom associated with a separate axis of rotation.[77] Two primary arthrokinematic movements (rotation and anterior translation) occur at this joint around three planes: sagittal, horizontal, and frontal.

The two major motions of the TMJ occur as rotations:

- Mouth opening and closing result from a rotation of the mandible about a horizontal axis
- Lateral deviation results from a rotation of the mandible about a vertical axis.

The motions of protrusion and retrusion are planar glides. In addition to the rotational motions during mouth opening and closing and lateral deviations, movements at the TMJ involve arthrokinematic rolls and slides. Thus:

- Mouth opening, contralateral deviation, and protrusion all involve an anterior osteokinematic rotation of the mandible and an anterior, inferior, and lateral glide of the mandibular head and disc.
- Mouth closing, ipsilateral deviation, and retrusion all involve a posterior osteokinematic rotation of the mandible and an anterior, inferior, and lateral glide of the mandibular head and disc.

Occlusal Positions. Occlusal positions are functional positions of the TMJ, and are defined as the point at which contact between some or all of the teeth occur. Under normal circumstances, the upper molars rest directly on the lower molars and the upper incisors slightly override the lower incisors. The ideal position provides mutual protection of anterior and posterior teeth, comfortable and painless mandibular function, and stability.[78]

- The *median occlusal* position: corresponds to the position in which all of the teeth are fully interdigitated,[79]and is considered the start position for all mandibular motions.
- The *centric* position is considered to be the position that implies the most retruded, unstrained position of the mandible from which lateral movements are possible and the components of the oral apparatus are the most balanced.[80]

The Close-Pack and Resting Positions. The joints close-packed position is difficult to determine because the position of maximal muscle tightness is also the position of least joint surface congruity and vice versa. Rocabado[81] considers there to be two close-packed positions named according to the end position of the mandibular head in the fossa: an anterior close-packed position and a posterior close-packed position:[81]

- Anterior close-packed position: This position is the position of maximum opening of the joint.
- Posterior close-packed position: This position is the maximum retruded position of the joint.

Under this premise, the open-packed, or "rest" position is any position away from the anterior or posterior close-packed positions of the joint.[81] The rest position, or "freeway space" corresponds to the position where the residual tension of the muscles are at rest and no contact occurs between maxillary and mandibular teeth. In this position, the tongue is against the palate of the mouth with its most anterior-superior tip in the area against the palate, just posterior to the rear of the upper central incisors.

THORACIC SPINE AND RIB CAGE

The primary function of the thoracic spine and rib cage is protection and function of the thoracic viscera. Each thoracic vertebra is involved in at least six articulations. In addition, the posterior thoracic muscles, spinous processes, anterior and posterior longitudinal ligaments, vertebral bodies, zygapophyseal and costotransverse joints, inferior articular process, pars interarticularis, intervertebral disk, nerve root, joint meniscus, and dura mater are all capable of producing pain in this region.

Biomechanics. The thoracic spinal segments possess the potential for a unique array of movements. However, there is very little agreement in the literature with regards to the biomechanics of the thoracic spine and most of the understanding is based largely on the ex vivo studies of White,[82]and Panjabi et al.,[83,84] and a variety of "clinical models."[85,86]

The rib cage and its articulations provide a significant degree of stability at the cost of reduced mobility. This has the affect of influencing the motions available in other regions of the spine, and the shoulder girdle, and increasing the potential for postural impairments in this region, while providing an important weight-bearing mechanism for the vertebral column.[87-90] Indeed, the capacity of the spine to bear load has been found to be up to three times greater with an intact rib cage.[91,92]

Respiration. The main movement in the upper six ribs during respiration (see Chapter 10) and other movements is one of rotation of the neck of the rib, with only small amounts of superior and inferior motion. In the seventh to tenth ribs, the principal movement is upward, backward, and medially during inspiration with the reverse occurring during expiration.[85]

Because the anterior end of the ribs is lower than the posterior, when the ribs elevate, they rise upward while the rib neck drops down. In the upper ribs, this results in an anterior elevation (pump handle) and in the middle and lower ribs (excluding the free ribs), a lateral elevation (bucket handle), with the former movement increasing the anterior–posterior diameter of the thoracic cavity, and the latter increasing the transverse diameter.

Both kinds of rib motion are produced by the action of the diaphragm. The seventh to tenth ribs act to increase the abdominal cavity free space to afford space for the descending diaphragm.

Posture. A number of common kyphotic deformities are associated with this region, including Scheuermann's, neuromuscular dysfunctions, skeletal dysplasias, and collagen diseases.

Lumbar Spine

Generally, the five lumbar vertebral bodies are distinguished from the thoracic bodies by the absence of rib facets. The pedicles project from the upper portion of the vertebral body. The spinous process is primarily horizontal in orientation, while the posterior inferior border projects below the upper level of the spinous process below. The region between the superior articular process and the lamina is the pars interarticularis.

Ligamentous support for the lumbar spine is provided by the anterior longitudinal ligament, the posterior longitudinal ligament, the attachments of the annulus fibrosis, and the interosseous ligaments between the spinous processes.

Biomechanics. Motions at the lumbar spine joints can occur in three cardinal planes: sagittal (flexion and extension), coronal (side bending), and transverse (rotation). About 6 degrees of freedom are available at the lumbar spine.

The amount of segmental motion at each vertebral level varies. Most of the flexion and extension of the lumbar spine occurs in the lower segmental levels, whereas most of the side bending of the lumbar spine occurs in the mid-lumbar area. Rotation, which occurs with side bending as a coupled motion, is minimal, and occurs most at the lumbosacral junction. The amount of range available in the lumbar spine decreases with age.

Different trunk muscles play differing roles in the provision of dynamic stability to the spine. These muscles can be classified functionally as either *mobilizers* or *stabilizers.*

- Mobilizers function to produce movement in the sagittal plane using concentric acceleration. This particular muscle group can generate a tremendous amount of force.
- Stabilizers can be further divided into global and local stabilizers.[93] Global stabilizers have a role in eccentrically

decelerating momentum, and controlling rotation of the spine as a whole. In contrast, the local stabilizers function to maintain a continuous low-force activity at joints in all positions and directions, and thus provide segmental joint support.

The Global Muscle System. This system consists of muscles whose origins are on the pelvis and whose insertions are on the thoracic cage. These muscles include:

- The rectus abdominis
- The internal and external obliques
- The lateral fibers of the quadratus lumborum
- The thoracic part of lumbar iliocostalis

The global muscle system acts on the trunk and spine, without being directly attached to it. These muscles appear to provide general trunk stabilization, but are not capable of having a direct segmental influence on the spine.

The Local Muscle System. The local miuscle system consists of muscles that have insertions and/or origins at the lumbar vertebra or pelvis, and which are responsible for providing segmental stability and directly controlling the lumbar segments and sacroiliac joint. These muscles include:

- The lumbar portions of the iliocostalis and longissimus thoracis muscles
- The medial fibers of the quadratus lumborum
- The diaphragm
- The lumbar multifidus: considered to have the greatest potential to provide dynamic control to the motion segment, particularly in its neutral zone
- The pelvic floor muscles
- The transversus abdominis: primarily active in providing rotational and lateral control to the spine while maintaining adequate levels of intra-abdominal pressure, and imparting tension to the thoracolumbar fascia
- The posterior fibers of the internal oblique that attach to the tensor fascia latae

The local muscle system is important for the provision of segmental control to the spine, and provides an important stiffening effect on the lumbar spine, thereby enhancing its dynamic stability.

SACROILIAC JOINT

The sacroiliac joint (SIJ) forms a junction between the sacrum and the pelvis. In this joint, hyaline cartilage on the sacral side moves against fibrocartilage on the iliac side. The joint is generally C-shaped with two lever arms that interlock at the second sacral level. Much of the stability for the SIJ is provided by numerous ridges and depressions. Stability at the SIJ is also provided by the presence of ligaments, which offer resistance to shear and loading. The deep anterior, posterior, and interosseous ligaments resist the load of the sacrum relative to the ilium. The more superficial ligaments (eg, sacrotuberous ligament) react to dynamic motions (eg, straight-leg raising during physical motion). The long dorsal sacroiliac ligament can become stretched in periods of reduced lumbar lordosis (eg, pregnancy).

Many large and small muscles have relationships with these ligaments and the SIJ. These include the piriformis, biceps femoris, gluteus maximus and minimus, erector spinae, latissimus dorsi, thoracolumbar fascia, and iliacus. Any of these muscles can be involved with a painful SIJ. As a true joint, the SIJ is a pain-sensitive structure richly innervated by a combination of unmyelinated free nerve endings and posterior primary rami of L2-S3. The wide possibility of innervation may explain why pain emanation from the joint can manifest in so many various ways, with different and unique referral patterns for individual patients.

Biomechanics. The results from the numerous studies on mobility of the sacroiliac joint have led to a variety of different hypotheses and models of pelvic mechanics over the years.

EXAMINATION OF THE MUSCULOSKELETAL SYSTEM

Patient History and Systems Review

Refer to Chapter 6.

Tests and Measures

The tests and measures component of the musculoskeletal examination serves as an adjunct to the history and systems review. This examination may be modified based on the history—the examination of an acutely injured patient differs greatly from that of a patient in less discomfort or distress. In addition, the examination of a child differs in some respects to that of an adult. An overview of the examination of each of the major joints is provided in Tables 8-24 through 8-32.

TABLE 8-24. EXAMINATION OF THE CERVICAL SPINE

Observation and inspection	
Upper quarter and peripheral joint scan	Temporomandibular joint, shoulder complex, elbow, forearm, and wrist and hand Dermatomes and key muscle tests as appropriate
Examination of movements. Active range of motion with passive overpressure (except extension and rotation)	a. Flexion, extension, side bending (right and left), rotation (right and left) b. Combined movements as appropriate c. Repetitive movements as appropriate d. Sustained positions as appropriate e. Craniovertebral joint movement testing
Resisted isometric movements	All AROM directions
Palpation	
Neurological tests as appropriate	Reflexes, key muscle tests, sensory scan, peripheral nerve assessment Neurodynamic mobility tests (upper limb tension tests, Slump test)
Joint mobility tests	a. Side glides b. Anterior and posterior glides c. Traction and compression
Special tests (refer to "Special Tests" section).	As indicated
Diagnostic imaging	As appropriate

TABLE 8-25. EXAMINATION OF THE LUMBAR SPINE

Observation and inspection	
Lower quarter and peripheral joint scan	SIJ, Hip, knee, ankle, and foot Dermatomes and key muscle tests as appropriate
Examination of movements. Active range of motion with passive overpressure	a. Flexion, extension, side bending (right and left), rotation (right and left) b. Combined movements as appropriate c. Repetitive movements as appropriate d. Sustained positions as appropriate e. Sacroiliac joint movement testing
Resisted isometric movements	All AROM directions Rectus abdominis, internal and external obliques, quadratus lumborum, back and hip extensors
Palpation	
Neurological tests as appropriate	Reflexes, key muscle tests, sensory scan, peripheral nerve assessment Neurodynamic mobility tests (straight leg raise, slump test, prone knee flexion)
Joint mobility tests	a. Side glides b. Anterior and posterior glides c. Traction and compression
Special tests (refer to "Special Tests" section)	As indicated
Diagnostic imaging	As appropriate

Observation. The patient's general posture and ability to perform functional tasks provides information about the severity of symptoms, willingness to move, range of motion, and gross muscle strength.[94] Postural assessment is typically the first component of the test and measures of any patient with a musculoskeletal dysfunction (see Chapter 7).

TABLE 8-26. EXAMINATION OF THE THORACIC SPINE

Observation and inspection	
Upper quarter and peripheral joint scan	Temporomandibular joint, shoulder complex, elbow, forearm, and wrist and hand Dermatomes and key muscle tests as appropriate
Examination of movements. Active range of motion with passive overpressure	a. Flexion, extension, side bending (right and left), rotation (right and left) b. Bucket handle and pump handle rib motions c. Combined movements as appropriate d. Repetitive movements as appropriate e. Sustained positions as appropriate
Resisted isometric movements	All AROM directions Rectus abdominis, internal and external obliques, quadratus lumborum, back and hip extensors
Palpation	
Neurological tests as appropriate	Reflexes, key muscle tests, sensory scan, peripheral nerve assessment Neurodynamic mobility tests (straight leg raise, slump test) as appropriate
Joint mobility tests	a. Distraction and compression b. Flexion and extension of the zygapophysial joints c. Rib springing d. Posteroanterior unilateral vertebral pressure
Special tests (refer to "Special Tests" section)	As indicated
Diagnostic imaging	As appropriate

TABLE 8-27. EXAMINATION OF THE SHOULDER

I. History
II. Observation and inspection
III. Upper quarter scan as appropriate
IV. Examination of movements. Active range of motion with passive overpressure of the following movements:
  a. Elevation (forward flexion, abduction, scaption)—painful arc
  b. Adduction, extension horizontal adduction and abduction, circumduction, external rotation, and internal rotation
  c. Scapulohumeral range of abduction—scapulohumeral rhythm
V. Resisted isometric movements
  a. Elevation (forward flexion, abduction, scaption)
  b. Extension
  c. Adduction
  d. Abduction
  e. External rotation
  f. Internal rotation
  g. Elbow flexion
  h. Elbow extension
VI. Palpation
VII. Neurological tests as appropriate (reflexes, sensory scan, peripheral nerve assessment)
VIII. Joint mobility tests
  a. Glenohumeral joint
    a. Distraction
    b. Inferior glide of the humeral head
    c. Posterior glide of the humeral head
    d. Anterior glide of the humeral head
  b. Sternoclavicular joint
    a. Superior glide of the clavicle on the sternum
    b. Inferior glide of the clavicle on the sternum
    c. Posterior glide of the clavicle on the sternum
    d. Anterior glide of the clavicle
  c. Acromioclavicular joint
    a. Compression/distraction
    b. Anterior glide of the clavicle on the acromion
    c. Posterior glide of the clavicle
  d. Scapulothoracic joint
    a. Rotation of the scapula on the thoracic wall
    b. Elevation of the scapula on the thoracic wall
    c. Depression of the scapula on the thoracic wall
    d. Retraction of the scapula on the thoracic wall
    e. Protraction of the scapula on the thoracic wall
    f. Distraction of the scapula from the thoracic wall
IX. Special tests (refer to "Special Tests" section)
X. Diagnostic imaging as appropriate

Palpation. It is suggested that palpation immediately follow or be integrated with observation, and occur prior to other testing procedures.[94] Palpation, using varying levels of tactile pressure, requires a detailed knowledge of anatomy and a systematic approach. The following should be noted during palpation:

- Myofascial mobility
- Skin temperature
- Areas of localized tenderness and/or asymmetry
- Skin and soft tissue density and extensibility
- Peripheral pulses as indicated
- Areas of edema

TABLE 8-28. EXAMINATION OF THE ELBOW, FOREARM, WRIST, AND HAND

I. History
II. Observation and inspection
III. Upper quarter scan as appropriate
IV. Examination of movements. Active range of motion with passive overpressure of the following movements:
   a. Flexion and extension of the elbow
   b. Pronation and supination of the forearm
   c. Wrist flexion and extension
   d. Radial deviation and ulnar deviation of the wrist
   e. Finger flexion and finger extension (MCP, PIP, and DIP joints)
   f. Finger abduction and adduction
   g. Thumb flexion, extension, abduction, and adduction
   h. Opposition of the thumb and little finger
V. Resisted isometric movements:
   a. Elbow flexion and extension
   b. Pronation and supination of the forearm
   c. Wrist flexion and extension
   d. Radial deviation and ulnar deviation of the wrist
   e. Finger flexion and finger extension (MCP, PIP, and DIP joints)
   f. Finger abduction and adduction
   g. Thumb flexion, extension, abduction, and adduction
   h. Opposition of the thumb and little finger
VI. Palpation
VII. Neurological tests as appropriate (reflexes, sensory scan, peripheral nerve assessment)
VIII. Joint mobility tests:
   a. Distraction/compression of the ulnohumeral joint
   b. Medial and lateral glide of the ulnohumeral joint
   c. Distraction of the radiohumeral joint
   d. Anterior and posterior glide of the radial head
   e. Anterior and posterior glide of the proximal radioulnar joint
   f. Anterior and posterior glide of the distal radioulnar joint
   g. Long-axis extension at the wrist and fingers (MCP, PIP, and DIP joints)
   h. Anteroposterior glide at the wrist and fingers (MCP, PIP, and DIP joints)
   i. Side glide at the wrist and fingers (MCP, PIP, and DIP joints)
   j. Anteroposterior glides of the intermetacarpal joints
   k. Rotation of the MCP, PIP, and DIP joints
   l. Individual carpal bone mobility
IX. Special tests, including functional testing (refer to "Special Tests" section).
X. Diagnostic imaging as appropriate.

Range of Motion. Within the field of physical therapy, goniometry is commonly used to measure the total amount of available motion at a specific joint. Goniometry can be used to measure both active and passive range of motion.

Active Range of Motion. Active range of motion testing gives the clinician information about:

- The quantity of available physiological motion
- The presence of muscle substitutions
- The willingness of the patient to move
- The integrity of the contractile and inert tissues
- The quality of motion
- Symptom reproduction
- The pattern of motion restriction (capsular/non-capsular—see Chapter 5)

TABLE 8-29. EXAMINATION OF THE SACROILIAC JOINT

I. History
II. Observation and inspection
III. Lower quarter scan as appropriate
IV. Examination of movements. Active range of motion with passive overpressure of the following movements:
  a. Lumbar spine flexion, extension, side bending (right and left), rotation (right and left)
  b. Hip flexion, extension, abduction, adduction, internal rotation, external rotation
  c. Weight-bearing kinetic tests (ipsilateral and contralateral)
V. Resisted isometric movements:
  a. Lumbar spine flexion
  b. Hip flexion, extension, abduction, adduction, internal rotation, external rotation
VI. Palpation
VII. Neurological tests as appropriate (reflexes, sensory scan, peripheral nerve assessment)
VIII. Joint mobility tests:
  a. Anterior and posterior joint distraction
  b. Anterior and posterior joint compression
  c. Short and long arm tests
IX. Special tests, including ligament stress tests (refer to "Special Tests" section)
X. Diagnostic imaging as appropriate

TABLE 8-30. EXAMINATION OF THE KNEE JOINT COMPLEX

I. History
II. Observation and inspection
III. Lower quarter scan as appropriate
IV. Examination of movements. Active range of motion with passive overpressure of the following movements:
  a. Hip flexion, extension, abduction, adduction, internal rotation, external rotation
  b. Knee flexion, extension
  c. Ankle dorsiflexion, plantar flexion
  d. Internal rotation of the tibia on the femur, external rotation of the tibia on the femur
V. Resisted isometric movements:
  a. Hip flexion, extension, abduction, adduction, internal rotation, external rotation
  b. Knee flexion, extension
  c. Ankle dorsiflexion, plantar flexion
VI. Ligament stability tests:
  a. One plane medial instability
  b. One plane lateral instability
  c. One plane anterior and posterior instability
  d. Anteromedial and anterolateral rotary instability
  e. Posteromedial and posterolateral rotary instability
VII. Palpation
VIII. Neurological tests as appropriate (reflexes, sensory scan, peripheral nerve assessment)
IX. Joint mobility tests:
  a. Anterior and posterior glides of the tibia on the femur
  b. Medial and lateral translation of the tibia on the femur
  c. Patellar glides
  d. Anteroposterior glides of the proximal tibiofibular joint
X. Special tests (refer to "Special Tests" section) and diagnostic imaging as appropriate

TABLE 8-31. EXAMINATION OF THE LOWER LEG ANKLE AND FOOT

I. History
II. Observation and inspection
III. Lower quarter scan as appropriate
IV. Examination of movements. Active range of motion with passive overpressure of the following movements:
  a. Plantar flexion, dorsiflexion in weight bearing and non-weight bearing
  b. Supination, pronation in weight bearing and non-weight bearing
  c. Toe extension, flexion in weight bearing and non-weight bearing
V. Resisted isometric movements:
  a. Knee flexion, extension
  b. Plantar flexion, dorsiflexion
  c. Supination, pronation
  d. Toe extension, flexion
VI. Palpation
VII. Neurological tests as appropriate (reflexes, sensory scan, peripheral nerve assessment).
VIII. Joint mobility tests:
  a. Inversion and eversion at the subtalar joint
  b. Adduction and abduction at the midtarsal joints
  c. Anteroposterior glide at the talocrural joint
  d. Tarsal bone mobility
IX. Special tests (refer to "Special Tests" section)
X. Diagnostic imaging as appropriate

Active range of motion testing may be deferred if small and unguarded motions provoke intense pain as this may indicate a high degree of joint irritability. The normal active range of motion for each of the joints is depicted in Table 8-33.

Dynamic and static testing in the cardinal planes follows if the single motions do not provoke symptoms. Dynamic testing involves repeated movements in specific directions. Repeated movements can give the clinician some valuable insight into the patient's condition:[96]

- Internal derangements tend to worsen with repeated motions.
- The symptoms of a postural dysfunction remain unchanged with repeated motions

Study Pearl

Full and pain-free active range of motion suggests normalcy for that movement, although it is important to remember that normal *range* of motion is not synonymous with normal motion.[95] Normal motion implies that the control of motion must also be present.

TABLE 8-32. EXAMINATION OF THE TEMPOROMANDIBULAR JOINT

I. History
II. Observation and inspection
III. Upper quarter scan as appropriate
IV. Examination of movements. Active range of motion with passive overpressure of the following movements:
  a. Cervical flexion, extension, side bending (right and left), rotation (right and left)
  b. Mouth opening, closing (occlusion), protrusion, retrusion, lateral deviation (left and right)
V. Resisted isometric movements:
  a. Mouth opening, closing (occlusion), lateral deviation
VI. Palpation.
VII. Neurological tests as appropriate (reflexes, sensory scan, cranial nerve assessment)
VIII. Joint mobility tests:
  a. Distraction and anterior glide of the mandible
  b. Lateral glide of the mandible
  c. Medial glide of the mandible
  d. Posterior glide of the mandible
IX. Special tests (refer to "Special Tests" section)
X. Diagnostic imaging as appropriate

TABLE 8-33. ACTIVE RANGES OF THE MAJOR JOINTS

JOINT	ACTION	DEGREES OF MOTION
Shoulder	Flexion	0-180
	Extension	0-40
	Abduction	0-180
	Internal rotation	0-80
	External rotation	0-90
Elbow	Flexion	0-150
Forearm	Pronation	0-80
	Supination	0-80
Wrist	Flexion	0-60
	Extension	0-60
	Radial deviation	0-20
	Ulnar deviation	0-30
Hip	Flexion	0-100
	Extension	0-30
	Abduction	0-40
	Adduction	0-20
	Internal rotation	0-40
	External rotation	0-50
Knee	Flexion	0-150
Ankle	Plantar flexion	0-40
	Dorsiflexion	0-20
Foot	Inversion	0-30
	Eversion	0-20

- ▶ Pain from a dysfunction syndrome is increased with tissue loading, but ceases at rest.
- ▶ Repeated motions can indicate the irritability of the condition.
- ▶ Repeated motions can indicate to the clinician the direction of motion to be used as part of the intervention. If pain increases during repeated motion in a particular direction, exercising in that direction is not indicated. If pain only worsens in part of the range, repeated motion exercises can be used for that part of the range that is pain-free, or which does not worsen the symptoms.
- ▶ Pain that is increased after the repeated motions may indicate a re-triggering of the inflammatory response, and repeated motions in the opposite direction should be explored.

Sustained static positions may be used to help detect postural syndromes.[97]

Combined motion testing may be used when the symptoms are not reproduced with the cardinal plane motion tests. Combined motions, as their name suggests, use single plane motions with other motions superimposed. For example at the elbow, the single plane motion of elbow flexion is tested together with forearm supination and then forearm pronation. As with the single plane tests, the combined motions are tested statically and then dynamically in an effort to reproduce the patient's symptoms.

The active range of motion can be found to be either abnormal or normal. Abnormal motion is typically described as being reduced. It must be remembered though, that abnormal motion may also be excessive. Excessive motion is often missed and is erroneously classified as normal motion. To help determine whether the motion is normal or excessive, passive range of motion, in the form of passive overpressure, and the end feel are assessed.

Passive Range of Motion. Passive range of motion testing gives the clinician information about the integrity of the contractile and inert tissues, and the end-feel. It is important to perform gentle passive range of motion, and overpressure, at the end of the active range in order to fully test the motion. The passive overpressure should be applied carefully in the presence of pain. The barrier to active motion should occur earlier in the range than the barrier to passive motion. Pain that occurs at the end range of active and passive movement is suggestive of hypermobility or instability, a capsular contraction, or scar tissue that has not been adequately remodeled.[96]

Cyriax[33] introduced the concept of the end-feel, which is the quality of resistance at end range. The end-feel can indicate to the clinician the cause of the motion restriction (Tables 5-21 and 5-22). For example, a hard, capsular end-feel indicates a pericapsular hypomobility, while a jammed or pathomechanical end-feel indicates a pathomechanical hypomobility. A normal end-feel would indicate normal range, whereas an abnormal end-feel would suggest abnormal range, either hypomobile or hypermobile. An association between an increase in pain and abnormal-pathological end-feels compared to normal end-feels has been demonstrated.[98]

The planned intervention, and its intensity, is based on the type of tissue resistance to movement demonstrated by the end-feel, and the acuteness of the condition (Table 18-20).[33]

Study Pearl

- If active and passive motions are limited/painful in the same direction, the injured tissue is likely inert in nature.
- If active and passive motions are limited/painful in the opposite direction, the injured tissue is likely contractile in nature.

The exception to this generalization occurs with tenosynovitis.

Manual Muscle Testing. An important component of an examination is the assessment of muscle strength. The assessment of strength provides the clinician with information about the ability of the musculotendinous units to act across a bone-joint lever-arm system to actively generate motion, or passively resist movement against gravity and variable resistance.[99] Manual muscle testing is traditionally used by the clinician to assess the strength of a muscle or muscle group. The *Guide to Physical Therapist Practice*[100] lists both manual muscle testing (MMT) and dynamometry as appropriate measures of muscle strength.

- Manual muscle testing is a procedure for the evaluation of the function and strength of individual muscles and muscle groups based on the effective performance of a movement in relation to the forces of gravity and manual resistance.[101]
- Dynamometry is a method of strength testing using sophisticated strength measuring devices (eg, hand-grip, hand-held, fixed, and isokinetic dynamometry).

Valuable information can be gleaned from these tests, including:

- The amount of force the muscle is capable of producing and whether the amount of force produced varies with the joint angle.
- Whether any pain or weakness is produced with the contraction (Table 8-34).
- The endurance of the muscle, and how much substitution occurs during the test.

TABLE 8-34. FINDINGS FROM MUSCLE TESTING

FINDING	POSSIBLE EXPLANATION
Strong and painless contraction	Normal finding
Strong and painful contraction	Grade I contractile lesion
Weak and painless contraction	-Palsy (nerve compression, neuropathy) -Complete rupture of the muscle-tendon unit/avulsion
Weak and painful contraction	Serious pathology such as a significant muscle tear, fracture, tumor, etc

Study Pearl

Make test: an evaluation procedure where the patient is asked to apply a force against the clinician or dynamometer.
Break test: an evaluation procedure where the patient is asked to hold a contraction against pressure that is applied in the opposite direction to the contraction.

Manual muscle testing is an ordinal level of measurement[102] and has been found to have both interrater and intrarater reliability, especially when the scale is expanded to include plus or minus a half or a full grade.[103-105]

Examples of common grading scales used with manual muscle testing are depicted in Table 8-35. Choosing a particular grading system is based on the skill level of the clinician while ensuring consistency for each patient, so that coworkers who may be reexamining the patient are using the same testing methods.

To be a valid test, strength testing must elicit a maximum contraction of the muscle being tested. Five strategies ensure this:

1. Placing the joint which the muscle to be tested crosses in, or close to, its open packed position.
2. Placing the muscle to be tested in a shortened position. This puts the muscle in an ineffective physiological position, which has the effect of increasing motor neuron activity.
3. Having the patient perform an eccentric muscle contraction by using the command: "Don't let me move you." As the tension at each cross-bridge and the number of active cross-bridges is greater during an eccentric contraction, the maximum eccentric muscle tension developed is greater with an eccentric contraction than a concentric one.
4. Breaking the contraction: It is important to break the patient's muscle contraction in order to ensure that the patient is making a maximal effort and that the full power of the muscle is being tested.
5. Holding the contraction for at least 5 seconds: Weakness due to nerve palsy has a distinct fatigability. If a muscle appears to be weaker than normal, further investigation is required.

Study Pearl

In addition to examining the integrity of the contractile and inert structures, strength testing may be used to examine the integrity of the myotomes. A myotome is defined as a muscle or group of muscles served by a single nerve root. *Key muscle* is a better, more accurate term, as the muscles tested are the most representative of the supply from a particular segment.

The test is repeated three times. Muscle weakness, resulting from disuse will be consistently weak and should therefore not get weaker with several repeated contractions.

Another muscle that shares the same innervation (spinal nerve or peripheral nerve) is tested. Knowledge of both spinal nerve and peripheral nerve innervation will aid the clinician in determining which muscle to select.

Substitutions by other muscle groups during testing indicates the presence of weakness. It does not, however, tell the clinician the cause of the weakness. Whenever possible, the same muscle is tested on the opposite side, using the same testing procedure, and a comparison is made.

TABLE 8-35. COMPARISON OF MMT GRADES[a]

MEDICAL RESEARCH COUNCIL[b]	DANIELS AND WORTHINGHAM[c]	KENDALL AND MCCREARY[d]	EXPLANATION
5	Normal (N)	100%	Holds test position against maximal resistance
4+	Good + (G+)		Holds test position against moderate to strong pressure
4	Good (G)	80%	Holds test position against moderate resistance
4–	Good– (G–)		Holds test position against slight to moderate pressure
3+	Fair + (F+)		Holds test position against slight resistance
3	Fair (F)	50%	Holds test position against gravity
3–	Fair– (F–)		Gradual release from test position
2+	Poor + (P+)		Moves through partial ROM against gravity OR Moves through complete ROM gravity eliminated and holds against pressure
2	Poor (P)	20%	Able to move through full ROM gravity eliminated
2–	Poor – (P–)		Moves through partial ROM gravity eliminated
1	Trace (T)	5%	No visible movement; palpable or observable tendon prominence/flicker contraction
0	0	0%	No palpable or observable muscle contraction
The grades of 0, 1, and 2 are tested in the gravity-minimized position (contraction is perpendicular to the gravitational force). All other grades are tested in the anti-gravity position.	The more functional of the three grading systems because it tests a motion that utilizes all of the agonists and synergists involved in the motion.[1]	Designed to test a specific muscle rather than the motion, and requires both selective recruitment of a muscle by the patient and a sound knowledge of anatomy and kinesiology on the part of the clinician to determine the correct alignment of the muscle fibers.[1]	

[a]Data from Palmer ML, Epler M: Principles of examination techniques. In: Palmer ML, Epler M, eds. *Clinical Assessment Procedures in Physical Therapy*. Philadelphia, PA: Lippincott. 1990:8-36.
[b]Data from Frese E, Brown M, Norton B: Clinical reliability of manual muscle testing: middle trapezius and gluteus medius muscles. *Phys Ther.* 1987;67:1072-1076.
[c]Data from Daniels K, Worthingham C: *Muscle Testing Techniques of Manual Examination, 5th ed.* Philadelphia, PA: WB Saunders. 1986.
[d]Data from Kendall FP, McCreary EK, Provance PG: *Muscles: Testing and Function*. Baltimore: Williams & Wilkins. 1993.

Interpretation of Findings. Cyriax reasoned that if you isolate, and then apply tension to a structure, you could make a conclusion as to the integrity of that structure.[33] According to Cyriax, pain with a contraction generally indicates an injury to the muscle or a capsular structure (see Chapter 5).[33] This can be confirmed by combining the findings from the isometric test with the findings of the passive motion and the joint distraction and compression.

Cyriax also introduced the concept of tissue reactivity. Tissue reactivity is the manner in which different stresses and movements can alter the clinical signs and symptoms. This knowledge can be used to gauge any subtle changes to the patient's condition.[106]

Pain that occurs consistently with resistance, at whatever the length of the muscle, may indicate a tear of the muscle belly. Pain with muscle testing may indicate a muscle injury, a joint injury, or a combination of both.

Pain that does not occur during the test, but occurs upon the release of the contraction, is thought to have an articular source, produced by the joint glide that occurs following the release of tension.

The degree of significance with the findings in resisted testing depends on the position of the muscle, and the force applied. For example, pain reproduced with a minimal contraction in the rest position for the muscle is more strongly suggestive of a contractile lesion than pain reproduced with a maximal contraction in the lengthened position for the muscle.

Accessory Joint Motion. A variety of different measurement scales have been proposed for judging the amount of accessory joint motion present between two joint surfaces, most of which are based on a comparison with a comparable contralateral joint using manually applied forces in a logical and precise manner.[107] Using these techniques to assess the joint glide (arthrokinematic—see Chapter 5), joint motion is described as hypomobile (restricted), normal (unrestricted but not excessive), or hypermobile (excessive). The joint glides are tested in the loose (open) pack position of a peripheral joint (see Chapter 5) and at the end of available range in the spinal joints to avoid soft tissue tension affecting the results. The information gathered from these tests will help determine the integrity of the inert structures:

- The joint glide is unrestricted. An unrestricted joint glide indicates two differing conclusions:
  - The integrity of both the joint surface and the periarticular tissue is good. If this is the case, the patient's loss of motion must be due to a contractile tissue. With this scenario, the intervention should emphasize soft tissue mobilization techniques designed to change the length of a contractile tissue.
  - The joint glide is both unrestricted and excessive. Stress tests are then used to assess the integrity of the inert tissues, particularly the ligaments, and to determine whether instability exists at the joint. Instability at a joint may occur if the joint has undergone significant degenerative changes or trauma. The intervention for excessive motion that is impeding function focuses on stabilizing techniques designed to give secondary support to the joint through muscle action.
- The joint glide is restricted. If the joint glide is restricted, the joint surface and periarticular tissues are implicated as the cause for the patient's loss of motion, although, as mentioned above, the contractile tissues cannot definitively be ruled out. The intervention for this type of finding initially involves a specific joint mobilization to restore the glide.

Once the joint glide is restored following these mobilizations, the osteokinematic motion can be assessed again. If it is still reduced, the surrounding tissues have likely adaptively shortened. Distraction and compression can be used to help differentiate the cause of the restriction.

- Distraction: Traction is a force imparted passively by the clinician that results in a distraction of the joint surfaces.
  - If the distraction is limited, a contracture of connective tissue should be suspected.
  - If the distraction increases the symptoms, it may indicate a tear of connective tissue, and may be associated with increased range.
  - If the distraction eases the symptoms, it may indicate an involvement of the joint surface.
- Compression: Compression is the opposite force to distraction and involves an approximation of joint surfaces.
  - If the compression increases the symptoms, a loose body or internal derangement of the joint may be present.
  - If the compression decreases the symptoms, it may implicate the joint capsule.

NEUROLOGICAL TESTING

The evaluation of the transmission capability of the nervous system is performed to detect the presence of either upper motor neuron (UMN) lesion or lower motor neuron (LMN) lesion. In addition, the neurological examination (see Chapter 9) can often determine the exact site of the lesion.

Special Tests of the Upper Extremity. Special tests are merely confirmatory tests and should not be used alone to form a diagnosis. Selection for their use is at the discretion of the clinician and is based on a complete patient history. The results from these tests are used in conjunction with the other clinical findings and should not be used alone to form a diagnosis. To assure accuracy with these tests, both sides should be tested for comparison.

Special Tests of the Shoulder Complex. The special tests for the shoulder are divided into diagnostic categories.

Subacromial Impingement Tests. Patients with subacromial impingement syndrome usually perceive pain when a compressing force is applied on the greater tuberosity and rotator cuff region.[108] Pain may also be elicited with shoulder abduction in internal or external rotation.[108]

Neer impingement test. While scapular rotation is prevented with one hand of the clinician, the arm of the patient is passively forced into elevation at an angle between flexion and abduction, by the clinician's other hand. Overpressure (in neutral, internal rotation, external rotation) is applied. Post and Cohen[109] found the Neer test to have a sensitivity of 93% in the confirmation of subacromial impingement.

Hawkins-Kennedy impingement test. The arm of the patient is passively flexed up to 90 degrees in the plane of the scapula. The elbow is stabilized and the arm is forced into internal rotation.[110] Ure and colleagues[111] found that the sensitivity of the Hawkins-Kennedy test to be 62% for diagnosing subacromial impingement.

Yocum test. The Yocum test is performed by having the patient lift the elbow to shoulder height while resting the hand on the opposite shoulder. A study[112] comparing the Neer, Hawkins-Kennedy, and Yocum tests found all three to demonstrate a high sensitivity for diagnosing subacromial impingement.

Patte test ("hornblower's sign").[113,114] The patient's arm is supported in 90 degrees of abduction in the scapular plane, with the elbow flexed to 90 degrees. The patient is then asked to rotate the forearm externally against the resistance of the clinician's hand. If the patient is unable to externally rotate the shoulder in this position, the "hornblower's sign" is said to be present. The Patte test has demonstrated high sensitivity (92%), but poor specificity (30%) for the detection of impingment.

Lock test.[115,116] The Lock test is used to help differentiate the cause of symptoms when the patient complains of localized catching shoulder pain and pain or restricted movement when attempting to place the hand behind the back.

The patient is positioned in supine with the shoulder at the edge of the table, positioned in 45 degrees abduction, 30 degrees internal rotation, and the elbow positioned 10 degrees posterior to the frontal plane. The clinician stabilizes the scapula with one hand and grasps the patient's right elbow with the other hand. The clinician slowly glides the patient's elbow anteriorly. The end position for the test is achieved when the patient's right shoulder is in maximal humeral abduction with overpressure, and neither the patient nor clinician can externally rotate the arm while at this end range. Positive findings for this test include reproduction of the patient's symptoms and a decrease in range of motion compared to the uninvolved shoulder.

Dropping sign.[117] The "dropping sign" is performed with the patient sitting or standing. The clinician places the patient's elbow in 90 degrees of flexion with the arm by the side. The shoulder is externally rotated to 45 degrees and the patient is then asked to externally rotate the shoulder against resistance. If the patient is unable to maintain the externally rotated position, the arm drops back to the neutral position of shoulder rotation. This is called the "dropping sign."

Rotator Cuff Rupture Tests

Drop arm test. The clinician passively raises the patient's arm to an overhead position. The patient is asked to lower their arm with their palm down. If at any point in the descent, the patient's arm drops, this is indicative of a full thickness tear.

Biceps and Superior Labral Tears

Clunk test. The clunk test is the traditional test for diagnosing labral tears. The patient is positioned in supine. One hand of the clinician is placed on the posterior aspect of the shoulder over the humeral head, while the other hand grasps the humerus above the elbow. The clinician fully abducts the arm over the patient's head. Using the hand placed posterior to the humeral head, the clinician pushes anteriorly while the other hand externally rotates the humerus. A clunk-like sensation may be felt if a free labral fragment is caught in the joint. [118]

Crank test. The "crank" test[119] is performed with the patient positioned in supine. Their arm is elevated to 160 degrees in the scapular plane of the body and is in maximal internal or external rotation. The clinician then applies an axial load along the humerus. A positive test is indicated by the reproduction of a painful click in the shoulder during the maneuver.

Speed's test. The patient's arm is positioned in shoulder flexion, full external rotation, full elbow extension, and full forearm supination. Manual resistance is applied by the clinician. The test is positive if localized pain at the bicipital groove is reproduced.

The Speed's test suggests a superior labral tear when resisted forward flexion of the shoulder causes bicipital groove pain. The Speed's test is also used to detect bicipital tendonitis (see Yergason's test).

Yergason's test.[120] The patient's arm is positioned in 90 degrees of elbow flexion. The patient is asked to supinate their forearm, and externally rotate their arm against the manual resistance of the clinician. The Speed's and Yergason's tests more probably discriminate bicipital tendon disorders.[108] However, irritation and edema may occur in the long head of biceps, in any stage of subacromial impingement syndrome.

O'Brien's test. The O'Brien's test is performed with the patient's arm adducted 10 degrees in the front of the chest with the shoulder flexed to 90 degrees and fully internally rotated. In this position, the arm is flexed upward against the clinician's downward-directed force. The test is then repeated in the same manner except that the arm is positioned in maximum external rotation. Pain with this maneuver is typical in patients with superior labral tears.

Anterior slide test. The "anterior slide test"[121] is another clinical test designed to stress the superior labrum.[118] The patient stands with hands on the hips such that the thumbs are positioned posteriorly. One of the clinician's hands is placed over the patient's shoulder and the other hand behind the elbow. A force is then applied anteriorly and superiorly, and the patient is asked to push back against the force. The test is considered positive if pain is localized to the anterior-superior aspect of the shoulder, if there is a pop or a click in the anterior-superior region, or if the maneuver reproduces the symptoms.

The remaining tests are reserved for when the clinician needs to differentiate the structure causing the symptoms, when the provocation of symptoms during the examination has been minimal, or to rule out the possibility of instability.

Study Pearl

Two acronyms are commonly used to describe shoulder instability, TUBS (Traumatic, Unidirectional instability with Bankart lesion requiring Surgery) and AMBRII (Atraumatic onset of Multidirectional instability that is accompanied by Bilateral laxity or hypermobility. Rehabilitation is the primary course of intervention to restore glenohumeral stability. However, if an operation is necessary, a procedure such as a capsulorraphy is performed to tighten the Inferior capsule and the rotator Interval).[122]

Acromioclavicular Tests

Acromioclavicular shear test. The clinician cups their hands together and applies a compressive force with the hands over the AC joint, creating a posterior to anterior glide (shear) of the AC joint.

Stability Testing. It is important to remember that there is no correlation between the amount of joint laxity/mobility and joint instability at the shoulder. Joint stability is more likely a function of connective tissue support and an intact neuromuscular system.

The reproduction of symptoms is important because laxity alone does not indicate instability. Pain and muscle spasm can make the examination challenging.

Glenohumeral load and shift test. The patient is seated on the table with their arm supported in their lap. The clinician sits beside the patient with the inside of the hand over the patient's shoulder and their forearm stabilizing the scapula to the thorax. The clinician places their thumb across the posterior GH joint line and humeral head, and the web space across the patient's acromion. The clinician's index finger is placed across the anterior GH joint line and humeral head, and the long finger over the coracoid process. The clinician then applies a "load and shift" of the humeral head across the stabilized scapula in an anterior-medial direction to assess anterior stability, and in a posterior-lateral direction to assess posterior instability. The normal motion anteriorly is half of the distance of the humeral head.

Apprehension Test. The patient is positioned in supine with the arm in 90 degrees of abduction and full external rotation. The clinician holds the patient's wrist with one hand, while the other hand stabilizes the patient's elbow. The clinician applies overpressure into external rotation. Patient apprehension from this maneuver, rather than pain, is considered a positive test for anterior instability. Pain with this maneuver, but without apprehension, may indicate pathology other than instability, such as posterior impingement of the rotator cuff.

Sulcus Sign for Inferior Instability.[123] The sulcus sign is used to detect inferior instability due to a laxity of the superior glenohumeral and coracohumeral ligaments. The patient's arm is positioned in 20 to 50 degrees of abduction and neutral rotation. A positive test results in the presence of a sulcus sign (a depression greater than a finger width between the lateral acromion and the head of the humerus) when longitudinal traction is applied to the dependent arm in more than one position.

The sulcus sign can be graded by measuring the distance from the inferior margin of the acromion to the humeral head. A distance of less than 1 cm is graded as 1+ sulcus, 1 to 2 cm as a 2+ sulcus, and greater than 2 cm as a grade 3+ sulcus.

Jobe subluxation/relocation test. This test is similar to the apprehension test, except that manual pressure is applied anteriorly by the clinician in an attempt to provoke a subluxation, before using manual pressure in the opposite direction to relocate the subluxation. The patient is positioned in supine with their arm in 90 degrees of abduction and full external rotation. The clinician grasps the patient's forearm with one hand to maintain the testing position, and grasps the humeral head with the other hand. The clinician gently applies an anterior push to the posterior aspect of the subluxed humeral head. Pain and apprehension from the patient indicate a positive test for a superior labral tear. After pushing the humeral head anteriorly and demonstrating pain and apprehension, the clinician should then push the humeral head posteriorly while maintaining the shoulder in the same position (relocation part of the test). Reduction of pain and apprehension further substantiates the clinical finding of anterior instability and may indicate a positive test.

Rockwood test for anterior instability.[124] The patient is positioned in sitting with the clinician standing behind. With the arm by the patient's side, the clinician passively externally rotates the shoulder. The patient then abducts the arm to approximately 45 degrees and the test is repeated. The same maneuver is again repeated with the arm abducted to 90 degrees and then 120 degrees, in order to assess the different stabilizing structures. A positive test is indicated when apprehension is noted in the latter three positions (45, 90, and 120 degrees).

Anterior release test. The anterior release test is performed with the patient in supine and their shoulder positioned in 90 degrees of abduction and maximally externally rotated while a posteriorly directed force is applied to the proximal humerus. A positive test produces an increase or reproduction in the patient's symptoms upon release of the posteriorly directed force on the humerus.

Special Tests of the Elbow Complex

Tennis Elbow. A number of tests exist for tennis elbow (lateral epicondylitis). Two are described here:

Cozen's test. The clinician stabilizes the patient's elbow with one hand and the patient is asked to pronate the forearm, extend and radially deviate the wrist against the manual resistance of the clinician. A reproduction of pain in the area of the lateral epicondyle indicates a positive test.

Mill's test. The clinician palpates the patient's lateral epicondyle with one hand, while pronating the patient's forearm, fully flexing the wrist, and extending the elbow. A reproduction of pain in the area of the lateral epicondyle indicates a positive test.

Golfer's Elbow (Medial epicondylitis). The clinician palpates the medial epicondyle with one hand, while supinating the forearm, and extending the wrist and elbow with the other hand. A reproduction of pain in the area of the medial epicondyle indicates a positive test.

Elbow Flexion Test for Cubital Tunnel Syndrome. The patient is positioned in sitting. The patient is asked to depress both shoulders, flex both elbows maximally, supinate the forearms, and extend the wrists. This position is maintained for 3 to 5 minutes. Tingling or paresthesia in the ulnar distribution of the forearm and hand indicates a positive test.

Pressure Provocative Test for Cubital Tunnel Syndrome. Manual pressure is applied by the clinician, proximal to the cubital tunnel, with the elbow held in 20 degrees of flexion and the forearm in supination. Tingling or paresthesia in the ulnar distribution of the forearm and hand indicates a positive test.

Tinel's Sign (at the elbow). The clinician locates the groove between the olecranon process and the medial epicondyle through which the ulnar nerve passes. This groove is tapped by the index finger of the clinician. A positive sign is indicated by a tingling sensation in the ulnar distribution of the forearm and hand distal to the tapping point.

Special Tests of the Wrist and Hand. A number of tests can be used to document the neurovascular status of the wrist and hand.

Neurological and Autonomic Tests

Tinel tign at the carpal tunnel. The clinician taps over the carpal tunnel at wrist. Positive test causes tingling or paresthesia into thumb, index, middle and lateral half of ring finger (median nerve distribution), indicating carpal tunnel syndrome.

Phalen's (wrist flexion) test. The clinician maximally flexes patient's wrists and holds the position for 1 minute. A positive test causes tingling or paresthesia into the thumb, index, middle and lateral half of ring finger (median nerve distribution), indicating carpal tunnel syndrome.

Reverse Phalen's (prayer test). The clinician extends the patient's wrist while asking the patient to grip the clincian's hand. The clincian then applies direct pressure over the carpal tunnel for 1 minute. A positive test produces the same symptoms as seen in the Phalen's test and indicates median nerve pathology.

Carpal compression test. The clinician uses both thumbs to apply direct pressure on the carpal tunnel and the underlying median nerve for 30 seconds. If positive, an onset of median nerve symptoms should occur within 15 to 30 seconds

Froment's sign. The patient attempts to grasp a piece of paper between the thumb and index finger. When the clinician attempts to pull away the paper, the terminal phalanx of thumb flexes because of paralysis of the adductor pollicis muscle, indicating a positive test. If, at same time, the MCP of the thumb hyperextends, the hyperextension is noted as a positive Jeanne's sign. If both tests are positive it indicates ulnar nerve palsy.

Egawa's sign. The patient flexes the middle digit and then alternately deviates the wrist radially and ulnarly. If the patient is unable to do this, the interossei are affected. A positive sign is indicative of ulnar nerve palsy.

Wrinkle (Shrivel) test. The patient's finger is placed in warm water for 5 to 20 minutes. The finger is then removed and observed as to whether the skin over the pulp is wrinkled. Normally, it should wrinkle, but in the presence of denervation it will not. This test is only valid in the first few months after injury.

Ninhydrin sweat test. The patient's hand is cleaned thoroughly and wiped with alcohol. The patient is asked to wait 5 to 30 minutes keeping their fingertips from contacting any surface to allow time for the sweating process to ensue. After waiting, the fingertips are pressed with moderate pressure against good quality bond paper that has not been touched. The fingertips are held in place for 15 seconds and traced with a pencil. The paper is then sprayed with a spray reagent and allowed to dry (24 hours). Sweat areas stain purple. If the change in color (from white to purple) does not occur, it is considered positive for a nerve lesion.

Weber's (Moberg's) two-point discrimination test. The clinician uses a paper clip, two-point discriminator, or calipers to simultaneously apply pressure on two adjacent points in a longitudinal direction or perpendicular to the long axis of the finger. The clinician moves proximal to distal in an attempt to find the minimal distance at which patient can distinguish between the two stimuli. The patient must concentrate and not be allowed to see the area and the hand should be immobile on a hard surface. Starting with a distance that can be easily distinguished, the clinician ensures that the two points are touched simultaneously. There should be no blanching of the skin when points are applied. About 7 to 8 trials are attempted before the distance is narrowed. Normal discrimination is less than 6 mm. Fair = 6 to 10 mm. Poor = 11 to 15 mm. Protective = 1 point perceived. Winding a watch = 6 mm. Sewing = 6 to 8 mm. Handling precision tools = 12 mm. Gross tool handling > 15mm.

"O" test. The patient attempts to make an "O" with thumb and index finger. If unable to perform this, an anterior interosseus nerve syndrome is indicated. Inability to make "O" is caused by paralysis of flexor pollicis longus, pronator quadratus, and flexor digitorum profundus to the index finger.

Vascular Tests

Allen test. The patient is asked to open and close the fist quickly several times and then to squeeze tightly so that venous return is forced out. The clinician places a thumb over the radial artery and the index and middle finger over the ulnar artery to occlude them. The patient is then asked to open the hand. The palm should appear pale. The clinician releases the pressure from one artery and observes for filling on the respective side. The hand should flush immediately. If it flushes slowly, the artery is partially or completely occluded.

Ligament, Capsule, and Joint Instability Tests. The ligamentous instability tests for the fingers are described below:

MP collateral ligament test. The patient is positioned so that the pronated forearm and hand are supported in a relaxed position on the table surface. The clinician grasps the distal aspect of the metacarpals to provide stabilization. The thumb and index finger of the other hand is used to grip the medial and lateral aspect of the proximal phalanx and to maintain the joint in 30 degrees of flexion. To enhance examination and visualization, the patient is asked to slightly flex the uninvolved fingers further into flexion than the involved finger. The clinician radially distracts the proximal phalanx, which stresses the ulnar collateral ligament of the MCP joint, and asseses the end feel. Normally, there should be a slight opening with a firm end feel. The absence of a firm end feel, accompanied by associated sensations of pain or instability, indicate an ulnar collateral ligament sprain. This same test may then be reversed by distracting the proximal phalanx ulnarly to stress the radial collateral ligament. As before, the joint is maintained in 30 degrees of flexion while stabilizing the metacarpals with one hand. The clinician then ulnarly distracts the proximal phalanx which stresses the radial collateral ligament of the MCP joint. While applying the stress, the clinician visualizes and feels for an abnormal opening of the joint as compared to the uninvolved contralateral joint. Again, there should be a slight opening with a firm end feel. A sprain of the radial collateral ligament is indicated by the absence of a firm end feel accompanied by associated sensations of pain or instability. The tests are repeated on the other hand and comparisons are made.

PIP collateral ligament test. The patient is positioned so that the pronated forearm and hand are supported in a relaxed position on the table. The clinician grasps the medial and lateral aspect of the proximal phalanx with the thumb and index finger of one hand. Using the thumb and index finger of the other hand the clinician grips the medial and lateral aspect of the intermediate phalanx. While stabilizing the proximal phalanx with one hand, and maintaining the joint in 15 to 20 degrees of flexion, the clinician uses the other hand to radially distract the intermediate phalanx, which stresses the ulnar collateral ligament of the proximal interphalangeal joint, and assesses the end feel. Normally, there should be a slight opening with a firm end feel. The absence of a firm end feel accompanied by associated sensations of pain or instability indicates a sprain of the ulnar collateral ligament. This same test may then be reversed by distracting the intermediate phalanx ulnarly to stress the radial collateral ligament. Again, the joint is maintained in 15 to 20 degrees of flexion while stabilizing the proximal phalanx with one hand. Using the other hand, the clinician ulnarly distracts the intermediate phalanx, which stresses the radial collateral ligament of the PIP joint, and assesses the end feel. Again, there should be a slight opening with a firm end feel. The absence of a firm end feel accompanied by associated sensations of pain or instability indicates a radial collateral ligament sprain.

DIP collateral ligament test. The PIP tests may be repeated in similar fashions to assess the collateral stability of the DIP joints.

Test for tight retinacular ligaments (retinacular test). The PIP joint is held in full extension and the clinician moves the DIP joint into flexion. If the joint does not flex, the limitation is due to either contracture of the joint capsule or to retinacular tightness. To distinguish between these two, the clinician flexes the PIP joint slightly to relax the retinaculum. If the DIP joint then flexes, the retinacular ligaments are tight. If the joint does not flex, the DIP joint capsule is probably contracted.

Lunatotriquetral ballotement (Reagan's) test. The clinician grasps the triquetrum between the thumb and second finger of one hand and the lunate with the thumb and second finger of the other hand. The clinician then moves the lunate up and down (anteriorly and posteriorly), noting any laxity, crepitus, or pain, which indicates a positive test for lunatotriquetral instability.

Murphy's sign. The patient is asked to make a fist. If the head of the third metacarpal is level with the second and forth metacarpals, this is a positive sign, indicating a lunate dislocation.

Watson (Scaphoid shift) test. The patient sits with the elbow resting on their lap and with the forearm pronated. With one hand, the clinician takes the patient's wrist into full ulnar deviation and slight extension. The clinician presses the thumb of other hand against the distal pole of scaphoid to prevent it from moving toward the palm. Using the first hand, the clinician radially deviates and slightly flexes the patient's hand. If the scaphoid (and lunate) are unstable, the dorsal pole of the scaphoid subluxes over the dorsal rim of the radius and patient complains of pain, indicating a positive test for scapholunate dissociation.

Scaphoid stress test. The patient sits and the clinician holds the patient's wrist with one hand, so that the thumb applies pressure over the distal pole of scaphoid. The patient then attempts to radially deviate the wrist. Normally, the patient should be unable to deviate the wrist. If excessive laxity is present, the scaphoid is forced dorsally out of scaphoid fossa of radius with a resulting clunk and pain, indicating a positive test for scaphoid instability. This is an active modification of the Watson test.

"*Piano Keys*" *test.* The patient sits with both arms in pronation. The clincian stabilizes the patient's arms with one hand so that the clinician's index finger can push down on the distal ulna. The clinician's other hand supports the patient's hand. The clinician then pushes down on the distal ulna as if it is a piano key and compares this motion with the asymptomatic side. A positive test is indicated by a difference in mobility and production of pain/tenderness, indicating distal radioulnar jont instability.

Axial load test. The patient sits while the clinician stabilizes the patient's wrist with one hand. With the other hand, the clinician carefully grasps the patient's thumb and applies axial compression. Pain and/or crepitation indicates a positive test for a fracture of a metacarpal or adjacent carpal bones, or joint arthrosis. It may also be done for the fingers.

Pivot shift test of the midcarpal joint. The patient is seated with their elbow flexed to 90 degrees and resting on a firm surface with the hand fully supinated. The clincian stabilizes the forearm with one hand and uses the other hand to take the patient's hand into full radial deviation with the wrist maintained in neutral. The clincian maintains the patient's hand position and takes it into full ulnar deviation. The test is positive if the capitate is felt to "shift" away from the lunate, indicating injury to the anterior capsule and interosseous ligaments.

Grind test. The clincian holds the patient's hand with one hand and grasps the patient's thumb below the MCP joint with other hand. The clincian then applies axial compression and rotation to the MCP joint. If pain is elicited, the test is positive, and indicates degenerative joint disease in the MCP or metacarpotrapezial joint.

Tests for Tendons and Muscles

Finkelstein's test. The Finkelstein's test is used to determine the presence of de Quervain's or Hoffman's disease, tenosynovitis in the abductor pollicis longus, and the extensor pollicis brevis tendons of the thumb. The patient sits with the forearm supported on the table in a neutral position. The hand should be free to hang over the table edge. The patient is instructed to make a fist with the thumb inside the fingers, and then to deviate the wrist to the ulnar side. This motion can be accentuated by using one hand to stabilize the distal forearm while placing the other hand over the fist's radial side to gently push the wrist into further ulnar deviation. This manuever will cause a stretching in these tendons which is painful if tenosynovitis is present. Additional positive findings may be accomplished by asking the patient to begin with the wrist in full ulnar deviation and then to actively abduct or radially flex the wrist against manual resistance.

Flexor digitorum profundus.

Test for Jersey (Sweater) Finger Sign. The patient is asked to make a fist. Inability to flex or close distal phalanx indicates that the FDP is ruptured.

Flexor digitorum superficialis test. The patient is asked to flex the finger while holding the MCP in neutral. Inability to flex or close the middle phalanx indicates a rupture of the FDS.

Test for extensor hood rupture. The tested finger is flexed 90 degrees at the PIP joint over edge of table. The finger is held in position by the clincian and the middle phalanx is palpated while the patient carefully extends the PIP joint. A positive test, indicating a torn central extensor hood, is demonstrated by a lack of pressure from the middle phalanx while the distal phalanx is extending.

Bunnell–Littler (Finochietto–Bunnell) test. The clinician holds the MCP in slight extension while flexing the PIP. If the PIP cannot be flexed, tightness of the intrinsics or capsule should be suspected. The test is repeated in slight MCP flexion. If there is tightness of the intrinsics, the PIP will now be able to flex fully, but will not fully flex if the capsule is tight.

Linburg's sign. The patient flexes the thumb maximally onto the hypothenar eminence and actively extends the index finger as far as possible. If limited index finger extension and pain are noted, the test is positive for tendinitis at the interconnection between the FPL and flexor indicis (seen in 10%-15% of hands).

Mallet finger test. The clinician holds the patient's middle phalanx with the thumb and index finger. The patient is asked to extend the DIP joint. Inability to extend the distal phalanx indicates an extensor tendon rupture or avulsion of the distal phalanx.

Special Tests of the Lower Extremity

Special Tests of the Hip

Quadrant (Scour) test. The quadrant or scour test is a dynamic test of the inner quadrant and outer quadrant of the hip joint surface.

The patient is positioned in supine, close to the edge of the bed, with their hip flexed and foot resting on the bed. The clinician interlocks the fingers of both hands and places them over the top of the patient's knee. The patient's hip is then placed in 90 degrees of flexion with the knee allowed to flex comfortably. From this point, the clinician adducts the hip to the point when the patient's pelvis is felt to begin to lift on the bed to assess the inner quadrant. The position of flexion and adduction of the hip has the potential to compress or stress a number of structures including:

- The articular surfaces of the hip joint
- The insertion of the tensor fascia latae and the sartorius
- The iliopsoas muscle
- The iliopsoas bursa and neurovascular bundle
- The insertion of the pectineus
- The insertion of the adductor longus
- The femoral neck

Care must be taken when interpreting the results from this test. At the end range of flexion and adduction, a compression force is applied at the knee along the longitudinal axis of the femur. From this point, the clinician moves the hip into a position of flexion and abduction to examine the outer quadrant. Throughout the entire movement, the femur is held midway between internal and external rotation, and the movement at the hip joint should follow the smooth arc of a circle. An abnormal finding is resistance felt anywhere during the arc. The resistance may be caused by capsular tightness, an adhesion, a myofascial restriction, or a loss of joint congruity.

FABER (Flexion, abduction, external rotation) or Patrick's test. The FABER test is a screening test for hip, lumbar, or sacroiliac joint dysfunction, or an iliopsoas spasm.

The patient is positioned in supine. The clinician places the foot of the test leg on top of the knee of the opposite leg (placing the sole of the test leg foot against the medial aspect of the opposite thigh may be more comfortable for the patient with knee pathology). The clinician then slowly lowers the test leg into abduction, in the direction toward the examining table. A positive test results in pain and/or loss of motion as compared with the uninvolved side.

Having the patient demonstrate where the pain is with this test may assist with the interpretation of this test.

SI Provocation tests. A number of tests can be used to examine the sacroiliac joint. Unless the patient history or the physical examination highlights the presence of a sacroiliac dysfunction, the clinician relies on two simple stress tests to rule out sacroiliac pathology, the anterior gapping and posterior gapping tests.

In addition to the provocative tests, the passive motions of the hip can be examined with the innominate stabilized. The hip motions and their respective innominate motions, in parenthesis, are outlined in Table 8-17.

Craig's test. The Craig's test is used to assess femoral anteversion/retroversion. The patient is positioned in prone with the knee flexed to 90 degrees. The clinician rotates the hip through the full ranges of hip internal and external rotation while palpating the greater trochanter and determining the point in the range at which the greater trochanter is the most prominent laterally. If the angle is greater than 8 to 15 degrees in the direction of internal rotation when measured from the vertical and long axis of the tibia, the femur is considered to be in anteversion.

Flexion-Adduction test. This test is used as a screening test for early hip pathology. The patient is positioned in supine and the hip is passively flexed to 90 degrees and in neutral rotation. From this position, the clinician stabilizes the pelvis and the hip is passively adducted. The resultant end feel, restriction, discomfort, or pain is noted and compared with the normal side.

Trendelenburg's sign. The Trendelenburg's sign indicates weakness of the gluteus medius muscle during unilateral weight bearing. This position produces a strong contraction of the gluteus medius, which is powerfully assisted by the gluteus minimus and tensor fascia latae, in order to keep the pelvis horizontal. For example, when the body weight is supported by the right foot, the right hip abductors contract isometrically, and eccentrically, to prevent the left side of the pelvis from being pulled downward.

The clinician crouches or kneels behind the patient with their eyes level with the patient's pelvis, and ensures that the patient does not lean to one side during the testing. The patient is asked to stand on one limb for approximately 30 seconds and the clinician notes whether the pelvis remains level. If the hip remains level, the test is negative. A positive Trendelenburg sign is indicated when, during unilateral weight bearing, the pelvis drops toward the unsupported limb. A number of dysfunctions can produce the Trendelenburg sign. These include superior gluteal nerve palsy, a lumbar disc herniation, weakness of the gluteus medius, and advanced degeneration of the hip.

Pelvic drop test.[125] The patient is asked to place one foot on a 20 cm (8 in) stool or step and to stand up straight. The patient then lowers the non-weight bearing leg to the floor. On lowering the leg there should be no arm abduction, anterior or pelvic motion, or trunk flexion. Nor should there be any hip adduction or internal rotation of the weight-bearing hip. These compensations are indications of an unstable hip or weak external rotators.

Sign of the buttock. The patient is positioned in supine. The clinician performs a passive unilateral straight leg raise. If there is a unilateral restriction, the clinician flexes the knee and notes whether the hip flexion increases. If the restriction was due to the lumbar spine or hamstrings, hip flexion increases. If the hip flexion does not increase when the knee is flexed, it is a positive sign of the buttock test. If the sign of the buttock is encountered, the patient must be immediately returned to the physician for further investigation.

Muscle Length Tests

Thomas test and modified Thomas test. The original Thomas test was designed to test the flexibility of the iliopsoas complex, but has since been modified and expanded to assess a number of other soft tissue structures.

The original test involved positioning the patient in supine, with one knee held to the chest at the point when the lumbar spine begins to flex. The clinician assessed whether the thigh of the extended leg maintained full contact with the surface of the bed. If the thigh rose off the surface of the treatment table, the test was considered positive, indicating a decrease in flexibility in the rectus femoris or iliopsoas muscles or both.

A modified version to this test is commonly used. For the modified version, the patient is positioned in sitting at the end of the bed. From this position, the patient is asked to lie down, while bringing both knees against the chest. Once in this position, the patient is asked to perform a posterior pelvic tilt. While the contralateral hip is held in maximum hip flexion with the arms, the tested limb is lowered over the end of the bed, toward the floor. In this position, the thigh should be parallel with the bed, in neutral rotation, and neither abducted nor adducted, with the lower leg perpendicular to the thigh and in neutral rotation. Knee flexion of 100 to 110 degrees should be present with the thigh in full contact with the table.

If the thigh rises off the treatment table, a decrease in the flexibility of the iliopsoas muscle complex should be suspected. If the rectus femoris is adaptively shortened, the amount of knee extension should increase with the application of overpressure into hip extension. If the decrease in flexibility lies with the iliopsoas, attempts to correct the hip position should result in an increase in the external rotation of the thigh.

The application of overpressure into knee flexion can also be used. If the knee flexion produces an increase in hip flexion (the thigh rises higher off the bed), the rectus femoris is implicated, whereas if the overpressure produces no change in the degree of hip flexion, the iliopsoas is implicated.

This test can also be used to assess the flexibility of the tensor fascia latae, if the hip of the tested leg is maximally adducted while monitoring the ipsilateral ASIS for motion. Hip adduction of 20 degrees should be available.

Two things must be remembered when interpreting the results of this test.

1. The criteria are arbitrary and have been shown to vary between genders, limb dominance, and depend on the types and the levels of activity undertaken by the individual.

2. The apparent tightness might simply be normal tissue tension producing a deviation of the leg due to an increased flexibility of the antagonists.

As always, the cause of the asymmetry must be found (or at least looked for) and addressed.

Ely's test. This is a test to assess the flexibility of the rectus femoris. The patient is positioned in prone lying and the knee is flexed. If the rectus is tight, the pelvis is observed to anteriorly rotate early in the range of knee flexion, and the hip flexes.

Ober's test. The Ober's test is used to evaluate tightness of the iliotibial band and tensor fascia lata (see "Thomas test" also). The patient is placed in the side lying position, and, with the hip extended and abducted and the knee flexed, the proximal part of the leg is allowed to drop passively onto the contralateral limb. The test is considered positive when the leg fails to lower.

Straight leg raise test for hamstring length. The patient is positioned in supine with the legs together and extended. The clinician stands on the side of the leg to be tested and grasps the patient's ankle with one hand, while placing the other hand on the patient's opposite anterior superior iliac spine (ASIS). With the patient's knee extended, the clinician lifts the patient's leg, flexing the hip, until motion is felt at the opposite ASIS. The angle of flexion from the treatment table is measured. The clinician returns the leg to the table and repeats the maneuver from the other side of the table with the other leg. The hamstrings are considered shortened if a straight leg cannot be raised to an angle of 80 degrees from the horizontal, while the other leg is straight. Any limitation of flexion is interpreted as being caused by adaptively shortened hamstring muscles.

This straight leg raise test may also be used as a screen for adverse neural tension, particularly of the sciatic nerve.

90-90 Straight leg raise. The hamstring length can also be assessed with the patient positioned in supine and the tested leg flexed at the hip and knee to 90 degrees. From this position, the patient is asked to extend the knee of the involved side without extending the hip. The measurement is taken at the first resistance barrier.

Piriformis. The patient is positioned in supine. The clinician flexes the involved hip to 60 degrees. After stabilizing the patient's pelvis, the clinician applies a downward pressure through the femur, and maximally adducts the involved hip. From this position, the hip is moved into internal rotation and then external rotation. Internal rotation stresses the superior fibers, while external rotation stresses the inferior fibers. Normal range of motion should be 45 degrees into either rotation.

Hip adductors. The patient is positioned in supine with the leg to be tested close to the edge of the table. The leg not to be tested is positioned at 15 to 25 degrees abducted at the hip joint with the heel over the end of the table. Maintaining the tested knee in extension, the clinician passively abducts the tested leg. The normal range is 40 degrees. When the full range is reached, the knee of the tested leg is passively flexed, and the leg abducted further. If the maximum range does not increase when the knee is flexed, the one-joint adductors (pectineus, adductor magnus, adductor longus, adductor brevis) are shortened. If the range does increase with the knee passively flexed, the two-joint adductors (gracilis, biceps femoris, semimebranosus, and semitendinosus) are shortened.

Leg Length Discrepancy. The test for a leg length discrepancy is best performed radiographically. However, the following clinical test can be used to highlight the more significant discrepancies.

The patient is positioned in supine and the clinician palpates the ASIS. From this point, the clinician slides distally into the depression and then measures from this point to the tip of the malleolus making sure that the course of the tape follows the same route for both legs.

Fulcrum Test. The fulcrum test is used to test for the presence of a stress fracture of the femoral shaft. The patient is positioned in sitting with their knees bent over the edge of the bed, and feet dangling. A firm towel roll is placed under the involved thigh, and is moved proximal to distal as gentle pressure is applied to the anterior thigh with the clinician's hand. A positive test is when the patient reports sharp pain or expresses apprehension when the fulcrum arm is placed under the fracture site.

Special Tests of the Knee Complex

Stress Testing. The stress tests are used to determine the integrity of the joint, ligaments and the menisci. Serious functional instability of the knee appears to occur unpredictably. The reasons for such discrepancies are unknown, but they may be due to:

- Varying definitions of instability
- Varying degrees of damage of the anterior cruciate ligament (ACL)
- Different combinations of injuries
- Different mechanisms of compensation for the loss of the ACL
- Differences in rehabilitation
- The diverse physical demands and expectations of different populations

One-Plane Medial Instability

Abduction valgus stress. The patient is positioned in supine with their involved knee extended. The clinician applies a strong valgus force, with a counter force applied at the lateral femoral condyle. Normally, there is little or no valgus movement in the knee, and, if present, should be less than the amount of varus motion. Under normal conditions, the end-feel is firm. With degeneration of the medial or lateral compartments, varus and valgus motions may be increased, while the end feels will be normal.

With the knee tested in full extension, any demonstrable instability is usually very significant. Pain with this maneuver is caused by an increase in tension of the medial collateral structures, or the connection of these structures with the medial meniscus. If pain or an excessive amount of motion is detected compared with the other extremity, a hypermobility or instability should be suspected. The following structures may be implicated:

- Superficial and deep fibers of the medial collateral ligament (MCL)
- Posterior oblique ligament
- Posterior-medial capsule
- Medial capsular ligament
- ACL
- Posterior cruciate ligament (PCL)

The test is then repeated at 10 to 30 degrees of knee flexion, to further assess the MCL, the posterior oblique ligament, and the PCL. One-plane valgus instability in 30 degrees of flexion usually denotes a tearing, of at least a second degree, of the middle third of the capsular ligament, and the parallel fibers of the MCL.

The posterior fibers of the MCL can be isolated, by placing the knee in 90 degrees of flexion with full external rotation of the tibia. The femur is prevented from rotating by the clinician's shoulder. The clinician places one hand on the dorsum of the foot and the other on the heel, and an external rotation force is applied using the foot as a lever.

One-Plane Lateral Instability. The patient is positioned in supine with the involved knee in full extension. The clinician applies a strong varus force, with a counter force applied at the medial femoral condyle. To be able to assess the amount of varus movement, the clinician should repeat the maneuver several times, applying slight overpressure at the end of the range of motion. Under normal conditions, the end-feel is firm, after slight movement.

If this test is positive for pain or excessive motion as a compared with the other extremity the following structures may be implicated:

- Lateral collateral ligament (LCL)
- Lateral capsular ligament
- Arcuate-popliteus complex
- ACL
- PCL

If the instability is gross, one or both cruciate ligaments may be involved, as well as, occasionally, the biceps femoris tendon and the iliotibial band, leading to a rotary instability, if not in the short term, certainly over a period of time.

The test is then repeated at 10 to 30 degrees of knee flexion and the tibia in full external rotation to further assess the LCL, the posterior-lateral capsule and the arcuate-popliteus complex.

One-Plane Anterior Instability. A number of tests have been advocated for testing the integrity of the ACL. Two of the more commonly used ones are the Lachman's test and the anterior drawer test.

The Lachman's test. The Lachman's test is one of the easiest and most accurate diagnostic measures used to assess ACL injuries. A number of factors can influence the results of the Lachman test. These include:

- An inability of the patient to relax
- The degree of knee flexion
- The size of the clinician's hand
- The stabilization (and thus relaxation) of the patient's thigh

According to Weiss et al,[126] these factors can be minimized by the use of the modified Lachman's test. In this test, the patient is positioned supine with their feet resting firmly on the end of the table and their knees flexed 10 to 15 degrees. The clinician stabilizes the distal end of patient's femur using their thigh rather than their hand as in the Lachman's test, and then attempts to displace patient's tibia anteriorly. If the tibia moves forward, and the concavity of the patellar tendon/ligament becomes convex, the test is considered positive.

The grading of knee instability is as follows:[127-129]

- 1+ (mild): 5 mm or less
- 2+ (moderate): 5 to 10 mm
- 3+ (serious): more than 10 mm

False negatives with this test can occur. False negatives may be caused by a significant hemarthrosis, protective hamstring spasm, or a tear of the posterior horn of the medial meniscus.

Anterior drawer test. The aforementioned Lachman's test is a modification of the anterior drawer test, of which there are a number of variations.[130] The patient is positioned in supine with the knee to be tested flexed to approximately 80 degrees and in neutral rotation. The clinician fixates the patient's leg by sitting on the foot. The clinician grasps the lower leg of the patient just distal to the joint space of the knee. The clinician can place the thumbs, either in the joint space, or just distal to it, to assess mobility. The clinician tests the tension in the musculature. It is important that all muscles around the knee be relaxed so as to allow any translatory movement to occur. With both hands, the clinician now abruptly pulls the lower leg forward. This test is positive when an abnormal anterior movement of the tibia occurs compared with the other extremity.

One-Plane Posterior Instability. The PCL is very strong and is rarely completely torn. It is typically injured in a dashboard injury, or in knee flexion activities (kneeling on the patella). A number of tests have been advocated to test the integrity of the PCL:

Gravity (Godfrey) sign. The patient is positioned in supine with the knee flexed to about 90 degrees. The clinician assesses the contour of the tibial tuberosities. If there is a rupture (partial) of the PCL, the tibial tuberosity on the involved side will be less visible than on the noninvolved side. This is caused by an abnormal posterior translation, resulting from a rupture of the PCL. In cases of doubt, the patient can be asked to contract the hamstrings slightly by pushing their heels into the clinician's hands. This will usually result in an increase in the posterior translation of the tibia. This maneuver is often performed as a quick test for integrity of the PCL.

Posterior drawer. The patient is positioned in supine with the knee flexed to 90 degrees. The clinician attempts a posterior displacement of the tibia on the femur.

Rotary instabilities. Rotary or complex instabilities occur when the abnormal or pathological movement is present in two or more planes. The ligamentous laxities, present at the knee joint in these situations, allow motion to take place around the sagittal, coronal, and the horizontal axis.

Posterior-lateral instability. This type of instability is relatively rare, as it requires complete PCL laxity. It occurs when the lateral tibial plateau subluxes posteriorly on the femur, with the axis shifting posteriorly and medially to the medial joint area. With a hyperextension test, this posterior displacement is obvious and has been labeled the external rotation recurvatum sign.

Active posterolateral drawer test.[131] The patient sits with the foot on the floor in neutral rotation and the knee flexed to 80 to 90 degrees. The patient is asked to isometrically contract the hamstrings, while the clinician stabilizes the foot. A positive result for the test is a posterior subluxation of the lateral tibial plateau.

Hughston's posterior-lateral drawer test.[128,129] The patient is positioned in supine with the involved leg flexed at the hip to 45 degrees, the knee flexed to 80 to 90 degrees, and the lower leg in slight external rotation. The clinician pushes the lower leg posteriorly. If the tibia rotates posteriorly during the test, the test is positive for posterior-lateral instability, and indicates that the following structures may have been injured:

- PCL
- Arcuate-popliteus complex
- LCL
- Posterior-lateral capsule

The one-plane medial and lateral stability tests can be used to help differentiate further which lateral and posterior-lateral structures are affected.

Hughston's external rotational recurvatum test. This test is used to detect an abnormal relationship between the femur and tibia in knee extension. The patient is positioned in supine with their legs straight, and the clinician positioned at the foot of the table. The clinician gently grasps the great toes of both feet at the same time, and lifts the feet from the table, while focusing on the tibial tuberosities of both legs. The patient must be completely relaxed. In the presence of a posterior-lateral rotary instability, the knee moves into relative hyperextension at the lateral side of the knee, and the tibia externally rotates.

Posterior-Medial Rotary Instability

Hughston's posterior-medial drawer test. The patient is positioned in supine with the involved leg flexed at the hip to 45 degrees, the knee flexed to 80 to 90 degrees, and the lower leg in slight internal rotation. The clinician pushes the lower leg posteriorly. If the tibia rotates posteriorly during the test, the test is positive for posterior-medial instability, and indicates that the following structures may have been injured:

- PCL
- Posterior oblique ligament
- MCL
- Posterior-medial capsule
- ACL

The one-plane medial and lateral stability tests can be used to help differentiate further which medial and posterior-medial structures are affected.

Anterior-lateral rotary instability. The pathology for this condition almost certainly involves the PCL and, clinically, the instability allows the medial tibial condyle to sublux posteriorly, as the axis of motion has moved to the lateral joint compartment.

The diagnosis of anterior-lateral instability is based on the demonstration of a forward subluxation of the lateral tibial plateau as the knee approaches extension and the spontaneous reduction of the subluxation during flexion, in the lateral pivot shift test.

Pivot-shift test. The pivot shift is the anterior subluxation of the lateral tibial plateau that occurs when the lower leg is stabilized in (almost) full extension, whereby further flexion produces a palpable "spring-like" reduction. The pivot-shift is the most widely recognized dynamic instability of the knee, and it has been shown to correlate with reduced sports activity, degeneration of the cartilage, reinjury, meniscal damage, joint arthritis, and a history of instability symptoms.

Since the majority of patients with an ACL rupture complain of a "giving-way" sensation, the pivot shift test is regarded in current literature as capable of identifying rotational instability.

There are two main types of clinical tests to determine the presence of the pivot shift: the reduction test and the subluxation test.

1. In the reduction test, the knee is flexed from full extension under a valgus moment. A sudden reduction of the anteriorly subluxed lateral tibial plateau is seen as the pivot shift.
2. The subluxation test is effectively the reverse of the reduction test. However, only 35% to 75% of patients whose knees pivot while the patient is under anesthesia will experience such a pivot when awake. The test begins with the patient's knee extended. The clinician internally rotates the patient's tibia with one hand and applies a valgus stress to the patient's knee joint with the other. As the clinician gradually flexes the patient's ACL-deficient knee joint, the patient's subluxated anterior tibia is felt to snap back into normal alignment at 20 to 40 degrees of flexion.

There is little agreement in the literature with regard to the sensitivity of the pivot shift test, which varies between 0 and 98%.

The pivot shift can be positive with an isolated ACL injury, or a tear or stretching of the lateral capsule, although an injury to the MCL reduces the likelihood of a pivot shift even with ACL injury.

MacIntosh (True pivot-shift) test. The MacIntosh test is the most frequently used test to detect anterior-lateral instability, although

Hughston, Slocum, and Losee have all described variations, with the latter author having received credit for describing the instability simultaneously, and independently, from MacIntosh.

The clinician picks up the relaxed leg by grasping the ankle, and flexes the leg by placing the heel of the other hand over the lateral head of the gastrocnemius. The knee is then extended and a slight valgus stress is applied to its lateral aspect to support the tibia. Under the influence of gravity, the femur falls backward and, as the knee approaches extension, the tibial plateau subluxes forward. This subluxation can be accentuated by gently internally rotating the tibia with the hand that is cradling the foot and ankle. At this point, a strong valgus force is placed on the knee by the upper hand, thereby impinging the subluxed tibial plateau against the lateral femoral condyle, by jamming the two joint surfaces together. This will prevent easy reduction as the tibia is then flexed on the femur. At approximately 30 to 40 degrees of flexion, the displaced tibial plateau will suddenly reduce, often in a dramatic fashion.

Anterior-medial instability. Patients who demonstrate excessive anterior medial tibial condylar displacement during the anterior drawer test are exhibiting anterior-medial instability, as the axis of motion has moved to the lateral joint compartment. The pathology involves the ACL, the MCL, and the posterior medial capsule which, along with its reinforcing fibers, is termed the posterior oblique ligament.

Slocum's test. The Slocum's test is designed to assess for both rotary and anterior instabilities. The patient is positioned in supine and their knee is flexed to 80 degrees to 90 degrees, with the hip flexed to 45 degrees. The foot of the involved leg is first placed in 30 degrees of internal rotation. Excessive internal rotation results in a tightening of the remaining structures and can lead to false negatives. The clinician sits on the foot to maintain its position, and pulls the tibia forward. A positive test results from movement occurring primarily on the lateral side of the knee, and indicates a lesion to one or more of the following structures:

- ACL
- Posterior-lateral capsule
- Arcuate popliteus complex
- LCL
- PCL

If this test is positive, the second part of the test, which assesses anterior-medial rotary instability, is less reliable.

The second half of the test is similar to the first, except that the patient's foot is placed in about 15 degrees of external rotation. Again, by placing the foot in too much external rotation, the clinician runs the risk of false negatives during testing. Movement occurring primarily on the medial side of the knee during testing is a positive result, and indicates a lesion to one or more of the following structures:

- MCL
- Posterior oblique ligament
- Posterior-medial capsule
- ACL

Patellar stability tests. Patellar stability is assessed by gently pushing the patella medially and laterally while the knee is relaxed in a position of 90 degrees of flexion. This position is used because this is the position when all of the retinacula are on stretch. If this test is positive for laxity, further testing is needed, by applying isolated medial, and lateral, patellar glides, tilts, and rotations, with the knee in relaxed extension, and noting any limitations of motion, or excessive excursion.

- Glide: The glide component determines the amount of lateral deviation of the patella in the frontal plane. A 5 mm lateral displacement of the patella causes a 50% decrease in VMO tension. In the normal knee when fully extended and relaxed, the patella can be passively displaced medially and laterally approximately 1 cm in each direction or approximately 25% of the width of the patella. Displacement of more than half the patella over the medial or lateral aspect is considered abnormal. If the patient is apprehensive as this is being done, the problem is likely to be one of poor patellar engagement. A decreased medial glide of the patella has been found to be related to iliotibial band tightness.
- Tilt: The degree of patella tilt is assessed by comparing the height of the medial patellar border with the height of the lateral border, which helps to determine the degree of tightness in the deep retinacular fibers. A slight lateral tilt of patella is normal. An increased medial tilt results from a tight lateral retinaculum. If the passive lateral structures are too tight, the patella will tilt so that the medial border is higher than the lateral border (lateral tilt), making the posterior edge of the lateral border difficult to palpate. A posterior tilt results in fat pad irritation.
- Rotation: The rotation component determines if there is any deviation of the long axis of the patella from the long axis of the femur. If the inferior pole is sitting lateral to the long axis of the femur, the patient has an externally rotated patella, whereas if the inferior pole is sitting medial to the long axis, the patient has an internally rotated patella.

A patient may have one or more of these components present, but the clinician needs to determine which of them is abnormal.

Meniscal lesion tests. No single test provides predictive results for diagnosing meniscal tears. A combination of several positive results is highly predictive of meniscal tears.

Modified McMurray's test.[130] The McMurray's test was originally developed to diagnose posterior horn lesions of the medial meniscus. By modifying this test, it is possible to help diagnose other meniscus lesions as well.

The patient is positioned in supine and the clinician maximally flexes the hip and knee. This is performed by grasping the dorsum of the patient's foot in such a way that the thumb is lateral, the index and middle fingers are medial, and the ring and little fingers hold the medial edge of the foot. One hand is placed against the lateral aspect of the patient's knee. By rotating the patient's lower leg several times, the clinician can assess whether the patient is fully relaxed. While the lower leg is slightly externally rotated, the ipsilateral hand moves the patient's foot in a varus direction. The knee is flexed as far as comfortable, after which the foot is brought into a valgus direction with simultaneous internal rotation of the lower leg. The clinician then gently extends the knee to about 120 degrees, and at the same time exerts valgus pressure on the knee with the hand. This test is positive when a palpable click, or audible thump, is elicited that is also painful. It is thought that pain with passive external rotation implicates lesions of the posterior horn of the lateral meniscus, while pain with passive internal rotation implicates a lesion of the posterior horn of the medial meniscus, although false-positives are common.

If the test is negative, there still may be a meniscus lesion. One after the other, a similar maneuver can be repeated with valgus pressure and external rotation, then with varus pressure and external rotation, and finally with varus pressure and internal rotation.

Apley's test.[132] The patient is positioned in the prone position with their knee flexed to 90 degrees. The patient's thigh is stabilized by the clinician's knee. The clinician applies internal and external rotation with compression to the lower leg, noting any pain, and the quality of motion. Pain with this maneuver may indicate a meniscal lesion.

Anderson medial-lateral grind test. The Anderson medial-lateral grind test can be used to detect meniscal lesions. The patient is positioned in supine and the clinician grasps the uninvolved leg between the trunk and arm. The clinician places the index finger and thumb of the other hand over the anterior knee joint line. With the knee flexed at 45 degrees, a valgus stress is applied as the knee is simultaneously slightly flexed, followed by a varus component while the knee is extended, producing a circular motion of the knee. The maneuver is repeated, increasing the valgus and varus stresses with each rotation.

O'Donahue's test. The patient is positioned in supine, with their knee flexed to 90 degrees. The clinician stabilizes the thigh and rotates the tibia medially and laterally twice, and then fully flexes and rotates the tibia both ways again. Pain in either or both of the positions, is a positive sign for capsular irritation or a meniscal tear.

Boehler test. This test is performed in the same way as testing for stability of the collateral ligaments. Valgus stress results in pain with lateral meniscus (LM) tears. Varus stress results in pain with medial meniscus (MM) tears.

Payr test. The knee is flexed to 90 degrees. The application of varus stress compresses the posterior horn of the MM. Eliciting pain indicates a meniscal tear.

Special Tests for Specific Diagnoses.

Plical irritation. Plical irritation has a characteristic pattern of presentation. The anterior pain in the knee is episodic and associated with painful clicking, giving-way, and the feeling of something catching in the knee. Careful palpation of the patellar retinaculum and fat pad, with the knee extended and then flexed, can be used to detect tender plicae, and for the differentiation of tenderness within the fat pad, from tenderness over the anterior horn of the menisci.

- The patella bowstring test can be used to test for plical irritation. The patient is positioned in side lying, tested side up. Using the heel of the cranial hand, the clinician pushes the patella medially and maintains it there. While the patella is maintained in this position, the clinician flexes the knee and internally rotates the tibia with the other hand. The knee is then extended from the flexed position while the clinician palpates for any clunks.
- Medial shift at about 30 degrees of knee flexion (Mital–Hayden test): The patient is supine on the bed, with his/her knee supported in about 30 degrees flexion, by either a towel roll or the clinician's own thigh, which rests on the table. The clinician places both thumbs together at the lateral aspect of the patella and pushes the patella medially. If a painful click is elicited during this test, there is likely to be a symptomatic mediopatellar synovial plica.

Supra/infrapatellar tendonitis. The patient is positioned in supine with the lower extremity extended.

- Infrapatellar. The clinician pushes down on the suprapatellar aspect, palpates under the inferior pole of the patella, and checks for tenderness which may indicate infrapatellar tendonitis.
- Suprapatellar. The clinician pushes on the infrapatellar aspect of the patella, palpates under the superior pole of the patella, and checks for tenderness which may indicate suprapatellar tendinitis.

Integrity of Patellofemoral Articulating Surfaces. These tests involve the application of manual compression to the patella in an attempt to elicit pain.

The McConnell's test. This test involves manual compression to the patella with the palm of the hand at various angles of knee flexion to compress the articulating facets. While the findings have little bearing on the overall intervention, they can guide the clinician as to which knee flexion angles to avoid during exercise.

- 20 degrees flexion: inferior facet
- 45 degrees flexion: middle facet
- 90 degrees flexion: all facets except the odd facet
- Full flexion: odd facet (medial) and lateral facet

Zohler's test. The patient is supine on the bed with his/her knee extended and resting on the table. The clinician pushes the patient's patella in a distal direction. While continuing to exert pressure in a distal direction, the clinician instructs the patient to contract the quadriceps muscle. If this test is painful, there is likely to be a symptomatic patellar chondromalacia, although this test may be positive in a large proportion of asymptomatic individuals.

Clarke's test. This test is similar to the one above, except that the clinician applies an increasing compressive force to the base of the patella while the patient actively contracts the quadriceps. Like

Zohler's test, this test may also be positive in a large proportion of asymptomatic individuals.

Waldron test. The patient is positioned in standing. While the patient performs a series of slow deep knee bends, the clinician palpates the patella for crepitus, and its occurrence relative to the range.

Patellar Mobility and Retinaculum Tests. Patella glides can be used to examine for retinacular mobility. Inability to glide normally indicates tightness of the retinacula.

The lateral retinaculum is assessed by way of a patellar tilt and a medial-lateral displacement (glide). A number of patient positions can be used to assess the flexibility of the retinacular tissue.

Fairbank Apprehension Test for Patellar Instability. The Fairbank test is best performed with the patient's leg supported at approximately 30 degrees of knee flexion. The clinician applies a laterally directed force to the medial aspect of the patella, attempting to sublux it laterally while applying a small amount of passive flexion to the knee.

Wilson Test for Osteochondritis Dissecans. The following accessory test can be performed when osteochondritis dissecans of the knee is suspected. The clinician flexes the patient's hip and knee to 90 degrees. Axial compression is exerted at the knee by pushing proximally, in line with the tibia, with the distal hand. The lower leg is held in internal rotation while the knee is slowly extended, while the axial compression is maintained. In many cases of osteochondritis dissecans, the patient experiences pain because the pressure on the medial cartilaginous surfaces is increased significantly.

Hamstring Flexibility. The popliteal angle is the most popular method reported in the literature for assessing hamstring tightness especially in the presence of a knee flexion contracture. The patient is positioned in supine and the opposite leg lies on top of the table. The leg to be tested is positioned in 90 degrees of hip flexion. The popliteal angle is determined by measuring the angle that the tibia subtends with the extended line of the femur when the knee of the limb under examination is maximally passively extended to initial tissue resistance. The popliteal angle is at the maximum of 180 degrees from birth to age 2 years. This angle then decreases to average 155 degrees by age 6 years and remains steady thereafter. An angle <125 degrees suggests significant hamstring tightness.

Iliotibial Band Flexibility. The cardinal sign for iliotibial contracture is that in the supine patient an abduction contracture is present when the hip and knee are extended, but is eliminated by flexion of the hip and knee.

Tests for iliotibial tendinitis. Iliotibial band tendinitis may be classified by four grades based on pain and activity limitation:

I—Pain beginning after activity that neither restricts distance or speed of athletic activity

II—Pain beginning during activity that neither restricts distance or speed

III—Pain beginning during activity that may restrict either distance or speed
IV—Pain so severe as to preclude athletic participation

Renne's[133] *test.* The patient stands on the affected leg. As the patient flexes the knee to 30 degrees to 40 degrees, a positive test is indicated when a palpable "creak" is produced, as the maneuver brings the ITB into tight contact with the lateral femoral condyle.

Noble's compression[134] *test.* The patient is positioned in supine with the affected knee flexed to 90 degrees. Pressure is applied over the proximal, prominent part of the lateral femoral condyle as the knee is gradually extended. A positive test is indicated when pain is reproduced at 30 to 40 degrees.

Creak test. The patient stands on the involved leg. As the patient flexes the knee to approximately 30 degrees, the patient will notice a "creak" over the lateral femoral epicondyle.

Special Tests of the Ankle and Foot. The examination of the ligamentous structures of the ankle and foot is essential, not only because of their vast array, but also because of the amount of stability that they provide. Positive results for the ligamentous stability tests include excessive movement as compared with the same test on the uninvolved extremity, pain (depending on the severity), or apprehension.

Mortise/Syndesmosis

Clunk (Cotton) test. The patient is positioned in supine with his/her foot over the end of the bed. One hand is used to stabilize the distal leg (crus), while the clinician uses the other hand to grasp the heel and move the calcaneus medially and laterally. A clunk can be felt as the talus hits the tibia and fibula if there has been significant mortise widening.

Alternatively, the patient can be positioned in supine with their knee flexed to the point where the ankle is in the position of full dorsiflexion. The clinician applies over pressure into further dorsiflexion by grasping the femoral condyles with one hand and leaning down into the table. The clinician uses the other hand to pull the crus anteriorly. Because the ankle is in its close packed position, no movement should be felt.

Posterior drawer test. The posterior drawer test can also be used to test for the presence of instability at the inferior tibiofibular joint. The patient is supine. The hip and knee are fully flexed to provide as much dorsiflexion of the ankle as possible. This drives the wide anterior part of the talus back into the mortice. An anterior stabilizing force is then applied to the crus, and the foot and talus are translated posteriorly. If the inferior tibiofibular joint is stable, there will be no drawer available, but if there is instability, there will be a drawer.

Squeeze (Distal tibiofibular compression) test. In the squeeze test, the clinician squeezes the upper to middle third of the leg at a point about 6 to 8 in below the knee. Pain felt in the distal third of the leg may indicate a compromised syndesmosis, if the presence of a tibia and/or fibula fracture, calf contusion, or compartment syndrome have all been ruled out.

Lateral Collaterals. The lateral collaterals resist inversion and consist of the anterior talofibular, calcaneofibular, and posterior talofibular. An additional function of the lateral ligaments of the ankle is to prevent excessive varus movement, especially during plantar flexion. In extreme plantar flexion, the mortice no longer stabilizes the broader anterior part of the talus, and varus movement of the ankle is then possible.

Anterior talofibular ligament (ATFL). The patient is positioned in supine. The crus is gripped with the stabilizing hand, using a lumbrical grip, while the other hand grasps over the mortise and onto the neck of talus, so that the index fingers are together at the point between fibular and talus. The clinician moves the patient's foot into plantar flexion and full inversion, and a force is applied in an attempt to adduct (distract) the calcaneus, thereby gapping the lateral side of the ankle. Pain on the lateral aspect of the ankle with this test, and/or displacement depending on severity, may indicate a sprain of the ligament.

The anterior drawer test. The anterior drawer stress test is performed to estimate the stability of the ATFL. The test is performed with the patient sitting at the end of the bed or lying supine with their knee flexed to relax the gastrocnemius-soleus muscles and the foot supported perpendicular to the leg. The clinician uses one hand to stabilize the crus, while the other hand grasps the patient's heel and positions the ankle in 10 to 15 degrees of plantar flexion. The heel is very gently pulled forward, and, if the test is positive, the talus, and with it the foot, rotates anteriorly out of the ankle mortice, around the intact deltoid ligament, which serves as the center of rotation.

The dimple sign. Another positive sign for a rupture of the ATFL, if pain and spasm are minimal, is the presence of "a dimple" located just in front of the tip of the lateral malleolus, during the anterior drawer test. This results from a negative pressure created by the forward movement of the talus, which draws the skin inwards at the side of ligament rupture. This dimple sign is also seen with a combined rupture of the ATFL and calcaneofibular ligaments. However, the sign is only present within the first 48 hours of injury.

Calcaneofibular ligament (CFL). The inversion stress maneuver is a test that attempts to assess CFL integrity. The patient is positioned supine. The crus is gripped with the stabilizing hand while the moving hand cups the heel. The ankle is dorsiflexed via the calcaneus to a right angle (total dorsiflexion is impractical) and inverted. An adduction, and anterior-medial translation of the calcaneus is then applied tending to gap the lateral side of the joint. Pain on the lateral aspect of the ankle with this test, and/or displacement depending on severity, may indicate a sprain of the ligament.

Posterior talofibular. The patient is either prone or supine, and the crus is gripped or the fibula is stabilized. The patient's leg is stabilized in internal rotation, and the foot is placed in full dorsiflexion. The clinician externally rotates the heel/calcaneus, thereby moving the talar attachment of the ligament away from the malleolus. Pain on the lateral aspect of the ankle with this test, and/or displacement depending on severity, may indicate a sprain of the ligament.

Medial Collaterals (Deltoid Complex). The medial collaterals function to resist eversion. Given their strength, these ligaments are only usually injured as the result of major trauma.

Kleiger (External rotation) test. The Kleiger (external rotation) test is a general test to assess the integrity of the deltoid ligament complex, but can also implicate the syndesmosis if pain is produced over the anterior or posterior tibiofibular ligaments and the interosseous membrane. If this test is positive, further testing is necessary to determine the source of the symptoms.

The patient sits with their legs dangling over the end of the bed, with the knee flexed to 90 degrees, and the foot relaxed. The clinician stabilizes the lower leg with one hand and, using the other hand, grasps the foot and rotates it laterally. Pain on the medial and lateral aspect of the ankle, and/or displacement of the talus from the medial malleolus, depending on severity, with this test may indicate a tear of the deltoid ligament.

Thompson Test for Achilles Tendon Rupture. In this test, the patient is positioned in prone, or in kneeling with the feet over the edge of the bed. With the patient relaxed, the clinician gently squeezes the calf muscle and observes for the production of plantar flexion. An absence of plantar flexion indicates a complete rupture of the Achilles tendon.

Patla's test for tibialis posterior length.[135] The patient is positioned in prone, with the knee flexed to 90 degrees. The clinician stabilizes the calcaneus in eversion and the ankle in dorsiflexion with one hand. With the other hand, the clinician contacts the plantar surface of the bases of the second, third, and fourth metatarsals with the thumb, while the index and middle fingers contact the plantar surface of the navicular. The clinician then pushes the navicular and metatarsal heads dorsally and compares the end feel and patient response with the uninvolved side. A positive test is indicated with reproduction of the patient's symptoms.

Feiss line. The Feiss line test is used to assess the height of the medial arch, using the navicular position. With the patient non-weight bearing, the clinician marks the apex of the medial malleolus and the plantar aspect of the first MTP joint, and a line is drawn between the two points. The navicular is palpated on the medial aspect of the foot, and an assessment is made as to the position of the navicular relative to the imaginary line. The patient is then asked to stand with their feet about 3 to 6 in apart. In weight bearing the navicular normally lies on, or very close to the line. If the navicular falls one third of the distance to the floor, it represents a first-degree flatfoot; if it falls two thirds of the distance, it represents a second-degree flatfoot, and if it rests on the floor, it represents a third-degree flatfoot.

"Too Many Toes" sign. The patient is asked to stand in a normal relaxed position while the clinician views the patient from behind. If the heel is in valgus, the *forefoot is* abducted, or the tibia is externally

rotated more than normal, the clinician will observe more toes on the involved side than on the normal side.

Articular Stability Tests

Navicular drop test. The navicular drop test is a method to assess the degree to which the talus plantarflexes in space on a calcaneus that has been stabilized by the ground, during subtalar joint pronation.

The clinician palpates the position of the navicular tubercle as the patient's foot is non-weight bearing but resting on the floor surface with the subtalar joint maintained in neutral. The clinician then attempts to quantify inferior displacement of the navicular tubercle as the patient assumes 50% weight bearing on the tested foot. A navicular drop which is greater than 10 mm from the neutral position to the relaxed standing position suggests excessive medial longitudinal arch collapse associated with abnormal pronation.

Talar rock. The talar rock is an articular stability test for the subtalar joint. The test is performed with the patient positioned in side lying, with his or her hip and knee flexed. The clinician sits on the table with his or her back to the patient, and places both hands around the ankle just distal to the malleoli. The clinician applies a slight distraction force to the ankle, before applying a rocking movement to the foot in an upward or downward direction. A "clunk" should be felt at the end of each of the movements.

Passive foot rotation. This test assesses the integrity of the midtarsal and tarsometatarsal joints. A rotational movement is applied to the midtarsal and tarsometatarsal joints. At the midtarsal joint, the proximal row of the tarsal bones (navicular, calcaneus, and talus) is stabilized, and the distal row (cuneiforms and cuboid) is rotated in both directions. At the tarsometatarsal joints, the distal row of the tarsals is stabilized and the metatarsals are rotated in both directions.

Neurovascular Status

Homan's sign. The patient is positioned in supine with their knee extended. The clinician stabilizes the thigh with one hand, and passively dorsiflexes the patient's ankle with the other. Pain in the calf with this maneuver may indicate a positive Homan's sign for deep vein thrombophlebitis (DVT), especially if there are associated signs including pallor and swelling in the leg and a loss of the dorsal pedis pulse.

Buerger's test. The patient is positioned in supine with the knee extended. The clinician elevates the patient's leg to about 45 degrees and maintains it there for at least 3 minutes. Blanching of the foot is positive for poor arterial circulation, especially if the patient sits with the legs over the end of the bed and it takes 1 to 2 minutes for the limb color to be restored.

Morton's test. The patient is positioned in supine. The clinician grasps the foot around the metatarsal heads and squeezes the heads together. The reproduction of pain with this maneuver indicates the presence of a neuroma, or a stress fracture.

Duchenne's test. The patient is positioned in supine with his/her legs straight. The clinician pushes through the sole on the first metatarsal head, and pushes the foot into dorsiflexion. The patient is asked to planterflex the foot. If the medial border dorsiflexes and offers no resistance while the lateral border plantarflexes, a lesion of the superficial fibular nerve, or a lesion of the L4, L5, and S1 nerve root is indicated.

Tinel's sign. There are two locations around the ankle from where the Tinel's sign can be elicited. The anterior tibial branch of the deep fibular nerve can be tapped on the anterior aspect of the ankle. The posterior tibial nerve may be tapped behind the medial malleolus. Tingling or paresthesia with this test is considered a positive finding.

Dorsal pedis pulse. The dorsal pedis pulse can be palpated just lateral to the tendon of the extensor hallucis longus over the dorsum of the foot.

Special Tests of the Spine and SIJ

Special Tests of the Upper Cervical Spine

Vertebral artery tests. A positive vertebral artery test is one in which signs or symptoms change, especially if the changes evoked include upper motor neuron signs and symptoms. More subtle examination findings can include a significant delay in verbal responses to questions of orientation, with some inconsistency of answers; changes in pupil size; and nystagmus.[136] Clinical testing of the vertebral artery should stop once positive signs or symptoms are noted. Throughout the tests, the clinician should observe the patient's eyes for possible nystagmus or changes in pupil size, and should have the patient count backward to assess their quality of speech. The patient is asked to report any changes in symptoms, however insignificant he or she may feel the changes to be.

Initial test. The initial test consists of having the patient rotate the head to each side while in the sitting position. The longus colli and scalene muscles rotate the cervical spine and can squeeze the vertebral artery on the side contralateral to the rotation.[137] The presence of muscular compression of the artery can be further tested by combining cervical flexion with rotation to place the inferior oblique capitis on stretch.[137]

Barre's test. Barre's test can be used to test for vertebral artery insufficiency, especially if the patient is unable to lie supine.

The patient is seated with the arms outstretched, forearms supinated. The patient is asked to close his or her eyes and move his or her head and neck into maximum extension and rotation. A positive test is one in which one of the outstretched arms sinks toward the floor and pronates, indicating the side of the compromise.

Hautard's (Hautant's, Hautart, or Hautarth) test.[138,139] As with Barre's test, proprioceptive loss rather than dizziness is sought in Hautard's test. The test has two parts. The patient is seated. Both arms are actively flexed to 90 degrees at the shoulders. The eyes are then closed for a few seconds while the clinician observes for any loss of position of one or both arms. If the arms move, the proprioception loss has a nonvascular cause. If the first part of the test is negative, the patient is asked to extend and rotate the neck. Because the

Study Pearl

Following a positive vertebral artery test or positive responses in the history, the patient must be handled very carefully, and further intervention, particularly manipulation of the cervical spine, should not be delivered. The patient should not, under any circumstance, be allowed to leave the clinic until his or her physician has been contacted, and until the necessary arrangements have been made for the safe transport of the patient to an appropriate facility.

second part of the test is performed to elicit a vascular cause for the dizziness, the eyes can be open or closed. Having the eyes open allows the clinician to observe for nystagmus and changes in pupil size. Each position is held for 10 to 30 seconds. If wavering of the arms occurs with the second part of the test, a vascular cause for the symptoms is suspected.

Cervical quadrant test.[140] The patient is positioned in supine. The supine position is reported to result in an increase in passive motion at the cervical spine compared with sitting and may, therefore, better test the ability of the vertebral artery to sustain a stretch. The clinician passively moves the patient's head into extension and side bending. Maintaining this position, the clinician rotates the patient's head to the same side as the side bending and holds it there for 30 seconds. A positive test is one in which referring symptoms are produced if the opposite artery is involved.

DeKleyn-Nieuwenhuyse test.[141] The patient is positioned in supine. The clinician passively moves the patient's head into extension and rotation. A positive test is one in which referring symptoms are produced if the opposite artery is involved. Despite its widespread appearance in a number of texts, this test is not recommended because of the severe traction stresses it places on the vertebral artery.[139]

Dix-Hallpike test. This test can be used to help determine if the cause of the patient's dizziness is because of a vestibular impairment due to an accumulation of utricle debris (otoconia), which can move within the posterior semicircular canals, and stimulate the vestibular sense organ (cupula). This test is only usually performed if the vertebral artery test and instability tests do not provoke symptoms.

The test involves having the patient suddenly lie down from a sitting position with the head rotated in the direction that the clinician feels is the provocative position.[139] The end point of the test is when the patient's head overhangs the end of the table so that the cervical spine is extended. A positive test is the reproduction of the patient's symptoms.

Modified sharp–purser test. This test was originally designed to test the sagittal stability of the AA segment in rheumatoid arthritic patients, as a number of pathological conditions can affect the stability of the osseoligamentous ring of the median joints of this segment in this patient population. These changes result in degeneration and thinning of the articular cartilage between the odontoid process and the anterior arch of atlas, or the dens can become softened.

The aim of the test was to determine whether the instability was significant enough to provoke central nervous system signs and/or symptoms.

The patient is positioned in sitting. The patient is asked to segmentally flex the head and relate any signs or symptoms that this might evoke to the clinician. In addition, a positive test may be indicated by the patient hearing or feeling a clunk in the neck. Local symptoms such as soreness are ignored for the purposes of evaluating the test. If no serious signs or symptoms are provoked, the clinician stabilizes C2 with one hand, and applies a posteriorly oriented force to the forehead.

In the presence of a positive test, a provisional assumption is made that the symptoms are caused by excessive translation of the atlas compromising one or more of the sensitive structures listed above. The test is considered positive and the physical examination is terminated. No intervention should be attempted other than the issuing of a cervical collar to prevent craniovertebral flexion and an immediate physician referral.

Special Tests of the Cervical Spine and TMJ

Temporomandibular joint screen. As the temporomandibular joint can refer pain to the cervical region, the clinician is well-advised to rule out this joint as the cause for the patient's symptoms. The patient is asked to open and close the mouth, and to laterally deviate the jaw as the clinician observes the quality and quantity of motion, and notes any reproduction of symptoms.

Lhermitte's symptom or "phenomenon." This is not so much a test, as a symptom described as an electric shock-like sensation that radiates down the spinal column into the upper or lower limbs when flexing the neck. It can also be precipitated by extending the head, coughing, sneezing, or bending forward or by moving the limbs.[142] Lhermitte's symptom and abnormalities in the posterior part of the cervical spinal cord on MRI are strongly associated.[143]

Brachial Plexus Tests

Stretch test. This test is similar to the straight leg raise for the lower extremity as it stretches the brachial plexus. The patient is positioned in sitting. The patient is asked to side bend the head to the uninvolved side and to extend the shoulder and elbow on the involved side. Pain and paresthesia along the involved arm is indicative of a brachial plexus irritation.

Compression test. The patient is positioned in sitting. The patient is asked to side bend the head to the uninvolved side. The clinician applies firm pressure to the brachial plexus by squeezing the plexus between the thumb and fingers. Reproduction of shoulder or upper arm pain is positive for mechanical cervical lesions.[144]

Tinel's sign. The patient is positioned in sitting. The patient is asked to side bend the head to the uninvolved side. The clinician taps along the trunks of the brachial plexus using the fingertips. Local pain indicates a cervical plexus lesion. A tingling sensation in the distribution of one of the trunks may indicate a compression or neuroma of one or more trunks of the brachial plexus.[145]

Thoracic Outlet Tests. Despite their widespread use, no studies documenting the reliability of the common thoracic outlet maneuvers of Adson's, Allen's, or the costoclavicular maneuver have been performed.[105] The specificity of these tests, determined in asymptomatic patients, has been reported to be between 18% and 87%,[146-149] while the sensitivity has been documented at 94%.[105,148]

When performing thoracic outlet syndrome tests, evaluation for either the diminution or disappearance of pulse or reproduction of neurological symptoms indicates a positive test. However, the aim of the tests should be to reproduce the patient's symptoms rather than to obliterate the radial pulse, as more than 50% of normal, asymptomatic people will exhibit obliteration of the radial pulse during classic provocative testing.[150]

A baseline pulse should be established first, before performing the respective test maneuvers.

Adson's vascular test. The patient extends their neck, turns their head toward the side being examined, and takes a deep breath. This test, if positive, tends to implicate the scalenes because this test increases the tension of the anterior and middle scalenes, and compromises the interscalene triangle.[151]

Allen's pectoralis minor test. The Allen's test increases the tone of the pectoralis minor muscle. The shoulder of the seated patient is positioned in 90 degrees of glenohumeral abduction, 90 degrees of glenohumeral external rotation, and 90 degrees of elbow flexion on the tested side. While the radial pulse is monitored, the patient is asked to turn their head away from the tested side. This test, if positive, tends to implicate pectoralis tightness as the cause for the symptoms.

Costoclavicular. During this test, the shoulders are drawn back and downward in an exaggerated military position to reduce the volume of the costoclavicular space.

Hallstead maneuver. The patient is positioned in sitting on the edge of a table. The clinician grasps the arm on the symptomatic side, passively depresses its shoulder girdle and then pulls the arm down toward the floor, while palpating the radial pulse. The patient is asked to extend the head and to turn away from the tested side. A positive test for thoracic outlet syndrome (TOS) is indicated if there is an absence or diminishing of the pulse.

Roos test.[152] The patient is positioned in sitting. The arm is positioned in 90 degrees of shoulder abduction, and 90 degrees of elbow flexion. The patient is asked to perform slow finger clenching for 3 minutes. The radial pulse may be reduced or obliterated during this maneuver, and an infraclavicular bruit may be heard. If the patient is unable to maintain the arms in the start position for 3 minutes or reports pain heaviness or numbness and tingling, the test is considered positive for TOS on the involved side. This test is also referred to as the hands-up test or the elevated arm stress test (EAST).

Overhead test. The overhead exercise test is useful to detect thoracic outlet arterial compression. The patient elevates both arms overhead, and then rapidly flexes and extends the fingers. A positive test is achieved if the patient experiences heaviness, fatigue, numbness, tingling, blanching, or discoloration of a limb within 20 seconds.[151]

Hyperabduction maneuver (Wright test).[146] This test is considered by many to be the best provocative test for thoracic outlet compression caused by compression in the costoclavicular space. The test is performed by asking the patient to turn the head away from the side being examined, and take a deep breath while the clincian passively abducts and externally rotates the patient's arm.

Passive shoulder shrug. This simple but effective test is used with patients who present with TOS symptoms to help rule out thoracic outlet syndrome. The patient is seated with their arms folded and the clinician stands behind. The clinician grasps the patient's elbows and passively elevates the shoulders up and forward. This position is maintained for 30 seconds. Any changes in the patient's symptoms are noted. The maneuver has the affect of slackening the soft tissues and the plexus.

Upper Limb Tension Tests

Special Tests of the Lumbar Spine and SIJ

Neurodynamic Mobility Testing

Straight Leg Raise Test. The straight leg raise (SLR) test should be a routine test during the examination of the lumbar spine among patients with sciatica or pseudoclaudication. However, the test is often negative in patients with spinal stenosis.[153] A leg elevation of less than 60 degrees is abnormal, suggesting compression or irritation of the nerve roots. A positive test reproduces the symptoms of sciatica, with pain that radiates below the knee, not merely back or hamstring pain.[153] Ipsilateral straight-leg raising has sensitivity but not specificity for a herniated intervertebral disk (IVD), whereas crossed straight-leg raising is insensitive but highly specific. The clinician must remember that the SLR test stresses a number of structures including:

- The lumbosacral nerve roots
- The hamstrings
- The hip joint
- The sacroiliac joint

The following guidelines can be used to interpret the results from the test[154]:

- Symptoms reproduced in the 0 to 30 degrees range may indicate hip pathology or a severely inflamed nerve root.
- Symptoms reproduced in the 30 to 50 degrees range may indicate sciatic nerve root involvement.
- Symptoms reproduced in the 50 to 70 degrees range may indicate hamstring involvement.
- Symptoms reproduced in the 70 to 90 degrees range may indicate involvement of the sacroiliac joint.

Pheasant's test. The patient is positioned in prone. While monitoring for motion at the patient's pelvis, the clinician passively flexes the patient's knees. The Pheasant's test introduces an anterior pelvic tilt/increase in lordosis through the pull of the rectus femoris. Once motion occurs at the pelvis, the clinician determines whether the low back symptoms have been reproduced.[155] A pulling sensation on the anterior aspect of the thighs is a normal finding. If full knee flexion is achieved before the tilting occurs, the patient is positioned in the prone on elbows position and the test is repeated. Patients who test positive for this maneuver tend to have the following subjective complaints:

- Pain with supine lying with the legs straight, unless the rectus and hip flexors are especially flexible
- Pain with prone lying

- Pain with sitting erect
- Pain with prolonged standing

The cause of the pain is thought to be due to the passive stretching or compression of pain sensitive structures. These structures include the zygapophyseal joints, the segmental ligaments and the anterior aspect of the IVD.

Anterior SI joint stress test. The anterior stress test, also called the gapping test, is performed with the patient supine. The clinician stands to one side of the patient and, crossing their arms, places the palm of their hands on the patient's anterior superior iliac spines. The crossing of the arms ensures that the applied force is in a lateral direction, thereby gapping the anterior aspect of the sacroiliac joint. The stress is maintained for 7 to 10 seconds, or until an end feel is felt. The procedure stresses the anterior (ventral) ligament and compresses the posterior aspect of the joint. A positive test is one in which the patient's groin and/or SIJ pain is reproduced either anteriorly, posteriorly, unilaterally, or bilaterally.[156]

The anterior gapping test, and its posterior counterpart (see below), are believed to be sensitive for severe arthritis or ventral ligament tears,[33] although they have been shown to be poorly reproducible.[157]

Posterior sacroiliac joint stress test. The posterior stress test, also called the compression test, is performed with the patient in side lying. The clinician, standing behind the patient, applies a downward force on the side of the patient's uppermost innominate using both hands. The procedure creates a medial force that tends to gap the posterior aspect of the joint while compressing its anterior aspect. The reproduction of pain over one or both of the sacroiliac joints is considered positive.

FADE (Flexion, adduction, extension) positional test[158]. The set up for the FADE test is similar to that of the FABER test, except that the start position involves moving the patient's hip into flexion and adduction. From that position, the clinician moves the patient's hip into extension and slight abduction. A positive test is indicated by pain or loss of motion as compared with the uninvolved side.

Posterior–anterior pressures. Posterior-anterior pressures, advocated by Maitland,[140] are applied over the spinous, mammillary, and transverse processes of this region. The clinician should apply the posterior–anterior force in a slow and gentle fashion using the index and middle finger of one hand, while monitoring the paravertebrals with the other hand.

While these maneuvers are capable of eliciting pain, restricted movement and/or muscle spasm, they are fairly nonspecific in determining the exact level involved, or the exact cause of the symptoms, and have been found to have poor inter-rater reliability in the absence of corroborating clinical data.[159] However, as a screening tool, the PA pressures have their uses, and help detect the presence of excessive motion, and/or spasm.

COMMON ORTHOPEDIC CONDITIONS

There are a number of orthopedic conditions frequently encountered, descriptions of which follow. The intervention strategies for many of these conditions are described in the "Intervention Principles for Musculoskeletal Injuries" section. Treatments specific to certain conditions are included with the descriptions.

ACHILLES TENDINITIS

Achilles tendinitis, the most common overuse syndrome of the lower leg, can be caused by a number of factors[160]:

- Adverse biomechanics: The brisk and frequent transitions from pronation to supination cause the Achilles tendon to undergo a "bow-string" action.[160] In addition, if the foot remains in a pronated position after knee extension has begun, a twisting action of the tendon occurs due to the external tibial rotation at the knee and the internal tibial rotation at the foot.[161] Inflexibility of the cavus foot can be a precursor to Achilles tendinitis due to the compensatory overpronation.
- Training variables: These include a lack of a stretching programs, an increase in training pace, and hill training.[160] Overtraining has been found to be associated with calf muscle fatigue and microtears of the tendon.[161,162]
- Muscular insufficiency: Muscle weakness can lead to an inability to eccentrically control dorsiflexion during the beginning of the support phase of running.[160,163-165]
- Shoe type: Spike shoes lock the feet on the surface during the single support phase in running and increase the athlete's foot grip but also transfer lateral and torque shear forces directly to the foot and ankle and through to the Achilles tendon.
- Sacroiliac joint dysfunction. Changes in sacroiliac joint mechanics as compared with the contralateral side.[166]

Achilles tendinitis typically occurs as one of two types[167]:

1. Insertional: involving the tendon-bone interface
2. Noninsertional: occurs just proximal to the tendon insertion on the calcaneus in or around the tendon substance. Can be referred to as peritendinitis, peritendinitis with tendinosis, and tendinosis.[167,168]

Clinical symptoms of Achilles tendinitis consist of a gradual onset of pain and swelling in the Achilles tendon, 2 to 3 cm proximal to its insertion, which is exacerbated by weight bearing activity. Some patients will present with pain and stiffness along the Achilles tendon when rising in the morning or pain at the start of activity that improves as the activity progresses.

Upon observation, the patient will often be found to have pronated feet and the presence of swelling is common. Observation during gait may reveal an antalgic gait, with the involved leg held in external rotation both during stance and swing phase.

- Localization of the tenderness with palpation is extremely important.
  - Tenderness that is located 2 to 6 cm proximal to the insertion is indicative of noninsertional tendonitis.
  - Pain at the bone-tendon junction, is more indicative of insertional tendinitis.
  - If there is an area in the tendon itself, which is discrete and painful with side to side pressure of the fingers, this often indicates an area of mucoid degeneration or a small partial rupture of the tendon.
  - If the tenderness is in the area of the retrocalcaneal bursa, which is noted by side-to-side pressure in that area, this is the primary area of involvement.

A lack of 20 to 30 degrees of dorsiflexion in knee extension signifies gastrocnemius tightness, and inability to dorsiflex 30 to 35 degrees in knee flexion implicates the soleus as well.

There is often pain with resisted testing of the gastocnemius/soleus complex.

The intervention for Achilles tendonitis varies depending on the severity of the symptoms. The condition can be diagnosed according to the following types[169]:

- Type I: Characterized by pain that is only experienced after activity. These patients should reduce their exercise by approximately 25%.
- Type II: Characterized by pain that occurs during and after activity but does not affect performance. These patients should reduce their training by approximately 50%.
- Type III: Characterized by pain during and after activity but has no affect on performance. These patients should discontinue running temporarily.

The intervention strategies for tendon injuries are outlined in "Intervention Principles for Musculoskeletal Injuries" section.

ACROMIOCLAVICULAR JOINT INJURIES

Injuries to the AC joint were originally classified by Tossy and colleagues[170] and Allman[171] as incomplete (grades I and II) and complete (grade III). This classification has been expanded to include six types of injuries based on the direction and amount of displacement (Table 8-36).[3,4,172,173]

- Types I, II, III, and V all involve inferior displacement of the acromion with respect to the clavicle. They differ based on severity of injury to the ligaments and the amount of resultant displacement.[174]
- Types I and II usually result from a fall or a blow to the point on the lateral aspect of the shoulder, or a fall on an outstretched hand (FOOSH), producing a sprain.
- Types III and IV usually involve a dislocation (commonly called AC separations) and a distal clavicle fracture, both of which commonly disrupt the coracoclavicular ligaments.[2] In addition, damage to the deltoid and trapezius fascia, and

TABLE 8-36. CLASSIFICATION OF AC INJURIES AND CLINICAL FINDINGS

Type I	Isolated sprain of acromioclavicular ligaments Coracoclavicular ligaments intact Deltoid and trapezoid muscles intact Tenderness and mild pain at AC joint High (160-180 degrees) painful arc Resisted adduction is often painful Intervention is with TFM, ice, and pain-free AROM
Type II	AC ligament is disrupted Sprain of coracoclavicular ligament AC joint is wider; may be a slight vertical separation when compared to the normal shoulder Coracoclavicular interspace may be slightly increased Deltoid and trapezoid muscles intact Moderate to severe local pain Tenderness in coracoclavicular space PROM all painful at end range with horizontal adduction being the most painful Resisted abduction and abduction are often painful Intervention initiated with ice and pain-free AROM/PROM; TFM introduced on day 4
Type III	AC ligament is disrupted AC joint dislocated and the shoulder complex displaced inferiorly Coracoclavicular interspace 25%-100% greater than normal shoulder Coracoclavicular ligament is disrupted Deltoid and trapezoid muscles are usually detached from the distal end of the clavicle A fracture of the clavicle is usually present in patients under 13 years of age Arm held by patient in adducted position Obvious gap visible between acromion and clavicle AROM all painful; PROM painless if done carefully Piano key phenomenon (clavicle springs back after being pushed caudally) present
Type IV	AC ligament is disrupted AC joint dislocated and the clavicle anatomically displaced posteriorly into or through the trapezius muscle Coracoclavicular ligaments completely disrupted Coracoclavicular interspace may be displaced but may appear normal Deltoid and trapezoid muscles are detached from the distal end of the clavicle Clavicle displaced posteriorly; surgery indicated for types IV-VI
Type V	AC ligaments disrupted Coracoclavicular ligaments completely disrupted AC joint dislocated and gross disparity between the clavicle and the scapula (300%-500% greater than normal) Deltoid and trapezoid muscles are detached from the distal end of the clavicle Tenderness over entire lateral half of the clavicle
Type VI	AC ligaments disrupted Coracoclavicular ligaments completely disrupted AC joint dislocated and the clavicle anatomically displaced inferiorly to the clavicle or the coracoid process Coracoclavicular interspace reversed with the clavicle being inferior to the acromion or the coracoid process Deltoid and trapezoid muscles are detached from the distal end of the clavicle Cranial aspect of shoulder is flatter than opposite side. Often accompanied with clavicle or upper rib fracture and/or brachial plexus injury

AROM, active range of motion; PROM, passive range of motion; TFM, transverse friction massage.

Data from Allman FL Jr: Fractures and ligamentous injuries of the clavicle and its articulation. J Bone Joint Surg. 1967;49A:774-784; Rockwood CA Jr: Injuries to the acromioclavicular joint. In: Rockwood CA Jr., Green DP, eds. *Fractures in Adults, 2nd ed.* Philadelphia, PA: Lippincott. 1984:860-910; and Rockwood CA Jr., Young DC: Disorders of the acromioclavicular joint. In: Rockwood CA Jr., Matsen FA III, eds. *The Shoulder.* Philadelphia, PA: W.B. B Saunders. 1990:413-468.

TABLE 8-37. PHYSICAL THERAPY INTERVENTION FOR AC JOINT INJURIES

INJURY TYPE	INTERVENTION
Type I	Does not require immobilization Ice is recommended for pain. If return to sport involves contact or impact forces, a donut pad placed over the shoulder helps to protect the joint.
Type II	Patients are typically prescribed a sling as desired. ROM exercises are initiated as tolerated, often beginning with PROM to minimize muscle activation of the trapezius and deltoid. However, because the deltoid and trapezius fibers reinforce the AC joint capsule, specific strengthening exercises for these muscles are part of the long-term rehabilitation program. Return to function usually occurs within 2-3 weeks after injury
Type III	The most appropriate intervention is somewhat controversial and can be either surgical or conservative. The most commonly used device for reduction is the Kenny-Howard Harness.

rarely the skin, can occur.[2] Type IV injuries are characterized by posterior displacement of the clavicle.

- Type VI injuries have a clavicle inferiorly displaced into either a subacromial or subcoracoid position. These types (IV, V, VI) also have complete rupture of all the ligament complexes and are much rarer injuries than types I through III.[2]

Physical therapy intervention varies according to injury severity (Table 8-37).

ADHESIVE CAPSULITIS

Adhesive capsulitis, commonly referred to as *frozen shoulder* is associated with a number of factors, including:

- Female gender
- Age older than 40 years
- Post-trauma
- Diabetes
- Prolonged immobilization
- Thyroid disease
- Post-stroke or myocardial infarction
- Certain psychiatric conditions
- The presence of certain autoimmune diseases[175]

Nash and Hazelman[176] have described the concept of primary and secondary frozen shoulder:

- Primary: idiopathic in origin and insidious onset
- Secondary: either traumatic in origin, or related to a disease process, neurological, or cardiac condition

Adhesive capsulitis is diagnosed primarily by physical examination—patients demonstrate limited active and passive range of motion with a capsular pattern of restriction. The six ROM measurements that should be taken include flexion, external rotation at the side, external rotation in abduction, internal rotation in abduction, horizontal abduction, and functional internal rotation up the back.

The three classic stages of adhesive capsulitis include[177]:

1. The early painful stage (freezing): lasts 2 to 9 months. Patients have diffuse pain, difficulty with sleeping on the affected side, and restricted movement secondary to pain.
2. The stiffening stage (freezing): lasts 4 to 12 months. Characterized by progressive loss of ROM and decreased function.
3. Recovery stage (thawing): lasts 5 to 24 months. Characterized by gradual increases in ROM and decreased pain.

The primary goal of physical therapy is the restoration of the range of motion and focuses on the application of controlled tensile stresses using stretching and joint mobilizations to produce elongation of the restricting tissues.

- The patient with capsular restriction and low irritability may require aggressive soft tissue and joint mobilization.
- The patient with high irritability may require pain-easing manual therapy techniques.
- The patient with limited ROM due to nonstructural changes requires addressing the cause of the pain.

Surgical intervention (manipulation) is reserved for those patients that do not respond to conservative intervention.

Ankle Sprains

An ankle sprain, the most common injury in sports and recreational activities, can lead to chronic instability and impairment if left untreated. Most acute ankle injuries occur in people 21 to 30 years old, although injuries in the younger and older age groups tend to be more serious.

Lateral Ankle (Inversion) Sprain. Sprains of the lateral ligamentous complex represent 85% of ankle ligament sprains.[178,179] Lateral ligament sprains are more common than medial ligament sprains for two major reasons[180]:

1. The lateral malleolus projects more distally than the medial malleolus producing less bony obstruction to inversion than eversion
2. The deltoid ligament is much stronger than the lateral ligaments.

Lateral ankle sprains can be graded according to severity:

- Grade I sprains are characterized by minimum to no swelling and localized tenderness over the ATFL. These sprains require on the average 11.7 days before the full resumption of athletic activities.[181]
- Grade II sprains are characterized by localized swelling and more diffuse lateral tenderness. These sprains require approximately 2 to 6 weeks for return to full athletic function.[182,183]

Study Pearl

The ankle is stable in the neutral position or in dorsiflexion because the widest part of the talus is in the mortise. However ankle stability is decreased in plantar flexion as the narrow posterior portion of the talus is in the mortise. Thus, the most common mechanism of an ankle sprain is one of inversion and plantar flexion.

Study Pearl

The high ankle sprain (syndesmotic sprain), which occurs less frequently than the lateral ankle sprain, involves disruption of the ligamentous structures between the distal fibula and tibia, just proximal to the ankle joint.

- Grade III sprains are characterized by significant swelling, pain, and ecchymosis and should be referred to a specialist.[184] Grade III injuries may require greater than 6 weeks to return to full function. For acute grade III ankle sprains, the average duration of disability has been reported anywhere from 4.5 to 26 weeks, and only 25% to 60% of patients are symptom-free 1 to 4 years after injury.[185]

Once pain and inflammation are under control (4-14 days), the patient begins dynamic balance and proprioceptive exercises, with or without an external support. Exercises that promote ankle dorsiflexion past the neutral position, enabling a closer to normal walking pattern are introduced. Open chain (non-weight bearing) progressive resistive exercises with rubber tubing resistance are performed (2 sets of 30 reps each) for isolated plantar flexion, dorsiflexion, inversion, and eversion. Stationary cycling can also be performed (at a comfortable intensity for up to 30 minutes) to provide cardiovascular endurance training and controlled ankle range of motion.[186] Plyometric activities are introduced during the return to activity phase.

Anterior Cruciate Ligament Tear. Causes for an ACL injury have been divided into intrinsic and extrinsic factors.[187]

- Intrinsic factors include:
  - A narrow intercondylar notch
  - A weak ACL
  - Generalized overall joint laxity
  - Lower extremity malalignment
- Extrinsic factors include:
  - Abnormal quadriceps and hamstring relationships
  - Altered neuromuscular control
  - The shoe-surface interface
  - The playing surface
  - The athlete's playing style

ACL injury rates are two to eight times higher in women than in men participating in the same sports.[187,188]

All ACL tears (ie, sprains) are categorized as grade I, II, or III injuries. Ligament tears are classified according to the degree of injury, which ranges from overstretched ligament fibers (ie, partial or moderate tears) to ligament ruptures (ie, complete tears or disruptions).

Young athletes are more likely to sustain growth plate injuries (eg, avulsion fractures) rather than midsubstance tears because the epiphyseal cartilage in their growth plates is structurally weaker than their ligaments.[191,192]

Symptomatic ACL deficiencies in young athletes' knee joints are subject to the same long-term detrimental effects that occur in adult athletes.[193] Young athletes also may be more predisposed to more long-term degenerative knee conditions as the result of more years of chronic rotary knee instabilities from ACL deficiencies.[194]

Isolated ACL injuries are rare because the ACL functions in conjunction with the collateral ligaments of the knee. When the outer aspect of the knee receives a direct blow that causes valgus stress, the MCL often is torn first, followed by the ACL, which becomes the second component of a sports-related ACL injury.[195] Meniscal injuries

Study Pearl

A midsubstance tear indicates a central ligament tear as opposed to a tear at one of the ligament's bony attachment sites. Nearly all ACL tears are complete midsubstance tears.[189,190]

also can occur in conjunction with ACL tears. Approximately 49% of patients with sports-related ACL injuries have meniscal tears.[196]

Diagnoses of sports-related ACL injuries can be difficult. Thorough patient histories and physical examinations are essential for accurate diagnoses of ACL injuries. Patients commonly describe the sensation of their knee "popping" or "giving out" as their tibia subluxes anteriorly. Other signs and symptoms of ACL injuries include pain, immediate dysfunction, and instability in the involved knee, and the inability to walk without assistance. A classic sign of ACL injuries is acute hemarthrosis (ie, extravasation of blood into a joint or synovial cavity).[197] Atrophy of the quadriceps is an almost constant finding with patients who have a torn ACL.[198-202] During the examination, it is important for clinicians to examine the patient's contralateral knee for baseline comparisons. This especially is true in children who have inherent or congenital laxities (eg, knock-knee [genu valgum], back-knee [genu recurvatum]). It also is important to remember that the pain the patient experiences during the examination may affect the accuracy of the test results.

Magnetic resonance imaging (MRI) scans are useful for diagnosing ACL injuries, although their use in discriminating between complete and partial ACL tears is limited.[191] Diagnostic MRI scans, however, can detect associated meniscal tears that routine radiographs cannot show.[191]

Study Pearl

A noninvasive mechanical testing device, such as a KT-1000, can be used to highlight anterior–posterior knee ligament instability. These arthrometers assess the amount of displacement between the femur and the tibia at a given force. Although most patients who have a complete tear of the ACL have increased tibial translation on instrumented testing,[203] it is not known exactly how many of these patients will have "giving-way" of the knee or how many knees will have overt or latent damage of the cartilage within a few years.[204-206]

Avascular Necrosis of the Femoral Head

Avascular necrosis (AVN) of the femoral head is also known as aseptic necrosis or osteonecrosis. AVN results from a mechanical interruption of the circulation of the femoral head. The systemic administration of steroids and an excessive intake of alcohol are the two factors most often associated with non-traumatic avascular necrosis.

The clinical findings for AVN vary, and it is only when the femoral head becomes deformed, that limitations of motion in a non-capsular pattern occur. The pain, which is typically felt in the groin, proximal thigh, or buttock area, is usually exacerbated by weight bearing, but it is often present at rest. Axial loading of the joint as in the scour test, may reproduce the symptoms. A limp or antalgic gait is typically a late finding, and the functional disability is proportionate to the level of pain.

Although conservative intervention is aimed at limiting the stresses through the hip joint, and the use of a support, operative intervention (joint replacement) is generally recommended.

Bursitis

A bursitis is an inflammation of a bursa that occurs when the synovial fluid within the bursa becomes infected or irritated. Symptoms of bursitis include localized tenderness, warmth, edema, erythema, and loss of function. Common forms of bursitis include:

- Subacromial (subdeltoid) bursitis: Repetitive activities with an elevated arm most frequently cause inflammation of this bursa. Difficulty in GH abduction may occur, specifically from 70 to 100 degrees.

- Olecranon bursitis: Because of its superficial location, this bursa is easily traumatized from acute blows or chronic stress. Trauma of the skin and surrounding tissues makes the olecranon a frequent location for infectious bursitis.
- Iliopsoas bursitis: This type of bursitis is often associated with hip pathology (eg, rheumatoid arthritis, osteoarthritis) or recreational injury (eg, running). Pain from iliopsoas bursitis radiates down the anteromedial side of the thigh to the knee and is increased on extension, adduction, and internal rotation of the hip.
- Trochanteric bursitis: Trochanteric bursitis is the second most frequent cause of lateral hip pain.[207] The bursae become inflamed through either friction or direct trauma, such as a fall on the side of the hip. The reproduction of pain with palpation, or by stretching the iliotibial band (ITB) across the trochanter with hip adduction, or the extremes of internal or external hip rotation.[208] Resisted abduction, extension, or external rotation of the hip, are also painful.
- Ischial bursitis: Inflammation of this bursa commonly arises as a result of trauma, prolonged sitting on a hard surface (weaver bottom), or prolonged sitting in the same position (spinal cord injury).
- Prepatellar bursitis: Inflammation arises secondary to trauma or constant friction between the skin and the patella, most commonly when frequent forward kneeling is performed.
- Infrapatellar bursitis: The symptoms are often caused by frequent kneeling in an upright position and are located more distally than those of prepatellar bursitis.
- Pes anserine bursitis: This type of bursitis can result from an abnormal pull of any of the three tendons or to repetitive friction from a dysfunctional gait. Patients with anserine bursitis are commonly obese, older females with a history of osteoarthritis of the knees.

Study Pearl

The compression of the median nerve may result from a wide-variety of factors, several of which can easily be remembered using the pneumonic P.R.A.G.M.A.T.I.C.:

Pregnancy secondary to fluid retention.
Renal dysfunction.
Acromegaly.
Gout and pseudogout.
Myxedema or mass.
Amyotrophy. Neuralgic amyotrophy is the most likely diagnosis in patients who suddenly develop arm pain followed within a few days by arm paralysis in the distribution of single or multiple nerves or extending over multiple myotomes.
Trauma (repetitive or direct). About half of the cases of CTS are related to repetitive and cumulative trauma in the workplace, making it the occupational epidemic syndrome of our time.
Infection.
Collagen disorders. The incidence of carpal tunnel syndrome in patients with polyarthritis is high.

Other causes include rheumatoid arthritis, diabetes, hypothyroidism, and hemodialysis. Less common causes include incursion of the lumbrical muscles within the tunnel during finger movements, and hypertrophy of the lumbricales.

Carpal Tunnel Syndrome

Carpal tunnel syndrome (CTS), which is caused by entrapment of the median nerve within the carpal tunnel, may result in numbness, pain, or paresthesia of the thumb, index, and middle fingers (the median nerve distribution). CTS more commonly occurs between the fourth and sixth decades.

The diagnosis of carpal tunnel syndrome is most reliably made by an experienced clinician after a review of the patient's history and a physical examination.[209] The clinical features of this syndrome include:

- Intermittent pain and paresthesias in the median nerve distribution of the hand, which may become constant as the condition progresses.[210-213] The symptoms are typically worse at night, exacerbated by strenuous wrist movements, and can be associated with morning stiffness. The pain may radiate proximally into the forearm and arm.
- Muscle weakness and paralysis can occur on occasion.

The physical assessment focuses on an examination of the motor and sensory functions of the hand as compared to the uninvolved hand and includes Phalen's test, Tinel's sign, and the upper limb tension test (ULTT) for the median nerve.[210,214-216]

A number of medical tests can be used to help diagnose CTS. These include the median nerve conduction study and electromyogram (EMG) study. A carpal tunnel view radiograph may be the only view that shows abnormalities within the carpal tunnel.[217]

The conservative intervention for mild cases typically includes the use of splints, activity and ergonomic modification, isolated tendon excursion exercises, diuretics, and nonsteroidal anti-inflammatory drugs (NSAIDs).[218] Night splints appear to help reduce the nocturnal symptoms and allow the wrist to rest fully, although one study found that night splints did not significantly reduce intracarpal pressure when compared to controls who did not wear them.[219] Patient education is also important to avoid sustained pinching or gripping, repetitive wrist motions, and sustained positions of full wrist flexion.

Evaluation for surgical management is necessary for patients with atrophy of the thenar muscles, decreased sensation, and persistent symptoms that are intolerable despite conservative therapy.[220]

De Quervain's Tenosynovitis

De Quervain's disease is a form of stenosing tenosynovitis that occurs progressively and which affects the tendon sheaths of the first dorsal compartment of the wrist. The problems associated with this condition include a thickening of the extensor retinaculum, a narrowing of the fibro-osseus canal, and an eventual entrapment and compression of the tendons, especially during radial deviation.[221] The most common predisposing factors include[222,223]:

Overuse, repetitive tasks which involve overexertion of the thumb, or radial and ulnar deviation of the wrist. Such activities include golf, fly-fishing, typing, sewing, knitting, and scissor cutting.

Arthritis

Frequently, patients report a gradual and insidious onset of a dull ache over the radial aspect of the wrist made worse by turning doorknobs or keys. Examination of the wrist may reveal:

- A localized swelling and tenderness in the region of the radial styloid process and wrist pain radiating proximally into the forearm and distally into the thumb.
- Severe pain with wrist ulnar deviation and thumb flexion and adduction. A reproduction of the pain can also be reported with thumb extension and abduction.
- Crepitus of the tendons moving through the extensor sheath.
- Palpable thickening of the extensor sheath and of the tendons distal to the extensor tunnel.
- A loss of abduction of the carpometacarpal (CMC) joint of the thumb.
- A positive Finklestein's test (see "Special Tests of the Wrist and Hand").

Although the diagnosis is mostly clinical, posterior–anterior and lateral radiographs of the wrist can be obtained to rule out any bony pathology, such as a scaphoid fracture, radioscaphoid, or triscaphoid arthritis; and Kienböck's disease.

Conservative intervention includes rest, continuous immobilization through splinting with a thumb spica for 3 weeks, and anti-inflammatory medication. Following the removal of the splint, ROM exercises are prescribed, with a gradual progression to strengthening.

The more invasive intervention begins with cortisone injections. If two to three injections do not give relief, surgical tendon sheath release is an option.

DUPUYTREN'S CONTRACTURE

Dupuytren's disease, an active cellular process in the fascia of the hand, is characterized by the development of nodules in the palmar and digital fascia. These nodules occur in specific locations along longitudinal tension lines.[224,225] The appearance of the nodules is followed by the formation of tendon-like cords, which are due to the pathologic change in normal fascia.[226-228] The contractures form at the MCP joint, the PIP joint, and, occasionally, the DIP joint.[229]

The diagnosis of Dupuytren's disease in its early stages may be difficult, and is based on the palpable nodule, characteristic skin changes, changes in the fascia, and progressive joint contracture. The skin changes are caused by a retraction of the skin, resulting in dimples or pits. The disease is usually bilateral, with one hand being more severely involved. However, there appears to be no association with hand dominance. The patient may have one, two, or three rays involved in the more severely affected hand. The most commonly involved digit is the little finger, which is involved in approximately 70% of patients.

Conservative interventions have not yet proven to be clinically useful or of any long-term value in the treatment of established contractures. Surgery is the intervention of choice when the MCP joint contracts to 30 degrees and the deformity becomes a functional problem.[230] Scar management and splinting are an important part of the postoperative management. Active, active-assisted, and passive exercises are usually initiated at the first treatment session.

EPICONDYLITIS

Lateral Epicondylitis (Tennis Elbow). Lateral epicondylitis, which involves the muscles that control wrist extension and radial deviation, results in pain on the lateral aspect of the elbow, which is aggravated with movements of the wrist, by palpation over the tendon insertion site, or with use of the exensor muscles of the wrist.

> **Study Pearl**
>
> Histopathological studies have demonstrated that tennis elbow is not an inflammatory condition; rather, it is a degenerative condition.[231,232]

Tennis elbow is usually the result of overuse, but can be traumatic in origin. For example, participants of tennis, baseball, javelin, golf, squash, racquetball, swimming, and weightlifting who perform repetitive wrist extension against resistance are particularly at risk.

The pain of tennis elbow is often activity-related. Diffuse achiness and morning stiffness are also common complaints. Occasionally the pain is experienced at night and the patient may report frequent dropping of objects, especially if they are carried with the palm facing down.

Tenderness is usually found over the extensor carpi radialis brevis (ECRB) and extensor carpi radialis longus (ECRL), especially at the lateral epicondyle. The site of maximum tenderness is most commonly over the anterior aspect of the lateral epicondyle.

Lateral epicondylitis is a self-limiting complaint; without intervention, the symptoms will usually resolve within 8 to 12 months.[233] Poor technique, particularly with racket sports, is the cause of many elbow problems. Emphasis should be placed on recruiting the whole of the shoulder and trunk when hitting the ball, so as to dissipate the forces as widely as possible. In addition to correcting poor technique, patient education should address racket size, grip size, and string tension.

An exercise regimen consisting of progressive resistance exercise to the wrist extensors, with the elbow flexed to 90 degrees and also with the elbow straight is recommended.[234] This should be performed as a ten repetition maximum, morning and night. Gradually the weight must be increased so that the ten-repetition maximum is always maintained. Counterforce bracing[235] (such as the Count-R-Force brace from Medical Sports, Arlington, Virginia) has been shown to:

- Have a beneficial effect on the force couple imbalances, and altered movements associated with tennis elbow.[236-238]
- Decrease elbow angular acceleration.[239]
- Decrease electromyographic activity.[239]

However, contrary to popular belief, tennis elbow braces have been shown to have little effect in vibrational dampening.[240]

Surgery is indicated if the symptoms do not resolve despite properly performed nonoperative treatments lasting 6 months.

MEDIAL EPICONDYLITIS (GOLFER'S ELBOW)

Medial epicondylitis, which is less common than lateral epicondylitis, primarily involves a tendinopathy of some or all of the following structures: the common flexor origin, specifically the flexor carpi radialis, and the humeral head of the pronator teres.[241] the palmaris longus, flexor carpi ulnaris, and flexor digitorum superficialis.[242]

The mechanism for medial epicondylitis is not usually related to direct trauma, but rather to overuse. This commonly occurs for three reasons:

1. The flexor-pronator tissues fatigue in response to repeated stress.
2. There is a sudden change in the level of stress that predisposes the elbow to medial ligamentous injury.[243]
3. The ulnar collateral ligament fails to stabilize the valgus forces sufficiently.[244]

Chronic symptoms result from a loss of extensibility of the tissues, leaving the tendon unable to attenuate tensile loads.

The typical clinical presentation for medial epicondylitis is pain and tenderness over the flexor-pronator origin, slightly distal and anterior to the medial epicondyle, in a aggressive advanced-level athlete. The symptoms are typically exacerbated with either, resisted wrist flexion and pronation, or passive wrist extension and supination.

The conservative intervention for this condition initially involves rest, activity modification, and local modalities. Once the acute phase has passed, the focus is to restore the range of motion, and correct imbalances of flexibility and strength. The strengthening program is progressed to include concentric and eccentric exercises of the flexor pronator muscles. Splinting, or the use of a counterforce brace, may be a useful adjunct.

Finger Injuries

Boutonnière Deformity. The boutonnière or "buttonhole" deformity occurs with damage to the common extensor tendon that inserts on the base of the middle phalanx. Biomechanical factors then produce a deformity of extension of the MCP and DIP joints, and flexion of the PIP joint.

The conservative approach to this condition is based on severity. A mobile correctable deformity requires little more than immobilizing the PIP in full extension for 6 to 8 weeks, with the DIP and MCP joints held free. Gentle AROM exercises can begin for flexion and extension of the PIP joint at 4 to 8 weeks, with the splint being reapplied between exercises. General strengthening usually begins at 10 to 12 weeks.

Swan-Neck (Recurvatum) Deformity. The swan-neck deformity is characterized by a flexion deformity at the DIP, and hyperextension of the PIP joint, which results in an increased extensor force across the PIP joint and hyperextension at the PIP joint. The resultant loss of function includes an inability to bring the tips of the fingers into a grasp position.

The conservative intervention for swan-neck deformity is based on severity. If there is no loss of PIP joint flexion, a silver ring splint used for the correction of the PIP hyperextension.

Mallet Finger. A mallet finger deformity, one of the most common hand injuries sustained by the athletic population, involves a traumatic disruption of the terminal tendon with a resultant loss of active extension of the DIP joint.

The physical examination reveals a flexion deformity of the DIP joint, which can be extended passively but not actively due to a combination of zero tension being provided by the extensor digitorum communis (EDC) and the increased tone in the FDP.

Mallet deformities with an associated large fracture fragment are typically treated with 6 weeks of immobilization following open reduction and internal fixation.[245] The approach for other types includes closed reduction followed by 6 weeks of continuous dorsal splinting of the DIP in 0 degree of extension to 15 degrees of hyperextension (the PIP joint should be free to move).[245] Gentle progressive resistive exercises (PREs) for the hand are initiated at week 8. Unrestricted use usually occurs after 12 weeks.

Rupture of the Terminal Phalangeal Flexor (Jersey Finger). A Jersey finger, which involves a rupture of the FDP tendon from its insertion on the distal phalanx, is often misdiagnosed as it has no characteristic deformity.[245] The typical cause is forceful passive extension during simultaneous contraction of the FDP.

To test the integrity of the tendon, the clinician isolates the FDP by holding the MCP and PIP joints of the affected finger in full extension, and asks the patient to attempt to flex the DIP. If it flexes, it is intact. If not, it is ruptured.

The intervention varies from doing nothing, if function is not seriously affected, to surgical reattachment of the tendon.

Groin Strain

The hip adductor muscles are the most frequent causes of a groin starin, with the adductor longus being the most commonly injured.[246,247] Adductor strains are associated with jumping, running, kicking, and twisting activities.

The signs and symptoms associated with this condition include[248]:

- Twinging or stabbing pain in the groin area with quick starts and stops
- Edema or ecchymosis several days post injury
- Pain with manual resistance to hip adduction
- A palpable defect in severe ruptures
- Muscle guarding

The intervention involves the principles of PRICEMEM in the acute stage, followed by heat applications, hip adductor isometrics, and gentle stretching during the subacute phase to address any imbalance between the adductors and the abdominals. The intervention is progressed to a graded resistive program as tolerated and then a gradual return to full activity.

Hallux Valgus

Hallux valgus, a deformity of the first MTP joint in which the proximal phalanx is deviated laterally with respect to the first metatarsal, has been observed to occur almost exclusively in populations that wear shoes. Women have been observed to have hallux valgus in a rate of 9:1 compared with men.[249]

With increasing lateral deviation of the hallux, the sesamoids subluxate laterally, the hallux pronates, and the medial aspect of the first metatarsal head becomes more prominent. As a result, weight-bearing shifts from the first metatarsal head to the second metatarsal, and occasionally the third.

The intervention includes for the use of wider shoes and orthotics, or a toe spacer between the first and second toes.

Structural realignment of the first metatarsal varus may be necessary if pain persists.

Lumbar Herniated Nucleus Pulposus

A herniated nucleus pulposus (HNP) can occur due to a number of factors that cause a progressive decline in the water-retaining ability of the nucleus pulposus, and a decrease in the mechanical stiffness of the disk, which allows the annulus to bulge with a corresponding loss of disk and foramina height. Further degeneration may result in radial tears and leakage from the nuclear material. The resultant inflammatory response may cause a number of signs and symptoms including radiating pain without numbness, weakness, or loss of reflex.

The pertinent historical information begins with an analysis of the chief complaint:

- Does the patient's complaint concern dominant leg pain, dominant back pain, or a mixture of significant problems with both?
- Is the onset acute, subacute, or chronic?
- Under what circumstances did onset occur?
- What positions or actions cause an increase in symptoms? It is important to specifically exclude red flags, such as nonmechanical pain—pain at night unrelated to activity or movement, which may be indicative of a tumor or infection.
- Which activities is the patient unable or less able to perform and which activities exacerbate or moderate the pain?
- What is the patient's prior history, particularly of similar symptoms or response to treatment?
- What are the physical demands of the patient's occupation and daily activities?

The intervention focuses on the reduction of inflammation while encouraging the patient to perform activities of daily living as tolerated. The McKenzie exercise progression is recommended in most cases.

Iliotibial Band Friction Syndrome

ITBFS is a repetitive stress injury caused by friction of the iliotibial band as it slides over the prominent lateral femoral epicondyle at approximately 30 degrees of knee flexion.

Subjectively, the patient reports diffuse lateral knee pain with the repetitive motions of the knee (eg, climbing or descending stairs, cycling, and running). The progression of symptoms is often associated with changes in training surfaces, increased mileage, or training on crowned roads.

Objectively, there is localized tenderness to palpation at the lateral femoral condyle and/or on the anterior-lateral portion of the proximal tibia. The special tests for the ITB (Ober's test, prone lying test, and retinacular test) should be positive.

The intervention for ITBFS consists of activity modification, heat or ice applications, stretching of the iliotibial band and related structures, and strengthening of the hip abductors.

Surgical intervention is reserved for the more recalcitrant cases.

Little Leaguer's Elbow

Little Leaguer's elbow involves an avulsion lesion to the medial apophysis. The repetitive motions involved in the various phases of throwing, particularly during the late cocking and acceleration phases, place enormous strains on the immature elbow, which can result in the more serious conditions of osteochondritis, or an avulsion fracture.

Clinical findings include a history of pain on the medial side of the elbow, with and without throwing. Physical findings commonly include a persistent elbow discomfort or stiffness due to aggravation by the injury. A locking or "catching" sensation indicates a loose body.

Management is conservative and ranges from rest and elimination of the offending activity for 3 to 6 weeks to joint protection for several months if osteochondritis dissecans is present.

Surgical intervention is reserved for those patients with symptoms of a loose body, osteochondritis, or who fail to respond to conservative therapy.

Meniscal Injuries

Meniscal injuries are especially prevalent among those who play soccer, football, and basketball. Meniscal tears can be classified into two types, traumatic and degenerative:

1. Traumatic tears: most commonly found in young, athletically active individuals, and are frequently associated with ACL tears or, less commonly, with PCL tears. Injuries to the healthy meniscus are usually produced by a combination of compressive forces coupled with rotation of the flexed knee as it starts to move into extension. The type and location of the tear is determined by the magnitude and direction of the forces acting on the knee and the position of the knee when injured.
2. Degenerative tears: tend to occur in patients older than 40 years with no history of a traumatic event. These tears have minimal to no healing capacity.

The most common report following menical injury is one of joint-line pain, joint clicking or locking, and the knee giving way. Tests to evaluate the menisci are outlined in the "Special Tests of the Knee" section.

The treatment options for meniscal tears include no intervention, partial menisectomy, or meniscal repair depending on knowledge of the exact type, location, and extent of the meniscal tear. Determinations as to the course of treatment are based on several variables. These include the patient's age, the chronicity of the injury, the patient's activity requirements, and arthroscopic findings as to the location and length of the tear.

The outer 25% to 30% of the menisci is known to be vascular.[250] Tears in the vascular region are repairable as well as tears extending into the avascular midsubstance if vascularity is stimulated through abrasion of the perimeniscal synovium and/or implantation of a fibrin clot.[251-254] Next to an adequate blood supply, the most important factor influencing the prognosis of the meniscus repair is ACL stability.

Muscle Injury

The various types of muscle injury are outlined in Table 8-38.

Myosistis Ossificans. Myositis ossificans is an aberrant reparative process that causes benign heterotopic (ie, extraskeletal)

TABLE 8-38. CLASSIFICATION OF MUSCLE INJURY

TYPE	RELATED FACTORS
Exercise-induced muscle injury (delayed muscle soreness)	Increased activity Unaccustomed activity Excessive eccentric work Viral infections Secondary to muscle cell damage Onset at 24-48 hours after exercise
Strains First degree (mild): minimal structural damage; minimal hemorrhage; early resolution Second degree (moderate): partial tear; large spectrum of injury; significant early functional loss	Sudden overstretch Sudden contraction Decelerating limb Insufficient warm-up Lack of flexibility
Third degree (severe): complete tear; may require aspiration; may require surgery	Increasing severity of strain associated with greater muscle fiber death, more hemorrhage, and more eventual scarring Steroid use or abuse
Contusions Mild, moderate, severe Intramuscular vs intermuscular	Previous muscle injury Collagen disease
Avulsions Bony	Direct blow, associated with increasing muscle trauma and tearing of fiber proportionate to severity
Apophyseal Muscle	Specific sites vulnerable May be complication of stress fractures Osteoporosis Skeletally immature but well-developed muscle strength Associated with steroid injection or generalized collagen disorders

Data from Reid DC: *Sports Injury Assessment and Rehabilitation.* New York, NY: Churchill Livingstone; 1992.

ossification in soft tissue.[255-259] Myositis ossificans manifests in two forms.

- Myositis ossificans circumscripta: can develop either in response to soft tissue injury (eg, blunt trauma, stab wound, fracture/dislocation, or surgical incision) or can occur without known injury. Proposed mechanisms for atraumatic myositis ossificans include nondocumented trauma, repeated small mechanical injuries, and nonmechanical injuries caused by ischemia or inflammation. Most ossifications (ie, 80%) arise in the thigh or arm. Other sites include intercostal spaces, erector spinae, pectoralis muscles, glutei, and the chest.
- Myositis ossificans progressive: an autosomal dominant genetic disorder. While there is no proven medical therapy, patients with this condition may be administered cortisone and adrenocorticotropin during acute episodes.

Once diagnosed, the body part is immediately immobilized for about 2 to 4 weeks. Following the immobilization a regime of gradually increased exercise is initiated to promote a greater range of motion. Pain medications may be indicated, as are other supportive measures, especially occupational therapy, to facilitate functioning.

Osteoarthritis

Historically, osteoarthritis has been divided into primary and secondary forms:

- Primary. Primary osteoarthritis (OA) is an idiopathic phenomenon, occurring in previously intact joints, that is related to the aging process and typically occurs in older individuals. Most investigators believe that degenerative alterations primarily begin in the articular cartilage, as a result of either excessive loading of a healthy joint or relatively normal loading of a previously disturbed joint. These alterations appear to occur in the following sequence:
  - External forces accelerate the catabolic effects of the chondrocytes and disrupt the cartilaginous matrix.
  - Enzymatic destruction increases cartilage degradation, which is accompanied by decreased proteoglycans and collagen synthesis.
  - Changes in the proteoglycans render the cartilage less resistant to compressive forces in the joint and more susceptible to the effects of stress.
  - The decreased strength of the cartilage is compounded by adverse alterations of the collagen.
  - Elevated levels of collagen degradation place excessive stresses on the remaining fibers, eventually leading to mechanical failure.
  - The diminished elastic return and reduced contact area of the cartilage, coupled with the cyclic nature of joint loading, causes the situation to worsen over time.
  - Microscopic flaking and fibrillations develop along the normally smooth articular cartilage surface. The loss of cartilage results in a loss of the joint space.
  - Progressive erosion of the damaged cartilage occurs until the underlying bone is exposed. Bone denuded of its protective cartilage continues to articulate with the opposing surface.
  - Eventually, the increasing stresses exceed the biomechanical yield strength of the bone.

The subchondral bone responds with vascular invasion and increased cellularity, becoming thickened and dense (eburnation) at areas of pressure. Furthermore, the traumatized subchondral bone may undergo cystic degeneration, due to either osseous necrosis secondary to chronic impaction or the intrusion of synovial fluid. At nonpressure areas along the articular margin, vascularization of subchondral marrow, osseous metaplasia of synovial CT, and ossifying cartilaginous protrusions lead to irregular outgrowth of new bone (osteophytes). Fragmentation of these osteophytes or of the articular cartilage itself results in intra-articular loose bodies (joint mice).

Primary OA occurs most commonly in the hands, particularly in the distal interphalangeal (DIP) joints, proximal interphalangeal (PIP) joints, and first carpometacarpal joints. Deep, achy, joint pain exacerbated by extensive use is the primary symptom. Also, reduced range of motion and crepitus are frequently present. Joint malalignment may be visible. Heberden nodes, which represent palpable osteophytes in the DIP joints, are characteristic in women but not men. (Heberden nodes are features of OA, not rheumatoid arthritis, and they have no known association with glenohumeral disease or inguinal lymphadenopathy.) Inflammatory changes are typically absent or at least not pronounced.

- Secondary. Secondary OA is a degenerative disease of the synovial joints that results from some predisposing condition, usually trauma that has adversely altered the articular cartilage and/or subchondral bone of the affected joints. Secondary OA often occurs in relatively young individuals.

The medical intervention for OA includes:

- Nonsteroidal anti-inflammatory drugs (NSAIDs)
- Corticosteroid injections
- Topical analgesics
- Surgical joint replacement

The goals of a physical therapy intervention include:

- The reduction of pain and muscle spasm through the use of modalities and relaxation training
- Therapeutic exercises to:
  - Maintain or improve range of motion
  - Correct muscle imbalances
  - Strengthening exercises
  - Flexibility exercises
  - Improve balance and ambulation
- Provide assistive devices as needed (canes, walkers, orthotics, reachers etc.)
- Aerobic conditioning using low to nonimpact exercises (walking program, pool exercises)
- Patient education and empowerment:
  - Joint protection strategies
  - Energy conservation techniques
  - Activities to avoid
- Promotion of healthy lifestyle, eg, weight reduction

Osteochondritis Dissecans. Osteochondritis dissecans (OCD) is a term for osteochondral fracture. OCD is caused by blood deprivation in the subchondral bone. This loss of blood flow causes the subchondral bone to die in a process called avascular necrosis. The bone is then reabsorbed by the body, leaving the articular cartilage it supported prone to damage. Although rare, OCD is an important cause of joint pain in physically active adolescents, but because their bones are still growing, adolescents are more likely than adults to recover from OCD.[260-267]

Clinical findings include pain and swelling of the affected joint which catches and locks during movement. Physical examination typically reveals an effusion, tenderness, and crepitus.

Nonsurgical treatment is rarely an option as the capacity for articular cartilage to heal is limited. As a result, even moderate cases require some form of surgery. Postoperative rehabilitation involves a period of immobilization while maintaining muscle strength using isometric exercises that help restore muscle lost to atrophy without disturbing the cartilage of the affected joint. Once the immobilization period has ended, continuous passive motion (CPM) and/or low impact activities, such as walking or swimming are introduced.

Osteomyelitis. Osteomyelitis is an infectious process of the bone and its marrow. The term can refer to infections caused by pyogenic microorganisms, but can also be used to describe other sources of infection such as tuberculosis, or specific fungal infections (mycotic osteomyelitis), parasitic infections (Hydatid disease), viral infections, or syphilitic infections (Charcot arthropathy).[268-272]

Findings at physical examination may include the following:

- Fever or no fever
- Edema
- Warmth
- Tenderness to palpation
- Reduction in the use of the extremity

Diagnosis of osteomyelitis is often based on radiologic results showing a lytic center with a ring of sclerosis, but a culture of material taken from a bone biopsy is needed to identify the specific pathogen. Osteomyelitis often requires prolonged antibiotic therapy, with a course lasting a matter of weeks or months. Osteomyelitis also may require surgical debridement. Severe cases may lead to the loss of a limb.

Paget's Disease. Paget's disease (osteitis deformans) of bone is an osteometabolic disorder. The disease is described as a focal disorder of accelerated skeletal remodeling that may affect one or more bones.[273-282] This produces a slowly progressive enlargement and deformity of multiple bones. Despite intensive studies and widespread interest, its etiology remains obscure. Complications include pathological fractures, delayed union, progressive skeletal deformities, chronic bone pain, neurological compromise of the peripheral and central nervous systems with facial or ocular nerve compression and spinal stenosis, and Pagetic arthritis.

- Involvement of the lumbar spine may produce symptoms of clinical spinal stenosis.
- Involvement of the cervical and thoracic spine may predispose to myelopathy.

Although this disorder may be asymptomatic, when symptoms do occur, they occur insidiously. Paget's disease is managed either medically or surgically.

PATELLAR TENDINITIS

Patellar tendinitis (Jumper's knee) is an overuse condition frequently associated with eccentric overloading during deceleration activities such as repeated jumping and landing, or downhill running.

The diagnosis of patellar tendinitis is based on a detailed history, and careful palpation of the tendons.

Study Pearl

Some feel that the term "patellar tendinitis" is a misnomer because the patellar "tendon," which connects two bones, is technically a ligament.

A number of protocols have been recommended for the conservative intervention of patellar tendonitis:

- Grade I lesions, characterized by no significant functional impairment and pain only after the activity, are addressed with an adequate warm-up and ice massage after the activity.
- Grade II-III strains: activity modification, thermal modalites to the area.[283]

Surgical intervention, which is only usually required if significant tendinosis develops, is successful in the majority of patients.

Patellofemoral Dysfunction

Anterior knee pain or patellofemoral pain syndrome (PFS) is characterized by pain in the vicinity of the patella, which is worsened by sitting and and during activities that require knee flexion and forceful contraction of the quadriceps (eg, during squats, ascending/descending stairs). The pain, which is characteristically located behind the kneecap (ie, retropatellar), may worsen if the aggravating activity is performed repeatedly.

Although PFS can occur in anyone, particularly athletes, women who are not athletic appear to be more prone to this problem than men who are not athletic. The impairments resulting from patellofemoral dysfunction have been related to problems that cannot be improved by physical therapy, and those that can. The former include anatomical variance (femoral trochlear dysplasia, patellar morphology and the amount of congruence of the patellofemoral, the natural positioning of the patella [alta/baja] joint), and gender (females are more predisposed).

The usual physical findings are localized around the knee:

- Tenderness along the facets of the patella.
- An apprehension sign may be elicited by manually fixing the position of the patella against the femur and having the patient contract the ipsilateral quadriceps.
- Crepitus may be present.
- An alteration in the Q-angle.
- Excessive foot pronation, excessive knee valgus, or an antalgic gait pattern.

The focus of the intervention is to control the pain and inflammation. The basic exercise principles for management of PFS are to restore muscle balance within the quadriceps group, and to improve flexibility of the iliotibial band, hip, hamstring, and gastrocnemius. Patellar taping techniques (McConnell method) or soft knee braces have been advocated to reduce the friction on the patella and to control the tracking position of the patella.

Plantar Fasciitis

Plantar fasciitis is an inflammatory process of the plantar fascia and is a common cause of inferior heel pain. Plantar fasciitis is usually unilateral, although both feet can be affected.

Common findings include a history of pain and tenderness on the plantar medial aspect of the heel, especially during initial weight bearing in the morning, at the end of the day, or after a period of sitting.

Upon palpation there is typically localized pain along the medial edge of the fascia or at its origin on the anterior edge of the calcaneus. To test for plantar fasciitis, the fascia needs to be put on stretch with a bowstring type test. The patient's heel is manually fixed in eversion. The clinician takes hold of the first metatarsal, and places it in dorsiflexion, before extending the big toe as far as possible. Pain should be elicited at the medial tubercle.

A number of interventions have been suggested over the years for the intervention of plantar fasciitis, which vary from night splinting and orthotics to stretching (gastrocnemius) and strengthening of the leg muscles and foot intrinsics, and extracorporeal shock wave lithotripsy[284]

RHEUMATOID DISEASES

Rheumatoid Arthritis. Rheumatoid arthritis (RA) is a disease that causes significant damage to the soft tissues and periarticular structures.[285]

The physical therapy examination of the patient with suspected rheumatoid arthritis involves[285]:

- Measurement of joint range of motion. Goniometric measurement of passive range of motion (PROM) is indicated at all affected joints following a gross range of motion screening.
- Measurement of strength: application of standard manual muscle tests to determine strength and pain at various points in the range.
- Measurement of independence with functional activities. Functional measures may include ADL, work, and leisure activities. The choice of a functional instrument is influenced by several factors including the characteristics and needs of the individual patient, the level and depth of information required, and its predictive value in gauging the efficacy of treatment.
- Measurement of joint stability: the ligamentous laxity of any affected joint should be fully investigated.
- Measurement of mobility and gait.
- Measurement of sensory integrity.
- Measurement of psychological status.
- Determination of level of impairment including deconditioning, pain, weakness, cardiopulmonary complications, neurological manifestations, environmental barriers, and fatigue.

Based on the pathomechanics of the rheumatoid process, the following concepts form the foundation of any intervention to manage RA[285]:

- Decrease pain.
- Control the inflammation.
- Increase or maintain the ROM of all joints sufficient for functional activities. Focus on joint systems rather than isolated joints.
- Increase or maintain muscle strength sufficient for functional activities.

Study Pearl

The signs and symptoms of rheumatoid arthritis include:

- Systemic manifestations: morning stiffness lasting for more than 3 minutes, anorexia, weight loss, and fatigue.
- Arthritis of three or more joint areas: the 14 more commonly involved joints include the right or left PIP, MCP, wrists, elbow, knee, ankle, and MTP joints. In the hand, many common deformities can be seen, such as ulnar deviation of the MCP joints, radial deviation of the carpometacarpal block, boutonnière deformity, and swan-neck deformities of the digits.
- Muscle atrophy and myositis
- Tenosynovitis
- Positive laboratory tests: elevated erythrocyte sedimentation rate (ESR) or C-reactive protein; synovial fluid analysis
- Radiographic findings

- Increase joint stability and decrease any mechanical stress on all affected joints. The clinician should target functional activities that require specific techniques of joint protection.
- Increase endurance for all functional activities.
- Promote independence in all ADL, including bed mobility and transfers.
- Improve efficiency and safety of gait pattern.
- Establish patterns of adequate physical activity or exercise to maintain or improve musculoskeletal and cardiovascular fitness and general health.
- Educate the patient, family, and other personnel to promote the individual's capacity for self-management.
- Consider the type of rheumatoid disease:
  - The type in which scarring outweighs the articular damage. Patients with stiff joints because of scarring do poorly after soft tissue surgery. Patients in this group require aggressive and sustained therapy, often for 3 to 4 months.
  - The type in which joint laxity and tissue laxity become difficult to stabilize after soft tissue procedures. The patients in this group require careful treatment and control of the ROM and the direction of motion by the use of splints for many months after surgery.

Juvenile Rheumatoid Arthritis

Refer to Chapter 16.

Gout. Gout (known as podagra when it involves the big toe) is the most common form of inflammatory arthritis in men older than 40 years of age, and appears to be on the increase.[286] Gout is caused by the accumulation of uric acid crystals in synovial joints. The rising prevalence of gout is thought to stem from dietary changes, environmental factors, increasing longevity, subclinical renal impairment, and the increased use of drugs causing hyperuricemia, particularly diuretics.[287]

Gout can present in a number of ways, although the most usual is a recurrent attack of acute inflammatory arthritis (red, tender, hot, swollen) of the involved joint. Diagnosis is confirmed clinically by the visualization of the characteristic crystals in joint fluid.

Ankylosing Spondylitis. Ankylosing spondylitis (AS, also known as Bekhterev's or Marie-Strümpell disease) is a chronic rheumatoid disorder. The patient is usually between 15 and 40 years of age.[288] Although males are affected more frequently than females, mild courses of AS are more common in the latter.[289]

The disease includes involvement of the anterior longitudinal ligament and ossification of the disk, thoracic zygapophysial joints, costovertebral joints, and manubriosternal joints. This multijoint involvement makes the checking of chest expansion measurements a required test in this region. In time, AS progresses to involve the whole spine and results in spinal deformities, including flattening of the lumbar lordosis, kyphosis of the thoracic spine, and hyperextension of the cervical spine. These changes, in turn, result in flexion contractures of the hips and knees, with significant morbidity and disability.[289]

The most characteristic feature of the back pain associated with AS is pain at night.[290] Patients often awaken in the early morning (between 2 and 5 am) with back pain and stiffness, and usually either take a shower or exercise before returning to sleep.[289] Back ache during the day is typically intermittent irrespective of exertion or rest.[289]

Calin and colleagues[291] describe five screening questions for AS:

1. Is there morning stiffness?
2. Is there improvement in discomfort with exercise?
3. Was the onset of back pain before age 40 years?
4. Did the problem begin slowly?
5. Has the pain persisted for at least 3 months?

Using at least four positive answers to define a "positive" result, the sensitivity of these questions was 0.95 and specificity, 0.85.[291] A human leukocyte antigen (HLA) haplotype association (HLA-B27) has been found with ankylosing spondylitis.[289]

Peripheral arthritis is uncommon in AS, but when it occurs, it is usually late in the course of the arthritis.[292] The arthritis usually occurs in the lower extremities in an asymmetric distribution, with involvement of the "axial" joints, including shoulders and hips, more common than involvement of more distal joints.[289,293]

Inspection usually reveals a flat lumbar spine and gross limitation of side bending in both directions. Mobility loss tends to be bilateral and symmetric. There is loss of spinal elongation on flexion (Schober's test), although this can occur in patients with chronic low back pain or spinal tumors and is thus not specific for inflammatory spondylopathies.[294] The patient may relate a history of costochondritis and, upon examination, rib springing may give a hard end-feel. Basal rib expansion often is decreased. The glides of the costotransverse joints and distraction of the sternoclavicular joints are decreased, and the lumbar spine exhibits a capsular pattern.

As the disease progresses, the pain and stiffness can spread up the entire spine, pulling it into forward flexion, so that the patient adopts the typical stooped-over position. The patient gazes downward, the entire back is rounded, the hips and knees are semiflexed, and the arms cannot be raised beyond a limited amount at the shoulders.[295]

Exercise is particularly important for these patients to maintain the mobility of the spine and involved joints for as long as possible, and to prevent the spine from stiffening in an unacceptable kyphotic position. A strict regimen of daily exercises, which include positioning and spinal extension exercises, breathing exercises, and exercises for the peripheral joints, must be followed.[296] Several times a day, patients should lie prone for 5 minutes, and they should be encouraged to sleep on a hard mattress and avoid the side lying position. Swimming is the best routine sport.

Systemic Lupus Erythematosus. Systemic lupus erythematosus (SLE) is a chronic inflammatory autoimmune disorder which can affect any organ or system of the body.

Clinical manifestations for the physical therapist to note include:

- Musculoskeletal involvement—arthralgias and arthritis constitute the most common presenting manifestations of SLE.
- Cardiopulmonary signs—pleuritis, pericarditis, and dyspnea.

Study Pearl

- Patients with psoriatic arthritis have less tenderness over both affected joints and tender points than patients with rheumatoid arthritis.[297]
- The spondyloarthropathy of psoriatic arthritis may be distinguished from ankylosing spondylitis (AS) by the pattern of the sacroiliitis.[298] Whereas sacroiliitis in AS tends to be symmetric, affecting both sacroiliac joints to the same degree, it tends to be asymmetric in psoriatic arthritis,[293] and patients with psoriatic arthritis do not have as severe a spondyloarthropathy as patients with AS.[288]

- Neurologic involvement—headaches, depression, seizures, peripheral neuropathy (Raynaud's phenomenon).
- Kidney dysfunction or failure.

Physical therapy goals include:

- Patient education on how to control and restrict activities—energy conservation.
- Careful observation for signs of a renal failure such as weight gain, edema, or hypertension.
- Patient education on how to warm and protect the hands and feet if Raynaud's phenomenon is present.

Psoriatic Arthritis. Psoriatic arthritis, an inflammatory arthritis, affects men and women with equal frequency.[293] Its peak onset is in the fourth decade of life, although it may occur in children and in older adults. Psoriatic arthritis can manifest in one of a number of patterns.

Another articular feature of psoriatic arthritis is the presence of dactylitis, tenosynovitis (often digital, in flexor and extensor tendons and in the Achilles tendon), and enthesitis.[298] The presence of erosive disease in the distal interphalangeal joints is typical.[298]

Nail lesions occur in more than 80% of the patients with psoriatic arthritis, and have been found to be the only clinical feature distinguishing patients with psoriatic arthritis from patients with uncomplicated psoriasis.[299] Other extra-articular features include iritis, urethritis, and cardiac impairments similar to those seen in AS, although less frequently.[298]

Psoriatic arthritis, which may result in significant joint damage and disability, is treated in a similar fashion to that of rheumatoid arthritis.

Reactive Arthritis. Reactive arthritis, formerly known as Reiter syndrome, refers to an acute nonpurulent arthritis that complicates an infection elsewhere in the body. Reactive arthritis falls under the rheumatic disease category of seronegative spondyloarthropathies, which includes ankylosing spondylitis, psoriatic arthritis and arthritis associated with inflammatory bowel disease.[300-304] Reactive arthritis is triggered following enteric or urogenital infections. The symptoms, which generally appear within 1 to 3 weeks from onset of inciting episode of urethritis/cervicitis or diarrhea, include eye inflammation, fatigue, fever (usually low grade), malaise, asymmetric joint stiffness (primarily involving the knees, ankles, and feet), enthesopathy, and cutaneous lesions.

Sjögren's Syndrome. Sjögren's syndrome (SS) is an autoimmune disorder primarily characterized by lymphocytic infiltrates in the exocrine glands. Typically, most patients present with sicca symptoms, such as xerophthalmia (dry eyes), xerostomia (dry mouth), and parotid gland enlargement.[305-311] Additional features include arthralgia, arthritis, Raynaud phenomenon, myalgia, pulmonary disease, gastrointestinal disease, leukopenia, anemia, lymphadenopathy, neuropathy, vasculitis, renal tubular acidosis, and lymphoma.

SS is sometimes called primary SS when no other underlying rheumatic disorder is present, whereas SS is sometimes called secondary SS if it is associated with another underlying rheumatic disease, such as systemic lupus erythematosus (SLE), rheumatoid arthritis (RA), or scleroderma (Scl). The pathogenesis of SS is not known.

Rotator Cuff Tendonitis

Rotator cuff tendon problems are the most frequent cause of shoulder problems. These problems occur because of trauma, attrition, and the anatomical structure of the subacromial space. The supraspinatus is the tendon most often affected. Rotator cuff tears are described by size, location, direction and depth.[312] Characteristic signs and symptoms include:

- Complaints of a dull ache radiating into the upper and lower arm. This ache is worse after activity, at night and with actions such as reaching above the head or putting on a coat.
- Painful arc: The pain may begin around 50 to 60 degrees of abduction in patients with shoulder immobility.
- Palpable anterior tenderness over the coracoacromial ligament, the biceps tendon, and at the supraspinatus insertion.
- Weakness: The amount of weakness is directly related to the size of the tear.[313]

The conservative intervention for patients with a partial tear varies, but typically involves a gradual progression of range of motion, and strengthening exercises for the rotator cuff muscles and the scapular stabilizers.[317-320]

The indications for a surgical repair are persistent pain that interferes with activities of daily living, work, or sports; patients who are unresponsive to a 4- to 6-month period of conservative care; or active young patients (younger than 50 years of age) with an acute full-thickness tear.[321]

Study Pearl

Subacromial impingement syndrome (SIS) is closely related to rotator cuff disease of which there are a number of variants:.

- Anterior (external) impingement, of which there are two types:
  - Primary impingement: structural impingement of the rotator cuff beneath the coracromial arch as a result of subacromial overcrowding.
  - Secondary impingement: results from glenohumeral instability and/or tensile overload of the rotator cuff and subsequent poor control of the humeral head during overhead activities.[314-316]
- Posterior (internal) impingement: abnormal contact between the rotator cuff undersurface and the posterosuperior glenoid rim.

A glenohumeral internal rotation deficit (GIRD) is created by progressive contracture of the posterior glenohumeral capsule and decreased static and dynamic flexibility of the posterior shoulder muscles.

Scaphoid Fracture

The scaphoid is the most commonly fractured carpal bone.[322-325] Accurate early diagnosis of scaphoid fracture is critical to avoid long-term pain, loss of mobility, and decreased function.[326]

There is a high incidence of delayed healing or nonunion with scaphoid fractures due to its scant blood supply.

The most common cause of a scaphoid fracture is from a fall on an outstretched hand (FOOSH) with the wrist positioned in pronation. Patients typically complain of localized dorsal wrist pain with tenderness over the anatomic snuffbox. On physical examination, little swelling may be noted, although loss of the concavity of the anatomic snuff box is frequently seen.[327] A reliable test for scaphoid injury is axial compression of the thumb along its longitudinal axis.[328,329] This test translates force directly across the scaphoid, and should elicit pain if there is a fracture.[328]

Current management for a scaphoid fracture is immobilization in a long-arm or short-arm thumb spica cast, with the wrist position, and length of immobilization dependent on the location of the fracture.

Once the splint is removed, AROM exercises for wrist flexion and extension, and radial and ulnar deviation are initiated, with PROM to the same motions and gentle strengthening exercises beginning after approximately 2 weeks. The exercise program is progressed to include weight-bearing activities, plyometrics, open- and closed-chain exercises and neuromuscular reeducation, before finally progressing to functional and sports specific exercises and activities. A wrist and thumb immobilization splint can be fabricated to wear between exercises and at night.

Study Pearl

Skeletal demineralization, caused by an imbalance between bone formation and bone resorption, may be a primary disorder or may be secondary to a variety of other diseases or disorders such as osteomalacia and hyperparathyroidism.

Skeletal Demineralization. Skeletal demineralization refers to a loss of mass and calcium content from the bones. Skeletal demineralization can vary in severity:

- Less severe bone loss: osteopenia
- More severe bone loss: osteoporosis

Risk factors for skeletal demineralization include those that are modifiable and those that are non-modifiable. The non-modifiable risk factors include:

- Gender
- Race
- Age
- Family history
- Body size
- Early menopause

The modifiable risk factors include:

- Use of specific medications
- Low calcium intake
- Low vitamin D levels
- Estrogen deficiency
- Excessive alcohol intake
- Cigarette smoking
- Physical inactivity
- Prolonged overuse of thyroid hormone

Study Pearl

Osteoporosis accounts for the largest number of fractures among the elderly.

Osteoporosis. Osteoporosis is a systemic skeletal disorder characterized by decreased bone mass and deterioration of bony microarchitecture.[331-341] Osteoporosis results from a combination of genetic and environmental factors that affect both peak bone mass and the rate of bone loss. These factors include medications, diet, race, sex, lifestyle, and physical activity.

Osteoporosis may be either primary or secondary.

- Primary: Primary osteoporosis is subdivided into types 1 and 2.
  - Type 1, or postmenopausal, osteoporosis is thought to result from gonadal (ie, estrogen, testosterone) deficiency, resulting in accelerated bone loss. An increased recruitment and responsiveness of osteoclast precursors and an

increase in bone resorption, which outpaces bone formation, occurs. After menopause, women experience an accelerated bone loss of 1% to 5% per year for the first 5 to 7 years. The end result is a decrease in trabecular bone and an increased risk of Colles and vertebral fractures.
- Type 2, or senile, osteoporosis occurs in women and men because of decreased formation of bone and decreased renal production of 1,25(OH)2 D3 occurring late in life. The consequence is a loss of cortical and trabecular bone and increased risk for fractures of the hip, long bones, and vertebrae.

- Secondary: Secondary osteoporosis, also called type 3 occurs secondary to medications, especially glucocorticoids, or other conditions that cause increased bone loss by various mechanisms.

Osteoporosis can occur in either a generalized or a regional form. The cardinal feature is a fracture, and the clinical picture depends on the fracture site. Vertebral fracture often manifests as acute back pain after bending, lifting, or coughing or as asymptomatic progressive kyphosis with loss of height. Most fractures occur in the mid-to-lower thoracic or upper lumbar spine. The pain is described variably as sharp, nagging, or dull; movement may exacerbate pain; and, sometimes, pain radiates to the abdomen.

Acute pain usually resolves after 4 to 6 weeks. When kyphosis becomes severe, the patient may develop a restrictive pattern of respiratory impairment.

Forearm, hip, and proximal femoral fractures usually occur after falls, with forward falls often resulting in Colles fractures and backward falls resulting in hip fractures. Rib fractures are most often associated with osteoporosis secondary to corticosteroid use or Cushing's syndrome, but they can also be observed with other etiologies.

To definitively diagnose osteoporosis, one must perform some type of quantitative imaging study on the bone in question. Medical and screening tests of bone mineral density are available:

- Screening tests: include finger densitometry and heel (calcaneal) ultrasonography.
- Medical tests: include single photon absorptiometry (SPA) and dual energy x-ray absorptiometry (DXA). Radiographs may show fractures or other conditions, such as osteoarthritis, disk disease, or spondylolisthesis. Osteopenia (low bone density) may be apparent as radiographic lucency but is not always noticeable until 30% of bone mineral is lost.

Bone mineral density (BMD) testing is the best predictor of fracture risk. Although measurement at any site can be used to assess overall fracture risk, measurement at a particular site is the best predictor of fracture risk at that site.

Osteomalacia. Osteomalacia is characterized by incomplete mineralization of normal osteoid tissue following closure of the growth plates. Rickets is defined as the failure of osteoid to calcify in a growing person or animal. Failure of osteoid to calcify in the adult is called

Study Pearl

Osteopenia (low bone density) may be apparent as radiographic lucency but is not always noticeable until 30% of bone mineral is lost.[342,343]

Study Pearl

Cushing's syndrome is a hormonal disorder caused by prolonged exposure of the body's tissues to high levels of the hormone cortisol. Symptoms vary, but most people have upper body obesity, rounded (moon) face, increased fat around the neck, and thinning arms and legs. In addition Cushing's syndrome is associated with severe fatigue, hypertension, and increased risk of fracture.

Study Pearl

BMD is reported as a T-score, which compares the patient's BMD to that of a healthy young adult.

Study Pearl

Effective medical therapy is available to help prevent and treat osteoporosis, including gonadal hormone replacement, calcitonin, selective estrogen-receptor modulators, and bisphosphonates.[340] However, these agents reduce bone resorption with little, if any, effect on bone formation.[340]

Study Pearl

Vitamin D maintains calcium and phosphate homeostasis through its action on bone, the GI tract, kidneys, and parathyroid glands. Vitamin D may be supplied in the diet or produced from a sterol precursor in the skin following exposure to ultraviolet light. Sequential hydroxylation then is required to produce the metabolically active form of vitamin D.

osteomalacia. Normal bone mineralization depends on interdependent factors that supply adequate calcium and phosphate to the bones. Clinically, osteomalacia is manifested by progressive generalized bone pain, muscle weakness, hypocalcemia, pseudofractures. In its late stages, osteomalacia is characterized by a waddling gait.[344]

Because anyone can be at risk for developing osteopenia or osteoporosis, every patient should be questioned regarding family history of bone disease and risk factors for low peak bone mass.

The physical therapy interevntion for skeletal demineralization includes:

- Weight-bearing and aerobic exercise, which have been shown to have a positive effect on BMD, although the exact mechanism is not known.[339,345,346] Regular exercise should be encouraged in all patients, including children and adolescents in order to strengthen the skeleton during the maturation process. In addition, exercise also improves agility and balance, thereby reducing the risk of falls.
- Postural correction and training: should address walking, standing, and sitting.
- Pain control methods: use of adjunctive interventions (see Chapter 18).

Spinal Stenosis (Degenerative). Degenerative spinal stenosis (DSS) involves a narrowing of the spinal canal, nerve root canal (lateral recess), or intervertebral foramina of the lumbar spine. DSS is predominantly a disorder of patients older than 65 years.[347] Lumbar spinal stenosis may be classified as central or lateral[348]:

- Central stenosis is characterized by a narrowing of the spinal canal around the thecal sac containing the cauda equina.
- Lateral stenosis is characterized by encroachment of the spinal nerve in the lateral recess of the spinal canal or in the intervertebral foramen.[349]

Patients with lumbar spinal stenosis, who are symptomatic, often relate a long history of low back pain, with an increase in symptoms related to lumbar extension activities such as walking, and prolonged standing.

Lumbar flexion exercises have been proposed for the conservative treatment of patients with lumbar spinal stenosis, in addition to hip flexor, rectus femoris and lumbar paraspinal stretching. As appropriate, lumbar (core) stabilization exercises, aerobic conditioning, and positioning through a posterior pelvic tilt are introduced.[350-352] Failure to respond to a conservative approach is an indication for nerve root and sinuvertebral nerve infiltration.[353] Permanent relief in lateral recess stenosis has been reported with an injection of local anesthetic around the nerve root.[354] When nerve root infiltration fails, surgical decompression of the nerve root is indicated.

SPONDYLOLYSIS/SPONDYLOLISTHESIS

Spondylylosis involves a defect of the pars interarticularis of the spine. Such defects can range from a stress fracture to a traumatic bony fracture with separation.

Spondylolisthesis, which usually occurs in the lumbar spine, is a term used to identify anterior slippage and inability to resist shear forces of a vertebral segment in relation to the vertebral segment immediately below it. Five groups have been described based on etiology:[355]

1. Congenital
2. Isthmic
3. Degenerative[356]
4. Traumatic
5. Pathologic

Spondylolisthesis aquisita is a term used to describe the slip caused by the surgical disruption of ligaments, bone, and disc.

The typical presentation is one of low back pain that is mechanical in nature and which is worsened with activity but alleviated with rest. The patient may complain of leg pain. If neurogenic claudication is present, the patient may complain of leg tiredness, aches, and fatigue.[357]

Range of motion of lumbar spine flexion frequently is normal with both types of claudication. Some patients will be able to touch their toes without difficulty. Strength is usually intact in the lower extremities. Sensation also is usually intact. A check of distal pulses is important to rule out any coexisting vascular insufficiency. Findings such as hairless lower extremities, coldness of the feet, or absent pulses are signs of peripheral vascular disease. Sensory defects in a stocking glove distribution are more suggestive of diabetic neuropathy. The muscle stretch reflexes generally will be normal or diminished. If hyperreflexic symptoms and other upper motor neuron signs such as clonus or a positive Babinski test are found, the cervical, thoracic, and lumbar spine should be investigated to rule out a spinal cord or cauda equina lesion. The therapeutic exercise progression for this population is similar to that of DSS.[358-360]

Temporomandibular Joint Disorders (TMD)

TMD is associated with pain, joint sounds, and irregular or deviating jaw function due to an abnormal positional relationship of the articular disc to the mandibular condyle and the articular eminence,[361-363] which can result in mechanical interference and restriction of the normal range of mandibular activity.[364-366] Due to the close proximity, the cervical spine must be thoroughly examined in conjunction with the TMJ.

The conservative intervention for this condition depends on the causative factors. Typically, the focus is on[367]:

- Control of pain and inflammation.
- Postural education.
- The correction of any occlusal disharmony and any adverse parafunctional habits (nail biting, pencil chewing, teeth clenching, or bruxism).

Thoracic Outlet Syndrome

Thoracic outlet syndrome (TOS) is characterized by symptoms related to compression of the neural or vascular structures that pass through the thoracic outlet. The other names used for TOS are based on descriptions of the potential sources for its compression. These names include cervical rib syndrome, scalenus anticus syndrome, hyperabduction syndrome, costoclavicular syndrome, pectoralis minor syndrome, and first thoracic rib syndrome.

The lowest trunk of the brachial plexus (C8 and T1 nerve roots), is the most commonly compressed neural structure in TOS. There may be multiple points of compression of the peripheral nerves between the cervical spine and hand, in addition to the thoracic outlet.

The chief complaint is usually one of diffuse arm and shoulder pain, especially with arm elevation beyond 90 degrees. Other symptoms may include pain localized in the neck, face, head, chest, axilla; and upper extremity paresthesias, numbness, weakness, heaviness, swelling, discoloration, or Raynaud phenomenon.[368] Neural compression symptoms occur more commonly than vascular symptoms.[369]

Thoracic outlet syndrome is a clinical diagnosis, made almost entirely on the history and physical examination. To help rule out other conditions that can mimic thoracic outlet syndrome, the physical examination should include:

- A careful inspection of the spine, thorax, shoulder girdles, and upper extremities for postural abnormalities, shoulder asymmetry, muscle atrophy, excessively large breasts, obesity, and drooping of the shoulder girdle.
- The supraclavicular fossa should be palpated for fibromuscular bands, percussed for brachial plexus irritability, and auscultated for vascular bruits that appear by placing the upper extremity in the position of vascular compression.
- The neck and shoulder girdle should be assessed for active and passive ranges of motion, areas of tenderness, or other signs of intrinsic disease.
- A thorough neurologic examination of the upper extremity should include a search for sensory and motor deficits and abnormalities of muscle stretch reflexes.
- Respiration is assessed to ensure patient is using correct abdominodiaphragmatic breathing.
- Assessment of the *suspensory* muscles—the middle and upper trapezius, levator scapulae and sternocleidomastoid (thoracic outlet "openers"). These muscles are typically found to be weak.
- Assessment of the scapulothoracic muscles—the anterior and middle scalenes, subclavius, pectoralis minor and major (thoracic outlet "closers"). These muscles are typically found to be adaptively shortened.
- First rib position or presence of cervical rib.
- Clavicle position and history of prior fracture, producing abnormal callous formation or malalignment.
- Scapula position, acromioclavicular joint mobility and sternoclavicular joint mobility.
- Neurophysiological tests are useful to exclude coexistent pathologies such as peripheral nerve entrapment or cervical radiculopathy; an abnormal reflex F wave conduction and decreased sensory action potentials in the medial antebrachial cutaneous nerve may be diagnostic.[370]

Conservative intervention should be attempted before surgery and should be directed toward muscle relaxation, relief of inflammation and attention to posture. The focus of the intervention is the correction of postural abnormalities of the neck and shoulder girdle, strengthening of the scapular suspensory muscles, stretching of the scapulothoracic muscles, and mobilization of the whole shoulder complex and first and second ribs.

If symptoms progress or fail to respond within 4 months, surgical intervention should be considered.[371] Lower plexus thoracic outlet syndrome is surgically treated by first rib and (if present) cervical rib excision.[372] Although it has been suggested that the insured patient is more likely to have an operation, results are independent of any associated litigation.[373]

TORTICOLLIS

Torticollis is not a specific diagnosis but rather a sign of an underlying disorder resulting in the characteristic tilting of the head to one side.[374] The neuromuscular causes of torticollis may be classified as congenital or acquired.

- Congenital muscular torticollis (CMT): the most common type of torticollis.[375] Several causes are implicated, including fetal positioning, difficult labor and delivery, cervical muscle abnormalities, Sprengel's deformity, and Klippel-Feil syndrome.[376]
- Acquired torticollis, which includes spasmodic torticollis, is clinically similar but has different etiologies.[377]
  - Acquired torticollis in children may be related to trauma or infections, as in Grisel's syndrome, which occurs after head, neck, and pharyngeal infections.[378]
- Spasmodic torticollis is the involuntary hyperkinesis of neck musculature, causing turning of the head on the trunk, sometimes with additional forward flexion (anterocollis), backwards extension (retrocollis), or lateral flexion (laterocollis).[379] It is also marked by abnormal head postures.[380] The sternocleidomastoid muscle is involved in 75% of cases and the trapezius in 50%.[381]

Various treatments for torticollis have been described. Spencer et al[382] described a single-subject study using behavioral therapies that consisted of progressive relaxation, positive practice, and visual feedback. Their patient had significant improvements in all areas, which were maintained at a 2-year follow-up examination.

Agras and Marshall[383] used massed negative practice (ie, repeating the spasmodic positioning), 200 to 400 repetitions of the movement daily, which achieved full resolution of symptoms in 1 of 2 patients. Results persisted for 22 months.

Another single-case study used positive practice (exercising against the spasmed muscle groups) in a bed-ridden woman who had 8 years of spasmodic torticollis symptoms. After 3 months of positive practice, she was able to ambulate unassisted; her therapeutic gains were maintained at a 1-year follow-up examination.[384]

Biofeedback has also been used successfully in the intervention of torticollis.[385]

Volkmann's Ischemic Contracture.

An acute compartment syndrome that can be caused by constrictive casts or dressings, limb placement during surgery, blunt trauma, hematoma, burns, frostbite, snake bite, strenuous exercise, and fractures.[386] Clinical findings include[387]:

- A swollen and tense tender compartment
- Severe pain, exacerbated with passive stretch of the forearm muscles
- Sensibility deficits
- Motor weakness or paralysis
- No absence of radial and ulnar pulses at the wrist

The clinical diagnosis is confirmed by measuring the intracompartmental tissue fluid pressure.

Conservative intervention involves the removal of the constricting splint, dressing, or cast. Surgical intervention, by performing a fasciotomy, is reserved for patients whose symptoms do not resolve quickly.[388]

Wrist Fractures

Colles' Fracture.[389] A colles' fracture involves a complete fracture of the distal radius with a posterior displacement of the distal fragment, which are evident on the lateral film—the Colles' fracture has the characteristic dorsiflexion or "silver fork" deformity. The typical mechanism of injury is a FOOSH.

Management of this fracture requires an accurate reduction with maintenance of the normal length of the radius. Loss of full rotation of the forearm is a common consequence of this type of fracture.

Smith Fracture. A Smith fracture, or reverse Colles' fracture, is a complete fracture of the distal radius with anterior displacement of the distal fragment.[390] The usual mechanism for this type of fracture is a fall on the back of a flexed hand.

The typical intervention for a Smith's fracture is with closed reduction and long-arm casting in supination, followed by a short arm cast.[391] Unstable fractures require an open reduction and internal fixation (ORIF).

Barton's Fracture. A Barton's fracture involves a posterior or anterior articular fracture of the distal radius and subluxation of the wrist.[392] The mechanism of injury for this type of fracture usually includes some form of traumatic injury to the wrist, or from a sudden pronation of the distal forearm on a fixed wrist. The fracture is reduced and an above elbow cast is then applied, followed by a forearm cast with the wrist in ulnar deviation.

Buckle Fracture. A buckle fracture is an incomplete, undisplaced fracture of the distal radius. Immobilization for 3 to 4 weeks in a short-arm cast or palmar splint is typically adequate.[322]

ZYGAPOPHYSEAL JOINT DYSFUNCTION

Facet joint syndrome is a term used to describe a pain-provoking dysfunction of the zygapophyseal joint.[393] This pain is the result of a lesion to the joint and its pain-sensitive structures. Zygapophyseal movement dysfunctions can result from a hypomobility, or a hypermobility/instability. Hypomobility in the lumbar spine can have a variety of causes including ligament tears,[394] muscle tears or contusions,[395] lumbago,[33] intra-articular meniscoid entrapment,[396] zygapophyseal joint capsular tightness, and zygapophyseal joint fixation or subluxation.[397]

Theoretically, the signs and symptoms that present with a hypomobility include unilateral low back pain with is aggravated with certain movements. These movements are tested with AROM and the combined motion tests.

The intervention for a zygapophyseal dysfunction includes specific joint mobilizations, postural education, correction of muscle imbalances, and core stabilization exercises.

INTERVENTION PRINCIPLES FOR MUSCULOSKELETAL INJURIES

A number of principles should guide the intervention through the various stages of musculoskeletal tissue healing. These include:

- Control pain, inflammation, and swelling (edema)
- Promote and progress healing
- Instructions to the patient on a therapeutic exercise program that:
  - Corrects any imbalances between strength and flexibility
  - Addresses postural and movement dysfunctions
  - Integrates the open and closed kinetic chains
  - Incorporates neuromuscular reeducation
  - Maintains or improves the overall strength and fitness
  - Improves the functional outcome of the patient

CONTROL PAIN AND INFLAMMATION

The clinician's has a number of tools at his or her disposal to help to control pain, inflammation, and swelling (edema). These include the application of electrotherapeutic and physical modalities (refer to Chapter 18), gentle range of motion exercises, and graded manual techniques. During the acute stage of healing the principles of PRICEMEM (Protection, Rest, Ice, Compression, Elevation, Manual therapy, Early motion, and Medications) are recommended. The modalities used during the acute phase involve the application of cryotherapy, electrical stimulation, pulsed ultrasound, and iontophoresis. Modalities used during the later stages of healing include thermotherapy, phonophoresis, electrical stimulation, ultrasound (US), iontophoresis, and diathermy. The applications of cold and heat are taught to the patient at the earliest opportunity.

Gentle manual techniques (grade I or II joint mobilizations) may also be used to help with pain (refer to Chapter 18). As the patient progresses, gentle passive muscle stretching may be introduced. Self-stretching and self-mobilization techniques are taught to the patient at the earliest and appropriate opportunity.

The goals of the acute phase should include:

- Maximizing patient comfort by decreasing pain and inflammation
- Protection of the injury site
- Restoration of pain-free range of motion throughout the entire kinetic chain
- Retardation of muscle atrophy
- Minimizing the detrimental effects of immobilization and activity restriction[398-400]
- Attainment of early neuromuscular control
- Improving soft tissue extensibility
- Increasing functional tolerance
- Maintaining general fitness
- Appropriate management of scar tissue
- Encouraging the patient toward independence with the home exercise program
- Progression of the patient to the functional stage

PROMOTE AND PROGRESS HEALING

The promotion and progression of tissue repair involves a delicate balance between protection, and the application of controlled functional stresses to the damaged structure. Tissue repair can be viewed as an adaptive live process in response to both intrinsic and extrinsic stimuli.[401] These stimuli can be in the form of manual techniques and/or therapeutic exercises. Although physical therapy cannot accelerate the healing process, it can ensure that the healing process is not delayed or disrupted, and that it occurs in an optimal environment.[402] In addition to excess stress, detrimental environments include prolonged immobilization, which must be avoided. The rehabilitation procedures chosen to progress the patient will depend on the type of tissue involved, the extent of the damage, and the stage of healing. The intervention must be related to the signs and symptoms present rather than the actual diagnosis.

The functional phase addresses any tissue overload problems and functional biomechanical deficits. The goals of the functional phase should address:

- Attainment of full range of pain-free motion
- Restoration of normal joint kinematics
- Improvement of muscle strength to within normal limits
- Improvement of neuromuscular control
- Restoration of normal muscle force couples
- Correction of any deficits in the whole kinetic chain that are involved in an activity to which the patient is planning to return
- Performance of activity-specific progressions before full return to function

The selection of intervention procedures, and the intervention progression, must be guided by continuous reexamination of the patient's response to a given procedure, making the reexamination of patient dysfunction before, during, and after each intervention, essential.[32] There are three possible scenarios following a reexamination:

1. The patient's function has improved. In this scenario, the intensity of the intervention may be incrementally increased.
2. The patient's function has diminished. In this scenario, the intensity and the focus of the intervention must be changed. Further review of the home exercise program may be needed. The patient may require further education on activity modification and the use of heat and ice at home. The working hypothesis must be reviewed. Further investigation is needed.
3. There is no change in the patient's function. Depending on the elapse of time since the last visit, there may be a reason for the lack of change. This finding may indicate the need for a change in the intensity of the intervention. If the patient is in the acute or subacute stage of healing, a decrease in the intensity may be warranted, to allow the tissues more of an opportunity to heal. In the chronic stage, an increase in intensity may be warranted.

Questions for this chapter and the entire book appear on the included CD-ROM, with additional questions at www.DuttonNPTE.com.

REFERENCES

1. Wiater JM: Functional anatomy of the shoulder. In: Placzek JD, Boyce DA, eds. *Orthopaedic Physical Therapy Secrets.* Philadelphia, PA: Hanley & Belfus; 2001:243-248.
2. Turnbull JR: Acromioclavicular joint disorders. *Med Sci Sports Exerc.* 1998;30:S26-S32.
3. Rockwood CA Jr: Injuries to the acromioclavicular joint. In: Rockwood CA Jr, Green DP, eds. *Fractures in Adults.* 2nd ed. Philadelphia, PA: Lippincott; 1984:860-910.
4. Rockwood CA Jr, Young DC: Disorders of the acromioclavicular joint. In: Rockwood CA Jr, Matsen FA III, eds. *The Shoulder.* Philadelphia, PA: Saunders; 1990:413-468.
5. Keele CA, Neil E: *Samson Wright's Applied Physiology.* 12th ed. London: Oxford University Press; 1971.
6. Cohen MS, Bruno RJ: The collateral ligaments of the elbow: anatomy and clinical correlation. *Clin Orthop Rel Res.* 2001;1: 123-130.
7. An KN, Morrey BF: Biomechanics of the elbow. In: Morrey BF, ed. *The Elbow and Its Disorders.* 2nd ed. Philadelphia, PA: Saunders; 1993:53-73.
8. Morrey BF, An KN: Functional anatomy of the ligaments of the elbow. *Clin Orthop.* 1985;201:84-90.
9. Regan WD, Korinek SL, Morrey BF, et al: Biomechanical study of ligaments around the elbow joint. *Clin Orthop.* 1991;271: 170-179.
10. Cummings GS: Comparison of muscle to other soft tissue in limiting elbow extension. *J Orthop Sports Phys Ther.* 1984;5:170.

11. Kapandji IA: *The Physiology of the Joints: Upper Limb.* New York, NY: Churchill Livingstone; 1991.
12. Hammer WI: *Functional Soft Tissue Examination and Treatment by Manual Methods.* Gaithersburg, MD: Aspen; 1991.
13. Patterson RM, Nicodemus CL, Viegas SF, et al: High-speed, threedimensional kinematic analysis of the normal wrist. *J Hand Surg [Am].* 1998;23:446-453.
14. Sun JS, Shih TT, Ko CM, et al: In vivo kinematic study of normal wrist motion: an ultrafast computed tomographic study. *Clin Biomech.* 2000;15:212-216.
15. Moore JS: De Quervain's tenosynovitis: stenosing tenosynovits of the first dorsal compartment. *J Occup Environ Med.* 1997;39: 990-1002.
16. Tubiana R, Thomine J-M, Mackin E: *Examination of the Hand and Wrist.* London: Mosby; 1996.
17. Sarrafian SK, Melamed JL, Goshgarian GM: Study of wrist motion in flexion and extension. *Clin Orthop Rel Res.* 1977;126:153-159.
18. Crowninshield RD, Johnston RC, Andrews JG, et al: A biomechanical investigation of the human hip. *J Biomech.* 1978;11:75-85.
19. Cibulka MT, Sinacore DR, Cromer GS, et al: Unilateral hip rotation range of motion asymmetry in patients with sacroiliac joint regional pain. *Spine.* 1998;23:1009-1015.
20. Afoke NYP, Byers PD, Hutton WC: Contact pressures in the human hip joint. *J Bone Joint Surg [Am].* 1987;69B:536.
21. Oatis CA: Biomechanics of the hip. In: Echternach J, ed. *Clinics* in Physical Therapy: Physical Therapy of the Hip. New York, NY: Churchill Livingstone; 1990:37-50.
22. Kapandji IA: *The Physiology of the Joints: Lower Limb.* New York, NY: Churchill Livingstone; 1991.
23. Pauwels F: *Biomechanics of the Normal and Diseased Hip.* Berlin: Springer-Verlag; 1976.
24. Maquet PGJ: *Biomechanics of the Hip as Applied to Osteoarthritis and Related Conditions.* Berlin: Springer-Verlag; 1985.
25. Menke W, Schmitz B, Schild H, et al: Transversale Skelettachsen der unteren Extremität bei Coxarthrose. *Z Orthop Ihre Grenzgeb.* 1991;129:255-259.
26. Pizzutillo PT, MacEwen GD, Shands AR: Anteversion of the femur. In: Tonzo RG, ed. *Surgery of the Hip Joint.* New York, NY: Springer-Verlag; 1984.
27. Lausten GS, Jorgensen F, Boesen J: Measurement of anteversion of the femoral neck, ultrasound and CT compared. *J Bone Joint Surg [Am].* 1989;71B:237.
28. Gross MT: Lower quarter screening for skeletal malalignment—suggestions for orthotics and shoewear. *J Orthop Sports Phys Ther.* 1995;21:389-405.
29. Deusinger R: Validity of pelvic tilt measurements in anatomical neutral position. *J Biomech.* 1992;25:764.
30. Kaltenborn FM: *Manual Mobilization of the Extremity Joints: Basic Examination and Treatment Techniques.* 4th ed. Oslo: Olaf Norlis Bokhandel; 1989.
31. Williams PL, Warwick R, Dyson M, et al: *Gray's Anatomy.* 37th ed. London: Churchill Livingstone; 1989.
32. Yoder E: Physical therapy management of nonsurgical hip problems in adults. In: Echternach JL, ed. *Physical Therapy of the Hip.* New York, NY: Churchill Livingstone; 1990:103-137.

33. Cyriax J: *Textbook of Orthopaedic Medicine: Diagnosis of Soft Tissue Lesions.* 8th ed. London: Bailliere Tindall; 1982.
34. Cyriax JH, Cyriax PJ: *Illustrated Manual of Orthopaedic Medicine.* London: Butterworth; 1983.
35. Dye SF: An evolutionary perspective of the knee. *J Bone Joint Surg.* 1987;69A:976-983.
36. Davids JR: Pediatric knee. Clinical assessment and common disorders. *Pediatr Clin North Am.* 1996;43:1067-1090.
37. McGinty G, Irrgang JJ, Pezzullo D: Biomechanical considerations for rehabilitation of the knee. *Clin Biomech.* 2000;15: 160-166.
38. Kendall FP, McCreary EK, Provance PG: *Muscles: Testing and Function.* Baltimore, MD: Williams & Wilkins; 1993.
39. Brownstein B, Noyes FR, Mangine RE, et al: Anatomy and biomechanics. In: Mangine RE, ed. *Physical Therapy of the Knee.* New York, NY: Churchill Livingstone; 1988:1-30.
40. Desio SM, Burks RT, Bachus KN: Soft tissue restraints to lateral patellar translation in the human knee. *Am J Sports Med.* 1998;26: 59-65.
41. Fulkerson JP: *Disorders of the Patellofemoral Joint.* Baltimore, MD: Williams & Wilkins; 1997.
42. Grelsamer RP, McConnell J: *The Patella: A Team Approach.* Gaithersburg, MD: Aspen; 1998.
43. Woodland LH, Francis RS: Parameters and comparisons of the quadriceps angle of college aged men and women in the supine and standing positions. *Am J Sports Med.* 1992;20:208-211.
44. Olerud C, Berg P: The variation of the quadriceps angle with different positions of the foot. *Clin Orthop.* 1984;191:162-165.
45. Rand JA: The patellofemoral joint in total knee arthroplasty. *J Bone Joint Surg [Am].* 1994;76:612-620.
46. Aglietti P, Insall JN, Walker PS, et al: A new patella prosthesis. *Clin Orthop.* 1975;107:175-187.
47. McConnell J, Fulkerson JP: The knee: patellofemoral and soft tissue injuries. In: Zachazewski JE, Magee DJ, Quillen WS, eds. *Athletic Injuries and Rehabilitation.* Philadelphia, PA: Saunders; 1996:693-728.
48. Fujikawa K, Seedholm BB, Wright V: Biomechanics of the patellofemoral joint. Parts 1 and 2. Study of the patellofemoral compartment and movement of the patella. *Eng Med.* 1983; 12:3-21.
49. Goodfellow JW, Hungerford DS, Woods C: Patellofemoral joint mechanics and pathology: I and II. *J Bone Joint Surg.* 1976;58B: 287-299.
50. Hehne H-J: Biomechanics of the patellofemoral joint and its clinical relevance. *Clin Orthop.* 1990;258:73-85.
51. Huberti HH, Hayes WC: Patellofemoral contact pressures. The influence of Q-angle and tendofemoral contact. *J Bone Joint Surg.* 1984;66A:715-724.
52. Carson WG, James SL, Larson RL, et al: Patellofemoral disorders—physical and radiographic examination. Part I. Physical examination. *Clin Orthop.* 1984;185:178-186.
53. Hungerford DS, Barry M: Biomechanics of the patellofemoral joint. *Clin Orthop.* 1979;144:9-15.
54. Steinkamp LA, Dilligham MF, Markel MD, et al: Biomechanical considerations in patellofemoral joint rehabilitation. *Am J Sports Med.* 1993;21:438-444.

55. Grelsamer RP, McConnell J: *Applied Mechanics of the Patellofemoral Joint. The Patella: A Team Approach.* Gaithersburg, MD: Aspen; 1998:25-41.
56. Beynnon BD, Fleming BC, Johnson RJ, et al: Anterior cruciate ligament strain behavior during rehabilitation exercises in vivo. *Am J Sports Med.* 1995;23:24-34.
57. Lutz GE, Palmitier RA, An KN, et al: Comparison of tibiofemoral joint forces during open-kinetic-chain and closed-kinetic-chain exercises. *Am J Bone Joint Surg.* 1993;75:732-739.
58. Reilly DT, Martens M: Experimental analysis of the quadriceps muscle force and patello-femoral joint reaction force for various activities. *Acta Orthop Scand.* 1972;43:126-137.
59. Lundberg A, Goldie I, Kalin B, et al. Kinematics of the ankle/foot complex: plantar flexion and dorsiflexion. *Foot Ankle.* 1989;9: 194-200.
60. Levens AS, Inman VT, Blosser JA: Transverse rotations of the lower extremity in locomotion. *J Bone Joint Surg.*1948;30A: 859-872.
61. Oatis CA: Biomechanics of the foot and ankle under static conditions. *Phys Ther.* 1988;68:1815-1821.
62. Subotnick SI: Biomechanics of the subtalar and midtarsal joints. *J Am Podiatry Assoc.* 1975;65:756-764.
63. Elftman H: The transverse tarsal joint and its control. *Clin Orthop Rel Res.* 1960;16:41-45.
64. White AA, Johnson RM, Panjabi MM, et al: Biomechanical analysis of clinical stability in the cervical spine. *Clin Orthop.* 1975;109: 85-96.
65. Panjabi M, Dvorak J, Crisco J, et al: Flexion, extension, and lateral bending of the upper cervical spine in response to alar ligament transections. *J Spinal Disord.* 1991;4:157-167.
66. Vangilder JC, Menezes AH, Dolan KD: *The Craniovertebral Junction and Its Abnormalities.* Mount Kisco, NY: Futura; 1987.
67. Buckworth J: Anatomy of the suboccipital region. In: Vernon H, ed. *Upper Cervical Syndrome.* Baltimore: MD, Williams & Wilkins; 1988.
68. Bogduk N: Innervation and pain patterns of the cervical spine. In: Grant R, ed. *Physical Therapy of the Cervical and Thoracic Spine.* New York, NY: Churchill Livingstone; 1988.
69. Swash M, Fox K: Muscle spindle innervation in man. *J Anat.* 1972;112:61-80.
70. Lazorthes G: Pathology, classification and clinical aspects of vascular diseases of the spinal cord. In: Vinken PJ, Bruyn GW, eds. *Handbook of Clinical Neurology.* Oxford: Elsevier; 1972: 494-506.
71. Penning L: *Functional Pathology of the Cervical Spine.* Baltimore, MD: Williams & Wilkins; 1968.
72. Janda V: Muscles and motor control in cervicogenic disorders: assessment and management. In: Grant R, ed. *Physical Therapy of the Cervical and Thoracic Spine.* New York, NY: Churchill Livingstone; 1994:195-216.
73. Jull GA, Janda V: Muscle and motor control in low back pain. In: Twomey LT, Taylor JR, eds. *Physical Therapy of the Low Back: Clinics in Physical Therapy.* New York, NY: Churchill Livingstone; 1987:258.

74. Bergmark A: Stability of the lumbar spine. *Acta Orthop Scand.* 1989;60:1-54.
75. Mayoux-Benhamou MA, Revel M, Valle C, et al: Longus colli has a postural function on cervical curvature. *Surg Radiol Anat.* 1994;16:367-371.
76. Conley MS, Meyer RA, Bloomberg JJ, et al: Noninvasive analysis of human neck muscle function. *Spine.* 1995;20:2505-2512.
77. Viener AE: Oral surgery. In: Garliner D, ed. *Myofunctional Therapy.* Philadelphia, PA: Saunders; 1976.
78. Castaneda R: Occlusion. In: Kaplan AS, Assael LA, eds. Temporomandibular Disorders: Diagnosis and Treatment. Philadelphia: Saunders; 1991:40-49.
79. Sicher H, Du Brul EL: *Oral Anatomy.* 8th ed. St. Louis, MD: Mosby; 1988.
80. Hertling D: The temporomandibular joint. In: Hertling D, Kessler RM, eds. *Management of Common Musculoskeletal Disorders.* 3rd ed. Philadelphia, PA: Lippincott-Raven; 1996:444-485.
81. Rocabado M: Arthrokinemetics of the temporomandibular joint. In: Gelb H, ed. *Clinical Management of Head, Neck and TMJ Pain and Dysfunction.* Philadelphia, PA: Saunders; 1985.
82. White AA: An analysis of the mechanics of the thoracic spine in man. *Acta Orthop Scand Suppl.* 1969;127:8-92.
83. Panjabi MM, Hausfeld JN, White AA: A biomechanical study of the ligamentous stability of the thoracic spine in man. *Acta Orthop Scand.* 1981;52:315-326.
84. Panjabi MM, Brand RA, White AA: Mechanical properties of the human thoracic spine. *J BoneJoint Surg.* 1976;58A:642-652.
85. Lee DG: Biomechanics of the thorax. In: Grant R, ed. *Physical Therapy of the Cervical and Thoracic Spine.* New York: Churchill Livingstone; 1988:47-76.
86. Flynn TW: Thoracic spine and chest wall. In: Wadsworth C, ed. *Current Concepts of Orthopedic Physical Therapy—Home Study Course.* La Crosse, WI: Orthopaedic Section, APTA; 2001.
87. Refshauge KM, Bolst L, Goodsell M: The relationship between cervicothoracic posture and the presence of pain. *J Man Manip Ther.* 1995;3:21-24.
88. Edmondston SJ, Singer KP: Thoracic spine: anatomical and biomechanical considerations for manual therapy. *Man Ther.* 1997;2:132-143.
89. Raine S, Twomey LT: Attributes and qualities of human posture and their relationship to dysfunction or musculoskeletal pain. *Crit Rev Phys Rehabil Med.* 1994;6:409-437.
90. Singer KP, Malmivaara A: Pathoanatomical characteristics of the thoracolumbar junctional region. In: Giles LGF, Singer KP, eds. *Clinical Anatomy and Management of the Thoracic Spine.* Oxford: Butterworth-Heinemann; 2000:100-113.
91. Andriacchi T, Schultz A, Belytschko T, et al: A model for studies of mechanical interactions between the human spine and rib cage. *J Biomech.* 1974;7:497-505.
92. Shea KG, Schlegel JD, Bachus KN, et al: *The Contribution of the Rib Cage to Thoracic Spine Stability.* Burlington: International Society for the Study of the Lumbar Spine; 1996:150.
93. Bergmark A: Stability of the lumbar spine. A study in mechanical engineering. *Acta Orthop Scand.* 1989;230:20-24.

94. White DJ: Musculoskeletal examination. In: O'Sullivan SB, Schmitz TJ, eds. *Physical Rehabilitation.* 5th ed. Philadelphia, PA: Davis; 2007:159-192.
95. Farfan HF: The scientific basis of manipulative procedures. *Clin Rheum Dis.* 1980;6:159-177.
96. McKenzie R, May S: Physical examination. In: McKenzie R, May S, eds. *The Human Extremities: Mechanical Diagnosis and Therapy.* Waikanae, New Zealand: Spinal Publications; 2000: 105-121.
97. McKenzie RA: The lumbar spine: mechanical diagnosis and therapy. Waikanae, New Zealand: Spinal Publications; 1981.
98. Petersen CM, Hayes KW: Construct validity of Cyriax's selective tension examination: association of end-feels with pain at the knee and shoulder. *J Orthop Sports Phys Ther.* 2000;30:512-527.
99. American Medical Association. *Guides to the Evaluation of Permanent Impairment.* 5th ed. Chicago: American Medical Association; 2001.
100. APTA: Guide to physical therapist practice. *Phys Ther.* 2001;81: S13-S95.
101. Wintz MN: Variations in current manual muscle testing. *Phys Ther Rev.* 1959;39:466-475.
102. Sapega AA. Muscle performance evaluation in orthopedic practice. *J Bone Joint Surg.* 1990;72A:15620-1574.
103. Iddings DM, Smith LK, Spencer WA: Muscle testing: part 2. Reliability in clinical use. *Phys Ther Rev.* 1961;41:249-256.
104. Silver M, McElroy A, Morrow L, et al: Further standardization of manual muscle test for clinical study: applied in chronic renal disease. *Phys Ther.* 1970;50:1456-1465.
105. Marx RG, Bombardier C, Wright JG: What do we know about the reliability and validity of physical examination tests used to examine the upper extremity? *J Hand Surg.* 1999;24A: 185-193.
106. Tovin BJ, Greenfield BH: Impairment-based diagnosis for the shoulder girdle. In: *Evaluation and Treatment of the Shoulder: An Integration of the Guide to Physical Therapist Practice.* Philadelphia, PA: Davis; 2001:55-74.
107. Riddle DL: Measurement of accessory motion: critical issues and related concepts. *Phys Ther.* 1992;72:865-874.
108. Calis M, Akgun K, Birtane M, et al: Diagnostic values of clinical diagnostic tests in subacromial impingement syndrome. *Ann Rheum Dis.* 2000;59:44-47.
109. Post M, Cohen J: Impingement syndrome: a review of late stage II and early stage III lesions. *Clin Orthop Rel Res.* 1986; 207:127-132.
110. Hawkins RJ, Kennedy JC: Impingement syndrome in athletics. *Am J Sports Med.* 1980;8:151-163.
111. Ure BM, Tiling T, Kirchner R, et al: Zuverlassigkeit der klinischen untersuchung der schulter im vergleich zur arthroskopie. *Unfallchirurg.* 1993;96:382-386.
112. Leroux JL, Thomas E, Bonnel F, et al: Diagnostic value of clinical tests for shoulder impingement. *Rev Rheum.* 1995;62:423-428.
113. Patte D, Goutallier D, Monpierre H, et al: Over-extension lesions. *Rev Chir Orthop.* 1988;74:314-318.
114. Arthuis M: Obstetrical paralysis of the brachial plexus I. Diagnosis: clinical study of the initial period. *Rev Chir Orthop Reparatrice Appar Mot.* 1972;58:124-136.

115. Maitland G: *Peripheral Manipulation.* 3rd ed. London: Butterworth; 1991.
116. Mullen F: Locking and quadrant of the shoulder: relationships of the humerus and scapula during locking and quadrant. In: Proceedings of the Sixth Biennial Conference, Manipulative Therapist Association of Australia. Adelaide: MTAA; 1989: 130-137.
117. Neer CS: Anatomy of shoulder reconstruction. In: Neer CS, ed. *Shoulder Reconstruction.* Philadelphia, PA: Saunders; 1990:1-39.
118. Clarnette RG, Miniaci A. Clinical exam of the shoulder. *Med Sci Sports Exerc.* 1998;30:1-6.
119. Liu SH, Henry MH, Nuccion SL: A prospective evaluation of a new physical examination in predicting glenoid labral tears. *Am J Sports Med.* 1996;24:721-725.
120. Yergason RM: Rupture of biceps. *J Bone Joint Surg.* 1931;13:160.
121. Kibler WB: Specificity and sensitivity of the anterior slide test in throwing athletes with superior glenoid labral tears. *Arthroscopy.* 1995;11:296-300.
122. Lippitt S: Diagnosis and management of AMBRII syndrome. *Tech Orthop.* 1991;6:61.
123. Neer CSI, Foster CR: Inferior capsular shift for involuntary inferior and multidirectional instability of the shoulder. *J Bone Joint Surg.* 1980;62A:897-908.
124. Rockwood CA: Subluxations and dislocations about the shoulder. In: Rockwood CA, Green DP, eds. *Fractures in Adults.* Vol. 1. Philadelphia, PA: Lippincott; 1984.
125. Zimney NJ: Clinical reasoning in the evaluation and management of undiagnosed chronic hip pain in young adult. *Phys Ther.* 1998;78:62-73.
126. Weiss JR, Irrgang JJ, Sawhney R, et al: A functional assessment of anterior cruciate ligament deficiency in an acute and clinical setting. *J Orthop Sports Phys Ther.* 1990;11:372-373.
127. Hanten WP, Pace MB. Reliability of measuring anterior laxity of the knee joint using a knee ligament arthrometer. *Phys Ther.* 1987;67:357-359.
128. Hughston JC, Andrews JR, Cross MJ, et al: Classification of knee ligament instabilities. Part 2. *J Bone Joint Surg.* 1976;58A:173-179.
129. Hughston JC, Andrews JR, Cross MJ, et al: Classification of knee ligament instabilities. Part 1. *J Bone Joint Surg.* 1976;58A:159-172.
130. Winkel D, Matthijs O, Phelps V. *Examination of the Knee.* Gaithersburg, MD: Aspen; 1997.
131. Shino K, Horibe S, Ono K: The voluntary evoked posterolateral drawer sign in the knee with posterolateral instability. *Clin Orthop.* 1987;215:179-186.
132. Apley AG: The diagnosis of meniscus injuries: some new clinical methods. *J Bone Joint Surg.* 1947;29B:78-84.
133. Renne JW: The iliotibial band friction syndrome. *J Bone Joint Surg.* 1975;57:1110-1111.
134. Noble HB, Hajek MR, Porter M: Diagnosis and treatment of iliotibial band tightness in runners. *Phys Sports Med.* 1982;10: 67-74.
135. Patla CE, Abbott JH: Tibialis posterior myofascial tightness as a source of heel pain: diagnosis and treatment. *J Orthop Sports Phys Ther.* 2000;30:624-632.
136. Feudale F, Liebelt E: Recognizing vertebral artery dissection in children: a case report. *Pediatr Emerg Care.* 2000;16:184-188.

137. Aspinall W: Clinical testing for cervical mechanical disorders which produce ischemic vertigo. *J Orthop Sports Phys Ther.* 1989; 11:176-182.
138. Evans RC: *Illustrated Essentials in Orthopedic Physical Assessment.* St. Louis, MD: Mosby-Year Book; 1994.
139. Meadows J: *Orthopedic Differential Diagnosis in Physical Therapy.* New York, NY: McGraw-Hill; 1999.
140. Maitland G: *Vertebral Manipulation.* Sydney: Butterworth; 1986.
141. Ombregt L, Bisschop P, ter Veer HJ, et al: *A System of Orthopaedic Medicine.* London: Saunders; 1995.
142. Kanchandani R, Howe JG: Lhermitte's sign in multiple sclerosis: a clinical survey and review of the literature. *J Neurol Neurosurg Psychiatry.* 1982;45:308-312.
143. Smith KJ, McDonald WI: Spontaneous and mechanically evoked activity due to central demyelinating lesion. *Nature.* 1980;286: 154-155.
144. Uchihara T, Furukawa T, Tsukagoshi H: Compression of brachial plexus as a diagnostic test of a cervical cord lesion. *Spine.* 1994;19:2170-2173.
145. Landi A, Copeland S: Value of the Tinel sign in brachial plexus lesions. *Ann R Coll Surg Engl.* 1979;61:470-471.
146. Wright IS: The neurovascular syndrome produced by hyperabduction of the arms. *Am Heart J.* 1945;29:1-19.
147. Telford ED, Mottershead S: Pressure at the cervico-brachial junction: an operative and anatomical study. *J Bone Joint Surg.* 1948; 30B:249-265.
148. Winsor T, Brow R: Costoclavicular syndrome: its diagnosis and treatment. *JAMA.* 1966;196:697-699.
149. Rayan GM, Jensen C: Thoracic outlet syndrome: provocative examination maneuvers in a typical population. *J Shoulder Elbow Surg.* 1995;4:113-117.
150. Selke FW, Kelly TR: Thoracic outlet syndrome. *Am J Surg.* 1988; 156:54-57.
151. Nichols AW: The thoracic outlet syndrome in athletes. *J Am Board Fam Pract.* 1996;9:346-355.
152. Roos DB: Congenital anomalies associated with thoracic outlet syndrome. *J Surg.* 1976;132:771-778.
153. Deyo RA, Weinstein JN: Low back pain. *N Engl J Med.* 2001;344:363-370.
154. Fahrni WH: Observations on straight leg raising with special reference to nerve root adhesions. *Can J Surg.* 1966;9:44-48.
155. Kirkaldy-Willis WH: *Managing Low Back Pain.* 2nd ed. New York, NY: Churchill Livingstone; 1988.
156. Lee DG: *The Pelvic Girdle: An Approach to the Examination and Treatment of the Lumbo-Pelvic-Hip Region.* 2nd ed. Edinburgh: Churchill Livingstone; 1999.
157. Potter NA, Rothstein JM: Intertester reliability for selected clinical tests of the sacroiliac joint. *Phys Ther.* 1985;65:1671.
158. Meadows J, Pettman E, Fowler C: *Manual Therapy, NAIOMT Level II & III Course Notes.* Denver: North American Institute of Manual Therapy; 1995.
159. Binkley J, Stratford PW, Gill C: Interrater reliability of lumbar accessory motion mobility testing. *Phys Ther Rev.* 1995;75:786–792, discussion 793-795.

160. McCrory JL, Martin DF, Lowery RB, et al: Etiologic factors associated with Achilles tendinitis in runners. *Med Sci Sports Exerc.* 1999;31:1374-1381.
161. Clement DB, Taunton JE, Smart GW. Achilles tendinitis and peritendinitis: etiology and treatment. *Am J Sports Med.* 1984; 12:179-183.
162. James SL, Bates BT, Osternig LR. Injuries to runners. *Am J Sports Med.* 1978;6:40-49.
163. Clement DB, Taunton JE, Smart GW, et al: A survey of overuse running injuries. *Physician Sports Med.* 1981;9:47-58.
164. Renstrom P, Johnson RJ. Overuse injuries in sports: a review. *Sports Med.* 1985;2:316-333.
165. Hess GP, Cappiello WL, Poole RM, et al: Prevention and treatment of overuse tendon injuries. *Sports Med.* 1989;8:371-384.
166. Voorn R. Case report: can sacroiliac joint dysfunction cause chronic Achilles tendinitis? *J Orthop Sports Phys Ther.* 1998;27: 436-443.
167. Clain MR, Baxter DE. Achilles tendinitis. *Foot Ankle.* 1992;13: 482-487.
168. Puddu G, Ippolito E, Postacchini F. A classification of Achilles tendon disease. *Am J Sports Med.* 1976;4:145-150.
169. Nichols AW: Achilles tendinitis in running athletes. *J Am Bd Fam Pract.* 1989;2:196-203.
170. Tossy JD, Mead MC, Simond HM: Acromioclavicular separations: useful and practical classification for treatment. *Clin Orthop.* 1963;28:111-119.
171. Allman, F.L., Jr.: Fractures and ligamentous injuries of the clavicle and its articulation. *J Bone Joint Surg.* 1967;49A:774-784.
172. Williams GR, Nguyen VD, Rockwood CA Jr: Classification and radiographic analysis of acromioclavicular dislocations. *Appl Radiol.* 1989;15:29-34.
173. Wirth MA, Rockwood CA Jr: Chronic conditions of the acromioclavicular and sternoclavicular joints. In: Chapman MW, ed. *Operative Orthopaedics.* 2nd ed. Philadelphia, PA: Lippincott; 1993: 1673-1683.
174. Rockwood CA: *Rockwood and Green's Fractures in Adults.* Philadelphia, PA: Lippincott; 1991:1181-1239.
175. Brue S, Valentin A, Forssblad M, et al: Idiopathic adhesive capsulitis of the shoulder: a review. *Knee Surg Sports Traumatol Arthrosc.* 2007;15:1048-1054.
176. Nash P, Hazelman BD: Frozen shoulder. *Baillieres Clin Rheumatol.* 1989;3:551.
177. Reeves B: The natural history of the frozen shoulder syndrome. *Scand J Rheumatol.* 1975;4:193-196.
178. Garrick JG: The frequency of injury, mechanism of injury, and epidemiology of ankle sprains. *Am J Sports Med.* 1977;5:241-242.
179. O'Donoghue DH: Treatment of ankle injuries. *Northwest Med.* 1958;57:1277-1286.
180. Attarian DE, McCracken HJ, Devito DP, et al: Biomechanical characteristics of human ankle ligaments. *Foot Ankle.* 1985;6:54-58.
181. Thorndike A: *Athletic Injuries: Prevention, Diagnosis and Treatment.* Philadelphia, PA: Lea and Febiger; 1962.
182. Inman VT: Sprains of the ankle. In: Chapman MW, ed. *AAOS Instructional Course Lectures*; 1975:294-308.

183. O'Donoghue DH: *Treatment of Injuries to Athletes.* Philadelphia, PA: Saunders; 1976:698-746.
184. Gronmark T, Johnson O, Kogstad O: Rupture of the lateral ligaments of the ankle. *Foot Ankle.* 1980;1:84-89.
185. Iversen LD, Clawson DK: *Manual of Acute Orthopaedics.* Boston: Little, Brown; 1982.
186. Roy S, Irvin R: *Sports Medicine—Prevention, Evaluation, Management, and Rehabilitation.* Englewood Cliffs, NJ: Prentice-Hall; 1983.
187. Arendt E, Dick R: Knee injury patterns among men and women in collegiate basketball and soccer. NCAA data and review of literature. *Am J Sports Med.* 1995;23:694-701.
188. Bjordal JM, Arnly F, Hannestad B, et al: Epidemiology of anterior cruciate ligament injuries in soccer. *Am J Sports Med.* 1997; 25:341-345.
189. Arnoczky SP: Anatomy of the anterior cruciate ligament. In: Urist MR, ed. *Clinical Orthopedics and Related Research.* Philadelphia, PA: Lippincott; 1983:19-20, 26-30.
190. Cabaud HE: Biomechanics of the anterior cruciate ligament. In: Urist MR, ed. *Clinical Orthopedics and Related Research.* Philadelphia, PA: Lippincott; 1983:26-30.
191. Clasby L, Young MA: Management of sports-related anterior cruciate ligament injuries. *AORN J.* 1997;66:609-625, 628, 630; quiz 632-636.
192. Mizuta H, et al: The conservative treatment of complete tears of the anterior cruciate ligament in skeletally immature patients. *J Bone Joint Surg.* 1995;77:890.
193. Parker AW, Drez D, Cooper JL: Anterior cruciate injuries in patients with open physes. *Am J Sports Med.* 1994;22:47.
194. Micheli LJ, Jenkins M: Knee injuries. In: Micheli LJ, ed. *The Sports Medicine Bible.* Scranton: Harper & Row; 1995:130.
195. Stanish WD, Lai A: New concepts of rehabilitation following anterior cruciate reconstruction. *Clin Sports Med.* 1993;12:25-58.
196. Daniel DM, Stone ML, Dobson BE, et al. Fate of the ACL-injured patient. *Am J Sports Med.* 1994;22:642.
197. Liu SH, Osti L, Henry M, et al: The diagnosis of acute complete tears of the anterior cruciate ligament. *J Bone Joint Surg.* 1995;77:586.
198. Gerber C, Hoppeler H, Claassen H, et al: The lower-extremity musculature in chronic symptomatic instability of the anterior cruciate ligament. *J Bone Joint Surg.* 1985;67A:1034-1043.
199. Kariya Y, Itoh M, Nakamura T, et al: Magnetic resonance imaging and spectroscopy of thigh muscles in cruciate ligament insufficiency. *Acta Orthop Scand.* 1989;60:322-325.
200. Lorentzon R, Elmqvist LG, Sjostrom M, et al: Thigh musculature in relation to chronic anterior cruciate ligament tear: muscle size, morphology, and mechanical output before reconstruction. *Am J Sports Med.* 1989;17:423-429.
201. Noyes FR, Mangine RE, Barber S. Early knee motion after open and arthroscopic anterior cruciate ligament reconstruction. *Am J Sports Med.* 1987;15:149-160.
202. Yasuda K, Ohkoshi Y, Tanabe Y, et al: Quantitative evaluation of knee instability and muscle strength after anterior cruciate ligament reconstruction using patellar and quadriceps tendon. *Am J Sports Med.* 1992;20:471-475.

203. Daniel DM, Malcom LL, Losse G, et al: Instrumented measurement of anterior laxity of the knee. *J Bone Joint Surg*. 1985;67A: 720-725.
204. Indelicato PA, Bittar ES. A perspective of lesions associated with ACL insufficiency of the knee. A review of 100 cases. *Clin Orthop*. 1985;198:77-80.
205. Irvine GB, Glasgow MMS. The natural history of the meniscus in anterior cruciate insufficiency. Arthroscopic analysis. *J Bone Joint Surg*. 1992;74B:403-405.
206. Frank CB, Jackson DW: The science of reconstruction of the anterior cruciate ligament. *J Bone Joint Surg*. 1997;79:1556-1576.
207. Roberts WN, Williams RB: Hip pain. *Primary Care*. 1988; 15:783-793.
208. Hammer WI: The use of transverse friction massage in the management of chronic bursitis of the hip or shoulder. *J Man Physiol Ther*. 1993;16:107-111.
209. Katz JN, Larson MG, Sabra A, et al: The carpal tunnel syndrome: diagnostic utility of the history and physical examination findings. *Ann Intern Med*. 1990;112:321-327.
210. D'Arcy CA, McGee S: Does this patient have carpal tunnel syndrome? *JAMA*. 2000;283:3110-3117.
211. Barnes CG, Curry HLE: Carpal tunnel syndrome in rheumatoid arthritis: a clinical and electrodiagnostic survey. *Ann Rheum Dis*. 1970;26:226-233.
212. Feuerstein M, Burrell LM, Miller VI, et al: Clinical management of carpal tunnel syndrome: a 12 year review of outcomes. *Am J Ind Med*. 1999;35:232-245.
213. Szabo RM: Carpal tunnel syndrome-general. In: Gelberman RH, ed. *Operative Nerve Repair and Reconstruction*. Philadelphia, PA: J. B. Lippincott; 1991;882-883.
214. Heller L, Ring H, Costeff H, et al: Evaluation of Tinel's and Phalen's signs in diagnosis of the carpal tunnel syndrome. *Eur Neurol*. 1986;25:40-42.
215. Kenneally M, Rubenach H, Elvey R: The upper limb tension test: the SLR of the arm. In: Grant R, ed. *Physical Therapy of the Cervical and Thoracic Spine*. New York, NY: Churchill Livingstone; 1988.
216. Kleinrensink GJ, Stoeckart R, Vleeming A, et al: Mechanical tension in the median nerve. The effects of joint positions. *Clin Biomech*. 1995;10:240-244.
217. Taleisnik J: Classification of carpal instability. In: Taleisnik J, ed. *The Wrist*. New York, NY: Churchill Livingstone; 1985:229-238.
218. Chang MH, Chiang HT, Lee SSJ, et al: Oral drug of choice in carpal tunnel syndrome. *Neurology*. 1998;51:390-393.
219. Luchetti R, Schoenhuber R, Alfarano M, et al: Serial overnight recordings of intracarpal canal pressure in carpal tunnel syndrome patients with and without wrist splinting. *J Hand Surg*. 1994;19:35-37.
220. Von Schroeder HP, Botte MJ: Carpal tunnel syndrome. *Hand Clin*. 1996;12:643-655.
221. Lapidus PW, Fenton R: Stenosing tenovaginitis at the wrist and fingers: report of 423 cases in 269 patients. *Arch Surg*. 1952;64:475-487.
222. Muckart RD: Stenosing tendovaginitis of abductor pollicis brevis at the radial styloid (de Quervain's disease). *Clin Orthop*. 1964;33:201-208.

223. Finkelstein H: Stenosing tenovaginitis at the radial styloid process. *J Bone and Joint Surg*. 1930;12A:509.
224. McFarlane RM, Albion U: Dupuytren's disease. In: Hunter JM, Schneider LH, Mackin EJ, et al (eds). *Rehabilitation of the Hand*. 3rd ed. St. Louis, MO: CV Mosby; 1990:867.
225. Saar JD, Grothaus PC: dupuytren's disease: an overview. *Plastic & Reconstructive Surgery*. 2000;106:125-136.
226. Hill NA, Hurst LC: Dupuytren's contracture. In: Doyle JR, ed. *Landmark Advances in Hand Surgery. Hand Clinics*. Philadelphia, PA: WB Saunders; 1989:349.
227. Luck JV: Dupuytren's contracture: a new concept of the pathogenesis correlated with surgical management. *J Bone Joint Surg (Am)*. 1959;41:635.
228. Rayan GM: Clinical presentation and types of Dupuytren's disease. *Hand Clin*. 1999;15:87.
229. Strickland JW, Leibovic SJ: Anatomy and pathogenesis of the digital cords and nodules. *Hand Clin*. 1991;7:645.
230. Eckhaus D: Dupuytren's disease. In: Clark GL, Aiello B, Eckhaus D, et al, eds. *Hand Rehabilitation*. Edinburgh: Churchill Livingstone; 1993:37-42.
231. Nirschl RP: Elbow tendinosis: tennis elbow. *Clin. Sports Med*. 1992;11:851-870.
232. Nirschl RP: Tennis elbow tendinosis: pathoanatomy, nonsurgical and surgical management. In: Gordon SL, Blair SJ, Fine LJ, eds. *Repetitive Motion Disorders of the Upper Extremity*. Rosemont, IL: American Academy of Orthopaedic Surgeons. 1995;467-479.
233. Bailey RA, Brock BH: Hydrocortisone in tennis-elbow: a controlled series. *J R Soc Med*. 1957;50:389-390.
234. Johnson EW: Tennis elbow. Misconceptions and widespread mythology. *AM J Phys Med Rehabil*. 2000;79:113.
235. Nirschl RP, Pettrone FA: Tennis elbow. *J Bone Joint Surg [Am]*. 1979;61-A:832-839.
236. Kibler WB: Concepts in exercise rehabilitation of athletic injury. In: Leadbetter WB, Buckwalter JA, Gordon SL, eds. *Sports-Induced Inflammation: Clinical and Basic Science Concepts*. Park Ridge, IL: American Academy of Orthopaedic Surgeons. 1990;759-769.
237. Froimson A: Treatment of tennis elbow with forearm support. *J Bone Joint Surg*. 1961;43:100-103.
238. Ilfeld FW, Field SM: Treatment of tennis elbow: use of special brace. *JAMA*. 1966;195:67-71.
239. Groppel J, Nirschl RP: A biomechanical and electromyographical analysis of the effects of counter force braces on the tennis player. *Am J Sports Med*. 1986;14:195-200.
240. Chiumento AB, Bauer JA, Fiolkowski P: A comparison of the dampening properties of tennis elbow braces. *MSSE*. 1997; 29:123.
241. Jobe FW, Ciccotti MG: Lateral and medial epicondylitis of the elbow. *J Am Acad Orthop Surgeons*. 1994;2:1-8.
242. Nirschl RP: Prevention and treatment of elbow and shoulder injuries in the tennis player. *Clin Sports Med*. 1988;7:289-308.
243. Krischek O, Hopf C, Nafe B, et al: Shock-wave therapy for tennis and golfer's elbow—1 year follow-up. *Arch Orthop Trauma Surg*. 1999;119:62-66.

244. Glousman RE, Barron J, Jobe FW, et al: An electromyographic analysis of the elbow in normal and injured pitchers with medial collateral ligament insufficiency. *Am J Sports Med.* 1992; 20:311-317.
245. Burton RI, Eaton RG: Common hand injuries in the athlete. *Orthop Clin North Am.* 1973;4:809-838.
246. Hasselman CT, Best TM, Garrett WE: When groin pain signals an adductor strain. *Physician Sports Med.* 1995;23:53-60.
247. Lovell G: The diagnosis of chronic groin pain in athletes: a review of 189 cases. *Aust J Sci Med Sport.* 1995;27:76-79.
248. Casperson PC, Kauerman D: Groin and hamstring injuries. *Athletic Training.* 1982;17:43.
249. Frey C: Foot health and shoewear for women. *CORR.* 2000;372: 32-44.
250. Arnoczky SP, Warren RF: Microvasculature of the human meniscus. *Am J Sports Med.* 1982;10:90-95.
251. Arnoczky SP, McDevitt CA, Schmidt MB, et al: The effect of cryopreservation on canine menisci: a biochemical, morphologic, biomechanical evaluation. *J Orthop Res.* 1988;6:1-12.
252. Henning CE, Lynch MA, Yearout KM: Arthroscopic meniscal repair using an exogenous fibrin clot. *Clin Orthop.* 1990;252:64-72.
253. Henning CE, Lynch MA, Glick C: An in vivo strain gauge study of elongation of the anterior cruciate ligament. *Am J Sports Med.* 1985;13:22-26.
254. Henning CE: Current status of meniscal salvage. *Clin Sports Med.* 1990;9:567-576.
255. Beauchesne RP, Schutzer SF: Myositis ossificans of the piriformis muscle: an unusual cause of piriformis syndrome. A case report. *J Bone Joint Surg Am.* 1997;79:906-910.
256. Weider D: Treatment of traumatic myositis ossificans with acetic acid iontophoresis. *Phys Ther.* 1992;72:133-137.
257. Waller SL, Porter DE, Huntley JS: Myositis ossificans progressiva. *Br J Hosp Med (Lond).* 2006;67:606-607.
258. Hendifar AE, Johnson D, Arkfeld DG: Myositis ossificans: a case report. *Arthritis Rheum.* 2005;53:793-795.
259. Waldridge BM, Beard D, Livesey LC: What is your diagnosis? Myositis ossificans. *J Am Vet Med Assoc.* 2004;225:1533-1534.
260. Ronga M, Zappala G, Cherubino M, et al: Osteochondritis dissecans of the entire femoral trochlea. *Am J Sports Med.* 2006 34:1508-1511. Epub 2006 Mar 27.
261. Crawford DC, Safran MR: Osteochondritis dissecans of the knee. *J Am Acad Orthop Surg.* 2006;14:90-100.
262. Fortier LA, Nixon AJ: New surgical treatments for osteochondritis dissecans and subchondral bone cysts. *Vet Clin North Am Equine Pract.* 2005;21:673-690, vii.
263. Debeer P, Brys P: Osteochondritis dissecans of the humeral head: clinical and radiological findings. *Acta Orthop Belg.* 2005;71:484-488.
264. Johnson MP: Physical therapist management of an adult with osteochondritis dissecans of the knee. *Phys Ther.* 2005; 85:665-675.
265. Campos PS, Freitas CE, Pena N, et al: Osteochondritis dissecans of the temporomandibular joint. *Dentomaxillofac Radiol.* 2005;34:193-197.
266. Flynn JM, Kocher MS, Ganley TJ: Osteochondritis dissecans of the knee. *J Pediatr Orthop.* 2004;24:434-443.

267. Schenck RC Jr, Goodnight JM: Osteochondritis dissecans. *J Bone Joint Surg Am.* 1996;78:439-456.
268. Kankate RK, Selvan TP: Primary haematogenous osteomyelitis of the patella: a rare cause for anterior knee pain in an adult. *PMJ.* 2000;76:707-709.
269. Dich VQ, Nelson JD, Haltalin KC: Osteomyelitis in infants and children: a review of 163 cases. *Am J Dis Child.* 1975;129: 1273-1278.
270. Roy DR: Osteomyelitis of the patella. *CORR.* 2001;389:30-34.
271. Lew DP, Waldvogel FA: Osteomyelitis. *Lancet.* 2004;364: 369-379.
272. Lew DP, Waldvogel FA: Osteomyelitis. *N Engl J Med.* 1997;336: 999-1007.
273. Siris ES, Lyles KW, Singer FR, et al: Medical management of Paget's disease of bone: indications for treatment and review of current therapies. *J Bone Miner Res.* 2006;21 (suppl 2): P94-P98.
274. Bone HG: Nonmalignant complications of Paget's disease. *J Bone Miner Res.* 2006;21 (suppl 2):P64-P98.
275. Shankar S, Hosking DJ: Biochemical assessment of Paget's disease of bone. *J Bone Miner Res.* 2006;21 (suppl 2):P22-27.
276. Langston AL, Campbell MK, Fraser WD, et al: Clinical determinants of quality of life in Paget's disease of bone. *Calcif Tissue Int.* 2007;80:1-9. Epub 2007 Jan 4.
277. Griz L, Caldas G, Bandeira C, et al: Paget's disease of bone. *Arq Bras Endocrinol Metabol.* 2006;50:814-822.
278. Palkar S, Mohan V: Paget's disease in diabetic subjects. *J Assoc Physicians India.* 2006;54:585.
279. Bhatt K, Balakrishnan C, Mangat G, et al: Paget's disease of the bone: a report of three cases. *J Assoc Physicians India.* 2006; 54:571-574.
280. Klein GR, Parvizi J: Surgical manifestations of Paget's disease. *J Am Acad Orthop Surg.* 2006;14:577-586.
281. Takata S, Hashimoto J, Nakatsuka K, et al: Guidelines for diagnosis and management of Paget's disease of bone in Japan. *J Bone Miner Metab.* 2006;24:359-367.
282. Whyte MP: Clinical practice. Paget's disease of bone. *N Engl J Med.* 2006;355:593-600.
283. Black JE, Alten SR: How I manage infrapatellar tendinitis. *Physician Sports Med.* 1984;12:86-90.
284. Rompe JD, Schoellner C, Nafe B: Evaluation of low-energy extracorporeal shock-wave application for treatment of chronic plantar fasciitis. *J Bone Joint Surg.* 2002;84-A:335-341.
285. Guccione AA, Minor MA: Arthritis. In: O'Sullivan SB, Schmitz TJ, eds. *Physical Rehabilitation, 5th ed.* Philadelphia, PA: FA Davis. 2007:1057-1085.
286. Roubenoff R: Gout and hyperuricaemia. *Rheum Dis Clin North Am.* 1990;16:539-550.
287. Isomaki H, von Essen R, Ruutsalo H-M: Gout, particularly diuretics-induced, is on the increase in Finland. *Scand J Rheumatol.* 1977;6:213-216.
288. Gladman DD, Brubacher B, Buskila D, et al: Differences in the expression of spondyloarthropathy: a comparison between ankylosing spondylitis and psoriatic arthritis: genetic and gender effects. *Clin Invest Med.* 1993;16:1-7.

289. Haslock I: Ankylosing spondylitis. *Baillieres Clin Rheumatol.* 1993;7:99.
290. Gran JT: An epidemiologic survey of the signs and symptoms of ankylosing spondylitis. *Clin Rheumatol.* 1985;4:161-169.
291. Calin A, Porta J, Fries JF, et al: Clinical history as a screening test for ankylosing spondylitis. *JAMA.* 1977;237:2613-2614.
292. Cohen MD, Ginsurg WW: Late onset peripheral joint disease in ankylosing spondylitis. *Arthritis Rheum.* 1983;26:186-190.
293. Gladman DD: Clinical aspects of the spondyloarthropathies. *Am J Med Sci.* 1998;316:234-238.
294. Deyo RA, Rainville J, Kent DL: What can the history and physical examination tell us about low back pain? *JAMA.* 1992; 268:760-765.
295. Turek SL: *Orthopaedics—Principles and Their Application*, 4th ed. Philadelphia, PA: JB Lippincott. 1984.
296. Kraag G, Stokes B, Groh J, et al: The effects of comprehensive home physiotherapy and supervision on patients with ankylosing spondylitis: an 8-month follow-up. *J Rheumatol.* 1994;21:261-263.
297. Buskila D, Langevitz P, Gladman DD, et al: Patients with rheumatoid arthritis are more tender than those with psoriatic arthritis. *J Rheumatol.* 1992;19:1115-1119.
298. Gladman DD: Psoriatic arthritis. In: Kelley WN, Harris ED, Ruddy S, et al eds. *Textbook of Rheumatology, 5th ed.* Philadelphia, PA: WB Saunders. 1997:999-1005.
299. Gladman DD, Anhorn KB, Schachter RK, et al: HLA antigens in psoriatic arthritis. *J Rheumatol.* 1986;13:586-592.
300. Leirisalo-Repo M: Reactive arthritis. *Scand J Rheumatol.* 2005; 34:251-259.
301. Colmegna I, Espinoza LR: Recent advances in reactive arthritis. *Curr Rheumatol Rep.* 2005;7:201-207.
302. Toivanen A, Toivanen P: Reactive arthritis. *Best Pract Res Clin Rheumatol.* 2004;18:689-703.
303. Kohnke SJ: Reactive arthritis. A clinical approach. *Orthop Nurs.* 2004;23:274-280.
304. Childs SG: Reactive arthritis. Immune-mediated synovitis or joint infection. *Orthop Nurs.* 2004;23:267-273.
305. Haga HJ, Peen E: A study of the arthritis pattern in primary Sjogren's syndrome. *Clin Exp Rheumatol.* 2007;25:88-91.
306. Binard A, Devauchelle-Pensec V, Fautrel B, et al: Epidemiology of Sjogren's syndrome: where are we now? *Clin Exp Rheumatol.* 2007;25:1-4.
307. Amarasena R, Bowman S: Sjogren's syndrome. *Clin Med.* 2007; 7:53-56.
308. Mitsias DI, Kapsogeorgou EK, Moutsopoulos HM: Sjogren's syndrome: why autoimmune epithelitis? *Oral Dis.* 2006;12:523-532.
309. Garcia-Carrasco M, Fuentes-Alexandro S, Escarcega RO, et al: Pathophysiology of Sjogren's syndrome. *Arch Med Res.* 2006; 37:921-932.
310. Fox RI, Liu AY: Sjogren's syndrome in dermatology. *Clin Dermatol.* 2006;24:393-413.
311. Mavragani CP, Moutsopoulos NM, Moutsopoulos HM: The management of Sjogren's syndrome. *Nat Clin Pract Rheumatol.* 2006;2:252-261.
312. Burkhart SS: A stepwise approach to arthroscopic rotator cuff repair based on biomechanical principles. *Arthroscopy.* 2000;16:82-90.

313. Burkhart SS: A 26-year-old woman with shoulder pain. *JAMA.* 2000;284:1559-1567.
314. Jobe FW, Kvitne RS, Giangarra CE: Shoulder pain in the overhand and throwing athlete: the relationship of anterior instability and rotator cuff impingement. *Orthop. Rev.* 1989;18:963-975.
315. Jobe CM, et al: Anterior shoulder instability, impingement and rotator cuff tear. In: Jobe FW ed. *Operative Techniques in Upper Extremity Sports Injuries.* St Louis, MO: Mosby-Year Book. 1996.
316. Jobe FW, Pink M: Classification and treatment of shoulder dysfunction in the overhead athlete. *J Orthop Sports Phys Ther.* 1993;18:427-431.
317. Gordon EJ: Diagnosis and treatment of common shoulder disorders. *Med Trial Tech Q.* 1981;28:25-73.
318. Nixon JE, DiStefano V: Ruptures of the rotator cuff. *Orthop Clin North Am.* 1975;6:423-445.
319. Ellman H: Diagnosis and treatment of incomplete rotator cuff tears. *Clin Orthop.* 1990;254:64-74.
320. Goldberg BA, Nowinski RJ, Matsen FA III: Outcome of nonoperative management of full-thickness rotator cuff tears. *CORR.* 2001;1:99-107.
321. Gartsman GM: Arthroscopic rotator cuff repair. *CORR.* 2001;390: 95-106.
322. Onieal M-E: *Essentials of Musculoskeletal Care,* Rosemont, IL: American Academy of Orthopaedic Surgeons. 1997.
323. Onieal M-E: The hand: examination and diagnosis. *American Society for Surgery of the Hand, 3rd ed.* New York, NY: Churchill Livingstone. 1990.
324. Onieal M-E: Common wrist and ankle injuries. *ADVANCE for Nurse Practitioners.* 1996;4:31-36.
325. Gates SJ, Mooar PA: *Orthopaedics and Sports Medicine for Nurses: Common Problems in Management.* Baltimore, MD: Williams & Wilkins. 1999.
326. Wackerle JF: A prospective study identifying the sensitivity of radiographic findings and the efficacy of clinical findings in carpal navicular fractures. *Ann Emerg Med.* 1987;16:733-737.
327. Perron AD, Brady WJ, Keats TE, et al: Orthopedic pitfalls in the ED: scaphoid fracture. *Am J Emerg Med,.* 2001;19:310-316.
328. Chen SC: The scaphoid compression test. *J Hand Surg.* 1989;14:323-325.
329. Waizenegger M, Barton NJ, Davis TR, et al: Clinical signs in scaphoid fractures. *J Hand Surg.* 1994;19B:743-747.
330. Watson HK, Kao SD: Degenerative disorders of the carpus. In: Lichtman DM, Alexander AH, eds. *The Wrist and Its Disorders, 2nd ed.* Philadelphia, PA: W. B. Saunders. 1997;583-591.
331. Bukata SV, Rosier RN: Diagnosis and treatment of osteoporosis. *Curr Opin Orthop.* 2000;11:336-340.
332. Lane JM, Russell L, Khan SN: Osteoporosis. *Clin Orthop.* 2000; 372:139-150.
333. Eisman JA: Genetics of osteoporosis. *Endocrine Rev.* 1999; 20:788-804.
334. Scheiber LB, Torregrosa L: Early intervention for postmenopausal osteoporosis. *J Musculoskel Med.* 1999;16:146-157.
335. Lane JM, Riley EH, Wirganowicz PZ: Osteoporosis: diagnosis and treatment. *J Bone Joint Surg.* 1996;78A:618-632.

336. Block J, Smith R, Black D, et al: Does exercise prevent osteoporosis. *JAMA.* 1987;257:345.
337. NIH Consensus Development Panel on Osteoporosis Prevention D, and Therapy: Osteoporosis prevention, diagnosis, and therapy. *JAMA.* 2001;285:785-795.
338. Sran MM, Khan KM: Is spinal mobilization safe in severe secondary osteoporosis?—a case report. *Man Ther.* 2005;29:29.
339. Shea B, Bonaiuti D, Iovine R, et al: Cochrane review on exercise for preventing and treating osteoporosis in postmenopausal women. *Eura Medicophys.* 2004;40:199-209.
340. O'Connell MB: Prescription drug therapies for prevention and treatment of postmenopausal osteoporosis. *J Manag Care Pharm.* 2006;12:S10-S19; quiz S26-S28.
341. Compston J: Does parathyroid hormone treatment affect fracture risk or bone mineral density in patients with osteoporosis? *Nat Clin Pract Rheumatol.* 2007;1:1.
342. Cummings SR: A 55-year-old woman with osteopenia. *JAMA.* 2006;296:2601-2610.
343. Dupree K, Dobs A: Osteopenia and male hypogonadism. *Rev Urol.* 2004;6:S30-S34.
344. Basha B, Rao DS, Han ZH, et al: Osteomalacia due to vitamin D depletion: a neglected consequence of intestinal malabsorption. *Am J Med.* 2000;108:296-300.
345. Bonaiuti D, Shea B, Iovine R, et al: Exercise for preventing and treating osteoporosis in postmenopausal women. *Cochrane Database Syst Rev.* 2002:3.
346. Marcus R: Role of exercise in preventing and treating osteoporosis. *Rheum Dis Clin North Am.* 2001;27:131-141, vi.
347. Turner JA, Ersek M, Herron L, et al: Surgery for lumbar spinal stenosis: attempted meta-analysis of the literature. *Spine.* 1992;17:1-8.
348. Arnoldi CC, Brodsky AE, Cauchoix J: Lumbar spinal stenosis and nerve root encroachment syndromes: definition and classification. *Clin Orthop.* 1976;115:4-5.
349. Verbiest H: A radicular syndrome from developmental narrowing of the lumbar vertebral canal. *J Bone Joint Surg.* 1954; 26B:230.
350. Huijbregts PA: Lumbopelvic region: aging, disease, examination, diagnosis, and treatment. In: Wadsworth C, ed. *Current Concepts of Orthopaedic Physical Therapy—Home Study Course.* La Crosse, WI: *Orthopaedic Section, APTA.* 2001.
351. Cailliet R: *Low Back Pain Syndrome, 4th ed.* Philadelphia, PA: FA Davis Co. 1991:263-268.
352. Katz JN, Dalgas M, Stucki G, et al: Degenerative lumbar spinal stenosis: diagnostic value of the history and physical examination. *Arthritis Rheum.* 1995;38:1236-1241.
353. Weinstein SM, Herring SA: Rehabilitation of the patient with low back pain. In: DeLisa JA, Gans BM, eds. *Rehabilitation Medicine: Principles and Practice, 2nd ed.* Philadelphia, PA: JB Lippincott Company. 1993:996-1017.
354. Fast A: Low back disorders: conservative management. *Arch Phys Med Rehabil.* 1988;69:880-891.
355. Fritz JM, Erhard RE, Vignovic M: A nonsurgical treatment approach to patients with lumbar spinal stenosis. *Phys Ther.* 1997;77:962-973.

356. Bodack MP, Monteiro M: Therapeutic exercise in the treatment of patients with lumbar spinal stenosis. *CORR.* 2001;384:144-152.
357. Dooley JF, McBroom RJ, Taguchi T, et al: Nerve root infiltration in the diagnosis of radicular pain. *Spine.* 1988;13:79-83.
358. Tajima T, Furakawa K, Kuramochi E: Selective lumbosacral radiculography and block. *Spine.* 1980;5:68-77.
359. Newman PH: The etiology of spondylolisthesis. *J Bone Joint Surg.* 1963;45B:39-59.
360. Yang K, King A: Mechanism of facet load transmission as a hypothesis for low back pain. *Spine.* 1984;9:557-565.
361. Laus M, Tigani D, Alfonso C, et al: Degenerative spondylolisthesis: lumbar stenosis and instability. *Chir Organi Mov.* 1992; 77:39-49.
362. Isacsson G, Linde C, Isberg A: Subjective symptoms in patients with temporomandibular disk displacement versus patients with myogenic craniomandibular disorders. *J Prosthet Dent.* 1989; 61:70-77.
363. Paesani D, Westesson P-L, Hatala M, et al: Prevalence of temporomandibular joint internal derangement in patients with craniomandibular disorders. *Am J Orthod Dentofacial Orthop.* 1992;101:41-47.
364. Dolwick MF: Clinical diagnosis of temporomandibular joint internal derangement and myofascial pain and dysfunction. *Oral Maxillofac Surg Clin North Am.* 1989;1:1-6.
365. Juniper RP: Temporomandibular joint dysfunction: a theory based upon electromyographic studies of the lateral pterygoid muscle. *Br J Oral Maxillofac Surg.* 1984;22:1-8.
366. Porter MR: The attachment of the lateral pterygoid muscle to the meniscus. *J Prosthet Dent.* 1970;24:555-562.
367. Wongwatana S, Kronman JH, Clark RE, et al: Anatomic basis for disk displacement in temporomandibular joint (TMJ) dysfunction. *Am J Orthod Dentofacial Orthop.* 1994;105:257-264.
368. Bell WE: *Orofacial Pains: Classification, Diagnosis, Management, 3rd ed.* Chicago: New Year Medical Publishers. 1985.
369. Thompson JF, Jannsen F: Thoracic outlet syndromes. *Br J Surg.* 1996;83:435-436.
370. Roos DB: The place for scalenectomy and first-rib resection in thoracic outlet syndrome. *Surgery.* 1982;92:1077-1085.
371. Nishida T, Price SJ, Minieka MM: Medial antebrachial cutaneous nerve conduction in true neurogenic thoracic outlet syndrome. *Electromyogr Clin Neurophysiol.* 1993;33:285-288.
372. Silver D: Thoracic outlet syndrome. In: Sabiston DC, ed. *Textbook of Surgery: The Biological Basis of Modern Surgical Practice, 13th ed.* Philadelphia: WB Saunders Company. 1986.
373. Crawford FA: Thoracic outlet syndrome. *Surg Clin North Am.* 1980;60:947-956.
374. Sanders RJ, Johnson RF: Medico-legal matters. In: Sanders RJ, Haug CE, eds. *Thoracic Outlet Syndrome: A Common Sequela of Neck Injuries.* Philadelphia, PA: JB Lippincott. 1991:271-277.
375. Kiwak KJ: Establishing an etiology for torticollis. *Postgrad Med.* 1984;75:126-134.
376. Kiesewetter WB, Nelson PK, Pallandino VS, et al: Neonatal torticollis. *JAMA.* 1955;157:1281-1285.
377. Gorlin RJ, Cohen MM, Levin LS: *Syndromes of the Head and Neck, 3rd ed.* New York, NY: Oxford University Press. 1990.
378. Smith DL, DeMario MC: Spasmodic torticollis: a case report and review of therapies. *J Am Board Fam Pract.* 1996;9:435-441.

379. Wilson BC, Jarvis BL, Haydon RC: Nontraumatic subluxation of the atlantoaxial joint: Grisel's syndrome. *Larynoscope.* 1987; 96:705-708.
380. Britton TC: Torticollis—what is straight ahead? *Lancet.* 1998; 351:1223-1224.
381. Spencer J, Goetsch VL, Brugnoli RJ, et al: Behavior therapy for spasmodic torticollis: a case study suggesting a causal role for anxiety. *J Behav Ther Exp Psychiatry.* 1191;22:305-311.
382. Agras S, Marshall C: The application of negative practice to spasmodic torticollis. *Am J Psychiatry.* 1965;121:579-582.
383. Leplow B: Heterogeneity of biofeedback training effects in spasmodic torticollis: a single-case approach. *Behav Res Ther.* 1990;28:359-365.
384. Botte MJ, Gelberman RH: Acute compartment syndrome of the forearm. *Hand Clin.* 1998;14:391-403.
385. Onieal M-E: Common wrist and elbow injuries in primary care. Lippincott's primary care practice. *Musculoskeletal Conditions.* 1999;3:441-450.
386. Wilson RL, Carter MS: Management of hand fractures. In: Hunter J, Schneider LH, Mackin EJ, et al eds. *Rehabilitation of the Hand.* St Louis, MO: CV Mosby. 1990:284.
387. Mooney V, Robertson J: The facet syndrome. *Clin Orthop.* 1976;115:149-156.
388. Burnell A: Injection techniques in low back pain. In: Twomey LT, ed. *Symposium: Low Back Pain.* Perth: Western Australian Institute of Technology. 1974:111.
389. Strange FG: Debunking the disc. *Proc R Soc Med.* 1966;9: 952-956.
390. Kraft GL, Levinthal DH: Facet synovial impingement. *Surg Gynecol Obstet.* 1951;93:439-443.
391. Seimons LP: *Low Back Pain: Clinical Diagnosis and Management.* Norwalk, CT: Appleton-Century-Crofts. 1983.
392. Booth FW: Physiologic and biochemical effects of immobilization on muscle. *Clin Orthop Relat Res.* 1987;219:15-21.
393. Eiff MP, Smith AT, Smith GE: Early mobilization versus immobilization in the treatment of lateral ankle sprains. *Am Sports Med.* 1994;22:83-88.
394. Akeson WH, et al: Collagen cross-linking alterations in the joint contractures: changes in the reducible cross-links in periarticular connective tissue after 9 weeks immobilization. *Connect Tissue Res.* 1977;5:15.
395. Akeson WH, Amiel D, Abel MF, et al: Effects of immobilization on joints. *Clin Orthop.* 1987;219:28-37.
396. Akeson WH, Amiel D, Woo SL-Y: Immobility effects on synovial joints: the pathomechanics of joint contracture. *Biorheology.* 1980;17:95-110.
397. Woo SL-Y, Matthews J, Akeson WH, et al: Connective tissue response to immobility: a correlative study of biochemical and biomechanical measurements of normal and immobilized rabbit knee. *Arthritis Rheum.* 1975;18:257-264.
398. Dehne E, Tory R: Treatment of joint injuries by immediate mobilization based upon the spiral adaption concept. *Clin Orthop.* 1971;77:218-232.
399. McKenzie R, May S: Introduction. In: McKenzie R, May S, eds. *The Human Extremities: Mechanical Diagnosis and Therapy.* Waikanae, New Zealand: Spinal Publications New Zealand Ltd. 2000:1-5.

Neuromuscular Physical Therapy

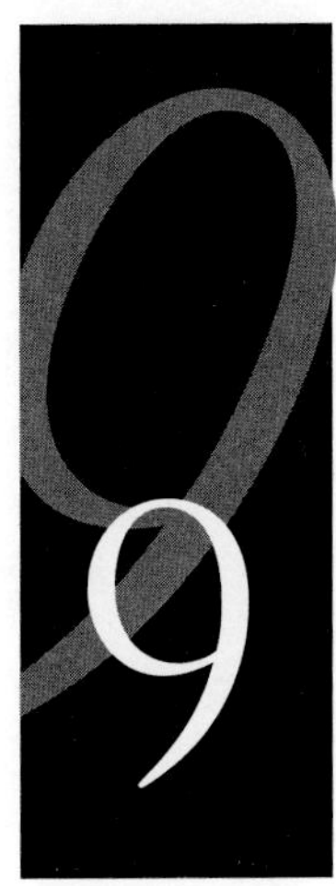

BASIC ANATOMY AND PHYSIOLOGY

The nerve cell, or neuron, which serves to store and process information, is the functional unit of the nervous system. The other cellular constituent include[1]:

- The neuroglial cell, or glia, which functions to provide structural and metabolic support for the neurons.[2] Glial cells outnumber the neurons 10:1.[3]
- Microglia: phagocytize pathogens and cellular debris within the CNS.
- Schwann cells: surround axons of all peripheral nerve fibers, forming a neurolemmal sheath; wrap around many peripheral fibers to form myelin sheaths.
- Satellite cells (ganglionic gliocytes): support ganglia within the PNS.
- Oligodendrocytes: form myelin sheaths around axons, producing white matter of the CNS.
- Astrocytes: vascular processes that cover capillaries within the brain and contribute to the blood-brain barrier.
- Ependymal cells: form the epithelial lining of brain cavities (ventricles) and the central canal of the spinal cord.

Although neurons come in a variety of sizes and shapes, there are four functional parts to each nerve (Table 9-1, Figure 9-1).

The communication of information from one nerve cell to another occurs at junctions called synapses, where a chemical is released in the form of a neurotransmitter (Figure 9-2). A synapse is the functional connection between a neuron and a second cell.[1] In the CNS this other cell is also a neuron. In the PNS, the other cell may be either a neuron or effector cell within a muscle or gland. Neuron-neuron synapses usually involve a connection between the axon of one neuron and the dendrites, cell body, or axon of a second neuron. In almost all synapses, transmission is in one direction only—from the axon of the

TABLE 9-1. FUNCTIONAL PARTS OF A NERVE

CELL TYPE	FUNCTIONS
Dendrite	Serves a receptive function, receiving information from other nerve cells or the environment.
Axon	Conducts information to other nerve cells.
Cell body	Contains the nucleus of the cell and has important integrative functions.
Axon terminal	The transmission site for action potentials, the messengers of the nerve cell.

first (or presynaptic) neuron to the second (or postsynaptic) neuron. Synaptic transmission can be either electrical or chemical.

- Electrical synapses: in order for two cells to be electrically coupled, they must be joined by areas of contact with low electrical resistance. Adjacent cells that are electrically coupled are joined together by gap junctions. Gap junctions are present in cardiac muscle, some smooth muscles, and in various regions of the brain, although the functional significance of the latter is presently unknown.

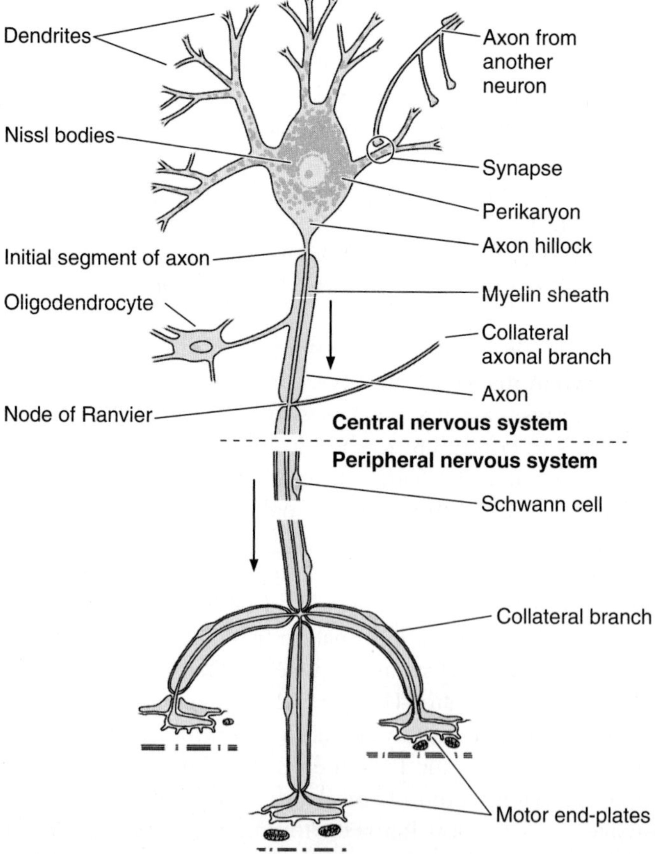

Figure 9-1. The motor neuron. (Reproduced, with permission, from Junqueira LC, Carneiro J: *Basic Histology: Text and Atlas, 10th ed.* New York, NY: McGraw-Hill. 2003:162.)

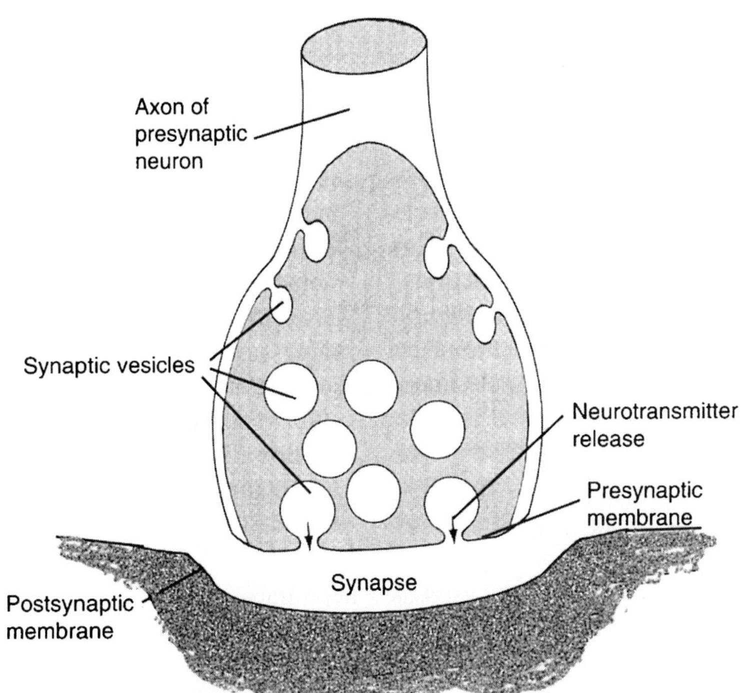

Figure 9-2. Nerve ending and synapse. (Reproduced, with permission, from Luttgens K, Hamilton N: *Kinesiology: Scientific Basis of Human Motion, 10th ed.* New York, NY: McGraw-Hill. 2002:73.)

- Chemical synapses: transmission across the majority of synapses in the nervous system is one way and occurs through the release of chemical neurotransmitters from presynaptic axon endings called axon terminals. The presynaptic endings are separated from the postsynaptic cell by a synaptic cleft.

The neurotransmitter molecules within the presynaptic neuron endings are contained within many small, membrane-enclosed synaptic vesicles. Voltage-regulated calcium (Ca^{2+}) channels are located in the axon terminal adjacent to the docking sites. The arrival of action potentials at the axon terminal open these voltage-regulated Ca^{2+} channels and it is the inward diffusion of Ca^{2+} that triggers the rapid fusion of the synaptic vesicle with the axon membrane and the release of neurotransmitter through a process called exocytosis.

Once the neurotransmitter molecules have been released from the presynaptic axon terminals, they diffuse rapidly across the synaptic cleft and reach the membrane of the postsynaptic cell where they bind to specific receptor proteins that are located within the postsynaptic membrane. Receptor proteins have high specificity for their neurotransmitter, which is the ligand of the receptor protein, and binding of the neurotransmitter ligand to its receptor protein causes ion channels to open in the postsynaptic membrane.

The opening of ion channels often produces a depolarization called an excitatory postsynaptic potential (EPSP), which in turn stimulate the postsynaptic cell to produce an action potential. In other cases a hyperpolarization occurs, called an inhibitory postsynaptic potential (IPSP), which antagonize this effect.

Study Pearl

The great majority of drugs that act on the nervous system do so by altering synaptic mechanisms (refer to Chapter 19).

NEUROTRANSMITTERS

Acetylcholine. Those neurons that use acetylcholine as a neurotransmitter are called cholinergic neurons. Acetylcholine (Ach) is used as an excitatory neurotransmitter by some neurons in the CNS and by somatic motor neurons at the neuromuscular junction.[1] At autonomic nerve endings, ACh maybe even excitatory or inhibitory, depending on the organ involved.

Monoamines. The regulatory molecules epinephrine, norepinephrine, dopamine, and serotonin are in the chemical family known as monoamines. Of these, epinephrine is a hormone but not a transmitter, while norepinephrine is also a hormone but also a neurotransmitter. As with acetylcholine, monoamine neurotransmitters are released by exocytosis from presynaptic vesicles, diffuse across the synaptic cleft, and interact with specific receptor proteins in the membrane of the postsynaptic cell.

Serotonin. Serotonin is used as a neurotransmitter by neurons with cell bodies in the raphe nuclei that are located along the midline of the brainstem. Physiological functions attributed to serotonin include a role in the regulation of mood and behavior, appetite, and cerebral circulation. Drugs that block the reuptake of serotonin into the presynaptic axons (selective serotonin reuptake inhibitors [SSRIs]) have been developed in the treatment of depression (refer to Chapter 19).

Dopamine. Neurons that use dopamine as a neurotransmitter are called dopaminergic neurons. The cell bodies of dopaminergic neurons are highly concentrated in the midbrain and their axons can be subdivided into two systems:

- Nigrostriatal system: the cell bodies of this system are located in a part of the midbrain called the substantia nigra, which send fibers to the caudate nucleus and the putamen (centers for motor control that are part of the basal nuclei). There is much evidence that in Parkinson disease there is degeneration of these neurons in the substantia nigra.
- Mesolimbic system: involves neurons that originate in the midbrain and send axons to structures in the forebrain that are part of the limbic system. The dopamine release by these neurons may be involved in behavior and reward.

Norepinephrine. Norepinephrine is used as a neurotransmitter in both the PNS (smooth muscles, cardiac muscle, and glands) and CNS (general behavioral arousal). Mental arousal can be elicited by amphetamines and other such drugs that stimulate pathways in which norepinephrine is used as a neurotransmitter (refer to Chapter 19).

Amino Acids

- Glutamic acid and aspartic acid: function as excitatory neurotransmitters in the CNS. Glutamic acid has been implicated in the physiology of memory.
- Gamma-aminobutyric acid (GABA): a derivative of glutamic acid is the most prevalent neurotransmitter in the brain (as many as one third of all the neurons in the brain use GABA

as a neurotransmitter). GABA, which has an inhibitory function, is involved in motor control. A deficiency of GABA releasing neurons is responsible for the uncontrolled movements seen in people with Huntington's chorea.

- Glycine: inhibitory neurotransmitters which have very important functions in the spinal cord, where they help in the control of skeletal movements.

Peptides/Neuropeptides. More than 25 peptides of various sizes are found in the synapses of the brain and are often called neuropeptides.

THE NEUROMUSCULAR JUNCTION

As the nerve impulse reaches its effector organ or another nerve cell, the impulse is transferred between the two at a motor endplate or synapse. At this junction, a transmitter substance is released from the nerve (see above), which causes the other excitable tissue to discharge. Most axons of the peripheral nerves terminate on muscle cells. Whereas terminals of autonomic nerve fibers do not come in intimate contact with smooth muscle or gland cells, terminals of motor fibers form large synapses with muscle fibers, called neuromuscular junctions (NMJs) or motor end plates—the point of contact between the motor nerve and the muscle. All skeletal muscle contains a NMJ. The polarization at the presynaptic motor nerve increases the entry of calcium ions through voltage gated calcium channels, causing fusion of acetylcholine (ACh)-containing vesicles with the presynaptic membrane. The nerve terminal releases ACh into the synapse. ACh diffuses across the synapse, activating the postsynaptic ACh receptor, and thus opening sodium channels with resultant depolarization of the muscle membrane, release of calcium from the sarcoplasmic reticulum, and muscle contraction. Normally, the ACh released is more than is needed for activation of all of the receptors providing a margin of safety in the NMJ transmission. Disease-related loss of the safety margin provides the basis for clinical testing of NMJ function.

NERVOUS SYSTEM ORGANIZATION

The nervous system can be divided into two anatomical divisions, with their own subdivisions:

- The central nervous system (CNS)
  - Brain
  - Spinal cord
- Peripheral nervous system (PNS)
  - Cranial nerves
  - Spinal nerves

The PNS can be divided into two major divisions: the afferent division, and the efferent division.

- Afferent division: the neurons of this division (sometimes referred to as primary afferents or first-order neurons) convey information from receptors in the periphery to the CNS. The cell bodies of afferent neurons are located outside of the brain or spinal cord in structures called ganglia.

- Efferent division: this division is further divided into a somatic nervous system and an autonomic nervous system.
  - Somatic division: innervates the skin, muscles and joints.
  - Autonomic system: the autonomic system (ANS) is the division of the PNS that functions primarily at a subconscious level. The ANS innervates the glands and smooth muscle of the viscera.[2] Fibers within this system are further subdivided into two components: parasympathetic and sympathetic. In general, these two systems have antagonist effects on their end organs.
    - Sympathetic: fight or flight, or fight or freeze, system (Figure 9-3)
    - Parasympathetic: rest and digest system (Figure 9-4)

MYELIN

Myelin coats, protects, and insulates most of the axons of the PNS and CNS. Myelin is divided into segments about 1 mm long by small gaps where the myelin is absent (nodes of Ranvier). As impulses are sent along the nerves, the impulses jump from node to node through a process called *salutatory conduction.* The myelin, which has a high electrical resistance and low capacitance, functions to increase the nerve conduction velocity (NCV) of neural transmissions. Destruction of the myelin in the CNS triggers many of the symptoms of diseases such as multiple sclerosis (MS).

CENTRAL NERVOUS SYSTEM

Nerves within the central nervous system (CNS) are referred to as upper motor neurons (UMN).

Study Pearl

Running through the entire brainstem is a core of tissue called the reticular formation, the neurons of which receive and integrate information from a wide range of areas including many areas of the brain, many afferent pathways, and the cardiovascular, respiratory, swallowing, and vomiting centers.

Brain. During embryonic development, the brain, contained within the skull (cranium), rapidly grows and differentiates into three distinct swellings: the prosencephalon, the mesencephalon, and the rhombencephalon (Table 9-2).[1]

Brainstem. The brainstem attaches to the spinal cord and includes the mesencephalon (midbrain), pons, and medulla oblongata (Table 9-2), and contains nuclei for autonomic functions of the body and their connecting tracts. The brain stem gives rise to 10 of the 12 pairs of cranial nerves.

White Matter of the Cerebrum. The thick white matter of the cerebrum consists of dendrites, myelinated axons, and associated neuroglia. The three types of fiber tracts within the white matter are named according to their location and the direction in which they conduct impulses:

- Association fibers: located in a given cerebral hemisphere and conduct impulses between neurons within that hemisphere.
- Commissural (transverse) fibers: connect the neurons and gyri of one hemisphere with those of the other (eg, corpus callosum, anterior commissure).
- Projection fibers: form the ascending and descending tracks that transmit impulses from the cerebrum to other parts of the brain and spinal cord.

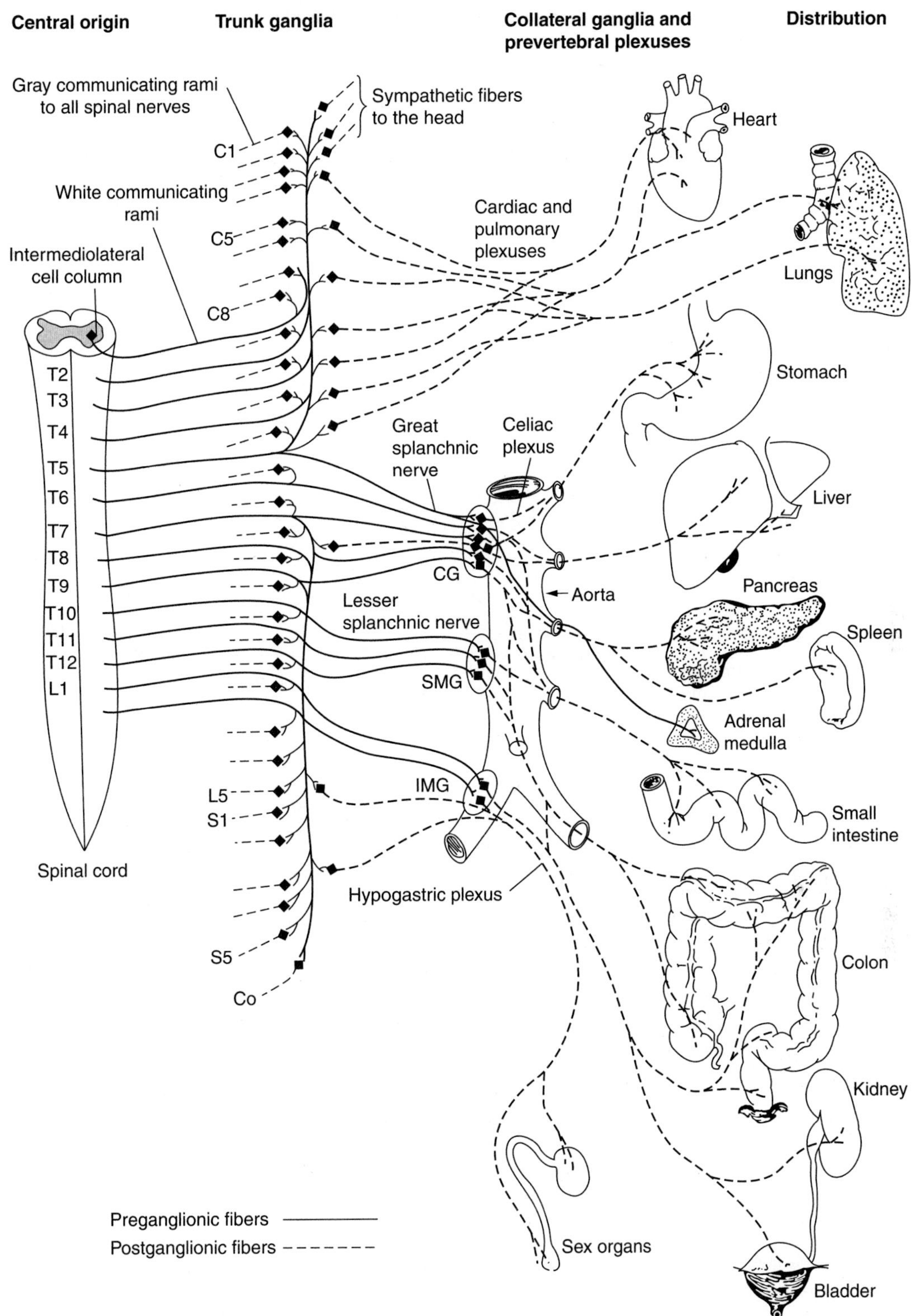

Figure 9-3. Sympathetic division of the autonomic nervous system. (Reproduced, with permission, from Waxman, SG: *Correlative Neuroanatomy, 24th ed.* New York: McGraw-Hill. 2000:250.)

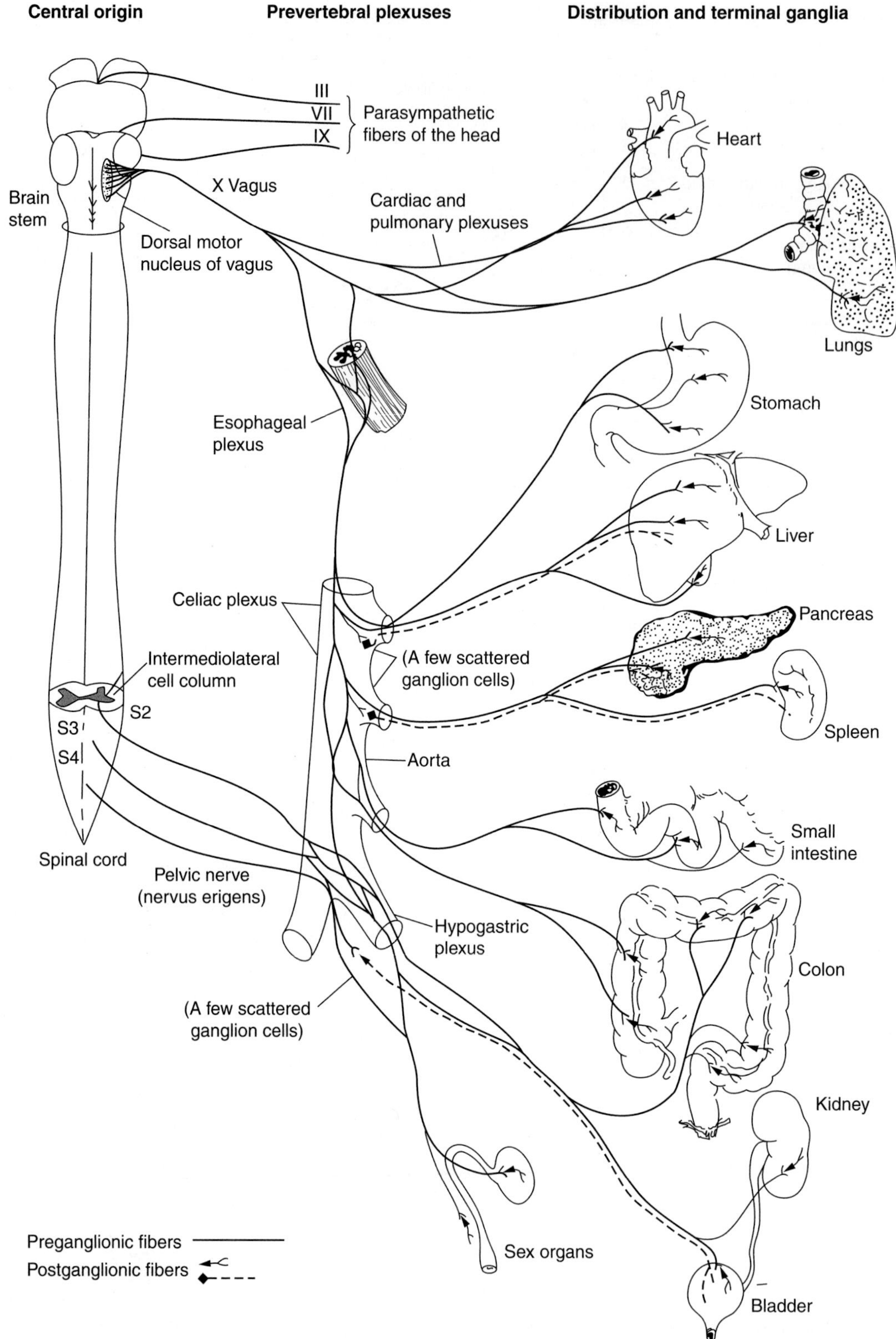

Figure 9-4. Parasympathetic division of the autonomic nervous system. (Reproduced, with permission, from Waxman, SG: *Correlative Neuroanatomy, 24th ed.* New York: McGraw-Hill. 2000:253.)

TABLE 9-2. DERIVATION AND FUNCTIONS OF THE MAJOR BRAIN STRUCTURES

	REGION	STRUCTURE	DESCRIPTION/FUNCTION
Prosencephalon (Forebrain)	Telencephalon	Cerebrum	Consists of six paired lobes within two convoluted hemispheres. The outer part of the cerebral hemispheres is called the cerebral cortex. The elevated folds of the convolutions (crests) are called the cerebral gyri, and the depressed grooves (fissures) are the cerebral sulci.
	Diencephalon	Limbic system	Phylogenetically, the oldest part of the brain. Controls most sensory and motor activities; reasoning, memory, intelligence, etc. Instinctual and limbic functions include basic emotional behavior, such as anger, fear, sex, and hunger.
		Thalamus	The principal function of the thalamus is to act as a relay center for all sensory impulses, except smell, to the cerebral cortex and subcortical regions. Also performs initial autonomic response to pain and crude awareness.
		Hypothalamus	Regulation of food and water intake, body temperature, heartbeat, etc; control of secretory activity in the anterior pituitary; instinctual and limbic functions.
		Epithalamus	Production of cerebrospinal fluid by the choroid plexus (see Meninges of the Central Nervous System). Influence of the circadian rhythm through the release of hormones from the pineal gland. Integration of olfactory, visceral and somatic afferent pathways via the habenular nuclei.
		Pituitary gland	Regulation of various endocrine functions.
Mesencephalon (Midbrain)	Mesencephalon	Corpora quadrigemina	Consists of the superior colliculi (visual reflexes, hand-eye coordination) and the inferior colliculi (auditory reflexes).
		Cerebral peduncles	Cylindrical structures composed of ascending and descending projection fiber tracts that support and connect the cerebrum to other regions of the brain to allow reflex coordination.
		The mesencephalic aqueduct (Sylvius)	Connects the third and fourth ventricle.
		Red nucleus	Functions in reflexes concerned with motor coordination and maintenance of posture.
		Substantia nigra	Functions to inhibit involuntary movements. It is a major element of the basal ganglia. Degeneration of pigmented neurons in the substantia nigra region is the principal pathology that underlies Parkinson disease.
Rhombencephalon (Hindbrain)	Metencephalon	Pons	Balance and motor coordination The nuclei of the pons serve a number of important functions: ▶ Some of the nuclei function with nuclei of the medulla oblongata to regulate the rate and depth of breathing. ▶ Several nuclei (tegmentum) within the pons are associated with specific cranial nerves (trigeminal [V], abducens [VI], facial [VII], and vestibulocochlear [VIII]). ▶ The surface fibers extend transversely to connect with the cerebellum through the middle cerebellar peduncles. ▶ Raphe nuclei are involved with pain modulation and the control of arousal.
		Cerebellum	The principal functions of the cerebellum include: ▶ Coordination of skeletal muscle contractions by recruiting precise motor units within the muscles such as accurate force, direction and extent of movement, and sequencing of movements (neocerebellum). ▶ Equilibrium, and regulation of muscle tone via the floculonodular lobe and proprioceptive input. ▶ Modification of muscle tone and synergistic actions of muscles.

(*Continued*)

TABLE 9-2. DERIVATION AND FUNCTIONS OF THE MAJOR BRAIN STRUCTURES (*Continued*)

	REGION	STRUCTURE	DESCRIPTION/FUNCTION
	Myelencephalon	Medulla oblongata	Relay center that connects the spinal cord with the pons; contains many nuclei; visceral autonomic center (eg, respiration, heart rate, vasoconstriction): ▶ Composed of vital nuclei and white matter that form all of the descending and ascending tracks communicating between the spinal cord and various parts of the brain. ▶ Most of the fibers within these tracks cross over (decussate) to the opposite side through the pyramidal region of the medulla oblongata permitting one side of the brain to receive information from, and send information to, the opposite side of the body.

Data from Van de Graaff KM, Fox SI: Central nervous system. In: Van de Graaff KM, Fox SI, eds. *Concepts of Human Anatomy and Physiology*. New York, NY: WCB/McGraw-Hill; 1999:407-446.

Basal Nuclei. The basal nuclei include the corpus striatum (caudate nucleus, claustrum, and lenticular nuclei [putamen, globus pallidus]), and the amygdaloid nucleus. The basal nuclei (ganglia) are associated with other structures of the brain, particularly within the mesencephalon. The functions of the basal nuclei include:

- Control of unconscious contractions of certain skeletal muscles, such as those of the upper extremities involved in involuntary arm movements during walking—caudate nucleus and putamen.
- The regulation (amplitude and velocity) of muscle tone necessary for specific and intentional body movements—globus pallidus. Muscle tone refers to firmness of the tissue and is the resistance to passive elongation or stretch.[4] It is a function of both the mechanical-elastic properties of muscle and neural drive.[4]
- Provision of three main circuits:
  - Oculomotor: functions with saccadic movements.
  - Skeletomotor: reinforces selected motor patterns while suppressing conflicting patterns, and makes preparations for movements.

Study Pearl

The blood-brain barrier, a capillary barrier comprising both anatomical and physiological transport systems, precisely regulates the chemical composition of the extracellular fluid (ECF) of the brain, and closely monitors both the substances that enter the ECF and the rate at which they enter.

Study Pearl

There are no connective tissue components in the spinal nerves comparable to the epineurium and perineurium of the peripheral nerve (see later) (at least they are not developed to the same degree).[5] As a result, the spinal nerve roots are more sensitive to both tension and compression. The spinal nerve roots are also devoid of lymphatics, and are thus predisposed to prolonged inflammation.[6]

Blood Supply. The brain is completely dependent upon a continuous supply of arterial blood to provide it with glucose and oxygen (Figures 9-5 and 9-6).

Meninges of the Central Nervous System. Three membranes, or meninges, and related spaces, are important for nutrition of the spinal cord (Table 9-3). The meninges envelop the structures of the CNS, and form barriers that resist the entrance of a variety of noxious organisms.

Cerebrospinal Fluid. The cerebrospinal fluid (CSF) that flows through the meningeal spaces, and within the four ventricles of the brain, functions to:

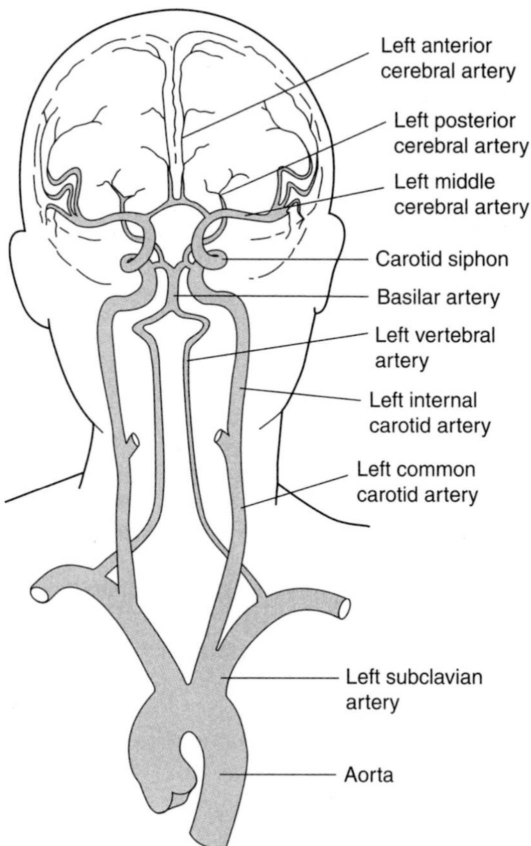

Figure 9-5. Major cerebral arteries. (Reproduced, with permission, from Waxman, SG: *Correlative Neuroanatomy, 24th ed.* New York: McGraw-Hill. 2000:169.)

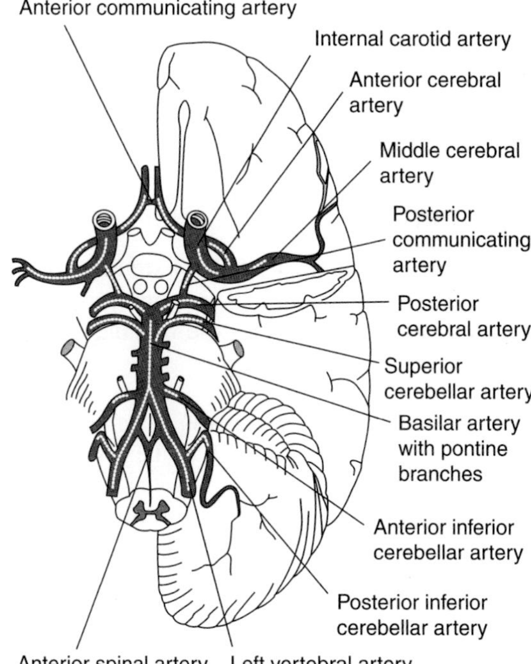

Figure 9-6. Circle of Willis and principal arteries of the brainstem. (Reproduced, with permission, from Waxman, SG. *Correlative Neuroanatomy, 24th ed.* New York: McGraw-Hill. 2000:169.)

TABLE 9-3. MENINGES OF THE CNS

Dura mater	The outermost and strongest of the layers. Composed of an inner meningeal layer, and an outermost periosteal layer. The dura runs uninterrupted from the interior of the cranium, through the foramen magnum, and surrounds the spinal cord throughout its distribution from the cranium to the coccyx at the second sacral level (S 2).[a] The dura is also attached to the posterior surfaces of C 2 and C 3.[b] The dura forms a vertical sac (dural sac) around the spinal cord, and its short lateral projections blend with the epineurium of the spinal nerves. The dura is separated from the bones and ligaments that form the walls of the vertebral canal by an epidural space, which can become partly calcified or even ossified with age.[c]
Arachnoid	A thin and delicate avascular layer, coextensive with the dura mater and the pia mater. Even though the arachnoid and pia mater are interconnected by trabeculae, there is a space between them called the subarachnoid space, which contains the cerebrospinal fluid. It is the supposed rhythmic flow of this cerebrospinal fluid, which is used by craniosacral therapists to explain the rationale behind their techniques, although this has yet to be substantiated in the literature.
Pia mater	The deepest of the layers. It is intimately related and firmly attached via connective tissue investments, to the outer surface of the spinal cord and nerve roots. The pia mater conveys the blood vessels that supply the spinal cord, and has a series of lateral specializations, the denticulate (dentate) ligaments, which anchor the spinal cord to the dura mater.[a] These ligaments, which derive their name from their tooth-like appearance, extend the whole length of the spinal cord.

[a]Data from Pratt N: *Anatomy of the Cervical Spine.* La Crosse, WI: Orthopaedic Section, APTA. 1996.
[b]Data from Sunderland S: Anatomical perivertebral influences on the intervertebral foramen. In: Goldstein MN, ed: *The Research Status of Spinal Manipulative Therapy.* Bethesda, Maryland, HEW Publication No (NIH). 1975:76-998.
[c]Data from Waxman SG: *Correlative Neuroanatomy, 24th ed.* New York, NY: McGraw-Hill. 1996.

- Provide a cushion for the spinal cord, allowing the CNS to literally float in the fluid.
- Provide a type of blood-brain barrier through selective secretion between the capillaries of the choroids plexus and the CSF that flows next to the neural tissue.
- Control brain excitability by regulating ionic composition.
- Aid in the exchange of nutrients and waste products.

Study Pearl

The normal pressure for CSF, which varies according to body position, ranges from 70 to 180 mm/H_2O.

The CSF flow is aided by circulatory, respiratory, and postural pressure changes. Most of the CSF is secreted into the ventricles by highly vascular tissues, the choroid plexuses. The CSF returns to the venous blood through the arachnoid villi.

THE SPINAL CORD

The spinal cord is the part of the CNS that extends down through the foramen magnum of the skull into the vertebral canal of the vertebral column and which is continuous with the medulla and brain stem at its upper end.

- The conus medullaris serves as the lower end of the cord. In adults, the conus end at the L1 or L2 level of the vertebral column.
- A series of specializations, the filum terminales and the coccygeal ligament, anchor the spinal cord and dural sac inferiorly, and ensure that tensile forces applied to the spinal cord are distributed throughout its entire length.[7]

Study Pearl

The cauda equina (CE) is formed by nerve roots caudal to the level of spinal cord termination.

Two prominent enlargements can be seen in a posterior view of the spinal cord: the cervical enlargement located between C3 and T2; the lumbar enlargement lies between T9 and T12.

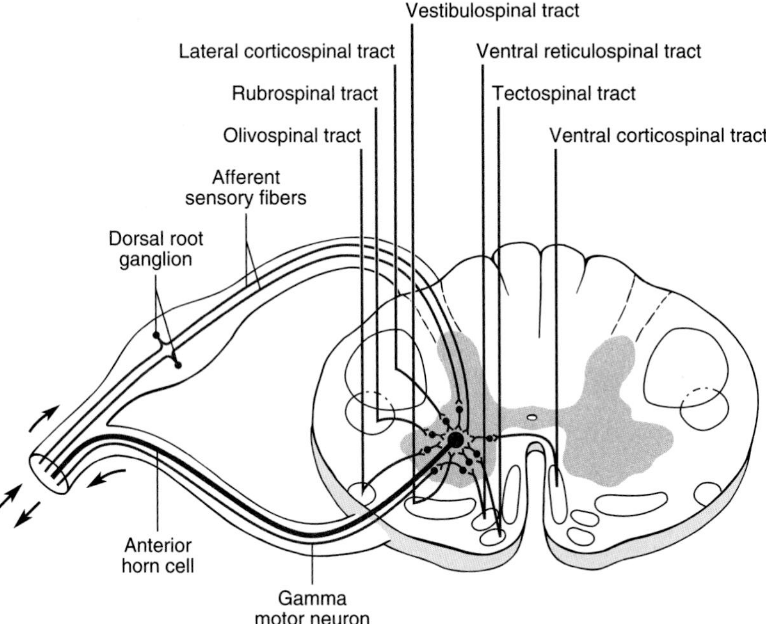

Figure 9-7. Spinal cord, cross section. (Reproduced, with permission, from Gilman, S: *Clinical Examination of the Nervous Tissue*. New York: McGraw-Hill. 2000:141.)

Gray Matter. The central gray matter of the spinal cord, which roughly resembles the letter H (Figure 9-7), contains two anterior (ventral) and two posterior (dorsal) horns united by gray commissure within the central canal.

- Anterior horns: contain cell bodies that give rise to motor (efferent) neurons.
- Gamma motor neurons to muscle spindles (Table 9-4).
- Alpha motor neurons to effect muscles.
- Posterior horns: contain sensory (afferent) neurons located in the posterior (dorsal) root ganglia, a swelling that contains nerve cell bodies.[3]

White Matter. The white matter of the spinal cord consists of bundles or tracts of myelinated fibers of sensory and motor neurons (Tables 9-5 and 9-6).

Study Pearl

The spinal cord has a segmental organization. Each of the 31 pairs of spinal nerves that arise from the spinal cord has an anterior (ventral) root and a posteior (dorsal) root.[3]

Study Pearl

Aggregates of tracts are referred to as columns, or lemnisci.

TABLE 9-4. THE MUSCLE SPINDLE

MUSCLE SPINDLE
Muscle spindles are sensory receptors within the belly of a muscle, which primarily detect changes in the length of the muscle. Within each muscle spindle there are specialized skeletal muscle fibers called *intrafusal fibers*. The central portion of the intrafusal fiber is unable to contract. When the muscle spindle is stimulated by a quick stretch, its receptors are polarized and an impulse volley enters the spinal cord and synapses with alpha motor neurons that innervate the extrafusal fibers of the stretched muscle and its synergistic muscles. The same afferent supplies inhibitory input to the antagonist muscles by way of interneurons so that as the agonist contracts, the antagonist will be relaxed in the process of reciprocal inhibition. This has the effect of producing a smooth contraction and relaxation of muscle and eliminating any jerkiness during movement under normal circumstances. The firing of the alpha motor neuron fibers is influenced by the rate of stretch; the faster and greater the stimulus, the greater the effect of the associated extrafusal fibers.

TABLE 9-5. MAJOR ASCENDING TRACTS OF THE SPINAL CORD

TRACTS	FUNCTION
Dorsal Medial Lemniscus ▶ Fasciculus gracilis: contains fibers from sacral, lumbar, and the lower six thoracic segments. These axons are located in the medial ipsilateral part of the dorsal column. ▶ Fasciculus cuneatus: appears at the level of T6 and contains the axons that enter the cord ipsilaterally at the upper six thoracic and cervical levels and that are located in the lateral part of the dorsal column.	▶ Convey proprioception, fine touch, position (kinesthesia) and vibratory senses to the *medulla oblongata* where the axons terminate respectively in the *nucleus gracilis* and the *nucleus cuneatus*. Conveys impulses concerned with well-localized touch and with the sense of movement and position. ▶ Important in moment-to-moment (temporal) and point-to-point (spatial) discrimination. ▶ Make it possible for you to put a key in a door lock without light or visualize the position of any part of your body without looking. ▶ Lesions to the tract from destructive tumors, hemorrhage, scar tissue, swelling, infections, direct trauma, etc. abolish or diminish tactile sensations and movement or position sense. The cell bodies of the primary neurons in the dorsal column pathway are in the spinal ganglion. The peripheral processes of these neurons begin at receptors in the joint capsule, muscles, and skin (tactile and pressure receptors).
Spinothalamic Tracts Helps mediate the sensations of pain, cold, warmth, and touch from receptors throughout the body (except the face) to the brain.[a-d]	Most of the cells project to the contralateral thalamus, although a small fraction project ipsilaterally.[e]
▶ Lateral spinothalamic tract	Conveys information about pain and temperature sensations.
▶ Ventral spinothalamic tract	Conveys information about pressure and simple touch. As the spinothalamic tract ascends, it migrates from a lateral position to a posterior-lateral position. In the midbrain, the tract lies adjacent to the medial lemniscus. The axons of the secondary neurons terminate in one of a number of centers in the thalamus.
Spinoreticular Tracts	Convey messages with regard to deep and chronic pain to reticular formation of the brainstem by diffuse, polysynaptic pathways.
Spinocerebellar Tracts	The spinocerebellar tract conducts impulses related to the position and movement of muscles to the cerebellum. This information enables the cerebellum to add smoothness and precision to patterns of movement initiated in the cerebral hemispheres. Spinocerebellar impulses do not reach the cerebrum directly and, therefore, have no conscious representation.
Posterior Spinocerebellar Tracts ▶ Uncrossed and more numerous than those of the anterior spinocerebellar tract. They arise from the dorsal nucleus of Clarke and ascend as a posterolateral tract to enter the cerebellum through the inferior cerebellar peduncle and terminate in the anterior lobe and part of the pyramis.	Mostly concerned with proprioceptive information from the upper limbs and with the control of posture.
Anterior Spinocerebellar Tracts ▶ Fibers from the anterior spinocerebellar tract ascend from the lower cord and are divided into a few ipsilateral (uncrossed) and a majority of contralateral (crossed) fibers.	Mostly concerned with proprioceptive information from the lower limbs and with the control of posture.
Corticopontocerebellar Tracts ▶ Afferent fibers from the temporal, parietal, occipital and frontal lobes of the cerebral cortex pass through the internal capsule and crus cerebri and synapse in the pontine nuclei. From here, the fibers enter the cerebellum through the middle cerebellar peduncle and terminate in the contralateral cerebellar hemisphere.	Provide motor information to the cerebellum from the frontal lobe.

(*Continued*)

TABLE 9-5. MAJOR ASCENDING TRACTS OF THE SPINAL CORD (*Continued*)

TRACTS	FUNCTION
Cerebro-olivocerebellar Tract	
▶ Afferent fibers from the temporal, parietal, occipital, and frontal lobes of the cerebral cortex pass through the internal capsule and synapse in both the ipsilateral and contralateral inferior olivary nuclei. From here, the fibers enter the cerebellum through the inferior cerebellar peduncle and terminate in the contralateral cerebellar hemisphere. Note: This pathway differs from all other afferents in that its fibers terminate in the cerebellum as climbing fibers, whereas all other afferents terminate as mossy fibers.	Concerned with muscle joint information
Cerebroreticulocerebellar Tract	
▶ Afferent fibers from all over the cerebral cortex terminate in the pontine and medullary reticular formation, both ipsilaterally and contralaterally. From here, the fibers enter the cerebellum through the middle cerebellar peduncle and terminate in the ipsilateral cerebellar hemisphere.	Concerned with muscle joint information
Cuneocerebellar Tract	
▶ Afferent fibers from the lateral cuneate nucleus in the medulla enter the cerebellum through the inferior cerebellar peduncle and terminate in the ipsilateral cerebellar hemisphere.	Concerned with muscle joint information
Vestibulocerebellar Tract	
▶ Afferent fibers of the vestibular system project to the cerebellum in two ways. Primary vestibular afferents project directly to the ipsilateral cerebellar hemisphere (primarily to the flocculonodular lobe) through the inferior cerebellar peduncle. Other vestibular afferents first synapse in the vestibular nuclei, and then also enter the cerebellum through the inferior cerebellar peduncle.	Conveys information from the semi-circular canals of the inner ear to the cerebellum via the vestibular nucleus located in the lower pons and medulla. These fibers travel to the flocculi on the inferior cerebellar peduncle.

[a]Data from Willis WD: *The Pain System*. Basel: Karger; 1985.
[b]Data from Spiller WG, Martin E: The treatment of persistent pain of organic origin in the lower part of the body by division of the anterior-lateral column of the spinal cord. *JAMA*. 1912;58:1489-1490.
[c]Data from Gowers WR: A case of unilateral gunshot injury to the spinal cord. *Trans Clin Lond.* 1878;11:24-32.
[d]Data from Vierck CJ, Greenspan JD, Ritz LA: Long-term changes in purposive and reflexive responses to nociceptive stimulation following anterior-lateral chordotomy. *J Neurosci.* 1990;10:2077-2095.
[e]Data from Willis WD, Coggeshall RE: *Sensory Mechanisms of the Spinal Cord.* 2nd ed. New York, NY: Plenum Press; 1991.

Blood Supply. The blood supply of the spinal cord consists of one anterior, and two posterior spinal arteries. The anterior and posterior spinal arteries arise from the vertebral arteries in the neck and descend from the base of the skull. Various radicular arteries branch off the thoracic and abdominal aorta to provide collateral flow:

- ▶ Anterior spinal artery: supplies the anterior two thirds of the cord.
  - Ischemic injury to this vessel results in dysfunction of the corticospinal, lateral spinothalamic, and autonomic interomedial pathways.
  - Anterior spinal artery syndrome involves paraplegia, loss of pain and temperature sensation, and autonomic dysfunction.
- ▶ Posterior spinal arteries: primarily supply the posterior (dorsal) columns.

TABLE 9-6. MAJOR DESCENDING TRACTS OF THE SPINAL CORD

TRACT	FUNCTION
Corticospinal Tract Originates in part from the pyramidal cells in the cortex of each cerebral hemisphere and courses through the internal capsule, then through the medullary pyramids. At this point some 80% of the fibers from each hemisphere, decussate in the pyramidal decussation, and continue to descend in the lateral white column of the opposite side. The remaining 20% continue down ipsilaterally, in the anteromedial white column, to innervate bilaterally, the more medially located motor neurones of the axial and proximal muscles.	Has a strong influence on the musculature of the extremities, particularly on the distal hands and feet. It is especially important in the regulation of fine skilled movements. Although not its exclusive action, it tends to have a facilitative action upon anterior horn cells which innervate flexor muscles, and an inhibitory influence on those that innervate extensor musculature.
Rubrospinal Tract Fibers of the rubrospinal tract have their cell bodies in the red nucleus, situated in the tegmentum of the midbrain. All fibers decussate immediately on leaving the red nucleus and descend through the pons, medulla and spinal cord as the rubrospinal tract. The red nucleus receives afferents from the cerebellum and the cerebral cortex, and therefore they both have an influence on the rubrospinal tract.	Involved in large movements of proximal musculature of the limbs. It inhibits activity of extensors, and increases activity of flexors.
Reticulospinal Tract Fibers have cell bodies in the pontine and medullary reticular formation. The fibers from the pons descend in the pontine reticulospinal tract and are mainly ipsilateral. The fibers from the medulla descend in the medullary reticulospinal tract, and are both ipsilateral and contralateral.	Involved in the influence of muscle spindles, making them more or less sensitive, and hence altering muscle reflexes. The reticulospinal tract is also involved in the control of sympathetic and sacral parasympathetic outflow by the hypothalamus.
Vestibulospinal Tract The fibers have their cell bodies in the vestibular nuclei situated in the pons. There are two spinal pathways to note. The first is the lateral vestibulospinal tract which has cell bodies in the lateral vestibular nucleus, and whose axons descend ipsilaterally in the spinal cord. The second is the medial vestibulospinal tract (medial longitudinal fasciculus), which has cell bodies in the medial vestibular nucleus and projects mainly to ipsilateral cervical regions of the spinal cord. The vestibular nuclei receive afferents from the vestibular apparatus, which includes the semicircular canals, and the otolith organs (utricle and saccule). The medial longitudinal fasciculus, which in addition receives inputs from the superior and inferior vestibular nuclei, ascends cranially through the brainstem for coordination of head and eye movements.	The lateral vestibulospinal tract is involved in postural control (especially related to movements of the head) by inhibiting axial flexor muscles, and stimulating axial extensor muscles. The medial longitudinal fasciculus is involved in the coordination of head and eye movements.
Tectospinal Tract Fibers have their cell bodies in the deep layers of the superior colliculus in the midbrain. The fibers decussate just caudally to their origin in the midbrain, and descend close to the medial longitudinal fasciculus in the tectospinal tract.	Plays an important role in mediating contralateral movements of the head in response to auditory, visual and somatic stimuli. This is a protective reflex.

PERIPHERAL NERVOUS SYSTEM

Peripheral nerves are referred to as lower motor neurons (LMN). The peripheral nervous system (PNS) consists of 12 pairs of nerves that connect with the brain (cranial nerves that are referred to by the Roman numerals I through XII), and 31 pairs of nerves that connect with the spinal cord as the spinal nerves.

Cranial Nerves. The cranial nerve roots enter and exit the brain stem to provide sensory and motor innervation to the head and muscles of the face. CN I and II (olfactory and optic, respectively) are

TABLE 9-7. CRANIAL NERVES AND THEIR FUNCTION

CRANIAL NERVE	ANATOMY AND FUNCTION
I—Olfactory	The olfactory nerve is responsible for the sense of smell.
II—Optic	The fibers of the optic nerve arise from the inner layer of the retina and proceed posteriorly to enter the cranial cavity via the optic foramen, to form the optic chiasm. The fibers from the nasal half of the retina decussate within the optic chiasm, while those from the lateral half do not. The optic nerve is responsible for vision.
III—Oculomotor	The somatic portion of the oculomotor nerve supplies the levator palpabrae superioris muscle, the superior, medial and inferior rectus muscles, and the inferior oblique muscles. These muscles are responsible for some eye movements. The visceral efferent portion of this nerve innervates two smooth intraocular muscles: the ciliary and the constrictor pupillae. These muscles are responsible for papillary constriction.
IV—Trochlear	The trochlear nerve supplies the superior oblique muscle of the eye.
V—Trigeminal	All three of the branches (maxillary, ophthalmic and mandibular) contain sensory cells. The ophthalmic and maxillary are exclusively sensory, the latter supplying the soft and hard palate, maxillary sinuses, upper teeth and upper lip and the mucous membrane of the pharynx. The mandibular branch carries sensory information but also represents the motor component of the nerve, supplying the muscles of mastication, both pterygoids, the anterior belly of digastric, tensor tympani, tensor veli palatini and mylohyoid.
VI—Abducens	The abducens nerve innervates the lateral rectus muscle of the eye.
VII—Facial	The facial nerve is comprised of a sensory (intermediate) root, which conveys taste, and a motor root, the facial nerve proper, which supplies the muscles of facial expression, the platysma muscle, and the stapedius muscle of the inner ear.
VIII—Vestibulocochlear	The cochlear portion is concerned with the sense of hearing. The tympanic membrane is connected to a 3-bone chain (malleus, incus, and stapes). The ossicular chain transfers the acoustic stimulus to the fluid-filled cochlea. The vestibular portion is part of the system of equilibrium, the vestibular system.
IX—Glossopharyngeal	The glossopharyngeal nerve serves a number of functions. ▶ It receives sensory fibres from the posterior one-third of the tongue, the tonsils, the pharynx, the middle ear and the carotid body. ▶ It supplies parasympathetic fibres to the parotid gland via the otic ganglion. ▶ It supplies motor fibres to stylopharyngeus muscle. ▶ It contributes to the pharyngeal plexus.
X—Vagus	The vagus nerve contains somatic motor, visceral efferent, visceral sensory, and somatic sensory fibers. The functions of the vagus nerve are numerous.
XI—Accessory	The cranial root is often viewed as an aberrant portion of the vagus nerve. The spinal portion of the nerve supplies the sternocleidomastoid and the trapezius muscles.
XII—Hypoglossal	The hypoglossal nerve is the motor nerve of the tongue, innervating the ipsilateral side of the tongue, as well as forming the descendens hypoglossi, which anastomosis with other cervical branches to form the ansa hypoglossi, which in turn innervates the infrahyoid muscles.

not true nerves but are fiber tracts of the brain. The anatomy and function of the cranial nerve system are described in Table 9-7.

The Spinal Nerves. A total of 31 pairs of spinal nerves, exit from all levels of the vertebral column, except for those of C1 and C2,[8] each derived from the spinal cord. The spinal nerves are divided into 8 cervical pairs (C1-8), 12 thoracic pairs (T1-12), 5 lumbar pairs (L1-5), 5 sacral pairs (S1-5), and a coccygeal pair (Figure 9-8).

The posterior (dorsal) and anterior (ventral) roots of the spinal nerves are located within the vertebral canal.

As the nerve roots exit the vertebral canal, they penetrate the dura mater, before passing through dural sleeves within the intervertebral foramen. The dural sleeves are continuous with the epineurium of the nerves.

Study Pearl

The primary watershed area of the spinal cord is the midthoracic region. Vascular injury may cause a cord lesion at a level several segments higher than the level of spinal injury. For example, a lower cervical spine fracture may result in disruption of the vertebral artery that ascends through the affected vertebra. The resulting vascular injury may cause an ischemic high cervical cord injury. At any given level of the spinal cord, the central part is a watershed area. Cervical hyperextension injuries may cause ischemic injury to the central part of the cord, causing a central cord syndrome (see later).

Study Pearl

The portion of the spinal nerve that is not within the vertebral canal, and which usually occupies the intervertebral foramen, is referred to as a peripheral nerve.

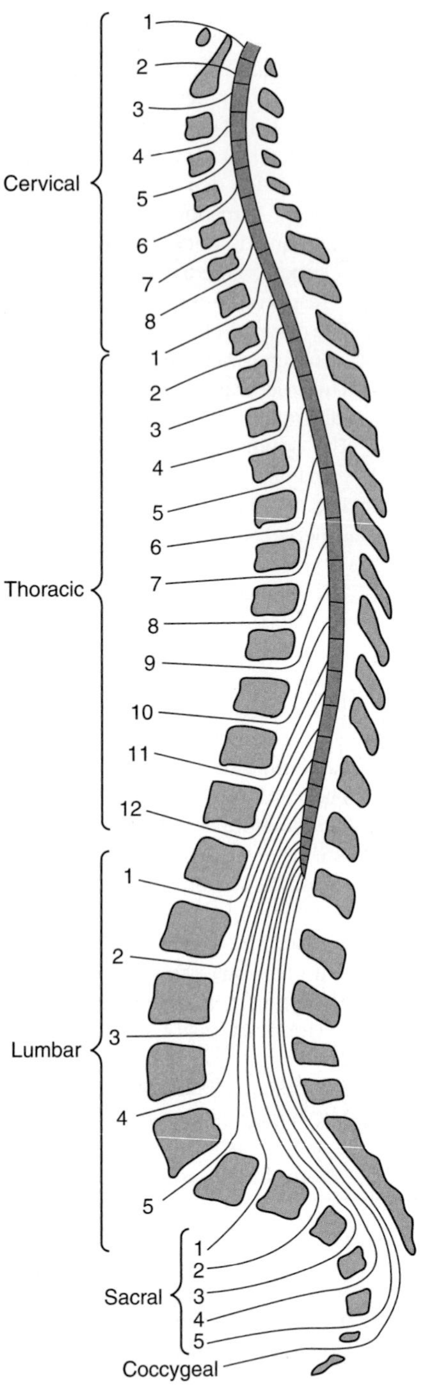

Figure 9-8. Schematic illustration of the relationships between the vertebral column, the spinal cord, and the spinal nerves. (Reproduced, with permission, from Waxman, SG: *Correlative Neuroanatomy, 24th ed.* New York: McGraw-Hill. 2000:47.)

Essentially, there are three types of spinal nerves[3]:

- Primary posterior (dorsal). This typically consists of a medial sensory branch, and a lateral motor branch. The posterior roots of the spinal nerves are represented by restricted peripheral sensory regions called dermatomes (Figure 9-9).

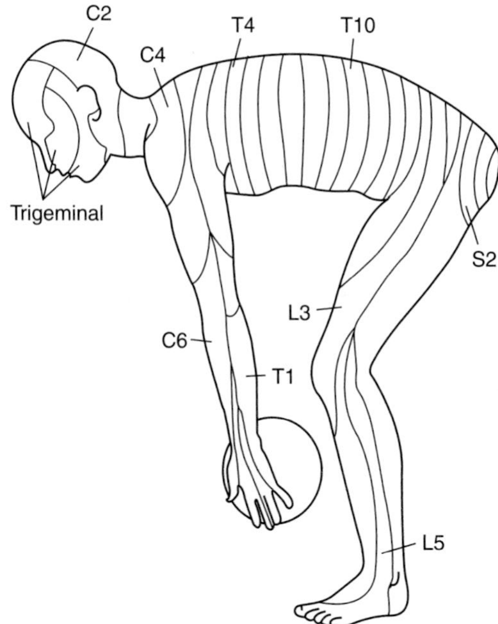

Figure 9-9. Segmental distribution of the body viewed in the approximate quadruped position. (Reproduced, with permission, from Waxman, SG: *Correlative Neuroanatomy, 24th ed.* New York: McGraw-Hill. 2000:50.)

The peripheral sensory nerves are represented by more distinct and circumscribed areas (Figures 9-10 through 9-13).

- Primary anterior (ventral). The primary anterior division forms the cervical, brachial and lumbosacral plexuses.
- Communicating ramus. The rami serve as a connection between the spinal nerves and the sympathetic trunk.

> **Study Pearl**
>
> Only the thoracic and upper lumbar nerves contain a white ramus communicans, but the gray ramus is present in all spinal nerves.

Nerve fibers can be categorized according to function: sensory, motor, or mixed (Table 9-8).

Peripheral Nerves. Peripheral nerves are enclosed in layers of tissue. From the inside outward, these are the endoneurium, perineurium, and epineurium.[9] Compression of a peripheral nerve can result in paresthesia. Paresthesia is a symptom of direct involvement of the nerve root. Further irritation and destruction of the neural fibers interfere with conduction, resulting in a motor and/or sensory deficit. It is therefore possible for a nerve root compression to cause pure motor paresis, a pure sensory deficit, or both, depending on which aspect of the nerve root is being compressed. If pressure is exerted from above the nerve root, sensory impairment may result, whereas compression from below can induce motor paresis.

Cervical Nerves. The eight pairs of cervical nerves are derived from cord segments between the level of the foramen magnum and the middle of the seventh cervical vertebra.[10]

Posterior Primary Divisions. The C1 (suboccipital) nerve is the only branch of the first posterior primary divisions and it serves the muscles of the suboccipital triangle, with very few sensory fibers.[10]

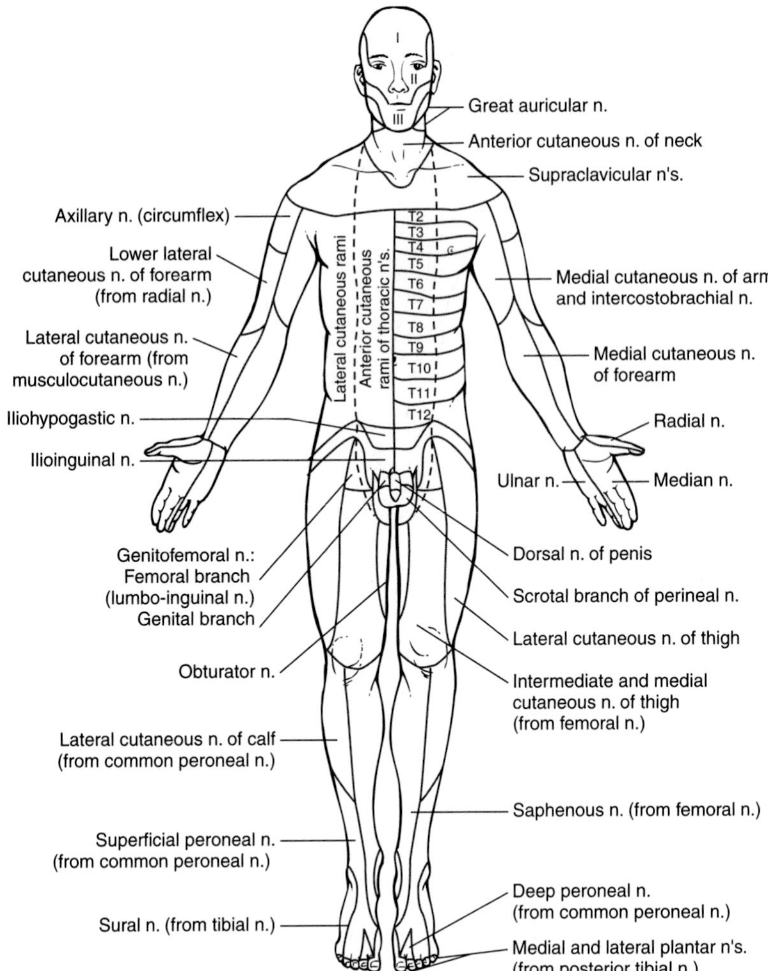

Figure 9-10. Peripheral nerve sensory distribution—anterior view. (Reproduced, with permission, from Gilman, S: *Clinical Examination of the Nervous Tissue.* New York: McGraw-Hill. 2000:179.)

Study Pearl

The phrenic nerve, the largest branch of the cervical plexus, plays a critical role in respiration.

Anterior Primary Divisions. The anterior primary divisions of the first four cervical nerves (C1-4) form the cervical plexus.

Cervical Plexus (C1-4). See Figure 9-14.

The symptoms of phrenic nerve compression depend largely on the degree of involvement, and whether one or both of the nerves are involved.[10-12]

- Unilateral paralysis of the diaphragm causes few or no symptoms except with heavy exertion.
- Bilateral paralysis of the diaphragm is characterized by dyspnea upon the slightest exertion, and difficulty with coughing and sneezing.[11,12]
- Phrenic neuralgia, which results from neck tumors, aortic aneurysm, and pericardial or other mediastinal infections, is characterized by pain near the free border of the ribs, beneath the clavicle, and deep in the neck.[11,12]

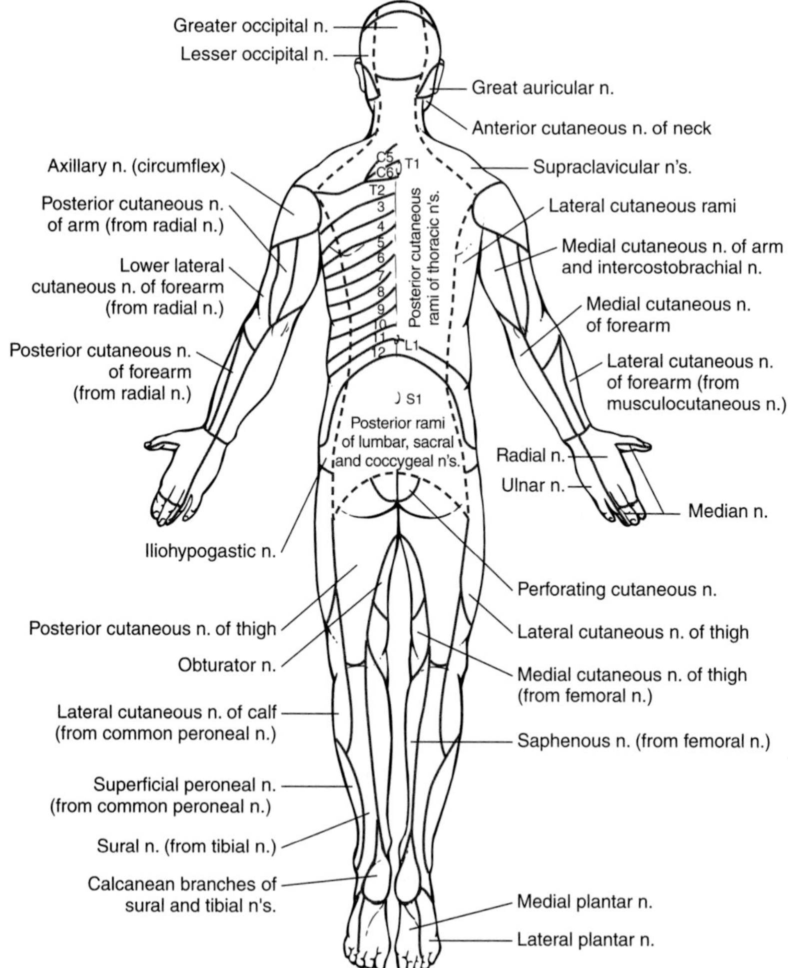

Figure 9-11. Peripheral nerve sensory distribution—posterior view. (Reproduced, with permission, from Gilman, S: *Clinical Examination of the Nervous Tissue*. New York: McGraw-Hill. 2000:180.)

Brachial Plexus. See Figure 9-15.

From the Trunks. A nerve extends to the subclavius muscle (C5-6) from the upper trunk (fifth root).[18]

The suprascapular nerve is derived from the upper trunk of the brachial plexus formed by the roots of C5 and C6 and supplies the supraspinatus and infraspinatus muscles, and articular branches to the glenohumeral and acromioclavicular joints. It also provides sensory and sympathetic fibers to two-thirds of the shoulder capsule, and to the glenohumeral and acromioclavicular joints.

From the Cords

- The medial and lateral pectoral nerves originate from the medial and lateral cords respectively. They supply the pectoralis major and pectoralis minor muscles. The pectoralis major muscle has dual innervation.[19]
- The three subscapular nerves from the posterior cord consist of:
  - The upper subscapular nerve (C5-6), which supplies the subscapularis muscle.

Study Pearl

The long and relatively superficial course of the long thoracic nerve makes it susceptible to injury. Injury to the long thoracic nerve can occur from any of the following causes.[5,13-15]

- Entrapment of the fifth and sixth cervical roots as they pass through the scalenus medius muscle.
- Compression of the nerve during traction to the upper extremity by the undersurface of the scapula as the nerve crosses over the second rib.
- Compression and traction to the nerve by the inferior angle of the scapula during general anesthesia or with passive abduction of the arm.

An injury to the long thoracic nerve may cause scapular winging; that is, the scapula assumes a position of medial translation and upward rotation of the inferior angle.[16,17]

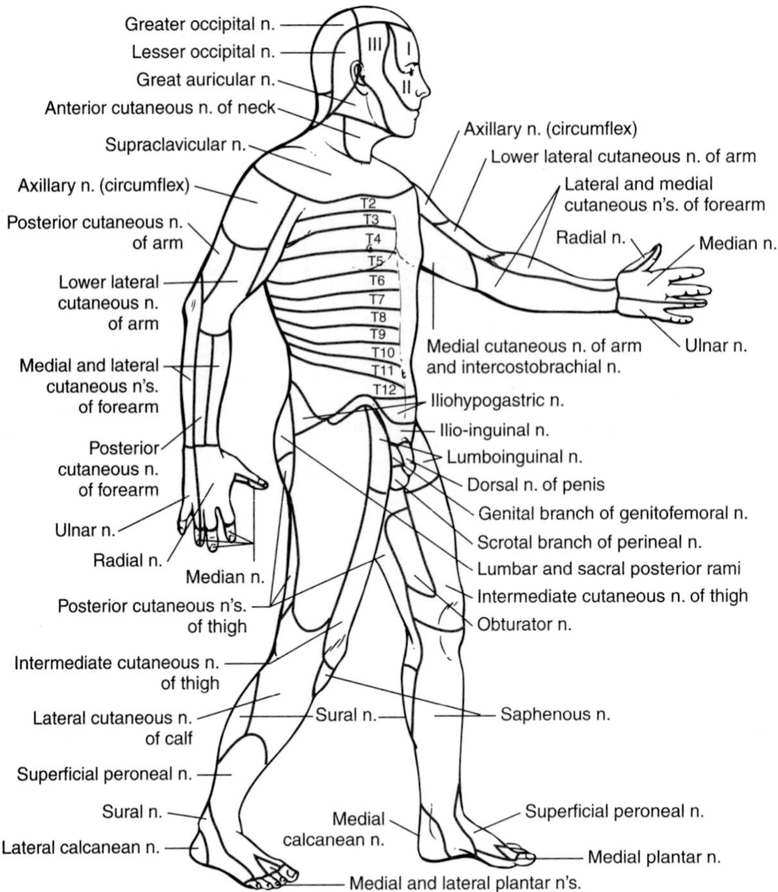

Figure 9-12. Peripheral nerve sensory distribution—lateral view. (Reproduced, with permission, from Gilman, S: *Clinical Examination of the Nervous Tissue.* New York: McGraw-Hill. 2000:181.)

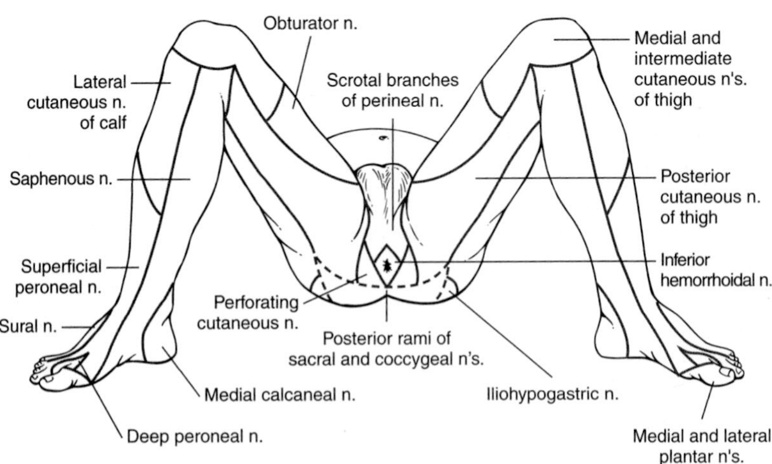

Figure 9-13. Peripheral nerve sensory distribution of pelvis and lower extremities. (Reproduced, with permission, from Gilman, S: *Clinical Examination of the Nervous Tissue.* New York: McGraw-Hill. 2000:181.)

TABLE 9-8. SENSORY, MOTOR, AND MIXED NERVES

TYPE	DESCRIPTION/FUNCTION	EXAMPLES
Sensory	Sensory nerves carry afferents from a portion of the skin. They also carry efferents to the skin structures. When a sensory nerve is compressed, the symptoms occur in the area of the nerve distribution. This area of distribution is called a dermatome, which is a well-defined segmental portion of the skin, and generally follows the segmental distribution of the underlying muscle innervation.[a]	Lateral (femoral) cutaneous nerve of the thigh, the saphenous nerve and the interdigital nerves
Motor	Carry efferents to muscles, and return sensation from muscles, and associated ligamentous structures. Any nerve that innervates a muscle, also mediates the sensation from the joint upon which that muscle acts. The symptoms produced as the result of a motor nerve involvement are not well localized. The muscle is usually tender to palpation and there may be atrophy.	The ulnar nerve, the suprascapular nerve, and the dorsal scapular nerve
Mixed	A combination of skin, sensory, and motor fibers to one trunk. Involvement of a mixed nerve presents with a combination of sensory and motor findings.	The median nerve, the ulnar nerve at the elbow as it enters the tunnel of Guyon, the fibular (peroneal) nerve at the knee, and the ilioinguinal nerve

[a]Data from Waxman SG: *Correlative Neuroanatomy*. 24th ed. New York, NY: McGraw-Hill; 1996.

- The thoracodorsal nerve, or middle subscapular nerve (C6, C7, and C8), which supplies the latissimus dorsi.
- The lower subscapular nerve (C5-6) to the teres major and part of the subscapularis muscle.

▶ Sensory branches of the medial cord (C8-T1) form the medial brachial cutaneous nerve to the medial surface of the arm and the medial antebrachial cutaneous nerve to the medial surface of the forearm.

Nerves of the Brachial Plexus

Musculocutaneous Nerve (C5-6). The musculocutaneous nerve originates from the anterior division of the upper and middle trunks of the C5-7 roots,[20,21] and supplies the coracobrachialis, biceps brachii, and brachialis muscles, before emerging between the biceps brachii and the brachioradialis muscles just proximal to the elbow.[21-23] The sensory branch, called the lateral antebrachial cutaneous nerve, divides into anterior and posterior divisions to innervate the anterior-lateral aspect of the forearm.[21]

Axillary Nerve (C5-6). The axillary nerve gives a branch to the teres minor muscle and the posterior deltoid muscle before terminating as the superior lateral brachial cutaneous nerve. The axillary nerve also gives branches to supply the middle and anterior deltoid muscle.

Radial Nerve (C6-8, T1). The radial nerve, the largest branch of the brachial plexus, supplies the triceps, the anconeus, and the upper portion of the extensor-supinator group of forearm muscles.

In the forearm, a branch of the radial nerve, the posterior interosseous nerve, innervates all of the muscles of the six extensor compartments of the wrist, with the exception of the extensor carpi radialis brevis (ECRB) and extensor carpi radialis longus (ECRL).

Study Pearl

The radial nerve is frequently entrapped at its bifurcation in the region of the elbow, where the common radial nerve becomes the sensory branch and a deep or posterior interosseous branch.

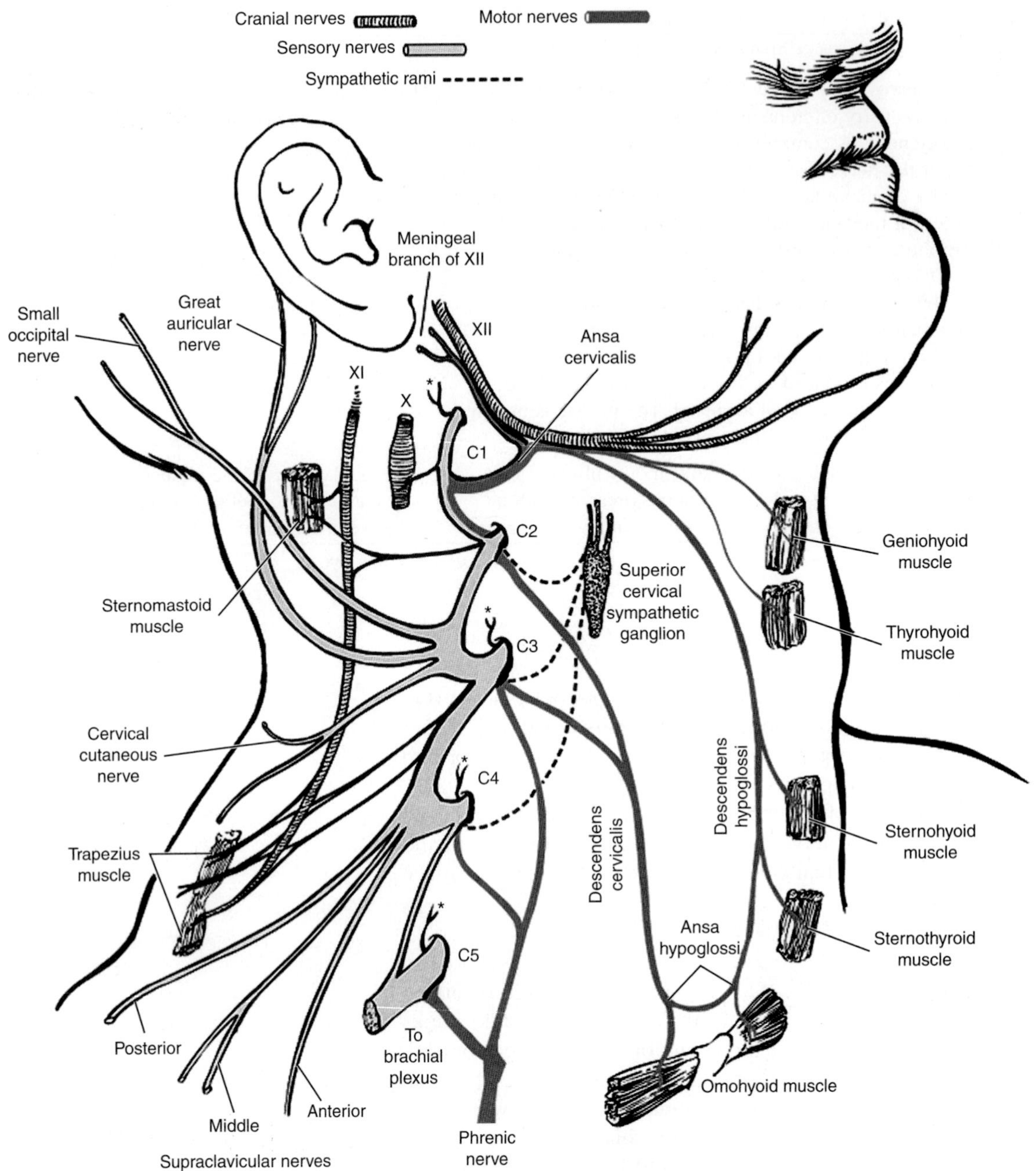

Figure 9-14. The cervical plexus. (Reproduced, with permission, from Waxman, SG: *Correlative Neuroanatomy, 24th ed.* New York: McGraw-Hill. 2000:356.)

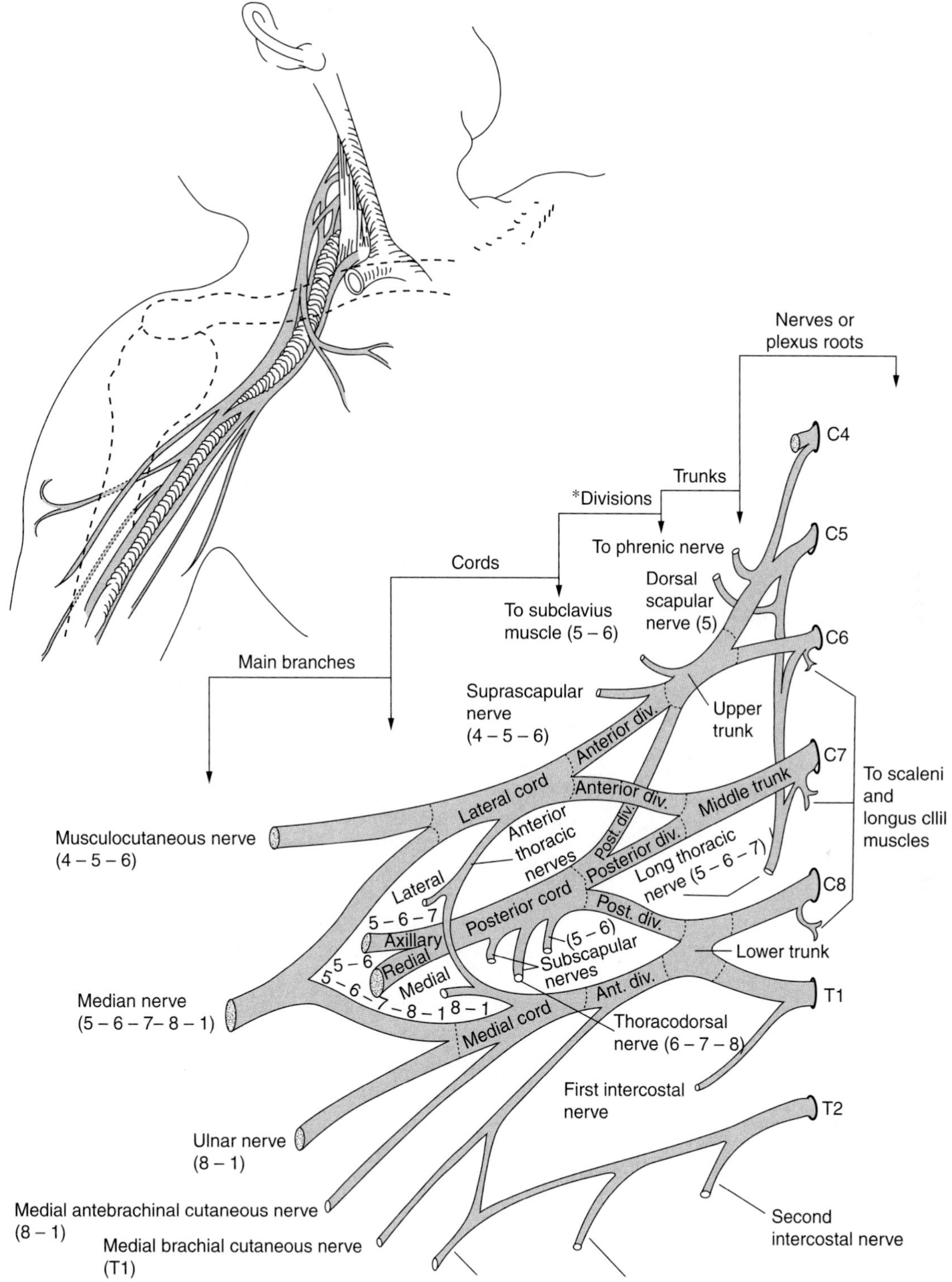

Figure 9-15. The brachial plexus. (Reproduced, with permission, from Waxman, SG: *Correlative Neuroanatomy, 24th ed.* New York: McGraw-Hill. 2000:358.)

Study Pearl

The site of the entrapment of the radial nerve can often be determined by the clinical findings, as follows:

- If the impairment occurs at a point below the triceps innervation, the strength of the triceps remains intact.
- If the impairment occurs at a point below the brachioradialis branch, some supination is retained.
- If the impairment occurs at a point in the forearm, the branches to the small muscle groups, extensors of the thumb, extensors of the index finger, extensors of the other fingers, and extensor carpi ulnaris may be affected.
- If the impairment occurs at a point on the posterior aspect of the wrist, only sensory loss of the hand is affected.

The sensory distribution of the radial nerve include the posterior brachial cutaneous nerve, to the posterior aspect of the arm; the posterior antebrachial cutaneous nerve, to the posterior surface of the forearm; and the superficial radial nerve, to the posterior aspect of the radial half of the hand. The isolated area of supply is a small patch of skin over the posterior aspect of the first interosseous space.

The major disability associated with radial nerve injury is a weak grip, which is weakened because of poor stabilization of the wrist and finger joints. In addition, the patient demonstrates an inability to extend the thumb, wrist, and elbow, as well as the proximal phalanges. Pronation of the forearm and adduction of the thumb also are affected, and the wrist and fingers adopt a position termed wrist drop. The triceps and other radial reflexes are absent, but the sensory loss is often slight, owing to overlapping innervation.

Median Nerve (C5-T1). The median nerve trunk derives its fibers from the lower three (sometimes four) cervical and the first thoracic segment of the spinal cord. The nerve trunk descends along with the brachial artery, and passes onto the anterior aspect of the forearm, where it gives off muscular branches, including the anterior interosseous nerve. It then enters the hand, terminating in both muscular and cutaneous branches. The sensory branches of the median nerve supply the skin of the palmar aspect of the thumb and the lateral 2½ fingers, and the distal ends of the same fingers.

The anterior interosseous nerve provides motor innervation to the flexor pollicis longus (FPL); the medial part of flexor digitorum profundus (FDP) (it may supply all or none of the flexor digitorum profundus and part of the flexor digitorum superficialis),involving the index and sometimes the middle finger; and to the pronator quadratus. It also sends sensory fibers to the distal radioulnar, radiocarpal, intercarpal, and carpometacarpal joints.[24,25]

Ulnar Nerve (C8, T1). The ulnar nerve is the largest branch of the medial cord. In the forearm, the ulnar nerve supplies the flexor carpi ulnaris (FCU) and the ulnar head of the FDP muscles. Proximal to the wrist, the anterior (palmar) cutaneous branch of the ulnar nerve arises. This branch runs across the anterior aspect of the forearm and wrist outside of the tunnel of Guyon to supply the proximal part of the ulnar side of the palm. A few centimeters more distally to the tunnel, a posterior cutaneous branch arises and supplies the ulnar side of the posterior aspect of the hand, the posterior aspect of the fifth finger, and the ulnar half of the forefinger. The ulnar nerve also supplies all of the small muscles deep and medial to the long flexor tendon of the thumb, except the first two lumbricales.

Thoracic Nerves

Posterior (Dorsal) Rami. The thoracic posterior rami travel posteriorly, close to the vertebral zygapophysial joints, before dividing into medial and lateral branches.

- The medial branches supply the short, medially placed back muscles and the skin of the back as far as the midscapular line.[26] The medial branches of the upper six thoracic posterior rami penetrate the rhomboids and trapezius, reaching the skin in close proximity to the vertebral spines, which they occasionally supply.

- The lateral branches supply the sacrospinalis muscles, the longissimus thoracis, the iliocostalis cervicis, and the levatores costarum.[26]

Anterior (Ventral) Rami. There are 12 pairs of thoracic anterior rami, and all but the 12th are located between the ribs where they serve as intercostal nerves, providing sensory distribution to the skin of the lateral aspect of the trunk, the intercostal muscles, parietal pleura, and the skin over the anterior aspect of the thorax and abdomen.

Lumbar Plexus. The lumbar plexus is formed from the anterior (ventral) nerve roots of the second through fifth lumbar nerves. (Figure 9-16). It then travels anteriorly into the body of the psoas muscle to form the lateral femoral cutaneous, femoral, and obturator nerves. The lower branch of L2, all of L3, and the upper branch of L4 split into a small anterior and a large posterior division. The three anterior divisions unite to form the obturator nerve; the three posterior divisions unite to form the femoral nerve, and the lateral femoral cutaneous nerve.

L1, L2, and L4 divide into upper and lower branches. The upper branch of L1 forms the iliohypogastric and ilioinguinal nerves. The lower branch of L1 joins the upper branch of L2 to form the genitofemoral nerve. The lower branch of L4 joins L5 to form the lumbosacral trunk.

- ***Iliohypogastric nerve (T12, L1).*** This nerve divides into lateral and anterior cutaneous branches. The lateral, or iliac, branch supplies the skin of the upper lateral part of the thigh, while the anterior, or hypogastric branch, descends anteriorly to supply the skin over the symphysis.
- ***Ilioinguinal nerve (L1).*** This nerve penetrates the internal oblique, which it supplies, before emerging from the superficial inguinal ring to supply the skin of the upper medial part of the thigh and the root of the penis and scrotum or mons pubis and labium majores.
- ***Genitofemoral nerve (L1, 2).*** This nerve divides into genital and femoral branches. The genital branch supplies the cremasteric muscle and the skin of the scrotum or labia, while the femoral branch supplies the skin of the middle upper part of the thigh and the femoral artery.

Collateral muscular branches supply the quadratus lumborum and intertransversarii from L1 and L4 and the psoas muscle from L2 and L3.

Femoral nerve (L2-4). The femoral nerve is the largest branch of the lumbar plexus. It arises from the lateral border of the psoas just superior to the inguinal ligament. The nerve supplies the sartorius, pectineus, and quadriceps femoris muscles. The sensory distribution of the femoral nerve includes the anterior and medial surfaces of the thigh via the anterior femoral cutaneous nerve, and the medial aspect

Study Pearl

The clinical features of median nerve impairment, depending on the level of injury, include the following[10]:

1. Paralysis is noted in the flexor-pronator muscles of the forearm, all of the superficial palmar muscles except the flexor carpi ulnaris, and all of the deep palmar muscles, except the ulnar half of the flexor digitorum profundus and the thenar muscles that lie superficial to the tendon of the flexor pollices longus.
2. In the forearm, pronation is weak or lost.
3. At the wrist, there is weak flexion and radial deviation, and the hand inclines to the ulnar side.
4. In the hand, an ape-hand deformity can be present. This deformity is associated with:
   a. An inability to oppose or flex the thumb, or abduct it in its own plane.
   b. A weakened grip, especially in thumb and index finger, with a tendency for these digits to become hyperextended, and the thumb adducted.
   c. An inability to flex the distal phalanx of the thumb and index finger.
   d. Weakness of middle finger flexion.
   e. Atrophy of the thenar muscles.
5. There is a loss of sensation to a variable degree over the cutaneous distribution of the median nerve, most constantly over the distal phalanges of the first two fingers.
6. Pain is present in many median nerve impairments.
7. Atrophy of the thenar eminence is seen early. Atrophy of the flexor-pronator groups of muscles in the forearm is seen after a few months.
8. The skin of the palm is frequently dry, cold, discolored, chapped, and at times keratotic.

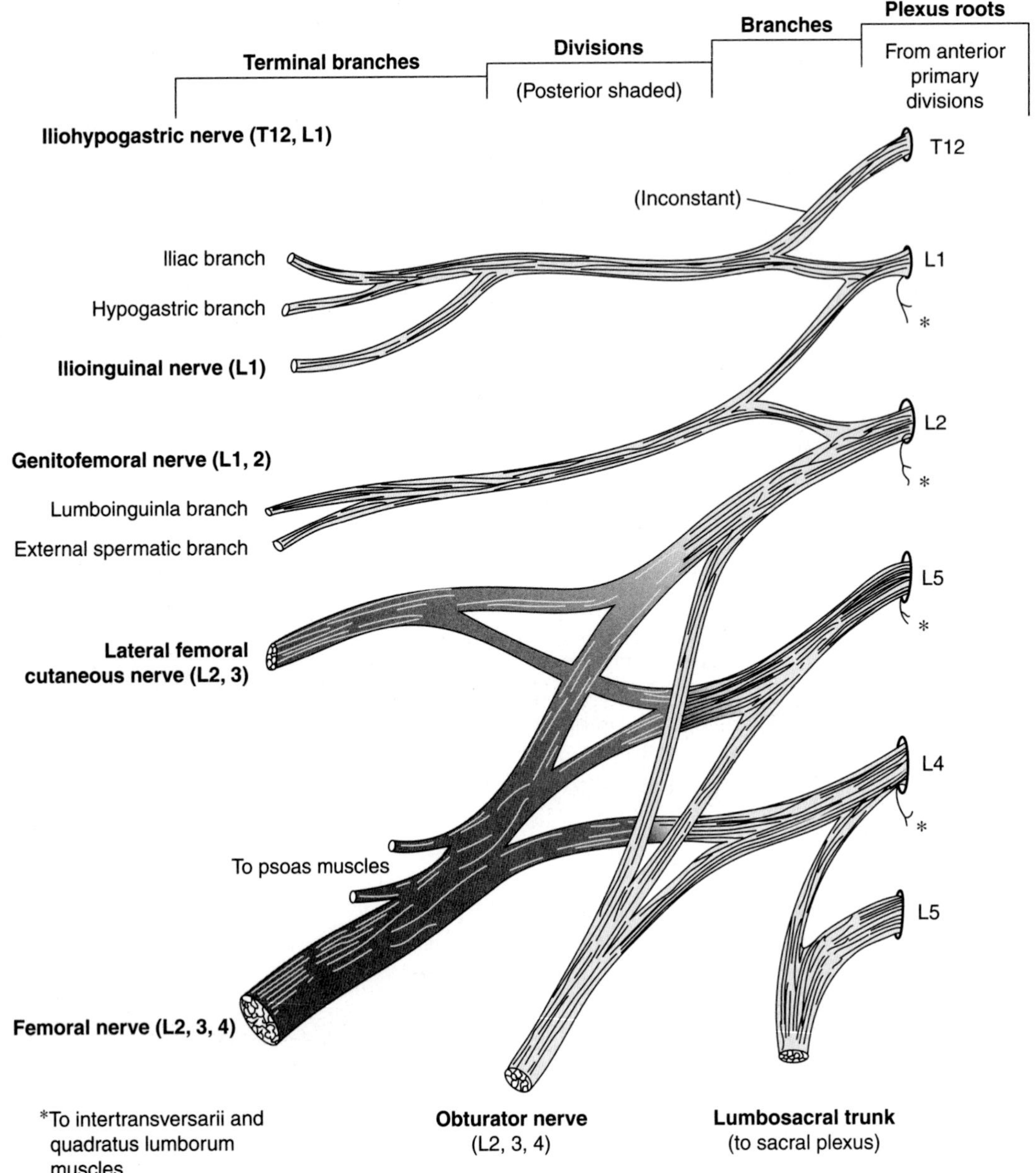

Figure 9-16. The lumbar plexus. (Reproduced, with permission, from Waxman, SG: *Correlative Neuroanatomy, 24th ed.* New York: McGraw-Hill. 2000:364.)

of the knee, the proximal leg, and articular branches to the knee via the saphenous nerve.

Femoral nerve palsy has been reported after acetabular fracture, cardiac catheterization, total hip arthroplasty, or anterior lumbar spinal fusion, and spontaneously in hemophilia.[30-32]

Obturator Nerve (L2-4). The obturator nerve splits into anterior and posterior branches.

- The anterior division of the obturator nerve gives an articular branch to the hip joint near its origin. The anterior division divides into numerous named and unnamed branches, including the cutaneous branches to the subsartorial plexus and directly to a small area of skin on the middle internal part of the thigh, vascular branches to the femoral artery, and communicating branches to the femoral cutaneous and accessory obturator nerves.

- The posterior division of the obturator nerve penetrates the anterior part of the obturator externus, which it supplies, and descends deep to the adductor brevis. It also supplies the adductors magnus and brevis (if it has not received supply from the anterior division) and gives an articular branch to the knee joint.
- ***Lateral (femoral) cutaneous nerve of the thigh.*** The lateral (femoral) cutaneous nerve of the thigh is purely sensory and is derived primarily from the second and third lumbar nerve roots, with occasional contributions from the first lumbar nerve root.[34-37]

SACRAL PLEXUS

The lumbosacral trunk (L4, 5) descends into the pelvis, where it enters the formation of the sacral plexus (Figure 9-17).

The sacral plexus is formed by the anterior (ventral) rami of the L4 and L5 and the S1 through S4 nerves. The L4 and L5 nerves join to become the lumbosacral trunk. The S1 through S4 nerves converge to form the triangular band of the sacral plexus.

Collateral Branches of the Posterior Division

Superior Gluteal Nerve. The roots of the superior gluteal nerve (L4,5; S1) originate within the pelvis from the sacral plexus, and innervate the gluteus medius and gluteus minimus.[38]

Inferior Gluteal Nerve. The inferior gluteal nerve (L5; S1,2) innervates the gluteus maximus muscle. Nerves to the piriformis consist of short smaller branches from S1 and S2.

Superior Cluneal Nerve. The medial branch of the superior cluneal nerve passes superficially over the iliac crest, where it is covered by two layers of dense fibrous fascia.

Posterior Femoral Cutaneous Nerve. The posterior femoral cutaneous nerve constitutes a collateral branch, with roots from both anterior and posterior divisions of S1 and S2, and the anterior divisions of S2 and S3. Perineal branches pass to the skin of the superior medial aspect of the thigh and the skin of the scrotum or labium majores.

Collateral Branches of the Anterior Division. Collateral branches from the anterior divisions extend to the quadratus femoris and gemellus inferior muscles (from L4, L5, and S1) and to the obturator internus and gemellus superior muscles (from L5, S1, and S2).

Sciatic Nerve. The sciatic nerve arises from the L4, L5, and S1 through S3 nerve roots as a continuation of the lumbosacral plexus. The nerve is composed of the independent tibial (medial) and common fibular (peroneal) (lateral) divisions, which are usually united as

Study Pearl

The thoracic nerves may be involved in the same types of impairments that affect other peripheral nerves. A loss of function of one, or more of the thoracic nerves may produce partial or complete paralysis of the abdominal muscles and a loss of the abdominal reflexes in the affected quadrant. With unilateral impairments of the nerve, the umbilicus usually is drawn toward the unaffected side when the abdomen is tensed (Beevor's sign), indicating a paralysis of the lower abdominal muscles as a result of a lesion at the level of the 10th thoracic segment.

A specific syndrome called the T4 syndrome[27-29] has been shown to cause vague pain, numbness, and paresthesia in the upper extremity and generalized posterior head and neck pain.

Study Pearl

An entrapment of the femoral nerve by an iliopsoas hematoma is the most likely cause of femoral nerve palsy.[33] Direct blows to the abdomen or a hyperextension moment at the hip that tears the iliacus muscle may produce an iliacus hematoma.

Study Pearl

The obturator nerve may be involved by the same pathologic processes that affect the femoral nerve. Disability is usually minimal, although external rotation and adduction of the thigh are impaired, and crossing of the legs is difficult. The patient also may complain of severe pain, which radiates from the groin down the inner aspect of the thigh.

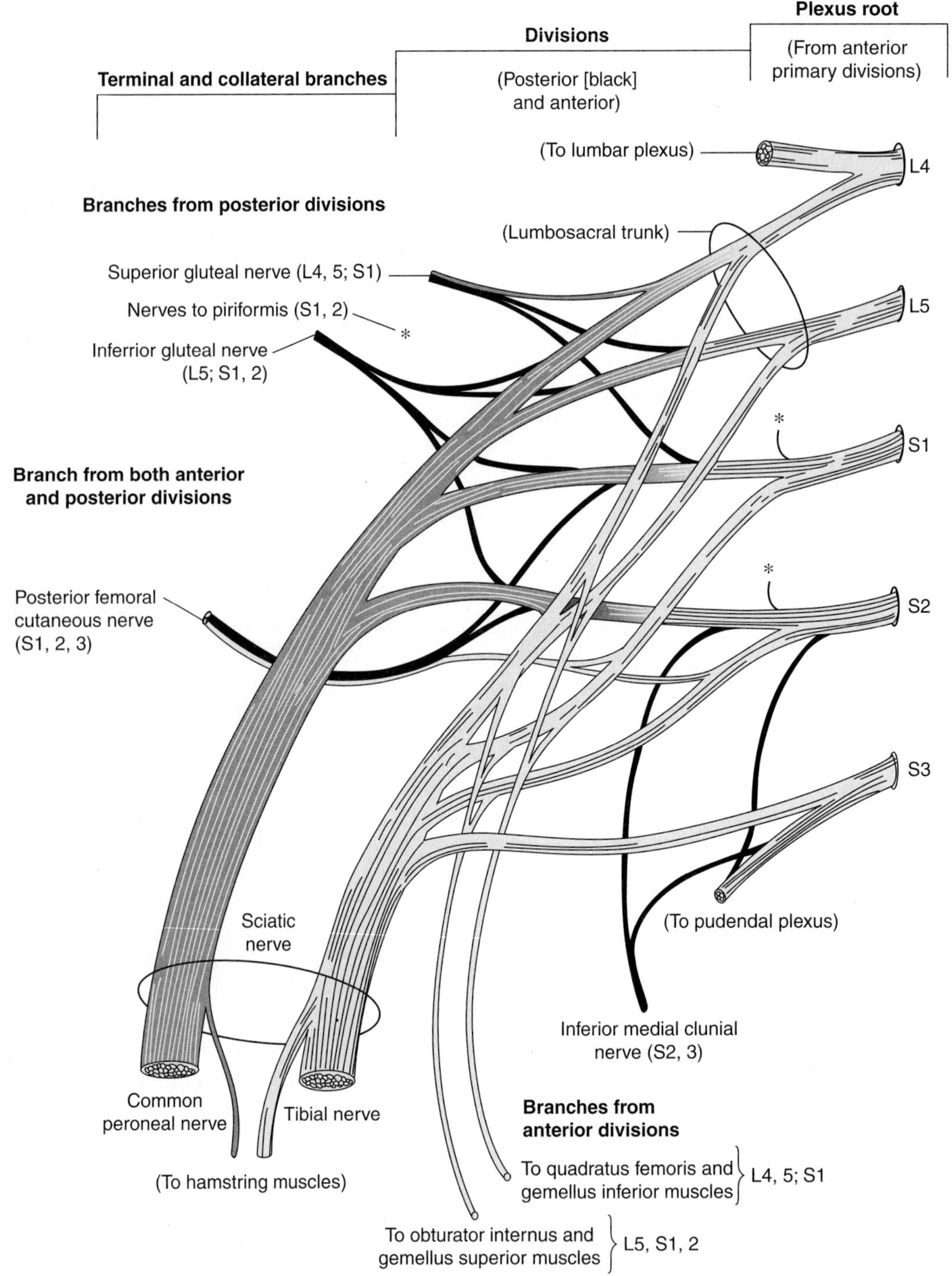

Figure 9-17. The sacral plexus. (Reproduced, with permission, from Waxman, SG: *Correlative Neuroanatomy, 24th ed.* New York: McGraw-Hill. 2000:366.)

a single nerve down to the distal aspect of the thigh. The tibial division is the larger of the two divisions. The common fibular (peroneal) nerve is formed by the upper four posterior divisions (L4,5; S1,2) of the sacral plexus, and the tibial nerve, is formed from all five anterior divisions (L4,5; S1-3).

Innervation for the short head of the biceps comes from the common fibular (peroneal) division. Rami from the tibial trunk pass to the semitendinosus and semimembranosus muscles, the long head of the biceps, and the adductor magnus muscle.

Tibial Nerve. The part of the tibial trunk below the popliteal space is called the *posterior tibial nerve*; the part within the space is called the internal *popliteal nerve*. The tibial nerve supplies the gastrocnemius, plantaris, soleus, popliteus, tibialis posterior, flexor digitorum longus (FDL), and flexor halluces longus (FHL) muscles.

Sural Nerve. The sural nerve, a sensory branch of the tibial nerve, is formed by the lateral sural cutaneous nerve from the common fibular (peroneal) nerve and the medial calcaneal nerve from the tibial nerve. The sural nerve supplies the skin on the posterior-lateral aspect of the lower one third of the leg and the lateral side of the foot.

Terminal Branches of the Tibial Nerve. In the distal leg, the tibial nerve lies laterally to the posterior tibial vessels, and it supplies articular branches to the ankle joint and to the posterior-medial aspect of the ankle. From this point, its terminal branches include:

- ***Medial plantar nerve*** (comparable to the median nerve in the hand). This nerve supplies the flexor digitorum brevis, abductor halluces, flexor halluces brevis, and first lumbrical muscles; and sensory branches to the medial side of the sole, the plantar surfaces of the medial 3½ toes, and the distal phalanges of the same toes.
- ***Lateral plantar nerve*** (comparable to the ulnar nerve in the hand). This nerve supplies the small muscles of the foot, except those innervated by the medial plantar nerve; and sensory branches to the lateral portions of the sole, the plantar surface of the lateral 1½ toes, and the distal phalanges of these toes.
- ***Medial calcaneal nerve.*** As it passes beneath the flexor retinaculum, the tibial nerve gives off medial calcanean branches to the skin of the heel.

Common Fibular (Peroneal) Nerve. The common fibular (peroneal) nerve gives off sensory branches in the popliteal space, including the superior and inferior articular branches to the knee joint, and the lateral sural cutaneous nerve.

At the top of the popliteal fossa, the common fibular (peroneal) nerve begins its descent along the posterior border of the biceps femoris, then crosses the posterior aspect of the knee joint to the upper and outside portion of the leg near the head of the fibula. The nerve curves around the lateral aspect of the fibula and then anteriorly before passing deep to the two heads of the fibularis (peroneus) longus muscle, where it divides into three terminal rami: the recurrent articular, superficial, and deep fibular (peroneal) nerves.

- The recurrent articular nerve accompanies the anterior tibial recurrent artery, supplying the tibiofibular and knee joints, and a small branch to the tibialis anterior muscle.
- The superficial fibular (peroneal) nerve originates deep to the fibularis (peroneus) longus before supplying the fibularis longus and brevis muscles and sensory distribution to the

Study Pearl

When the medial branch of the superior cluneal nerve passes through the fascia against the posterior iliac crest and the osteofibrous tunnel consisting of the two layers of the fascia and the superior rim of the iliac crest, the possibility of irritation or trauma to the nerve is increased, making this a potential site of nerve compression or constriction.[39]

Study Pearl

Injury to the sciatic nerve may result indirectly from a herniated intervertebral disk (protruded nucleus pulposus), or more directly from a hip dislocation, local aneurysm, or direct external trauma of the sciatic notch, the latter of which can be confused with a compressive radiculopathy of the lumbar or sacral nerve root.[40] Following are some useful clues to help distinguish the two conditions:

- Pain from radiculopathy should not significantly change with hip motion except in the case of a straight leg raise, whereas with a sciatic entrapment by the piriformis pain is accentuated with hip internal rotation and relieved by hip external rotation.
- Sciatic neuropathy produces sensory changes on the sole of the foot, whereas radiculopathy generally does not, unless there is a predominant S1 involvement.
- Compressive radiculopathy below the L4 level causes palpable atrophy of the gluteal muscles, whereas a sciatic entrapment spares these muscles.
- The sciatic trunk is frequently tender from root compression at the foraminal level, whereas it is not normally tender in a sciatic nerve entrapment.[41]

Study Pearl

An insidious entrapment of the common fibular (peroneal) nerve (and it is very vulnerable, especially at the fibular neck) can be confused with symptoms of a herniated disk, tendinitis of the popliteus tendon, mononeuritis, idiopathic peroneal palsy, intrinsic and extrinsic nerve tumors, and extraneural compression by a synovial cyst, ganglion cyst, soft tissue tumor, osseous mass, or a large fabella.[42] Traumatic injury of the nerve may occur secondary to a fracture, dislocation, surgical procedure, application of skeletal traction, or a tight cast.[42] The pain from an entrapment of the common fibular (peroneal) nerve is typically on the lateral surface of the knee, leg, and foot. Lateral knee pain is a common problem among patients seeking medical attention, and entrapment of the common fibular (peroneal) nerve is frequently overlooked in the differential diagnostic considerations, especially in the absence of trauma or the presence of a palpable mass at the neck of the fibula.

Study Pearl

The common fibular (peroneal) division is relatively tethered at the sciatic notch and the neck of the fibula as compared with the tibial division and is therefore less able to tolerate or distribute tension.

lower anterior aspect of the leg, the posterior aspect of the foot, part of the big toe, and adjacent sides of the second to fifth toes up to the second phalanges.

- The deep fibular (peroneal) nerve supplies the tibialis anterior, extensor digitorum longus, extensor hallucis longus, and fibularis (peroneus) tertius muscles. The deep fibular (peroneal) nerve divides into a medial and lateral branch approximately 1.5 cm above the ankle joint. These branches extend to the skin of the adjacent sides of the medial two toes (medial branch), to the extensor digitorum brevis muscle (lateral branch), and to the adjacent joints.

Pudendal and Coccygeal Plexuses. The pudendal and coccygeal plexuses are the most inferior portions of the lumbosacral plexus and serve to supply nerves to the perineal structures.

- The pudendal plexus supplies the coccygeus, levator ani, and sphincter ani externus muscles. A lesion to the pudendal nerve can result in voiding and erectile dysfunctions.[43]

The pudendal nerve divides into:

- The inferior hemorrhoidal nerves to the external anal sphincter and adjacent skin.
- The perineal nerve.
- The posterior nerve of the penis.
- The nerves of the coccygeal plexus are the small sensory anococcygeal nerves derived from the last three segments (S4,5; C). They pierce the sacrotuberous ligament and supply the skin in the region of the coccyx.

Nerve Fiber Types

- A fibers (Table 9-9): large, myelinated, fast conducting.
- Alpha: responsible for proprioception, somatic motor.
- Beta: responsible for touch, pressure.
- Gamma: responsible for motor to the muscle spindles.
- Delta: responsible for pain, temperature, touch.
- B fibers: small, myelinated, conduct less rapidly—preganglionic autonomic.
- C fibers: smallest, unmyelinated, slowest conducting.
- Posterior root: pain, reflex responses.
- Sympathetic: postganglionic sympathetics.

Reflexes

A reflex response can be a simple behavior, movement or activity. The circuitry that generates these patterns varies greatly in complexity, depending on the nature of the reflex.

Reflexes can be controlled by spinal or supraspinal (brain stem) pathways. Reflexes are classified on the basis of the relevant pathways and central connections as follows:

- Segmental reflexes: the stimulus and the response have a fixed spatial relationship.
- Monosynaptic reflexes: the stretch (myotatic) reflex. The term deep tendon reflex is a misnomer—there are no deep tendons

TABLE 9-9. CLASSIFICATION OF AFFERENT NEURONS

SIZE	TYPE	GROUP	SUBGROUP	DIAMETER (MICROMETERS)	CONDUCTION VELOCITY (M/S)	RECEPTOR	STIMULUS
Large	Aα	I	1a	12-20 (22)	70-120	Proprioceptive mechanoreceptor	Muscle velocity and length change, muscle shortening of rapid speed
	Aα	I	1b			Proprioceptive mechanoreceptor	Muscle length information from touch and Pacinian corpuscles
	Aα	II	Muscle	6-12	36-72		
	Aβ	II	Skin			Cutaneous receptors	Touch, vibration, hair receptors
	Aδ	III	Muscle	1-5 (6)	6(12)-36(80)	75% mechanoreceptors and thermoreceptors	Temperature change
Small	Aδ	III	Skin			25% nociceptors, mechanoreceptors, and thermoreceptors (hot and cold)	Noxious, mechanical, and temperature (> 45°C, < 10°C)
	C	IV	Muscle	0.3-1.0	0.4-1.0	50% mechanoreceptors and thermoreceptors	Touch and temperature
	C	IV	Skin			50% nociceptors, 20% mechanoreceptors, and 30% thermoreceptors (hot and cold)	Noxious, mechanical, and temperature (> 45°C, < 10°C)

that we use and no reflexes that are conversely superficial. A muscle stretch reflex is a better term that is widely gaining acceptance.

- Polysynaptic and oligosynaptic (superficial) reflexes: the plantar response (sign of Babinski) and the blink reflex.

Monosynaptic Reflex. The stretch or myotatic reflex consists of just two neurons and one synapse. A brief tap of the reflex hammer on the tendon produces a stretch of the tendon (afferent Ia reflex arc involving the muscle spindle—Table 9-4) which in turn, causes a contraction of the tendon and muscle belly—the inverse stretch reflex (afferent Ib reflex arc involving the Golgi tendon organ—Table 9-10). The gamma reflex loop, forms part of this loop and allows the muscle tension to come under the control of descending pathways (reticulospinal, vestibulospinal, and others), which excite gamma motor neurons, causing contraction of the muscle spindle, and in turn increased stretch sensitivity and increased rate of firing of spindle afferents to the alpha motor neurons.

TABLE 9-10. GOLGI TENDON ORGANS

GOLGI TENDON ORGANS
Golgi tendon organs (GTOs) function to protect muscle attachments from strain or avulsion by using a postsynaptic inhibitory synapse of the muscle in which they are located. The GTO receptors are arranged in series with the extrafusal muscle fibers and, therefore, become activated by stretch. The signals from the GTO may go both to local areas within the spinal cord and through the spinal cerebellar tracts to the cerebellum. The local signals result in excitation of interneurons, which in turn inhibit the anterior α motor neurons of the GTO's own muscle and synergist, while facilitating the antagonists. This is theorized to prevent overcontraction, or stretch, of a muscle.

TABLE 9-11. SUPERFICIAL (CUTANEOUS) REFLEXES

REFLEX		NORMAL RESPONSE	PERTINENT CENTRAL NERVOUS SYSTEM SEGMENT
Upper abdominal	Lateral to medial scratching of the skin toward the umbilicus in each of the two upper quadrants	Umbilicus moves up and toward area being stroked	T7-T9
Lower abdominal	Lateral to medial scratching of the skin toward the umbilicus in each of the two lower quadrants	Umbilicus moves down and toward area being stroked	T11-T12
Cremasteric	Stroking the skin on the proximal and medial thigh	Scrotum/testicle elevates	T12, L1
Plantar	Stroking lateral sole of foot from calcaneus to base of fifth metatarsal and medially across the metatarsal heads	Plantar flexion of toes	S1-S2
Gluteal	A stroke over the skin of the buttocks	Skin tenses in gluteal area	L4-L5, S1-S3
Anal	Scratching the perianal skin	Contraction of anal sphincter muscles	S2-S4

Reproduced, with permission, from Magee DJ: *Orthopedic Physical Assessment.* 4th ed. Philadelphia, PA: WB Saunders. 2002. Copyright © Elsevier.

Superficial Reflexes. A superficial reflex is typically elicited by cutaneous sensory (nociceptive) stimuli and results in a withdrawal (protective) response. The presence of an abnormal superficial reflex is suggestive of CNS (upper motor neuron) impairment, and requires an appropriate referral.

Examples of superficial reflexes include those listed in Table 9-11 and the Babinski.

Babinski. The Babinski sign is the single most meaningful clinically evoked reflex. It is sensitive, specific, and reproducible. In this test, the clinician applies noxious stimuli to sole of the patient's foot by running a pointed object along the plantar aspect (Figure 9-18).[44]

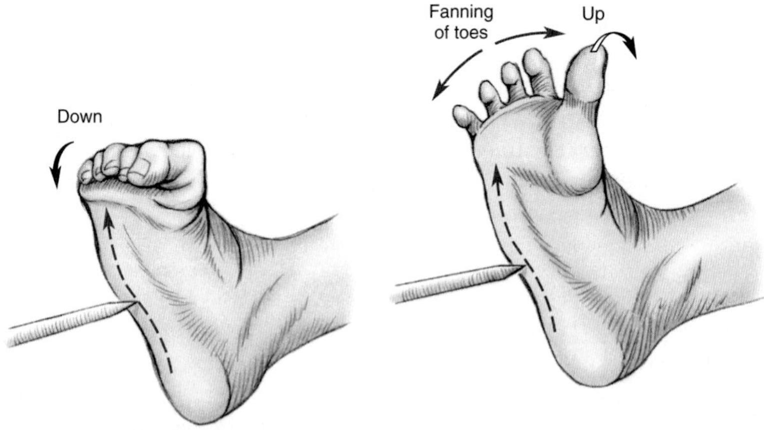

Figure 9-18. The plantar response. (Reproduced, with permission, from Gilman, S: *Clinical Examination of the Nervous Tissue.* New York: McGraw-Hill. 2000:170.)

A positive test, demonstrated by extension of the big toe and a splaying (abduction) of the other toes, is indicative of an injury to the corticospinal tract.

Primitive Reflexes. The presence of superficial reflexes under circumstances in which they should be absent makes them abnormal/pathologic as they are normally integrated by individuals as they develop. Injury or disease can prevent this normal suppression by the cerebrum, resulting in a release of the primitive reflex under abnormal circumstances.[45] Some reflexes occur only in specific periods of development and are not evident later in development as they become integrated by the CNS (see Chapter 16).

Study Pearl

As a general rule, influence of the primitive reflexes is not readily observed in the healthy, normally developing child after 6 months of age (exceptions include the symmetric tonic neck reflex and the plantar grasp reflex).

Patterned Behavioral Reflexes. A number of reflex responses to tactile stimuli occur in association with lesions to the brain.

- Grasp reflex of the hand: the application of a light tactile stimulus applied to the lateral margin of the ulna or radial side of the hand produces an instinctive or orienting grasp reflex.
- Grasp reflex of the foot: firm pressure on the metatarsal head produces sustained flexion of all the toes.
- Suck reflex: a light stroking of the lip with a tongue blade or finger produces a pursing of the lips and an opening of the mouth.

Supraspinal Reflexes. A number of processes involved in locomotor function are oriented around the supraspinal reflexes.

Postural reflexes constantly react and compensate for changes in balance require input from the somatosensory, vestibular, and visual systems. Voluntary control of these compensatory movements would be impossible and highly inefficient, so these reactions must be reflex in nature.

Head movements must be regulated in order to maintain normal eye-head-neck-trunk relationships, and to allow for visual fixation. There are three main control mechanisms for maintaining steady-gaze fixation; the vestibulo-ocular reflex (VOR); and a gaze-holding system (the neural integrator), which operates whenever the eyes are required to hold an eccentric gaze position. The cervico-ocular reflex (COR) also plays a role.

Cervico-ocular and Vestibulo-ocular Reflexes. For vision to be effectively integrated with balance, the subject must be capable of selecting an object for inspection and to fix the gaze on the object, regardless of head or object movement. The cervico-ocular reflexes (COR) and vestibulo-ocular reflexes (VOR) work together to maintain the position and visual fixation of the eyes during movements of the head and neck. Mechanoreceptors in the cervical muscles, particularly the short-range rotators (ie, the obliquus capitis posterior inferior, rectus capitis posterior major, splenius capitis, and sternocleidomastoid) are the primary source of afferent input in the elicitation of the COR. The VOR is stimulated by movement of the head in space and has a strong influence on eye movement and positioning.

Visual fixation at higher speeds requires the contraction of the extraocular muscles to allow eye movements to counteract the effect of the head movements, even if the head is turning in the opposite direction. The ability to track and focus on a moving target that is moving across a visual field is termed smooth pursuit, and requires a greater degree of voluntary control than the COR and VOR can provide. The area in the brain stem where this integration of horizontal eye movements takes place is the paramedian pontine reticular formation (PPRF).

The ability to read a book or to scan a page requires quick movements of the eyes called saccades. Unlike smooth pursuit, saccades can occur with a visual stimulus, by sound, verbal command, or tactile stimuli. However, like smooth pursuit, saccades are generated in the PPRF.

Protective Reflexes. Protective reflexes are a function of the midbrain/cortical regions (refer to Chapter 16). They include:

- Righting reactions
- Protective extension
- Equilibrium reactions

Neuromuscular Control

Success in skilled performance depends upon how effectively the individual detects, perceives, and uses relevant sensory information.[46] Patients cannot succeed in functional and recreational activities if their neuromuscular system has not been prepared to meet the proprioceptive and balance demands of their specific activities.[47] The terms proprioception and balance are not synonymous. Proprioception can be viewed as the precursor of good balance.[48]

Proprioception. Proprioception plays an important role in coordinating muscle activity through the integration of sensory input.[49,50] Proprioception can be both conscious and unconscious.[50,51]

Fatigue can play a part in injury particularly if the fatigue produces a dominance of the agonists or antagonists over the other.[54,55] Fatigue also reduces a muscle's capability to absorb or dissipate loads. It seems plausible that some form of muscle spindle desensitization, or perhaps ligament relaxation and Golgi tendon desensitization, occurs with excessive fatigue.[56] This may then lead to a decreased efferent muscle response, and poorer ability to maintain balance.

Proprioceptive deficits can also be found with aging,[57] arthrosis,[58] and joint instability.[48,51,53,59-63]

Balance. The visual system, which involves CN II, III, IV, and VI, assists in balance control by providing input about the position of the head and/or the body in space. The coordination of eye movements during gaze is a complex affair, and is controlled by efferent signals from the trochlear, abducens and oculomotor nuclei via the fourth, sixth and third cranial nerves, respectively (refer to cervico-ocular and vestibular reflexes).[64] Coordination of these nuclei is achieved by gaze centers in the reticular formation, midbrain and cortex, and by the cerebellum, which have fibers that project into the three eye muscle nuclei and control the orbital movements concerned with slow and rapid eye movements.[64]

Position and Movement Sense. Kinesthesia refers to the sense of position and movement. While the articular receptors quite clearly play a very active role in kinesthesia, two other sensors, the muscle spindle and the Golgi tendon organ (GTO), are also important.

The Transmission of Pain

Pain, at some point or other, is felt by everyone. Acute pain can be defined as the normal, predicted physiological response to an adverse chemical, thermal or mechanical stimulus . . . associated with surgery, trauma and acute illness.[65,66]

Any tissue, which contains free nerve endings that are involved with nociception, is capable of being a source of pain. In the cutaneous tissue of man the existence of unmyelinated polymodal nociceptors, which are responsive to thermal, mechanical, and chemical stimuli have been established.[67,68] Common free nerve endings have two distinct pathways into the CNS, which correspond to the two different types of pain:

- Fast conducting—A-delta fibers
- Slow conducting—C fibers

A-delta, and C-fiber nociceptors have been clearly identified in fibers that innervate joints and muscles, but not in viscerae where the situation is much more complicated.[68] Thus, although certain fibers are undoubtedly nociceptors, others are activated by non-noxious stimuli but then increase their activity as the intensity of the stimulus increases.

Each of the two fiber types has different pain characteristics: A-delta fibers evoke a rapid, sharp, lancinating pain reaction, and C-fibers cause a slow, dull, crawling pain.

- The fast signals of the C fibers terminate in laminae I and V of the posterior (dorsal) horn. Lamina V is the area for convergence, summation and projection. The response of the cells in lamina V depends largely on the intensity of the stimulus. High intensity stimulation leads to facilitation of the cell and relatively easy transmission across the cord to the other side and, from here, upward to the brain in the lateral division of the anterior-lateral sensory pathway (lateral spinothalamic tract). More gentle stimulation inhibits this transmission.
- The slow signals of the C fibers terminate in laminae II and III of the posterior horn. Most of the signal then passes through another short fiber neuron to terminate in lamina V. Here the neuron gives off a long axon, most of which joins with the fast signal axons to cross the spinal cord, and continue upward in the brain in the same spinal tract. About 75% to 90% of all pain fibers terminate in the reticular formation of the medulla, pons and mesencephalon. From here, other neurons transmit the signal to the thalamus, hypothalamus (pituitary), limbic system and the cerebral cortex.

The central pathways for processing nociceptive information begin at the level of the spinal cord (and medullary) posterior horn. As with the periphery, the posterior horn of the spinal cord contains

Study Pearl

Patients' attitudes, beliefs, and personalities may strongly affect their immediate experience of acute pain.

many transmitters and receptors both identified and alleged including: several peptides (substance P, calcitonin gene related peptide, somatostatin, neuropeptide Y, and galanin); excitatory aminoacids (aspartate, glutamate); inhibitory aminoacids (γ-aminobytyric acid [GABA] and glycine); nitric oxide; the arachidonic acid metabolites; the endogenous opioids; adenosine; and the monoamines (serotonin and noradrenaline).[68] This diverse list illustrates the complexities faced with pain control (see later).

Interneuronal networks in the posterior horn are responsible not only for the transmission of nociceptive information to neurons that project to the brain, but also for the modulation of that information. The information is passed on to other spinal cord neurons, including the flexor motoneurons, and the nociceptive projection neurons; eg, certain patterns of stimulation can lead to enhanced reflex actions and to the sensitization of projection neurons, and increased nociceptive transmission. Other inputs result in the inhibition of projection neurons.

A small number of fast fibers are passed directly to the thalamus, and then to the cerebral cortex, bypassing the brain stem. It is believed that these signals are important for recognizing and localizing pain, but not for analyzing it. Of the slow signals, none, or at least very few, avoid the reticular system.

Study Pearl

- Referred pain: pain that is felt at a site removed from the source of involvement.
- Radicular pain: a specific type of referred pain that is felt in a dermatome, myotome, or sclerotome of an involved peripheral nerve root.

The Control of Pain. Melzack and Wall[69] postulated that interneurons in the substantia gelatinosa act as a gate to modulate sensory input. They proposed that the substantia gelatinosa interneuron projected to the second order neuron of the pain-temperature pathway located in lamina V, which they called the transmission cell. It was reasoned that if the substantia gelatinosa interneuron were depolarized, it would inhibit transmission cell firing, and thus decrease further transmission of input ascending in the spinothalamic tract. The degree of modulation appeared to depend upon the proportion of input from the large A fibers, and the small C fibers, so that the gate could be closed by either decreasing C fiber input, or by increasing A fiber, or mechanoreceptive input.

Melzack and Wall also believed that the gate could be modified by a descending inhibitory pathway from the brain, or brain stem,[70] suggesting that the CNS apparently plays a part in this modulation in a mechanism called central biasing.

The gate theory was, and is, supported by practical evidence, although the experimental evidence for the theory is lacking. Researchers have identified many clinical pain states that cannot be fully explained by the gate control theory.[71] The likelihood is that the reality of pain perception is much more complicated, even at the spinal cord level, and further research will alter our perception.

Numerous investigations have been made of what is known as the "descending analgesia systems." These pathways have been shown to utilize several different neurotransmitters, including opioids, serotonin, and/or catecholamines.

The peri-aquaductal grey (PAG) area of the upper pons is believed to be involved in complex behavioral responses to stressful or life-threatening situations, or to promote recuperative behavior after a defense reaction. The nerve fibers derived from the grey area secrete enkephalin (a substance that is believed to produce pre-synaptic inhibition of the incoming pain signals to lamina I through V) and serotonin while the raphe magnus releases enkephalin only.[72]

NEUROLOGICAL EXAMINATION

The examination begins when the clinician establishes essential facts about the patient beginning with the chief complaint and continuing through a full, logic sequence of the patient's history of the present illness (see also Examination of a Comatose Patient). This is supplemented with a history of past medical disorders, a review of systems, family history, and social history, focusing principally on the current problem but also assessing the risk factors for neurologic diseases.[73,74] Following an evaluation of the findings, a diagnosis is made using the neuromuscular preferred practice patterns (Table 9-12).

HISTORY

In addition to those areas to be covered in the "history" that are mentioned in Chapter 6, the history specific to the neurological examination should include details about:

- Chief complaint: recorded in the patient's own words (as appropriate) with quotations. If there is no complaint because of a cognitive disorder or other reasons, information can be obtained from the family or referring physician.
- History of the presenting symptoms: onset, progression, nature of symptoms, any specific mechanism of injury (Table 9-13).
- Family and psychiatric history: anxiety, depression, difficulties with concentration, sleep disorders, mood swings, obsessive thoughts, and compulsive behavior.
- Inherited disorders. Examples include, but are not limited to:
  - Autosomal dominant: Huntington disease
  - Autosomal recessive: Friedrich's ataxia
  - Alzheimer's

REVIEW OF SYSTEMS

The review of systems specific to the patient with a neurologic dysfunction should include an investigation of:

TABLE 9-12. NEUROMUSCULAR PREFERRED PRACTICE PATTERNS

PATTERN	DESCRIPTION
A	Primary prevention/risk reduction for loss of balance and falling
B	Impaired neuromotor development
C	Impaired motor function and sensory integrity associated with nonprogressive disorders of the central nervous system—congenital origin or acquired in infancy or childhood
D	Impaired motor function and sensory integrity associated with nonprogressive disorders of the central nervous system—acquired in adolescence or adulthood
E	Impaired motor function and sensory integrity associated with progressive disorders of the central nervous system
F	Impaired peripheral nerve integrity and muscle performance associated with peripheral nerve injury
G	Impaired motor function and sensory integrity associated with acute or chronic polyneuropathies
H	Impaired motor function, peripheral nerve integrity, and sensory integrity associated with nonprogressive disorders of the spinal cord
I	Impaired arousal, range of motion, and motor control associated with coma, near coma or vegetative state

Data from Guide to physical therapist practice. *Phys Ther.* 2001;81:S13-S95.

TABLE 9-13. SPECIFIC AREAS OF INQUIRY ORGANIZED BY FUNCTIONAL SYSTEMS

Higher cerebral functions	Disorders of memory, judgment, insight, concentration
	Disorientation in time and space
	Disturbances of consciousness, including blackouts or seizures and head injury
	Speech disorders (difficulty understanding spoken or written language, trouble finding correct words, irrelevant or meaningless speech)
	Sleep disturbances
	Psychologic disturbances (anxiety, depression, etc)
Cranial nerve and brainstem functions	Visual disorders, including loss of vision and double vision
	Headache
	Dizziness (as opposed to vertigo)
	Deafness
	Tinnitus
	Difficulty with articulation
Motor functions	Weakness or paralysis
	Slowness or stiffness of movement
	Involuntary movements, including tremors or twitches
	Unsteadiness in standing and walking
	Falling
Sensory functions	Loss of sensation
	Numbness, including decreased sensation or tingling
	Pain
Autonomic functions	Disturbances in the control of urination and defecation
	Lightheadedness upon standing
	Nausea and vomiting

Reproduced, with permission, from Gilman S: The neurologic history. In: Gilman S, ed. *Clinical Examination of the Nervous System.* New York, NY: McGraw-Hill; 2000:1-14.

- Constitutional symptoms: changes in personality or mood, fatigue, lassitude, weight loss or gain, and sleep disorders.
- Head, eyes, ears, nose, mouth, and throat.
- Cardiovascular and respiratory: exercise tolerance, shortness of breath, wheezing, respiratory infections, difficulty lying in bed, ankle swelling, irregular heartbeat, previously detected heart murmurs, chest pain, and myocardial infarction.
- Gastrointestinal: abdominal pain, indigestion, nausea, vomiting, constipation, diarrhea, bloody or black stools, and use of medications such as antacids.
- Genitourinary: urinary frequency, dysuria, infections, incontinence, dribbling, difficulty starting or stopping the stream, and nocturia.
- Musculoskeletal: muscle weakness, stiffness, difficulty walking, and joint pain.
- Integumentary: skin lesions, changes in the size of moles and the resultant biopsies of such lesions, itching or flaking of skin.
- Endocrine system: generalized weakness, changes in skin texture, skin pigmentation, hair loss, and discomfort in cold or warm environments.
- Hematologic/lymphatic systems: pallor, fatigue, easy bruising, excessive bleeding, and any history of anemia.
- Psychologic: emotional responses/behaviors.
- Arousal, orientation, and cognition (see also Examination of a Comatose Patient).

- Arousal: the physiological readiness of the human system for activity.
- Orientation: the patient's awareness of time, person, and place.
- Cognition (see Examination of Cognition)

- ▶ Memory: as for the patient's date of birth, dates of completing various schools, descriptions of the events of the past couple of days and previous 3 to 5 years.
- ▶ Safety, judgment, impulsiveness.
- ▶ Affect, mood.
- ▶ Level of attention, length of attention span, ability to attend to task without redirection.
- ▶ Level of frustration/tolerance.
- ▶ Insight into disability (anosognosia: severe denial of awareness of severity of condition).

TESTS AND MEASURES

The appropriateness and extent of each of the following components will vary according to the information already available and the severity of the patient's presenting condition. It should be obvious that not all of the following tests and measures will be used every time and with every patient.

Observation

- ▶ Position of head: tilted to the right or left, whether the chin is rotated to the right or left (torticollis).
- ▶ Facial expression: signs of distress, anger, depression, asymmetry, poverty of expression (masking—Parkinson's), ptosis, or apathy.
- ▶ Does the patient appear younger or older than the stated age?
- ▶ Premature balding in males may be hereditary, but frontal balding occurs with myotonic dystrophy and early graying can be seen in pernicious anemia.
- ▶ Overall grooming: hair, nails.
- ▶ Skin: color, temperature and moisture, and dryness.
- ▶ Dysmorphic features: an excessively large head, short neck, or short legs.
- ▶ Posture of the trunk and limbs. Observation of sitting posture should focus on the ability to remain upright against gravity, symmetry (difference in preservation of motor function between right and left sides, weight distribution), scapular position (early indicator of muscle balance and control in the scapular region), use of upper extremities to assist with and maintain posture, and position of lower trunk and pelvis.[75]
- ▶ Quality of gait: ataxic, shuffling, or spastic.
- ▶ Speech: clarity and fluency.
- ▶ Presence of CNS infection: patient may display irritability (photophobia, disorientation, restlessness), slowed mental function, lethargy, persistent headache, or altered vital signs.
- ▶ Vital signs: height, weight, blood pressure, pulse rate, respiratory rate, oral temperature (as appropriate).
- ▶ Signs of meningeal irritation: limitation and guarding of neck flexion (nuchal rigidity) resulting from spasm of posterior neck muscles.

- Kernig's sign: patient supine, clinician flexes thigh and knee fully to the chest, then extends the knee; positive sign is spasm of the hamstring, resistance, and pain.
- Brudzinski's sign: patient supine, clinician flexes head to chest; positive test causes flexion of both legs (drawing up).

Anthropometric Characteristics

- Relationship of limb length to trunk length is important, especially with spinal cord injuries, since longer limbs will provide the advantage of a longer lever arm for closed chain upper activities but will also necessitate increased control for management of flaccid or spastic lower extremities.[75]
- Obesity will increase the demand on extremities during mobility and may prevent achievement of the range of motion of the pelvis and hips required for many mobility skills.
- Very thin individuals have an increased susceptibility to pressure ulcers due to their more prominent bony prominences.

Examination of Cognition. Cognition is defined as the process of knowing and includes both awareness and judgment. Cognition dependent functions include:

- Retention and immediate recall: the clinician verbally presents three digits at a rate of about one per second and asks the patient to repeat the digits forward and backward.
- Executive functions, calculations: present the following problems—subtract 7 from 100, count from 1 to 20 and backward to 1.
- Grasp of general information: name of the US president, the name of five large cities in the United States.
- Proverb interpretation: the clinician verbally presents a proverb and asks for an interpretation of the proverb.
- Similarities: the clinician verbally presents an object such as an apple and lemon and asks what way they are similar.
- Insight: describe finding a stamped, addressed, sealed envelope on the street and ask what should be done with it.
- Higher-level cognitive abilities:
  - Judgment
  - Abstract reasoning
  - Problem-solving
  - Wealth of general knowledge

Assessment of Speech and Language. Assess fluency of speech, speech production.

- Aphasia.[76-79] Aphasia is a symptom not a disease—it is an acquired disorder of language caused by brain damage, usually involving the left cerebral hemisphere. Many specific aphasic syndromes have been reported (Table 9-14).
- Verbal apraxia[80-82]: impairment of volitional articulatory control secondary to a cortical, dominant hemisphere lesion.
- Dysarthria: impairment of speech production.
- Receptive function (comprehension).

TABLE 9-14. TYPES OF APHASIA

TYPE	DESCRIPTION
Non-fluent aphasia (Broca's, motor aphasia, expressive aphasia)	Lesion of the frontal region of the dominant hemisphere. Speech is typically awkward, restricted, and produced with effort. Typical lesions occur in the dorsolateral frontal cortex, operculum, anterior parietal cortex, and lateral striate and periventricular white matter.
Fluent aphasia (Wernicke's aphasia, receptive aphasia)	Lesion of the posterior region of the superior temporal gyrus. Spontaneous speech is preserved while auditory comprehension is impaired. Despite the fluency, the speech is full of emptiness and gibberish jargon, which may include invented words known as neologisms.
Conduction aphasia	Lesion of the supramarginal gyrus and arcuate fasciculus. Language output is fluent, but naming and repetition are impaired. Hesitations and word-finding pauses are frequent.
Global aphasia	Marked impairment in the comprehension and production of language. The patient has deficits in repeating, naming, understanding, and producing fluent speech.
Transcortical aphasia	By definition, patients with transcortical aphasia can repeat, but they have difficulty naming or producing spontaneous speech or understanding spoken speech.
Anomic aphasia	Lesion of the angular gyrus. Patients with anomic aphasia present with intact repetition, fluent speech, intact or mostly intact repetition, and an inability to name things.

Assessment of Visiospatial Function. The physical therapist can assess for a number of visiospatial or perception deficits (Table 9-15):

- Homonymous hemianopsia: loss of half of visual field in each eye contralateral to the side of a cerebral hemisphere lesion.
- Body scheme/body image: have patient identify body parts or their relationship to each other.
- Visual spatial neglect: whether patient ignores one side of the body and stimuli coming from that side.

TABLE 9-15. COMMON CONCEPTUAL AND COMMUNICATION PROBLEMS IN HEMIPLEGIC PATIENTS

LEFT HEMISPHERE LESIONS	COMMON FUNCTIONAL DEFICIT
Aphasias	Lacks functional speech
Ideomotor and ideational apraxias	Cannot plan and execute serial steps in performances
Number alexia	Cannot recognize symbols to do simple computations
Right-left discrimination	Unable to distinguish right from left on self or reverse on others
Slow in organization and performance	Cannot remember what he or she intended to do next
RIGHT HEMISPHERE LESIONS	**COMMON FUNCTIONAL DEFICIT**
Visuospatial	Cannot orient self to changes in environment while going from one treatment area to another
Left unilateral neglect of self	Generally unaware of objects to left and propels wheelchair into them
Body image	Distorted awareness and impression of self
Dressing apraxia	Applies shirt to right side, but unable to do left side application
Constructional apraxia	Unable to transpose two dimensional instructions into three-dimensional structure, as per "do-it-yourself" kits
Illusions of shortening of time	Patient arrives extremely early for appointments
Number concepts—spatial type	Unable to align columns and rows of digits
Rapid organization and performance	Errors from haste; may cause accidents
Depth of language skills	May mention tasks related to pre-stroke occupation, but cannot go into details

Reproduced, with permission, from Rothstein JM, Roy SH, Wolf SL: Perceptual and communication problems in hemiplegia. In: *The Rehabilitation Specialists Handbook*. Philadelphia, PA: FA Davis; 1991:548-550.

TABLE 9-16. MINI MENTAL STATE EXAMINATION

FUNCTION	SCORE	METHOD OR QUERY
Arousal		Is the patient responsive to you upon entering the exam room?
Affect		Does the patient look depressed or despondent, admit to being depressed, and demonstrate psychomotor retardation?
Orientation	1	Name of facility
	1	Floor
	1	Town/city
	1	County
	1	Day of week (exact)
	1	Month (exact)
	1	Date (plus or minus one day only)
	1	Year (exact)
Registration	3	Repeat three words: ball, tree, flag
Sentence repetition	1	Repeat "no ifs, ands, or buts"
Auditory comprehension	3	Follow three-step command: "Take this paper in your (non-dominant) hand, fold it in half, and place it on your lap"
Naming	2	Ask patient to name: pencil, watch
Writing	1	Ask patient to write a sentence
Construction	1	Copy a figure (intersecting pentagons)
Attention/concentration	5	Spell "world" backwards or count backwards from 100 by 7s (take best score)
Read	1	Read and execute "close your eyes"
Recall	3	Recall the three words (see Registration above)

Data from Galea M, Woodward M: Mini-mental state examination (MMSE). *Aust J Physiother.* 2005;51:198.
Mossello E, Boncinelli M: Mini-mental state examination: a 30-year story. *Aging Clin Exp Res.* 2006;18:271-273.

Study Pearl

Agnosia is the inability to recognize familiar objects with one sensory modality, while retaining the ability to recognize the same object with another sensory modality.

- Right/left discrimination.
- Vertical disorientation: patient unable to determine whether an object is upright or vertical.
- Topographical disorientation: patient unable to navigate a familiar route on own.
- Figure-ground discrimination: whether the patient can pick out an object from an array of objects, eg, choosing a knife from the cutlery drawer.
- Form constancy: whether the patient can pick out an object from an array of similarly shaped but different sized objects.
- Depth and distance perception.

Mini Mental State Examination. The mini mental state examination (MMSE)[83,84] is the most widely used screening tool for items such as orientation, registration, attention and calculation, recall, and language (Table 9-16). Maximum score is 30; scores between 21 and 24 indicate mild cognitive impairment, scores between 16 and 20 reflect moderate impairment, and a score of 15 and below indicates severe impairment.

Levels of Cognitive Function: Rancho Los Amigos Cognitive Functioning Scale. This assessment scale was designed to evaluate cognitive recovery following traumatic brain injury.[85] The assessment tool includes eight levels of behavior, and delineates emerging behaviors (Table 9-17). A modified version is also available (Table 9-18).

Assessment of Righting Reactions. The patient's ability to perform automatic adjustments to restore normal alignment of the

TABLE 9-17. RANCHO LOS AMIGOS COGNITIVE FUNCTIONING SCALE

I—No response	Patient appears to be in a deep sleep and is completely unresponsive to any stimuli.
II—Generalized response	Patiently acts inconsistently and purposely to stimuli in a nonspecific manner. Responses are limited and often the same regardless of stimulus presented. Responses may be physiological changes, gross body movements, and/or vocalization.
III—Localized responses	Patient reacts specifically but inconsistently to stimuli. Response is not directly related to the type of stimulus presented. May follow simple commands in an inconsistent, delayed manner, such as closing eyes or squeezing hands.
IV—Confused-agitated	Patient is in heightened state of activity. Behavior is bizarre and non-purposeful relative to immediate environment. Does not discriminate among persons or objects; is unable to cooperate directly with treatment efforts. Verbalizations frequently are incoherent and/or inappropriate to the environment; confabulation may be present. Gross attention to environment is very brief. Patient lacks short-term and long-term recall.
V—Confused-inappropriate	Patient is able to respond to simple commands fairly consistently. However, with increased complexity of commands or lack of any external structure, responses are non-purposeful, random, or fragmented. Demonstrates gross attention to the environment that is highly distractible and lacks ability to focus attention on a specific task. With structure, may be able to converse on a social automatic level for short periods of time. The vocalization is often inappropriate and confabulatory. Memory is severely impaired; often shows inappropriate use of objects; may perform previously learned tasks with structure but is unable to learn new information.
VI—Confused-appropriate	Patient shows goal-directed behavior but is dependent on external input or direction. Follows simple directions consistently and shows carryover for relearned problems but appropriate to the situation; past memories show more depth and detail than recent memory.
VII—Automatic-appropriate	Patient appears appropriate and oriented within hospital and home settings: goes through daily routine automatically, but frequently robot-like with minimal to absent confusion and has shallow recall of activities. Shows carryover for new learning but at a decreased rate. With structure is able to initiate social or recreational activities; judgment remains impaired.
VIII—Purposeful and appropriate.	Patient is able to recall and to integrate past and recent events and is aware of and responsive to environment. Shows carryover for new learning and needs no supervision once activities are learned. May continue to show a decreased ability relative to premorbid abilities, abstract reasoning, tolerance for stress, and judgment in emergencies or unusual circumstances.
IX—Purposeful, appropriate	Stand-by assistance on request.
X—Purposeful, appropriate	Modified independent.

Data from Hagen C, Malkmus D, Durham P: *Rancho Los Amigos Cognitive Scale.* Rancho Los Amigos Hospital; California. Downey. 1972.

head and trunk when changing position. This can be performed with or without perturbations, or by displacing the base of support by using a movable surface (eg, Swiss ball), to assess the patient's ability to:

- Maintain and restore the normal position of the head in space.
- To maintain and restore the normal position of the head with regard to trunk alignment.
- To maintain and restore a normal position of the head and the four extremities.
- To align the body as necessary for various motor activities.
- To adjust posture appropriately.
- Overlap with the equilibrium reactions.

Assessment of Equilibrium Reactions. Equilibrium reactions enable the patient to alter the body's center of mass and/or base

TABLE 9-18. MODIFIED RANCHO LOSS AMIGOS COGNITIVE FUNCTIONING SCALE

Level	Description	Characteristics
Level I	**No response: total assistance**	Complete absence of observable change in behavior when presented visual, auditory, tactile, proprioceptive, vestibular or painful stimuli.
Level II	**Generalized response: total assistance**	Demonstrates generalized reflex response to painful stimuli. Responds to repeated auditory stimuli with increased or decreased activity. Responds to external stimuli with physiological changes generalized, gross body movement and/or not purposeful vocalization. Responses noted above may be same regardless of type and location of stimulation. Responses may be significantly delayed.
Level III	**Localized response: total assistance**	Demonstrates withdrawal or vocalization to painful stimuli. Turns toward or away from auditory stimuli. Blinks when strong light crosses visual field. Follows moving object passed within visual field. Responds to discomfort by pulling tubes or restraints. Responds inconsistently to simple commands. Responses directly related to type of stimulus. May respond to some persons (especially family and friends) but not to others.
Level IV	**Confused/agitated: maximal assistance**	Alert and in heightened state of activity. Purposeful attempts to remove restraints or tubes or crawl out of bed. May perform motor activities such as sitting, reaching and walking but without any apparent purpose or upon another's request. Very brief and usually non-purposeful moments of sustained alternatives and divided attention. Absent short-term memory. May cry out or scream out of proportion to stimulus even after its removal. May exhibit aggressive or flight behavior. Mood may swing from euphoric to hostile with no apparent relationship to environmental events. Unable to cooperate with treatment efforts. Verbalizations are frequently incoherent and/or inappropriate to activity or environment.
Level V	**Confused, inappropriate non-agitated: maximal assistance**	Alert, not agitated but may wander randomly or with a vague intention of going home. May become agitated in response to external stimulation, and/or lack of environmental structure. Not oriented to person, place or time. Frequent brief periods, non-purposeful sustained attention. Severely impaired recent memory, with confusion of past and present in reaction to ongoing activity. Absent goal directed, problem solving, self-monitoring behavior. Often demonstrates inappropriate use of objects without external direction. May be able to perform previously learned tasks when structured and cues provided. Unable to learn new information. Able to respond appropriately to simple commands fairly consistently with external structures and cues. Responses to simple commands without external structure are random and non-purposeful in relation to command. Able to converse on a social, automatic level for brief periods of time when provided external structure and cues. Verbalizations about present events become inappropriate and confabulatory when external structure and cues are not provided.
Level VI	**Confused, appropriate: moderate assistance**	Inconsistently oriented to person, time and place. Able to attend to highly familiar tasks in non-distracting environment for 30 min with moderate redirection. Remote memory has more depth and detail than recent memory. Vague recognition of some staff. Able to use assistive memory aide with maximum assistance. Emerging awareness of appropriate response to self, family and basic needs. Moderate assist to problem solve barriers to task completion. Supervised for old learning (eg, self care). Shows carry over for relearned familiar tasks (eg, self care). Maximum assistance for new learning with little or nor carry over. Unaware of impairments, disabilities and safety risks. Consistently follows simple directions. Verbal expressions are appropriate in highly familiar and structured situations.

(Continued)

TABLE 9-18. MODIFIED RANCHO LOSS AMIGOS COGNITIVE FUNCTIONING SCALE (*Continued*)

Level VII	**Automatic, appropriate: minimal assistance for daily living skills**	Consistently oriented to person and place, within highly familiar environments. Moderate assistance for orientation to time. Able to attend to highly familiar tasks in a non-distraction environment for at least 30 min with minimal assist to complete tasks. Minimal supervision for new learning. Demonstrates carry over of new learning. Initiates and carries out steps to complete familiar personal and household routine but has shallow recall of what he/she has been doing. Able to monitor accuracy and completeness of each step in routine personal and household ADLs and modify plan with minimal assistance. Superficial awareness of his/her condition but unaware of specific impairments and disabilities and the limits they place on his/her ability to safely, accurately and completely carry out his/her household, community, work and leisure ADLs. Minimal supervision for safety in routine home and community activities. Unrealistic planning for the future. Unable to think about consequences of a decision or action. Overestimates abilities. Unaware of others' needs and feelings. Oppositional/uncooperative. Unable to recognize inappropriate social interaction behavior.
Level VIII	**Purposeful, appropriate: stand-by assistance**	Consistently oriented to person, place and time. Independently attends to and completes familiar tasks for 1 h in distracting environments. Able to recall and integrate past and recent events. Uses assistive memory devices to recall daily schedule, "to do" lists and record critical information for later use with stand-by assistance. Initiates and carries out steps to complete familiar personal, household, community, work and leisure routines with stand-by assistance and can modify the plan when needed with minimal assistance. Requires no assistance once new tasks/activities are learned. Aware of and acknowledges impairments and disabilities when they interfere with task completion but requires stand-by assistance to take appropriate corrective action. Thinks about consequences of a decision or action with minimal assistance. Overestimates or underestimates abilities. Acknowledges others' needs and feelings and responds appropriately with minimal assistance. Depressed. Irritable. Low frustration tolerance/easily angered. Argumentative. Self-centered. Uncharacteristically dependent/independent. Able to recognize and acknowledge inappropriate social interaction behavior while it is occurring and takes corrective action with minimal assistance.
Level IX	**Purposeful, appropriate: stand-by assistance on request**	Independently shifts back and forth between tasks and completes them accurately for at least two consecutive hours. Uses assistive memory devices to recall daily schedule, "to do" lists and record critical information for later use with assistance when requested. Initiates and carries out steps to complete familiar personal, household, work and leisure tasks independently and unfamiliar personal, household, work and leisure tasks with assistance when requested. Aware of and acknowledges impairments and disabilities when they interfere with task completion and takes appropriate corrective action but requires stand-by assist to anticipate a problem before it occurs and take action to avoid it. Able to think about consequences of decisions or actions with assistance when requested. Accurately estimates abilities but requires stand-by assistance to adjust to task demands. Acknowledges others' needs and feelings and responds appropriately with stand-by assistance. Depression may continue. May be easily irritable. May have low frustration tolerance. Able to self-monitor appropriateness of social interaction with stand-by assistance.

(*Continued*)

TABLE 9-18. MODIFIED RANCHO LOSS AMIGOS COGNITIVE FUNCTIONING SCALE (*Continued*)

Level X	**Purposeful, appropriate: modified independent**	Able to handle multiple tasks simultaneously in all environments but may require periodic breaks. Able to independently procure, create and maintain own assistive memory devices. Independently initiates and carries out steps to complete familiar and unfamiliar personal, household, community, work and leisure tasks but may require more than usual amount of time and/or compensatory strategies to complete them. Anticipates impact of impairments and disabilities on ability to complete daily living tasks and takes action to avoid problems before they occur but may require more than usual amount of time and/or compensatory strategies. Able to independently think about consequences of decisions or actions but may require more than usual amount of time and/or compensatory strategies to select the appropriate decision or action. Accurately estimates abilities and independently adjusts to task demands. Able to recognize the needs and feelings of others and automatically respond in appropriate manner. Periodic periods of depression may occur. Irritability and low frustration tolerance when sick, fatigued and/or under emotional stress. Social interaction behavior is consistently appropriate.

Data from Malkmus D, Stenderup K: *Rancho Los Amigos Cognitive Scale Revised.* Rancho Los Amigos Hospital; California: Downey; 1972.

of support to maintain balance. As appropriate, the clinician can assess for the presence of:

- Movement strategies: the timing, sequencing, or scaling of ankle and hip strategies, the appropriateness of the chosen strategy, and the number of strategies in the patient's repertoire.
- The ankle strategy is the first strategy to be elicited by a small range and low velocity perturbation when the feet are on the ground.
- The hip strategy is elicited by a greater force, challenge or perturbation through the pelvis and hips. The hips should move in the opposite direction to the head in order to maintain balance.
- Suspensory strategy: lowering the body's center of gravity.
- Stepping strategy: rapid steps are taken in an effort to realign the body's center of gravity over the base of support.

It is important to assess the patient's ability to perform active weight shifts in multiple directions in both standing and sitting. A number of clinical tests have been devised to assess sensory interaction/organization:

- Simple (static) sitting balance test: the patient is asked to hold a steady position, first with arm support and then with no arm support.
- Simple (static) standing balance test: the patient is asked to hold a steady position, first with double limb support and then with single limb support.
- Clinical test for sensory interaction in balance (CTSIB): foam and dome (Shumway-Cook and Horak), or the modified version.[86,87] Consists of six different sensory conditions, progressing in difficulty:
  - Eyes open, fixed support surface (platform or dense foam).
  - Eyes closed, fixed support.

- Visual conflict (patient wears a dome over the head in such a manner that it moves when the head moves, or stands in front of a moving surround screen), fixed support surface.
- Eyes open, moving support surface.
- Eyes closed, moving support surface.
- Visual conflict, moving support surface.

- ▶ Nystagmus tests (electronystagmography).
- ▶ Romberg test[88]: static balance test used to detect posterior column (sensory) ataxia. The patient stands with feet in normal stance position, first with eyes open, then with eyes closed. To increase the sensitivity of this test, the patient is asked to stand in a tandem heel to toe position, first with the eyes open, and then with the eyes closed (Sharpened or Tandem Romberg).
- ▶ Functional balance test: the patient performs functional movements such as standing up and sitting down, walking, changing direction, walking through an obstacle course. The test can be made more challenging by asking the patient to perform two functions at the same time—walk and talk, obey commands.

Standardized Tests for Functional Balance

- ▶ Dynamic gait index.[89,90]
- ▶ Get up and go test.[91,92]
- ▶ Functional reach test.[93-95]
- ▶ The Berg Balance Scale.[96-100]
- ▶ Performance-oriented mobility assessment (POMA).[101,102]

Assessment of Protective Reactions. The patient's ability to stabilize and support the body by performing an automatic adjustment of the arms and/or legs in response to a displacing stimulus in which the center of gravity exceeds the base of support (eg, extension of arms to protect against fall). This can be performed with or without perturbations, or by displacing the base of support by using a movable surface (eg, Swiss ball).

- ▶ Postural reflex mechanisms
- ▶ Postural adaptation to growth

Assessment of:

- ▶ Balance
- ▶ Postural reactions
- ▶ Postural tone—refers to the overall level of tension in the body musculature necessary to maintain body posture against gravity[4]
- ▶ Range of motion
- ▶ Proprioception
- ▶ Placing
- ▶ Quality of motion
- ▶ Sensation
- ▶ Stereognosis

Examination of a Comatose Patient. Coma is a mental state defined by no eye opening even to pain, failure to obey commands, and inability to speak with recognizable words.

TABLE 9-19. LEVELS OF CONSCIOUSNESS: A CONTINUUM OF PHYSIOLOGICAL READINESS FOR ACTIVITY

TERM	DESCRIPTION
Alert	A quality of mind characterized by attentiveness to normal levels of stimulation, self-awareness, subjectivity, sapience, and sentience.
Lethargic	The patient appears drowsy and may fall asleep if not stimulated in some way. Patient has difficulty in focusing or maintaining attention on the question or task.
Obtunded	A state of consciousness characterized by a state of sleep, reduced alertness to arousal, and delayed responses to stimuli.
Stupor (semicoma)	The patient responds only to strong, generally noxious stimuli and returns to the unconscious state when stimulation is stopped. When aroused, the patient is unable to interact with the therapist.
Vegetative state (unresponsive vigilance)	Absence of the capacity for self-aware mental activity due to overwhelming damage or dysfunction of the cerebral hemispheres with sufficient sparing of the diencephalon and brain stem to preserve autonomic and motor reflexes as well as normal sleep-wake cycles. Characterized by a lack of cognitive responsiveness but with the return of sleep/wake cycles, and normalization of vegetative functions (respiration, heart rate, blood pressure, digestion).
Coma	The patient is unarousable and unresponsive and any response to repeated stimuli is only primitive avoidance reflexes; in profound coma, all brain stem and myotatic reflexes may be absent.

Consciousness requires the integrity of the reticular formation located in the rostral pons and the midbrain and at least one cerebral hemisphere. The various levels of consciousness are outlined in Table 9-19. The most commonly used standardized examination of comatose patients is the Glasgow Coma Scale (GCS) (Table 9-20). The GCS scale is intended for grading coma severity and establishing prognosis following head injury. Scoring range is from 3 to 15:

- Score of 8 or less: severe brain injury.
- Score of 9 to 12: moderate brain injury.
- Score of 13 to 15: minor brain injury.

Signs and Symptoms of Cerebral Edema and Increased Intracranial Pressure

- Changes in level of consciousness—progressing from restlessness and confusion to decreasing level of consciousness, and unresponsiveness.

TABLE 9-20. GLASGOW COMA SCALE (GCS)

	TEST	PATIENT RESPONSE	SCORE
Eye-opening	Spontaneous	Opens eyes	4
	To speech	Opens eyes	3
	To pain	Opens eyes	2
	To pain	Doesn't open	1
Best verbal response	Speech	Conversation carried out correctly	5
		Confused, disoriented	4
		Inappropriate words	3
		Unintelligible sounds only	2
		Mute	1
Best motor response	Commands	Follows simple commands	6
	To pain	Pulls examiner's hand away	5
	To pain	Pulls part of body away	4
	To pain	Flexes body to pain	3
	To pain	Decerebrates	2
	To pain	No motor response	1

- Fluctuations in vital signs—increased blood pressure; widening pulse pressure and slowing of pulse, irregular respirations including periods of apnea; elevated temperature.
- Decorticate or decerebrate rigidity (see Examination of Motor Function).
- Pupillary changes (Figure 9-19).
- Headache.
- Vomiting/nausea.
- Progressive impairment of motor function.
- Seizures.
- Pathological reflexes.

CRANIAL NERVE EXAMINATION

With practice, the entire cranial nerve (Table 9-21) examination[103] can be performed in approximately 5 minutes.[104]

CN I —The Olfactory Nerve. The sense of smell is tested by having the patient identify familiar odors (coffee, lavender, vanilla) with each nostril. The clinician should avoid irritant odors that can stimulate the trigeminal nerve.

CN II—The Optic Nerve. The optic nerve is tested by examining visual acuity, and confrontation. Although, the formal testing of visual acuity is presented here, in reality, it is sufficient to test this aspect of cranial nerve II at the same time that cranial nerves III, IV, and VI are being tested.

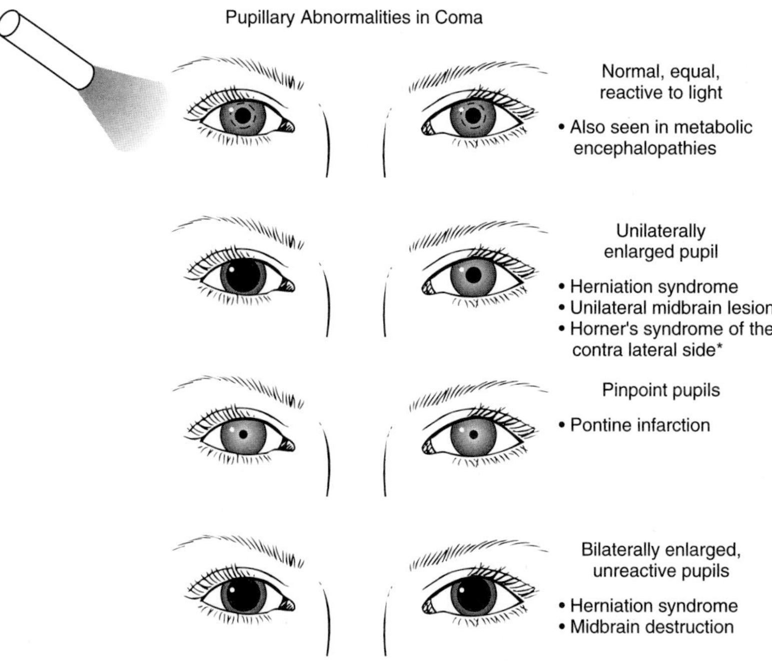

Figure 9-19. Pupillary abnormalities. (Reproduced, with permission, from Gilman, S: *Clinical Examination of the Nervous Tissue.* New York: McGraw-Hill. 2000:58.)

TABLE 9-21. CRANIAL NERVES AND METHODS OF TESTING

NERVES	FUNCTION: AFFERENT (SENSORY)	FUNCTION: EFFERENT (MOTOR)	TESTS
I—Olfactory	Smell	—	Unilateral identification of familiar odors (eg, chocolate, coffee)
II—Optic	Sight	—	Visual acuity; peripheral vision; pupillary light reflex
III—Oculomotor	—	*Voluntary motor:* levator of eyelid; superior, medial, and inferior recti; inferior oblique muscle of eyeball *Autonomic:* smooth muscle of eyeball	Upward, downward, and medial gaze; reaction to light
IV—Trochlear	—	*Voluntary motor:* superior oblique muscle of eyeball	Extraocular eye movements: downward and lateral gaze
V—Trigeminal	Touch, pain: skin of face, mucous membranes of nose, sinuses, mouth, anterior tongue	*Voluntary motor:* muscles of mastication	Corneal reflex; sensation above eye, between eye and mouth, below mouth to angle of jaw; clench teeth, push down on chin to separate jaws
VI—Abducens	—	*Voluntary motor:* lateral rectus muscle of eyeball	Lateral gaze (eye abduction)
VII—Facial	Taste: anterior two thirds of tongue	*Voluntary motor:* facial muscles *Autonomic:* lacrimal, submandibular, and sublingual glands	Facial expressions (Close eyes tight; smile and show teeth; whistle and puff cheeks); identify familiar tastes (eg, sweet, sour)
VIII—Vestibulocochlear (acoustic nerve)	Hearing/equilibrium	— —	Hearing tests; balance and coordination tests
IX—Glossopharyngeal	Visceral sensibility (pharynx, tongue, tonsils); taste	*Voluntary motor:* unimportant muscle of pharynx *Autonomic:* parotid gland	Gag reflex; ability to swallow; phonation
X—Vagus	Touch, pain; pharynx, larynx, trachea, bronchi and lungs Taste: tongue, epiglottis	*Voluntary motor:* muscles of palate, pharynx, and larynx *Autonomic:* involuntary muscle and gland control	Gag reflex; ability to swallow; speech (phonation)
XI—Accessory	—	*Voluntary motor:* Movement of head and shoulders-sternocleidomastoid and trapezius muscles	Resisted head; shoulder shrug
XII—Hypoglossal	—	*Voluntary motor:* movement of tongue	Tongue protrusion (if injured, tongue deviates toward injured side); inspection of tongue for atrophy

Visual Acuity. This is a test of central vision. If possible, the clinician should use a well-lit Snellen eye chart. The patient is positioned 20 ft from the chart. Patients who use corrective lenses other than reading glasses should be instructed to use them. The patient is asked to cover one eye and to read the smallest line possible. A patient who cannot read the largest letter should be positioned closer to the chart and the new distance noted. The clinician determines the smallest line of print from which the patient can identify more than half the letters. The visual acuity designated at the side of this line, together with the use of glasses, if any, is recorded.

Study Pearl

Visual acuity is expressed as a fraction (eg, 20/20), in which the numerator indicates the distance of the patient from the chart, the denominator the distance at which a normal eye can read the letters.

Confrontation test. This is a rough clinical test of peripheral vision and to highlight a loss of vision in one of the visual fields. The patient and clinician sit facing each other, with their eyes level. Both the lateral and medial fields of vision are tested. The entire lateral field is tested with both eyes open, and the medial field is tested by covering one eye. When testing the medial field of vision the clinician covers the patient's eye directly opposite their own (not diagonally opposite).

With their arms outstretched and the hands holding a small object such as a pencil, the clinician slowly brings the object into the peripheral field of vision of the patient. This is performed from eight separate directions. Each time the patient is asked to say "now" as soon as they see the object. During the examination, the clinician should keep the object equidistant between his or her own eye and the patient's so that the patient's visual field can be compared to the clinician's own.

CN III—Oculomotor; CN IV—Trochlear; CN VI—Abducens. These three cranial nerves are tested together. The clinician:

- Inspects the size and shape of each pupil for symmetry.
- Tests the consensual pupillary response to light. This is tested by having the patient cover one eye, while the clinician observes the uncovered eye. The uncovered eye should undergo the same changes as the covered by first dilating, and then constricting, when the covered eye is uncovered.
- Looks for the ability of the eyes to track movement in the six fields of gaze. The standard test is to smoothly move a target in a "H" configuration, and then in midline just above eye level toward the base of the nose (convergence).[105,106] The patient should be able to smoothly track a target at moderate speed, without evidence of nystagmus.
- Looks for ptosis of the upper eyelids.

CN V—Trigeminal. The patient is asked to clench the teeth, and the clinician palpates the temporal and masseter muscles. The three sensory branches of the trigeminal nerve are tested, with pinprick, close to the mid-line of the face, because the skin that is more lateral is overlapped by the nerves of the face.[106]

The jaw tendon reflex is assessed for hyperreflexia, which would indicate the presence of an upper motor neuron lesion.

Study Pearl

Loss or reduced ability to smile and frown is caused by a peripheral palsy, whereas the loss of the smile only is caused by a supranuclear lesion.[106]

CN VII—Facial. The clinician inspects the face at rest and in conversation with the patient, and notes any asymmetry. The patient is asked to smile. If there is asymmetry, the patient is asked to frown, or wrinkle the forehead.

CN VIII—Vestibulocochlear. The vestibular nerve can be tested in a number of ways depending on the objective.

- Balance testing assesses the vestibulospinal reflexes (VSR). The VSR serves to stabilize the body while the head is moving and helps control coordination and movement.
- Caloric stimulation can be used to assess the vestibulo-ocular reflex. The vestibulo-ocular reflex can also be assessed by testing the ability of the eyes to follow a moving object (see Supraspinal Reflex Testing later in this chapter).

The clinician assesses the function of the cochlear component of the nerve-hearing. There are three basic types of hearing loss[105]:

- Conductive. This type of hearing loss applies to any disturbance in the conduction of the sound impulse as it passes through the ear canal (Figure 9-20), tympanic membrane, middle ear, and ossicular chain to the footplate of the stapes, which is situated in the oval window (Figure 9-21). As a general rule, an individual with conductive hearing loss speaks softly, hears well on the telephone, and hears best in a noisy environment.
- Sensorineural. This type of hearing loss applies to a disturbance anywhere from the cochlea, through the auditory nerve, and on to the hearing center in the cerebral cortex. As a general rule, an individual with a perceptive hearing loss usually

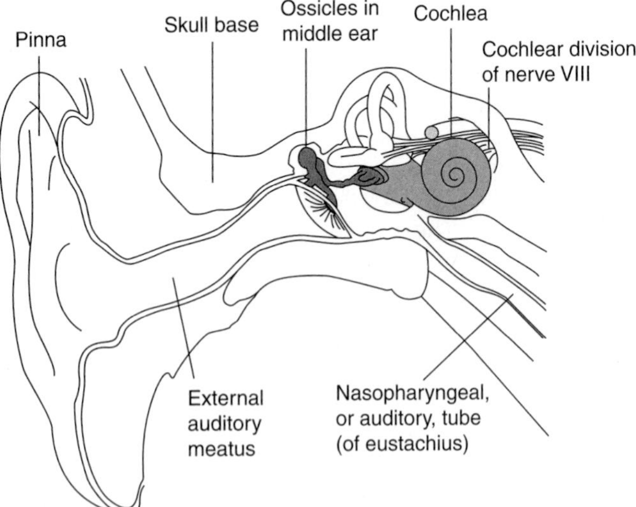

Figure 9-20. The human ear. The cochlea has been turned slightly, and the middle ear muscles have been omitted to make the relationship clear. (Reproduced, with permission, from Waxman, SG: *Correlative Neuroanatomy, 24th ed.* New York: McGraw-Hill. 2000:222.)

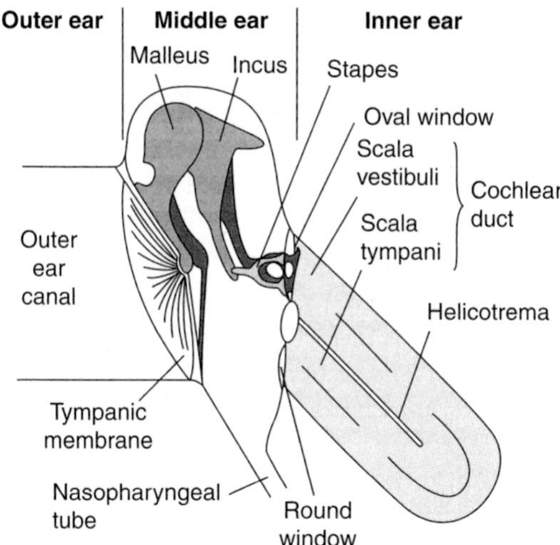

Figure 9-21. Schematic view of the ear. (Reproduced, with permission, from Waxman, SG: *Correlative Neuroanatomy, 24th ed.* New York: McGraw-Hill. 2000:223.)

speaks loudly, hears better in a quiet environment, and hears poorly in a crowd and on the telephone.

- Mixed. This type of hearing loss is a combination of conductive and sensorineural.

Two quick tests can be used to test hearing, by gently rubbing two fingers equidistant from each of the patient's ears simultaneously, or using a 256-Hz tuning fork and asking the patient to identify in which ear the noise appears to be the loudest. If a hearing deficit is present, then the clinician should test for lateralization, and compare air and bone conduction.

Lateralization. The clinician places a tuning fork over the vertex, middle of the forehead, or front teeth. The patient is asked whether the vibration is heard more in one ear (Weber's test). Normal individuals cannot lateralize the vibration to either ear. In conduction deafness (eg, that caused by middle ear disease), the vibration is heard more in the affected ear. In sensorineural deafness, the vibration is heard better in the normal ear.

Air and Bone Conduction. Air conduction is assessed by placing the tuning fork in front of the external auditory meatus, while bone conduction is assessed by placing the tuning fork on the mastoid process (Rinne's test). In a normal individual, the tuning fork is heard louder and longer by air than by bone conduction.[106] In conduction deafness, bone conduction hearing is better.[106] In sensorineural deafness, both air and bone conduction are reduced although air conduction is the better of the two.[106]

CN IX—Glossopharyngeal. The gag reflex is used to test this nerve, but is only reserved for the severely affected patients.

CN X—Vagus. The clinician listens to the patient's voice and notes any hoarseness and/or nasal quality. The patient is asked to open their mouth and say "aah." The clinician watches the movements of the soft palate and pharynx. The soft palate should rise symmetrically, the uvula should remain in the midline, and each side of the posterior pharynx should move medially.

CN XI—Spinal Accessory. From behind the patient, the clinician notes any atrophy or fasciculation in the trapezius muscles and compares side to side. The patient is asked to shrug both shoulders upward against the clinician's hand. The strength of contraction should be noted.

The patient is asked to attempt to turn his or her head to each side against the clinician's hand. The contraction of the opposite side sternocleidomastoid, and the force of contraction should be noted.

CN XII—Hypoglossal. The clinician inspects the tongue as it lies on the floor of the mouth looking for fasciculation. The patient is asked to stick out the tongue. The clinician looks for asymmetry, atrophy, or deviation from the midline. The patient is asked to move the tongue from side to side and the symmetry of movement should be noted.

Study Pearl

The causes of generalized hyporeflexia run the gamut from neurological disease, chromosomal metabolic conditions, and hypothyroidism to schizophrenia and anxiety.[107]

Reflex Testing. Muscle stretch reflexes (Table 9-22) may be graded in a variety of ways, including the following:

0 Absent (areflexia)
1+ Decreased (hyporeflexia)
2+ Normal
3+ Hyperactive (brisk)
4+ Hyperactive with clonus (hyperreflexive)

Each of these categories can occur as a generalized, or local, phenomenon. The absence of a reflex signifies an interruption of the

TABLE 9-22. COMMON DEEP TENDON REFLEXES

REFLEX	SITE OF STIMULUS	NORMAL RESPONSE	PERTINENT CENTRAL NERVOUS SYSTEM SEGMENT
Jaw	Mandible	Mouth closes	Cranial nerve V
Biceps	Biceps tendon	Biceps contraction	C5-C6
Brachioradialis	Brachioradialis tendon or just distal to the musculotendinous junction	Flexion of elbow and/or pronation of forearm	C5-C6
Triceps	Distal triceps tendon above the olecranon process	Elbow extension	C7-C8
Patella	Patellar tendon	Leg extension	L3-L4
Medial hamstrings	Semimembranosus tendon	Knee flexion	L5, S1
Lateral hamstrings	Biceps femoris tendon	Knee flexion	S1-S2
Tibialis posterior	Tibialis posterior tendon behind medial malleolus	Plantar flexion of foot with inversion	L4-L5
Achilles	Achilles tendon	Plantar flexion of foot	S1-S2

Reproduced, with permission, from Magee DJ: *Orthopedic Physical Assessment, 4th ed.* Philadelphia, PA: WB Saunders. 2002. Table 1-24:46.

reflex arc. A hyperactive reflex denotes a release from cortical inhibitory influences. Reflex asymmetry has more pathological significance than the absolute activity of the reflex. For example a bilateral patella reflex of 3+ is less significant than a 3+ on the left and a 2+ on the right.

Nongeneralized hyporeflexia can result from peripheral neuropathy, spinal nerve root compression and cauda equina syndrome, or the patient's physiological make-up. It is thus important to test more than one reflex, and to evaluate all the information gleaned from the examination, before reaching a conclusion as to the relevance of the findings.

True neurological hyperreflexia contains a clonic component, and is suggestive of CNS (upper motor neuron) impairment such as a brainstem or cerebral impairment, spinal cord compression, or a neurological disease.[106] As with hyporeflexia, the clinician should assess more than one reflex before coming to a conclusion about a hyperreflexia. Additional findings would include weakness, spasticity, postural abnormalities, and extensor plantar (see Superficial Reflexes) responses. Spasticity is a velocity-dependent (resistance increases with velocity) hypertonia and hyperactive muscle stretch reflex resulting from hyper-excitability of the stretch reflex. The presence of spasticity typically indicates an injury to the corticospinal system (suprasegmental/UMN lesions).[108-110]

The Jendrassik maneuver can be used during testing to enhance a muscle reflex that is difficult to elicit.[111]

- For the upper extremity reflexes, the patient is asked to cross the ankles and then to isometrically attempt to abduct the legs.
- For the lower extremity reflexes, the patient is asked to interlock the fingers and then to isometrically attempt to pull the elbows apart.

The superficial (cutaneous) and pathological reflexes (Table 9-23) can also be tested. Various substitutes for the Babinski have

Study Pearl

Hyporeflexia, if not generalized to the whole body, indicates a lower motor neuron (LMN) or sensory paresis.

TABLE 9-23. PATHOLOGIC REFLEXES

REFLEX	ELICITATION	POSITIVE RESPONSE	PATHOLOGY
Babinski's	Stroking of lateral aspect of side of foot	Extension of big toe and fanning of four small toes	Pyramidal tract lesion
		Normal reaction in newborns	Organic hemiplegia
Chaddock's	Stroking of lateral side of foot beneath lateral malleolus	Same response as above	Pyramidal tract lesion
Oppenheim's	Stroking of anteromedial tibial surface	Same response as above	Pyramidal tract lesion
Gordon's	Squeezing of calf muscles firmly	Same response as above	Pyramidal tract lesion
Brudzinski's	Passive flexion of one lower limb	Similar movement occurs in opposite limb	Meningitis
Hoffmann's	"Flicking" of terminal phalanx of index, middle, or ring finger	Reflex flexion of distal phalanx of thumb and of distal phalanx of index or middle finger (whichever one was not "flicked")	Increased irritability of sensory nerves in tetany Pyramidal tract lesion
Lhermitte's	Neck flexion	An electric shock-like sensation that radiates down the spinal column into the upper or lower limbs	Abnormalities (de-myelination) in the posterior part of the cervical spinal cord

Data from Magee DJ: *Orthopedic Physical Assessment.* Philadelphia, PA: WB Saunders; 2002.

been described, and some are occasionally useful. They are listed as follows.

Oppenheim. The clinician applies noxious stimuli to the crest of the patient's tibia by running a fingernail along the crest. A positive test, demonstrated by the Babinski sign, is indicative of an UMN impairment.

Clonus. The clinician passively applies a sudden dorsiflexion of the patient's ankle and the stretch is maintained during the test. The clinician notes a gradual increase in tone and then the transient occurrence of ankle clonus. In some patients, there is a more sustained clonus, and in others there is only a very short-lived finding. During the testing, the patient should not flex their neck as this can often increase the number of beats. A positive test, demonstrated by four or five reflex twitches of the plantar flexors (2 to 3 twitches are considered normal), is indicative of an upper motor neuron impairment.

Hoffmann's Sign. Hoffmann's sign is the upper limb equivalent of the Babinski. However, unlike the Babinski, some normal individuals can exhibit a present Hoffmann's sign.[73] The clinician holds the patient's middle finger and briskly pinches the distal phalanx thereby applying a noxious stimulus to the nail bed of the middle finger.[73] Denno and Meadows[112] devised a dynamic version of the Hoffman sign, which involves the patient performing repeated flexion and extension of the head before being tested for the Hoffmann's sign. A positive response for this test is the presence of the Hoffman's sign.

Supraspinal Reflex Testing

- Visual fixation of a stationary target can be tested using the tip of a pencil. The patient is seated and is asked to look straight ahead and focus on the tip of the pencil, which is held by the clinician at arms-length from the patient. The test is repeated with the patient's eyes turned to the extremes of horizontal and vertical gaze, and the pencil tip positioned accordingly.
- The VOR can be tested by asking the patient to fix vision on a distant object. The clinician holds the patients head firmly with the palms of the hands against their cheeks, and produces a rapid but small head turn. If the reflex movement of the eyes is too big or too small, the inappropriate eye movement will be followed by a corrective (saccadic) movement. Presence of this corrective action may indicate a lesion of the vestibular nerve.[113]
- Smooth pursuit can be tested by having the patient fix their gaze on an object placed in front of them. The object is then moved to the right while the patient follows it with their eyes. The clinician looks for the presence of corrective saccades, which indicate that the pursuit is not holding the eye on the moving target. The object is then moved back to the start position before being moved to the left while the patient follows it with their eyes. The object can then be moved in a variety of directions, combining horizontal, vertical and diagonal

movements to test if the patient can follow the object with their eyes without saccadic movements. Difficulty with smooth pursuit may indicate a lesion of the cerebellum, reticular formation, or cerebral cortex, or a cranial nerve lesion (oculomotor, trochlear, or abducens).[113]

EXAMINATION OF MOTOR FUNCTION

- Posture: observe the patient while sitting, standing, or walking. Note where the patient is erect, bent forward, or leaning to either side and whether changes in position alter posture. While patients are standing, they can be asked to place their feet together and close the eyes, while the clinician observes their ability to maintain normal posture (Romberg's sign).
- Apraxia: the inability to perform voluntary learned movement in the absence of loss of sensation, strength, coordination, attention, or comprehension. The presence of apraxia indicates the breakdown in the conceptual and/or motor production systems. A number of variations are recognized:
  - Ideomotor apraxia: patient cannot perform the task upon command but can do the task when left on own.
  - Ideational apraxia: patient cannot perform the task at all, either on command or on own.
- Muscle atrophy: determine muscle bulk, and firmness. If atrophy is present:
  - Determine whether it is due to denervation, disuse, or primary atrophy.
  - Check for the presence of persistent fasciculations.
- Resistance to passive movement of the limbs: muscle tone is the term is used for the resistance felt when the patient's joint is passively moved with the muscles of the limb relaxed. Even when relaxed, all muscle groups and joints possess a certain amount of intrinsic resistance to passive movement. Neurologic disease produces both increases (hypertonia) and decreases (hypotonia) in muscle tone.
- Flaccidity (absent tone), hypotonia (reduced tone): characteristic of segmental/lower motor neuron lesions (spinal nerve root and peripheral nerve injury), but may also be seen briefly with upper motor neuron lesions (spinal shock, cerebral shock).
- Presence of spasticity:
  - Clasped knife phenomenon. This phenomenon is reflected by a sudden letting go by the patient when resistance is applied.
  - Clonus—an exaggeration of the stretch reflex. A maintained stretch stimulus produces a cyclical, spasmodic contraction.
  - Hyperactive cutaneous/superficial reflexes (Babinski's sign).
  - Hyperreflexia.
  - Muscle weakness.
  - Spasticity can be graded using the Modified Ashworth scale[114-118]:
    - 0: no increase in muscle tone.
    - 1: slight increase in muscle tone, minimal resistance at end of range of motion.

  - 1+: slight increase in muscle tone, minimal resistance through less than half of range of motion.
  - 2: more marked increase in muscle tone, through most of range of motion, affected part easily moved.
  - 3: considerable increase in muscle tone, passive movement difficult.
  - 4: affected part rigid in flexion or extension.
- Rigidity: characteristic of lesions of the basal ganglia. In contrast to spasticity increased resistance is encountered throughout the range of the joint regardless of the velocity of passive movement.
  - Cogwheel phenomenon: a ratchet-like response to passive movement characterized by an alternate giving way and increased resistance to movement.
  - Leadpipe: characterized by constant rigidity. Leadpipe rigidity is common in patients with Parkinson disease.
- Opisthotonos[119,120]: prolonged severe spasm of muscles causing the head, back and heels to arch backward; arms and hands are held rigidly flexed. Seen in severe meningitis, tetanus, and epilepsy.
- Posturing:
  - Decorticate: upper extremities are held in flexion and the lower extremities in extension (Figure 9-22).
  - Decerebrate: upper and lower extremities are held in extension (Figure 9-22).

Posturing in Comatose States

Decortication
The arm, wrist, fingers are flexed with thumb trapped in palm. The arms are adducted and in position resting on chest. Legs are extended pronated. Seen in lesions of the thalamus.

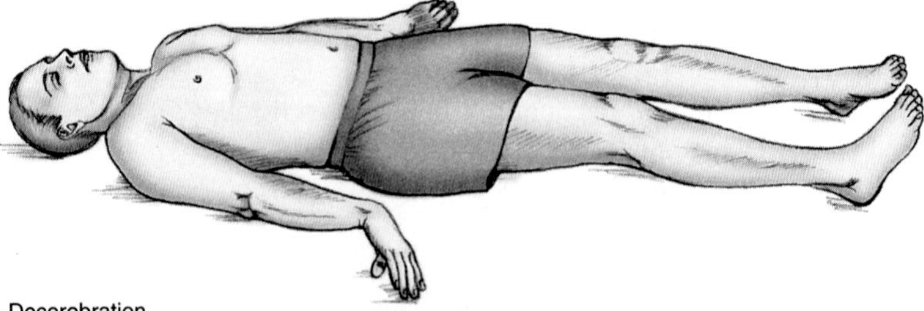

Decerebration
The arms are extended, pronated. Legs extended. Seen in lesions of the midbrain.

Figure 9-22. The appearance of decorticate and decerebrate posturing. (Reproduced, with permission, from Gilman, S: *Clinical Examination of the Nervous Tissue*. New York: McGraw-Hill; 2000:60.)

- Muscle strength: manual muscle testing can be used to assess muscle strength with neurological patients with the following provisos:
  - Passive restraint: soft tissue changes (contractures) can restrict ability to move throughout the full range of motion.
  - Active restraint: spastic muscles can restrict ability to move.
  - Abnormal reflex activity can restrict ability to move.
  - Muscle recruitment problems.

Examination of Coordination

Coordination is the ability to execute smooth, accurate, controlled motor responses. Efficient motor control includes normal muscle tone and postural response mechanisms, selective movement, and coordination. Abnormalities of coordination are common in motor system disorders. Coordinated movements are characterized by appropriate speed, distance, direction, timing, and muscular tension. Two terms often associated with coordination are dexterity and agility:

- Dexterity: refers to the skillful use of the fingers during fine motor tasks.
- Agility: refers to the ability to rapidly and smoothly initiate, stop, or modify movement while maintaining postural control.[121]

As the cerebellum, basal ganglia, and posterior (dorsal) column medial lemniscal pathway provide input to, and act together with, the cortex in the production of coordinated movement, lesions in any of these areas impact higher level processing and execution of coordinated motor responses (Table 9-24).[121] The examination of coordination involves the assessment of:

- Finger opposition: the patient is asked to tap the index finger on the thumb. Standardized tests and measures for finger dexterity include, but are not limited to, the Jebsen-Taylor Hand Function Test,[122] the Minnesota Rate of Manipulation Test,[123-125] the Purdue pegboard, and the O'Connor Tweezer test.
- Pronation/supination: the patient is asked to alternate between pronation and supination of the forearm in a rapid fashion.
- Mass grasp: the patient is asked to open and close a fist.
- Circle drawing: the patient is asked to draw a circle in the air with either the upper extremity or lower extremity.
- Finger-nose-finger movements. The clinician holds an object about 1 m from the patient's face and asks the patient to use an index finger to touch repeatedly and alternately.
- Heel-knee-shin test. The patient is positioned in supine, and asked to place the heel of one foot on the knee of the opposite leg and run the heel down the shin across the posterior aspect of the foot to the great toe.
- Rebound test. The patient is positioned with the elbow flexed. The clinician applies sufficient manual resistance to produce an isometric contraction of the biceps before suddenly releasing the tension.

TABLE 9-24. MANIFESTATIONS OF CEREBELLAR, BASAL GANGLIA, AND DORSAL COLUMN-MEDIAL LEMNISCAL PATHOLOGY

AREA OF PATHOLOGY	MANIFESTATION	DESCRIPTION
Cerebellum	Asthenia	Generalized muscle weakness associated with cerebellar lesions
	Dysarthria	Disorder of the motor component of speech articulation
	Dysdiadochokinesia	An impaired ability to perform rapid alternating movements
	Dysmetria	An inability to judge the distance or range of a movement
	Gait ataxia	Ambulatory patterns that typically demonstrate a broad base of support
	Hypotonia	A decrease in muscle tone
	Nystagmus	A rhythmic, quick, oscillatory, back-and-forth movement of the eyes
	Rebound phenomenon	The loss of the check reflex, or check factor, which functions to halt forceful active movements when resistance is eliminated
	Tremor	An involuntary oscillatory movement resulting from alternate contractions of opposing muscle groups
Basal ganglia	Akinesia	An inability to initiate movement
	Athetosis	Characterized by slow, involuntary, writhing, twisting, movements.
	Bradykinesia	Decreased amplitude and velocity of voluntary movement
	Chorea	Characterized by involuntary, rapid, irregular, and jerky movements involving multiple joints
	Dystonia	Sustained involuntary contractions of agonists and antagonists muscles causing abnormal posturing or twisting movements
	Hemiballismus	Characterized by large amplitude sudden, violent, flailing motions of the arm and leg of one side of the body
	Rigidity	An increase in muscle tone causing greater resistance to passive movement
	Resting tremor	Involuntary, rhythmic, oscillatory movements observed at rest
Dorsal column-medial lemniscal	Varied	Coordination and equilibrium impairments related to the patient's lack of joint position sense and awareness of movement, and impaired localized sensation

Data from Schmitz TJ: Examination of coordination. In: O'Sullivan SB, Schmitz TJ, eds: *Physical Rehabilitation, 5th ed.* Philadelphia, PA: FA Davis. 2007:193-225.

For each of the above tests, the clinician should note:

- Speed/rate versus control
- Precision of movement
- Degree of steadiness
- Consistency
- Correctness and accuracy of response

Assessment of Gait

One of the most important aspects of the neurologic examination as walking is a highly demanding activity that requires the coordinated activity of the entire nervous system (see Chapter 7).

Neurodynamic Mobility

The examination of the neurodynamic mobility of the peripheral nervous system is performed using the theoretical concepts and techniques of adverse neural tension.

Examination of Sensory Function

Indications for examination of sensory function are based on the history and systems review (Table 9-25). Sensory dysfunction may be associated with any pathology or injury affecting either the PNS or CNS, or with a combined involvement of both systems:

TABLE 9-25. TERMINOLOGY OF COMMON SENSORY IMPAIRMENTS

TERM	DEFINITION
Allodynia	Pain produced by a non-noxious stimulus
Analgesia	Complete loss of pain sensitivity
Astereognosis	Inability to recognize the form and shape of objects by touch
Causalgia	Painful, burning sensations, usually along the distribution of a nerve
Dysesthesia	Touch sensation experienced as pain
Hypalgesia	Decreased sensitivity to pain
Hyperalgesia	Increased sensitivity to pain
Paresthesia	Abnormal sensation such as numbness, occurring, or tingling, without apparent cause

Data from Schmitz TJ: Examination of sensory function. In: O'Sullivan SB, Schmitz TJ, eds: *Physical Rehabilitation*. 5th ed. Philadelphia, PA: FA Davis; 2007:121-157.

- Pathology, disease, or injury to the peripheral nerves such as trauma, metabolic disturbances (diabetes, hypothyroidism, alcoholism), infections, impingement or compression, toxins, and nutritional deficits (vitamin B_{12}).
- Cerebral vascular accident, transient ischemic attack, tumors, multiple sclerosis.

A full examination of the sensory system involves testing pain, temperature, light touch, vibration, position, and discriminative sensations. For patients with no apparent neurological symptoms or signs, an abbreviated examination may be substituted.

Study Pearl

It is worth remembering that few systematic reports addressing the reliability of traditional sensory tests appear in the literature.

Description of Tests

Pain

- Origin: lateral spinothalamic tract.
- Test: pinprick. This test is performed using a sharp safety pin, occasionally substituting the blunt end for the point as a stimulus. When investigating an area of cutaneous sensory loss, it is recommended that the clinician begin the pinprick test in the area of anesthesia and work outward until the border of normal sensation is located.

The clinician stimulates in the aforementioned patterns, and asks the patient "Is this sharp or dull?" or, when making comparisons using the sharp stimulus, "Does this feel the same as this?" (Note: It is important that the clinician use as light a touch as the patient can perceive and not, under any circumstances, press hard enough to draw blood.)

Temperature

- Origin: lateral spinothalamic tract.
- Test: using two test tubes, filled with hot and cold water, the clinician touches the skin and asks the patient to identify "hot" or "cold." The impulses for temperature sensation travel together with pain sensation in the lateral spinothalamic tract.

Pressure

- Origin: spinothalamic tract.
- Test: firm pressure is applied to the patient's muscle belly.

Vibration

- Origin: posterior column/medial lemniscal tract.
- Test: using a relatively low-pitched tuning fork, preferably of 128 Hz, the clinician taps it on the heel of their hand and places it firmly over a bony process of the patient such as the malleoli, patellae, epicondyles, vertebral spinous processes, and iliac crest. The patient is asked what he or she feels. To be certain, the patient is asked to inform the clinician when the vibration stops, and then the clinician touches the fork to stop the vibration. At this point, the patient should indicate that the vibration has stopped. If vibration sense is absent, then the clinician should move proximally along the extremity and re-test.

Position Sense (Proprioception)

- Origin: posterior column/medial lemniscal tract.
- Test: the patient is tested for their ability to perceive passive movements of the extremities, especially the distal portions. It is awareness of the position of joints at rest. The clinician grasps the patient's big toe, holding it by its sides between the thumb and index finger, and then pulls it away from the other toes to avoid friction, and to prevent extraneous tactile stimulation from indicating a change of position. "Down" and "up" are demonstrated to the patient as the clinician moves the patient's toe clearly upward and downward. Then, with the patient's eyes closed, the patient is asked for an "up" or "down" response, as the clinician moves the toe in a small arc. This is repeated several times on each side, avoiding simple alternation of the stimuli. If position sense is impaired, then the clinician should move proximally along the extremity and re-test. Alternatively, the patient is asked to duplicate the position with the opposite extremity.

Movement sense (Kinesthesia)

- Origin: posterior column/medial lemniscal tract.
- Test: the patient is asked to indicate verbally the direction of movement while the extremity is in motion. The clinician must grip the patient's extremity over neutral borders.

Stereognosis

- Origin: posterior column/medial lemniscal tract.
- Test: the patient is asked to recognize, through touch alone, a variety of small objects such as comb, coins, pencils, safety pins that are placed in the hand.

Graphesthesia

- Origin: posterior column/medial lemniscal tract.
- Test: the patient is asked to recognize letters, numbers or designs traced on the skin. Using a blunt object, the clinician draws a large number in the patient's palm, asking the patient to identify the number, letter, or design.

Two point discrimination

- Origin: posterior column/medial lemniscal tract.
- Test: a measure is taken of the smallest distance between two stimuli that can still be perceived by the patient as two distinct stimuli.

EXAMINATION OF AUTONOMIC NERVOUS SYSTEM FUNCTION

- Pupils: loss of function of the sympathetic innervation of the pupil leads to papillary constriction; Horner's syndrome, which consists of anihidrosis on the ipsilateral side of the face, ptosis, a small pupil, and enopthalmos. Loss of parasympathetic function results in a dilated pupil and possible blurred vision.
- Cardiovascular system: disorders of blood pressure, heart rate (see Chapter 11):
  - Sympathetic stimulation results in increased heart rate, force ofcontractionandincreasedbloodpressureandrespiratory rate.
  - Parasympathetic stimulation results in decreased heart rate, force of contraction and decreased blood pressure and respiratory rate.
- Integumentary changes. Sympathetic stimulation results in increased sweating.
- Urinary function. Parasympathetic stimulation causes detrusor contraction and bladder emptying.
- Sexual dysfunction. This may be the earliest manifestation of autonomic insufficiency. In males, the parasympathetic system functions principally in achieving erection and the sympathetic system in performing ejaculation.
- Gastrointestinal dysfunction: dysphagia, reflex, nausea, vomiting, and upper abdominal pain.
- Sympathetic stimulation inhibits peristalsis and tone and causes contraction of the upper and lower esophageal, ileocecal, and anal sphincters.

NEUROLOGIC DYSFUNCTION

The two major types of neurologic dysfunction can be classified as either an upper motor neuron lesion, or a lower motor neuron lesion, or a combination of both.

UPPER MOTOR NEURON LESION

The upper motor neuron (UMN) is located in the white columns of the spinal cord and the cerebral hemispheres. An UMN lesion, also known as a central palsy, is characterized by spastic paralysis or paresis, little or no muscle atrophy, hyperreflexive stretch reflexes in a nonsegmental distribution, and the presence of pathological signs and reflexes, such as the following:

- Nystagmus. In health, nystagmus occurs during self-rotation in order to hold images of the visual world steady on the retina and maintain clear vision[127-129]. The more serious causes of nystagmus include lesions to the brain stem or cerebellum, and a characteristic sign of vertebrobasilar compromise.
- Dysphasia. A problem with vocabulary that results from a cerebral lesion in the speech areas of the frontal or temporal lobes.

- Wallenberg's syndrome. This is the result of a lateral medullary infarction and is characterized by selective involvement of the spinothalamic sensory modalities with dissociated distribution (ipsilateral trigeminal and contralateral hemibody/limbs), contralateral or bilateral trigeminal sensory impairment, restricted sensory involvement, and a concomitant deficit of lemniscal sensations.[189,190]
- Ataxia. Ataxia is often most marked in the extremities. In the lower extremities, it is characterized by the so-called "drunken-sailor" gait pattern, with the patient veering from one side to the other, and having a tendency to fall toward the side of the lesion (see Chapter 7). Ataxia of the upper extremities is characterized by a loss of accuracy in the reaching for, or placing of objects. Although ataxia can have a number of causes, it generally suggests CNS disturbance, specifically a cerebellar disorder, or a lesion of the posterior columns.[191-193]

Study Pearl

It must be remembered that not all spasticity is problematic—it can be harnessed for transfers, ambulation, prevention of osteopenia, and improvement of bowel and bladder continence. Management strategies for spasticity are described in the Interventions for Neurologic Dysfunction section.

- Spasticity. Spasticity occurs because the reflex arc to the muscle remains anatomically intact despite the loss of cerebral innervation and control via the long tracts. *Spinal or neurogenic shock* occurs immediately following any trauma to the spinal cord sufficient to cause tetraplegia or paraplegia (refer to Spinal/Neurogenic Shock).[194-196] This shock results in the loss of reflexes innervated by the portion of the cord below the site of the lesion—the muscles innervated by the traumatized portion of the cord, the portion below the lesion, as well as the bladder, become flaccid. Spinal shock, which wears off between 24 hours and approximately 3 months after injury, can be replaced by spasticity in some, or all of these muscles. During spinal shock, the reflex arc does not function, but as the spine recovers from the shock, the reflex arc begins to function without the inhibitory or regulatory impulses from the brain, creating local spasticity and clonus
- Drop attack. This is described as a loss of balance resulting in a fall, but with no loss of consciousness. The patient, usually elderly, will fall forward with the precipitating factor being extension of the head. Recovery is usually immediate. Causes include:
  - A vestibular system impairment[197]
  - Neoplastic and other impairments of the cerebellum[198]
  - Vertebrobasilar compromise[199]
  - Sudden spinal cord compression
  - Type 1 Chiari malformation[200]
- Wernicke's encephalopathy. This is an impairment, which is typically localized to the posterior part of the midbrain,[201] and which produces the classic triad of Wernicke's encephalopathy: abnormal mental state, ophthalmoplegia, and gait ataxia.[202]
- Vertical diplopia.[203] Patients with vertical diplopia complain of seeing two images ("double vision"), one atop or diagonally displaced from the other.
- Dysphonia. Dysphonia presents as a hoarseness of the voice. Usually no pain is reported. Painless dysphonia is a common symptom of Wallenberg's syndrome.[189]
- Hemianopia. This is defined as a loss in half of the visual field and is always bilateral. A visual field defect describes sensory loss restricted to the visual field and arises from damage to the primary visual pathways linking the optic tract and striate cortex.

- Ptosis. Ptosis is defined as a pathological depression of the superior eyelid such that it covers part of the pupil due to a palsy of the levator palpabrae and Muller's muscles.
- Miosis. Miosis is defined as the inability to dilate the pupil (damage to sympathetic ganglia). It is one of the symptoms of Horner's syndrome.
- Horner's syndrome. This is caused by an interference to the cervicothoracic sympathetic outflow due to a lesion of: (1) the reticular formation, (2) the descending sympathetic system and, (3) the oculomotor nerve caused by a sympathetic paralysis.[204] The other clinical signs of Horner's syndrome are ptosis, enopthalamus, facial reddening, and anhydrosis. If Horner's syndrome is identified, the patient should immediately be returned or referred to a physician for further examination.
- Dysarthria. Dysarthria is defined as an undiagnosed change in articulation. Dominant or nondominant hemispheric ischemia as well as brainstem and cerebellar impairments may result in altered articulation.

LOWER MOTOR NEURON LESION

The lower motor neuron begins at the alpha motor neuron and includes the posterior and anterior roots, the spinal nerve, the peripheral nerve, the neuromuscular junction, and the muscle fiber complex.[205] The lower motor neuron (LMN) consists of a cell body located in the anterior gray column, and its axon, which travels to a muscle by way of the cranial or peripheral nerve. A lesion to the LMN, also known as a peripheral palsy, can occur in the cell body or anywhere along the axon. These lesions can be due to direct trauma, toxins, infections, ischemia and compression. The characteristics of a LMN lesion include muscle atrophy and hypotonus, a diminished or absent stretch reflex of the areas served by a spinal nerve root, or a peripheral nerve and an absence of pathological signs or reflexes.

> **Study Pearl**
>
> The differing symptoms between a UMN and a LMN are the result of injuries to different parts of the nervous system: LMN impairment involves damage to a neurological structure distal to the anterior horn cell, whereas the UMN impairment involves damage to a neurological structure proximal to the anterior horn cell, namely the spinal cord and/or CNS.

INFECTIOUS DISEASES

Meningitis. Meningitis is an infection of the membranes covering the brain and spinal cord and the cerebrospinal fluid (CSF).[206-214] Once in the CSF, exudates proliferate, damaging cranial nerves (eg, cranial nerve VIII, with resultant hearing loss),[215,216] obliterating CSF pathways, and inducing vasculitis and thrombophlebitis, and brain edema. As the brain edema progresses, intracranial pressure (ICP) rises. Without medical intervention, the cerebral edema worsens and the increasing ICP proceeds unchecked, the CNS autoregulatory processes begin to fail, resulting in decreased alertness and changes in mental status.

Swift identification by the physical therapist can be lifesaving. Classic symptoms (not evident in infants or seen often in the elderly) include: headache; discomfort on neck flexion (nuchal rigidity); fever and chills; photophobia; vomiting; seizures; focal neurologic symptoms; mental confusion. Objectively, both the Kernig's sign and Brudzinski sign are typically positive.

- Kernig sign: passive knee extension in supine patient elicits neck pain and hamstring resistance.
- Brudzinski sign: passive neck or single hip flexion is accompanied by involuntary flexion of both hips

Encephalitis. Encephalitis involves an irritation and inflammation of the brain parenchyma. It is usually infectious, but can be noninfectious (acute disseminated encephalitis). As with meningitis, swift identification by the physical therapist can be lifesaving. The classic presentation includes behavioral and personality changes, photophobia, lethargy, and acute confusion or decreased level of consciousness.

CEREBRAL VASCULAR ACCIDENT

For description of the cerebrovascular accident (CVA), its etiology and manifestations refer to Chapter 14. Refer also to Interventions for Neurological Dysfunction section.

TRANSIENT ISCHEMIC ATTACK

A transient ischemic attack (TIA) is a temporary loss of blood flow to a part of the brain that produces stroke-like symptoms.[217-223] TIAs are rapid in onset, occurring in fewer than 5 minutes (usually < 1 minute) and with a variable duration that typically lasts 2 to 15 minutes (rarely as long as 24 hours), with most being less than 1 hour. Significant medical history questions to the patient or relatives include recent surgery (eg, carotid, cardiac), previous strokes, seizures, and use of illicit drugs. The clinician should carefully investigate onset, duration, fluctuation, and intensity of symptoms. Contacting the patient's primary physician is important. Ideally, severity of neurologic deficits should be recorded with the aid of stroke scales (Table 9-26).

Study Pearl

Common locations for aneurysms in the brain are:

- The circle of Willis or the middle cerebral artery (MCA) bifurcation, anterior communicating artery, the internal carotid artery (ICA) at the posterior communicating artery origin, and the MCA bifurcation.
- The superior cerebellar artery and the vertebral artery (VA) at the origin of the posterior inferior cerebellar artery (PICA).
- Anterior inferior cerebellar artery (AICA) aneurysms are rare.

CEREBRAL ANEURYSM

An aneurysm is an abnormal local dilatation in the wall of a blood vessel due to a defect, disease, or injury.[224-230] The aneurysmal sac itself is usually composed only of intima and adventitia. The intima is typically normal, although subintimal cellular proliferation is common. Lymphocytes and phagocytes may infiltrate the adventitia. Atherosclerotic changes in the parent vessel are also common. Common causes of an aneurysm include developmental/congenital or inherited conditions, trauma, infection, tumor, and vasculopathies such as fibromuscular dysplasia (FMD).

Most aneurysms do not cause symptoms until they rupture; when they rupture, they are associated with significant morbidity and mortality.

TRAUMATIC BRAIN INJURY

Traumatic brain injury (TBI) is an insult to the brain from an external mechanical force, which has the potential to produce permanent or temporary impairments of cognitive, physical, and psychosocial functions.[231-243] The risk of TBI is highest for individuals aged 15 to 24 years. In individuals aged 75 years and older, falls are the most common cause of TBI.

Injuries are divided into a number of categories:

- Focal injuries: tend to be caused by contact forces.
- Hypoxic-ischemic injury: results from a lack of oxygenated blood flow to the brain tissue. For example, increased intracranial pressure (ICP): can lead to cerebral hypoxia.

TABLE 9-26. NIH STROKE SCALE

Time: ___ ___:___ ___ 1[ ]am 2[ ]pm

Administer stroke scale items in the order listed. Record performance in each category after each subscale exam. Do not go back and change scores. Follow directions provided for each exam technique. Scores should reflect what the patient does, not what the clinician thinks the patient can do. The clinician should record answers while administering the exam and work quickly. Except where indicated, the patient should not be coached (ie, repeated requests to patient to make a special effort).

IF ANY ITEM IS LEFT UNTESTED, A DETAILED EXPLANATION MUST BE CLEARLY WRITTEN ON THE FORM. ALL UNTESTED ITEMS WILL BE REVIEWED BY THE MEDICAL MONITOR, AND DISCUSSED WITH THE EXAMINER BY TELEPHONE.

INSTRUCTIONS	SCALE DEFINITION	SCORE
1a. Level of Consciousness: The investigator must choose a response, even if a full evaluation is prevented by such obstacles as an endotracheal tube, language barrier, orotracheal trauma/bandages. A 3 is scored only if the patient makes no movement (other than eflexive posturing) in response to noxious stimulation.	0 = Alert; keenly responsive. 1 = Not alert, but arousable by minor stimulation to obey, answer, or respond. 2 = Not alert, requires repeated stimulation to attend, or is obtunded and requires strong or painful stimulation to make movements (not stereotyped). 3 = Responds only with reflex motor or autonomic effects or totally unresponsive, flaccid, areflexic.	_____
1b. LOC Questions: The patient is asked the month and his/her age. The answer must be correct—there is no partial credit for being close. Aphasic and stuporous patients who do not comprehend the questions will score 2. Patients unable to speak because of endotracheal intubation, orotracheal trauma, severe dysarthria from any cause, language barrier or any other problem not secondary to aphasia are given a 1. It is important that only the initial answer be graded and that the examiner not "help" the patient with verbal or non-verbal cues.	0 = Answers both questions correctly. 1 = Answers one question correctly. 2 = Answers neither question correctly.	_____
1c. LOC Commands: The patient is asked to open and close the eyes and then to grip and release the non-paretic hand. Substitute another one step command if the hands cannot be used. Credit is given if an unequivocal attempt is made but not completed due to weakness. If the patient does not respond to command, the task should be demonstrated to them (pantomime) and score the result (ie, follows none, one or two commands). Patients with trauma, amputation, or other physical impediments should be given suitable one-step commands. Only the first attempt is scored.	0 = Performs both tasks correctly 1 = Performs one task correctly 2 = Performs neither task correctly	_____
2. Best Gaze: Only horizontal eye movements will be tested. Voluntary or reflexive (oculocephalic) eye movements will be scored but caloric testing is not done. If the patient has a conjugate deviation of the eyes that can be overcome by voluntary or reflexive activity, the score will be 1. If a patient has an isolated peripheral nerve paresis (CN III, IV or VI) score a 1. Gaze is testable in all aphasic patients. Patients with ocular trauma, bandages, pre-existing blindness or other disorder of visual acuity or fields should be tested with reflexive movements and a choice made by the investigator. Establishing eye contact and then moving about the patient from side to side will occasionally clarify the presence of a partial gaze palsy.	0 = Normal 1 = Partial gaze palsy. This score is given when gaze is abnormal in one or both eyes, but where forced deviation or total gaze paresis are not present. 2 = Forced deviation, or total gaze paresis not overcome by the oculocephalic maneuver.	_____

(*Continued*)

TABLE 9-26. NIH STROKE SCALE (*Continued*)

INSTRUCTIONS	SCALE DEFINITION	SCORE
3. Visual: Visual fields (upper and lower quadrants) are tested by confrontation, using finger counting or visual threat as appropriate. Patient must be encouraged, but if they look at the side of the moving fingers appropriately, this can be scored as normal. If there is unilateral blindness or enucleation, visual fields in the remaining eye are scored. Score 1 only if a clear-cut asymmetry, including quadrantanopia is found. If patient is blind from any cause score 3. Double simultaneous stimulation is performed at this point. If there is extinction patient receives a 1 and the results are used to answer question 11.	0 = No visual loss 1 = Partial hemianopia 2 = Complete hemianopia 3 = Bilateral hemianopia (blind including cortical blindness)	______
4. Facial Palsy: Ask, or use pantomime to encourage the patient to show teeth or raise eyebrows and close eyes. Score symmetry of grimace in response to noxious stimuli in the poorly responsive or non-comprehending patient. If facial trauma/bandages, orotracheal tube, tape or other physical barrier obscures the face, these should be removed to the extent possible.	0 = Normal symmetrical movement 1 = Minor paralysis (flattened nasolabial fold, asymmetry on smiling) 2 = Partial paralysis (total or near total paralysis of lower face) 3 = Complete paralysis of one or both sides (absence of facial movement in the upper and lower face)	______
5 & 6. Motor Arm and Leg: The limb is placed in the appropriate position: extend the arms (palms down) 90 degrees (if sitting) or 45 degrees (if supine) and the leg 30 degrees (always tested supine). Drift is scored if the arm falls before 10 seconds or the leg before 5 seconds. The aphasic patient is encouraged using urgency in the voice and pantomime but not noxious stimulation. Each limb is tested in turn, beginning with the non-paretic arm. Only in the case of amputation or joint fusion at the shoulder or hip may the score be "9" and the examiner must clearly write the explanation for scoring as a "9".	0 = No drift, limb holds 90 (or 45) degrees for full 10 seconds. 1 = Drift, Limb holds 90 (or 45) degrees, but drifts down before full 10 seconds; does not hit bed or other support. 2 = Some effort against gravity, limb cannot get to or maintain (if cued) 90 (or 45) degrees, drifts down to bed, but has some effort against gravity. 3 = No effort against gravity, limb falls. 4 = No movement 9 = Amputation, joint fusion explain: ____________________ **5a. Left Arm** **5b. Right Arm**	______ ______
	0 = No drift, leg holds 30 degrees position for full 5 seconds. 1 = Drift, leg falls by the end of the 5 second period but does not hit bed. 2 = Some effort against gravity; leg falls to bed by 5 seconds, but has some effort against gravity. 3 = No effort against gravity, leg falls to bed immediately. 4 = No movement 9 = Amputation, joint fusion explain: ____________________ **6a. Left Leg** **6b. Right Leg**	______ ______

(*Continued*)

TABLE 9-26. NIH STROKE SCALE (*Continued*)

INSTRUCTIONS	SCALE DEFINITION	SCORE
7. Limb Ataxia: This item is aimed at finding evidence of a unilateral cerebellar lesion. Test with eyes open. In case of visual defect, insure testing is done in intact visual field. The finger-nose-finger and heel-shin tests are performed on both sides, and ataxia is scored only if present out of proportion to weakness. Ataxia is absent in the patient who cannot understand or is paralyzed. Only in the case of amputation or joint fusion may the item be scored "9", and the examiner must clearly write the explanation for not scoring. In case of blindness test by touching nose from extended arm position.	0 = Absent 1 = Present in one limb 2 = Present in two limbs If present, is ataxia in Right arm 1 = Yes 2 = No 9 = amputation or joint fusion, explain ____________ Left arm 1 = Yes 2 = No 9 = amputation or joint fusion, explain ____________ Right leg 1 = Yes 2 = No 9 = amputation or joint fusion, explain ____________ Left leg 1 = Yes 2 = No 9 = amputation or joint fusion, explain ____________	_____ _____ _____ _____ _____
8. Sensory: Sensation or grimace to pin prick when tested, or withdrawal from noxious stimulus in the obtunded or aphasic patient. Only sensory loss attributed to stroke is scored as abnormal and the examiner should test as many body areas [arms (not hands), legs, trunk, face] as needed to accurately check for hemisensory loss. A score of 2, "severe or total," should only be given when a severe or total loss of sensation can be clearly demonstrated. Stuporous and aphasic patients will therefore probably score 1 or 0. The patient with brain stem stroke who has bilateral loss of sensation is scored 2. If the patient does not respond and is quadriplegic score 2. Patients in coma (item 1a=3) are arbitrarily given a 2 on this item.	0 = Normal; no sensory loss. 1 = Mild to moderate sensory loss; patient feels pinprick is less sharp or is dull on the affected side; or there is a loss of superficial pain with pinprick but patient is aware he/she is being touched. 2 = Severe to total sensory loss; patient is not aware of being touched in the face, arm, and leg.	_____
9. Best Language: A great deal of information about comprehension will be obtained during the preceding sections of the examination. The patient is asked to describe what is happening in the attached picture, to name the items on the attached naming sheet, and to read from the attached list of sentences. Comprehension is judged from responses here as well as to all of the commands in the preceding general neurological exam. If visual loss interferes with the tests, ask the patient to identify objects placed in the hand, repeat, and produce speech. The intubated patient should be asked to write. The patient in coma (question 1a=3) will arbitrarily score 3 on this item. The examiner must choose a score in the patient with stupor or limited cooperation but a score of 3 should be used only if the patient is mute and follows no one step commands.	0 = No aphasia, normal 1 = Mild to moderate aphasia; some obvious loss of fluency or facility of comprehension, without significant limitation on ideas expressed or form of expression. Reduction of speech and/or comprehension, however, makes conversation about provided material difficult or impossible. For example in conversation about provided materials examiner can identify picture or naming card from patient's response. 2 = Severe aphasia; all communication is through fragmentary expression; great need for inference, questioning, and guessing by the listener. Range of information that can be exchanged is limited; listener carries burden of communication. Examiner cannot identify materials provided from patient response. 3 = Mute, global aphasia; no usable speech or auditory comprehension.	_____

(*Continued*)

TABLE 9-26. NIH STROKE SCALE (*Continued*)

INSTRUCTIONS	SCALE DEFINITION	SCORE
10. Dysarthria: If patient is thought to be normal an adequate sample of speech must be obtained by asking patient to read or repeat words from the attached list. If the patient has severe aphasia, the clarity of articulation of spontaneous speech can be rated. Only if the patient is intubated or has other physical barrier to producing speech, may the item be scored "9", and the examiner must clearly write an explanation for not scoring. Do not tell the patient why he/she is being tested.	0 = Normal 1 = Mild to moderate; patient slurs at least some words and, at worst, can be understood with some difficulty. 2 = Severe; patient's speech is so slurred as to be unintelligible in the absence of or out of proportion to any dysphasia, or is mute/anarthric. 9 = Intubated or other physical barrier, explain ______	______
11. Extinction and Inattention (formerly Neglect): Sufficient information to identify neglect may be obtained during the prior testing. If the patient has a severe visual loss preventing visual double simultaneous stimulation, and the cutaneous stimuli are normal, the score is normal. If the patient has aphasia but does appear to attend to both sides, the score is normal. The presence of visual spatial neglect or anosagnosia may also be taken as evidence of abnormality. Since the abnormality is scored only if present, the item is never untestable.	0 = No abnormality. 1 = Visual, tactile, auditory, spatial, or personal inattention or extinction to bilateral simultaneous stimulation in one of the sensory modalities. 2 = Profound hemi-inattention or hemi-inattention to more than one modality. Does not recognize own hand or orients to only one side of space.	______
Additional item, not a part of the NIH Stroke Scale score.		
A. Distal Motor Function: The patient's hand is held up at the forearm by the examiner and patient is asked to extend his/her fingers as much as possible. If the patient can't or doesn't extend the fingers the examiner places the fingers in full extension and observes for any flexion movement for 5 seconds. The patient's first attempts only are graded. Repetition of the instructions or of the testing is prohibited.	0 = Normal (No flexion after 5 seconds) 1 = At least some extension after 5 seconds, but not fully extended. Any movement of the fingers which is not command is not scored. 2 = No voluntary extension after 5 seconds. Movements of the fingers at another time are not scored. **a. Left Arm** **b. Right Arm**	____ ____

- Diffuse injuries. Diffuse axonal injury (DAI) is typically caused by forces associated with acceleration-deceleration or rotational injuries, eg, high-impact collisions of MVAs, contact sports, and shaken-baby syndrome. The collision of the head with a solid object can cause brain injury through a combination of contact forces and inertial forces:
  - Inertial force occurs when the head is set in motion with or without any contact force, leading to acceleration of the head.
  - Coup contusions occur at the area of direct impact to the skull because of the creation of negative pressure when the skull, distorted at the site of impact, returns to its normal shape.

- Contrecoup contusions are similar to coup contusions but are located opposite the site of direct impact. The three basic types of tissue deformation include the following:
  - Compressive—tissue compression
  - Tensile—tissue stretching
  - Shear—tissue distortion produced when tissue slides over other tissue
  - Impulsive loading (ie, sudden motion without significant physical contact)

Complications associated with TBI include:

- Epidural or subdural hematoma
- Intracerebral hemorrhage
- Subarachnoid hemorrhage
- Increased intracranial pressure (ICP)

Direct impairments associated with TBI include cognitive (Table 9-19), behavioral, perceptual and communication impairments. Secondary impairments include soft tissue contractures/atrophy, skin breakdown, deep vein thrombosis, heterotropic ossification, and pneumonia.

A number of clinical rating scales exist that can be used to evaluate change in the patient over time. Two of the more commonly used scales are the Glasgow Coma Scale (GCS) (Table 9-20), and the Ranchos Los Amigos Cognitive Functioning Scale (Table 9-16).

The goals of the physical therapy intervention include[244]:

- The prevention of the aforementioned secondary impairments through proper positioning both in bed and in a chair/wheelchair.[245,246] The patient should be turned every two hours when in bed.
- Improving arousal through sensory stimulation involving the presentation of sensory stimulation in a highly structured and consistent manner.[244]
- Patient and family education.

Managing the effects of abnormal tone and spasticity (refer to Strategies to Manage Hypertonia and Strategies to Manage Hypotonia).

- Early transition to sitting postures as tolerated.

CONCUSSIONS

Concussion is caused by a diffuse axonal injury of the deep structures of the brain, leading to widespread neurologic dysfunction, including impaired consciousness or coma. Neuropathologic findings in patients with diffuse axonal injury can be graded by as follows:

- Grade 1: axonal injury mainly in parasagittal white matter of the cerebral hemispheres.
- Grade 2: as in grade 1, plus lesions in the corpus callosum.
- Grade 3: as in grade 2, plus a focal lesion in the cerebral peduncle.

SPINAL CORD INJURY

The extent and seriousness of the consequences of a spinal cord injury (SCI) depends on the location and severity of the lesion.

- Injury to the corticospinal tract or posterior columns, respectively, produces ipsilateral paralysis or loss of sensation of light touch, proprioception, and vibration.
- Injury to the lateral spinothalamic tract produces contralateral loss of pain and temperature sensation.
- Injury to the posterior columns may produce complete loss of vibration sensation and proprioception, but only partial loss of light touch sensation because the anterior spinothalamic tract also transmits light touch information.

Spinal cord injuries can be categorized as complete or incomplete. A complete cord syndrome is characterized clinically as complete loss of motor and sensory function below the level of the lesion.

Incomplete cord syndromes (Table 9-27) have variable neurologic findings with partial loss of sensory and/or motor function below the level of injury (Table 9-28).

A spinal cord concussion is characterized by a temporary neurologic lesion localized to the spinal cord that fully recovers without any apparent structural damage.

Study Pearl

- Tetraplegia is defined as complete paralysis of all four extremities and trunk, including the respiratory muscles, and results from lesions of the cervical cord.
- Paraplegia is defined as complete paralysis of all or part of the trunk and both lower extremities resulting from lesions of the thoracic or lumbar spinal cord or cauda equina.

Study Pearl

The term sacral sparing can be defined as an incomplete lesion of the spinal cord where some of the innermost (long) tracts with the sacral fibers remain intact and innervated. Signs and symptoms of sacral sparing include sensation of the saddle area, movement of the toe flexors, and rectal sphincter contraction.

Complications Associated with Spinal Cord Injury

Autonomic Dysreflexia. Autonomic dysreflexia (AD) is a potentially life-threatening condition caused by a reflex sympathetic discharge that occurs in patients with spinal cord injury above the splanchnic sympathetic outflow (T5-T6), resulting in a sudden and significant rise in both systolic and diastolic blood pressures.[247-253] Progressively higher spinal cord lesions or injury causes increasing degrees of autonomic dysfunction.

Below the injury, intact peripheral sensory nerves transmit impulses that ascend in the spinothalamic and posterior columns to stimulate sympathetic neurons located in the intermediolateral gray matter of the spinal cord. The inhibitory outflow above the SCI from cerebral vasomotor centers is increased, but it is unable to pass below the block of the SCI. The result is sudden elevation in blood pressure and vasodilation above the level of injury. Clinical manifestations of AD may include:

- Bradycardia.
- Profuse sweating above the level of lesion, especially in the face, neck, and shoulders.
- Complaints of a headache.
- Piloerection above, or possibly below, the level of the lesion.
- Flushing of the skin above the level of the lesion.

The potential triggers for AD are numerous and include:

- Bladder distension/urinary catheter blockage from twisting.
- Urinary tract infection.

Study Pearl

The neurological level refers to the most caudal level of the spinal cord with normal motor and sensory function on both the left and right sides of the body.

- Motor level: the most caudal segment of the spinal cord with normal motor function bilaterally.
- Sensory level: the most caudal segment of the spinal cord with normal sensory function bilaterally.

For example, a patient with C4 quadriplegia has, by definition, abnormal motor and sensory function from C5 down.

TABLE 9-27. THE INCOMPLETE SCI SYNDROMES

SYNDROME	DESCRIPTION	CHARACTERISTIC FINDINGS
Anterior cord	Usually seen as a result of compression of the anterior spinal artery from bone fragments or a large disc herniation.	Manifested by complete motor paralysis (corticospinal function) and sensory anesthesia (spinothalamic function); sparing of the dorsal column (deep pressure and proprioception are only retained sensibilities of the trunk and lower extremities); greater motor loss in the legs than arms.
Posterior cord	A rare incomplete lesion with primary damage to the posterior sensory cortex and posterior columns as a result of impact injuries or an hyperextension force.	Loss of deep touch, position and vibration below the level of the lesion, with preservation of motor function, pain and temperature sensation. Unfortunately, the sense of proprioception is lost, which can limit the patient's potential for functional gait.
Central cord	Usually involves a cervical lesion. Most often occurs after hyperextension injury in an individual with long-standing cervical spondylosis. Injury may result from both posterior pinching of the cord by buckled ligamentum flavum or from anterior compression by osteophytes.	Greater motor weakness in the upper extremities than in the lower extremities. The pattern of motor weakness shows greater distal involvement in the affected extremity than proximal muscle weakness. Sensory loss is variable, and the patient is more likely to lose pain and/or temperature sensation than proprioception and/or vibration. Dysesthesias, especially those in the upper extremities (eg, sensation of burning in the hands or arms), are common. Sacral sensory sparing usually exists.
Brown-Séquard	Hemisection of the spinal cord, often in the cervical region resulting in interruption of the lateral corticospinal tracts, the lateral spinal thalamic tract, and at times the posterior columns.	Interruption of the lateral corticospinal tracts resulting in ipsilateral spastic paralysis below the level of the lesion, Babinski sign ipsilateral to lesion (abnormal reflexes and Babinski's sign may not be present in acute injury). Interruption of lateral spinothalamic tracts resulting in contralateral loss of pain and temperature sensation. This usually occurs 2-3 segments below the level of the lesion. Interruption of posterior white column resulting in ipsilateral loss of tactile discrimination, vibratory, and position sensation below the level of the lesion.
Conus medullaris syndrome	A sacral cord injury involving the most distal bulbous part of the spinal cord (conus medullaris) with or without involvement of the lumbar nerve roots.	A combination of upper motor neuron (UMN) and lower motor neuron (LMN) symptoms. Areflexia in the bladder, bowel, and to a lesser degree, lower limbs. Motor and sensory loss in the lower limbs is variable.
Cauda equina	An injury to the lumbosacral nerve roots caudal to the level of spinal cord termination. Causes include trauma, lumbar disk disease, abscess, spinal anesthesia, tumor, metastatic, or CNS elements, late-stage ankylosing spondylitis, or idiopathic.	Areflexic bowel and/or bladder, with variable motor and sensory loss in the lower limbs. Because this syndrome is a nerve root injury rather than a true SCI, the affected limbs are areflexic. This injury is usually caused by a central lumbar disk herniation.

- Bowel distension or impaction.
- Hemorrhoids.
- Deep vein thrombosis.
- Pulmonary emboli.
- Pressure ulcers.
- Ingrown toenail.

Spinal/Neurogenic Shock. Spinal shock is associated with autonomic dysfunction. In addition it is characterized by hypotension, relative bradycardia, peripheral vasodilation, and hypothermia. Neurogenic shock, which may last for several days to several weeks, does not usually occur with SCI below the level of T6.

Study Pearl

Physical therapists who treat SCI patients need to be familiar with established protocols for medical management within his/her particular setting. The patient should be placed in an upright position immediately, rather than remain in a supine or reclining position, before completing a careful inspection to identify the source of the potential trigger.

TABLE 9-28. SYMPTOMS AND SIGNS OF CONUS MEDULLARIS AND CAUDA EQUINA SYNDROMES

	CONUS MEDULLARIS SYNDROME	CAUDA EQUINA SYNDROME
Presentation	Sudden and bilateral	Gradual and unilateral
Reflexes	Knee jerks preserved but ankle jerks affected	Both ankle and knee jerks affected
Radicular pain	Less severe	More severe
Low back pain	More	Less
Sensory symptoms and signs	Numbness tends to be more localized to perianal area; symmetrical and bilateral; sensory dissociation occurs	Numbness tends to be more localized to saddle area; asymmetrical, may be unilateral; no sensory dissociation; loss of sensation in specific dermatomes in lower extremities with numbness and paresthesia; possible numbness in pubic area, including glans penis or clitoris
Motor strength	Typically symmetric, hyperreflexic distal paresis of lower limbs that is less marked; fasciculations may be present	Asymmetric areflexic paraplegia that is more marked; fasciculations rare; atrophy more common
Impotence	Frequent	Less frequent; erectile dysfunction that includes inability to have erection, inability to maintain erection, lack of sensation in pubic area (including glans penis or clitoris), and inability to ejaculate
Sphincter dysfunction	Urinary retention and atonic anal sphincter cause overflow urinary incontinence and fecal incontinence; tend to present early in course of disease	Urinary retention; tends to present late in course of disease

Study Pearl

One of the first indicators that spinal shock is resolving is the presence of a positive bulbocavernosus reflex. During a digital rectal examination, this reflex is elicited by pressure applied to the glans penis or glans clitoris or by intermittently "tugging" on an indwelling catheter.[254]

Spasticity. Refer to Strategies to Manage Hypertonia.

Heterotopic Ossification. A strong association exists between heterotopic ossification and spinal cord injury, with lesions occurring at multiple sites and showing a strong propensity to recur. The condition originates when osteoprogenitor stem cells, lying dormant within the affected soft tissues, are stimulated to differentiate into osteoblasts, beginning the process of osteoid formation, and eventually leading to mature heterotopic bone. Heterotopic ossification often begins as a painful palpable mass that gradually becomes nontender and smaller but firmer to palpation.

Orthostatic Hypotension. Orthostatic hypotension (refer to Chapter 11) is a sign of autonomic dysfunction and dysautonomia. Upper thoracic and cervical SCI, especially complete injuries, leave individuals with an inability to control all or most of their sympathetic nervous system (SNS) function. Immediately after SCI occurs, blood pressure rises acutely. This brief response is followed by a period of decreased SNS activity because of interruption of the descending sympathetic tracts. Lack of supraspinal input develops, causing cutaneous vasodilatation, lack of sympathetic vasoconstrictor activity, and absent sympathetic input to the heart.

Pressure Ulcers. Refer to Chapter 13.

Deep Vein Thrombosis. Factors predisposing individuals with acute SCI to DVT include venous stasis secondary to muscle paralysis and transient hypercoagulable state with reduced fibrinolytic activity along with increased factor VIII activity.[255-258]

Impaired Temperature Control. After damage to the spinal cord, the hypothalamus can no longer control cutaneous blood flow or the level of sweating.[254] This lack of sweating is often associated with excessive compensatory diaphoresis above the level of the lesion.[254]

Respiratory Impairment. Respiratory function depends on the level of the lesion. Between C1 and C3, phrenic nerve innervation and spontaneous respiration are significantly impaired or lost.[254]

Bladder and Bowel and Sexual Dysfunction. Urinary tract infections are among the most frequent medical complications during the initial medical-rehabilitation period.[254] The spinal integration center for micturition is the conus medullaris. The primary reflex control originates from the sacral segments of S2, S3, and S4 within the conus medullaris.[254]

One of two types of bladder conditions can develop following spinal shock, depending on the location of the lesion:

- Lesions that occur within the spinal cord above the conus medullaris: spastic or reflex (automatic) bladder.
- A lesion of the conus medullaris or cauda equina: flaccid or nonreflex (autonomous) bladder.

As with the bladder, the neurogenic bowel condition that develops after spinal shock subsides can be of two types based on the site of the lesion.

- A lesion that occurs within the spinal cord above the conus medullaris: spastic or reflex (automatic) bowel.
- A lesion of the conus medullaris or cauda equina: flaccid or nonreflex (autonomous) bowel.

As with bowel and bladder function, sexual capabilities are broadly divided between UMN and LMN lesions.

Physical Therapy Examination. SCI is a dynamic process. In all acute cord syndromes, the full extent of injury may not be apparent initially and therefore requires a thorough neurologic examination (see Neurological Examination).[254] This section summarizes the tests and measures most frequently used with the SCI population.

- Strength. The American Spinal Injury Association (ASIA) and the International Medical Society of Paraplegia[259] recommends testing the strength of the designated key muscle group on each side in each of the designated 10 paired myotomes, using a head to toe sequence.[75] It is important to palpate the tested muscle during the manual muscle test to rule out the presence of muscle substitution.
- Range of motion. Assessment of range of motion is important as extremes of range of motion often play important roles in compensating for strength deficits in the spinal cord-injured population.

Study Pearl

The presence of neurologic deficits that indicate multilevel involvement suggests SCI rather than a nerve root injury. In the absence of spinal shock, motor weakness with intact reflexes indicates SCI, while motor weakness with absent reflexes indicates a nerve root lesion.

- Joint integrity and mobility. The integrity of the scapulothoracic, shoulder, elbow, and wrist joints are of particular concern in this population because of the increased demand for upper extremity weight-bearing during mobility tasks.[75]
- Sensory integrity. Assessment of sensory function helps to identify the different pathways for light touch, proprioception, vibration, and pain (pinprick). Differentiating a nerve root injury from SCI can be difficult.
- Pain. The presence, intensity, and location of pain are noted. Pain after spinal cord injury can generally be categorized as nociceptive pain or neuropathic pain.[75]
- Motor function—control and learning.[75]
  - Complete SCI causes total loss of voluntary movement below the level of injury but spasticity, which produces an involuntary increase in muscle tone, can still occur and may interfere, or be used to assist, with motor control and mobility skills.
  - Incomplete SCI injuries may provide some overlap of voluntary control and spasticity across spinal levels making the result of motor function more difficult to predict.
- Cardiovascular/pulmonary.
  - Circulation, particularly with its relevance to orthostatic hypotension.
  - Function of respiratory muscles.
- Chest shape, symmetry, and expansion.
  - Breathing pattern, especially the presence of paradoxical breathing.
  - Ability to cough.
  - Length of vocalization and syllables per breath.
  - Aerobic capacity and endurance.
- Integumentary system. During the acute phase, meticulous and regular skin inspection is a shared responsibility of the patient and the entire medical/rehabilitative team. As management progresses into the active rehabilitation phase, the patient will gradually assume greater responsibility for this activity.
- Function:
  - Basic mobility and self-care: a review of the following functional mobility skills—rolling in bed to both sides, rolling from supine to prone and returning to supine, moving supine to/from long sitting, transitioning from supine to/from sitting at edge of bed, and transferring from bed or mat to/from a wheelchair.
  - Locomotion and gait: wheelchair mobility, ability to perform an effective pressure relief technique when seated in a wheelchair, standard gait assessment as appropriate. The spinal cord injury functional ambulation inventory (SCI-FAI)[260] is an observational gate assessment instrument with three domains:
    - Gait parameters.
    - Assistive device used.
    - Walking mobility score.

Physical Therapy Intervention. The following goals should act as guidelines in the acute care setting (Table 9-29):

- Respiratory management as appropriate, including deep breathing exercises, assisted coughing, airway clearance, and abdominal support.

TABLE 9-29. FUNCTIONAL OUTCOMES RELATED TO LEVEL OF SPINAL CORD INJURY

LEVEL OF LESION	FUNCTION/MOTION	CARE NEEDS	ADLS	EQUIPMENT NEEDS
C1-C3	Limited head/neck movement Rotate/flex neck (sternocleidomastoid) Extend neck (cervical paraspinals) Speech and swallowing (neck accessories) Total paralysis of trunk, UE and LE	24 hour care needs Able to direct care needs	Ventilator dependent Impaired communication Dependent for all care needs Mobility: Power wheelchair Hoyer lift	Adapted computer Bedside/portable ventilator Suction machine Specialty bed Hoyer Reclining shower chair
C4	Head and neck control (cervical paraspinals) Shoulder shrug (upper traps) Inspiration(diaphragm) Lack of shoulder control (deltoids) Paralysis of trunk, UE, and LE Inability to cough, low respiratory reserve	24 hours care needs Able to direct care needs	May or may not be vent dependent Improved communication Assisted cough Dependent for all care needs Mobility: Power wheelchair Hoyer lift	Adapted computer Bedside/portable ventilator as needed Suction machine Specialty bed Hoyer Reclining shower chair
C5	Shoulder control (deltoids) Elbow flexion (biceps/elbow flexors) Supinate hands (brachialis and brachioradialis) Lack elbow extension and hand pronation Paralysis of trunk and LE	10 hours personal care need 6 hours homemaking assistance	Set-up/equipment: eating, drinking, face wash and teeth Assisted cough Dependent for bowel, bladder and lower body hygiene Dependent for bed mobility and transfers Mobility: Hoyer or stand pivot Power wheelchair w/ hand controls Manual wheelchair Drive motor vehicle w/ hand controls	Power and manual wheelchairs Adaptive splints/braces Page turners/computer adaptations
C6	Wrist extension (extensor carpi ulnaris and extensor carpi radialis longus/ brevis) Arm across chest (clavicular pectoralis) Lack elbow extension (triceps) Lack wrist flexion Lack hand control Paralysis of trunk and LE	6 hours personal care needs 4 hours homemaking assistance	Assisted cough Set-up for feeding, bathing and dressing Independent pressure relief, turns and skin assessment May be independent for bowel/bladder care	Independent slide board transfer Manual wheelchair Drive with adaptive equipment
C7	Elbow flexion and extension (biceps/triceps) Arm toward body (sternal pectoralis) Lack finger function Lack trunk stability	6 hours personal care needs 2 hours homemaking assistance	More effective cough Fewer adaptive aids Independent w/ all ADLs May need adaptive aids for bowel care	Manual wheelchair Transfers without adaptive equipment

(*Continued*)

TABLE 9-29. FUNCTIONAL OUTCOMES RELATED TO LEVEL OF SPINAL CORD INJURY (*Continued*)

LEVEL OF LESION	FUNCTION/MOTION	CARE NEEDS	ADLS	EQUIPMENT NEEDS
C8-T1	Increased finger and hand strength Finger flexion (flexor digitorum) Finger extension (extensor communis) Thumb movement (policus longis brevis) Separate fingers (interossei separates)	4 hours personal care needs 2 hours homemaking assistance	Independent w/ or w/o assistive devices Assist w/ complex meal prep and home management	Manual wheelchair
T2-T6	Normal motor function of head, neck, shoulders, arms, hands and fingers Increased use of intercostals Increase trunk control (erector spinae)	3 hours personal care needs/ homemaking	Independent in personal care	Manual wheelchair May have limited walking with extensive bracing Drive with hand controls
T7-T12	Added motor function Increased abdominal control Increased trunk stability	2 hours personal care needs/ homemaking	Independent Improved cough Improved balance control	Manual wheelchair May have limited walking with bracing Driving with hand controls
L2-L5	Added motor function in hips and knees L2 Hip flexors (iliopsas) L3 Knee extensors (quadriceps) L4 Ankle dorsiflexors (tibialis anterior) L5 Long toe extensors (ext hallucis longus)	May need 1 hour personal care/ homemaking	Independent	Manual wheelchair May walk short distance with braces and assistive devices Driving with hand controls
S1-S5	Ankle plantar flexors (gastrocnemius) Various degrees of bowel, bladder and sexual function Lower level equals greater function	No personal or home-maker needs	Independent	Increased ability to walk with less adaptive/supportive devices Manual wheelchair for distance

- Pain management.
- Maintenance of joint range of motion and prevention of contractures while remembering that patients with spinal cord injury do not require full range of motion in all joints—some joints benefit from allowing tightness to develop in certain muscles to enhance function.[254]
- Selective strengthening.
- Gradual orientation to the vertical position and increased sitting tolerance. The ability to transfer to a sitting position from a supine position assists with ADLs, bed mobility, and for transfer preparation.
- Independence with bed mobility as appropriate. The ability to roll is essential for many ADLs, for independence in bed mobility and bed positioning and is a building block for other

mobility skills.[75] The following functional postures are important to emphasize[75]:

- Prone on elbow.
- Supine on elbows.
- Quadruped and tall kneeling.
- Long sitting.
- Short sitting.

- Independence in pressure relief as appropriate. Pressure relief should initially be performed for 15 seconds or more, at least every 15 to 30 minutes.[75]
- Independence in wheelchair transfers to mat, bed, car, toilet, bathtub, and floor, as appropriate.
- Independence in wheelchair mobility as appropriate.
- Independence in preventative measures (self skin inspection; self lower extremity range of motion exercises) as appropriate.
- Gait training as appropriate.[75]
- Plan for discharge.

Syringomyelia

Syringomyelia is the development of a fluid-filled cavity or syrinx within the spinal cord of unknown etiology.[261-265] Syringomyelia usually progresses slowly but it may have a more acute course, especially when the brain stem is affected (ie, syringobulbia). Clinical manifestations include the following:

- Dissociated sensory loss. Syrinx interrupts the decussating spinothalamic fibers that mediate pain and temperature sensibility, resulting in loss of these sensations, while light touch, vibration, and position senses are preserved.
- Motor changes.
- Diminished upper extremity reflexes.
- Lower limb spasticity.
- Respiratory insufficiency.
- Impaired bowel and bladder functions.

Cauda Equina Syndrome

Cauda equina syndrome (CES) may result from any lesion that compresses the CE nerve roots. The findings associated with CES include some or all of the following: low back pain; acute or chronic radiating pain; unilateral or bilateral lower extremity motor and/or sensory abnormality; bowel and/or bladder dysfunction; saddle (perineal) anesthesia (the clinician can inquire if toilet paper feels different when wiping); bladder dysfunction (may present as incontinence, but often presents earlier as difficulty starting or stopping a stream of urine).[266-270] Reflex abnormalities may be present; they typically include loss or diminution of reflexes. Hyperactive reflexes may signal spinal cord involvement and exclude the diagnosis of CES. CES is a medical emergency.

Neurodegenerative and Inflammatory Disorders

Alzheimer Disease. Refer to Chapter 14.

Multiple Sclerosis. Multiple sclerosis (MS) is an idiopathic/autoimmune inflammatory demyelinating disease of the CNS (inflammation and demyelination), which tends to progress over years to decades.[271-283] Classic MS symptoms include:

- Sensory changes
- Pain
- Motor (eg, muscle cramping) and autonomic (eg, bladder, bowel, sexual dysfunction) spinal cord symptoms (eg, spasticity)
- Balance and coordination deficits and dizziness
- Bowel, bladder and sexual dysfunction
- Constitutional symptoms, especially fatigue and dizziness
- Subjective reports of difficulties with attention span, concentration, memory, and judgment
- Depression and affective changes
- Eye symptoms, including optic neuritis (ie, inflammation or demyelination of optic nerve), and diplopia on lateral gaze

Medical management includes disease modifying medications, and management of relapses and symptoms through the use of corticosteroids, antispasticity medications, and pain medications.

The physical therapy intervention is based on the impairments identified in the examination.

Myasthenia Gravis. Myasthenia gravis (MG) is an autoimmune disorder of peripheral nerves in which antibodies form against acetylcholine (ACh) nicotinic postsynaptic receptors at the myoneural junction.[284-295] A reduction in the number of skeletal muscle ACh receptors results in a pattern of progressively reduced muscle strength with repeated use of the muscle and recovery of muscle strength following a period of rest. The bulbar muscles (muscles of the throat, tongue, jaw, and face) are affected most commonly and most severely, which can lead to ptosis, diplopia, blurred vision, difficulty swallowing, or dysarthria. Patients with MG can present with a wide range of signs and symptoms, depending on the severity of the disease.

Mild presentations of MG involve subtle findings, such as ptosis. Severe exacerbations of MG have a more dramatic presentation. The patient's ability to generate adequate ventilation and to clear bronchial secretions are of utmost concern with severe exacerbations of MG. An inability to cough leads to an accumulation of secretions; therefore, rales, rhonchi, and wheezes may be auscultated locally or diffusely.

The role of physical therapy with MG encompasses the following:

- Monitor changes in the patient's condition for complications.
- Maintain or improve cardiovascular endurance without exacerbating fatigue.
- Promote independence in functional mobility skills and activities of daily living.
- Teach energy conservation techniques.
- Provide psychological and emotional support.
- Family/caregiver education.

Polymyositis. Polymyositis (PM), dermatomyositis (DM), and inclusion body myositis (IBM) are the major members of a group of skeletal muscle diseases called the idiopathic (the specific etiology is unknown but is thought to be autoimmune) inflammatory myopathies.[296-307]

- PM: the immune system is prepared to act against previously unrecognized muscle antigens.
- DM: complement-mediated damage to endomysial vessels and microvasculature of the dermis occurs.
- Although classified as an inflammatory myopathy, IBM shows minimal evidence of inflammation. This is the most common inflammatory myopathy in patients older than 50 years.

The history and examination findings of patients with PM or DM typically includes the following:

- Symmetric proximal muscle weakness with insidious onset.
- Muscle tenderness on palpation.
- Dysphagia.
- Aspiration (if pharyngeal and esophageal muscles are involved).
- Arthralgias.
- Functional loss: difficulty kneeling, climbing or descending stairs, and arising from a seated position.
- Characteristic rash of face, trunk, and hands (seen in DM only).
- Normal sensory test results and reflexes, although reflexes may be abnormal with advanced disease.
- Congestive heart failure (CHF), arrhythmia, interstitial lung disease, pneumonia/aspiration.

Epilepsy. The International Classification of Seizures divides epileptic seizures into two categories: partial seizures (ie, focal or localization-related seizures) and generalized seizures.

- Partial seizures, which result from a seizure discharge within a particular brain region
- Generalized convulsive seizures, which are classified on the basis of clinical symptoms and EEG abnormalities.

Seizures typically are divided into tonic, clonic, and postictal phases.

- Tonic phase. The tonic phase begins with flexion of the trunk and elevation and abduction of the elbows. Subsequent extension of the back and neck is followed by extension of arms and legs. Autonomic signs are common during this phase.
- Clonic phase. The tonic stage gives way to clonic convulsive movements, in which the tonic muscles relax intermittently for a variable period of time. During the clonic stage, a generalized tremor occurs at a rate of 8 tremors per second, which may slow down to about 4 tremors per second.

Voiding may occur at the end of the clonic phase as sphincter muscles relax. The convulsion, including tonic and clonic phases, lasts for 1 to 2 minutes.

- Postictal state. The postictal state includes a variable period of unconsciousness during which the patient becomes quiet and breathing resumes.

Physical Therapy Intervention. It is important to note the time of onset, duration, type of seizure, and sequence of events. The role of a physical therapist during a seizure event is as follows:

- Remain with the patient to protect the patient from injury.
- Remove any potentially harmful nearby objects, and loosen restrictive clothing.
- Do not restrain the limbs.
- Establish an airway and prevent aspiration. It is important to remember that artificial ventilation should not be initiated during tonic-clonic activity.

Cerebellar Disorders. Lesions to the cerebellum are associated with intention tremor, ataxia, poor coordination of trunk and extremities, athetosis, dysmetria, balance deficits, and dysdiadochokinesia. A number of cerebellar disorders are recognized:

- Ataxia-telangiectasia (A-T): an autosomal recessive, complex, multisystem disorder characterized by progressive neurologic impairment, cerebellar ataxia, and a predisposition to malignancy.
- Friedreich ataxia (FA): The major pathophysiologic finding in FA is a "dying back phenomena" of axons, which begins in the periphery with a loss of neurons, and a secondary fibrous gliosis that does not replace the bulk of the lost fibers.[318-327] The primary sites of these changes are the posterior columns and corticospinal, anterior, and lateral spinocerebellar tracts and spinal roots. This results in loss of large myelinated axons in peripheral nerves, which increases with age and disease duration.
- Unmyelinated fibers in sensory roots and peripheral sensory nerves are spared.
- The posterior column degeneration accounts for the loss of position and vibration senses and the sensory ataxia.
- The loss of large neurons in the sensory ganglia causes extinction of tendon reflexes.
- The cerebellar ataxia is explained by loss of the lateral and anterior spinocerebellar tracts and involvement of the Clarke column, dentate nucleus, superior vermis, and dentatorubral pathways.
- Loss of cells in the nuclei of cranial nerves VIII, X, and XII results in facial weakness and speech and swallowing difficulties.
- Myocardial muscle fibers also show degeneration and are replaced by macrophages and fibroblasts.
- Kyphoscoliosis is likely; it is secondary to spinal muscular imbalance.

Onset of FA is early, with gait ataxia (both of a sensory and cerebellar type) being the usual presenting symptom—tabetocerebellar gait. Typically, both lower extremities are affected equally. The features of gait in FA include a wide-based gait with constant shifting of position to maintain balance. Sitting and standing are associated with titubation.

The sensory ataxia resulting from a loss of joint position sense contributes to the wide-based stance and gait but a steppage gait also is present, characterized by uneven and irregular striking of the floor by the bottom of the feet. Attempts to correct any imbalance typically result in abrupt and wild movements.

As the disease progresses, ataxia affects the trunk, legs, and arms. Titubation of the trunk may appear.

Patients with advanced FA may have profound distal weakness of the legs and feet. Eventually, the patient is unable to walk.

With disease progression, dysarthria and dysphagia appear. Speech becomes slurred, slow, and eventually incomprehensible. Incoordination of breathing, swallowing, and laughing may result in the patient nearly choking while speaking.

The goals of a physical therapy intervention are determined from the findings from the clinical examination but will likely include some or all of the following:

- Functional mobility and safety.
- Assistive and adaptive equipment as appropriate.
- Postural stability (static and dynamic).
- Weight-bearing postures.
- Weight shifting progressions.
- Reaching and pointing activities.
- Promotion of control during movement transitions (eg, sit to stand) and reversals of movement.
- Coordination—accuracy and precision of limb movements:
  - Eye-hand coordination exercises.
  - Eye-head coordination exercises.
  - Upper extremity coordination—Frenkel exercises (see Table 9-30).
  - Lower extremity coordination (Table 9-30).
- Activities involving reciprocal movement (gait, stationary bike, etc).
- Balance, including standing balance and gait activities.
- Patient education regarding energy conservation techniques.

Vestibular Disorders. The three main categories of dizziness that patients describe include:

- Vertigo: an illusion of motion. Of the various causes of vertigo, benign positional vertigo (BPV) is the most common cause (see next section).
- Near-syncope: due to reduced blood flow to the entire brain.
- Dysequilibrium: essentially a gait disorder, most often caused by cervical spondylosis.

Balance disorders are significant risk factors for falls in elderly individuals. The physical therapy examination specific to identifying vestibular disorders includes the following assessments[329]:

- History to identify the symptoms as well as their duration and the circumstances under which the symptoms occur. The clinician should elicit a clear description of the type of symptoms

TABLE 9-30. FRENKEL EXERCISES FOR COORDINATION

Techniques for lower extremities	Supine position	Flexion and extension at each leg at hip and knee joint, heel sliding on bed.
		Abduction and adduction of each leg with knee bent, heel sliding on bed. Repeat same with knee extended.
		Flexion and extension of one knee at the time with heel raised.
		Place heel upon some definite part of the opposite leg, for example on the patella, mid tibia, ankle, or toes.
		Slide heel from contralateral knee joint down along shin and back to knee.
		Flexion and extension of both legs simultaneously, holding knees and ankles together.
		Draw up one extremity while extending the other: reciprocal flexion and extension.
		Flexion and extension of one leg and simultaneous abduction and adduction of the other. Reverse procedure.
	Sitting position	Alternately raise each leg, then place foot firmly on a footprint on the floor.
		Glide each foot alternately over a cross marked on the floor: forward, backward, to left, to right.
		With a foot in footprint, raise heel, lift foot off floor; in this position extend and flex knee, and bring toes back to original position; bring heel down in corresponding part of footprint.
		Practice sitting down on chair: avoid falling into chair; allow muscles of hips and knees to ease the body down. Stand in front of chair, with knee slightly flexed and body bent slightly forward. Sit down by continuing the flexion of knees, hips and trunk.
		Practice standing up: feet are drawn back until partly under the chair so that the whole foot can be firmly planted. Bend body forward and rise slowly, extending the knees and hips and straightening the body.
	Standing position	Encourage walking on entire foot.
		Stand on tiptoe, then on the heel of one leg.
		Walk sideways a few steps in each direction.
		Walk between two parallel bars 14 inches apart, keeping a distance of 6 inches between the feet. Avoid outward rotation of legs.
		Walk on straight line; avoid toeing out.
		Take one half step and bring other foot in apposition. Continue taking several alternate half steps. Repeat with quarter steps.
		Alternate half and quarter steps, bringing each foot in apposition after each step. Then walk by alternate half steps and quarter steps.
		Make a complete turn to the left, using left heel as a pivot. Repeat to right.
		Walk along a circle on the floor, first in one direction, then in the other.
Techniques for extremities	Reaching activities	Placing it on marks at different levels on the wall.
		Add marks with chalk to symbols on blackboard, eg, change minus to plus, cross "t," dot "i," play tic-tac-toe.
		Place small, readily grasped objects on squares of check board which has been numbered.
		Practice writing.
		Practice drawing geometric figures.

experienced by the patient (eg, vertigo, imbalance, disequilibrium, presyncopal sensations, gait ataxia). Specific activities, head or body positions that provoke symptoms should be determined. Visual disturbances, such as oscillopsia (blurred vision with head movement), should be documented.

- Assessment of eye movements. The key tests include observation for nystagmus, examination of the VOR at high acceleration (head thrust test) head-shaking induced nystagmus (HSN), positional testing (benign paroxysmal positional vertigo [BPPV] test, and Hallpike-Dix test), and the dynamic visual acuity (DVA) test.
- Gait assessment: including ambulation with head movement.
- Balance testing: balance with altered sensory cues, and balance under static (eg, sitting, standing) and dynamic conditions.

- Sensory assessment: should include visual and proprioceptive abilities.
- Vestibular function tests: semicircular canal tests and otolith tests.
- Function assessment: the patient's perception of the impact of the symptoms on daily activities. A number of tools have been devised to help the clinician assess vestibular disorders. These include[330]:
  - The Dizziness Handicap Inventory (DHI)[331]: used to measure a patient's self perceived handicap as a result of their vestibular disorder, has excellent test-retest reliability (r=0.97) and good internal consistency reliability (r = 0 .89). Patients respond to 25 questions, subgrouped into functional, emotional, and physical components.
  - Motion Sensitivity Quotient (MSQ)[329]: provides a subjective score of an individual's dizziness. The test involves placing patients into positions incorporating head or entire body motion to determine whether the movement reproduces dizziness.
  - Hallpike maneuver: requires the patient to lie back from the sitting to supine position 3 times. The first time, the patient is asked to lie back with the head facing forward and the neck slightly extended; this movement is repeated with the patient's head turned 45 degrees to the right and a third time with the head turned 45 degrees to the left. The patient is instructed to keep both eyes open each time he or she lies back. The clinician checks for nystagmus and asks the patient about any symptoms of vertigo. Failure either to observe or to provoke unidirectional nystagmus casts doubt on whether the process is localized to the peripheral vestibular system. Either finding suggests a need to consider other diagnostic alternatives.

Refer to Management Strategies for Specific Conditions for details with regard to vestibular rehabilitation therapy, which include:

- Habituation training: repetition of movement and positions that provoke dizziness and vertigo.
- Activities that engage the VOR and VSR.
- Eye exercises: involving up and down and side to side movements of the eyes, progressing from slow to fast movements.
- Head motions in all directions, progressing from slow to fast movements.

The more common types of vestibular disorders include:

- Vestibular neuronitis. Vestibular neuronitis can be defined as an acute, sustained dysfunction of the peripheral vestibular system with secondary nausea, vomiting, and vertigo.[332-339] Patients usually complain of abrupt onset of severe, debilitating vertigo. Common findings include:
  - Symptoms that increases with head movement.
  - Spontaneous, unidirectional, horizontal nystagmus.
  - The patient tends to fall toward his or her involved side when attempting ambulation or during Romberg tests.
  - The involved side has either unilaterally impaired or no response to caloric stimulation.

The physical therapist should perform the Hallpike maneuver on all patients who complain of vertigo but do not exhibit nystagmus on routine examination of the extraocular muscles.

- Central vertigo. Central vertigo is due to a disease originating from the CNS usually including lesions of cranial nerve VIII as well.[340-346] A thorough neurologic and cardiologic examination is important to identify patients with central vertigo.
- Benign positional vertigo. Benign positional vertigo (BPV) is caused by calcium carbonate particles called otoliths (or otoconia) that are improperly displaced into the semicircular canals of the vestibular labyrinth of the inner ear.[347-357] These otoliths are normally attached to hair cells on a membrane inside the utricle and saccule. Because they are denser than the surrounding endolymph, vertical changes in head movement cause the otoliths to tilt the hair cells. The otoliths may become displaced from the utricle by aging, head trauma, or labyrinthine disease. When this occurs, the otoliths have the potential to enter the semicircular canals. When they do, they almost always enter the posterior semicircular canal because this is the most dependent (inferior) of the three canals. Changing head position causes the otoliths to move through the canal. Endolymph is dragged along with the movement of the otoliths, and this stimulates the hair cells of the cupula of the affected semicircular canal, causing vertigo. When the otoliths stop moving, the endolymph also stops moving and the hair cells return to their baseline position, thus terminating the vertigo and nystagmus. Reversing the head maneuver causes the particles to move in the opposite direction, producing nystagmus in the same axis but reversed in direction of rotation. Symptoms of BPV are usually worse in the morning (the otoliths are more likely to clump together as the patient sleeps) and mitigate as the day progresses (the otoliths become more dispersed with head movement).

In addition to the patient's history, a diagnosis of BPV is indicated by a positive Hallpike test (rotatory nystagmus and reproduction of symptoms). In the head-hanging position, the fast phase should beat toward the forehead (upbeat) and in the same direction as the affected side (ipsilateral). The neurologic examination is otherwise unremarkable.

- Labyrinthitis. Labyrinthitis is an inflammation or dysfunction of the vestibular labyrinth, which is characterized by the acute onset of vertigo, commonly associated with head or body movement. Vertigo is often accompanied by nausea, vomiting, or malaise.
- Ménière syndrome. Ménière syndrome is a labyrinthine disorder in which there is an increase in volume and pressure of the endolymph of the inner ear.[358-360] It typically presents with waxing and waning hearing loss and tinnitus associated with vertigo. Patients may report an abnormal sensation of pressure or fullness in the ears.

A complete neurological examination is necessary to rule out other conditions. Vestibular maneuvers may be helpful in diagnosing this syndrome. Interpretation of either of the following maneuvers is identical.

- Nylen-Bárány maneuver: the patient sits at the end of the examining table and is laid back quickly, while the head is supported and the neck is carefully hyperextended. The head is first turned toward one shoulder; then, the maneuver is repeated with the head turned toward the other shoulder.
- Hallpike maneuver: previously described.

In the interpretation of these maneuvers, the reproducibility of the vestibular symptoms, including vertigo, nausea, and malaise, should be noted. Typically, these symptoms are worse with the head in a particular position; that position should be noted.

The maneuvers should be repeated several times over a 5 to 10 minute period, as tolerated by the patient. Fatigue and extinction of the vestibular symptoms (ie, whether or not the severity of the symptoms decreases with successive repetition of the maneuvers) should be noted. Evaluation of hearing is important in these patients (Rinne test and Weber test).

Basal Ganglia Disorders

Parkinson Disease. For details about the pathogenesis, examination and intervention of Parkinson disease, refer to Chapter 14.

Huntington Chorea. Huntington chorea (HC), also known as Huntington disease (HD), is an autosomal dominant inherited disease characterized by choreiform movements and progressive dementia.[361-363] Symptoms arising from a typical presentation of HD usually do not develop until a person is aged 35 years or older. The majority of patients affected by HD complain of involuntary movements or rigidity. In the remainder of cases, there may be early and subtle mental status changes that initially appear as increased irritability, moodiness, or antisocial behavior. Dementia develops as the disease progresses.

The pathognomonic feature of HD is the movement disorder that often begins as a piano-playing motion of the fingers or as facial twitching or grimaces, and twitching and writhing of the distal extremities. As the disease progresses, the movement disorder becomes more generalized and involves the trunk producing the characteristic dancing gait. Although patients appear to be off-balance, the ability to balance is actually well preserved. Eventually, the patient's gait is impaired. Symptoms become worse with anxiety or stress.

No specific pharmacologic therapy for HD exists. Chorea sometimes may be suppressed with drugs, but the associated adverse effects can be severe. Most patients are actually untroubled by the choreic movements. Suppression of the movements does not result in improved function.

Cranial and Peripheral Nerve Disorders

Bell's Palsy. Bell's palsy is one of the most common neurologic disorders affecting the cranial nerves. Although it is commonly believed that Bell's palsy is an inflammation of the facial nerve

(CN VII), other cranial nerves are probably also affected. The actual cause is unknown, although vascular, infectious, genetic, and immunologic factors have all been proposed.[364-369] The most common signs and symptoms include:

- An abrupt, unilateral, peripheral facial paresis or paralysis with no explainable reason. A careful, complete examination should be able to exclude other possible causes of facial paralysis.
- In supranuclear lesions such as a cortical stroke (upper motor neuron; above the facial nucleus in the pons), the upper third of the face is spared while the lower two thirds are paralyzed. The orbicularis, frontalis, and corrugator muscles are innervated bilaterally, which explains the pattern of facial paralysis.
- The results of the other cranial nerve tests should be normal.

Most patients recover fully from his condition in several weeks or months. The physical intervention in these patients is typically supportive, and includes:

- Electrical stimulation of specific motor points of the facial muscles to maintain tone and support function.
- Facial muscle exercises: forehead wrinkling, eyebrow raises, frowning, smiling, eye closing, cheek puffing.
- Functional training: teaching the patient to chew on one side of the mouth.

Peripheral Nerve Injury. Peripheral nerve injuries may occur due to trauma (eg, a blunt or penetrating wound) or acute compression,[370-377] with subsequent demyelination and axonal degeneration that results in disruption of the sensory and/or motor function of the injured nerve (Table 9-31). The clinical appearance of an injured nerve depends on the nerve affected. In general, the temporal sequence of neurological manifestations is as follows: irritative sensory symptoms, such as pain and paresthesia; ablative sensory symptoms of numbness; and, finally, ablative motor signs, such as weakness and atrophy. In a major mixed nerve, such as the sciatic or median, signs of sympathetic dystrophy, which include dry, thin, hairless skin, ridged, thickened, crackly nails, and recurrent ulcerations, may be prominent features in chronic cases.

The classification of nerve injury described by Seddon in 1943 comprised neurapraxia, axonotmesis, and neurotmesis. Sunderland, in 1951, expanded this classification system to 5 degrees of nerve injury.

- A first-degree injury or neurapraxia involves a temporary conduction block with demyelination of the nerve at the site of injury. Electrodiagnostic study results are normal above and below the level of injury, and no denervation muscle changes are present. No Tinel sign is present. Once the nerve has remyelinated at that area, complete recovery occurs. Recovery may take up to 12 weeks.
- A second-degree injury or axonotmesis results from a more severe trauma or compression. This causes Wallerian degeneration distal

TABLE 9-31. PERIPHERAL NERVE INJURY LOCATION AND FINDINGS OF THE UPPER EXTREMITY

CORD AND NERVE	LEVEL OF INJURY	MOTOR LOSS	CUTANEOUS LOSS
Posterior cord: radial (C5-T1)	Plexus—proximal to axillary nerve	All muscles innervated by radial nerve All muscles innervated by Axillary nerve	Throughout radial and axillary distribution
	Axilla (brachio-axillary angle)	Triceps (medial and lateral heads), anconeus	Posterior brachial cutaneous
	Spiral groove	All muscles innervated by radial nerve except medial head of triceps	Posterior antebrachial cutaneous
	Proximal to lateral epicondyle	Brachialis, brachioradialis, ECRL, ECRB	
	Arcade of Frohse	Supinator, all muscles innervated by posterior interosseous nerve	Superficial radial (Wartenberg's syndrome)
Posterior cord: axillary nerve (C5-6)	Axilla (quadrangular space)	Teres minor, deltoid	Lateral arm
Medial and lateral cord: median nerve (C5-T1)	Plexus (proximal to the joining of the medial and lateral cords)—thoracic outlet syndrome	All muscles innervated by median, musculocutaneous, and ulnar nerves	Throughout median, musculocutaneous, and ulnar distributions
	Ligament of Struthers—proximal to medial epicondyle)	Pronator teres	
	Cubital fossa exit—between two heads of the pronator teres	Pronator teres, FCR, FDS, PL, lumbricales I and II	
	Forearm	Anterior interosseous: FDP (I and II), FPL, PQ Median muscular branch: Thenar muscles (APB, FPB, OP), lumbricales I and II.	Palmar branch: radial half of thumb Digital branch: Dorsal tips of thumb, index and middle finger, and radial half of ring finger
Lateral: musculocutaneous nerve (C5-7)	Coracobrachialis	Coracobrachialis Biceps Brachialis	
	Elbow		Lateral antebrachial cutaneous nerve: lateral forearm
Medial: ulnar nerve (C8-T1)	Cubital tunnel	FCU, FDP, Adductor pollicis, lumbricales and interossei	Dorsal and palmar aspects on the ulnar side of the hand
	Between the two heads of the FCU	FDP, FCU	
	Proximal to wrist	Deep branch: all hand muscles innervated by the ulnar nerve Superficial branch: palmaris brevis	Dorsal cutaneous: medial aspect of ring and little finger; dorsum of hand Dorsal digital: DIP aspect of little finger, PIP aspect of ring and middle finger. Palmar cutaneous: medial third of palm
	Guyon canal	Muscles of the hypothenar eminence (Hand of Benediction), interossei	Ulnar aspect of the hand

APB, adductor pollicis brevis; DIP, distal interphalangeal; ECRB, extensor carpi radialis brevis; ECRL, extensor carpi radialis longus; FCR, flexor carpi radialis; FCU, flexor carpi ulnaris; FDP, flexor digitorum profundus; FDS, flexor digitorum superficialis; FPB, flexor pollicis brevis; FPL, flexor pollicis longus; OP, opponens pollicis; PIP, proximal interphalangeal; PL, palmaris longus; PQ, pronator quadratus.

to the level of injury and proximal axonal degeneration to at least the next node of Ranvier. In more severe traumatic injuries, the proximal degeneration may extend beyond the next node of Ranvier. Electrodiagnostic studies demonstrate denervation changes in the affected muscles, and in cases of reinnervation, motor unit potentials (MUPs) are present. Axonal regeneration occurs at the rate of 1 mm/d or 1 in/mo and can be monitored with an advancing Tinel sign. The endoneurial tubes remain intact, and, therefore, recovery is complete with axons reinnervating their original motor and sensory targets.

- A third-degree injury was introduced by Sunderland to describe an injury more severe than second-degree injury. Similar to a second-degree injury, Wallerian degeneration occurs, and electrodiagnostic studies demonstrate denervation changes with fibrillations in the affected muscles. In cases of reinnervation, MUPs are present. Regeneration occurs at 1 mm/d, and progress may be monitored with an advancing Tinel sign. However, with the increased severity of the injury, the endoneurial tubes are not intact, and regenerating axons therefore may not reinnervate their original motor and sensory targets. The pattern of recovery is mixed and incomplete. Reinnervation occurs only if sensory fibers reach their sensory end organs and motor fibers reach their muscle targets. Even within a sensory nerve, recovery can be mismatched if sensory fibers reinnervate a different sensory area within the nerve's sensory distribution. If the muscle target is a long distance from the site of injury, nerve regeneration may occur, but the muscle may not be completely reinnervated due to the long period of denervation.
- A fourth-degree injury results in a large area of scar at the site of nerve injury and precludes any axons from advancing distal to the level of nerve injury. Electrodiagnostic studies reveal denervation changes in the affected muscles, and no MUPs are present. A Tinel sign is noted at the level of the injury, but it does not advance beyond that level. No improvement in function is noted, and the patient requires surgery to restore neural continuity, thus permitting axonal regeneration and motor and sensory reinnervation.
- A fifth-degree injury is a complete transection of the nerve. Similar to a fourth-degree injury, it requires surgery to restore neural continuity. Electrodiagnostic findings are the same as those for a fourth-degree injury.
- A sixth-degree injury was introduced by Mackinnon to describe a mixed nerve injury that combines the other degrees of injury. This commonly occurs when some fascicles of the nerve are working normally while other fascicles may be recovering, and other fascicles may require surgical intervention to permit axonal regeneration.

Nerve injuries are frequently overlooked as a source of acute or, more usually, chronic symptomatology. Loss of vibration sensibility has been suggested as an early indicator of peripheral compression neuropathy. Nerve conduction studies may be performed, focusing on the sites of interest. Diabetes, with its associated neuropathies or cheiroarthropathy, may be an underlying cause (see Chapter 12).

The conservative intervention for mild cases of peripheral nerve injury typically includes protection of the joints including the surrounding ligaments and tendons, activity modification, passive range of motion and NSAIDs. Splints, slings or both (as appropriate) may be prescribed. For example, a radial nerve injury results in a loss of wrist and finger extension, and wrist drop. A wrist-resting splint may be used to support the hand in a neutral wrist position and place the hand in a more functional position. In patients with brachial plexus nerve injuries, particularly when C5-6 is affected, or in patients who have suffered a stroke, continued downward stress at the glenohumeral joint may cause the glenohumeral joint to subluxate without the muscle support of the rotator cuff muscles. A sling is helpful to unload this joint, prevent complete shoulder dislocation, and decrease pain. Night splints appear to help to reduce the nocturnal symptoms associated with carpal tunnel syndrome and allow the wrist to rest fully. Splints worn during the day are helpful only if they do not interfere with normal activity.

Ergonomic modifications can help reduce the incidence of peripheral nerve injuries and alleviate symptoms in the already symptomatic patient. Patient education is also important to avoid sustained activities and positions/postures, and repetitive motions.

No definitive studies have been done to support the use of electrical muscle stimulation to prevent muscle degeneration. If the nerve does not regenerate in time to reinnervate the muscle, there is no need to stimulate the muscle. With reinnervated muscle, it is theoretically possible to use alternating current stimulation. However, it is necessary to have a large number of reinnervated muscle fibers to stimulate the muscle with alternating current.

LACERATIONS

In patients with neurologic deficits following a laceration, an operative procedure to explore the nerve should be performed as soon after injury as possible. With clean sharp injuries to the nerve, a direct repair is performed. With more crushing or avulsion injuries, the nerve ends are reapproximated so that motor and sensory topography can be aligned. The definitive reconstruction is done at 3 weeks or when the wound permits.

CLOSED INJURIES

In patients with closed traction injuries, surgical intervention is recommended 3 months following nerve injury. These patients are reexamined both clinically and with electrodiagnostic studies. With no evidence of reinnervation clinically or electrically, surgical intervention is necessary.

PERIPHERAL NERVE ENTRAPMENTS

The majority of peripheral nerve entrapments result from chronic injury to a nerve as it travels through an osseoligamentous tunnel; the compression usually is between ligamentous and bony surfaces. The only exceptions to this anatomical generalization are found in entrapment of the posterior interosseous nerve by the muscular arcade of the supinator, compression of the sciatic nerve by the opposing aponeurotic edges of the piriformis and gemelli muscles, and some cases of thoracic outlet syndrome. Peripheral nerve entrapments are the most common in the upper extremity, particularly in the forearm, and wrist. Neurogenic syndromes are usually incomplete, indicating the absence of severe motor or sensory deficits, but in the typical case they are accompanied by a history of pain or vague sensory disturbances (Table 9-32).

HERPES ZOSTER

The varicella-zoster virus is responsible for chickenpox. After the chickenpox has run its course, the virus lies dormant in the posterior root ganglia. On occasion, a focal reactivation along a ganglion's distribution can result in herpes zoster (shingles).[378-385] Herpes zoster (refer to Chapter 13) manifests as a vesicular rash, usually restricted to a single dermatome. Development of the rash may be preceded by unilateral-sided trunk pain, tingling, or burning. Additional symptoms may include abdominal pain, difficulty using the muscles of facial expression, fever and chills, and headache. Treatment involves a prescription of an antiviral medication and/or corticosteroids. Herpes zoster usually clears in 2 to 3 weeks and rarely recurs, but can last from months to years (postherpetic neuralgia).

TRIGEMINAL NEURALGIA

Trigeminal neuralgia (TN), or tic douloureux, is a syndrome characterized by pain often accompanied by a brief facial spasm or tic.[386-396] The distribution of symptoms is unilateral and follows the sensory distribution of the trigeminal nerve (CN V), typically radiating throughout the maxillary (V2) or mandibular (V3) area. Although no known cause exists, aneurysms, tumors, chronic meningeal inflammation, or other lesions may result in irritation of the trigeminal nerve roots. In addition, an abnormal vascular course of the superior cerebellar artery may be causative. However, in most cases, the etiology is labeled idiopathic by default.

Pateint history is the most important factor in the diagnosis of TN.

- ▶ Pain is typically described as unilateral, stabbing or shock-like and, although often occurring in brief attacks, may occur in volleys of multiple attacks.
- ▶ Activities such as face washing, or chewing may be reported to trigger an episode.

In most cases, there is a normal neurologic examination, although a CN examination may reveal symptoms, particularly the corneal reflex.

SPINAL MUSCULAR ATROPHY

The spinal muscular atrophies (SMAs) are a heterogeneous group of disorders, which are characterized by primary degeneration of the anterior horn cells of the spinal cord and occasionally the bulbar motor nuclei.[397-403] Because bulbar features can be present, the term SMA does not technically describe the disorder; thus alternative

TABLE 9-32. PERIPHERAL NERVE ENTRAPMENT SYNDROMES OF THE UPPER EXTREMITY

SYNDROME	ENTRAPMENT SITE	DESCRIPTION OF FINDINGS
Axillary	The axillary nerve is susceptible to injury at several sites, including the origin of the nerve from the posterior cord, the anterior-inferior aspect of the subscapularis muscle and shoulder capsule, the quadrilateral space, and within the subfascial surface of the deltoid muscle.	A deltoid paralysis causes an inability to protract or retract the arm or raise it to the horizontal position, although after some time, supplementary movements may partially take over these functions. Teres minor paralysis causes weakness of shoulder external rotation. Sensation is lost over the deltoid prominence.
Suprascapular nerve entrapment	The suprascapular nerve arises from the lateral aspect of the upper trunk of the brachial plexus, runs across the posterior triangle of the neck together with the suprascapular artery and the omohyoid muscle, dips under the trapezius, and then passes through the suprascapular notch at the superior border of the scapula. As the nerve enters the supraspinous fossa, it supplies the supraspinatus muscle, then curls tightly around the base of the spine of the scapula, enters the infraspinous fossa, and supplies the infraspinatus. A stout, strong suprascapular ligament closes over the free upper margins of the suprascapular notch. Suprascapular nerve entrapment is by this ligament, often in conjunction with a tight, bony notch. The only sensory fibers in the suprascapular nerve supply the posterior aspect of the shoulder joint. These articular fibers are the source of the ill-localized, dull shoulder pain of the syndrome.	The syndrome often afflicts athletes, particularly those in basketball, volleyball, weight lifting, and gymnastics. The chief complaint is the insidious onset of a deep, dull aching pain in the posterior part of the shoulder and upper periscapular region. The pain is noncircumscribed and does not involve the neck or radiate down the arm. Weakness is confined to the supraspinatus (ie, in the initiation of shoulder abduction) and to the infraspinatus, the only muscle responsible for external rotation of the humerus. Atrophy of these muscles causes hollowing of the infraspinous fossa and prominence of the scapular spine. (Atrophy of the supraspinatus is not obvious due to the overlying trapezius.) Deep pressure over the midpoint of the superior scapular border may produce discomfort.
Musculocutaneous	Atraumatic isolated musculocutaneous neuropathies are rare. Reported cases have been associated with positioning during general anesthesia, peripheral nerve tumors, and strenuous upper extremity exercise without apparent underlying disease. Mechanisms proposed for these exercise-related cases include entrapment within the coracobrachialis, as well as traction between a proximal fixation point at the coracobrachialis and a distal fixation point at the deep fascia at the elbow.	Although a musculocutaneous lesion would be expected to demonstrate weakness of elbow flexion, one would not expect to see weakness in all shoulder motions with an injury isolated to the proximal musculocutaneous nerve. Other clinical features of musculocutaneous involvement include a loss of the biceps jerk, muscle atrophy, and loss of sensation to the anterior-lateral surface of the forearm.

(*Continued*)

TABLE 9-32. PERIPHERAL NERVE ENTRAPMENT SYNDROMES OF THE UPPER EXTREMITY (*Continued*)

SYNDROME	ENTRAPMENT SITE	DESCRIPTION OF FINDINGS
Cubital tunnel (ulnar entrapment at the elbow)	Five potential areas of ulnar nerve injury exist within its course to and out of the elbow. ▶ In 70% of the population, a tense sheet of fascia (the arcade of Struthers) stretches from the medial head of the triceps to insert into the medial intermuscular septum, arching over, and often compressing, the ulnar nerve approximately 6-8 cm above the medial epicondyle. ▶ The medial intermuscular septum presents a sharp edge that can indent the nerve, especially following anterior transposition where the nerve may be kinked. ▶ The cubital tunnel, floored by the medial collateral ligament of the elbow, is roofed by the strong arcuate ligament (retinaculum) stretching between the medial humeral epicondyle and the medial aspect of the olecranon. Compression and scarring frequently occur within this tunnel. ▶ The arching band of aponeurosis between the two heads of the flexor carpi ulnaris (Osborne band) often compresses the nerve, especially during repetitive contraction of the muscle. ▶ The aponeurotic covering between the flexors digitorum profundus and superficialis is an occasional site of compression. ▶ Other causes include: an increased carrying angle at the elbow, repetitive trauma to the flexed elbow, ruptured ulnar collateral ligament permitting the nerve to sublux.	Ulnar neuropathy at the elbow may be posttraumatic or nontraumatic. Trauma may be a single event or in mild repetitive form; the pathophysiological basis for the traumatic neuropathy likely is scarring and adhesion at the cubital tunnel or under the flexor carpi ulnaris aponeurosis. Patients with nontraumatic ulnar neuropathy often have jobs that require repetitive elbow flexion and extension or prolonged resting of the elbow on a hard surface, such as a desk. Elbow flexion narrows the cubital tunnel because of traction on the arcuate ligament and bulging of the medial collateral ligament. The nerve also elongates with elbow flexion, increasing intraneural pressure. With scarring and adhesion on the epineurium, elongation accentuates the tethering effect on the axons. Nocturnal paresthesia and pain usually are associated with sleeping with the elbow in flexion. A rare form of occupational ulnar neuropathy occurs in concert pianists, whose forceful and repetitive wrist flexion causes slamming of the nerve by the aponeurotic arch between the two heads of the flexor carpi ulnaris. Spontaneous subluxation of the ulnar nerve out of the cubital tunnel occurs in 15% of the population, which may aggravate symptoms of entrapment by the rubbing action exerted by the bony surfaces. Early symptoms include intermittent paresthesia along the ring and little fingers and discomfort along the medial aspect of the forearm. Pain usually comes later, as a deep ache around the elbow region, and often is exacerbated suddenly when the medial elbow is brushed accidentally. Gentle tapping of the nerve at and around the cubital tunnel elicits distressing electrical shock and/or tingling down the ulnar fingers. There may be diminished sensitivity to pinprick, light touch, and two-point discrimination on the ulnar pad of the fifth finger and along the ulnar split-half of the fourth finger. Provocative test with sustained elbow flexion or combined with gentle digital pressure on the cubital tunnel brings out the symptoms of paresthesia and pain. Weakness of finger abductors and adductors is variable. Late symptoms include dense numbness and profound weakness and atrophy of the intrinsic hand muscles. The last two digits assume the classic ulnar claw hand, with extension at the metacarpal phalangeal joints and flexion at the intraphalangeal joints. The old, "burnt out" neuropathic hand often is atrophic, weak, and thin-skinned but, surprisingly, painless and free of other sensory phenomena.

Pronator teres (median nerve)	Compromise of median nerve as it passes through the two heads of the pronator teres. Sites of compression include the lacertus fibrosus (bicipital aponeurosis, superficial forearm fascia), the Struthers ligament (thickened or aberrant origin of pronator teres from distal humerus), the pronator teres (musculofascial band or compression between 2 muscular heads), and the FDS proximal arch or the flexor digitorum superficialis.	Signs and symptoms: These include pain in the volar forearm that is exacerbated with activity and relieved by rest; decreased sensation in the thumb, index finger, long finger, and radial side of the ring finger; weakness of thenar muscles; and a positive Tinel or Phalen sign in the proximal forearm.
Anterior interosseous (median nerve)	Causative factors include tendinous bands, a deep head of the pronator teres, accessory muscles (including the Gantzer muscle, which is the accessory head of the FPL), aberrant radial artery branches, and fractures.	Symptoms include vague pain in the proximal forearm and weakness of the FPL and FDP to the index finger. Affected persons cannot form a circle by pinching their thumb and index finger (ie, hyperextension of index distal interphalangeal joint and thumb interphalangeal joint). Sensory involvement is not described.
Posterior interosseous (radial nerve)	PIN compression most commonly is associated with tendinous hypertrophy of the arcade of Frohse and fibrous thickening of the radiocapitellar joint capsule. Vascular compression by a hypertrophic leash of Henry has been reported. Lesions, such as lipoma, synovial cyst, rheumatoid synovitis, and vascular aneurysms, have been found in some cases. Hobbies or occupations associated with repetitive and forceful supination predispose to PIN neuropathy. Repetitive wrist flexion maneuvers compress the nerve as it enters the dorsal wrist capsule, inciting symptomatic inflammation. Chronic trauma to the flexion surface of the forearm likewise causes problems. For example, the constricting rings of the Canadian crutches, which exert direct pressure over the supinator surface, typically cause PIN neuropathy in paraplegic patients.	Because the posterior interosseous syndrome (PIN) purely affects a motor nerve, sensory symptoms are minor. A dull, aching pain sometimes is present over the front of the elbow, and palpation over the radiohumeral joint often aggravates the pain, probably due to irritation of the nervi nervorum of the PIN. Motor paralysis of the extensor muscles often is heralded by a feeling of fatigue during finger extension and elbow supination. Extension in the metacarpal phalangeal joints is weakened but not in the interphalangeal joints, since the latter is affected by the lumbricals. Because the index and fifth fingers receive both their own extensor tendon and tendon branch from the common extensor, they are less affected than extension of the third and fourth digits. Thus, in the early stage of entrapment, the hand exhibits a characteristic pattern on finger extension where the middle two fingers fail to extend, while the index and little fingers hold erect. Progression of paralysis eventually causes weakness in all of the finger extensors and in thumb abduction. Since the radial wrist extensors are spared because of their proximal innervation, wrist extension weakness usually is undetectable in spite of weakness of the ulnar wrist extensor.

(*Continued*)

TABLE 9-32. PERIPHERAL NERVE ENTRAPMENT SYNDROMES OF THE UPPER EXTREMITY *(Continued)*

SYNDROME	ENTRAPMENT SITE	DESCRIPTION OF FINDINGS
Radial tunnel	The deep branch of the radial nerve can be compressed by 5 structures within the radial tunnel. The most common site of compression is at the proximal fibrous edge of the supinator muscle, known as the arcade of Frohse. The most proximal structure that can compress the deep branch of the radial nerve is the fibrous fascia over the radiocapitellar joint. The next structures that can compress the deep branch of the radial nerve are the radial recurrent artery and the venae comitantes, known as the leash of Henry, although this is uncommon. Lastly, the deep branch of the radial nerve can also be compressed by the distal edge of the supinator muscle, which is known to be fibrous in 50%-70% of patients.	Symptoms: These may include pain in the upper extensor forearm; dysesthesia in a superficial radial nerve distribution; and weakening of the extension of the fingers, thumb, or wrist
Wartenberg's syndrome (superficial radial)	A compression of the superficial sensory radial nerve. Inflammation of the tendons of the first dorsal compartment can result in superficial radial neuritis.	Pain, paresthesias, and numbness of the radial aspects of the hand and wrist. In addition, the tendons of the brachioradialis and extensor carpi radialis longus (ECRL) muscles can press on the nerve in a scissor-like fashion when the forearm is pronated, causing a proximal tethering on the distal segment of the nerve at the wrist. Wartenberg's sign is described wherein the patient is asked to extend the fingers and abduction or clawing of the little finger occurs.
Guyon canal (deep ulnar nerve)	After entering the Guyon canal, the deep motor branch first supplies the abductor digiti minimi (ADM), then crosses under one head of the flexor digiti minimi (FDM), supplies this muscle, and crosses over to supply the opponens digiti minimi before rounding the hook of the hamate to enter the mid palmar space. Depending on the exact site of compression within the Guyon canal, the ADM or both the ADM and the FDM may be spared. The opponens always is affected, together with the interossei, ulnar lumbricals, and the adductor pollicis. Proximal compression within the Guyon canal often is attributed to thickening of the tendonous arch stretched between the pisiform and hamate. The hook of the hamate may be sharp-edged and forms an acute angle where the nerve turns radially. Injury to the nerve in this distal part of the canal may be accentuated by fibrous bands. The distal canal also is the common site for ganglions.	The vulnerable candidates include paraplegics using hand crutches that have a horizontal bar across the palm, motorcyclists who firmly grasp the hand bar control, weightlifters, and operators of pneumatic drills. The classic picture is a young man presenting with painless atrophy of the hypothenar muscles and interossei, with sparing of the thenar group. Variable sensory loss over the ulnar fingers or hypothenar eminence, together with aching pain in the palm, may be present in patients whose sensory branch is a recurrent nerve arising from within the proximal canal.

Carpal tunnel (median nerve)	Median nerve compression at the wrist is by the transverse carpal ligament (TCL), which attaches to and arches between the pisiform and hamate ulnarly and the scaphoid and trapezium radially. The palmar fascia is fused to the TCL proximally and then fans out to the soft tissue of the palmar skin as the palmar aponeurosis. The combined layers of the TCL and proximal palmar fascia form the flexor retinaculum. The palmaris longus tendon inserts in the palmar aponeurosis and lies directly over the median nerve just proximal to the TCL. It serves as the most reliable guide to the nerve at operation. The palmaris longus is absent in 25% of healthy individuals, in which case the nerve is beneath a fascial membrane midway between the flexor carpi radialis and the flexor digitorum superficialis tendons. Typically, the median palmar cutaneous nerve originates from the radial side of the median nerve proximal to or just deep to the flexor retinaculum, then tunnels through this structure to innervate the thenar eminence and the palm roughly up to the vertical line overlying the fourth metacarpal. The motor nerve to the thenar muscles also leaves the median nerve radially just beyond the distal edge of the flexor retinaculum, but variant nerves may pierce through the flexor retinaculum or arise from the ulnar aspect of the median nerve and an accessory motor branch may even emerge proximal to the flexor retinaculum. Ten percent of ulnar nerves and 4% of ulnar arteries lie radial to the hook of the hamate outside of the Guyon canal, which places them at risk for injury during carpal tunnel surgery.	Dull, aching pain at the wrist that extends up the forearm to the elbow. The pain typically is worse at night, disturbing sleep and is often associated with paresthesia in the median fingers and thumb on awakening. Sensation is decreased at the palmar pads of the thumb and index finger. In long-standing cases, the abductor pollicis brevis (APB) is weak and atrophic, causing thinning of the lateral contour of the thenar bulk. The flexor pollicis brevis is dually innervated by both the median and ulnar nerves and is unaffected. The opponens pollicis is affected very late. Forced wrist flexion causes increasing paresthesia and pain (Phalen sign), as does extreme wrist extension. Gentle tapping of the nerve over the flexor retinaculum sets off paresthesia (Tinel sign).

Data from Hollis MH, Lemay DE. *Nerve Entrapment Syndromes of the Lower Extremity.* Emedicine, 2005: http://www.emedicine.com/orthoped/topic422.htm; and Pang D. *Nerve Entrapment Syndromes.* Emedicine, 2004: http://www.emedicine.com/med/topic2909.htm.

designations, such as bulbospinal muscular atrophy, hereditary motor neuronopathy (HMN), and progressive muscular atrophy, have been used. The diversity of symptom distribution associated with this condition differ based on age of onset, the mode of inheritance, and its progression.

Patients with disorders of the motor unit present with predominantly LMN signs. Hypotonia can be demonstrated by a variety of bedside maneuvers. The traction response (pulling the patient upright to a sitting position by the hands) normally results in minimal head lag in term infants; hypotonic patients are unable to maintain an upright head position, falling forward. Vertical suspension (ie, lifting the patient upright with the clinician's hands under the axilla) also results in the patient's head falling forward. When a hypotonic infant is suspended horizontally (ie, held horizontally by supporting the trunk), the head and legs hang limply.

Arthrogryposis, or deformities of the limbs and joints at birth, results from in utero hypotonia. Skeletal deformities also can be seen. In the infant/newborn, fasciculations most often are restricted to the tongue, but they can be difficult to distinguish from normal random movements unless atrophy is also present. Atrophy suggests motor unit dysfunction but can occur in cerebral hypotonia. However, the combination of atrophy and fasciculations is strong evidence for denervation.

Pectus excavatum is present when the infant has longstanding weakness in the muscles of the chest wall, and as plantar flexor muscles become weaker, the foot everts into an equinovarus posture. In the SMAs, while bulbar symptoms may be present, sensory and corticospinal tract signs and sphincter abnormalities are absent.

Guillain-Barré Syndrome

Guillain-Barré syndrome (GBS) is a heterogeneous grouping of immune-mediated processes generally characterized by motor, sensory, and autonomic dysfunction.[404-415] Peripheral nerves and spinal roots are the major sites of demyelination, but cranial nerves also may be involved.

The typical GBS patient presents 2 to 4 weeks after a relatively benign respiratory or gastrointestinal illness complaining of dysesthesias of the fingers and lower extremity proximal muscle weakness. The weakness may progress over hours to days to involve the arms, truncal muscles, cranial nerves, and the muscles of respiration. The illness progresses from days to weeks. A plateau phase of persistent, unchanging symptoms then ensues followed days later by gradual symptom improvement. Up to one third of patients require mechanical ventilation during the course of their illness. Causes for this include cranial nerve involvement affecting airway maintenance and respiratory muscle paralysis.

The role of physical therapy includes:

- Maintain respiratory function using pulmonary physical therapy, and improve cardiovascular endurance.
- Prevent secondary impairments.
  - Skin breakdown.
  - Contractures.

- Prevent injury to denervated muscles.
- Splinting and positioning.

- Muscle reeducation through active assistance and active exercise progressing to resistive exercises.
- Energy conservation techniques.
- Functional progression as appropriate.

AMYOTROPHIC LATERAL SCLEROSIS

Amyotrophic lateral sclerosis (ALS), or Lou Gehrig's disease, is an idiopathic disease characterized by slowly progressive degeneration of upper and lower motor neurons.[416-423] While ALS is ultimately a diffuse disease, onset is often focal and asymmetric. At onset, bulbar motor neurons can be involved, resulting in:

- Progressive bulbar palsy, characterized by a slurring of words, or choking during a meal.
- Limb weakness (spinal muscular atrophy) if spinal cord anterior horn cells are affected.

Upper motor neuron involvement of spinal cord tracks results in spastic weakness of the limbs (primary lateral sclerosis). Later, spread to other motor areas produces the classic combination of upper and lower motor neuron dysfunction recognized as ALS:

- Arm weakness, charaterized by wrist drop that interferes with the patient's work performance.
- Leg weakness, charaterized by foot drop resulting in the patient stumbling or falling.
- Lower motor neuron signs.
- Ocular, sensory, or autonomic dysfunction occurs only very late in the disease course.
- Respiratory impairments, which eventually prove fatal.

The medical intervention includes the use of disease modifying agents for symptomatic management.

The physical therapy role with ALS is restorative intervention focusing on remediating or improving impairments and functional limitations. This includes:

- Maintenance of respiratory function (airway clearance techniques, cough facilitation, breathing exercises, chess stretching, suctioning, incentive spirometry).
- Prevention of secondary impairments.
  - Skin breakdown.
  - Contractures.
  - Injury to denervated muscles.
  - Splinting and positioning.
- Muscle reeducation.
- Energy conservation techniques and activity pacing.
- Improve or maintain cardiovascular endurance.
- Maintain maximal functional independence.
- Prescribe assistive devices and adaptive equipment as appropriate.
- Patient, family, caregiver education.

POSTPOLIO SYNDROME

Accepted criteria for diagnosis of postpolio syndrome (PPS) are a prior history of poliomyelitis, a stable period after recovery, a residual deficit of the initial polio, new muscle weakness, and, sometimes, new muscle atrophy.[424-434] Fatigue and muscle pain need not be present to meet the criteria for the syndrome. PPS symptoms tend to occur first in the weaker muscles. In individuals without polio or PPS, the functional consequences of aging and loss of motor units may be unnoticeable until a very advanced age. In the individual with PPS, any further loss of strength may be more readily apparent. A number of functional etiologies for weakness have been hypothesized, including disuse, overuse, and chronic weakness, as well as weight gain.

Difficulty with gait is caused by progressive weakness, pain, osteoarthritis, or joint instability; it is common in patients who previously used assistive devices but later discarded them.

Progressive weakness and atrophy may be observed in muscles that were affected initially by the poliovirus or in muscles that were spared clinically, which tends to happen in an asymmetric distribution. Fasciculations sometimes can be observed in atrophic muscles, as a result of the lower motor neuron injury.

The intervention for individuals with PPS include energy conservation and pacing one's activities. Reports on exercises are conflicting, but the key factor seems to be that strengthening exercises should be nonfatiguing. A specific suggestion is to exercise every other day, and the perceived rate of exertion should be less than "very hard" (see Chapter 17). Loads should be held for only 4 to 5 seconds, and there should be a 10-second rest between bouts and a 5-minute rest between sets. The patient should perform about 3 sets of 5 to 10 repetitions.

In addition to specifying exercises for those body areas experiencing the deleterious effects of disuse, the exercise prescription also should consider how to protect (1) muscles and joints that are experiencing the adverse effects of overuse and (2) body areas with very significant chronic weakness (generally, areas where the muscles have less than antigravity strength on manual muscle testing).

Electrical stimulation has been used to strengthen weakened muscles or to re-educate muscles weakened through disuse, as well as to decrease pain.

For myofascial pain, heat, electrical stimulation, trigger point injections, stretching exercises, biofeedback, and muscle relaxation exercises can be used.

For gait disturbances, assistive devices can be used, but sometimes patients refuse because of the philosophy of "not giving in." Treatment also can involve limitation of ambulation to shorter distances and the use of orthotics for joint protection.

Patients usually benefit from different adaptive techniques and equipment to perform any activities of daily living.

A speech therapy evaluation usually is recommended with any suggestion of swallowing problems.

NEUROLOGICAL REHABILITATION

Recovery is the reacquisition of movement skills lost through injury.[435] With complete recovery, the performance of the reacquired skills is identical in every way to preinjury performance.[436] Recovery can be categorized into two main types[436]:

- Spontaneous recovery: results from repair processes occurring immediately after the insult.
- Function-induced recovery: the neural reorganization that occurs as a result of increased use of involved body segments in behaviorally relevant tasks.

Study Pearl

- Compensation is defined as behavioral substitution, that is, alternative behavioral strategies are adopted to complete a task.[435]
- Neuroplasticity is the ability of the brain to change and repair itself. Mechanisms of neuroplasticity include neuroanatomical (neural regeneration via nerve growth factors and regenerative synaptogenesis), neurochemical, and neuroreceptive changes.[436]

Theories of Neurological Rehabilitation

Constraint-Induced Movement Therapy. Constraint-induced movement therapy has demonstrated significant improvements of upper extremity function.[437-442] Two factors, which are critical to successful outcomes achieved with these techniques include:

- The concentrated and repetitive practice of the involved upper extremity.
- The restriction of movement in the uninvolved upper extremity so that the patient is forced to use their involved side to perform functional movements.

Task-Oriented Approach. The task-oriented, or systems, approach is based on the current understanding of how movement arises. Central to this approach is the idea that specific task-oriented training combined with extensive practice is essential to reacquiring skill and enhancing recovery.[436] This approach views the entire body as a mechanical system with many interacting subsystems that all work together to manage and control internal and environmental influences. In this approach, the movement is organized around a behavioral goal (using behavioral shaping techniques) but is constrained by the environment. This encourages the predictive and adaptive control of movement.

Using observation of functional performance, analysis of the strategies or compensations used to accomplish tasks, and the assessment of impairments, the clinician focuses on resolving impairments, designing and implementing compensation strategies, and retraining the patient by means of functional activities.[443]

Impairment-Focused Interventions. Impairment-focused training includes training of developmental activity, the motor system, movement patterns, and neuromuscular reeducation.[436] A key concept of this approach is the use of sensory input to modify the CNS and to stimulate motor output. Two of the most popular approaches include neurodevelopmental treatment (NDT) and proprioceptive neuromuscular facilitation (PNF).

Neurodevelopmental Treatment. The neuromotor development treatment (NDT) approach, originated from the work of Karl and Berta Bobath who based their approach on the hierarchical model of neurophysiologic function. According to this approach, a maturational lag in the integration of primitive postural reflexes is often found in learning-disabled children. Based on this theory, it is assumed that abnormal postural reflex activity and abnormal muscle tone is caused by the loss of CNS control at the brainstem and spinal cord levels.

Thus the emphasis of NDT is on the inhibiting/integrating the primitive postural patterns (avoiding abnormal and compensatory patterns of movement), the promotion of the development of normal postural reactions, and the normalization of abnormal tone. The NDT approach uses facilitatory, inhibitory and reinforcement techniques:

- Inhibition: designed to decrease/inhibit the capacity to initiate a movement response to altered synaptic potential, using positioning and the use of specific movement patterns.
- Facilitation: designed to elicit voluntary muscular contraction through guided and assisted movement.
- Reinforcement of the inhibition of abnormal behavior through repeated use and development of the released normal movement.

The other key areas of treatment of this approach include:

- Normalization of postural alignment and stability.
- Normalization of sensory/perceptual experiences.
- Resumption of normal functional activities through meaningful and goal-oriented patterns of movement.

Proprioceptive Neuromuscular Facilitation. The concept of proprioceptive neuromuscular facilitation (PNF), also termed complex motions, was developed by Dr. Hermann Kabat, then by Sherrington, and finally by Margaret Knott and Dorothy Voss. The background and techniques of PNF are described in detail Chapter 17.

The Brunnstrom Approach. The Brunnstrom approach is based on the hierarchical model that uses a combination of very precise observations of the sequential changes in motor function that typically occur following stroke combined with an understanding of the reflex function of the nervous system. The Brunnstrom approach, which emphasizes synergy patterns, is rarely utilized these days, except for stroke patients, Brunnstrom's observations have enabled clinician's to document patient progress based on her 7 stages of recovery (see Table 14-3).

Integrated Approach. This approach considers a number of factors[444]:

- Variability in practice to facilitate skill transfer to a novel condition based on the constant practice.
- Intratask and in intertask organization performed randomly or serially, to create the regeneration of a motor plan which ultimately facilitates recall of the task.
- The use of functional activities and pre-gait activities (as appropriate):
  - Bed mobility:
    - Rolling to side lying
    - Rolling to prone
    - Scooting up in bed
    - Supine to short sitting
  - Repositioning in a chair:
    - Sit to stand
    - Lateral weight relief
    - Anterior/posterior weight relief

- Arising from the floor:
  - Pulling up on support (anterior approach)
  - Pushing up (posterior support)
  - Arising from the half-kneel position
  - Gait progression (see Chapter 7)

Cognitive Rehabilitation. Cognitive rehabilitation is designed to improve cognitive functions, functional abilities, and to increase levels of self-management and independence following damage to the CNS. The approach generally emphasizes restoring lost functions and teaching compensatory strategies to circumvent impaired cognitive functions, thereby improving competence in performing instrumental activities of daily living (IADLs). There are a number of treatment approaches to cognitive rehabilitation[445]:

- Retraining approach (transfer of training), which is based on the supposition that a disruption in one brain region can have a unconstructive impact on brain functioning as a whole. The approach focuses on the remediation of any underlying skills that the patient has lost by focusing on doing specifically selected perceptual exercises so that practicing one particular cognitive perceptual requirement will enhance performance in other tasks with similar perceptual demands.
- Restorative cognitive rehabilitation (RCR) is based on the theory that the performance of repetitive exercise can lead to the restoration of lost functions by targeting internal cognitive processes to produce improvements in real-world environments. Tasks include auditory, visual and verbal stimulation and practice, number manipulation, performance feedback, reinforcement, video feedback and behavior modification.
- Sensory integrative approach, which involves the integration of basic sensorimotor functions (tactile, proprioceptive, and vestibular) that proceed in a developmental sequence. The goal of the treatment is to stimulate sensorimotor responses and can include rubbing or icing to provide sensory input, resistance, and weight-bearing to impart proprioceptive input, and the use of spinning to provide vestibular input.
- Neurofunctional approach: the focus of this approach is on retraining life skills rather than on retraining specific cognitive and perceptual processes.
- Compensatory cognitive rehabilitation (CCR), which is designed to develop external prosthetic assistance for dysfunctions by employing visual cues, written instructions, memory notebooks, etc to trigger behavior.

MANAGEMENT STRATEGIES FOR SPECIFIC CONDITIONS

STRATEGIES TO MANAGE HYPERTONIA

Essential to the management of hypertonia (spasticity) is the avoidance of noxious stimuli by prompting intervention for urinary tract complications, proper skin care, and prevention of thrombophlebitis and heterotopic ossification.[446] The precise handling of a spastic limb is important and requires constant, firm manual contacts positioned over non-spastic areas.[4] Specific intervention techniques that can be used include[4]:

- Prolonged icing.
- Prolonged slow stretch.
- Inhibitory deep pressure.
- Retention of body heat.
- Relaxation through rhythmic rotation
- Neuromuscular electrical stimulation (NMES).[447]
- Transcutaneous electrical nerve stimulation (TENS).[448]

Serial Casting. This method by which a series of casts are applied to a joint to reduce contracture, is used when the patient is at risk for development of contractures and deformity, or demonstrates ineffective movement patterns or severe limitations in hygiene and skin care.[4] The limb is moved into its fully lengthened range using inhibitory and ROM techniques.[4] The cast is then applied. Each time a cast is removed (every 5 to 7 days), the joint is further stretched to its comfortable end-range and then recasted.[449-453]

Strategies to Manage Hypotonia

A number of approaches can be used to counteract hyotonia. These include:

- Range of motion exercises applied in conjunction with proper positioning and splinting. A daily program of stretching helps restore the resting length of a muscle and can prevent contracture.
- Strengthening exercises using active or resisted exercises, including proprioceptive neuromuscular facilitation (PNF) to strengthen limbs, and prevent imbalances between agonist and antagonist muscle groups.

Vestibular Rehabilitation Therapy

Vestibular rehabilitation therapy (VRT) has been a highly effective modality for most individuals with disorders of the vestibular or central balance system, and is designed to promote habituation and compensation for deficits related to a wide variety of balance disorders.[455]

VRT is based on the use of existing neural mechanisms for adaptation, plasticity, and compensation. VRT exercise protocols aim to improve vestibulo-ocular control, increase the gain of the vestibulo-ocular reflex (VOR), improve postural strategies, and increase levels of motor control for movement. The cervical-ocular reflex (COR) may be developed as a substitution strategy for visual stability for deficits in the VOR during head movements.

Several factors must be considered when designing a VRT program for an individual patient, including

- The status of visual and proprioceptive systems.
- Physical strength.

Study Pearl

An effective VRT program uses a team of healthcare providers to assess and treat patients with balance disorders. This team should include a physician trained in the evaluation and treatment of balance disorders (typically a neuro-otologist, otolaryngologist, or neurologist), a vestibular or physical therapist trained in balance testing and vestibular therapy, and an occupational therapist.

- Motor skills.
- Integrity of the cerebellum.
- General physical health.
- Decision-making and cognitive abilities.
- Age.
- Memory.
- Presence of psychological and anxiety disorders.

VRT is typically designed as a clinician-directed patient-motivated home-based exercise protocol, with individuals visiting the clinician on a limited basis until compensation and habituation are complete and optimal balance is attained.

The accurate diagnosis and assessment of a patient is critical for a successful individualized VRT program. Optimal candidates have stable central or peripheral vestibular deficits; symptoms provide specific activities or stimuli; and intact cognitive, cerebellar, visual, and proprioceptive systems. Patient motivation is a significant factor in successful implementation of a VRT program. Although some reports are conflicting, vestibular exercises are generally effective regardless of a patient's age and duration of symptoms.

Study Pearl

Examples of VRT include:
- Visual target is stationary and the subject moves his or head back and forth while trying to maintain visual fixation on the target
- The visual target and head move in opposite directions while the subject tries to keep the target in focus.

Questions for this chapter and the entire book appear on the included CD-ROM, with additional questions at www.DuttonNPTE.com.

REFERENCES

1. Van de Graaff KM, Fox SI: Functional organization of the nervous system. In: Van de Graaff KM, Fox SI, eds. *Concepts of Human Anatomy and Physiology.* New York, NY: WCB/McGraw-Hill. 1999:371-406.
2. Martin J: Introduction to the central nervous system. In: Martin J, ed. *Neuroanatomy: Text and Atlas, 2nd ed.* New York, NY: McGraw-Hill. 1996:1-32.
3. Waxman SG: *Correlative Neuroanatomy, 24th ed.* New York, NY: McGraw-Hill. 1996.
4. O'Sullivan SB: Strategies to improve motor function. In: O'Sullivan SB, Schmitz TJ, eds. *Physical Rehabilitation, 5th ed.* Philadelphia. PA: FA Davis. 2007:473-522.
5. Sunderland S: *Nerves and Nerve Injuries.* Edinburgh, UK: E & S Livingstone, Ltd. 1968.
6. Rydevik B, Garfin SR: Spinal nerve root compression. In: Szabo RM, ed. *Nerve Compression Syndromes: Diagnosis and Treatment.* Thorofare, NJ: Slack. 1989:247-261.
7. Pratt N: *Anatomy of the Cervical Spine.* La Crosse, WI: Orthopaedic Section, APTA. 1996.
8. Bogduk N: Innervation and pain patterns of the cervical spine. In: Grant R, ed. *Physical Therapy of the Cervical and Thoracic Spine.* New York, NY: Churchill Livingstone. 1988.
9. Fawcett DW: The nervous tissue. In: Fawcett DW, ed. *Bloom and Fawcett: A Textbook of Histology.* New York, NY: Chapman & Hall. 1984:336-339.

10. Chusid JG: *Correlative Neuroanatomy & Functional Neurology, 19th ed.* Norwalk, CT: Appleton-Century-Crofts. 1985: 144-148.
11. Carter GT, Kilmer DD, Bonekat HW, et al: Evaluation of phrenic nerve and pulmonary function in hereditary motor and sensory neuropathy type 1. *Muscle Nerve.* 1992;15:459-456.
12. Bolton CF: Clinical neurophysiology of the respiratory system. *Muscle Nerve.* 1993;16:809-818.
13. Gozna ER, Harris WR: Traumatic winging of the scapula. *J Bone Joint Surg.* 1979;61A:1230-1233.
14. Kauppila LI: The long thoracic nerve: possible mechanisms of injury based on autopsy study. *J Shoulder Elbow Surg.* 1993;2: 244-248.
15. Kauppila LI, Vastamaki M: Iatrogenic serratus anterior paralysis: long-term outcome in 26 patients. *Chest.* 1996;109:31-34.
16. Post M: Orthopaedic management of neuromuscular disorders. In: Post M, Bigliani LU, Flatow EL, et al, eds. *The Shoulder: Operative Technique.* Baltimore, MD: Williams and Wilkins. 1998:201-234.
17. Kuhn JE, Plancher KD, Hawkins RJ: Scapular winging. *J Am Acad Orthop Surgeons.* 1995;3:319-325.
18. Reis FP, de Camargo AM, Vitti M, et al: Electromyographic study of the subclavius muscle. *Acta Anatomica.* 1979;105: 284-290.
19. Hoffman GW, Elliott LF: The anatomy of the pectoral nerves and its significance to the general and plastic surgeon. *Ann Surg.* 1987;205:504-507.
20. Delagi EF, Perotto A: Arm. In: Delagi EF, Perotto A, eds. *Anatomic Guide for the Electromyographer, 2nd ed.* Springfield, IL: Charles C Thomas. 1981:66-71.
21. Sunderland S: The musculocutaneous nerve. In: Sunderland S, ed. *Nerves and Nerve Injuries, 2nd ed.* Edinburgh, UK: Churchill Livingstone. 1978:796-801.
22. de Moura WG, Jr: Surgical anatomy of the musculocutaneous nerve: a photographic essay. *J Reconstr Microsurg.* 1985; 1:291-297.
23. Flatow EL, Bigliani LU, April EW: An anatomic study of the musculocutaneous nerve and its relationship to the coracoid process. *Clin Orthop.* 1989;244:166-171.
24. Stern PJ, Kutz JE: An unusual variant of the anterior interosseous nerve syndrome: a case report and review of the literature. *J Hand Surg.* 1980;5:32-34.
25. Hope PG: Anterior interosseous nerve palsy following internal fixation of the proximal radius. *J Bone and Joint Surg.* 1988; 70B:280-282.
26. Mannheimer JS, Lampe GN: *Clinical Transcutaneous Electrical Nerve Stimulation.* Philadelphia, PA: FA Davis. 1984:440-445.
27. McGuckin N: The T4 syndrome. In: Grieve GP, ed. *Modern Manual Therapy of the Vertebral Column.* New York, NY: Churchill Livingstone. 1986:370-376.
28. DeFranca GG, Levine LJ: The T4 syndrome. *J Manip Physiol Ther.* 1995;18:34-37.
29. Grieve GP: Thoracic musculoskeletal problems. In: Boyling JD, Palastanga N, eds. *Grieve's Modern Manual Therapy of the*

Vertebral Column, 2nd ed. Edinburgh, UK: Churchill Livingstone. 1994:401-428.

30. Warfel BS, Marini SG, Lachmann EA, et al: Delayed femoral nerve palsy following femoral vessel catheterization. *Arch Phys Med Rehabil.* 1993;74:1211-1215.
31. Hardy SL: Femoral nerve palsy associated with an associated posterior wall transverse acetabular fracture. *J Orthop Trauma.* 1997;11:40-42.
32. Papastefanou SL, Stevens K, Mulholland RC: Femoral nerve palsy: an unusual complication of anterior lumbar interbody fusion. *Spine.* 1994;19:2842-2844.
33. Fealy S, Paletta GA, Jr: Femoral nerve palsy secondary to traumatic iliacus muscle hematoma: course after nonoperative management. *J Trauma Inj Inf Crit Care.* 1999;47:1150-1152.
34. Ecker AD, Woltman HW: Meralgia paresthetica: a report of one hundred and fifty cases. *J Am Med Assn.* 1938;110:1650-1652.
35. Keegan JJ, Holyoke EA: Meralgia paresthetica: an anatomical and surgical study. *J Neurosurg.* 1962;19:341-345.
36. Reichert FL: Meralgia paresthetica; a form of causalgia relieved by interruption of the sympathetic fibers. *Surg Clin North Am.* 1933;13:1443.
37. Sunderland S: Traumatized nerves, roots and ganglia: musculoskeletal factors and neuropathological consequences. In: Knorr IM, Huntwork EH, eds. *The Neurobiologic Mechanisms in Manipulative Therapy.* New York, NY: Plenum Press. 1978:137-166.
38. Kenny P, O'Brien CP, Synnott K, et al: Damage to the superior gluteal nerve after two different approaches to the hip. *J Bone Joint Surg.* 1999;81B:979-981.
39. Lu J, Ebraheim NA, Huntoon M, et al: Anatomic considerations of superior cluneal nerve at posterior iliac crest region. *Clin Orthop Relat Res.* 1998;347:224-228.
40. Sogaard I: Sciatic nerve entrapment: case report. *J Neurosurg.* 1983;58:275-276.
41. Robinson DR: Pyriformis syndrome in relation to sciatic pain. *Am J Surg.* 1947;73:355-358.
42. Resnick D: *Diagnosis of Bone and Joint Disorders.* Philadelphia, PA: Saunders. 1995.
43. Ohsawa K, Nishida T, Kurohmaru M, et al: Distribution pattern of pudendal nerve plexus for the phallus retractor muscles in the cock. *Okajimas Folia Anatomica Japonica.* 1991;67:439-441.
44. Dommisse GF, Grobler L: Arteries and veins of the lumbar nerve roots and cauda equina. *Clin Orthop.* 1976;115:22-29.
45. Halle JS: Neuromusculoskeletal scan examination with selected related topics. In: Flynn TW, ed. *The Thoracic Spine and Rib Cage: Musculoskeletal Evaluation and Treatment.* Boston, MA: Butterworth-Heinemann. 1996:121-146.
46. Voight ML, Cook G: Impaired neuromuscular control: reactive neuromuscular training. In: Prentice WE, Voight ML, eds. *Techniques in Musculoskeletal Rehabilitation.* New York, McGraw-Hill, 2001:93-124.
47. Voight ML, Cook G, Blackburn TA: Functional lower quarter exercises through reactive neuromuscular training. In: Bandy WD, ed. *Current Trends for the Rehabilitation of the Athlete—Home Study Course.* La. Crosse, WI: Sports Physical Therapy Section, APTA, Inc. 1997.

48. Lephart SM, Henry TJ: Functional rehabilitation for the upper and lower extremity. *Orthop Clin North Am.* 1995;26:579-592.
49. McCloskey DI: Kinesthetic sensibility. *Physiol Rev.* 1978; 58:763-820.
50. Borsa PA, Lephart SM, Kocher MS, et al: Functional assessment and rehabilitation of shoulder proprioception for glenohumeral instability. *J Sport Rehabil.* 1994;3:84-104.
51. Lephart SM, Warner JJP, Borsa PA, et al: Proprioception of the shoulder joint in healthy, unstable and surgically repaired shoulders. *J Shoulder Elbow Surg.* 1994;3:371-380.
52. Lee WA: Anticipatory control of postural and task muscles during rapid arm flexion. *J Mot Behav.* 1980;12:185-196.
53. Barrack RL, Skinner HB, Buckley SL: Proprioception in the anterior cruciate deficient knee. *Am J Sports Med.* 1989;17:1-6.
54. Skinner HB, Wyatt MP, Hodgdon JA, et al: Effect of fatigue on joint position sense of the knee. *J Orthop Res.* 1986;4:112-118.
55. Williams GR, Chmielewski T, Rudolph KS, et al: Dynamic knee stability: current theory and implications for clinicians and scientists. *J Orthop Sports Phys Ther.* 2001;31:546-566.
56. Johnston RB, III., Howard ME, Cawley PW, et al: Effect of lower extremity muscular fatigue on motor control performance. *Med Sci Sports Exerc.* 1998;30:1703-1707.
57. Skinner HB, Barrack RL, Cook SD: Age-related decline in proprioception. *Clin Orthop.* 1984;184:208-211.
58. Barrett DS, Cobb AG, Bentley G: Joint proprioception in normal, osteoarthritic and replaced knees. *J Bone Joint Surg.* 1991;73-B: 53-56.
59. Barrett DS: Proprioception and function after anterior cruciate ligament reconstruction. *J Bone Joint Surg.* 1991;73B:833-837.
60. Beard DJ, Kyberd PJ, Fergusson CM, et al: Proprioception after rupture of the anterior cruciate ligament. An objective indication of the need for surgery? *J Bone Joint Surg.* 1993;75-B: 311-315.
61. Corrigan JP, Cashman WF, Brady MP: Proprioception in the cruciate deficient knee. *J Bone Joint Surg.* 1992;74-B:247-250.
62. Fremerey RW, Lobenhoffer P, Zeichen J, et al: Proprioception after rehabilitation and reconstruction in knees with deficiency of the anterior cruciate ligament: a prospective, longitudinal study. *J Bone Joint Surg Br.* 2000;82:801-806.
63. Voight M, Blackburn T: Proprioception and balance training and testing following injury. In: Ellenbecker TS, ed. *Knee Ligament Rehabilitation.* Philadelphia, PA: Churchill Livingstone. 2000: 361-385.
64. Meadows J: *A Rationale and Complete Approach to the Sub-Acute Post-MVA Cervical Patient.* Calgary, AB: Swodeam Consulting. 1995.
65. Berg K: Balance and its measure in the elderly: a review. *Physiolother Can.* 1989;41:240-246.
66. Federation of State Medical Boards of the United States: Model *Guidelines for the Use of Controlled Substances for the Treatment of Pain.* Euless, TX: The Federation. 1998.
67. Bogduk N: The anatomy and physiology of nociception. In: Crosbie J, McConnell J, eds. *Key Issues in Physiotherapy.* Oxford, UK: Butterworth-Heinemann. 1993:48-87.

68. Besson JM: The neurobiology of pain. *Lancet.* 1999;353: 1610-1615.
69. Melzack R, Wall PD: On the nature of cutaneous sensory mechanisms. *Brain.* 1962;85:331-356.
70. Melzack R: The gate theory revisited. In: LeRoy PL, ed. *Current Concepts in the Management of Chronic Pain.* Miami, FL: Symposia Specialists. 1977.
71. Nathan PW: The gate-control theory of pain: a critical review. *Brain.* 1976;99:123-158.
72. Mayer DJ, Price DD: Central nervous system mechanisms of analgesia. *Pain.* 1976;2:379-404.
73. Gilman S: The physical and neurologic examination. In: Gilman S, ed. *Clinical Examination of the Nervous System.* New York, NY: McGraw-Hill. 2000:15-34.
74. Gilman S: The mental status examination. In: Gilman S, ed. *Clinical Examination of the Nervous System.* New York, NY: McGraw-Hill. 2000:35-64.
75. Spangler LL: Nonprogressive spinal cord disorders. In: Cameron MH, Monroe LG, eds. *Physical Rehabilitation: Evidence-Based Examination, Evaluation, and Intervention.* St Louis, MO: Saunders/Elsevier. 2007:538-579.
76. Jordan LC, Hillis AE: Disorders of speech and language: aphasia, apraxia and dysarthria. *Curr Opin Neurol.* 2006;19: 580-585.
77. Kanter SJ, Factora RM, Suh TT: Does this patient have primary progressive aphasia? *Cleve Clin J Med.* 2006;73: 1025-1027.
78. Ozeren A, Koc F, Demirkiran M, et al: Global aphasia due to left thalamic hemorrhage. *Neurol India.* 2006;54:415-417.
79. Perneczky R, Diehl-Schmid J, Pohl C, et al: Non-fluent progressive aphasia: cerebral metabolic patterns and brain reserve. *Brain Res.* 2007;1133:178-185.
80. Benowitz LI, Moya KL, Levine DN: Impaired verbal reasoning and constructional apraxia in subjects with right hemisphere damage. *Neuropsychologia.* 1990;28:231-241.
81. Freeman FJ, Sands ES, Harris KS: Temporal coordination of phonation and articulation in a case of verbal apraxia: a voice onset time study. *Brain Lang.* 1978;6:106-111.
82. Sands ES, Freeman FJ, Harris KS: Progressive changes in articulatory patterns in verbal apraxia: a longitudinal case study. *Brain Lang.* 1978;6:97-105.
83. Galea M, Woodward M: Mini-Mental State Examination (MMSE). *Aust J Physiother.* 2005;51:198.
84. Mossello E, Boncinelli M: Mini-Mental State Examination: a 30-year story. *Aging Clin Exp Res.* 2006;18:271-273.
85. Hagen C, Malkmus D, Durham P: *Rancho Los Amigos Cognitive Scale.* Rancho Los Amigos Hospital, US. 1972.
86. Shumway-Cook A, Horak FB: Rehabilitation strategies for patients with vestibular deficits. *Neurol Clin.* 1990;8:441-457.
87. Shumway-Cook A, Horak FB: Assessing the influence of sensory interaction of balance. Suggestion from the field. *Phys Ther.* 1986;66:1548-1550.
88. Rogers JH: Romberg and his test. *J Laryngol Otol.* 1980;94: 1401-1404.

89. Wrisley DM, Walker ML, Echternach JL, èt al: Reliability of the dynamic gait index in people with vestibular disorders. *Arch Phys Med Rehabil.* 2003;84:1528-1533.
90. Whitney SL, Hudak MT, Marchetti GF: The dynamic gait index relates to self-reported fall history in individuals with vestibular dysfunction. *J Vestib Res.* 2000;10:99-105.
91. Piva SR, Fitzgerald GK, Irrgang JJ, et al: Get up and go test in patients with knee osteoarthritis. *Arch Phys Med Rehabil.* 2004;85:284-289.
92. Mathias S, Nayak US, Isaacs B: Balance in elderly patients: the "get-up and go" test. *Arch Phys Med Rehabil.* 1986;67:387-389.
93. Volkman KG, Stergiou N, Stuberg W, et al: Methods to improve the reliability of the functional reach test in children and adolescents with typical development. *Pediatr Phys Ther.* 2007;19:20-27.
94. Sousa N, Sampaio J: Effects of progressive strength training on the performance of the Functional Reach Test and the Timed Get-Up-and-Go Test in an elderly population from the rural north of Portugal. *Am J Hum Biol.* 2005;17:746-751.
95. Takahashi T, Ishida K, Yamamoto H, et al: Modification of the functional reach test: analysis of lateral and anterior functional reach in community-dwelling older people. *Arch Gerontol Geriatr.* 2006;42:167-173.
96. Franchignoni F, Velozo CA: Use of the Berg balance scale in rehabilitation evaluation of patients with Parkinson's disease. *Arch Phys Med Rehabil.* 2005;86:2225-2226; author reply 2226.
97. Kornetti DL, Fritz SL, Chiu YP, et al: Rating scale analysis of the Berg balance scale. *Arch Phys Med Rehabil.* 2004;85: 1128-1135.
98. Whitney S, Wrisley D, Furman J: Concurrent validity of the Berg balance scale and the Dynamic Gait Index in people with vestibular dysfunction. *Physiother Res Int.* 2003;8:178-186.
99. Feld JA, Rabadi MH, Blau AD, et al: Berg balance scale and outcome measures in acquired brain injury. *Neurorehabil Neural Repair.* 2001;15:239-244.
100. Wee JY, Bagg SD, Palepu A: The Berg balance scale as a predictor of length of stay and discharge destination in an acute stroke rehabilitation setting. *Arch Phys Med Rehabil.* 1999;80:448-452.
101. Faber MJ, Bosscher RJ, van Wieringen PC: Clinimetric properties of the performance-oriented mobility assessment. *Phys Ther.* 2006;86:944-954.
102. Tinetti ME: Performance-oriented assessment of mobility problems in elderly patients. *J Am Geriatr Soc.* 1986;34:119-126.
103. Dutton M: The nervous system. In: Dutton M, ed. *Orthopedic Examination, Evaluation, and Intervention.* New York, NY: McGraw-Hill. 2004:7-19.
104. Goldberg S: The four minute neurological examination. Miami, FL: Medmaster Inc. 1992.
105. Judge RD, Zuidema GD, Fitzgerald FT: Head. In: Judge RD, Zuidema GD, Fitzgerald FT, eds. *Clinical Diagnosis, 4th ed.* Boston, MA: Little, Brown and Company. 1982:123-151.
106. Meadows J: *Orthopedic Differential Diagnosis in Physical Therapy.* New York, NY: McGraw-Hill. 1999.
107. Adams RD, Victor M: *Principles of Neurology.* 5th ed. New York, NY: McGraw-Hill, Health Professions Division. 1993.

108. Nielsen JB, Crone C, Hultborn H: The spinal pathophysiology of spasticity—from a basic science point of view. *Acta Physiol Oxf.* 2007;189:171-180.
109. Jellinger KA: Spasticity management: a practical multidisciplinary guide. *Eur J Neurol.* 2007;14:e50.
110. Dones I, Nazzi V, Broggi G: The guidelines for the diagnosis and treatment of spasticity. *J Neurosurg Sci.* 2006;50:101-105.
111. Currier RD, Fitzgerald FT: Nervous system. In: Judge RD, Zuidema GD, Fitzgerald FT, eds. *Clinical Diagnosis.* 4th ed. Boston, MA: Little, Brown and Company. 1982:405-445.
112. Denno JJ, Meadows GR: Early diagnosis of cervical spondylotic myelopathy: a useful clinical sign. *Spine.* 1991;16:1353-1355.
113. Kori AA, Leigh JL: The cranial nerve examination. In: Gilman S, ed. *Clinical Examination of the Nervous System.* New York, McGraw-Hill. 2000:65-111.
114. Mehrholz J, Wagner K, Meissner D, et al: Reliability of the modified Tardieu scale and the modified Ashworth scale in adult patients with severe brain injury: a comparison study. *Clin Rehabil.* 2005;19:751-759.
115. Haas BM, Bergstrom E, Jamous A, et al: The inter rater reliability of the original and of the modified Ashworth scale for the assessment of spasticity in patients with spinal cord injury. *Spinal Cord.* 1996;34:560-564.
116. Allison SC, Abraham LD, Petersen CL: Reliability of the modified Ashworth scale in the assessment of plantarflexor muscle spasticity in patients with traumatic brain injury. *Int J Rehabil Res.* 1996;19:67-78.
117. Sloan RL, Sinclair E, Thompson J, et al: Inter-rater reliability of the modified Ashworth scale for spasticity in hemiplegic patients. *Int J Rehabil Res.* 1992;15:158-161.
118. Bohannon RW, Smith MB: Interrater reliability of a modified Ashworth scale of muscle spasticity. *Phys Ther.* 1987;67:206-207.
119. Watanabe S, Satumae T, Takeshima R, et al: Opisthotonos after flumazenil administered to antagonize midazolam previously administered to treat developing local anesthetic toxicity. *Anesth Analg.* 1998;86:677-678.
120. Cameron AE: Opisthotonos again. *Anaesthesia.* 1987;42:1124.
121. Schmitz TJ: Examination of coordination. In: O'Sullivan SB, Schmitz TJ, eds. *Physical Rehabilitation, 5th ed.* Philadelphia, PA: FA Davis. 2007:193-225.
122. Stern EB: Stability of the Jebsen-Taylor Hand Function Test across three test sessions. *Am J Occup Ther.* 1992;46:647-649.
123. Surrey LR, Nelson K, Delelio C, et al: A comparison of performance outcomes between the Minnesota Rate of Manipulation Test and the Minnesota Manual Dexterity Test. *Work.* 2003; 20:97-102.
124. Clopton N, Schafer S, Clopton JR, et al: Examinee position and performance on the Minnesota Rate of Manipulation Test. *J Rehabil.* 1984;50:46-48.
125. Gloss DS, Wardle MG: Use of the Minnesota Rate of Manipulation Test for disability evaluation. *Percept Mot Skills.* 1982;55:527-532.
126. Tian J, Zee DS, Walker MF: Rotational and translational optokinetic nystagmus have different kinematics. *Vision Res.* 2007.

127. Buttner U, Kremmyda O: Smooth pursuit eye movements and optokinetic nystagmus. *Dev Ophthalmol.* 2007;40:76-89.
128. Lee AG, Brazis PW: Localizing forms of nystagmus: symptoms, diagnosis, and treatment. *Curr Neurol Neurosci Rep.* 2006;6:414-420.
129. Chia L-G, Shen W-C: Wallenberg's lateral medullary syndrome with loss of pain and temperature sensation on the contralateral face: clinical, MRI and electrophysiological studies. *J Neurol.* 1993;240:462-467.
130. Kim JS, Lee JH, Suh DC, et al: Spectrum of lateral medullary syndrome: correlation between clinical findings and magnetic resonance imaging in 33 subjects. *Stroke.* 1994;25:1405-1410.
131. Jenkins IH, Frackowiak RSJ: Functional studies of the human cerebellum with positron emission tomography. *Rev Neurol.* 1993;149:647-653.
132. Molinari M, Leggio MG, Solida A, et al: Cerebellum and procedural learning: evidence from focal cerebellar lesions. *Brain.* 1997;120:1753-1762.
133. Kim SG, Ugurbil K, Strick PL: Activation of a cerebellar output nucleus during cognitive processing. *Science.* 1994;265: 949-951.
134. Pierrot-Deseilligny E, Mazieres L: Spinal mechanisms underlying spasticity. In: Delwaide PJ, Young RR, eds. *Clinical Neurophysiology in Spasticity: Contribution to Assessment and Pathophysiology.* Amsterdam, Elsevier BV. 1985:63-76.
135. Hoppenfeld S: *Orthopedic Neurology—A Diagnostic Guide to Neurological Levels.* Philadelphia, PA: JB Lippincott. 1977.
136. Ashby P, McCrea D: Neurophysiology of spinal spasticity. In: Davidoff RA, ed. *Handbook of the Spinal Cord.* New York, NY: Marcel Decker. 1987:119-143.
137. Meissner I, Wiebers DO, Swanson JW, et al: The natural history of drop attacks. *Neurology.* 1986;36:1029-1034.
138. Zeiler K, Zeitlhofer J: Syncopal consciousness disorders and drop attacks from the neurologic viewpoint. *Wien Klin Wochenschr.* 1988;100:93-99.
139. Kameyama M: Vertigo and drop attack. With special reference to cerebrovascular disorders and atherosclerosis of the vertebral-basilar system. *Geriatrics.* 1965;20:892-900.
140. Bardella L, Maleci A, Di Lorenzo N: Drop attack as the only symptom of type 1 Chiari malformation. Illustration by a case. (Italian). *Rivista di Patologia Nervosa e Mentale.* 1984;105:217-222.
141. Schochet SS, Jr: Intoxications and metabolic diseases of the central nervous system. In: Nelson JS, Parisi JE, Schochet SS, Jr, eds. *Principles and Practice of Neuropathology.* St. Louis, MO, Mosby. 1993:302-343.
142. Harper CG, Giles M, Finlay-Jones R: Clinical signs in the Wernicke-Korsakoff complex: a retrospective analysis of 131 cases diagnosed at necropsy. *J Neurol Neurosurg Psychiatry.* 1986; 49:341-345.
143. Brazis PW, Lee AG: Binocular vertical diplopia. *Mayo Clinic Proceedings.* 1998;73:55-66.
144. Giles CL, Henderson JW: Horner's syndrome: an analysis of 216 cases. *Am J Ophthalmol.* 1958;46:289-296.
145. Jermyn RT: A nonsurgical approach to low back pain. *JAOA.* 2001;101(suppl 2):S6-S11.

146. Attia J, Hatala R, Cook DJ, et al: Does this adult patient have acute meningitis? *JAMA.* 1999;282:175-181.
147. Fitch MT, van de Beek D: Emergency diagnosis and treatment of adult meningitis. *Lancet Infect Dis.* 2007;7:191-200.
148. Al-Tawfiq JA: Haemophilus influenzae type e meningitis and bacteremia in a healthy adult. *Intern Med.* 2007;46:195-198.
149. Verhoff MA, Bollensen E, Oehmke S, et al: Acute bacterial meningitis as the cause of a traffic accident. *J Clin Forensic Med.* 2007;14:175-7.
150. Bleck TP: Nosocomial meningitis. *Curr Infect Dis Rep.* 2007;9:1-2.
151. Torpy JM, Lynm C, Glass RM: JAMA patient page. Meningitis. *JAMA.* 2007;297:122.
152. Nigrovic LE, Kuppermann N, Macias CG, et al: Clinical prediction rule for identifying children with cerebrospinal fluid pleocytosis at very low risk of bacterial meningitis. *JAMA.* 2007;297:52-60.
153. Roper JD: Get S.M.A.R.T. about meningitis. School meningitis awareness resource tools: vaccination clinic resource guide. *School Nurse News.* 2006;23:38-41.
154. Nagafuchi M, Nagafuchi Y, Sato R, et al: Adult meningism and viral meningitis, 1997-2004: clinical data and cerebrospinal fluid cytokines. *Intern Med.* 2006;45:1209-1212.
155. Parner ET, Reefhuis J, Schendel D, et al: Hearing loss diagnosis followed by meningitis in Danish children, 1995-2004. *Otolaryngol Head Neck Surg.* 2007;136:428-433.
156. Matos JO, Arruda AM, Tomita S, et al: Cryptococcus meningitis and reversible hearing loss. *Rev Bras Otorrinolaringol (Engl Ed).* 2006;72:849.
157. Hadjiev DI, Mineva PP: A reappraisal of the definition and pathophysiology of the transient ischemic attack. *Med Sci Monit.* 2007;13:RA50- RA53.
158. Harris DR: As simple as ABCD: identifying patients at high risk of stroke soon after a transient ischemic attack. *Can Fam Physician.* 2006;52:1553-1555.
159. Prabhakaran S: Reversible brain ischemia: lessons from transient ischemic attack. *Curr Opin Neurol.* 2007;20:65-70.
160. Barrett KM, Johnston KC: New transient ischemic attack guidelines: a step forward but journey just begun. *Ann Neurol.* 2006;60:273-274.
161. Borja J, Izquierdo I, Garcia-Rafanell J: Prevention of stroke in patients with ischemic stroke or transient ischemic attack. *Stroke.* 2006;37:2653; author reply 2654.
162. Caplan LR: Transient ischemic attack: definition and natural history. *Curr Atheroscler Rep.* 2006;8:276-280.
163. Pokorski RJ: Morbidity and mortality associated with transient ischemic attack (TIA). *J Insur Med.* 1996;28:136-141.
164. Kang SD: Ruptured anterior communicating artery aneurysm causing bilateral oculomotor nerve palsy: a case report. *J Korean Med Sci.* 2007;22:173-176.
165. Andaluz N, Tomsick TA, Keller JT, et al: Subdural hemorrhage in the posterior fossa caused by a ruptured cavernous carotid artery aneurysm after a balloon occlusion test. Case report. *J Neurosurg.* 2006;105:315-319.
166. Buckle C, Rabadi MH: Bilateral pontine infarction secondary to basilar trunk saccular aneurysm. *Arch Neurol.* 2006;63:1498-1499.

167. da Costa LB, Valiante T, Terbrugge K, et al: Anterior ethmoidal artery aneurysm and intracerebral hemorrhage. *AJNR Am J Neuroradiol.* 2006;27:1672-1674.
168. Fuse T, Umezu M, Yamamoto M, et al: External carotid artery aneurysm developing after embolization of a ruptured posterior inferior cerebellar artery aneurysm in a patient with cervicocephalic fibromuscular dysplasia—case report. *Neurol Med Chir (Tokyo).* 2006;46:290-293.
169. Saito H, Ogasawara K, Kubo Y, et al: Treatment of ruptured fusiform aneurysm in the posterior cerebral artery with posterior cerebral artery-superior cerebellar artery anastomosis combined with parent artery occlusion: case report. *Surg Neurol.* 2006;65:621-624.
170. Raghavan ML, Ma B, Harbaugh RE: Quantified aneurysm shape and rupture risk. *J Neurosurg.* 2005;102:355-362.
171. Agha A, Phillips J, Thompson CJ: Hypopituitarism following traumatic brain injury (TBI). *Br J Neurosurg.* 2007;21:210-216.
172. Kokiko ON, Hamm RJ: A review of pharmacological treatments used in experimental models of traumatic brain injury. *Brain Inj.* 2007;21:259-274.
173. Zehtabchi S, Sinert R, Soghoian S, et al: Identifying traumatic brain injury in patients with isolated head trauma: are arterial lactate and base deficit as helpful as in polytrauma? *Emerg Med J.* 2007;24:333-335.
174. Hartl R: Back to basics, or the evolution of traumatic brain injury management since Scipione Riva-Rocci. Crit Care Med. 2007; 35:1196-1197.
175. Irdesel J, Aydiner SB, Akgoz S: Rehabilitation outcome after traumatic brain injury. *Neurocirugia (Astur).* 2007;18:5-15.
176. Teasell R, Bayona N, Lippert C, et al: Post-traumatic seizure disorder following acquired brain injury. *Brain Inj.* 2007;21:201-214.
177. Scherer M: Gait rehabilitation with body weight-supported treadmill training for a blast injury survivor with traumatic brain injury. *Brain Inj.* 2007;21:93-100.
178. Pressman HT: Traumatic brain injury rehabilitation: case management and insurance-related issues. *Phys Med Rehabil Clin N Am.* 2007;18:165-174, viii.
179. Young JA: Pain and traumatic brain injury. *Phys Med Rehabil Clin N Am.* 2007;18:145-63, vii-viii.
180. Yen HL, Wong JT: Rehabilitation for traumatic brain injury in children and adolescents. *Ann Acad Med Singapore.* 2007;36:62-66.
181. Chua KS, Ng YS, Yap SG, et al: A brief review of traumatic brain injury rehabilitation. *Ann Acad Med Singapore.* 2007;36:31-42.
182. Ducrocq SC, Meyer PG, Orliaguet GA, et al: Epidemiology and early predictive factors of mortality and outcome in children with traumatic severe brain injury: experience of a French pediatric trauma center. *Pediatr Crit Care Med.* 2006;7:461-467.
183. Chesnut RM: The evolving management of traumatic brain injury: Don't shoot the messenger. *Crit Care Med.* 2006;34:2262; author reply 2262-2263.
184. Fulk GD: Traumatic brain injury. In: O'Sullivan SB, Schmitz TJ, eds. *Physical Rehabilitation, 5th ed.* Philadelphia, PA: FA Davis; 2007:895-935.
185. de Jong LD, Nieuwboer A, Aufdemkampe G: Contracture preventive positioning of the hemiplegic arm in subacute stroke

patients: a pilot randomized controlled trial. *Clin Rehabil.* 2006;20:656-667.

186. Chatterton HJ, Pomeroy VM, Gratton J: Positioning for stroke patients: a survey of physiotherapists' aims and practices. *Disabil Rehabil.* 2001;23:413-421.
187. Osgood SL, Kuczkowski KM: Autonomic dysreflexia in a parturient with spinal cord injury. *Acta Anaesthesiol Belg.* 2006;57:161-162.
188. Wu KP, Lai PL, Lee LF, et al: Autonomic dysreflexia triggered by an unstable lumbar spine in a quadriplegic patient. *Chang Gung Med J.* 2005;28:508-511.
189. Adiga S: Further lessons in autonomic dysreflexia. *Arch Phys Med Rehabil.* 2005;86:1891; author reply 1891.
190. Sullivan-Tevault M: Autonomic dysreflexia in spinal cord injury. *Emerg Med Serv.* 2005;34:79-80, 85.
191. Jacob C, Thwaini A, Rao A, et al: Autonomic dysreflexia: the forgotten medical emergency. *Hosp Med.* 2005;66:294-296.
192. Bycroft J, Shergill IS, Chung EA, et al: Autonomic dysreflexia: a medical emergency. *Postgrad Med J.* 2005;81:232-235.
193. Taylor AG: Autonomic dysreflexia in spinal cord injury. *Nurs Clin North Am.* 1974;9:717-725.
194. Fulk GD, Schmitz TJ, Behrman AL: Traumatic spinal cord injury. In: O'Sullivan SB, Schmitz TJ, eds. *Physical Rehabilitation.* 5th ed. Philadelphia, PA: FA Davis. 2007:937-996.
195. Czell D, Schreier R, Rupp R, et al: Influence of passive leg movements on blood circulation on the tilt table in healthy adults. *J Neuroengineering Rehabil.* 2004;1:4.
196. Jacobs PL, Mahoney ET, Robbins A, et al: Hypokinetic circulation in persons with paraplegia. *Med Sci Sports Exerc.* 2002;34:1401-1407.
197. Houtman S, Colier WN, Oeseburg B, et al: Systemic circulation and cerebral oxygenation during head-up tilt in spinal cord injured individuals. *Spinal Cord.* 2000;38:158-163.
198. Johnson RH, Spaulding JM: Disorders of the autonomic nervous system. Chapter 7. Some disorders of regional circulation. *Contemp Neurol Ser.* 1974;11:114-128.
199. American Spinal Injury Association: *International Standards for Neurological Classification of Spinal Cord Injury.* Chicago, IL: American Spinal Injury Association; 2002.
200. Field-Fote EC, Fluet GG, Schafer SD, et al: The spinal cord injury functional ambulation inventory (SCI-FAI). *J Rehabil Med.* 2001;33:177-181.
201. Greitz D: Unraveling the riddle of syringomyelia. *Neurosurg Rev.* 2006;29:251-263; discussion 264.
202. Milhorat TH: Classification of syringomyelia. *Neurosurg Focus.* 2000;8:E1.
203. Pearce JM: Syringes and syringomyelia. *Eur Neurol.* 2005;54:243.
204. Todor DR, Mu HT, Milhorat TH: Pain and syringomyelia: a review. *Neurosurg Focus.* 2000;8:E11.
205. Wollman DE: Syringomyelia: an uncommon cause of myelopathy in the geriatric population. *J Am Geriatr Soc.* 2004;52:1033-1034.
206. Ahn UM, Ahn NU, Buchowski JM, et al: Cauda equina syndrome secondary to lumbar disc herniation: a meta-analysis of surgical outcomes. *Spine.* 2000;25:1515-1522.
207. Brown KL: Cauda equina syndrome. Implications for the orthopaedic nurse in a clinical setting. *Orthop Nurs.* 1998;17:31-35; quiz 36-37.

208. Kennedy JG, Soffe KE, McGrath A, et al: Predictors of outcome in cauda equina syndrome. *Eur Spine.* 1999;J 8:317-322.
209. Orendacova J, Cizkova D, Kafka J, et al: Cauda equina syndrome. *Prog Neurobiol.* 2001;64:613-637.
210. Small SA, Perron AD, Brady WJ: Orthopedic pitfalls: cauda equina syndrome. *Am J Emerg Med.* 2005;23:159-163.
211. Karceski S: Multiple sclerosis: what have we learned? *Neurology.* 2007;68:E9-E10.
212. Antel J, Arnold D: The search for the missing links in multiple sclerosis. *Curr Neurol Neurosci Rep.* 2007;7:93-94.
213. Vanderlocht J, Hellings N, Hendriks JJ, et al: Current trends in multiple sclerosis research: an update on pathogenic concepts. *Acta Neurol Belg.* 2006;106:180-190.
214. Bruck W: New insights into the pathology of multiple sclerosis: towards a unified concept? *J Neurol.* 2007;254(suppl 1):I3-I9.
215. Holberg C, Finlayson M: Factors influencing the use of energy conservation strategies by persons with multiple sclerosis. *Am J Occup Ther.* 2007;61:96-107.
216. Sayao AL, Devonshire V, Tremlett H: Longitudinal follow-up of "benign" multiple sclerosis at 20 years. *Neurology.* 2007;68:496-500.
217. Pittock SJ: Does benign multiple sclerosis today imply benign multiple sclerosis tomorrow?: implications for treatment. *Neurology.* 2007;68:480-481.
218. Phillips JT: What causes multiple sclerosis to worsen? *Arch Neurol.* 2007;64:167-168.
219. Nortvedt MW, Riise T, Frugard J, et al: Prevalence of bladder, bowel and sexual problems among multiple sclerosis patients two to five years after diagnosis. *Mult Scler.* 2007;13:106-112.
220. Julian L, Merluzzi NM, Mohr DC: The relationship among depression, subjective cognitive impairment, and neuropsychological performance in multiple sclerosis. *Mult Scler.* 2007; 13:81-86.
221. Korostil M, Feinstein A: Anxiety disorders and their clinical correlates in multiple sclerosis patients. *Mult Scler.* 2007;13:67-72.
222. Mills R, Yap L, Young C: Treatment for ataxia in multiple sclerosis. *Cochrane Database Syst Rev.* 2007;CD005029.
223. Benedict RH, Bobholz JH: Multiple sclerosis. *Semin Neurol.* 2007;27:78-85.
224. Costello F: Myasthenia gravis and multiple sclerosis: a review of the ocular manifestations. *Insight.* 2006;31:19-22; quiz 23-24.
225. Rajasekaran D, Chandrasekar S, Rajendran M: Drug related crisis in myasthenia gravis. *J Assoc Physicians India.* 2006; 54:820-821.
226. Hartl DM, Leboulleux S, Klap P, et al: Myasthenia gravis mimicking unilateral vocal fold paralysis at presentation. *J Laryngol Otol.* 2007;121:174-178.
227. Conti-Fine BM, Milani M, Kaminski HJ: Myasthenia gravis: past, present, and future. *J Clin Invest.* 2006;116:2843-2854.
228. Toyka KV: Ptosis in myasthenia gravis: extended fatigue and recovery bedside test. *Neurology.* 2006;67:1524.
229. Meenakshisundaram S: Myasthenia gravis in older patients. *Age Ageing.* 2006;35:542.
230. Benatar M: A systematic review of diagnostic studies in myasthenia gravis. *Neuromuscul Disord.* 2006;16:459-467.

231. Romi F, Gilhus NE, Aarli JA: Myasthenia gravis: disease severity and prognosis. *Acta Neurol Scand Suppl.* 2006;183:24-25.
232. Singh R, Pentland B: Myasthenia gravis masquerading as post-poliomyelitis syndrome. *J Rehabil Med.* 2006;38:136-137.
233. Cheesman M, Kessell G: First presentation of myasthenia gravis. *Anaesthesia.* 2006;61:66.
234. Budrys V: A portrait of myasthenia gravis? *Eur Neurol.* 2005; 54:240-241.
235. Poudel M, Angel GM, Neopane A, et al: A typical case of Myasthenia Gravis. *Kathmandu Univ Med J.* 2003;1:193-196.
236. Alarcon GS: Infections in systemic connective tissue diseases: systemic lupus erythematosus, scleroderma, and polymyositis/dermatomyositis. *Infect Dis Clin North Am.* 2006;20:849-875.
237. Yoshidome Y, Morimoto S, Tamura N, et al: A case of polymyositis complicated with myasthenic crisis. *Clin Rheumatol.* 2006;26:1569-70.
238. Pongratz D: Therapeutic options in autoimmune inflammatory myopathies (dermatomyositis, polymyositis, inclusion body myositis). *J Neurol.* 2006;253:v64-v65.
239. Lundberg IE: The heart in dermatomyositis and polymyositis. *Rheumatology (Oxford).* 2006;45(suppl 4):iv18-iv21.
240. Senechal M, Crete M, Couture C, et al: Myocardial dysfunction in polymyositis. *Can J Cardiol.* 2006;22:869-871.
241. Ytterberg SR: Treatment of refractory polymyositis and dermatomyositis. *Curr Rheumatol Rep.* 2006;8:167-173.
242. Zampieri S, Ghirardello A, Iaccarino L, et al: Polymyositis-dermatomyositis and infections. *Autoimmunity.* 2006;39:191-196.
243. Hui AC, Wong SM, Leung T: Prognosis of polymyositis and dermatomyositis. *Clin Rheumatol.* 2007;26:92.
244. Bronner IM, van der Meulen MF, de Visser M, et al: Long-term outcome in polymyositis and dermatomyositis. *Ann Rheum Dis.* 2006;65:1456-1461.
245. Airio A, Kautiainen H, Hakala M: Prognosis and mortality of polymyositis and dermatomyositis patients. *Clin Rheumatol.* 2006;25:234-239.
246. Schnabel A, Hellmich B, Gross WL: Interstitial lung disease in polymyositis and dermatomyositis. *Curr Rheumatol Rep.* 2005;7:99-105.
247. Dalakas MC: Inflammatory disorders of muscle: progress in polymyositis, dermatomyositis and inclusion body myositis. *Curr Opin Neurol.* 2004;17:561-567.
248. Hara H: Autism and epilepsy: a retrospective follow-up study. *Brain Dev.* 2007;29:486-90
249. Regis J, Bartolomei J, Chauvel P: Epilepsy. *Prog Neurol Surg.* 2007;20:267-278.
250. French JA: Refractory epilepsy: clinical overview. *Epilepsia.* 48(suppl 1):3-7, 2007
251. Abou-Khalil BW: Is epilepsy intractability predetermined or acquired? *Epilepsy Curr.* 2007;7:9-10.
252. Hermann B, Seidenberg M: Epilepsy and cognition. *Epilepsy Curr.* 2007;7:1-6.
253. When is it epilepsy? *Harv Ment Health Lett.* 2006;23:5-6.
254. Haut SR, Hall CB, LeValley AJ, et al: Can patients with epilepsy predict their seizures? *Neurology.* 2007;68:262-266.

255. Beghi E, De Maria G, Gobbi G, et al: Diagnosis and treatment of the first epileptic seizure: guidelines of the italian league against epilepsy. *Epilepsia.* 2006;47(suppl 5):2-8.
256. Harris-Love MO, Siegel KL, Paul SM, et al: Rehabilitation management of Friedreich ataxia: lower extremity force-control variability and gait performance. *Neurorehabil Neural Repair.* 2004;18:117-124.
257. Voncken M, Ioannou P, Delatycki MB: Friedreich ataxia-update on pathogenesis and possible therapies. *Neurogenetics.* 2004;5:1-8.
258. Pandolfo M: Friedreich ataxia. *Semin Pediatr Neurol.* 2003;10: 163-172.
259. Alldredge CD, Schlieve CR, Miller NR, et al: Pathophysiology of the optic neuropathy associated with Friedreich ataxia. *Arch Ophthalmol.* 2003;121:1582-1585.
260. Albin RL: Dominant ataxias and Friedreich ataxia: an update. *Curr Opin Neurol.* 2003;16:507-514.
261. Puccio H, Koenig M: Friedreich ataxia: a paradigm for mitochondrial diseases. *Curr Opin Genet Dev.* 2002;12:272-277.
262. Pandolfo M: Molecular basis of Friedreich ataxia. *Mov Disord.* 2001;16:815-821.
263. Pandolfo M: The molecular basis of Friedreich ataxia. *Neurologia.* 2000;15:325-329.
264. Delatycki MB, Williamson R, Forrest SM: Friedreich ataxia: an overview. *J Med Genet.* 2000;37:1-8.
265. Koenig M, Mandel JL: Deciphering the cause of Friedreich ataxia. *Curr Opin Neurobiol.* 1997;7:689-694.
266. Smith-Wheelock M, Shepard NT, Telian SA: Physical therapy program for vestibular rehabilitation. *Am J Otol.* 1991;12: 218-225.
267. Schubert MC: Vestibular disorders. In: O'Sullivan SB, Schmitz TJ, eds. *Physical Rehabilitation.* 5th ed. Philadelphia, PA: FA Davis; 2007:999-1029.
268. Jacobson GP, Newman CW: The development of the Dizziness Handicap Inventory. *Arch Otolaryngol Head Neck Surg.* 1990;116: 424-427.
269. Gacek RR: The pathology of facial and vestibular neuronitis. *Am J Otolaryngol.* 1999;20:202-210.
270. Gacek RR, Gacek MR: Vestibular neuronitis. *Am J Otol.* 1999; 20:553-554.
271. Gacek RR, Gacek MR: Vestibular neuronitis: a viral neuropathy. *Adv Otorhinolaryngol.* 2002;60:54-66.
272. Imate Y, Sekitani T, Okami M, et al: Central disorders in vestibular neuronitis. *Acta Otolaryngol Suppl.* 1995;519:204-205.
273. Ishikawa K, Edo M, Togawa K: Clinical observation of 32 cases of vestibular neuronitis. *Acta Otolaryngol Suppl.* 1993;503:13-15.
274. Lumio JS, Aho J: Vestibular Neuronitis. *Ann Otol Rhinol Laryngol.* 1965;74:264-270.
275. Ogata Y, Sekitani T, Shimogori H, et al: Bilateral vestibular neuronitis. *Acta Otolaryngol Suppl.* 1993;503:57-60.
276. Tahara T, Sekitani T, Imate Y, et al: Vestibular neuronitis in children. *Acta Otolaryngol Suppl.* 1993;503:49-52.
277. Baloh RW: Differentiating between peripheral and central causes of vertigo. *Otolaryngol Head Neck Surg.* 1998;119:55-59.
278. Baloh RW: Differentiating between peripheral and central causes of vertigo. *J Neurol Sci.* 2004;221:3.

279. Buttner U, Helmchen C, Brandt T: Diagnostic criteria for central versus peripheral positioning nystagmus and vertigo: a review. *Acta Otolaryngol.* 1999;119:1-5.
280. Drozd CE: Acute vertigo: peripheral versus central etiology. *Nurse Pract.* 1999;24:147-148.
281. Frederic MW: Central vertigo. *Otolaryngol Clin North Am.* 1973;6:267-285.
282. Williams D: Central vertigo. *Trans Med Soc Lond.* 1958;74:15-19.
283. Williams DJ: Central vertigo. *Proc R Soc Med.* 1967;60:961-964.
284. Di Girolamo S, Ottaviani F, Scarano E, et al: Postural control in horizontal benign paroxysmal positional vertigo. *Eur Arch Otorhinolaryngol.* 2000;257:372-375.
285. Dornhoffer JL, Colvin GB: Benign paroxysmal positional vertigo and canalith repositioning: clinical correlations. *Am J Otol.* 2000;21:230-233.
286. Furman JM, Cass SP: Benign paroxysmal positional vertigo. *N Engl J Med.* 1999;341:1590-1596.
287. Herdman SJ, Blatt PJ, Schubert MC: Vestibular rehabilitation of patients with vestibular hypofunction or with benign paroxysmal positional vertigo. *Curr Opin Neurol.* 2000;13:39-43.
288. Hilton M, Pinder D: Benign paroxysmal positional vertigo. *BMJ.* 2003;326:673.
289. Karlberg M, Hall K, Quickert N, et al: What inner ear diseases cause benign paroxysmal positional vertigo? *Acta Otolaryngol.* 2000;120:380-385.
290. Kentala E, Pyykko I: Vertigo in patients with benign paroxysmal positional vertigo. *Acta Otolaryngol Suppl.* 2000;543:20-22.
291. Kovar M, Jepson T, Jones S: Diagnosing and treating benign paroxysmal positional vertigo. *J Gerontol Nurs.* 2006;32:22-7; quiz 28-29.
292. Mosca F, Morano M: Benign paroxysmal positional vertigo, incidence and treatment. *Ann Otolaryngol Chir Cervicofac.* 2001;118:95-101.
293. Solomon D: Benign paroxysmal positional vertigo. *Curr Treat Options Neurol.* 2000;2:417-428.
294. von Brevern M, Lempert T: Benign paroxysmal positional vertigo. *Arch Neurol.* 2001;58:1491-1493.
295. Gussen R: Meniere syndrome. Compensatory collateral venous drainage with endolymphatic sac fibrosis. *Arch Otolaryngol.* 1974;99:414-418.
296. Haubrich WS: Meniere of Meniere's syndrome. *Gastroenterology.* 1998;114:1150.
297. Lee H, Yi HA, Lee SR, et al: Drop attacks in elderly patients secondary to otologic causes with Meniere's syndrome or non-Meniere peripheral vestibulopathy. *J Neurol Sci.* 2005;232:71-76.
298. Karagol U, Deda G, Kukner S, et al: Early-onset Huntington chorea. *Eur J Pediatr.* 1995;154:752-753.
299. Lanska DJ: George Huntington and hereditary chorea. *J Child Neurol.* 1995;10:46-48.
300. Tolosa ES, Sparber SB: Huntington chorea. *Arch Neurol.* 1977;34:58-59.
301. Patient information. Bell's palsy. *J Fam Pract.* 2003;52:160.
302. Managing Bell's palsy. *Drug Ther Bull.* 2006;44:49-53.
303. Cederwall E, Olsen MF, Hanner P, et al: Evaluation of a physiotherapeutic treatment intervention in "Bell's" facial palsy. *Physiother Theory Pract.* 22:43-52, 2006.

304. Holland J: Bell's palsy. *Clin Evid.* 2006;15:1745-1750.
305. Hutchinson M: The management of Bell's palsy. *Ir Med J.* 2005;98:165.
306. Salinas R: Bell's palsy. *Clin Evid.* 2002;8:1301-1304.
307. Burnett MG, Zager EL: Pathophysiology of peripheral nerve injury: a brief review. *Neurosurg Focus.* 2004;16:E1.
308. Costa J, Henriques R, Barroso C, et al: Upper limb tremor induced by peripheral nerve injury. *Neurology.* 2006;67:1884-1886.
309. Duff SV: Impact of peripheral nerve injury on sensorimotor control. *J Hand Ther.* 2005;18:277-2791.
310. Hirate H, Sobue K, Tsuda T, et al: Peripheral nerve injury caused by misuse of elastic stockings. *Anaesth Intensive Care.* 2007; 35:306-307.
311. Mohler LR, Hanel DP: Closed fractures complicated by peripheral nerve injury. *J Am Acad Orthop Surg.* 2006;14:32-37.
312. Reyes O, Sosa I, Kuffler DP: Promoting neurological recovery following a traumatic peripheral nerve injury. *P R Health Sci J.* 2005;24:215-223.
313. Tomaino MM: Upper extremity peripheral nerve injury. *Am J Orthop.* 2005;34:60-61.
314. Winfree CJ: Peripheral nerve injury evaluation and management. *Curr Surg.* 2005;62:469-476.
315. Heald PW: Current treatment practice of herpes zoster. *Expert Opin Pharmacother.* 2001;2:1283-1287.
316. Leung AK, Robson WL, Leong AG: Herpes zoster in childhood. *J Pediatr Health Care.* 2006;20:300-303.
317. Miller GG, Dummer JS: Herpes simplex and varicella zoster viruses: forgotten but not gone. *Am J Transplant.* 2007;7:741-747.
318. Morrow T: Herpes zoster vaccine brings relief for the elderly. *Manag Care.* 2006;15:57-58.
319. Raza N, Dar NR, Ejaz A: Simultaneous onset of herpes zoster in a father and son. *J Ayub Med Coll Abbottabad.* 2006;18:64-65.
320. Sauerbrei A, Wutzler P: Herpes simplex and varicella-zoster virus infections during pregnancy: current concepts of prevention, diagnosis and therapy. Part 2: Varicella-zoster virus infections. *Med Microbiol Immunol.* 2007;196:95-102.
321. Thyregod HG, Rowbotham MC, Peters M, et al: Natural history of pain following herpes zoster. *Pain.* 2007;128:148-156.
322. Volpi A, Gatti A, Serafini G, et al: Clinical and psychosocial correlates of acute pain in herpes zoster. *J Clin Virol.* 2007; 38:275-279.
323. Bagheri SC, Farhidvash F, Perciaccante VJ: Diagnosis and treatment of patients with trigeminal neuralgia. *J Am Dent Assoc.* 2004;135:1713-1717.
324. Bennetto L, Patel NK, Fuller G: Trigeminal neuralgia and its management. *BMJ.* 2007;334:201-205.
325. Cheshire WP: Trigeminal neuralgia: diagnosis and treatment. *Curr Neurol Neurosci Rep.* 2005;5:79-85.
326. Cheshire WP, Jr: Trigeminal neuralgia. *Curr Pain Headache Rep.* 2007;11:69-74.
327. Ecker AD: The cause of trigeminal neuralgia. *Med Hypotheses.* 2004;62:1023.
328. El Gammal T, Brooks BS: Trigeminal neuralgia. *Radiology.* 2004;231:284.

329. Liu JK, Apfelbaum RI: Treatment of trigeminal neuralgia. *Neurosurg Clin N Am.* 2004;15:319-334.
330. Rozen TD: Trigeminal neuralgia and glossopharyngeal neuralgia. *Neurol Clin.* 2004;22:185-206.
331. Scrivani SJ, Mehta N, Mathews ES, et al: Clinical criteria for trigeminal neuralgia. *Oral Surg Oral Med Oral Pathol Oral Radiol Endod.* 2004;97:544; author reply 544-545.
332. Zakrzewska JM: Trigeminal neuralgia. *Clin Evid.* 2003;9: 1490-1498.
333. Zakrzewska JM, Lopez BC: Trigeminal neuralgia. *Clin Evid.* 2003;10:1599-1609.
334. Briese M, Esmaeili B, Sattelle DB: Is spinal muscular atrophy the result of defects in motor neuron processes? *Bioessays.* 2005; 27:946-957.
335. Iannaccone ST, Smith SA, Simard LR: Spinal muscular atrophy. *Curr Neurol Neurosci Rep.* 2004;4:74-80.
336. Muthukrishnan J, Varadarajulu R, Mehta SR, et al: Distal spinal muscular atrophy. *J Assoc Physicians India.* 2003;51:1113-1115.
337. Scheffer H: Spinal muscular atrophy. *Methods Mol Med.* 2004;92:343-358.
338. Wang HY, Ju YH, Chen SM, et al: Joint range of motion limitations in children and young adults with spinal muscular atrophy. *Arch Phys Med Rehabil.* 2004;85:1689-1693.
339. Wirth B, Brichta L, Hahnen E: Spinal muscular atrophy and therapeutic prospects. *Prog Mol Subcell Biol.* 2006;44:109-132.
340. Yap SH: Spinal muscular atrophy. *Int J Obstet Anesth.* 2003;12:237.
341. Bartell JC, Hayney MS: In the spotlight: Guillain-Barre syndrome. *J Am Pharm Assoc (Wash DC).* 2006;46:104-106.
342. Chaudhuri A: Guillain-Barre syndrome. *Lancet.* 2006;367:472-473; author reply 473-474.
343. Cosi V, Versino M: Guillain-Barre syndrome. *Neurol Sci.* 2006; 27(suppl 1):S47-S51.
344. Douglas MR, Winer JB: Guillain-Barre syndrome and its treatment. *Expert Rev Neurother.* 2006;6:1569-1574.
345. Gurwood AS, Drake J: Guillain-Barre syndrome. *Optometry.* 2006; 77:540-546.
346. Kashyap AS, Anand KP, Kashyap S: Guillain-Barre syndrome. *Lancet.* 2006;367:472; author reply 473-474.
347. Kuwabara S: Guillain-barre syndrome. *Curr Neurol Neurosci Rep.* 2007;7:57-62.
348. Logullo F, Manicone M, Di Bella P, et al: Asymmetric Guillain-Barre syndrome. *Neurol Sci.* 2006;27:355-359.
349. Saxena AK: Guillain-Barre syndrome. *Lancet.* 2006;367:472; author reply 473-474.
350. Shahar E: Current therapeutic options in severe Guillain-Barre syndrome. *Clin Neuropharmacol.* 2006;29:45-51.
351. Tsang RS, Valdivieso-Garcia A: Pathogenesis of Guillain-Barre syndrome. *Expert Rev Anti Infect Ther.* 2003;1:597-608.
352. van Doorn PA, Jacobs BC: Predicting the course of Guillain-Barre syndrome. *Lancet Neurol.* 2006;5:991-993.
353. Logroscino G, Armon C: Amyotrophic lateral sclerosis: a global threat with a possible difference in risk across ethnicities. *Neurology.* 2007;68:E17.

354. Kurt A, Nijboer F, Matuz T, et al: Depression and anxiety in individuals with amyotrophic lateral sclerosis: epidemiology and management. *CNS Drugs.* 2007;21:279-291.
355. Grossman AB, Woolley-Levine S, Bradley WG, et al: Detecting neurobehavioral changes in amyotrophic lateral sclerosis. *Amyotroph Lateral Scler.* 2007;8:56-61.
356. Hardiman O, Greenway M: The complex genetics of amyotrophic lateral sclerosis. *Lancet Neurol.* 2007;6:291-292.
357. Lederer CW, Santama N: Amyotrophic lateral sclerosis—the tools of the trait. *Biotechnol J.* 2007 2: 608–621.
358. Pozza AM, Delamura MK, Ramirez C, et al: Physiotherapeutic conduct in amyotrophic lateral sclerosis. *Sao Paulo Med J.* 2006;124:350-354.
359. Shoesmith CL, Strong MJ: Amyotrophic lateral sclerosis: update for family physicians. *Can Fam Physician.* 2006;52:1563-1569.
360. Aguilar JL, Echaniz-Laguna A, Fergani A, et al: Amyotrophic lateral sclerosis: all roads lead to Rome. *J Neurochem.* 2007;101:1153–1160.
361. Postpolio syndrome. *J Indian Med Assoc.* 2000;98:24-25.
362. Carlson M, Hadlock T: Physical therapist management following rotator cuff repair for a patient with postpolio syndrome. *Phys Ther.* 2007;87:179-192.
363. Dalakas M: Postpolio syndrome. *Curr Opin Rheumatol.* 1990; 2:901-907.
364. Gevirtz C: Managing postpolio syndrome pain. *Nursing.* 2006; 36:17.
365. Hodges DL, Kumar VN: Postpolio syndrome. *Orthop Rev.* 1986; 15:218-222.
366. Howard RS: Poliomyelitis and the postpolio syndrome. *BMJ.* 2005;330:1314-1318.
367. Moskowitz E: Postpolio syndrome. *Arch Phys Med Rehabil.* 1987; 68:322.
368. Nollet F, de Visser M: Postpolio syndrome. *Arch Neurol.* 2004;61:1142-1144.
369. Owen RR: Postpolio syndrome and cardiopulmonary conditioning. *West J Med.* 1991;154:557-558.
370. Sliwa J: Postpolio syndrome and rehabilitation. *Am J Phys Med Rehabil.* 2004;83:909.
371. Winters R: Postpolio syndrome. *J Am Acad Nurse Pract.* 1991;3:69-74.
372. Shumway-Cook A, Woollacott M: *Motor Control—Theory and Practical Applications.* Baltimore, MD: Williams & Wilkins; 1995.
373. O'Sullivan SB: Strategies to improve motor function. In: O'Sullivan SB, Schmitz TJ, eds. *Physical Rehabilitation.* 5th ed. Philadelphia, PA: FA Davis; 2007:471-522.
374. Hoare B, Wasiak J, Imms C, et al: Constraint-induced movement therapy in the treatment of the upper limb in children with hemiplegic cerebral palsy. *Cochrane Database Syst Rev.* 2007;CD004149.
375. Wu CY, Chen CL, Tsai WC, et al: A randomized controlled trial of modified constraint-induced movement therapy for elderly stroke survivors: changes in motor impairment, daily functioning, and quality of life. *Arch Phys Med Rehabil.* 2007;88:273-278.

376. Boake C, Noser EA, Ro T, et al: Constraint-induced movement therapy during early stroke rehabilitation. *Neurorehabil Neural Repair.* 2007;21:14-24.
377. Mark VW, Taub E, Morris DM: Neuroplasticity and constraint-induced movement therapy. *Eura Medicophys.* 2006;42:269-284.
378. Morris DM, Taub E, Mark VW: Constraint-induced movement therapy: characterizing the intervention protocol. *Eura Medicophys.* 2006;42:257-268.
379. Smania N: Constraint-induced movement therapy: an original concept in rehabilitation. *Eura Medicophys.* 2006;42:239-240.
380. Clayton-Krasinski D, Klepper S: Impaired neuromotor development. In: Cameron MH, Monroe LG, eds. *Physical Rehabilitation: Evidence-Based Examination, Evaluation, and Intervention.* St Louis, MO: Saunders/Elsevier; 2007:333-366.
381. Winstein CJ: Motor learning considerations in stroke rehabilitation. In: Duncan PW, Badke MB, eds. *Stroke Rehabilitation: The Recovery of Motor Control.* Chicago, IL: Yearbook Medical Publishers, Inc.; 1987:109-134.
382. Unsworth CA: Cognitive and perceptual dysfunction. In: O'Sullivan SB, Schmitz TJ, eds. *Physical Rehabilitation.* 5th ed. Philadelphia, PA: FA Davis; 2007:1149-1188.
383. Parziale JR, Akelman E, Herz DA: Spasticity: pathophysiology and management. *Orthopedics.* 1993;16:801-811.
384. Vodovnik L, Bowman BR, Hufford P: Effects of electrical stimulation on spinal spasticity. *Scand J Rehabil Med.* 1984;16: 29-34.
385. Goulet C, Arsenault AB, Bourbonnais D, et al: Effects of transcutaneous electrical nerve stimulation on H-reflex and spinal spasticity. *Scand J Rehabil Med.* 1996;28:169-176.
386. Marshall S, Teasell R, Bayona N, et al: Motor impairment rehabilitation post acquired brain injury. *Brain Inj.* 2007;21:133-160.
387. Booth MY, Yates CC, Edgar TS, et al: Serial casting vs combined intervention with botulinum toxin A and serial casting in the treatment of spastic equinus in children. *Pediatr Phys Ther.* 2003;15:216-220.
388. Westberry DE, Davids JR, Jacobs JM, et al: Effectiveness of serial stretch casting for resistant or recurrent knee flexion contractures following hamstring lengthening in children with cerebral palsy. *J Pediatr Orthop.* 2006;26:109-114.
389. Singer BJ, Dunne JW, Singer KP, et al: Non-surgical management of ankle contracture following acquired brain injury. *Disabil Rehabil.* 2004;26:335-345.
390. Stoeckmann T: Casting for the person with spasticity. *Top Stroke Rehabil.* 2001;8:27-35.
391. Bauer CA, Girardi M: Vestibular rehabilitation, Available at: http://www.emedicine.com/ent/topic666.htm, 2005.

Pulmonary Physical Therapy

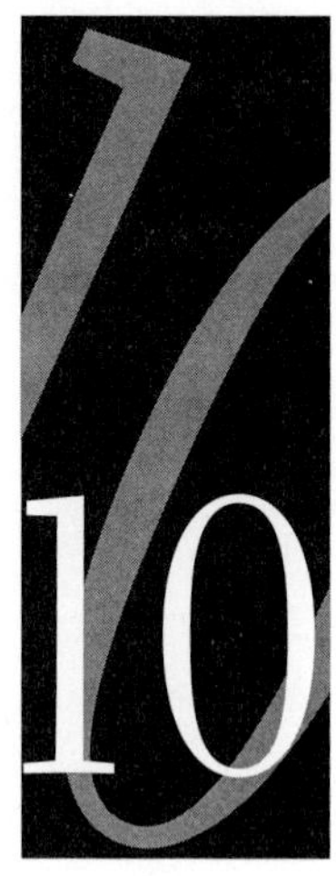

ANATOMY AND PHYSIOLOGY

The pulmonary or respiratory system (Figure 10-1) consists of the sternum, 12 pairs of ribs, the clavicle, and the vertebrae of the thoracic spine, which form the thoracic cage (Table 10-1).

The primary function of the respiratory system is to exchange gases between the environment and the tissues and blood so that arterial blood oxygen (O_2), carbon dioxide (CO_2), and pH levels remain within defined limits throughout many different physiological confines.[1] In addition, the pulmonary system contributes to temperature homeostasis via evaporative heat loss from the lungs, and protects the remainder of the respiratory system from damage caused by dry gases or harmful debris by filtering, humidifying, and warming or cooling the air to body temperature.[1]

The respiratory system (Table 10-2) can be divided into two main portions:[1]

1. The conducting portion, which includes the upper airway (Table 10-3) and the lower airway (trachea, bronchi and the bronchioles). Within this portion, air moves by bulk flow under the pressure gradients created by the respiratory muscles and the elastic recoil of the lungs. The left main bronchus branches at a more acute angle and is longer than the right main bronchus, which is more directly in line with the trachea.[1] This relationship predisposes to aspiration of material into the right rather than the left lung.[1]

2. The respiratory portion, which includes the terminal portion of the bronchial tree and alveoli, the site of gas exchange.[2] The total cross-sectional area rapidly increases at the respiratory zone. Forward velocity of air flow therefore decreases, and the gases readily move by diffusion through the alveoli into the pulmonary capillaries.

Study Pearl

- External respiration: the exchange of gases between the atmosphere and the blood.
- Internal respiration: the exchange of gases between the blood and the cells of the body.

Study Pearl

- Ventilation: The movement of air through the conducting airways (see "Pulmonary System Physiology").
- Respiration: A term used to describe the gas exchange within the body.

Study Pearl

The transitional zone, which consists of the respiratory bronchioles, separates the conducting and respiratory portions.

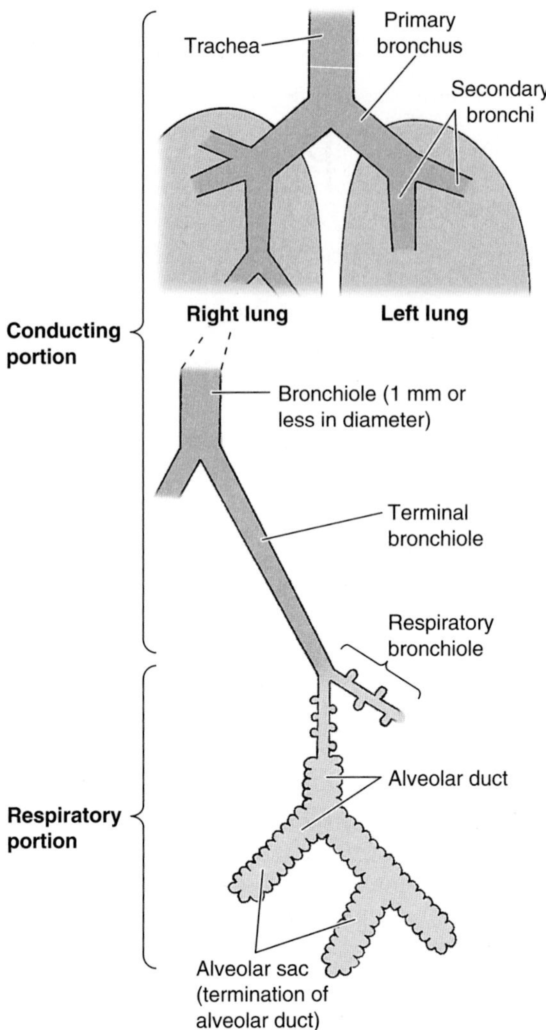

Figure 10-1. Schematic representation of the main divisions of the respiratory tract. (Reproduced, with permission, from Junqueira LC, Carneiro J: Basic Histology: Text and Atlas, *10th ed.* New York: McGraw-Hill. 2003:349.)

TABLE 10-1. BONY ANATOMY OF THE THORACIC CAGE

The Sternum	Consists of three parts: the manubrium, the body, and the xiphoid process. The articulation between the manubrium and the sternum serves to allow the *pump-handle* action of the sternal body during respiration.
The Rib cage	Formed by twelve pairs of ribs, each different from the others in size, width, and curvature, although they share some common characteristics. ▶ Ribs 1-7 are considered to be true ribs and have a single anterior costochondral attachment to the sternum. Approximately 32 structures attach to the first rib and body of T1. ▶ Ribs 8-10 are referred to as false ribs as they share costochondral attachments before attaching anteriorly to the sternum. ▶ Ribs 11 and 12 are termed floating or costovertebral ribs as they have no anterior attachment with the sternum. Based on the orientation of the joint axes of the thoracic vertebrae, movement of the upper ribs is primarily in an anterior and posterior direction (pump handle), whereas the transverse diameter increases for the lower ribs allowing movement primarily in the medial-lateral direction (bucket handle).
Costovertebral articulation	Forms an intimate relationship between the head of the rib and the lateral side of the vertebral body. ▶ The first, 11th, and 12th ribs articulate fully with their own vertebrae via a single costal facet, without any contact with the intervertebral disk (IVD). ▶ The remaining ribs articulate with both their own vertebra and the vertebra above, as well as to the IVD.

TABLE 10-2. VENTILATION TERMINOLOGY

TERM	DEFINITION
Air spaces	Alveolar ducts, alveolar sacs, and alveoli
Airways	Structures that conduct air from the mouth and nose to the respiratory bronchioles
Alveolar ventilation	Removal and replacement of gas in pulmonary alveoli; equal to the tidal volume minus the volume of dead space multiplied by the ventilation rate
Anatomical dead space	Volume of the conducting airways to the zone gas exchange occurs.
Apnea	Cessation of breathing
Dyspnea	Unpleasant subjective feeling of difficult or labored breathing.
Eupnea	Normal, comfortable breathing at rest
Hyperventilation	Alveolar ventilation that is excessive in relation to metabolic rate; results in abnormally low alveolar CO_2
Hypoventilation	An alveolar ventilation that is low in relation to metabolic rate; results in abnormally high alveolar CO_2
Physiological dead space	Combination of anatomical dead space and under ventilated or under perfused alveoli that do not contribute normally to blood-gas exchange
Pneumothorax	Presence of gas in the intrapleural space (the space between the visceral and parietal pleurae), causing lung collapse
Torr	Unit of pressure very nearly equal to the millimeter of mercury (760 mm Hg = 760 torr)

Data from Van de Graaff KM, Fox SI: Respiratory system. In: Van de Graaff KM, Fox SI, eds. *Concepts of Human Anatomy and Physiology.* New York: WCB/McGraw-Hill. 1999: 728-777.

Lungs

The lungs are located within the thoracic cavity, on either side of the mediastinum. The most superior aspect of each lung is called its apex.

- Right lung: divided into three lobes (right superior, right middle, and right inferior), separated by a series of oblique and horizontal fissure lines. Each lobe is subdivided by connective tissue into 10 independently functioning compartments, called bronchopulmonary segments.[2] Each bronchopulmonary segment is supplied by its own set of blood vessels and tertiary bronchus (or segmental bronchus). Thus, if one becomes infected or is damaged, other bronchopulmonary segments in the same lobe may not be affected.

TABLE 10-3. STRUCTURES OF THE UPPER AIRWAY

Nasal cavities	Serve as the entry point into the respiratory system. The upper airway is designed to filter and keep inspired air at 100% humidity and body temperature at 37°C (98.6°F).
Sinuses	Air pockets located inside the bones the form the skull. They are located beneath the maxillary, ethmoid, frontal, and sphenoid bones. The sinuses serve a number of functions including reducing the weight of the skull, protecting the face by deflecting the force of a direct blow to the sides, providing heat insulation for the base of the brain, creating resonance to the voice, facilitating facial growth and development, and aiding in smelling and breathing. The sinuses are lined with very fine hair-like projections called *cilia,* which function to move mucus (which is normally produced by the sinus) toward the ostium to allow drainage for the sinus.
Pharynx	A fibromuscular tube that extends from the base of the skull to the lower border of the cricoid cartilage (at which point it becomes the esophagus). The pharynx serves a dual role as it is used for both the respiratory and the digestive systems. The pharynx is divided by the soft palate into the nasopharynx, and the oropharynx.
Larynx (voice box)	Formed by cartilage, ligaments, muscles, and mucous membrane; connects the pharynx to the trachea, and houses the vocal cords. The larynx protects the entrance to the lower respiratory passages (trachea, bronchi, and lungs) from food and foreign bodies by acting as a valve.
Trachea	Begins at the level of the cricoid cartilage of the larynx (approximately at the level of C6) and terminates as the *carina,* a ridge at the bifurcation of the trachea into left and right bronchi. Considered as the differentiating structure between the upper and lower airways.

Study Pearl

The lungs both secrete and absorb fluid. Surface tension is created by the presence of the interface between air in the alveoli and the watery alveolar tissue. The surface tension, which is responsible for much of the lung's elastic recoil and for preventing the alveoli from collapsing during expiration, is kept at an optimal level because of a chemical called *surfactant*. The surfactant molecules reduce the attractive forces between the water molecules that produce the surface tension, thus reducing surface tension in the pulmonary alveoli.

Study Pearl

Even under normal conditions, the first breath of life is a difficult one because the newborn must overcome great surface tension forces in order to inflate his or her partially collapsed pulmonary alveoli. The transpulmonary pressure required for the first breath is 15 to 20 times that required for subsequent breaths.[2]

Study Pearl

The pleural cavity, the potential space between the two pleura, receives a small amount of pleural fluid that serves to hold the parietal and visceral pleurae together during ventilation while reducing friction between the lungs and the thoracic wall.[3]

- Left lung: divided into two lobes by a single oblique fissure line. Each lobe is divided into eight bronchopulmonary segments, which are self-contained functional units.

Physical Properties of the Lungs. In order for inspiration to occur, the lungs must be able to expand when stretched; they must have high compliance. In order for expiration to occur, the lungs must get smaller when this tension is released; they must have elasticity. The tendency to get smaller is also aided by surface tension forces within the pulmonary alveoli. The surface tension produces a force that is directed inward, raising the pressure within the alveolus.

Surfactant is produced in late fetal life.[2] Because no surfactant is produced until about the 8-months, premature babies are sometimes born with lungs that lack sufficient surfactant, and their alveoli are collapsed as a result.[2] This condition is called respiratory distress syndrome (RDS) or hyaline membrane disease (see Chapter 16).

PLEURAE

The two pleurae are dual-layered sacs that stabilize the lungs and separate them from the chest wall, diaphragm, and heart.[2]

- Parietal pleura: the parietal pleura lines the inside of the thoracic cage, diaphragm, the mediastinal border of the lung, and the great vessels of the superior mediastinum.
- Visceral pleura: the pleura that covers the outer surface of the lung, including the fissure lines.

MUSCLES OF RESPIRATION

The Diaphragm. The diaphragm, which is innervated by the phrenic nerve, is the primary muscle of inspiration. It is comprised of two hemidiaphragms, each with a central tendon. When the diaphragm is at rest, the hemidiaphragms are arched high into the thorax. When the diaphragm contracts it descends over the abdominal contents, flattening the dome, which causes the lower ribs to move outward, resulting in protrusion of the abdominal wall. In addition, the contracting diaphragm causes a decrease in intrathoracic pressure, which pulls air into the lungs.[3]

Intercostal Muscles. The intercostal muscles of the thoracic cage, which include the 11 pairs of internal and external intercostals, connect one rib to the next.[3]

- The external intercostals function to elevate the ribs thereby increasing thoracic volume.
- The internal intercostals function to lower the ribs, thereby decreasing thoracic volume.[3]

Accessory Muscles of Inspiration. The accessory muscles of inspiration are used when a more rapid or deep inhalation is required, or in disease states.

- The upper two ribs are raised by the scalenes and sternocleidomastoid.

- The remaining ribs are raised by the levator costarum and serratus.

In addition, the trapezius, pectorals, and serratus anterior can also become muscles of inspiration by fixing the shoulder girdle.

Pulmonary System Physiology

In order to inflate the lungs, the inspiratory muscles must perform two types of work: they must overcome the tendency of the lung to recoil inwards; and they must overcome the resistance to flow offered by the airways.[2] Fulfilling the needs of metabolizing tissues for oxygen (O_2) delivery and carbon dioxide (CO_2) elimination requires a high degree of coordination among several discrete functions.[4]

Study Pearl

Work of breathing (WOB) is the amount of energy or O_2 consumption needed by the respiratory muscles to produce enough ventilation and respiration to meet the metabolic demands of the body.

Terminology

Volumes and Capacities. There are four primary lung volumes (Table 10-4, Figure 10-2). These volumes can be combined to form four capacities (Table 10-4).

Flow Rates

- Forced expiratory volume in 1 second (FEV_1): the amount exhaled during the first second of forced vital capacity (FVC). In healthy individuals, at least 75% of the FVC is exhaled within the first second ($FEV_1/FVC \times 100 > 75\%$).
- Forced expiratory flow rate (FEF 25%-75%): the slope of a line drawn between the points 25% and 55% of exhaled volume on a forced vital capacity exhalation. This flow rate is more specific to the smaller airways, and shows a more dramatic change with disease than FEV_1.
- Peak expiratory flow (PEF): The maximum flow of air during the beginning of a forced expiratory breath.

Study Pearl

Dead space represents the volume of air in the respiratory system that does not participate in gas exchange. It is composed of several components:[1]

- Anatomic dead space: the volume of gas contained throughout the conducting airways.
- Alveolar dead space: the volume of gas within areas of "wasted ventilation"—alveoli that are ventilated but poorly or underperfused.
- Physiological dead space: the total volume of gas not involved in gas exchange – it represents the sum of the anatomic dead space and alveolar dead space. In health, this represents only about 30% of the tidal volume. In contrast, with non-uniform structural abnormalities of the lung, 60% to 70% of each tidal volume may be composed of dead-space volume.

Dead space volume increases as a function of lung volume, body height, bronchodilator drugs, diseases such as emphysema, and alveolar overdistention during mechanical ventilation. Anatomical dead space is decreased by reduction of the size of the airways, as occurs with bronchoconstriction or a tracheostomy.

Mechanics of Breathing. Inspiration and expiration are accomplished by alternately increasing and decreasing the volumes of the thorax and lungs. An increase in thoracic volume decreases intrapulmonary (intra-alveolar) pressure, thereby causing air to flow into the lungs.[2]

Inspiration. Normal, quiet inspiration results from contraction of the inspiratory muscles (diaphragm and intercostal muscles), which expands the chest wall while lowering the diaphragm. In a normal person, the mean pleural pressure is 3 to 5 cm H_2O below atmospheric pressure. Since the lungs tend to pull inward, this expansion results in a further reduction of pleural pressure. Therefore the more the chest wall is expanded during inspiration, the more subatmospheric is the resultant pleural pressure.

Expiration. During relaxed breathing, expiration is essentially a passive process.[5] The structure of the rib cage and associated cartilages provides continuous inelastic tension, so that when stretched by muscle contraction during inspiration, the rib cage can return passively to its resting dimensions when the muscles relax.[2] The resting position or lung volume (functional residual capacity),

TABLE 10-4. TERMS USED TO DESCRIBE LUNG VOLUMES AND CAPACITIES

TERM	DEFINITION	TERM	DEFINITION
Lung Volumes		Lung Capacities	
Tidal volume (TV)	Volume of gas inhaled or exhaled during a normal respiration. The average adult TV is 500 mL (range = 300-800mL). Given that the average breathing frequency is 15 breaths/min (range = 10-20 breaths/min), the product of tidal volume times frequency, termed *total minute ventilation*, averages 7.5L/min (range = 4-10 L/min).	Inspiratory capacity (IRV+TV)	The amount of air that can be inhaled from REEP. The average adult inspiratory capacity is 3000-4000 mL.
Inspiratory reserve volume (IRV)	The additional air that can be inhaled after a normal tidal breath in.	Vital capacity (IRV+TV+ERV)	The three volumes of air that are under volitional control: inspiratory reserve volume, expiratory reserve volume, and tidal volume, conventionally measured as a forced expiratory vital capacity (FVC). The average adult vital capacity is 4000-5000 mL.
Expiratory reserve volume (ERV)	The amount of additional air that can be breathed out after normal expiration. This is about 1-1.5 L for the average adult.	Functional residual capacity (ERV+RV)	The amount of air that resides in the lungs after a normal resting tidal exhalation.
Residual volume (RV)	The volume of gas that remains in the lungs after ERV has been exhaled.	Total lung capacity (IRV+TV+ERV+RV)	The total amount of air the lungs can hold (approximately 5 L).

Data from Van de Graaff KM, Fox SI: Respiratory system, in Van de Graaff KM, Fox SI (eds): Concepts of Human Anatomy and Physiology. New York, WCB/McGraw-Hill. 1999: 728-777.

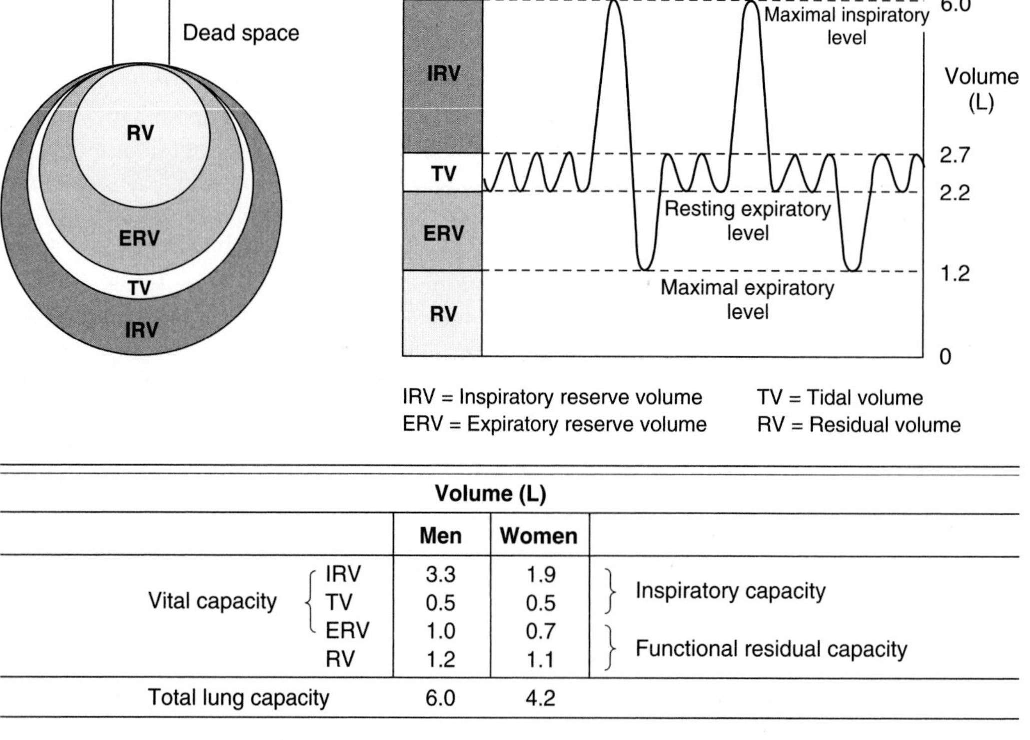

		Volume (L)		
		Men	Women	
Vital capacity	IRV	3.3	1.9	Inspiratory capacity
	TV	0.5	0.5	
	ERV	1.0	0.7	Functional residual capacity
	RV	1.2	1.1	
Total lung capacity		6.0	4.2	

Respiratory minute volume (rest): 6 L/min
Alveolar ventilation (rest): 4.2 L/min
Maximal voluntary ventilation (BTPS): 125–170 L/min
Timed vital capacity: 83% of total in 1 s; 97% in 3 s
Work of quiet breathing: 0.5 kg-m/min
Maximal work of breathing: 10 kg-m/breath

Figure 10-2. Lung volumes and some measurements related to the mechanics of breathing. The diagram at the upper right represents the excursions of a spirometer plotted against time. (Reproduced, with permission, from Ganong WF: Review of Medical Physiology. New York: McGraw-Hill. 2005:652.)

which occurs at the end of every normal expiration, is established when there is a balance of elastic forces. Under this condition, the elastic force of the lung tissues exactly equals those of the chest wall and diaphragm.[1] Since there is no air movement at the end of expiration, gas throughout the lungs is in equilibrium with atmospheric air. During forced exhalation, as in exercise or in disease states, the quadratus lumborum muscle, portions of the intercostals muscles, the abdominal muscles, and the triangularis sterni assist with exhalation.

Controls of Ventilation. Respiratory muscle activity involves multiple components of the neural, mechanical, and chemical control and is closely integrated with the cardiovascular system.[5] The spontaneous neuronal activity that produces cyclic breathing originates in the respiratory centers in the dorsal region of the medulla, which is influenced by two control centers in the pons:[1]

1. Apneustic: appears to promote inspiration by stimulating neurons in the medulla.
2. Pneumotaxic: seems to antagonize the apneustic center and inhibit inspiration.

CENTRAL AND PERIPHERAL CHEMORECEPTOR MECHANISMS

In addition to the neural and mechanical influences, the automatic control of breathing is also influenced by chemoreceptors.[1] Chemoreceptor input to the brainstem maintains the rate and depth of breathing at an efficient level. Of the two respiratory gases, CO_2 is the most tightly controlled.[1]

The central chemoreceptors monitor the CO_2 levels of both the arterial blood and cerebrospinal fluid.[1] A second group of chemoreceptors, the peripheral chemoreceptors, are located in the carotid and aortic bodies:[1]

- The carotid chemoreceptors are stimulated by low-arterial oxygen tensions, high-arterial CO_2 tensions, and acidosis (arterial pH below 7.35).
- The aortic chemoreceptors are not involved in ventilation, but produce reflex cardiovascular responses (ie, stimulation increases the heart rate and raises the blood pressure). In addition to responding to the same stimuli as the carotid chemoreceptors, they are also stimulated by a low oxygen content of the arterial blood.

The terms used to describe blood O_2 and CO_2 levels are outlined in Table 10-5.

Other factors that influence respiration include:[5]

- Age: the resting rate of the newborn is between 25 and 50 breaths per minute, a rate which gradually slows until adulthood, when it ranges between 12 and 20 breaths per minute.

Study Pearl

Lung compliance and pressure–volume relationships are attributable to the interdependence of elastic tissue elements (elastin and collagen ratio) and alveolar surface tension.[1] For example, in pulmonary fibrosis, collagen content is increased and lung compliance is decreased; in emphysema, elastin content is decreased (destruction of alveolar walls) and lung compliance is increased as compared to normal.[1]

Study Pearl

Three chemical levels in particular play a critical role in controlling respiration: the blood acid-base balance (pH—the concentration of free-floating hydrogen ions within the body), the partial pressure of CO_2 within the arterial blood bicarbonate ($PaCO_2$), and the amount of bicarbonate ions within the arterial blood (HCO_3^-).

Study Pearl

- The normal range for arterial pH is 7.36 to 7.44. Acidosis refers to an arterial pH below 7.35, and alkalosis refers to an arterial pH above 7.5
- The normal range of PCO_2 is 40 mm Hg. A rise in PCO_2, called hypercapnia, is caused by hypoventilation. Conversely, hyperventilation results in a fall in PCO_2, hypocapnia.

TABLE 10-5. TERMS USED TO DESCRIBE BLOOD OXYGEN AND CARBON DIOXIDE LEVELS

TERM	DEFINITION
Hypoxemia	A lower than normal oxygen content or PO_2 in arterial blood
Hypoxia	A lower than normal oxygen content or PO_2 in the lungs, blood, or tissues. This is a more general term than hypoxemia. Tissues can be hypoxic, for example, even though there is no hypoxemia (as when the blood flow is occluded).
Hypercapnia (hypercarbia)	An increase in the PCO_2 of systemic arteries to above 40 mm Hg. Usually this occurs when the ventilation is inadequate for a given metabolic rate (hypoventilation).

Data from Van de Graaff KM, Fox SI: Respiratory system. In: Van de Graaff KM, Fox SI, eds. *Concepts of Human Anatomy and Physiology*. New York: WCB/McGraw-Hill. 1999:728-777.

Study Pearl

The Hering-Breuer reflex, a protective mechanism, is stimulated by pulmonary stretch receptors. The activation of these receptors during inspiration inhibits the respiratory control centers, making further inspiration increasingly difficult. This helps to prevent undue distention of the lungs and may contribute to the smoothness of the ventilation cycles. The reflex appears to have a particularly significant impact on the breathing patterns of neonates.[6]

Study Pearl

The barometric pressure determines the total pressure of the air in the respiratory passages and the alveoli when the respiratory system is at rest.

- Body size and stature: men generally have a larger vital capacity than women, adults larger than adolescents and children. Tall, thin individuals generally have a larger vital capacity than stout or obese individuals.
- Exercise: resting rate and depth increase with exercise as a result of increased oxygen demand and CO_2 production.
- Body position: the recumbent position can significantly affect respiration through compression of the chest against the supporting surface and pressure from abdominal organs against the diaphragm.
- Environment: exposure to pollutants such as gas and particle emissions, asbestos, chemical waste products, or coal dust can diminish the ability to transport oxygen.
- Emotional stress: can result in an increased rate and depth of respirations.
- Pharmacological agents: any drug that depresses CNS function will result in respiratory depression. Examples include narcotic agents and barbiturates. Conversely, bronchodilators decreased airway resistance and residual volume with a resultant increase in vital capacity and air flow (refer to Chapter 19).

GAS EXCHANGE[1]

A number of structural elements are involved in the gas exchange process (Table 10-6). Respiratory gas exchange takes place in the

TABLE 10-6. STRUCTURAL ELEMENTS INVOLVED IN GAS EXCHANGE

STRUCTURE	DESCRIPTION
Alveoli	Alveoli are small evaginations of the respiratory bronchioles, alveolar ducts, and alveolar sacs. The alveolar wall consists of 2 thin layers of epithelial cells spread over a layer of connective tissue, which is particularly suited for gas exchange.
Capillaries	Capillaries are tiny blood vessels composed of a single layer of flattened endothelial cells that allow blood to be in close contact with tissues.
Alveolar-Capillary Membrane	It is at the alveolar-capillary interface that a common basement membrane is shared and where the journey that oxygen must take to get from the lung to the pulmonary capillaries bed begins.
Red Blood Cells	Red blood cells (erythrocytes) contain cytoplasm, protein, lipid substances, and hemoglobin (HgB).[1] Hemoglobin accounts for about 33% of the cellular volume. The biconcave structure maximizes the surface available for gas exchange in the capillaries.

Data from Collins SM, Cocanour B: Anatomy of the Cardiopulmonary System. In: DeTurk WE, Cahalin LP, eds. *Cardiovascular and Pulmonary Physical Therapy: An Evidence-Based Approach*. New York, McGraw-Hill. 2004:73-94.

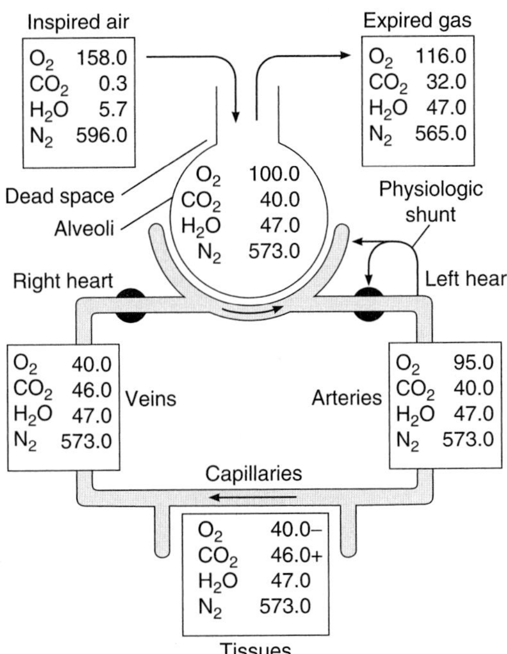

Figure 10-3. Partial pressures of gases (mm Hg) in various parts of the respiratory system and in the circulatory system. (Reproduced, with permission, from Ganong WF: Review of Medical Physiology. New York: McGraw-Hill. 2005:660.)

alveoli, by a process of diffusion.* Oxygen enters the blood from the alveolar air; CO_2 enters the alveolar air from the blood. If the concentration fraction of O_2 in a dry gas mixture is 21%, the partial pressure (PP) exerted by the O_2 is 21% of the total pressure (Figure 10-3). The total pressure of ambient (atmospheric) air is the barometric pressure. At sea level this is 1 atmosphere (atm) or 760 mm Hg.

Alveolar air is a mixture of nitrogen, O_2, CO_2, and water vapor. The concentrations and consequently the PPs of these gases in the alveolar air are different from their concentrations in ambient air. In ambient air, the water vapor content (humidity) is variable.

As air travels through the respiratory airways, it is warmed to 37°C and becomes completely saturated with water vapor.[4] At body temperature, water vapor exerts a pressure of 47 mm Hg (PH_2O). In order to represent accurately the PPs presented to the lung for gas exchange (ie, after warming and humidification), PH_2O is first subtracted from the barometric pressure. Thus, for inspired, tracheal gases at sea level: $PO_2 = 0.21 \times (760 - 47)$ mm Hg = 150 mm Hg.[4]

The concentration of O_2 in the alveoli (about 14%) is much less than in ambient air (21%). Although the oxygen supply to the alveolar is every so often renewed during inspiration, O_2 is constantly removed from the alveolar air by the blood. The average PP of O_2 in alveolar air (P_AO_2) at sea level is about 100 mm Hg. There is a negligible amount of CO_2 in ambient air and significant amounts (about 5.6%)

*Diffusion is the random movement of molecules down their concentration gradient. The term *partial pressure* can be substituted for *concentration* when speaking of gas mixtures because the contribution of each gas to the total pressure of a gas mixture is directly proportional to the concentration of that gas in the mixture (Dalton's Law).

Study Pearl

Atmospheric air consists primarily of nitrogen (78%) and O_2 (21%) with very small quantities of water vapor, CO_2 (0.4%), and inert gases such as argon (0.6%). Partial pressure (PP) is the individual pressure exerted independently by a particular gas within a mixture of gasses.[4] The PP exerted by each gas in a mixture equals the total pressure times the fractional composition of the gas in the mixture. Thus, given that the total atmospheric (barometric) pressure (at sea level) is about 760 mm Hg and, further, that air is about 21% oxygen, then the PP of O_2 (PO_2) in the air is 0.21 multiplied by 760 mm Hg which equals approximately 160 mm Hg.[4] The fraction of inspired oxygen (FiO_2) is defined as the concentration of O_2 in the air at a fraction of 1.0. Therefore the FiO_2 of room air, approximately 21% oxygen, is written as 0.21.[4]

Study Pearl

Inspired tracheal PO_2 is fixed unless

1. Supplemental O_2 is administered.
2. The individual changes altitude or rebreathes his or her own exhaled air.

In contrast, the PO_2 (and PCO_2) in alveolar gas and that in arterial, capillaries, and venous blood are affected by many factors in health and disease.

Study Pearl

If the CO_2 production by the tissues remains constant, a decrease in alveolar ventilation will result in an accumulation of CO_2 in the alveolus with an increase in its PP.[1]

Study Pearl

High breathing frequencies are commonly observed in the individual with a restrictive lung disease who has stiff (noncompliant) lungs that are difficult to expand to a normal tidal volume. Because a dead-space volume accompanies each breath, such breathing patterns provide less alveolar ventilation than the same total minute ventilation produced by slow, deep breathing.[4]

Study Pearl

As O_2 diffuses into the pulmonary blood, it combines with hemoglobin to form oxyhemoglobin. Blood in the systemic arteries has a percent oxyhemoglobin saturation of 97% (97% of the hemoglobin is in the form of oxyhemoglobin). This blood is delivered to the systemic capillaries, where O_2 diffuses into the cells where it is used in the production of energy (ATP). Blood leaving in the systemic veins is thus reduced in O_2; it has a PO_2 of about 40 mm Hg and a percent oxyhemoglobin saturation of about 75% when a person is at rest. Expressed another way, blood entering the tissues contains 20 ml O_2 per 100 ml blood, and blood leaving the tissues contains 15.5 ml O_2 per 100 ml blood. Thus, 22%, or 4.5 ml of O_2 out of the 20 ml of O_2 per 100 ml blood, is unloaded to the tissues.

in alveolar air because CO_2 is constantly being added to the alveolar air by the blood. During normal breathing, the average PP of alveolar CO_2 ($PACO_2$) is 40 mm Hg.

The values for alveolar gas pressures are basically the resultant of only two variables, both of which depend upon the integrity of the pulmonary and circulatory systems:

1. The relative magnitudes of the alveolar ventilation
2. The oxygen consumption and CO_2 production

When liquid is exposed to a gas mixture, as pulmonary capillary blood is to alveolar air, the molecules of each gas diffuse between air and liquid until the pressure of the dissolved molecules equals the PP of that gas in the gas mixture. The diffusion pathway between air and red blood cells consist of both tissue and blood. The tissue barrier is normally extremely thin, but in disease states, such as pulmonary fibrosis, the interstitial tissues may be thickened, widening the tissue barrier.[1]

The blood entering the pulmonary capillaries has come from the tissues and therefore has a high PCO_2 (46 mm Hg) and a low PO_2 (40 mm Hg). As it passes through the pulmonary capillaries, the blood is separated from the alveolar air by a tissue barrier which allows for the net diffusion of oxygen into the blood and carbon dioxide into the alveoli, which causes the capillary blood oxygen levels to rise and the carbon dioxide levels to fall. Once the alveolar and capillary partial pressures become equal, the net diffusion of these gases ceases.

Gas Transport

The various steps involved in O_2 and CO_2 transport are outlined in Table 10-7. After the diffusion of O_2 from the alveolar air into the blood, O_2 is transported by the blood to the tissue capillaries.[1]

When the hemoglobin is 100% saturated with O_2, each molecule is capable of combining with four molecules of O_2.

CO_2 is transported from the tissues to the lungs by way of the red blood cell. Carbon dioxide is carried by the blood as follows:[2]

1. Approximately 1/10 of the total blood CO_2 is dissolved in plasma.
2. Approximately 1/5 of the total blood CO_2 is carried attached to an amino acid in hemoglobin called carbaminohemoglobin.

Intrapulmonary Shunt

For ideal gas exchange to occur, equal volumes of fresh air entering the alveoli should come into contact with equal volumes of blood flowing through the alveolar capillaries. Put another way, alveolar ventilation (V_A) should match the pulmonary blood flow (Q). The relationship of the two flows is the ventilation/perfusion ratio, or the V/Q ratio.[1] Usually the V/Q ratio is considered for various areas of the lungs and not for the lungs as a whole. However, when considering the lungs as a whole, the ratio is 0.8. Alveolar ventilation and blood flow vary independently throughout the lung. In the upright position, blood flow is less than ventilation at the lung apex because some of the capillaries are compressed (the V/Q ratio is high). In contrast, at

TABLE 10-7. THE STEPS INVOLVED IN O_2 AND CO_2 TRANSPORT

Step One: Inspired (tracheal) to alveolar air gradient	The difference between tracheal and alveolar partial pressures is determined solely by the level of alveolar ventilation (V_A) in relation to metabolic requirements (O_2 consumed or CO_2 produced). Thus, for a given oxygen uptake (V_{O_2}) or carbon dioxide production (V_{CO_2}) the higher the ventilatory rate, the higher the alveolar PO_2 and the lower the alveolar PCO_2 and vice versa.
Step Two: Alveolar-to-arterial PO_2 difference	The difference in alveolar (PAO_2) and arterial (PaO_2) partial pressures of oxygen is determined by the ability of the lung to oxygenate and mix venous blood that is returned to the lung. This ability depends on the rate of diffusion between the alveoli in pulmonary capillaries and on the uniformity with which blood perfusing the pulmonary capillaries is matched with ventilation of the alveoli.
Step Three: Gas transport by the blood	Depends critically on the ability of hemoglobin to bind O_2 tightly at high PO_2 (ie, as blood leaves the lung) and also to release O_2 readily at lower PO_2 (ie, as blood transverses the capillaries of active tissue).
Step Four: Exchange of gases between capillary and tissue mitochondria	Occurs almost entirely by diffusion.

Data from Morgan BJ, Dempsey JA: Physiology of the cardiovascular and pulmonary systems. In: DeTurk WE, Cahalin LP, eds. *Cardiovascular and Pulmonary Physical Therapy: an Evidence-Based Approach*. New York: McGraw-Hill. 2004:95-122.

the base of the lung, ventilation is three times greater but blood flow is 10 times greater than that of the apex (the V/Q ratio is low).

Study Pearl

It is the PP of the dissolved oxygen molecules in the blood that primarily determines the volume of O_2 that combines with hemoglobin. As the PP of dissolved O_2 increases, the percent saturation of hemoglobin increases.

The Cough Mechanism

The major function of the cough mechanism or reflex is to help clear secretions from the airways, particularly to help expel them through the larynx. Normally, the cough is an involuntary reflex, which is controlled by a complex interaction of nerve fibers and receptor sites situated in the nose, nasopharynx, larynx, auditory canal, trachea, pulmonary bronchus and pleura, and the cough center which is located in the medulla of the brain. The movements resulting in a cough occur as follows: about 2.5 L of air are inspired, the epiglottis closes, and the vestibular folds and vocal cords close tightly to trap the inspired air in the lung; the abdominal muscles contract to force the abdominal contents up against the diaphragm; and the muscles of expiration contract forcefully. As a consequence, the pressure in the lungs increases to about 100 mm Hg. Then the vestibular folds, the vocal cords, and the epiglottis open suddenly, and the air rushes from the lungs at a high velocity, carrying foreign particles with it.

The cough reflex can be significantly compromised in the following patient populations:

- Spinal cord injuries above the T 10 level
- COPD
- Cystic fibrosis
- Postsurgical (abdominal/thoracic) due to pain

Study Pearl

Most of the CO_2 carried by the blood is in the form of bicarbonate.

Study Pearl

In lung disease blood flow is in excess of ventilation (the V/Q ratio is less than 1), resulting in low arterial oxygen (hypoxemia). The more severe the V/Q imbalance, the higher the concentration of inspired oxygen that is required to raise the arterial oxygen.

When ventilation exceeds blood flow, the V/Q ratio is high. There is excess alveolar ventilation, and not all of the ventilated air takes part in gas exchange, producing an alveolar dead space ("wasted" ventilation).

PHYSICAL THERAPY EXAMINATION

The examination of the patient's pulmonary status has several purposes:[7]

- To evaluate the appropriateness of the patient's participation in a pulmonary rehabilitation program

Study Pearl

The sneeze reflex differs in several ways to the cough reflex. The source of irritation that initiates the sneeze reflex is in the nasal passages instead of in the trachea and bronchi, and the action potentials are conducted along the trigeminal nerves to the medulla, where the reflex is triggered. During the sneeze reflex, the uvula and the soft palate are depressed so the air is directed primarily through the nasal passages, although a considerable amount passes through the oral cavity. The rapidly flowing air dislodges particulate matter from the nasal passages and propels it a considerable distance from the nose.

- To determine the therapeutic measures most appropriate for the participant's treatment program
- To monitor the participant's physiological response to exercise
- To appropriately progress the participant's treatment program over time.

History

The past medical history is an important part of the systems review of all patients, especially in those patients with known or suspected pulmonary disease. Previous medical problems that may predispose a person to pulmonary disorders include recurrent pulmonary infections, cardiac disease (eg, heart failure), musculoskeletal disorders (eg, scoliosis, ankylosing spondylitis), integumentary disorders (marked burns to thorax, scleroderma), obesity, premature birth, and neuromuscular disorders (eg, cerebrovascular accident, Guillain-Barré, muscular dystrophy).[8] Primary and secondary risk factors for pulmonary diseases are listed in Table 10-8.

The early signs of pulmonary disease include reports of marked shortness of breath (SOB) with exertion, a cough that won't go away, or frequent respiratory infections. Other signs and symptoms include reports of:

- Changes in the amount, consistency, and/or color of sputum
- An increase or decrease in the amount of sputum produced

TABLE 10-8. PRIMARY AND SECONDARY RISK FACTORS FOR PULMONARY DISORDERS

Obstructive lung disease	Smoking
	Occupational exposure to irritants or allergens (eg, asbestos, chemicals)
	Residing in locations with high levels of air pollution
	Premature birth— bronchopulmonary dysplasia
	Emphysema
	Asthma
	Bronchitis
	Bronchiectasis
	Cystic fibrosis
Restrictive lung disease	Occupational exposure to irritants or allergens (eg, asbestos, chemicals)
	Cardiovascular disorders (eg, pulmonary edema from heart failure, pulmonary emboli)
	Neuromuscular disorders (eg, spinal cord injury, cerebrovascular accident, Guillain-Barré, muscular dystrophy)
	Musculoskeletal disorders (eg, scoliosis, ankylosing spondylitis)
	Integumentary disorders (marked burns to thorax, scleroderma)
	Past oncologic disorder treated with chemotherapy or radiation therapy
	Trauma (eg, crush injuries).
	Surgical pain or scarring
	Obesity
	Pregnancy
	Premature births—hyaline membrane disease
Pulmonary hypertension	
Primary	Autoimmune dysfunction
	Vascular dysfunction
Secondary	Severe obstructive or restrictive lung disease
	Severe heart failure

Reproduced, with permission, from Cahalin LP: Pulmonary evaluation. In DeTurk WE, Cahalin LP, eds. *Cardiovascular and Pulmonary Physical Therapy: An Evidence-Based Approach*. New York: McGraw-Hill. 2004:221-269.

- An increase in the thickness or stickiness of sputum
- A change in sputum color to yellow or green or the presence of blood in the sputum
- An increase in the severity of shortness of breath, cough and/or wheezing
- A persistent feeling of malaise, fatigue, and lack of energy
- Ankle swelling
- Forgetfulness, confusion, slurring of speech, and sleepiness
- Trouble sleeping
- Using more pillows or sleeping in a chair instead of a bed to avoid shortness of breath (SOB)
- An unexplained increase or decrease in weight
- A lack of sexual drive
- Increasing morning headaches, dizzy spells, or restlessness

The clinician should also review the patient's occupational history (for exposures to chemicals and substances associated with asbestosis, silicosis and pneumoconiosis, or allergens), current medications, levels of activity and exercise, any family history of pulmonary disease, and social habits (smoking). A history of smoking is the greatest key to unlocking the likelihood and severity of pulmonary disease.[8]

Observation

A patient's appearance can suggest the presence and severity of several pulmonary disorders such as emphysema, chronic bronchitis, or restrictive lung disease.[8] Cyanosis (of the skin, lips, or extremities), digital clubbing, nasal flaring, and excessive use of the accessory muscles of respiration are all indications of a pulmonary disorder and potential hypoxia.

In addition, the clinician should observe for the presence of peripheral edema, and overall posture (stabilizing the shoulder girdle places the thorax in the inspiratory position and allows the additional recruitment of muscles for inspiration). The trachea should be in midline, superior to the suprasternal notch. The right and left thorax should be symmetrical. Asymmetry may be produced by scoliosis, scapular instability, or pain.

One of the most common subjective reports of patients with pulmonary disorders is dyspnea.[8] Dyspnea can be evaluated using a variety of different methods including listening to the breathing cycle using a stethoscope (Table 10-9), and observing the breathing patterns (Table 10-10). Focusing on the upper and the lower chest-wall movements can aid observation of the breathing pattern. A normal breathing pattern consists of an outward upper and lower chest-wall motion during inspiration and inward upper and lower chest wall-motion during expiration.

Tests and Measures

Auscultation. There are six to eight auscultatory sites on the posterior chest and four to six sites on the anterior chest (Figure 10-4).[8] Two sites are also present in the left and right axillary areas. It is recommended that the patient take two complete deep breaths while the diaphragm of the stethoscope is applied to each site followed by a short rest. (See Tables 10-11 to 10-13.)

Study Pearl

Listening to a patient's past history, habits, and complaints (and attempting to quantify these variables) is instrumental in understanding the absence or presence of disease, severity of disease, treatment choice, treatment effects, and quality-of-life.[8]

Study Pearl

Hypoxia is defined as a deficiency of oxygen at the tissue level or the body as a whole. The major causes of hypoxia are

- Reduced PO_2 (hypoxic hypoxia). Includes the following: breathing at high altitude, hypoventilation (eg, asthma, paralysis of respiratory muscles), deficient alveolar-capillary diffusion (eg, pneumonia), and abnormal matching of ventilation and blood flow (eg, emphysema)
- Inhibition of the mechanism by which hemoglobin binds oxygen (eg, carbon monoxide poisoning)
- Reduction in the total oxygen content of the blood due to an inadequate number of red blood cells (anemic hypoxia). Includes conditions of reduced hemoglobin and reduced hematocrit.
- Inability of the blood to carry oxygen (hypemic hypoxia)
- Insufficient blood flow to the tissues (ischemic hypoxia)
- Inefficient utilization of the oxygen due to the presence of a toxic agent (histotoxic hypoxia)

TABLE 10-9. BREATH SOUNDS AND OTHER EXAMINATION FINDINGS COMMONLY ASSOCIATED WITH SPECIFIC PATHOLOGIES

PATHOLOGY OR CONDITION	BREATH SOUNDS	ADVENTITIOUS BREATH SOUNDS	TRANSMITTED VOICE SOUNDS	PERCUSSION SOUNDS	FREMITUS	POSITION OF TRACHEA
Normal lung	Vesicular	Possibly late inspiratory crackles at bases which resolve with deep breaths	Absent	Resonant	Normal	Midline
Emphysema	Diminished vesicular	Usually absent	Absent	Hyperresonant	Decreased	Midline
Bronchitis	Vesicular	Early-inspiratory crackles and possible rhonchi and wheezing	Absent	Resonant to hyperresonant	Normal	Midline
Bronchiectasis	Vesicular	Mid-inspiratory crackles	Absent	Resonant	Normal	Midline
Pulmonary fibrosis	Bronchovesicular	Late inspiratory crackles	Absent	Resonant	Normal or increased	Midline
Status asthmaticus	Vesicular	Inspiratory and expiratory wheezing	Absent	Hyperresonant	Decreased	Midline
Large pleural effusion	Bronchial sounds immediately above the effusion and absent sounds over the effusion	Friction rub above the effusion	Possibly present above the effusion, but absent over the effusion	Flat	Absent	Shifted to the side opposite the pleural effusion
Pneumothorax	Absent	Absent	Absent	Tympanic	Absent	Shifted to the side opposite the pneumothorax
Atelectasis with patent bronchi	Bronchial	Absent	All are present	Dull	Increased	Shifted to the same side of the atelectasis
Atelectasis with plugged bronchi	Absent	Absent	Absent	Dull	Absent	Shifted to the same side of the atelectasis
Consolidation (eg pneumonia)	Bronchial	Late inspiratory crackles	All are present	Dull	Increased	Midline

Reproduced, with permission, from Cahalin LP: Pulmonary evaluation. In: DeTurk WE, Cahalin LP, eds. Cardiovascular and Pulmonary Physical Therapy: An Evidence Based Approach. New York: McGraw-Hill. 2004:221-269.

TABLE 10-10. CHARACTERISTICS AND EXAMINATION TECHNIQUES OF DIFFERENT BREATHING PATTERNS

BREATHING PATTERN	DISTINGUISHING CHARACTERISTIC	EXAMINATION TECHNIQUE
Normal	Synchronous upward and outward motion of the abdomen and upper chest	Visual, palpation, CWE
Abdominal-Paradox	Upward and outward motion of the upper chest and inward motion of the abdomen	Visual, palpation, CWE
Upper chest-Paradox	Upward and outward motion of the abdomen and inward motion of the upper chest	Visual, palpation, CWE
Excessive accessory muscle use	Excessive chest motion with increased use of the sternocleidomastoid muscle, scalenes, and other accessory muscles of inspiration	Visual, palpation, CWE

CWE, chest wall excursion via tape measure or ruler if the patient can assume a supine position.
Reproduced, with permission, from Cahalin LP: Pulmonary evaluation. In: DeTurk WE, Cahalin LP, eds. *Cardiovascular and Pulmonary Physical Therapy: An Evidence-Based Approach*. New York: McGraw-Hill. 2004:221-269.

Examining the Muscles of Breathing. Observation, palpation, and perturbation of the inspiratory muscles can provide important information to the clinician. For example, a patient with obstructive lung disease may demonstrate excessive use of the scalene and sternocleidomastoid muscles during respiration.

Placement of the hands on the upper and lower chest of the patient while breathing will yield valuable examination information about the principle breathing pattern.[8] Chest-wall excursion can be measured more objectively at three anatomical sites using a tape measure. The three anatomical sites include the sternal angle of Louis on the sternum (at the second rib), the xiphoid process, and a midpoint between the xiphoid process and the umbilicus. The difference between the resting position and the position of full inspiration, measured at the base of the lungs, should be between 2 and 3 in.

Study Pearl

Respiratory inductive plethysmography is considered by some to be the "gold standard" technique to evaluate chest-wall excursion and the relationship between upper and lower chest-wall excursion.[8]

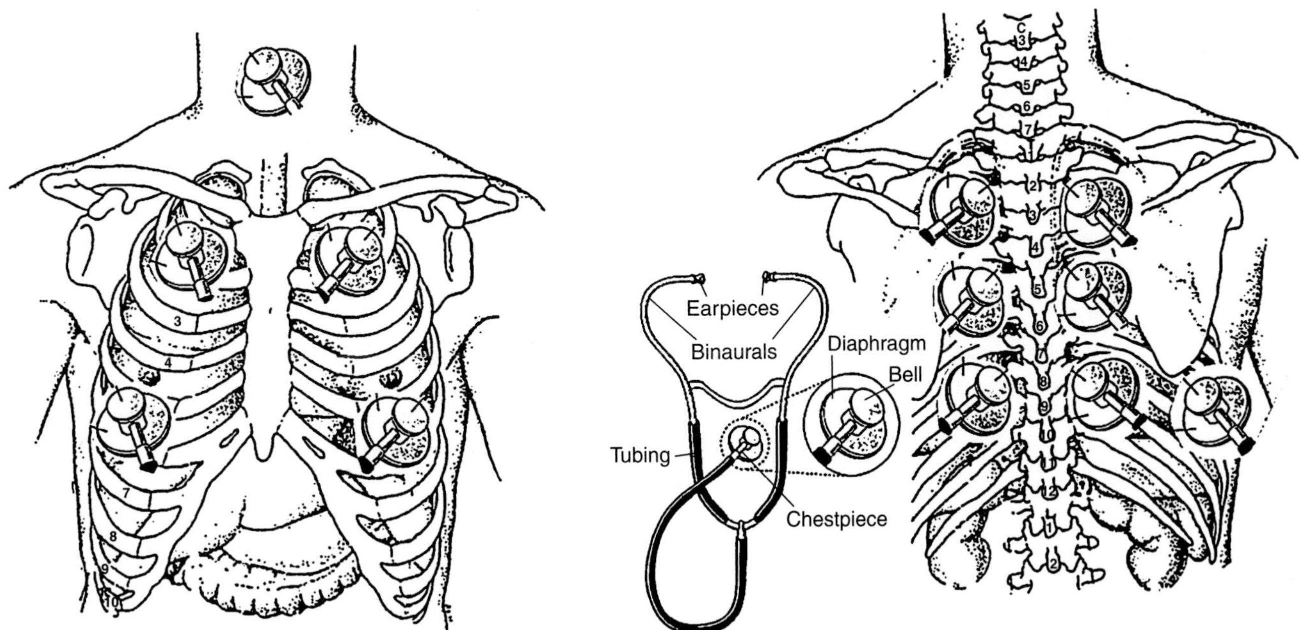

Figure 10-4. The stethoscope and sites for optimal auscultation with underlying lung segments. (Reproduced, with permission, from DeTurk WE, Cahalin LP: Cardiovascular and Pulmonary Physical Therapy: An Evidence-Based Approach. New York: McGraw-Hill. 2004:226.)

TABLE 10-11. DISTINGUISHING CHARACTERISTICS OF BREATH SOUNDS

SOUND	LOCATION OF SOUND	SOUND QUALITY	DISTINGUISHING CHARACTERISTIC
Vesicular	Periphery of lungs	Soft, low-pitched ("gentle rustling sound")	Inspiration is longer and louder than expiration **without** a pause
Bronchial	Sternum/manubrium	Loud, high-pitched ("hollow pipe sound")	Expiration is longer and louder than inspiration **with** a pause
Bronchovescular	1st and 2nd ICS and between scapulae (near main stem bronchus)	Medium pitched	Inspiration and expiration are equal in length and loudness
Tracheal	Over the trachea	Loud, harsh	Expiration is slightly longer than inspiration with similar loudness
Adventitious crackles (rales)	Over lungs with disease or disorders	Soft, high-pitched, discontinuous (like head rubbed between the fingers)	Occur early during inspiration with bronchitis, emphysema, asthma Occur late during inspiration with interstitial lung disease, pulmonary edema
Wheeze	Over lungs and airways that are constricted	High-pitched, continuous ("musical")	Heard most often during expiration, it may be heard during inspiration; the result of airway constriction
Transmitted voice sounds			
Egophony	Over consolidated lung tissue	"E" is heard as "A"	Mass/exudate in the lungs enables greater transmission of the sound of the patient repeating the letter "E"
Bronchophony	Over consolidated lung tissue	"99" is heard clearly	Mass/exudate in the lungs enables greater transmission of the sound of the patient repeating the number "99"
Whispered pectoriloquy	Over consolidated lung tissue	Whispered sound is heard clearly	Mass/exudate in the lungs enables greater transmission of the sound of the patient whispering

ICS, intercostal space
Reproduced, with permission, from Cahalin LP: Pulmonary evaluation. In: DeTurk WE, Cahalin LP, eds. *Cardiovascular and Pulmonary Physical Therapy: An Evidence-Based Approach*. New York: McGraw-Hill. 2004:221-269.

TABLE 10-12. NORMAL BREATH SOUNDS

SOUND	DESCRIPTION
Bronchial	Bronchial breath sounds consist of a full inspiratory and expiratory phase with the inspiratory phase usually being louder. They are normally heard over the trachea and larynx but may also be heard over the hilar region in individuals that are breathing hard (ie, after exercise) Bronchial sounds heard over the thorax suggest lung consolidation and pulmonary disease (pulmonary consolidation results in improved transmission of breath sounds originating in the trachea and primary bronchi that are then heard at increased intensity over the thorax).
Bronchovesicular	Bronchovesicular breath sounds consist of a full inspiratory phase with a shortened and softer expiratory phase. They are normally heard over the hilar region but should be quieter than the tracheal breath sounds. Increased intensity of bronchovesicular sounds is most often associated with increased ventilation or pulmonary consolidation.
Vesicular	Consist of a quiet, wispy inspiratory phase followed by a short, almost silent expiratory phase that is heard over the periphery of the lung field. These sounds are the result of attenuation of breath sounds produced in the bronchi at the hilar region of the lungs. Increased intensity may be associated with pulmonary consolidation.

Data from Cahalin LP: Pulmonary evaluation. In: DeTurk WE, Cahalin LP, eds. *Cardiovascular and Pulmonary Physical Therapy: An Evidence-Based Approach*. New York: McGraw-Hill. 2004:221-269.

TABLE 10-13. ABNORMAL BREATH SOUNDS

SOUND	DESCRIPTION
Crackles	Crackles are discontinuous, explosive, "popping" sounds that originate within the airways. They are heard when an obstructed airway suddenly opens and the pressures on either side of the obstruction suddenly equilibrate resulting in transient, distinct vibrations in the airway wall. The dynamic airway obstruction can be caused by either accumulation of secretions within the airway lumen or by airway collapse caused by pressure from inflammation or edema in surrounding pulmonary tissue. Crackles can be heard during inspiration when intrathoracic negative pressure results in opening of the airways or on expiration when thoracic positive pressure forces collapsed or blocked airways open. Crackles are heard more commonly during inspiration than expiration. They are significant as they imply either accumulation of fluid secretions or exudate within airways or inflammation and edema in the pulmonary tissue.
Wheezes	Continuous musical tones that are most commonly heard at end inspiration or early expiration. Result as a collapsed airway lumen gradually opens during inspiration or gradually closes during expiration. As the airway lumen becomes smaller, the air flow velocity increases resulting in harmonic vibration of the airway wall and thus the musical tonal quality. Can be classified as either high pitched or low pitched wheezes. May be monophonic (a single pitch and tonal quality heard over an isolated area) or polyphonic (multiple pitches and tones heard over a variable area of the lung). Wheezes are significant as they imply decreased airway lumen diameter either due to thickening of reactive airway walls or collapse of airways due to pressure from surrounding pulmonary disease.
Stridor	Intense continuous monophonic wheezes heard loudest over extrathoracic airways that can often be heard without the aid of a stethoscope. These extrathoracic sounds are often referred down the airways, can often be heard over the thorax, and are often mistaken as pulmonary wheezes. Tend to be accentuated during inspiration when extrathoracic airways collapse due to lower internal lumen pressure. Stridor is significant and indicates upper airway obstruction.
Stertor	A poorly defined and inconsistently used term to describe harsh discontinuous crackling sounds heard over the larynx or trachea. Also described as a sonorous snoring sound heard over extrathoracic airways. Stertor is significant as it is suggestive of accumulation of secretions within extrathoracic airways.
Rhonchi	Abnormal dry, leathery sounds heard in the lungs, which indicate inflammation of the bronchial tubes.

Examining Vital Signs. The following vital signs should be checked (refer to Chapter 11):

- Temperature.
- Heart rate.
- Blood pressure.
- Respirations—rate, rhythm (Table 10-14), and amplitude. Respiration rate is the number of breaths taken each minute (a breath is one inhalation and one exhalation). The rate is usually measured when a person is at rest and simply involves counting the number of breaths for 1 minute by counting how many times the chest rises. Normal respiration rates for an adult person at rest range from 15 to 20 breaths per minute (the normal rate for a newborn is between 30-60 breaths per minute). Respiration rates over 25 breaths per minute or under 12 breaths per minute (when at rest) may be considered abnormal. The expirations are normally approximately twice as long as the inspirations. The opposite occurs in conditions such as chronic obstructive pulmonary disease (COPD).

Chest Percussion. Chest percussion is an assessment technique that involves the creation of deliberate vibrations by tapping on the patient's chest wall. Just as lightly tapping on a container produces various sounds, so tapping on the chest wall produces sounds based on the amount of air in the lungs. Percussion helps to determine

TABLE 10-14. ABNORMAL BREATHING PATTERNS

PATTERN	DESCRIPTION
Cheyne-Stokes	A common and bizarre breathing pattern characterized by alternating periods of apnea and hyperpnea. Typically, over a period of 1 minute, a 10-20 second episode of apnea or hypopnea is observed followed by respirations of increasing depth and frequency. The cycle then repeats itself. Despite periods of apnea, significant hypoxia rarely occurs. Occurs in congestive heart failure, encephalitis, cerebral circulatory disturbances, and drug overdose, manifesting as a lesion of the bulbar center of respiration. The condition may also, however, be present as a normal finding in children, and in healthy adults following fast ascending to great altitudes, or in sleep.
Kussmaul's breathing	Rhythmic, gasping, and very deep type of respiration with normal or reduced frequency, associated with severe diabetes or renal acidosis or coma. Also known as air hunger syndrome.
Hyperventilation	Rapid breathing, often due to anxiety.
Biot (ataxic) breathing	Breathing that is irregular in timing and depth. It is indicative of meningitis or medullary lesions.
Apneustic breathing	This is an abnormal pattern of breathing characterized by a post-inspiratory pause. The usual cause of apneustic breathing is a pontine lesion.
Paradoxical respiration	This is an abnormal pattern of breathing in which the abdominal wall is sucked in during inspiration (it is usually pushed out). Paradoxical respiration is due to paralysis of the diaphragm.
Sleep apnea	Sleep apnea is defined as the cessation of breathing during sleep. There are three different types of sleep apnea: ▶ Obstructive: the most common. Characterized by repetitive pauses in breathing during sleep due to the obstruction and/or collapse of the upper airway (throat), usually accompanied by a reduction in blood oxygen saturation, and followed by an awakening to breathe. This is called an apnea event. Respiratory effort continues during the episodes of apnea. ▶ Central: a neurological condition causing cessation of all respiratory effort during sleep, usually with decreases in blood oxygen saturation. The person is aroused from sleep by an automatic breathing reflex, so may end up getting very little sleep at all. ▶ Mixed: a combination of the previous two. An episode of mixed sleep apnea usually starts with a central component and then becomes obstructive in nature. Generally the central component of the apnea becomes less troublesome once the obstructive apnea is treated.

whether the underlying tissues are filled with air, fluid, or solid material. While listening with a stethoscope, the clinician hyperextends the middle finger of one hand and places the distal interphalangeal joint firmly against the patient's chest. Using the end (not the pad) of the opposite middle finger, the clinician uses a quick flick of the wrist to strike the first finger. Five percussion tones are recognized:

- Resonance: low-pitched, hollow sound—a normal sound over healthy lungs.
- Hyperresonance: a normal finding in pediatric patients or very thin adults, but in normal adults it is suggestive of air trapped in the lungs (emphysema, asthma, chronic bronchitis, and pneumothorax).
- Dullness: indicates tissue consolidation (pneumonia, atelectasis, growth).
- Flatness: usually heard over bony areas, or dense areas such as the liver. If felt over the lungs, indicates pleural effusion.
- Tympanic: hollow, high, drum-like sounds. Tympany is normally heard over the stomach, but is not a normal chest sound. Tympanic sounds heard over the chest indicate excessive air in the chest, such as may occur with pneumothorax.

Exercise Tolerance Tests. Refer to Chapter 11.

Pulmonary Function Tests. Pulmonary function tests are a broad range of tests designed to assess a wide array of ventilation volumes including tidal volume, expiratory reserve volume (ERV),

TABLE 10-15. PULMONARY FUNCTION TESTS FOR THE PATIENT WITH DYSPNEA OF UNCERTAIN ETIOLOGY

	OBSTRUCTIVE		RESTRICTIVE
FUNCTION TEST	ASTHMA	EMPHYSEMA	FIBROSIS
FVC	Low	N or low	Low
FEV_1	Very low	Very low	Low
FEV_1/FVC %	Low	Low	N or high
TLC	Normal or high	High	Low

forced expiratory flow (FEF), forced vital capacity, functional residual capacity (FRC), inspiratory capacity, inspiratory reserve volume, peak expiratory flow (Tables 10-15 and 10-16).

Imaging Studies

Chest Radiographs. Refer to Table 10-17.

Computed Tomography. A computed tomography (CT) is simply digitized radiography and allows for numerous digital images of a tissue to be taken at many different angles. Using a CT, the degree of radiolucency and radiopacity are quantified, which then allows for the digitized radiograph to be computed and acquired.[8]

Magnetic Resonance Imaging. A magnetic resonance imaging (MRI) test quantifies and qualifies the tissue being scanned, which then allows for computation and acquisition of the MRI.

Bronchoscopy. Bronchoscopy allows visualization of the proximal airways of the lungs through a bronchoscope, a relatively large flexible scope that requires lubrication and some degree of anesthetic before insertion through the mouth into the trachea. A bronchoscopy is used to provide visualization of the proximal airways, and to remove secretions in the proximal airways.

Laboratory tests

Sputum Analysis. Laboratory analysis of a sputum sample includes many different tests for specific pathogens (Table 10-18).

Arterial Blood Gas (ABG) Analysis. An arterial blood gas (ABG) test measures the levels of oxygen and carbon dioxide in the blood to determine the effectiveness of alveolar ventilation. Values are expressed as the partial pressure of the gas (see Table 3-- Acid-based status tests in Appendix). An ABG measures:

- Partial pressure of O_2 (PaO_2): the O_2 level (normally at 105 mm Hg in the alveoli) indicates how well O_2 is able to move from the airspace of the lungs into the blood.

TABLE 10-16. DIFFERENCES BETWEEN RESTRICTIVE AND OBSTRUCTIVE DISEASE

RESTRICTIVE	OBSTRUCTIVE
Decreased TLC	~Increased TLC
Increased elastic recoil	Decreased elastic recoil
Decreased compliance	Increased compliance
Increased FEV_1% (ie, FEV_1/FVC)	Decreased FEV_1%

TABLE 10-17 METHODS TO EXAMINE CHEST RADIOGRAPHS

METHOD	DESCRIPTION
Begin examining the chest radiograph from the center of the film and examine it outwards.	
Identify the bones, soft tissues, and organs of the body.	a. Mediastinum from the larynx to the abdomen b. Heart, lungs, and vascular tree c. Hila d. Diaphragm/hemidiaphragm
Specific lung field examination: compare observed chest radiograph images to expected images.	a. Mediastinum should be a vertical translucent shadow overlying the cervical vertebra. b. Heart and great vessels should occupy the lower 2/3 of the mediastinum with two distinct visible curves on the right side and four distinct curves on the left side of the cardiovascular tree. On the right side, the first is formed by the right atrium and begins at the right cardiophrenic angle and proceeds superiorly as well as the inferior vena cava entering the right atrium, inferiorly. The second curve on the right side is the ascending aorta and the superior vena cava. The four distinct curves on the left side include the transverse arch and descending aorta, main pulmonary artery, left atrial appendage (which may or may not be visible), and the border of the left ventricle. c. Hila should be poorly defined areas of variable density in the medial part of the central portion of the lung fields. d. Diaphragm/hemidiaphragm should be visible and the dome of the right hemidiaphragm is normally 1-2 cm higher than the left. e. Lung fields should be examined in view of the different lobes of the lungs and the various bronchopulmonary segments of the different lobes. Lesions in the markings can be localized by a select sign (normal lines of demarcation between different structures are partially or completely obscured) or changed vascular markings (increased vascular markings are associated with venous dilation and decreased markings are often associated with hyperinflation of lungs).
Search for abnormal density within or lung fields.	Abnormal density is identified by radiopacity (white image) in areas where there should be radiolucency (dark image).
Examine the angle of the ribs and the intercostal spaces.	The ribs are normally oriented obliquely; maybe oriented horizontally with severe hyperinflation of the lungs as in chronic COPD

Reproduced, with permission, from Cahalin LP: Pulmonary evaluation. In: DeTurk WE, Cahalin LP, eds. *Cardiovascular and Pulmonary Physical Therapy: An Evidence-Based Approach*. New York: McGraw-Hill. 2004:221-269.

- Partial pressure of CO_2 ($PaCO_2$): the CO_2 level (normally 37-43 mm Hg) indicates how well CO_2 is able to move out of the blood into the airspace of the lungs and out with exhaled air.
- pH: the pH is a measure of hydrogen ion (H+) in blood that indicates the acid or base (alkaline) nature of blood. A pH of less than 7 is acidic, and a pH greater than 7 is called basic (alkaline). The pH of blood is usually close to 7.4. A pH of < 7.2 is indicative of severe acidemia, whereas a pH of > 7.6 is indicative of severe alkalemia.
- Bicarbonate (HCO_3): buffers are chemical substances that keep the pH of blood within a normal range. Bicarbonate is the most important buffer in the blood. Bicarbonate saturation levels, controlled chiefly by the kidneys, are normally at 22 to 28 mmole/L.
- O_2 content (O_2CT) and O_2 saturation (O_2Sat) values: like the PaO_2, these values provide information about the amount of oxygen in the blood.

A determination can be made as to whether the change in pH level is the result of a metabolic or respiratory condition (Table 10-19) and the state of compensation (if uncompensated the pH level is abnormal but the HCO_3 and $PaCO_2$ levels are normal; Table 10-20).

TABLE 10-18. CLINICAL AND LABORATORY ANALYSIS OF SPUTUM

Color:
- ▶ Red (blood)
- ▶ Pink (pulmonary edema)
- ▶ White or clear (may indicate chronic cough or cystic fibrosis or chronic bronchitis)
- ▶ Yellow (an improving infection)
- ▶ Brown/rust (pneumonia)
- ▶ Greenish-brown (acute infection)
- ▶ Gray (abscess)

Consistency:
- ▶ Thin—patient is often less sick
- ▶ Moderately thick—patient is often slightly more sick than the patient with thin consistency of sputum
- ▶ Thick—patient is often more sick than the patient with thin or moderately thick consistency of sputum

Smell:
- ▶ No striking smell—patient is often less sick
- ▶ Foul smell—patient is often more sick

Laboratory analysis: specific antigen recognition (via culturing of specimens in various cultural media with or without oxygen and carbon dioxide at different temperatures and durations) to diagnose respiratory infections including:

Bacterial Pathogens

Chlamydia
Enterobacteriaceae
Hemophilus influenzae
Klebsiella pneumonia
Legionella
Mycoplasma pneumoniae
Pseudomonas aeruginosa
Streptococcus pneumoniae
Staphylococcus aureus

Fungal Pathogens

Aspergillus
Blastomyces dermatitidis
Candida
Coccidioides immitis
Cryptococcus neoformans
Histoplasma capsulatum

Protozoa Pathogens

Pneumocystis carinii

Viral Pathogens

Adenoviruses
Influenza A
Influenza B
Parainfluenza viruses
Respiratory syncytial virus

Reproduced, with permission, from Cahalin LP: Pulmonary Evaluation. In: DeTurk WE, Cahalin LP (eds) *Cardiovascular and Pulmonary Physical Therapy: An Evidence-Based Approach.* New York: McGraw-Hill. 2004:221-269.

PULMONARY PATHOLOGY

Obstructive Diseases

Chronic Obstructive Pulmonary Disease. Chronic obstructive pulmonary disease (COPD) is a generic term that refers to lung diseases that result in air trapping in the lungs (Table 10-21), causing hyperinflation of the lungs and a barrel chest deformity.[9]

TABLE 10-19. ACID-BASE DISORDERS

TYPE	FINDINGS	CAUSES	RESPONSE
Respiratory acidosis	High PCO_2 levels	Alveolar hypoventilation (COPD, head injury, drug overdose, lung disease, pain)	The initial response is cellular buffering that occurs over minutes to hours, which elevates plasma bicarbonate (HCO_3^-) only slightly. The second step is renal compensation that occurs over 3-5 days. With renal compensation, renal excretion of carbonic acid is increased and bicarbonate reabsorption is increased.
Metabolic alkalosis	High HCO_3 levels	Loss of hydrogen ions (vomiting or nasogastric [NG] suction generates metabolic alkalosis by the loss of gastric secretions, which are rich in hydrochloric acid [HCl]). Renal losses of hydrogen ions occur whenever the distal delivery of sodium increases in the presence of excess aldosterone (hypokalemia). Alkali administration: Administration of sodium bicarbonate in amounts that exceed the capacity of the kidneys to excrete this excess bicarbonate may cause metabolic alkalosis. Contraction alkalosis: Loss of bicarbonate-poor, chloride-rich extracellular fluid, as observed with thiazide diuretic or loop diuretic therapy or chloride diarrhea concentration.	Alveolar hypoventilation with a rise in arterial carbon dioxide tension ($PaCO_2$), which diminishes the change in pH that would otherwise occur.
Respiratory alkalosis	Low PCO_2 levels	Alveolar hyperventilation: central nervous system disorder (pain, anxiety, fear, CVA, meningitis). Hypoxemia (high altitudes, severe anemia), mechanical ventilation	Increased renal excretion of bicarbonate.
Metabolic acidosis	Low HCO_3 levels	Inability to excrete the dietary H^+ load (chronic renal disease, hypoaldosteronism) Ketoacidosis (diabetes, alcoholism, and starvation), Lactic acidosis (circulatory failure, drugs and toxins, and hereditary causes) GI HCO_3^- loss (diarrhea)	Metabolic acidosis most commonly stimulates the central and peripheral chemoreceptors that control respiration, resulting in an increase in alveolar ventilation, which results in a compensatory respiratory alkalosis. In addition, extracellular buffering (carbonic acid [H_2CO_3]) and renal excretion of the H^+ ion occurs.

TABLE 10-20. ACID-BASE DISORDERS AND COMPENSATIONS

DISORDER	COMPENSATION
Respiratory acidosis (hypercapnia): PCO_2 increases	Metabolic alkalosis (HCO_3 increases)
Respiratory alkalosis (hypocapnia): PCO_2 decreases	Metabolic acidosis (HCO_3 decreases)
Metabolic acidosis (hypokalemia): HCO_3 decreases	Respiratory alkalosis (PCO_2 decreases)
Metabolic alkalosis (hyperkalemia): HCO_3 increases	Respiratory acidosis (PCO_2 increases)

TABLE 10-21. DISEASES OR CONDITIONS THAT MAY BE ASSOCIATED WITH OBSTRUCTION TO AIRFLOW

Lower airway obstruction:	Asthma Chronic bronchitis Emphysema Cystic fibrosis Sarcoidosis
Upper airway obstruction:	Croup Laryngotracheobronchitis Epiglottitis Various tumors and foreign bodies that may involve the upper airway

COPD is characterized by airway narrowing, parenchymal destruction, and pulmonary vascular thickening. COPD can be subdivided into:

- Nonseptic obstructive pulmonary diseases, including such diseases as asthma, chronic bronchitis, emphysema, and α_1 antitrypsin (α_1 ATD) deficiency.
- Septic obstructive pulmonary diseases, including cystic fibrosis and bronchiectasis.

Risk factors for the development of COPD include both host factors and environmental factors:

- Host factors: hyperreactivity of the airways, overall lung growth, and genetics.
- Environmental factors: Smoking is the primary risk factor for COPD, with approximately 80 to 90% of COPD deaths caused by smoking.[10-12] Other risk factors of COPD include air pollution, second-hand smoke, history of childhood respiratory infections and heredity.[10-12] Occupational exposure to certain industrial pollutants also increases the odds for COPD.[13] The quality of life for a person suffering from COPD diminishes as the disease progresses. At the onset, there is minimal shortness of breath, but as the disease progresses these people may eventually require supplemental oxygen and may have to rely on mechanical respiratory assistance.

The medical management of chronic pulmonary disease includes smoking cessation, pharmacological agents (see Chapter 19), and the use of supplemental oxygen. An absolute indication for use of long-term oxygen therapy is an arterial partial pressure of oxygen (PaO_2) of 55 mm Hg or less, which correlates with an SaO_2 of 88% or less.[14]

NONSEPTIC OBSTRUCTIVE PULMONARY DISEASES

Asthma. Asthma is a chronic pulmonary disease, characterized by reversible obstruction to airflow within the lungs, which is caused by increased reaction of the airways to various stimuli. An asthma episode is a series of events that result in narrowed airways. These include: swelling of the lining, tightening of the muscle, and increased secretion of mucus in the airway. Although the breathing problems associated with asthma usually happen in "episodes," the inflammation underlying asthma is continuous. Triggers range from respiratory infections, cigarette smoke, allergens such as pollen, air pollutants, and vigorous exercise (exercise-induced asthma) to exposure to cold air or sudden temperature change.

The characteristic symptoms of asthma are episodic wheezing (due to bronchoconstriction), dyspnea, chest pain, facial distress, and usually a non-productive cough.[15] The symptoms are more severe in children than adults.[9]

The primary intervention for asthma is prevention, including smoking cessation and minimizing exposure to any stimulants that precipitate an asthmatic episode. The goal of pharmacotherapy is to provide relief of symptoms by reducing underlying inflammation in the airways and prevent complications and/or progression with a minimum of side effects.[16] Two classes of medications have been used to treat asthma—anti-inflammatory agents and bronchodilators.

- Anti-inflammatory drugs interrupt the development of bronchial inflammation and have a preventive action. They may also modify or terminate ongoing inflammatory reactions in the airways. These agents include corticosteroids, cromolyn sodium, and other anti-inflammatory compounds.
- Bronchodilators act principally to open the airways by relaxing bronchial muscle. They include beta-adrenergic agonists, methylxanthines, and anticholinergics.

Establishment of a routine exercise program is also important.[9]

Chronic bronchitis. Chronic bronchitis is a clinical diagnosis based on the presence of a persistent productive cough that produces sputum for more than 3 months per year for at least two consecutive years in the absence of another definable medical cause.[9] Presenting symptoms include:[17,18]

- Patient may be obese
- Chronic cough with frequent clearing of the throat
- Low-grade fever
- Increased mucus
- Dyspnea on exertion
- Use of accessory muscles for breathing
- Coarse rhonchi and wheezing may be heard on auscultation
- May have signs of right heart failure (ie, cor pulmonale), such as edema and cyanosis (patients are sometimes referred to as *blue bloaters*)

Medical management includes supplemental oxygen therapy, antiviral medications, and corticosteroids to suppress the inflammatory process.[9] Bronchodilators may be utilized for the management of bronchospasm.[9]

Emphysema. Emphysema begins insidiously with the destruction of alveoli in the lungs, the walls of which become thin and fragile. Damage is irreversible and results in permanent destruction of the acini.* As the acini are destroyed, the lungs are able to transfer less and less oxygen to the bloodstream, causing shortness of breath/hyperinflation, and compensatory changes of the chest wall.

*Each acinus, the functional unit of the lung for gas exchange, is composed of 1 to 3 respiratory bronchioles and the alveolar ducts and sacs.

Hyperinflation causes shortening of the inspiratory muscles and flattening of the diaphragm with loss of sarcomeres.[9] The end result is a loss of diaphragmatic excursion, a decline in the mechanical effectiveness of the diaphragm, and other respiratory muscles to support the increased demand of ventilation.[19] Signs and symptoms of emphysema include:

- In later stages of the disease, the patient becomes emaciated, and may adopt the tripod sitting position.
- Barrel chest (enlarged anterior–posterior dimension), with an increased rib angle.
- The presence of a chronic cough and sputum production will vary and depend on the infectious history of the patient.
- Diminished breath sounds and wheezing.
- Shortness of breath, especially with exertion (dyspnea on exertion) assisted by pursed lips and use of accessory respiratory muscles (patients are sometimes referred to as *pink puffers*), the latter of which may be hypertrophied through overuse.
- Heart sounds appear very distant.

The diagnosis is made by pulmonary function tests, chest x-ray (reveals hyperinflation with flattened diaphragm, decreased vascular markings, and possibly enlargement of the right side of the heart), along with the patient's history, and physical examination.

There are a number of treatment options for the care of patients with emphysema:

- Smoking cessation is instrumental.
- Pharmacology (bronchodilators, anticholinergic drugs, corticosteroids).
- Long-term oxygen therapy, including the use of BiPap ventilation.
- Bullectomy: a bulla is a large airspace that is the result of destruction of the parenchyma, and which no longer participates in gas exchange or diffusion
- Lung volume reduction surgery.
- Lung transplantation (single or double): for those patients with end-stage disease who have maximized medical intervention.

α_1 Antitrypsin Deficiency. This condition is caused by the inherited deficiency of a protein called α_1-antitrypsin (AAT) or alpha1-protease inhibitor. AAT, an enzyme produced by the liver, counter balances the degradation of tissue caused by proto-lytic enzyme, protease.[9]

Symptoms usually begin before the age of 50 years with a mean onset of 46 years.[20] The key significance of ATD is the premature development of emphysema, occurring in the third or fourth decade of life.[20] SOB and decreased exercise capacity are typically the first symptoms.[21] Smoking significantly increases the severity of emphysema in AAT-deficient individuals.[20] Blood screening is primarily used to diagnose whether a person is a carrier or AAT-deficient. Most of the available treatment protocols are consistent with the treatments for emphysema with bronchodilators, corticosteroids, cessation of smoking, and preventative vaccinations.[9] Pulmonary rehabilitation and supplemental oxygen therapy also are effective.[9]

Septic Obstructive Pulmonary Diseases

Cystic Fibrosis. Refer to Chapter 16.

Bronchiectasis. Bronchiectasis, the permanent dilation of the bronchi, is caused by the destruction of the muscular and elastic properties of the lung, and is characterized by inflamed airways that are full of purulent sputum.[9,22] The accumulation of mucus and the accompanying infection cause inflammation, and subsequent weakening and widening of the passages. The weakened passages can become scarred and deformed, allowing more accumulations of mucus and bacteria, resulting in a cycle of infection and destruction. Symptom severity varies greatly from patient to patient and occasionally, a patient may be asymptomatic. Symptoms of bronchiectasis include coughing (worsened when lying down), persistent production of large volumes of secretions, recurrent hemoptysis, shortness of breath, abnormal chest sounds (crackles, rhonchi and pleural rubs), weakness, weight loss, and fatigue.[22] The diagnosis is usually confirmed with a chest x-ray, breathing tests, sputum culture or computed tomography (CT) scan.[22] The principle treatment for bronchiectasis commonly includes the use of antibiotics, corticosteroids, and bronchodilators.[9] Nutritional support, supplemental oxygen, pulmonary hygiene, and patient education are also key components.[9] Surgical resection of the involved lung tissue may be considered to minimize recurrent exacerbations and further loss of lung function.[9,23]

> **Study Pearl**
>
> Aspiration has been clearly identified as a common contributing factor to the development of pneumonia.[9] Aspiration is associated with malnutrition, tube feeding, contracture of the cervical extensors, and the use of depressant medications.[34]

Infectious and Inflammatory Diseases

Bronchiolitis. See Chapter 16.

Pneumonia. Pneumonia involves an invasion of the respiratory tract by infectious organisms that lead to an acute inflammatory response of the alveoli and terminal airspaces. The infectious agents are typically introduced into the lungs through hematogenous spread or inhalation.[24-33] The degree of inflammatory response differs according to the type of infectious agent present. The infectious agents have predilections for certain age groups (Table 10-22).

The classic presentation for pneumonia includes fever and a productive cough with sputum production that is usually yellowish-green or rust-colored.[9] Fatigue, weight loss, dyspnea, and tachycardia may also be present depending on the extent of the disease.[9] Radiography is the primary imaging study used to confirm the diagnosis of pneumonia. Several other diagnostic studies are available:

- Sputum culture
- Bronchoscopy
- Lung aspirate
- Thoracentesis
- Serology

Once the diagnosis of pneumonia is made, antibiotic decisions are made based on the offending organism, the age of the patient, the history of exposure, the possibility of resistance, and other pertinent history.

> **Study Pearl**
>
> Tuberculosis can develop after inhaling droplets sprayed into the air from a cough or sneeze by someone infected with *M. tuberculosis*. Although the usual site of the disease is the lung, other organs may be involved. The risk of contracting TB increases with the frequency of contact with people with the disease, crowded or unsanitary living conditions, and poor nutrition. Infants, the elderly, and individuals who are immunocompromised are at higher risk for progression to disease or reactivation of dormant disease. TB may also lie dormant for years and reappear after the initial infection is contained.

Mycobacterium Tuberculosis. Pulmonary tuberculosis (TB), in which the lungs are primarily involved, is a contagious bacterial infection caused by *Mycobacterium tuberculosis* (*M. tuberculosis*).[35-39]

TABLE 10-22. PREDILECTIONS OF PNEUMONIA IN CERTAIN AGE GROUPS

AGE GROUP	TYPE OF PNEUMONIA
Newborns (aged 0-30 d)	Bacterial pneumonia with group B Streptococcus, Listeria monocytogenes, or gram-negative rods (eg, Escherichia coli, Klebsiella pneumoniae) are a common cause. Pneumocystis carinii pneumonia (PCP): an opportunistic infection that occurs in immunosuppressed populations, primarily patients with advanced human immunodeficiency virus infection. The classic presentation is nonproductive cough, shortness of breath, and fever. Community-acquired viral infections: The most commonly isolated virus is respiratory syncytial virus (RSV).
Infants and Toddlers	Viruses are the most common cause of pneumonia. RSV is the most common viral pathogen followed by parainfluenza types 1, 2, 3, and influenza A or B. Bacterial infections in this age group are uncommon and attributable to Streptococcus pneumoniae, H influenzae type B, or Staphylococcus aureus.
Children younger than 5 years	Children enrolled in day care, or those with frequent ear infections are at increased risk for invasive pneumococcal disease and infection with resistant pneumococcal strains.
Children aged 5 years, ready to start school	Mycoplasma pneumoniae is the most common cause of community-acquired pneumonia. Chlamydia pneumoniae is also fairly common in this age group and presents similarly.
School-aged children and adolescents	Bacterial pneumonia (10%) is common, and these children are often febrile and look ill. Tuberculosis (TB) pneumonia in children warrants special mention. These children may present with fever, night sweats, chills, cough, and weight loss. If TB is not treated in the early stages of infection, approximately 25% of children younger than 15 years develop extrapulmonary disease. Viral pneumonias are still common in this age group and are usually mild and self-limited, although they are occasionally severe and can rapidly progress to respiratory failure.

Data from Coughlin AM: Combating community-acquired pneumonia. Nursing. 2007; 37:64hn1-3. Clark JE, Donna H, Spencer D, et al: Children with pneumonia—how do they present and how are they managed? Arch Dis Child. 2007; 29:29. Parienti JJ, Carrat F: Viral pneumonia and respiratory sepsis: association, causation, or it depends? Crit Care Med. 2007; 35:639-40. Hospital-acquired pneumonia. J Hosp Med. 2006; 1:26-7. Community-acquired pneumonia. J Hosp Med. 2006; 1:16-7. Flaherty KR, Martinez FJ: Nonspecific interstitial pneumonia. Semin Respir Crit Care Med. 2006; 27:652-8. Lynch JP, 3rd, Saggar R, Weigt SS, et al: Usual interstitial pneumonia. Semin Respir Crit Care Med. 2006; 27:634-51. Leong JR, Huang DT: Ventilator-associated pneumonia. Surg Clin North Am. 2006; 86:1409-29. Agusti C, Rano A, Aldabo I, et al: Fungal pneumonia, chronic respiratory diseases and glucocorticoids. Med Mycol. 2006; 44 Suppl:207-11. Scannapieco FA: Pneumonia in nonambulatory patients: The role of oral bacteria and oral hygiene. J Am Dent Assoc. 2006; 137 Suppl:21S-5S.

Clinical suspicion is aroused if there crackles when examining the lungs by stethoscope, and the presence of enlarged or tender lymph nodes in the neck or other areas. In addition to a chest x-ray, confirmatory tests may include:

- Sputum cultures.
- Tuberculin skin test. The Mantoux skin test (intradermal inoculation of 5 TU of purified protein derivative) should be read at 48 to 72 hours after placement.
- Bronchoscopy.
- Thoracentesis.
- Chest CT.
- Interferon (IFN)-gamma blood test. This type of test looks for an immune response to proteins produced by *M. tuberculosis.*
- Biopsy of the affected tissue (typically lungs, pleura, or lymph nodes)

The focus of treatment is to cure the infection with daily oral doses of multiple antitubercular drugs, which are continued until culture results show the drug sensitivity of the mycobacterial infection.

Restrictive Lung Disease

Restrictive lung disease is a group of diseases with differing etiologies that result in difficulty with lung expansion and a reduction in lung volume.[7]

> **Study Pearl**
>
> - When inflammation involves the bronchioles, it is called bronchiolitis.
> - When inflammation involves the alveoli, it is called alveolitis.
> - When inflammation involves the small blood vessels, it is called vasculitis.
> - When scarring of the lung tissue occurs, it is called pulmonary fibrosis. Fibrosis, or scarring of the lung tissue, results in permanent loss of that tissue's ability to transport oxygen.

> **Study Pearl**
>
> Collagen vascular diseases that demonstrate features of interstitial lung disease include systemic lupus erythematosus, rheumatoid arthritis, progressive systemic sclerosis, dermatomyositis and polymyositis, ankylosing spondylitis, Sjögren syndrome, and mixed connective tissue disease.

Interstitial Lung Disease/Pulmonary Fibrosis. Interstitial lung disease (ILD), or idiopathic pulmonary fibrosis, includes a variety of chronic lung disorders that involve damage to the alveolar and epithelial cells, which causes inflammatory cells to release cytokines, tumor necrosis factor (TNF), and platelet-derived growth factor.

The inflammatory chemicals result in smooth muscle proliferation, degradation of the alveoli, and the proliferation of fibroblasts and collagen deposition.[40]

The first symptoms of these diseases is usually an insidious onset of breathlessness and a nonproductive cough. The patient may also complain of systemic symptoms including low grade fever, malaise, arthralgias, weight loss, and clubbing of the fingers and toenails.[40]

The patient history should investigate environmental and occupational factors, hobbies, legal and illegal drug use, arthritis, and risk factors for diseases that affect the immune system. Specific tests include bronchoalveolar lavage (BAL), a test performed during bronchoscopy, which permits removal and examination of cells from the lower respiratory tract, and open lung biopsy.

Systemic Sclerosis. Systemic sclerosis (SSc) is a clinical disorder that affects the connective tissue of the skin and internal organs such as the gastrointestinal tract, lungs, heart, and kidneys.[41,42] It is characterized by alterations of the microvasculature, disturbances of the immune system and by large depositions of collagen.

Arthritis is the initial symptom in 66% of SSc patients, often preceding the classic skin changes, which are due to sclerotic changes of the overlying skin or surrounding connective tissue.[42] Bone alterations occur in approximately 6% of patients and consist of resorption of the tufts of the terminal phalanges, juxta-articular osteoporosis, erosions of the dorsal heads of metacarpal, and proximal phalangeal bones.[43] Neurological manifestations can include peripheral neuropathy with reduction in the conduction velocity.[43] Hematological abnormalities are mostly related to renal disease, microangiopathic hemolytic anemia or from bleeding gastrointestinal telangiectasias.[44]

Chest-Wall Disease or Injury

Environmental and Occupational Diseases

Pneumoconiosis. Coal worker's pneumoconiosis (CWP) is the accumulation of coal dust in the lungs, which enters the terminal bronchioles, and the tissue's reaction to its presence.[45] The carbon pigment of inhaled coal dust is engulfed by alveolar and interstitial macrophages, and the phagocytosed particles are transported up the mucociliary elevator before being expelled in the mucus or through the lymphatic system.[46,47] When this system becomes overwhelmed, an immune response may be triggered.[46,47]

Hypersensitivity pneumonitis. Hypersensitivity pneumonitis (HP), also referred to as extrinsic/external allergic alveolitis, is a complex syndrome involving sensitization to repeated inhalation of dusts containing organic antigens.[48,49] These dusts can be derived from a variety of sources, such as dairy and grain products, and animal dander and protein.[50-52]

Clinical presentations of HP are categorized as acute, subacute (intermittent), and chronic progressive based on the length and intensity of exposure and subsequent duration of illness.[52]

Parenchymal Disorders

Atelectasis. Atelectasis is a common pulmonary complication in patients following thoracic and upper abdominal procedures.[53-55] Atelectasis is defined as diminished volume affecting all or part of a lung. General anesthesia and surgical manipulation lead to atelectasis by causing dysfunction of the diaphragm and diminished surfactant activity.[53-55] Atelectasis is divided physiologically into obstructive and nonobstructive causes.

- Obstructive atelectasis is the most common type and it results from reabsorption of gas from the alveoli when communication between the alveoli and the trachea becomes obstructed. Causes of obstructive atelectasis include foreign body, tumor, and mucous plugging.
- Nonobstructive atelectasis can be caused by loss of contact between the parietal and visceral pleurae, compression, loss of surfactant, and replacement of parenchymal tissue by infiltrative disease or scarring.

Most symptoms and signs are determined by the rapidity with which the bronchial occlusion occurs, the size of the lung area affected, and the presence or absence of complicating infection. Rapid bronchial occlusion accompanied by a large area of lung collapse causes pain on the affected side, sudden onset of dyspnea, and cyanosis. Hypotension, tachycardia, fever, and shock may also occur.[53,54] Slowly developing atelectasis is often asymptomatic or may cause only minor symptoms. Middle lobe syndrome often is asymptomatic, although irritations may cause a severe, hacking, nonproductive cough.[53,54]

The physical examination findings show dullness to percussion over the affected area and diminished or absent breath sounds. Chest excursion is reduced or absent in the area. The trachea and the heart are deviated toward the affected side. Confirmation is achieved through laboratory studies and imaging.

Atelectasis of a noteworthy size results in hypoxemia as measured on ABG determinations. ABG evaluation shows that despite hypoxemia, the $PaCO_2$ level is usually normal or low as a result of the increased ventilation.[53,54]

Treatment of acute atelectasis requires removal of the underlying cause. Prevention of further atelectasis involves placing the patient in such a position that the unaffected side is dependent so as to promote increased drainage of the affected area, intermittent manual positive airway pressure,[56] and encouraging the patient to cough and to breathe deeply.[57]

Acute Respiratory Distress Syndrome. Acute respiratory distress syndrome (ARDS), which can occur in children as well as adults, is the presence of pulmonary edema in the absence of volume overload or depressed left ventricular function.[58] ARDS originates from a number of insults resulting in damage to the alveolocapillary membrane with subsequent fluid accumulation within the airspaces of the lung.[58] Damage to the surfactant-producing type II cells and the presence of protein-rich fluid in the alveolar space disrupts the production and function of pulmonary surfactant leading to microatelectasis and impaired gas exchange.[59] Mild tachypnea may be the only manifestation.[60,61]

PULMONARY ONCOLOGY

Cancer of the lung, also known as bronchogenic carcinoma, results from an abnormality in the body's system of checks and balances on cell growth so that cells divide in an uncontrolled fashion and the proliferation of cells eventually forms a tumor.[62] The lung is also a very common site for metastasis from tumors in other parts of the body.

Ninety to ninety-five percent of cancers of the lung are thought to arise from the epithelial, or lining cells, of the bronchi and bronchioles; for this reason lung cancers are sometimes called bronchogenic carcinomas.[62] Cancers can also arise from the pleura, called mesotheliomas, or rarely from supporting tissues within the lungs, for example, blood vessels.[62]

Common causes of lung cancer include:[62-65]

- Smoking, including passive smoking
- Exposure to asbestos fibers
- Radon gas exposure
- Familial predisposition
- Lung diseases (notably COPD)
- Prior history of lung cancer

Symptoms of lung cancer are varied dependent upon where and how widespread the tumor is[62,65]

- No symptoms
- Symptoms related to the cancer—cough, shortness of breath, wheezing, chest pain, and coughing up blood (hemoptysis)
- Symptoms related to metastasis—severe bone pain, neurologic symptoms
- Nonspecific symptoms—weight loss, weakness, and fatigue

As with other cancers, the treatment prescribed can be[66-69]

- Curative (removal or eradication of a cancer)
- Palliative (measures that are unable to cure a cancer but can reduce pain and suffering)

PULMONARY VASCULAR DISEASE

Pulmonary Embolism and Infarct. Pulmonary embolism (PE), which is closely linked to the presence of deep vein thrombosis (DVT), blood clots, or thrombus in the peripheral venous system, is a common and potentially fatal disease.[70] Unfortunately, the diagnosis is often missed because of its nonspecific signs and symptoms. The diagnosis of PE should be suspected in patients with respiratory symptoms (dyspnea, pleuritic chest pain, hemoptysis) unexplained by an alternate diagnosis, especially when a patient has risk factors, which include recent surgery, immobility (venous stasis), or a hypercoagulable state.[70] The prognosis of a PE episode is dependent on the size of the PE, its impact on the cardiopulmonary system, and the promise of medical care.

PULMONARY HYPERTENSION

Pulmonary hypertension can be defined as a mean pulmonary arterial pressure greater than 25 mm Hg at rest, and greater than 30 mm Hg during exercise.[71-74] Pulmonary hypertension is normally classified as primary or secondary:

- Primary pulmonary hypertension (PPH): a rare disease that chiefly affects women in their mid-30s, but children may also be affected.
- Secondary pulmonary hypertension (SPH): can be the sequela of a congenital heart defect, collagen vascular disease, lung disease with hypoxia, thromboembolic disease, and left heart failure.

Most patients present with nonspecific symptoms resulting in a delayed diagnosis. SOB is typically the first symptom but is usually attributed to physical deconditioning by both patient and physician. The diagnostic gold standard for determining the severity of pulmonary hypertension is heart catheterization.[9] Although there is no cure for PPH, many medical advances, including lung transplantation, have improved quality of life and prolonged survival.[9]

PULMONARY EDEMA

Pulmonary edema is an abnormal accumulation of fluid in the extravascular components of the lungs, commonly as a manifestation of congestive heart failure (CHF).[71] The edema build-up is the result of a breakdown in the barriers that protect the respiratory system.[72]

The clinical presentation of pulmonary edema varies. The patient could present with an acute or subacute onset of dyspnea, orthopnea, crackles, and peripheral cyanosis with hypoxemia.[73] The medical interventions for pulmonary edema include diuretics, medications to support cardiac function and blood pressure, and corticosteroids to minimize the inflammatory response.

PLEURAL DISEASES AND DISORDERS

Pneumothorax. A pneumothorax involves a collection of gas in the pleural space resulting in collapse of the lung on the affected side. Two major types exist:

1. Tension pneumothorax: air within the pleural space that is under pressure; displacing mediastinal structures and compromising cardiopulmonary function. The mediastinum impinges on and compresses the contralateral lung resulting in hypoxia, decreased venous return, decreased cardiac output, hypotension, and, ultimately, in hemodynamic collapse and death, if untreated.
2. Traumatic pneumothorax: results from a blunt or penetrating injury that disrupts the parietal or visceral pleura. If the pneumothorax is small and there is no underlying pulmonary disease, the patient may be asymptomatic. The most common symptom is acute dyspnea.

Pleural Effusion

Pleural enfusion is an excessive collection of fluid within the pleural space. An infected pleural effusion is called an empyema. Pleurisy, or pleuritis, occurs when the pleura that lines the chest cavity and surrounds each of the lungs becomes inflamed.

Central Disorders of the Pulmonary System

Sleep Disordered Breathing. Sleep disordered breathing (SDB) refers to a wide spectrum of sleep-related breathing abnormalities. SDB is likely a continuum of a spectrum of diseases. This concept suggests that an individual who snores may be exhibiting the first manifestation of SDB and that snoring should not be viewed as normal. A patient can move gradually through the continuum, for example, with weight gain and eventual development of Pickwickian syndrome. He or she also can move rapidly through the spectrum through alcohol or sedative use, which can cause an individual who snores to turn into a snorer with obstructive sleep apnea.

PHYSICAL THERAPY INTERVENTION

The physical therapy interventions for pulmonary conditions can be generally classified into primary prevention and secondary intervention.

- Primary prevention: the prevention of a pulmonary disease from developing, even among individuals with risk factors
- Secondary intervention: aimed at reducing symptoms and/or slowing the progression of a pulmonary disease.

The goals of a pulmonary physical intervention are to:[75]

- Increase understanding of the patient and family of the disease process, expectations, goals, and outcomes
- Increase cardiovascular endurance to enhance performance of physical tasks related to community and work integration
- Promote self-management of symptoms including independence in airway clearance, control of energy expenditure, and independence in activities of daily living (ADLs)
- Increase strength, power, and endurance of the peripheral muscles
- Reduce risks of secondary impairments
- Improve functional capacity

Physical Therapy Associated with Primary Prevention, Risk Reduction, and Deconditioning

A number of physical therapy interventions can be used to improve ventilation, respiration, and aerobic capacity (Table 10-23).

Therapeutic Exercise. The goal of therapeutic exercise is to help to increase aerobic endurance, improve functional capacity, improve physiologic response to increased oxygen demand, and

TABLE 10-23. DEAN'S HIERARCHY FOR TREATMENT OF PATIENTS WITH IMPAIRED OXYGEN TRANSPORT

Premise: Position of optimal physiological function is being upright and moving

I. Mobilization and Exercise

Goal: To elicit an exercise stimulus that addresses one of the three effects on the various steps in the oxygen transport pathway, or some combination

A. Acute effects
B. Long-term effects
C. Preventative effects

II. Body Positioning

Goal: To elicit a gravitational stimulus that simulates being upright and moving as much as possible (ie, active, active assisted, or passive)

A. Hemodynamic effects related to fluid shifts
B. Cardiopulmonary effects on ventilation and its distribution, perfusion, ventilation, and perfusion matching and gas exchange

III. Breathing Control Maneuvers

Goal: To augment alveolar ventilation, facilitate mucociliary transport, and stimulate coughing

A. Coordinated breathing with activity and exercise
B. Spontaneous eucapnic hyperventilation
C. Maximal tidal breaths and movement in three dimensions
D. Sustained maximal inspiration
E. Pursed lip breathing to end-tidal expiration
F. Incentive spirometry

IV. Coughing Maneuvers

Goal: To facilitate mucociliary clearance with the least effect on dynamic airway compression and adverse cardiovascular effects

A. Active and spontaneous cough with closed glottis
B. Active assist (self-supported or by other)
C. Modified coughing interventions with open glottis (eg, forced expiratory technique, huff)

V. Relaxation and Energy Conservation Interventions

Goal: To minimize the work of breathing, of the heart, and oxygen demand overall

A. Relaxation procedures at rest and during activity
B. Energy conservation (ie, balance of activity to rest, performing activities in an energy-efficient manner, improved movement economy during activity)
C. Pain control interventions

VI. ROM Exercises (Cardiopulmonary Indications)

Goal: To stimulate alveolar ventilation and alter its distribution

A. Active
B. Assisted active
C. Passive

VII. Postural Drainage Positioning

Goal: To facilitate airway clearance using gravitational effects

A. Bronchopulmonary segmental drainage positions

VIII. Manual Techniques

Goal: To facilitate airway clearance in conjunction with specific body positioning

A. Autogenic drainage
B. Manual percussion
C. Shaking and vibration
D. Deep breathing and coughing

IX. Suctioning

Goal: To facilitate the removal of airway secretions collected centrally

A. Open suction system
B. Closed suction system
C. Tracheal tickle
D. Instillation with saline
E. Use of manual inflation bag (bagging)

Reproduced, with permission, from Dean E: Optimizing treatment prescription: relating treatment to the underlying pathophysiology. In: Frownfelter D, Dean E, eds. *Principles and Practice of Cardiopulmonary Physical Therapy, 3rd ed.* St. Louis, Mosby-Year Book. 1996:251-263.

promote independence in ADLs.[76] In addition, aerobic exercise reduces bone loss during weight-bearing exercises, enhances the processing of free fatty acids and glucose, and improves skill and coordination.

Flexibility exercises can be incorporated to enhance chest-wall expansion, and to promote healthy postures.

Strength training is also an important consideration. Abdominal strengthening can be used when abdominal muscles are too weak to provide an effective cough.

Body mechanics and postural stabilization training have two potential benefits for the patient with airway clearance dysfunction and COPD:

- Reducing general body work
- Reducing the work of breathing and diminishing the effects of dyspnea

Functional Training. Functional training for the patient with a pulmonary disorder involves instruction in methods of energy conservation during daily activities, and a functional exercise progression. Simple activities like walking on level ground, getting out of a chair, or dressing are used initially and then progressed to more energy demanding activities like climbing stairs.

Physical Therapy Associated with Airway Clearance Dysfunction

Breathing Strategies and Exercises for Airway Clearance[77]

Forced Expiratory Technique. The patient is instructed to take a medium breath then tighten the abdominal muscles firmly while huffing, without contracting the throat muscles. The huff should be maintained long enough to mobilize and remove distal bronchial secretions without stimulating a spasmodic cough. The sound should be breathy and the mouth should be in the shape of an "O." The important part of this technique is the 15 to 30 seconds of relaxation with gentle diaphragmatic breathing following one or two huffs.

Active Cycle of Breathing Technique. This technique includes a 15 to 30 seconds breathing control (diaphragmatic breathing) phase, thoracic expansion exercises, a repeat of the breathing control phrase, a repeat of the thoracic expansion exercises, and then the FET technique and huffing to clear secretions from the smaller to the larger airways. The patient can assume a bronchial drainage position and focus on a quiet breathing pattern using the lower rib cage area without upper chest movement during the thoracic expansion phases.

Autogenic Drainage. The patient is instructed to breathe out through an O-shaped mouth and to listen during inhalation and exhalation for noises indicative of secretions such as high-pitched wheezes, gurgling, or popping sounds. The timing and pitch of the sounds give clues as to where the secretions may be located—sounds that are heard initially on inhalation and which are lower in pitch are most likely to be the result of secretions in the larger of the airways. These airways must be cleared with huffs or coughs prior to continuation of the technique. This technique can be broken down into four phases:

- The patient sits upright with a minimum of distractions in the room.
- Unstick phase: after a brief period of diaphragmatic breathing, the patient exhales to a low lung volume and breathes at a normal tidal volume at that low lung volume to affect peripheral secretions.
- Collect phase: as the patient becomes aware of secretions in the small airways, breathing becomes a bit deeper (at mid lung volumes) to affect the mobilization of the secretions proximally into the middle airways.
- Evacuation phase: at this point, breathing becomes deeper (from mid to high lung volumes).

The patient is asked to suppress coughing until it cannot be avoided. This phase enables secretions to accumulate in central airways, which can then be evacuated by huffing or a cough, using minimal effort.

The above steps, which correspond to the area of retained secretions, are repeated until all secretions are removed from the airways.

Assisted Cough/Huff Techniques. The huff or forced expiratory technique was explained previously. The assisted cough can be employed independently or with the help of an assistant. The technique can be as simple as placing a pillow over an incision to help splint the area, or as dynamic as using a manual technique at the time of the cough (see "Study Pearl"). Four types of manual assistance can be used: costophrenic (hand placement), abdominal thrust, anterior chest compression, and a counter rotation assist.[87]

Study Pearl

To perform the manual assisted cough, the patient is positioned in supine. The clinician places both hands flat against patient's upper abdomen directly below the xiphoid process. After taking a deep breath, the patient is instructed to cough two to three times. The cough is best performed using a flexed posture. With each cough the clinician applies manual pressure inwardly and superiorly. The amount of force used by the compression is dependent upon patient tolerance and abdominal sensation.

Segmental Breathing. During the technique the patient is asked to breathe in against the resistance of the clinician's hands. Segmental breathing is inappropriate in cases of intractable hypoventilation.

Diaphragmatic Breathing. Diaphragmatic breathing (lower rib cage breathing) involves using a tactile cue such as a hand, which is placed over the lower rib cage. On inhalation, the hand on the lower rib cage should rise, indicating air filling the lungs, and there should be little movement occurring at the upper chest. Initially, diaphragmatic breathing can be made easier with the bed declined 30 degrees at the head. To apply resistance, manual contact can be used, or the clinician can place a 5 to 10 lb sandbag over the patient's abdomen.

Pursed-Lip Breathing. Pursed-lip breathing is accomplished by breathing into the nose to a count of "1,2" and out via pursed lips to a count of "1,2,3,4." Purse lip breathing prolongs the expiratory phase, slows the respiratory rate, increases the excretion of carbon dioxide, and improves airflow by delaying small airway closure.

Paced Breathing. Paced breathing uses a combination of pursed-lip breathing and diaphragmatic breathing performed at the normal 1:2 ratio of inspiration to expiration during functional activities.

The patient is instructed to take a breath into the nose and walk two steps to a count of "1,2," followed by an exhalation to a count of"1,2,3,4" as they walk the next four steps.

Stacking Breaths. The technique of stacking breaths (inflation-hold) is used in situations when the volume of air a patient can inhale is limited. The technique involves taking a small to moderate sized breath and adding it to two or three additional sip-like breaths to increase inspiratory volume, thereby decreasing atelectasis, moving air behind the secretions, and increasing inspiratory volume to enhance a huff or cough.

Glossopharyngeal Breathing. Glossopharyngeal breathing (GPB) is a form of stacking breaths that is used with patients who cannot breathe independently due to weak inspiratory muscles. GPB requires cranial nerves V, VII, and IX-XII to be intact. The technique involves the use of the glottis (throat) to add to an inspiratory effort by projecting (gulping) boluses of air into the lungs. The glottis closes with each "gulp." One breath usually consists of 6 to 9 gulps of 40 to 200 mL each. During the training period the efficiency of GPB can be monitored by spirometrically measuring the milliliters of air per gulp, gulps per breath, and breaths per minute. GPB is rarely useful in the presence of an indwelling tracheotomy tube. It cannot be used when the tube is uncapped as it is during tracheotomy IPPV, and even when capped, the gulped air tends to leak around the outer walls of the tube and out the stoma as airway volumes and pressures increase during the GPB air stacking process. The safety and versatility afforded by GPB are key reasons to eliminate tracheotomy in favor of noninvasive aids.

Sustained Maximal Inspiration. Sustained maximal inspiration is a technique used to increase inhaled volume, sustain or improve alveolar inflation, and maintain or restore functional residual capacity. The patient is asked to inspire slowly through the nose or pursed-lips to the point of maximal inspiration. The maximal inspiration is held for three seconds and then the volume is passively exhaled.

Inspiratory Muscle Trainers. Inspiratory muscle trainers function by loading the muscles of inspiration using a series of graded aperture openings. The trainers are appropriate for patients with decreased compliance, decreased intrathoracic volume, resistance to airflow, an alteration in length tension relationship of the ventilatory muscles, and any patient who has decreased strength of the respiratory muscles.

Positioning for Airway Clearance

Bronchial drainage or postural drainage uses the shape and direction of the lung segments to drain the uppermost segment of the lung by placing the individual in gravity-enhancing postures or positions.[88-90] This requires that the area to be drained is uppermost, with the bronchus from the area in as close to a vertical position as possible or reasonable. The dependent areas of the lungs are those which are the best ventilated and perfused. Although the uppermost portion of the lungs have a large resting volume and are therefore better expanded, they have a decreased perfusion. Ten positions can be used to drain all of the segments of the lung, although it may not be necessary to use all 10 positions (Figure 10-5). These positions may need to be modified under certain conditions. The precautions for postural drainage are listed in Table 10-24.

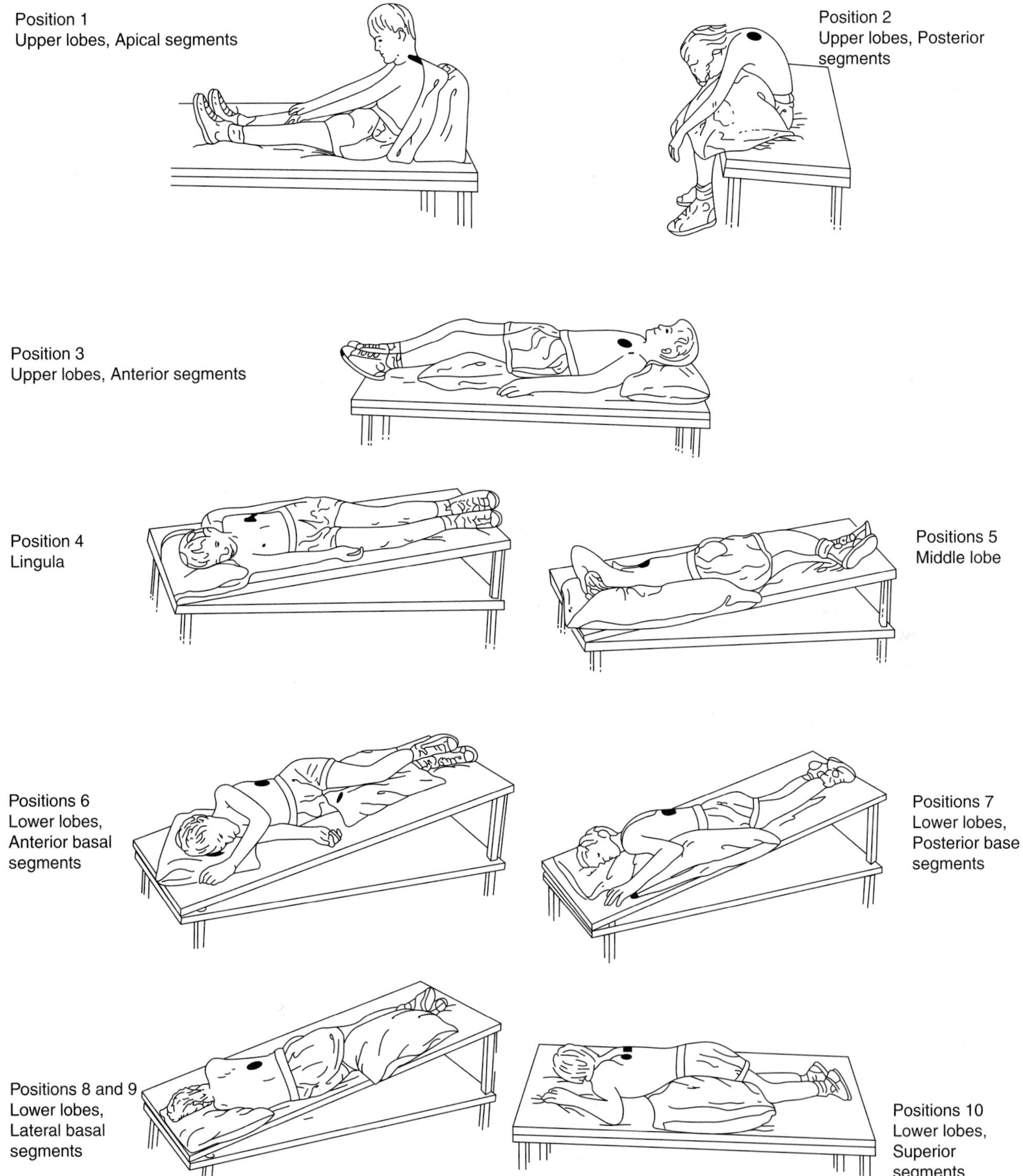

Figure 10-5. Postural drainage positions. (Reproduced with permission from DeTurk, WE, Cahalin, LP: Cardiovascular and Pulmonary Physical Therapy: An Evidence-Based Approach. New York: McGraw-Hill. 2004:226.)

TABLE 10-24. PRECAUTIONS FOR POSTURAL DRAINAGE AND MANUAL TECHNIQUES

Esophageal reflux
Hemoptysis
Dyspnea
Orthopnea
Bruising/rib fractures/flail chest
Coagulopathy
Cardiac arrhythmias
Desaturation/hemodynamic decompensation
Large pleural effusion
Bronchospasm
Spinal instability
Recent burn grafts
Osteopenia/osteoporosis
Requires assistance
Pain
Level of alertness
Risk for injury to caregiver and/or recipient
Nausea and vomiting
Untreated pneumothorax
Increased intracranial pressure
Recent surgery
Indwelling venous catheter
Feeding tubes

Reproduced, with permission, from Downs AM, Bishop Lindsay KL: Physical therapy associated with airway clearance dysfunction. In: DeTurk WE, Cahalin LP, eds: *Cardiovascular and pulmonary physical therapy: An evidence-based approach*. New York: McGraw-Hill. 2004:463-490.

Postural Drainage with Chest Percussion, Vibration, and Shaking

These techniques collectively referred to as traditional chest physical therapy, can be performed with an assistant, independently, or with mechanical devices.[76] For each of the manual techniques, hand placement should avoid bony prominences such as the scapula, spinous processes, and clavicles. In addition special care should be given to the ribs and breast tissue. Before these approaches are used to loosen and mobilize secretions, it is generally recommended that the patient be positioned to optimally drain a particular lung segment or lobe (see previous section).

Chest Percussion. Chest percussion involves the application of a cupped hand to a specific area of the chest wall in a rhythmic manner to loosen secretions. The technique may be done concurrently with a drainage position to enhance secretion mobilization. The area to be percussed is covered with a lightweight cloth to avoid erythema. The duration of percussion depends on the patient's needs and tolerance—the guideline is 3 to 5 minutes per postural drainage position. The force applied is sufficient to cause the patient's voice to quiver.

Shaking/Vibration. Shaking/vibration, which is commonly used following percussion, is a rhythmic technique applied to the rib cage throughout exhalation to hasten the removal of secretions from the tracheobronchial tree. As the patient exhales, the clinician makes a downward motion and a vibrating motion while maintaining full contact of the hands on the chest wall. The duration of the shaking depends on the patient's needs, tolerance, and clinical improvement—the guideline is five to seven trials of shaking.[7]

PHYSICAL THERAPY ASSOCIATED WITH RESPIRATORY FAILURE AND VENTILATORY PUMP DYSFUNCTION AND FAILURE

Respiratory failure can be classified as primarily hypoxic (known as type I) or as primarily hypercapnic (known as type II). Respiratory failure can also be classified as acute or chronic depending on its time course. It is important to distinguish between acute and chronic respiratory failure because individuals in the acute stages of respiratory failure should limit their activity since increasing the O_2 demand may worsen their condition.[91] However, early mobilization, positioning, and breathing exercises can help these patients by improving ventilation and stimulating respiratory drive.[91] For individuals with chronic respiratory failure or those at risk of developing failure, rehabilitation interventions should focus on improving breathing efficiency and improving overall conditioning through strength and aerobic training.[91]

Manual Therapy Techniques. Manual techniques for mobilization of the rib cage, thorax, pelvis, shoulder, and scapula can be utilized to enhance ventilation and improved respiration.[88-90] In addition, the clinician can apply the principles of proprioceptive neuromuscular facilitation (PNF) to the chest wall to enhance relaxation, stimulate enhanced tidal volume for inspiratory capacity, and improve mucous mobilization and clearance. Massage of the upper posterior thorax and neck area can be used to decrease muscle tension, anxiety, and enhance comfort. At present there are no well-controlled clinical research studies to support the use of manual techniques to enhance ventilation and respiration.

Breathing-Assist Technique. Breathing-assist techniques assist the patient's ventilation by passive or active-assist maneuvers performed by the clinician, which facilitates air entry into the thoracic cavity.[92] The patient is taught to decrease the cervical lordosis, close their mouth, lower their shoulders, and breathe at a slower, deeper rate.

Squeezing. Squeezing, a technique used to facilitate inspiration and exhalation, consists of manually compressing different areas on the thorax during expiration. The clinician pushes into areas of the thorax which have limited motion or under which retained secretions lie.

Assistive Devices

- Positive expiratory pressure (PEP): can be produced using pursed-lips, a mouthpiece, a face mask, or other device fitted with an exhalation port with a resistor, and a release-type valve.[76] Low-pressure PEP (10-20 cm H_2O) uses positive expiratory resistance via a face mask to assist in the removal of airway secretions. High-pressure PEP (50-120 cm H_2O) is used for patients with unstable airways.
- Oscillating positive pressure: an alternative to a stable level of pressure in PEP devices. Examples of these devices include the Flutter or Acapella.[93] These devices provide the benefits of a positive-pressure device plus the "interruptions" from the oscillations that promote changes in the viscosity of the secretions and enhance expiratory airflow.
- High-frequency chest-wall oscillation (vest airway clearance system):[94] an individually-sized chest-wall jacket powered by a generator which promotes secretion clearance of the entire lung fields while performed in the seated position.
- Intrapulmonary percussive ventilation: similar to the vest airway clearance system, but is delivered internally via a mouthpiece. The mouthpiece delivers a preset driving pressure and frequency of intra airway oscillations from a nebula-like apparatus.

MEDICAL MANAGEMENT OF RESPIRATORY FAILURE

Medical interventions for respiratory failure can provide supportive measures, mechanical ventilation, and supplemental O_2.

- Supplemental oxygen:[91] indicated when the patient can sustain sufficient work of breathing (WOB) to maintain ventilation independently but cannot maintain adequate levels of oxygenation. The amount of time a portable O_2 gas tank will provide depends on its size, how full it is, and the flow rate. O_2 tank sizes are letter coded. The most common tanks are small E-cylinders, with a volume of approximately 700 L, and large H-cylinders, with a volume of approximately 7000 L. Standard O_2 tanks are filled to a pressure of 2200 psi (pounds per square inch) of gaseous O_2 when full. The amount of time a tank has can be calculated using the following equation:

  $T = (P \times k)/\text{flow rate}$, where:

  T = time left in minutes

  P = pressure in psi

  K = 0.28 for an E-cylinder and 3.14 for an H-cylinder

  Flow rate = L/min
- Mechanical ventilation[91]: patients with respiratory insufficiency or those who cannot sustain the necessary work of breathing independently can have their breathing supported by mechanical ventilation. A mechanical ventilator substitutes for or assists the patient's ventilatory pump to allow breathing to occur. When examining a patient who is using a ventilator, the clinician should note the route of intubation, mode of ventilation, rate setting, tidal volume, amount of

positive end expiratory pressure (PEEP), pressure support, and the FiO_2.

SPECIAL CONSIDERATIONS FOR CERTAIN PATIENT POPULATIONS

Neurologic

- Subarachnoid hemorrhage: clinician should avoid activities involving incentive spirometry and forced coughing so as not to increase intracranial pressure (ICP).
- Traumatic brain injury: to minimize the risk of increasing the ICP, the clinician should avoid activities involving valsalva, coughing and suctioning, and postural drainage.

Neuromuscular Implications of Spinal Cord Injury[95] Immediately following a spinal cord injury there is often a period when the patient demonstrates paradoxical breathing—determined by placing a hand inferior to the xiphoid process and using the first three fingers to feel rib excursion.

The respiratory rate is usually increased due to a decrease in the tidal volume. Patients with long-standing spinal cord injury demonstrate a decrease of all lung volumes.

- Paraplegia (primarily T1 to T5): demonstrate weakened and/or absent abdominals, intercostals, erector spinae, a slight decrease in anterior and lateral expansion. These impairments result in a moderate decrease in chest expansion and vital capacity, decreased ability to build up intrathoracic and intra-abdominal pressures, and decreased cough effectiveness.
- Tetraplegia: C5-C8: missing the aforementioned muscles and weakened pectoralis, serratus anterior, and scalenes. Have a marked decrease in anterior expansion, upper and lower; marked decrease in lateral expansion; slight decrease in posterior expansion. These impairments result in significant decrease in chest expansion and vital capacity, significant decrease in FEV and cough effectiveness.
- Patients who have a lesion at C5-T1 can rely on both diaphragmatic and cervical muscles for breathing.
- Tetraplegia (C4): missing the aforementioned muscles and weakened scalenes, diaphragm. There is a marked decrease in anterior and lateral chest expansion and slight decrease in inferior and superior expansion. These impairments result in previously mentioned limitations but now more pronounced, including the possibility of a decrease in tidal volume. These patients may need mechanical ventilation.
- Tetraplegia (C3-C1): missing the aforementioned muscles and weakened and/or absent the last of the remaining accessory muscles. All planes of chest expansion severely limited. These impairments result in previously mentioned limitations, and significant decrease in tidal volume. Most will require mechanical ventilation 20 to 24 hours/day.
  - Patients with a lesion at the C2 to C3 levels can only rely on pharyngeal and laryngeal muscles for breathing, so only glossopharyngeal breathing exercises are appropriate.

TABLE 10-25. DEFINITION OF SURGICAL TERMS

TERM	DESCRIPTION
Lobectomy	The removal of a lobe, or section, of the lung performed to prevent the spread of cancer to other parts of the lung or other parts of the body, as well as to treat patients with such noncancerous diseases as chronic obstructive pulmonary disease (COPD).
Segmentectomy	The removal of a segment of the lung. The procedure has several variations and many names, including segmental resection, wide excision, lumpectomy, tumorectomy, quadrantectomy, and partial mastectomy.
Pneumonectomy (or pneumectomy)	The removal of a lung most commonly performed to excise a tumor. Other indications for lobectomy include solitary pulmonary nodule, bronchiectasis where other forms of treatment have failed, particularly if it is localized and recurrent hemoptysis is present.
Pleurectomy	Excision of the pleura—the most common surgery employed to manage patients with diffuse mesothelioma
Thoracotomy	Surgical incision of the chest wall, which is used primarily as a diagnostic tool when other procedures have failed to provide adequate diagnostic information.
Segmental resection or wedge resection	A resection is the removal of a part of the lung, often in order to remove a tumor. Wedge resection is removal of a wedge-shaped portion of lung tissue
Volume reduction surgery	Used to help relieve shortness of breath and increase tolerance for exercise in patients with chronic obstructive pulmonary disease, such as emphysema.

Medical and Surgical Intervention for Pulmonary Disorders

See Table 10-25.

Questions for this chapter and the entire book appear on the included CD-ROM, with additional questions at www.DuttonNPTE.com.

REFERENCES

1. Shaffer TH, Wolfson MR, Gault JH: Respiratory Physiology. In: Irwin S, Tecklin JS, eds. *Cardiopulmonary Physical Therapy,* 2nd ed. St Louis: Mosby. 1990: 217-244.
2. Van de Graaff KM, Fox SI: Respiratory system. In; Van de Graaff KM, Fox SI, eds. *Concepts of Human Anatomy and Physiology.* New York: WCB/McGraw-Hill. 1999: 728-777.
3. Collins SM, Cocanour B: Anatomy of the Cardiopulmonary System. In: DeTurk WE, Cahalin LP, eds. *Cardiovascular and Pulmonary Physical Therapy: an Evidence-Based Approach.* New York: McGraw-Hill. 2004: 73-94.
4. Morgan BJ, Dempsey JA: Physiology of the Cardiovascular and Pulmonary Systems. In: DeTurk WE, Cahalin LP, eds. *Cardiovascular and Pulmonary Physical Therapy: an Evidence-Based Approach.* New York: McGraw-Hill. 2004: 95-122.
5 .Schmitz TJ: Vital Signs. In: O'Sullivan SB, Schmitz TJ, eds. *Physical Rehabilitation, 5th ed.* Philadelphia: FA Davis. 2007: 81-120.
6. Hassan A, Gossage J, Ingram D, et al: Volume of activation of the Hering-Breuer inflation reflex in the newborn infant. *J Appl Physiol.* 2001; 90:763-769.
7. Starr JA: Chronic pulmonary dysfunction. In: O'Sullivan SB, Schmitz TJ, eds. *Physical Rehabilitation, 5th ed.* Philadelphia: FA Davis. 2007: 561-588.
8. Cahalin LP: Pulmonary Evaluation. In: DeTurk WE, Cahalin LP, eds. *Cardiovascular and pulmonary physical therapy: an evidence-based approach.* New York: McGraw-Hill. 2004: 221-269.

9. Wells C: Pulmonary Pathology. In: DeTurk WE, Cahalin LP, eds. *Cardiovascular and pulmonary physical therapy: an evidence-based approach.* New York: McGraw-Hill. 2004: 151-188.
10. Mahler DA, Barlow PB, Matthay RA: Chronic obstructive pulmonary disease. *Clin Geriatr Med.* 1986; 2:285-312.
11. Mulroy J: Chronic obstructive pulmonary disease in women. *Dimens Crit Care Nurs.* 2005;24:1-18; quiz 19-20.
12. Ong KC, Ong YY: Cardiopulmonary exercise testing in patients with chronic obstructive pulmonary disease. *Ann Acad Med Singapore.* 2000; 29:648-652.
13. Balmes JR: Occupational contribution to the burden of chronic obstructive pulmonary disease. *J Occup Environ Med.* 2005; 47:1 54-160.
14. Man SF, McAlister FA, Anthonisen NR, et al: Contemporary management of chronic obstructive pulmonary disease: clinical applications. *Jama.* 2003; 290:2313-2316.
15. Grimfeld A, Just J: Clinical characteristics of childhood asthma. *Clin Exp Allergy.* 1998; 28 (5):67-70; discussion 90-91.
16. Kemp JP: Comprehensive asthma management: guidelines for clinicians. *J Asthma.* 1998;35:601-620.
17. Chang AB, Masters IB, Everard ML: Re: membranous obliterative bronchitis: a proposed unifying model. *Pediatr Pulmonol.* 2006; 41:904; author reply 905-906.
18. Wang JS, Tseng HH, Lai RS, et al: Sauropus androgynus-constrictive obliterative bronchitis/bronchiolitis--histopathological study of pneumonectomy and biopsy specimens with emphasis on the inflammatory process and disease progression. *Histopathology.* 2000; 37:402-410.
19. Poole DC, Sexton WL, Farkas GA, et al: Diaphragm structure and function in health and disease. *Med Sci Sports Exerc.* 1997; 29:738-754.
20. Stoller JK: Clinical features and natural history of severe alpha 1-antitrypsin deficiency. Roger S. Mitchell Lecture. *Chest.* 1997; 111:123S-128S.
21. Schwaiblmair M, Vogelmeier C: Alpha 1-antitrypsin. Hope on the horizon for emphysema sufferers? *Drugs Aging.* 1998;12:429-440.
22. Jones A, Rowe BH: Bronchopulmonary hygiene physical therapy in bronchiectasis and chronic obstructive pulmonary disease: a systematic review. *Heart Lung.* 2000; 29:125-135.
23. Mysliwiec V, Pina JS: Bronchiectasis: the 'other' obstructive lung disease. *Postgrad Med.* 1999;106:123-126, 128-131.
24. Coughlin AM: Combating community-acquired pneumonia. *Nursing.* 2007;37:64:1-3.
25. Clark JE, Donna H, Spencer D, et al: Children with pneumonia—how do they present and how are they managed? *Arch Dis Child.* 2007;29:29.
26. Parienti JJ, Carrat F: Viral pneumonia and respiratory sepsis: association, causation, or it depends? *Crit Care Med.* 2007; 35:639-640.
27. Hospital-acquired pneumonia. *J Hosp Med.* 2006; 1:26-27.
28. Community-acquired pneumonia. *J Hosp Med.* 2006; 1:16-17.
29. Flaherty KR, Martinez FJ: Nonspecific interstitial pneumonia. *Semin Respir Crit Care Med.* 2006;27:652-658.
30. Lynch JP, 3rd, Saggar R, Weigt SS, et al: Usual interstitial pneumonia. *Semin Respir Crit Care Med.* 2006; 27:634-651.
31. Leong JR, Huang DT: Ventilator-associated pneumonia. *Surg Clin North Am.* 2006; 86:1409-1429.
32. Agusti C, Rano A, Aldabo I, et al: Fungal pneumonia, chronic respiratory diseases and glucocorticoids. *Med Mycol.* 2006;44 Suppl:207-211.

33. Scannapieco FA: Pneumonia in nonambulatory patients: The role of oral bacteria and oral hygiene. *J Am Dent Assoc.* 2006;137 Suppl:21S-5S.
34. Medina-Walpole AM, Katz PR: Nursing home-acquired pneumonia. *J Am Geriatr Soc.* 1999;47:1005-1015.
35. Richeldi L: Rapid identification of Mycobacterium tuberculosis infection. *Clin Microbiol Infect.* 2006; 12(9):34-36.
36. Yoshinaga Y, Kanamori T, Ota Y, et al: Clinical characteristics of Mycobacterium tuberculosis infection among rheumatoid arthritis patients. *Mod Rheumatol.* 2004; 14:143-148.
37. Johnson R, Streicher EM, Louw GE, et al: Drug resistance in Mycobacterium tuberculosis. *Curr Issues Mol Biol.* 2006; 8: 97-111.
38. Rotert R: Case of the month. Mycobacterium tuberculosis. *Jaapa.* 2006; 19:70.
39. Sterling TR, Haas DW: Transmission of Mycobacterium tuberculosis from health care workers. *N Engl J Med.* 2006; 355:118-121.
40. Nicod LP: Recognition and treatment of idiopathic pulmonary fibrosis. *Drugs.* 1998; 55:555-562.
41. Ong VH, Brough G, Denton CP: Management of systemic sclerosis. *Clin Med.* 2005; 5:214-219.
42. Haustein UF: Systemic sclerosis-scleroderma. *Dermatol Online J.* 2002; 8:3.
43. Casale R, Buonocore M, Matucci-Cerinic M: Systemic sclerosis (scleroderma): an integrated challenge in rehabilitation. *Arch Phys Med Rehabil.* 1997; 78:767-773.
44. Steen VD: Treatment of systemic sclerosis. *Am J Clin Dermatol.* 2001;2:315-325.
45. Tang WK, Lum CM, Ungvari GS, et al: Health-related quality of life in community-dwelling men with pneumoconiosis. *Respiration.* 2006;73:203-208.
46. Chong S, Lee KS, Chung MJ, et al: Pneumoconiosis: comparison of imaging and pathologic findings. *Radiographics.* 2006; 26:59-77.
47. Attfield MD, Kuempel ED: Pneumoconiosis, coalmine dust and the PFR. *Ann Occup Hyg.* 2003; 47:525-529.
48. Lacasse Y, Cormier Y: Hypersensitivity pneumonitis. *Orphanet J Rare Dis.* 2006; 1:25.
49. Kurup VP, Zacharisen MC, Fink JN: Hypersensitivity pneumonitis. *Indian J Chest Dis Allied Sci.* 2006; 48:115-128.
50. Navarro C, Mejia M, Gaxiola M, et al: Hypersensitivity pneumonitis: a broader perspective. *Treat Respir Med.* 2006;5:167-179.
51. Klote M: Hypersensitivity pneumonitis. *Allergy Asthma Proc.* 2005; 26:493-495.
52. Churg A, Muller NL, Flint J, et al: Chronic hypersensitivity pneumonitis. *Am J Surg Pathol.* 2006;30:201-218.
53. Igarashi A, Amagasa S, Oda S, et al: Pulmonary atelectasis manifested after induction of anesthesia: a contribution of sinobronchial syndrome? 2007; 21:66-68.
54. Duggan M, Kavanagh BP: Atelectasis in the perioperative patient. *Curr Opin Anaesthesiol.* 2007;20:37-42.
55. Wong AY, Fung LN: Pulmonary atelectasis following spinal anaesthesia for caesarean section. *Anaesth Intensive Care.* 2006; 34:687-688.
56. Schulz-Stubner S, Rickelman J: Intermittent manual positive airway pressure for the treatment and prevention of atelectasis. *Eur J Anaesthesiol.* 2005; 22:730-732.

57. Westerdahl E, Lindmark B, Eriksson T, et al: Deep-breathing exercises reduce atelectasis and improve pulmonary function after coronary artery bypass surgery. *Chest.* 2005; 128:3482-3488.
58. Hudson LD, Steinberg KP: Epidemiology of acute lung injury and ARDS. *Chest.* 1999;116:74S-82S.
59. Luh SP, Chiang CH: Acute lung injury/acute respiratory distress syndrome (ALI/ARDS): the mechanism, present strategies and future perspectives of therapies. *J Zhejiang Univ Sci B.* 2007; 8:60-69.
60. Singh N: AIP or ARDS? Not just semantics. *Crit Care.* 2006; 10:423.
61. Bautin A, Khubulava G, Kozlov I, et al: Surfactant therapy for patients with ARDS after cardiac surgery. *J Liposome Res.* 2006; 16:265-272.
62. Collins LG, Haines C, Perkel R, et al: Lung cancer: diagnosis and management. *Am Fam Physician.* 2007; 75:56-63.
63. Crevenna R, Marosi C, Schmidinger M, et al: Neuromuscular electrical stimulation for a patient with metastatic lung cancer—a case report. *Support Care Cancer.* 2006;14:970-973. Epub 2006 Mar 8.
64. Godtfredsen NS, Prescott E, Osler M: Effect of smoking reduction on lung cancer risk. *Jama.* 2005;294:1505-1510.
65. Buccheri G, Ferrigno D: Lung cancer: clinical presentation and specialist referral time. *Eur Respir J.* 2004; 24:898-904.66.
66. Hotta K, Fujiwara Y, Matsuo K, et al: Recent improvement in the survival of patients with advanced nonsmall cell lung cancer enrolled in phase III trials of first-line, systemic chemotherapy. *Cancer.* 2007;6:6.
67. Stewart DJ, Chiritescu G, Dahrouge S, et al: Chemotherapy dose-response relationships in non-small cell lung cancer and implied resistance mechanisms. *Cancer Treat Rev.* 2007; 2:2.
68. Barros JA, Valladares G, Faria AR, et al: Early diagnosis of lung cancer: the great challenge. Epidemiological variables, clinical variables, staging and treatment. *J Bras Pneumol.* 2006; 32:221-227.
69. Sugimura H, Nichols FC, Yang P, et al: Survival after recurrent nonsmall-cell lung cancer after complete pulmonary resection. *Ann Thorac Surg.* 2007;83:409-417; discussioin 417-418.
70. Alexander P, Giangola G: Deep venous thrombosis and pulmonary embolism: diagnosis, prophylaxis, and treatment. *Ann Vasc Surg.* 1999; 13:318-327.
71. Gluecker T, Capasso P, Schnyder P, et al: Clinical and radiologic features of pulmonary edema. *Radiographics.* 1999;19:1507-1531; discussion 1532-1533.
72. Ketai LH, Godwin JD: A new view of pulmonary edema and acute respiratory distress syndrome. *J Thorac Imaging.* 1998; 13:147-171.
73. Zwischenberger JB, Alpard SK, Bidani A: Early complications. Respiratory failure. *Chest Surg Clin N Am.* 1999; 9:543-564, viii.
74. Parfrey H, Chilvers ER: Pleural disease—diagnosis and management. *Practitioner.* 1999;243:412, 415-21.
75. Downs AM, Bishop-Lindsay KL: Physical therapy associated with airway clearance dysfunction. In: DeTurk WE, Cahalin LP, eds. *Cardiovascular and pulmonary physical therapy: an evidence-based approach.* New York: McGraw-Hill. 2004: 463-489.
76. Cohen M, Michel TH. *Cardiopulmonary symptoms in physical therapy practice.* New York: Churchill Livingstone. 1988.
77 Dutton M: Pulmonary Physical Therapy, in Dutton M (ed): Physical Therapist Assistant Exam Review Guide & JBTest Prep: PTA Exam Review. Sudbury, MA, Jones & Bartlett Learning, 2011: 263-289.

78. Placidi G, Cornacchia M, Polese G, et al: Chest physiotherapy with positive airway pressure: a pilot study of short-term effects on sputum clearance in patients with cystic fibrosis and severe airway obstruction. *Respir Care.* 2006; 51:1145-1153.
79. Boitano LJ: Management of airway clearance in neuromuscular disease. *Respir Care.* 2006;51:913-922; discussion 922-924.
80. McIlwaine M: Physiotherapy and airway clearance techniques and devices. *Paediatr Respir Rev.* 2006; 7:S220-222. Epub 2006 Jun 5.
81. Kendrick AH: Airway clearance techniques in cystic fibrosis. *Eur Respir J.* 2006; 27:1082-1083.
82. Panitch HB: Airway clearance in children with neuromuscular weakness. *Curr Opin Pediatr.* 2006; 18:277-281.
83. Alison JA: Clinical trials of airway clearance techniques. *Chron Respir Dis.* 2004; 1:123-124.
84. Flume PA: Airway clearance techniques. *Semin Respir Crit Care Med.* 2003; 24:727-736.
85. Tecklin JS: Airway clearance dysfunction. In: Cameron MH, Monroe LG, eds. *Physical Rehabilitation: Evidence-Based Examination, Evaluation, and Intervention.* St Louis, MO: Saunders/Elsevier. 2007: 642-668.
86. Eaton T, Young P, Zeng I, et al: A randomized evaluation of the acute efficacy, acceptability and tolerability of flutter and active cycle of breathing with and without postural drainage in non-cystic fibrosis bronchiectasis. *Chron Respir Dis.* 2007; 4:23-230.
87. Wilson GE: A comparison of traditional chest physiotherapy with the active cycle of breathing in patients with chronic supurative lung disease. *Eur Respir J.* 1995; 8:171S.
88. Massery M, Frownfelter D: Facilitating airway clearance with cough techniques. In: Frownfelter D, Dean E, eds. *Principles and Practice of Cardiopulmonary Physical Therapy, 3rd ed.* Philadelphia: Mosby-Yearbook. 1996: 367-382.
89. Spero K: Chest physical therapy. *Rehab Manag.* 2002;15:10.
90. Oberle GM: Chest physical therapy (CPT). *Rehab Manag.* 2002; 15:10.
91. Thomas J, Cook DJ, Brooks D: Chest physical therapy management of patients with cystic fibrosis. A meta-analysis. *Am J Respir Crit Care Med.* 1995; 151:846-850.
92. Dekerlegand J, Cahalin LP, Perme C: Respiratory failure. In: Cameron MH, Monroe LG, eds. *Physical Rehabilitation: Evidence-Based Examination, Evaluation, and Intervention.* St Louis, MO: Saunders/Elsevier. 2007: 689-717.
93. Kigin CM: Breathing exercises in chest physical therapy. *Chest.* 1987;92:190-191.
94. Thompson CS, Harrison S, Ashley J, et al: Randomised crossover study of the Flutter device and the active cycle of breathing technique in non-cystic fibrosis bronchiectasis. *Thorax.* 2002; 57:446-448.
95. Phillips GE, Pike SE, Jaffe A, et al: Comparison of active cycle of breathing and high-frequency oscillation jacket in children with cystic fibrosis. *Pediatr Pulmonol.* 2004; 37:71-75.
96. Massery M, Cahalin LP: Physical therapy associated with ventilatory pump dysfunction and failure. In: DeTurk WE, Cahalin LP, eds. *Cardiovascular and pulmonary physical therapy: an evidence-based approach.* New York: McGraw-Hill. 2004: 593-646.

Cardiovascular Physical Therapy

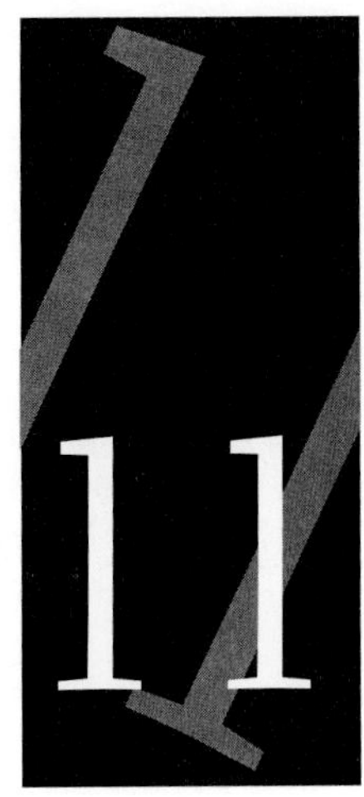

OVERVIEW

In states with direct access, examination and intervention procedures are being performed by physical therapists in all phases of cardiopulmonary rehabilitation.

Given the importance of the cardiopulmonary system to overall health and function, the examination of this system should be an integral component of every patient profile. Thus, every physical therapist should have, at a minimum, the knowledge and skills to be competent in cardiopulmonary care.[1]

> **Study Pearl**
>
> - The term cardiac (Greek kardia (καρδια) for "heart") means "related to the heart"; eg, cardiology, the study of diseases of the heart.
> - Medical terms related to blood often begin in hemo- or hemato- (haemo- and haemato-) from the Greek word "haima" for "blood"; eg, hematology: the science encompassing the medical study of the blood and blood-producing organs.

ANATOMY AND PHYSIOLOGY OF THE CARDIOVASCULAR SYSTEM

Anatomy and Physiology of Blood

Blood is a circulating tissue composed of several cells called corpuscles (Table 11-1), which constitute about 45% of whole blood. The other 55% is blood plasma, a yellowish fluid that is the blood's liquid medium. The functions of blood cells include:

- To supply nutrients (eg, oxygen, glucose) and constitutional elements to tissues and to remove waste products (eg, carbon dioxide, lactic acid)—main function.
- To enable cells (eg, leukocytes, abnormal tumor cells) and different substances (eg, amino acids, lipids, hormones) to be transported between tissues and organs.

> **Study Pearl**
>
> The normal pH of human arterial blood is approximately 7.40 (normal range is 7.35-7.45).
> Blood that has a pH below 7.35 is acidic, while blood pH above 7.45 is alkaline.
> Blood pH along with $paCO_2$ and HCO_3 readings are helpful in determining the acid-base balance of the body (Table 3—Appendix).

Blood plasma is essentially an aqueous solution containing 96% water, 4% blood plasma proteins, and trace amounts of other materials, including:

- Albumin (the most abundant constituent)
- Blood clotting factors (fibrinogen)

TABLE 11-1. BLOOD CORPUSCLES

Red blood cells or erythrocytes (96%)	In mammals, these biconcave disk-shaped corpuscles lack a nucleus and organelles, so are not cells strictly speaking. They contain the blood's hemoglobin and distribute oxygen. The red blood cells (together with endothelial vessel cells and some other cells) are also marked by proteins that define different blood types. The combined surface area of all the erythrocytes in the human anatomy would be roughly 2000 times as great as the body's exterior surface. The outstanding characteristic of erythrocytes is the presence of the iron-containing protein hemoglobin (see Transport of Oxygen). The percentage of total blood volume which is erythrocytes is called the hematocrit. The normal hematocrit level is approximately 45% in men and 42% in women.
White blood cells or leukocytes (3.0%)	Formed in the bone marrow and are part of the immune system (refer to chapter 5).
Thrombocytes (also known as platelets) (1.0%)	Metabolically active cell fragments that lack a nuclei, which have specific roles in the coagulation (blood clotting or hemostasis) process. They originate from large cells (megakaryocyte) in bone marrow.

Study Pearl

Plasma is distinguished from serum, which is plasma from which fibrinogen and several other proteins involved in clotting have been removed as a result of clotting.

- Immunoglobulins (antibodies)
- Hormones
- Various other proteins
- Various electrolytes (mainly sodium and chlorine)

Together, plasma and corpuscles form a non-Newtonian fluid (a fluid in which the viscosity changes with the applied strain rate and therefore has an ill-defined viscosity) whose flow properties are uniquely adapted to the architecture of the blood vessels.

Production and Degradation of Blood. The direct control of erythrocyte production (erythropoiesis) is exerted by a hormone called erythropoietin, which is secreted by the kidneys. Erythropoietin acts on the bone marrow to stimulate the maturation and proliferation of erythrocytes by a process called *hematopoiesis.* Erythrocytes usually live up to 120 days before they are degraded by the spleen and the Kupffer cells in the liver and then systematically replaced by new erythrocytes. The liver also clears proteins and amino acids (the kidney secretes many small proteins into the urine).

Study Pearl

Blood is about 7% of the human body weight, so the average adult has a blood volume of about 5 L, of which 2.7 to 3 L is plasma.

PERIPHERAL CIRCULATION—BLOOD VESSELS

Arteries. A normal artery wall consists of three layers: the intima, which is the innermost endothelial layer, is in direct contact with the flow of blood; the media, which surrounds the intima and consists of smooth muscle and elastic tissue; and the adventitia, the outermost layer, which consists of connective tissue. The inner diameter of the arteries through which the blood flows is the lumen.

Almost all arteries carry oxygenated blood away from the heart. The aorta is the root systemic artery. It receives blood directly from the left ventricle of the heart via the aortic valve. As the aorta branches, and these arteries branch in turn, they become successively smaller in diameter, down to the arteriole (Table 11-2).

Study Pearl

The size of the lumen is critical for adequate blood flow. A significant narrowing of the lumen, such as that which occurs with a fixed atherosclerotic lesion of coronary artery disease (CAD), will decrease the available blood supply to the myocardium.[2]

TABLE 11-2. SEGMENTS AND BRANCHES OF THE AORTA

SEGMENT OF AORTA	ARTERIAL BRANCH	GENERAL REGION OR ORGAN SERVED
Ascending portion of aorta	Right and left coronary arteries	Heart
Aortic arch	Brachiocephalic trunk	
	—Right common carotid artery	Right side of head and neck
	—Right subclavian artery	Right shoulder and right upper extremity
	Left common carotid artery	Left side of head and neck
	Left subclavian artery	Left shoulder and left upper extremity
Thoracic portion of aorta	Pericardial arteries	Pericardium of heart
	Posterior intercostal arteries	Intercostal and thoracic muscles, and pleurae
	Bronchial arteries	Bronchi of lungs
	Superior phrenic arteries	Superior surface of diaphragm
	Esophageal arteries	Esophagus
Abdominal portion of aorta	Inferior phrenic arteries	Inferior surface of diaphragm
	Celiac trunk	
	—Common hepatic artery	Liver, upper pancreas, and duodenum
	—Left gastric artery	Stomach and esophagus
	—Splenic artery	Spleen, pancreas, and stomach
	Superior mesenteric artery	Small intestine, pancreas, cecum, appendix, ascending colon, and transverse colon
	Suprarenal arteries	Adrenal (suprarenal) glands
	Lumbar arteries	Muscles and spinal cord of lumbar region
	Renal arteries	Kidneys
	Gonadal arteries	
	—Testicular arteries	Testes
	—Ovarian arteries	Ovaries
	Inferior mesenteric artery	Transverse colon, descending colon, sigmoid colon, and rectum
	Common iliac arteries	
	—External iliac arteries	Lower extremities
	—Internal iliac arteries	Genital organs and gluteal muscles

Data from Van de Graaff KM, Fox SI: Circulatory system. In: Van de Graaff KM, Fox SI, eds. *Concepts of Human Anatomy and Physiology.* New York, NY: WCB/McGraw-Hill. 1999:610-691.

- The arterial system is the higher-pressure portion of the circulatory system.
- Pulmonary arteries: carry oxygen- deficient blood that has just returned from the body to the lungs, where carbon dioxide is exchanged for oxygen.
- Systemic arteries: deliver blood to the arterioles, and then to the capillaries, where nutrients and gasses are exchanged.
- Arterioles: the smallest of the true arteries, arterioles have the greatest collective influence on both local blood flow and on overall blood pressure. They are the primary "adjustable nozzles" in the blood system, across which the greatest pressure drop occurs. The arterioles supply capillaries.
- Capillaries. Though not considered true arteries, the capillaries play an important role in the circulatory system. These vessels have no smooth muscle surrounding them and have a diameter less than that of a red blood cell. The red blood cells must distort in order to pass through the capillaries. This small diameter of the capillaries provides a relatively large surface area for the exchange of gases and nutrients. The specific role of the capillaries varies according to location.

- In the lungs, carbon dioxide is exchanged for oxygen (see later).
- In the tissues, oxygen (O_2), carbon dioxide (CO_2), and nutrients and wastes are exchanged.
- In the kidneys wastes are released to be eliminated from the body.
- In the intestine nutrients are picked up, and wastes released.

Veins. The veins carry the deoxygenated blood back to the heart (see later).

> **Study Pearl**
>
> It is the heme portions of the molecule which contain iron, and it is this iron that binds O_2.

TRANSPORT OF OXYGEN

The hemoglobin (Hb) molecule is the primary transporter of O_2 in mammals and many other species. Hemoglobin is made up of four subunits, each subunit consisting of an organic molecule known as *heme* attached to a polypeptide; the four polypeptides of each hemoglobin molecule are collectively called *globin*.

> **Study Pearl**
>
> The normal level of hemoglobin is 12 to 16 g/dL for women and 13.5 to 18 g/dL for men.

In the process of blood degradation, hemoglobin molecules are catabolized to yield heme and the polypeptide chains of globin. Iron is removed from the heme and the remainder of the heme is broken down in several steps to the yellow substance bilirubin, which is released into the blood, picked up by the Kupffer cells of the liver, and secreted into the bile.

> **Study Pearl**
>
> A fetus, receiving O_2 via the placenta, is exposed to much lower O_2 pressures (about 20% of the level found in an adult's lungs) and so fetuses produce another form of hemoglobin with a much higher affinity for O_2 (hemoglobin F) in order to extract as much O_2 as possible from this sparse supply.

With the exception of pulmonary and umbilical arteries, and their corresponding veins, arteries carry oxygenated blood away from the heart and deliver it to the body via arterioles and capillaries, where the O_2 is consumed; afterwards, venules and veins carry deoxygenated blood back to the heart.

Under normal conditions in humans, hemoglobin in blood leaving the lungs is about 96% to 97% saturated with O_2; "deoxygenated" blood returning to the lungs is still approximately 75% saturated (see Chapter 10).

LYMPHATIC SYSTEM

> **Study Pearl**
>
> The lymphatic system has four major purposes:
>
> - To return water, proteins, and lipids from the interstitium to the intravascular space.
> - To help keep edema from forming by acting as a safety valve for fluid overload.
> - To sustain the homeostasis of the extracellular environment.
> - To purify the interstitial fluid and provide a barrier to the spread of infection or malignant cells in the lymph nodes.

The lymphatic system is a network of tactically placed lymph nodes connected by an extensive network of lymphatic vessels, which act as the immune system's circulatory system (see Chapter 5). This system transports lymph but, unlike the circulatory system, has no pump. The fluids also transport foreign substances (such as bacteria), cancer cells, and dead or damaged cells that may be present in tissues into the lymphatic vessels. Lymph also contains many white blood cells.

The diameter of the lymph vessels increases as lymph fluid moves more centrally. Larger lymph collectors, known as trunks or ducts, deal with the larger volumes of lymph fluid.

The majority of the lymph produced by the body in a 24-hour period (2-4 L) returns to the left venous angle via the thoracic duct. Interstitial fluid normally contributes to the nourishment of tissues and about 90% of the fluid returns to the circulation via entry into venous capillaries. The remaining 10% is composed of high molecular weight proteins and their oncotically associated water, which is too large to readily pass through venous capillary walls. This leads to flow into the lymphatic capillaries where pressures are typically subatmospheric and can accommodate the large size of the proteins and their accompanying water. The proteins then travel as lymph through numerous filtering lymph nodes on their way to join the venous circulation. All substances transported by the lymph pass through at least one lymph node. Lymph nodes filter out and destroy foreign substances before the fluids return to the bloodstream. In the lymph nodes, white blood cells can collect, interact with one another and antigens, and create immune responses to foreign substances. Once through the lymph node, lymph then travels from lymphatic capillaries to lymphatic vessels to ducts to left subclavian vein.

Immune responses to infections cause the lymph nodes to swell after an infection.

Study Pearl

Lymph nodes often cluster in areas where the lymphatic vessels branch off, such as the neck, armpits, and groin. The major lymph nodes are the submaxillary, cervical, maxillary, mesenteric, iliac, inguinal, popliteal, and cubital nodes. Generally, the size of lymph nodes is dependent on the size of the drainage area. Usually, the closer the lymph node is to the spinal cord, the greater the size of the lymph node. The neck is the exception to the rule.

Study Pearl

- Lymph nodes, in conjunction with the spleen, tonsils, adenoids, and Peyer patches, are highly organized centers of immune cells that filter antigen from the extracellular fluid.
- Lymph nodes are also one of the first places that cancer cells can spread. Cancer cells in a lymph node can cause the node to swell.

THE HEART AND CIRCULATION

The Heart. The heart is a hollow, muscular organ that functions to pump blood around the body through the blood vessels using repeated, rhythmic contractions. The human heart (Latin *cor*) is derived embryologically from mesoderm that forms the heart tube. The muscle tissue of the heart; is comprised of striated muscle fibers called myocardium. Cardiac striated muscle fibers have numerous mitochondria; exhibit rhythmicity of contraction, and can work continuously without fatigue.

In the human body, the heart is normally situated slightly to the left of the sternum. It is enclosed by a sac and is surrounded by the lungs. The apex of the heart, located at the fifth intercostal space at the midclavicular line, is the blunted point at the inferior tip of the left ventricle. The base of the heart is located at the second intercostal space behind the sternum on the posterior aspect of the heart.

The heart wall is made of distinct layers. The first is the pericardium, a fibrous protective sac that encloses the heart. The epicardium, which is composed of a layer of flattened epithelial cells and connective tissue, forms the inner layer of the pericardium. The endocardium is a layer of flattened epithelial cells and connective tissue that lines the inner surface and cavities of the heart.

Heart Chambers and Valves. The heart consists of four chambers (Figure 11-1), the two upper atria (singular: atrium) and the two lower ventricles. Blood is pumped through the heart chambers (Table 11-3) aided by four heart valves.

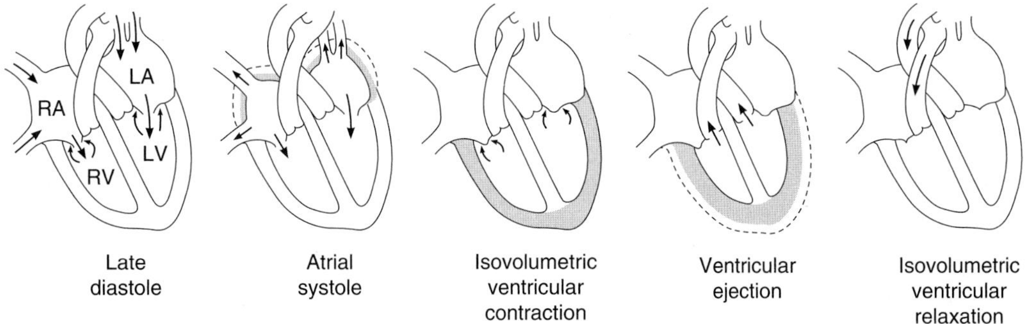

Figure 11-1. The four heart chambers and blood flow in the heart and great vessels. (Reproduced, with permission, from Ganong WF: *Review of Medical Physiology, 22nd ed.* New York, NY: McGraw-Hill. 2005:566.)

TABLE 11-3. CHAMBER PRESSURES

CHAMBER	CENTRAL VENOUS PRESSURE (MM HG)
Right atrium	0-5
Right ventricle	20-30
Left atrium	4-12
Left ventricle	120-140

Right Atrium. The right atrium (RA) receives blood from the systemic circulation via the superior vena cavae (Figure 11-2), which drains the upper component of the body and the inferior vena cava, which drains the lower component of the body. The coronary sinus, an additional venous return into the right atrium, receives blood from the heart itself. Blood passes from the right atrium into the right ventricle via the right atrioventricular (AV) valve (also known as the tricuspid valve as three triangular leaflets, or cusps form it).

Right Ventricle. The right ventricle (RV) receives blood from the RA. The ventricular contraction causes the right AV valve to close and the oxygen-depleted blood to leave the right ventricle via the pulmonary trunk to the lungs. The blood then enters the capillaries of the right and left pulmonary arteries where gaseous exchange takes places and the blood releases carbon dioxide into the lung cavity and picks up O_2. The oxygenated blood then flows through pulmonary veins to the left atrium.

Left Atrium. The left atrium (LA) receives the oxygenated blood from the lungs via four pulmonary veins (two left and two right pulmonary veins). From the LA the blood passes through the mitral (bicuspid) valve to enter the left ventricle.

Left Ventricle. The left ventricle (LV), which forms most of the diaphragmatic side of the heart, receives blood from the LA. The left ventricle is longer and more conical in shape than the right.

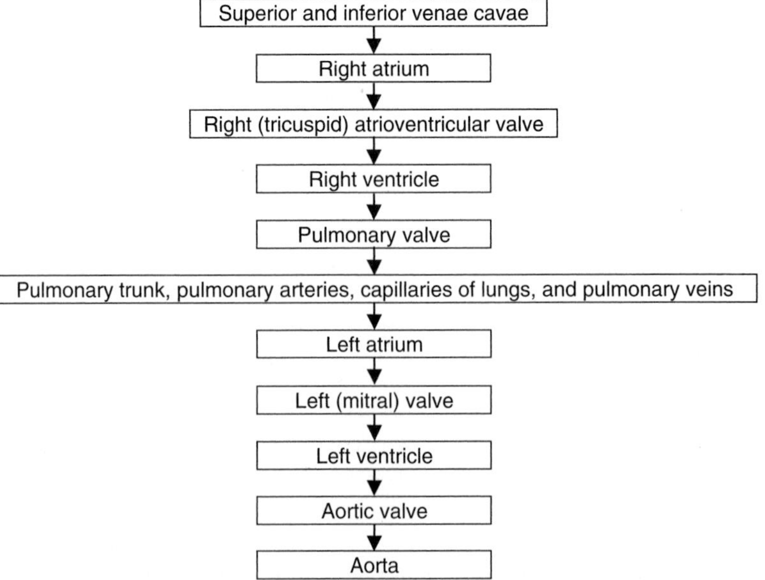

Figure 11-2. Systemic and pulmonary circulation.

Study Pearl

- Edema is an increase of water in the interstitial space, which can result from such things as immobility, chronic venous insufficiency, hypoproteinuria, cardiac insufficiencies or pregnancy.
- Lymphedema (refer to Pathology section) develops as a result of a mechanical insufficiency that arises in an area of functional and structural damage to the lymph collectors, resulting in the accumulation of hydrophilic proteins in the tissues.

Study Pearl

Cardiac muscle has a myogenic origin (an inherent source of contraction), whereas skeletal (striated) muscle has a neurogenic source for contraction (its motor nerve supply).

Study Pearl

- Myocardium: heart muscle, the major portion of the heart.

Study Pearl

Valves are flap-like structures that allow blood to flow in one direction. The heart has two kinds of valves, atrioventricular (tricuspid) and semilunar (the pulmonary valve and the aortic) valves.

The LV has more muscle (1.3-1.5 cm thick) than the right (0.3-0.5 cm thick) as it has to pump blood around the entire body (the right ventricle only needs to pump blood to the lungs), a task that involves exerting a considerable force to overcome the vascular pressure. The aortic valve allows blood to flow from the LV into the aorta, and then closes to prevent blood from leaking back into the LV.

A septum (also known as the fiber skeleton of the heart) divides the right atrium and ventricle from the left atrium and ventricle, preventing blood from passing between them. Even though the ventricles lie below the atria, the two vessels through which the blood exits the heart (the pulmonary artery and the aorta) leave the heart at its top side.

The function of the right side of the heart is to collect deoxygenated blood from the body and pump it into the lungs so that CO_2 can be dropped off and O_2 picked up. This happens through a process called diffusion (see Chapter 10). The left side collects oxygenated blood from the lungs and pumps it out to the body.

Coronary Circulation and the Cardiac Cycle.[2-7]

Myocardial metabolism is essentially aerobic, sustained by a system of continuous O_2 delivery. The blood supply to the heart itself (coronary circulation) is supplied by the left and right coronary arteries, which branch off directly from the aorta near the aortic valve (sinus of Valsalva).

Right Coronary Artery. The right coronary artery (RCA) arises from above the right cusp of the aortic valve where it is known as the conus artery.

- ▶ The RCA supplies blood to the right ventricle, and 25% to 35% of the left ventricle.
- ▶ In 85% of patients, the RCA gives off the posterior descending artery (PDA). In the other 15% of cases, the PDA is given off by the left circumflex artery.
- ▶ The PDA supplies blood to the inferior wall, ventricular septum, and the posteromedial papillary muscle.
- ▶ In 60% of patients the RCA supplies the SA nodal artery. The other 40% of the time, the SA nodal artery is supplied by the left circumflex artery.

Left Coronary Artery. The left coronary artery (LCA) originates from the aorta above the left cusp of the aortic valve. It typically bifurcates into the left anterior descending artery (supplies 45%-55% of the left ventricle, the anterolateral myocardium, apex, interventricular septum and the left circumflex artery) and the left circumflex artery (supplies the posterolateral aspect of the LV and the anterolateral papillary muscle).

The veins involved in the coronary circulation function in parallel to, and in balance with, the arterial system. The coronary sinus is the main drainage channel of venous blood from the myocardium. Located on the posterior surface of the heart between the left atrium and ventricle, it functions to empty the venous blood from the myocardium into the right atrium. The coronary veins and the coronary sinus are rarely the cause of significant heart disease.

Study Pearl

The AV valves are maintained in position by chordae tendineae, which in turn are held to the ventricular wall by papillary muscles.

- ▶ The papillary muscles serve to retain approximation of the valve leaflets during contraction of the ventricles.
- ▶ The chordae tendineae check the valves from everting when the ventricles contract thereby preventing any back flow of blood.

Study Pearl

- ▶ The blood that is pumped to the pulmonary trunk passes through the pulmonary semilunar valve, which lies at the base of the pulmonary trunk, and functions to prevent blood from leaking back into the right ventricle.
- ▶ Semilunar valves are half-moon-shaped flaps of endocardium and connective tissue reinforced by fibers that prevent the valves from turning inside out. Their main function is to prevent the back flow of blood from the aorta and pulmonary arteries into the ventricles when the heart relaxes between beats.

Study Pearl

When the left ventricle is relaxed, the mitral valve is open, allowing blood to flow from the atrium into the ventricle; when the left ventricle contracts, the mitral valve closes preventing the back flow of blood into the atrium.

Study Pearl

The majority of diseases primarily affect the LV (ie, ischemia, infarction, cardiomyopathy, and heart failure).[2]

Study Pearl

Lambl's excrescences are small thread-like strands on the ventricular surface of aortic (mitral) valve leaflets that are theorized of being capable of peripheral embolization.

Study Pearl

It is the closing of the valves that produces the familiar beating sounds of the heart, commonly referred to as the "lub-dub" sound—due to the closing of the semilunar and AV valves.

Study Pearl

The coronary arteries receive the majority of their blood flow during diastole, unlike the other arteries of the body that are perfused during systole.[2]

Study Pearl

Coronary artery disease (CAD) is associated with myocardial ischemia (angina pectoris) and to myocardial infarction (MI). As cardiac muscle is strictly aerobic, the myocardium begins to deteriorate if the blood flow is occluded for more than 8 to 12 beats.

Cardiac Cycle. Each single beat of the heart involves a sequence of interconnected events known as the cardiac cycle (Figure 11-1). The cardiac cycle consists of three major stages: atrial systole, ventricular systole and complete cardiac diastole.

- The atrial systole involves the contraction of the atria. This contraction occurs during the last third of diastole and complete ventricular filling.
- The ventricular systole involves the contraction of the ventricles and flow of blood into the circulatory system. Once all the blood empties from the ventricles, the pulmonary and aortic semilunar valves close. End systolic volume is the amount of blood in the ventricles after diastole, about 50 mL. When the aortic valve closes at the end of systole there is effective blood pressure and volume in the aorta to fill the coronary arteries. The coronary arteries are efficiently occluded during systole since the myocardium squeezes the vessels as the fibers contract.
- The complete cardiac diastole consists of relaxation of the atria (atrial diastole) and ventricles (ventricular diastole) in preparation for refilling with circulating blood. End diastolic volume is the amount of blood in the ventricles after diastole, about 120 mL.

ELECTRICAL CONDUCTION SYSTEM OF THE HEART

The electrical conduction system of the heart depends on specialized conduction tissue, which relays electrical impulses in the myocardium.

Sinoatrial Node. The sinoatrial (SA) node is the main pacemaker of the heart, and is located at the junction of the superior vena cava and right atrium. Under normal conditions, the SA node spontaneously generates an electrical impulse that is propagated to (and stimulates) the myocardium, causing a contraction (Figure 11-3). The electrical activity spreads throughout the atria via specialized pathways, known as internodal tracts, from the SA node to the atrioventricular (AV) node, a small mass of specialized cells. It is the ordered stimulation of the myocardium that allows efficient contraction of the heart, thereby allowing blood to be pumped throughout the body.

- Electrical activity that originates from the SA node at a rate of between 60 and 100 beats/min is known as normal sinus rhythm.
- If a rhythm originating from the sinus node is at a rate less than 60 beats/min, it is referred to as sinus bradycardia. Sinus bradycardia may pose a danger to the patient, particularly when the heart rate is very low—if the heart rate does not increase appropriately when VO_2 is increased.[2]
- If a rhythm originates from the sinus node at a rate of more than 100 beats/min, it is known as sinus tachycardia.

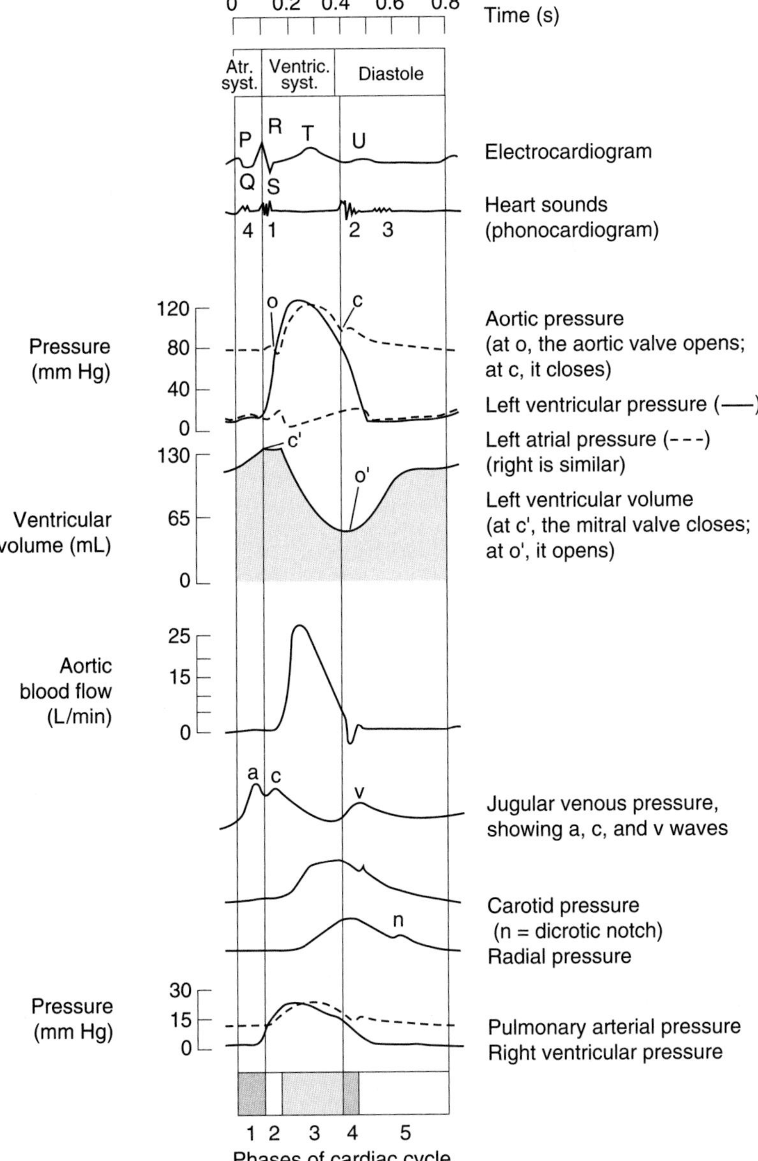

Figure 11-3. Events of the cardiac cycle at a heart rate of 75 beats/min. The phases of the cardiac cycle identified by the numbers at the bottom are as follows: 1, atrial systole; 2, isovolumetric ventricular contractions; 3, ventricular ejection; 4, isovolumetric ventricular relaxations; 5, ventricular filling. Note that late in systole, aortic pressure actually exceeds left ventricular pressure. However, the momentum of the blood keeps it flowing out of the ventricle for a short period. The pressure relationships in the right ventricle and pulmonary artery are similar. Abbreviations: Atr. Syst., atrial systole; Ventric. Syst., ventricular systole. (Reproduced, with permission, from Ganong WF: *Review of Medical Physiology, 22nd ed.* New York, NY: McGraw-Hill. 2005:566.)

Study Pearl

- The heart has a two-step pumping action—one action is involved in the pumping of blood from the right half of the heart through the lungs and back to the left half of the heart (pulmonary circulation); the other action is involved with pumping blood from the left half of the heart through all the tissues of the body (except, of course, the lungs) and back to the right half of the heart (systemic circulation).
- The ventricles are the pumps that produce the pressures which drive the blood through the entire pulmonary and systemic vascular systems and back to the heart (Figure 11-2) by contracting and relaxing.

Study Pearl

The inherent contraction rate heart cells differs according to location:

- Atrial muscle cells inherently contract at about 75/minute
- Ventricular muscle cells contract at about 30 to 40/minute

All of the heart muscle cells have a potential *emergency rate* of about 150 to 250 per minute that may be triggered by certain stimuli.

As the SA node has sympathetic and parasympathetic innervation, either of these systems can affect both the heart rate and its strength of contraction (see Chemical and Physical Influences on the Heart). The heart rate can also be changed by ischemic conditions of the myocardium, electrolyte imbalance, acidosis or alkalosis, hypoxemia, hypertension, emotional stress, drugs, alcohol, caffeine, hormonal influences, and exercise.

Atrioventricular Node. The atrioventricular (AV) node, situated at the junction of the right atrium and the right ventricle, serves as a critical delay in the conduction system. Without this delay, the atria and ventricles would contract simultaneously, and blood would not flow effectively from the atria to the ventricles. The distal portion of the AV node is known as the bundle of His. The bundle of His splits into the left bundle branch and the right bundle branch in the interventricular septum.

- The left bundle branch activates the left ventricle.
- The left bundle branch is short, splitting into the left anterior fascicle and the left posterior fascicle. The left posterior fascicle is relatively short and broad, with dual blood supply, making it particularly resistant to ischemic damage.
- The right bundle branch activates the right ventricle.

The two bundle branches thin out to produce numerous Purkinje fibers, which are the specialized conducting tissue of the ventricles and which stimulate individual groups of myocardial cells to contract. The normal rate of the AV node is between 40 and 60 beats/min.

Refractory Period. Ventricular muscle, unlike skeletal muscle, is incapable of any significant summation of contractions. A refractory period is the amount of time it takes for an excitable membrane to be stimulated and then be ready for stimulus again. The inability of the heart to generate summated contractions is the result of the long absolute refractory period (lasts almost as long as the contraction) of cardiac muscle.[9]

Study Pearl

A rhythm is either regular or irregular. Arrhythmias (dysrhythmias) are abnormal, dysordered rhythms (see Examination of Heart Rhythm). Causes of arrhythmias include ischemic conditions of the myocardium, electrolyte imbalance, acidosis or alkalosis, hypoxemia, hypertension, emotional stress, drugs, alcohol, and caffeine. A sinus arrhythmia may be caused by changes in intrathoracic pressure. Alterations between inspiration and expiration produce phasic increases and decreases in intrathoracic pressure which impacts on venous return, and thus heart rate.[8] Sinus arrhythmia is better thought of as a normal heart rhythm variant as it rarely has any clinical relevance because there is no hemodynamic compromise.

Study Pearl

In the event of severe cardiac pathology, the Purkinje fibers can function as pacemakers for the heart; under normal circumstances their rate of spontaneous firing is considerably lower (20-40 beats/min) than that of the main pacemakers and hence is overridden.[9]

Chemical and Physical Influences on the Heart

Although the heart is designed to continue beating according to the rhythm set by the SA node, the rate of this spontaneous depolarization can be modified by both sympathetic and vagus (parasympathetic) nerve (cranial nerve X) fibers to the heart. Autonomic innervation of the heart is mediated by cardiac control centers in the medulla oblongata of the brainstem, which in turn, are controlled by higher brain areas and by sensory feedback from pressure receptors (baroreceptors) in the aorta and carotid arteries.[10] In addition, surrounding the carotid sinus are the carotid bodies, small neurovascular organs that contain chemoreceptors which are sensitive to fluctuations in the blood levels of O_2, CO_2, potassium, calcium, and pH.

An increase in heart rate can result from:

- Increased CO_2 levels
- Decreased O_2 levels
- Decreased pH (elevated lactic acid and other metabolic products) levels

- Electrolyte imbalance
- Hypokalemia (a decrease in the concentration of potassium ion's)
- Hypercalcemia (an increase in calcium concentrations)

A decrease in heart rate results from:

- Increased O_2 levels
- Electrolyte imbalance
- Hyperkalemia (an increase in the concentration of potassium ion's)
- Hypocalcemia (a decrease in calcium concentrations)

Parasympathetic (Cholinergic) Stimulation

- Derived from the vagus nerve.
- The post-ganglionic parasympathetic nerves are cholinergic.
- Primary impact is on the resting heart, influencing resting heart rate substantially more than the sympathetic nervous system. Parasympathetic stimulation results in a depression of the heart rate, a decrease in the speed of the A-V node impulses (prolonged PR interval), and a decrease in the force of contraction of the atria and ventricles which prolongs systole. It also increases the permeability of the membrane to potassium, causing coronary artery vasoconstriction.
- Acetylcholine, released from parasympathetic endings, hyperpolarizes the SA node and thus decreases the rate of its spontaneous firing.

Sympathetic (Adrenergic) Stimulation

- Sympathetic nervous system neurons (which originate in the intermediolateral cell column at T1-L2 neurologic levels) control vasoconstriction and heart contractility. Sympathetic nervous system innervation of the heart comes from the T1-4 levels.
- The post ganglionic sympathetic nerves are adrenergic.
- Norepinephrine, released primarily by sympathetic nerve endings stimulates an increase in the spontaneous rate of firing at the SA node. This produces an increase in the rate (chronotropy) and force of myocardial contraction (inotropy), and coronary artery vasodilation by increasing the flow of calcium ions into the SA-nodal cells.
- Epinephrine, secreted by the adrenal medulla, speeds the rate of the A-V node impulses (resulting in a decreased PR interval) and increases the force of contraction of the atria and ventricles, allowing for a larger fraction of the cardiac cycle to be available for filling (increased diastole). This occurs as part of the normal exercise response (see Normal Exercise Response), especially when exercise is continued beyond a few minutes. During exercise, the effects of the sympathetic nervous system and catecholamine release significantly override any effect from the parasympathetic system.
- Sympathetic stimulation results in essentially the opposite reactions as to those listed under the parasympathetic stimulation.

Study Pearl

The smooth blood vessels of the heart, including the coronary arteries, have alpha-adrenergic and beta-adrenergic receptors.

- Many cardiovascular drugs either enhance or suppress sympathetic functioning. Those that mimic the action of the sympathetic nervous system are known as sympathomimetics (dopamine, epinephrine, and atropine); those that suppress sympathetic functioning are known as sympatholytics (beta-adrenergic antagonists).

Atrial Natriuretic Factor. Atrial natriuretic factor (ANF) is a powerful peptide hormone secreted by the heart that is involved in the homeostatic control of blood pressure and volume.[11] The secretion of ANF reduces blood volume and thus reduces central venous pressure, cardiac output, and arterial blood pressure.[11] ANF secretion also increases renal sodium secretion and excretion, and increases lipolysis.[11]

Bainbridge Reflex. The Bainbridge reflex, also called the atrial reflex, is an increase in heart rate due to an increase in central venous pressure. A stimulation of mechanoreceptors located within the right atrial myocardium occurs because of an increase in pressure and distension of the right atrium caused by an increase in venous return. The reflex acts to increase heart rate when blood pressure drops.

HEMODYNAMICS

Hemodynamics refers to the physical factors that govern blood flow within the circulatory system.

- Stroke volume (SV): the amount of blood pumped out by the left ventricle of the heart with each beat. The heart does not pump all the blood out of the ventricle—normally, only about two-thirds. The amount of blood pumped out is a factor of:
  - Exercise: prolonged aerobic exercise may increase stroke volume, producing a slower HR in a trained athlete. Reduced heart rate prolongs ventricular diastole (filling), increasing end-diastolic volume, and ultimately allowing more blood to be ejected.
  - Preload: this is the degree to which the ventricles are stretched prior to contracting. The greater the diastolic filling (preload) and thus ventricular stretching, the more forceful the ventricular contraction and thus the greater the quantity of blood pumped (Frank-Starling law). During diastole as muscle length increases (eg, the ventricular chamber size increases) the ability of the myocardium to develop force is increased, up to a point.[2] Beyond a certain length, however, force development is impaired owing to the inadequate alignment of actin and myosin.[2]
  - Left ventricular end diastolic volume: the amount of blood left in the ventricle at the end of diastole.
  - Contractility: the ability of the ventricle to contract.
  - Afterload: commonly measured as the aortic pressure during systole. It is the force the left ventricle must generate to overcome aortic pressure to open the aortic valve. Any increase in the afterload reduces the stroke volume.

- Cardiac output (CO): the amount of blood discharged by *each* ventricle (not both ventricles combined) per minute, usually expressed as liters per minute. Factors that influence CO includes venous pressure, HR, and left ventricular contractility.[2]
  - Calculated by multiplying stroke volume (SV) by the heart rate (HR). For example, if each ventricle has a rate of 75 beats/min and ejects 70 mL with each beat, the cardiac output = 75 beats/min × 0.07 L/beat = 5.25 L/min.
  - For the average adult at rest it is approximately 4 to 6 L/min. During periods of exercise, the cardiac output may reach 30 to 35 L/min.
  - Cardiac index: a valuable diagnostic and prognostic tool when treating patients with pulmonary hypertension (PH). Calculated as cardiac output (liters) per unit time (minutes) divided by body surface area (m^2); normally calculated in liters per minute per square meter. Normal cardiac index ranges between 2.5 and 40.0 L/min/m.
  - Ejection fraction (EF): percentage of blood NT from the ventricle during systole; a clinically useful measure of left ventricular function.
  - EF = stroke volume (SV)/left ventricular end diastolic volume (LVEDV).
  - Normal EF averages 60% to 70%; the lower the EF, the more impaired the left ventricle (LV).

Normal Exercise Response. An increase in $\dot{V}O_2$ occurs with an increase in external workload. There is a direct, almost linear relationship between HR and external workload (intensity). Therefore, if a physical therapy intervention requires an increase in systemic oxygen consumption expressed as either an increase in MET levels, kcal, L/O_2, or mL O_2 per kg of body weight per minute, then HR should also increase.[2]

In the normal heart, as workload increases, stroke volume (SV) increases linearly up to 50% of aerobic capacity. After this point, it increases only slightly. Factors that influence the magnitude of change in SV include ventricular function, body position, and exercise intensity. Cardiac output (CO) increases linearly with workload because of the increases in HR and SV in response to increasing exercise intensity. Factors that influence the degree of change in CO include age, posture, body size, presence of disease, and level of physical conditioning.

Study Pearl

The degree to which the HR increases with increasing workloads is influenced by many factors including age, fitness level, type of activity being performed, presence of disease, medications, blood volume, and environmental factors (eg, temperature, humidity, and altitude). An inability of the heart rate to increase with increasing workloads (chronotropic incompetence) should be of concern for the physical therapist (even if the patient is taking beta-blockers).[2]

Blood Pressure. Blood pressure is defined as the pressure exerted by the blood on the walls of the blood vessels, specifically *arterial blood pressure.* To withstand and adapt to the pressures within, arteries are surrounded by varying thicknesses of smooth muscle which have extensive elastic and inelastic connective tissues.

- Peak pressure in the arteries occurs during contraction of the left ventricle (systole) and provides the clinician with a measurement called the systolic pressure.
- The lowest pressure in the arteries occurs during cardiac relaxation when the heart is filling (diastole) and provides the clinician with a measurement called the diastolic pressure.

As with HR, a linear increase in systolic blood pressure should be expected with increasing levels of work. Diastolic pressure exhibits limited changes with exercise; it may not change, or either increase or decrease by 10 mm Hg.[2]

Factors Influencing Blood Pressure. There are many physical factors that influence blood pressure (see also Orthostatic Hypotension):

- Age: BP normally rises gradually after birth and reaches a peak during puberty. By late adolescence (18-19 years), adult BP is reached.[12] In older adults, the rise in blood pressure is primarily because of the degenerative effects of arteriosclerosis.[12]
- Rate of pumping (heart rate): the rate at which blood is pumped by the heart—the higher the heart rate, the higher (assuming no change in stroke volume) the blood pressure.
- Volume of blood: the amount of blood present in the body. The more blood present in the body, the higher the rate of blood returned to the heart and the resulting cardiac output.
- Cardiac output: the rate and volume of flow—product of the heart rate, or the rate of contraction, multiplied by the stroke volume, the amount of blood pumped out from the heart with each contraction—the efficiency with which the heart circulates the blood throughout the body.
- Resistance of the blood vessel walls (peripheral vascular resistance): the higher the resistance, the higher the blood pressure; the larger the blood vessel, the lower the resistance. Factors that influence peripheral vascular resistance include arteriolar tone, vasoconstriction, and to a lesser extent, blood viscosity.
- Viscosity, or thickness, of the blood: if the blood gets thicker, the result is an increase in blood pressure. Certain medical conditions can change the viscosity of the blood. For instance, low red blood cell concentration, anemia, reduces viscosity, whereas increased red blood cell concentration increases viscosity.
- Body temperature: an increase in body temperature causes the heart rate to increase. Conversely a decrease in body temperature causes the heart rate to decrease.
- Arm position: BP may vary as much as 20 mm Hg by altering arm position.[12] The pressure should be determined in both arms (see later). Causes of marked asymmetry in blood pressure of the arms are the following: errors in measurements, marked difference in arm size, thoracic outlet syndromes, embolic occlusion of an artery, dissection of an aorta, external arterial occlusion, coarctation of the aorta, and atheromatous occlusion.[13]
- Exercise: physical activity will increase cardiac output, with a consequent linear increase in blood pressure. Greater increases are noted in systolic pressure owing to proportional changes in the pressure gradient of peripheral vessels.[12]
- Valsalva maneuver: an attempt to exhale forcibly with the glottis, nose, and mouth closed.[12] This results in:
  - An increase in intrathoracic pressure with an accompanying collapse of the veins of the chest wall
  - A decrease in blood flow to the heart, and a decreased venous return
  - A drop in arterial blood pressure

Study Pearl

The so-called *blood thinners* (eg Coumadin) do not affect the viscosity of the blood, but rather the ability of the blood to clot (see Chapter 19).

When the breath is released, the intrathoracic pressure decreases, and venous return is suddenly reestablished as an *overshoot* mechanism to compensate for the drop in blood pressure. This causes a marked increase in heart rate and arterial blood pressure.[12]

- Orthostatic hypotension: a decrease in BP below normal (a systolic blood pressure decrease of at least 20 mm Hg or a diastolic blood pressure decrease of at least 10 mm Hg within three minutes of standing) to the point where the pressure is not adequate for normal oxygenation of the tissues when assuming an upright position (see Cardiovascular Conditions).[14]

Regulation of Blood Pressure. The CNS regulatory site for BP is located in the vasomotor center, which is located bilaterally in the lower pons and upper medulla. The vasomotor center is tonically active and produces a slow continual firing of nerve fibers, which in turn maintains a partial state of contraction of the blood vessels—vasomotor tone. The vasomotor center monitors sympathetic and vagal inputs and is influenced by neural impulses arising in the baroreceptors, chemoreceptors, hypothalamus, cerebral cortex, and skin.

Baroreceptor (Pressoreceptor) Reflex. Baroreceptors, which are located in the walls of the aortic arch and carotid sinus, are activated by either pressure or stretch receptors. Because these receptors are more responsive to continually changing pressure than to constant pressure, they play a key role in the short-term alteration of blood pressure. Alterationss are made in the mean arterial pressure by facilitating a compensatory decrease in CO and PVR.[2]

- An increase in BP results in a decrease in sympathetic activation of the heart, arterioles, and veins, and an increase in parasympathetic stimulation:
  - A decrease in CO
  - Vasodilation of peripheral blood vessels.
  - A decrease in blood pressure
- A decrease in BP, which results in a decreased firing of the arterial baroreceptors, and a subsequent increase in sympathetic activation of the heart, veins, and arterioles, and a decrease in parasympathetic activity of the heart:
  - Increased CO and PVR
  - Vasoconstriction of peripheral blood vessels.
  - Increase in blood pressure

Renin-Angiotensin System. The renin-angiotensin system (RAS) serves as a mechanism for long-term adjustment of blood pressure by allowing the kidney to compensate for loss in blood volume or drops in blood pressure through activation of an endogenous vasoconstrictor known as angiotensin II. Medications called afterload reducers (eg, ACE inhibitors, angiotensin receptor blockers) can block the effects of the renin-angiotensin system thereby reducing both preload and afterload.[2]

Aldosterone Release. Aldosterone, which is a steroid hormone, is released from the adrenal gland in response to either high serum potassium levels or if angiotensin II is present. The function of this hormone is to increase the excretion of potassium by the kidneys, while increasing sodium retention. Since sodium is the main ion which determines the amount of fluid in the blood vessels, aldosterone will increase fluid retention, and thus, indirectly, blood pressure.

Measurement of Blood Pressure

Arterial Pressure. There are a number of ways that arterial blood pressure (BP) can be measured. The most accurate method involves placing a cannula into a blood vessel and connecting it to an electronic pressure transducer. The less accurate, and less invasive method, uses manual measurement using a sphygmomanometer, an inflatable (Riva Rocci) cuff placed around the upper arm, at roughly the same vertical height as the heart in a sitting person, attached to a manometer (see Blood Pressure in Physical Examination section).

> **Study Pearl**
>
> The mean arterial pressure (MAP), which is an important clinical measure in critical care, is determined by the cardiac output (CO), systemic vascular resistance (SVR), and central venous pressure (CVP) and is based upon the relationship between flow, pressure and resistance. The following equation is used: MAP = CO × SVR.

Oscillometric methods for calculating BP are used in long-term measurement as well as in clinical practice. Oscillometric measurement (also termed NIBP for noninvasive blood pressure) is incorporated in many bedside patient monitors. It relies on a cuff similar to that of a sphygmomanometer, which is connected to an electric pump and a pressure transducer. The cuff is placed on the upper arm and is automatically inflated. When pressure is gradually released, the small oscillations in cuff pressure that are caused by the cyclic expansion of the brachial artery are recorded and used to calculate systolic and diastolic pressures.

Blood pressure values, measured with a sphygmomanometer, are usually given in millimeters of mercury (mm Hg).

- The systolic pressure: the pressure exerted on the brachial artery when the heart is contracting.[14]
- The diastolic pressure: the pressure exerted on the brachial artery during the relaxation phase of the heart contraction.[14]

The values for resting blood pressure in adults are

- Normal: systolic blood pressure < 120 mm Hg and diastolic blood pressure < 80 mm Hg
- Prehypertension: systolic blood pressure 120 to 139 mm Hg or diastolic blood pressure 80 to 90 mm Hg
- Stage 1 hypertension: systolic blood pressure 140 to 159 mm Hg or diastolic blood pressure 90 to 99 mm Hg
- Stage 2 hypertension: systolic blood pressure ≥ 160 mm Hg or diastolic blood pressure ≥ 100 mm Hg

> **Study Pearl**
>
> White coat hypertension (WCH), also known as the white coat effect or isolated office hypertension, is the presence of higher BP when measured in the physician's office than at other times.[15-17] Whether WCH is a benign phenomenon or carries increased cardiovascular risk is still not known.

The normal values for resting blood pressure in children are

- Systolic: birth to 1 month 60 to 90; up to 3 years of age 75 to 130; over 3 years of age 90 to 140
- Diastolic: birth to 1 month 30 to 60; up to 3 years of age 45 to 90; over 3 years of age 50 to 80

Venous Pressure. Venous pressure (VP) is the blood pressure in a vein. VP is much less than arterial blood pressure, eg, typically about 5 mm Hg in the right atrium, 8 mm Hg in the left atrium. Measurement of pressures in the venous system and the pulmonary vessels plays an important role in intensive care medicine but requires invasive techniques.

EXAMINATION OF THE CARDIOVASCULAR SYSTEM

A complete physical examination includes an evaluation of the general appearance of the patient, the patient history, the chief complaint, and a review of the specific organ systems. Cardinal symptoms of cardiac disease usually include chest, neck, or arm pain or discomfort; palpitations; dyspnea; syncope (fainting); fatigue; cough; and cyanosis.[18]

Health History

The clinical significance of heart disease is determined by the impact of the disease on cardiac output.[2] In addition to general questions about health, the clinician should ask questions related to the cardinal symptoms of cardiac disease, including any of the following:

- Chest pain: chest pain of systemic origin may be cardiac or noncardiac and may radiate to the neck, jaw, upper trapezius, upper back, shoulder, or arms (most commonly the left arm).[18]
- Dyspnea: generalized feeling of breathlessness or shortness of breath, can be cardiovascular in origin; it may also occur secondary to pulmonary pathologic conditions, trauma, fever, certain medications, or obesity.[18] Dyspnea can be graded using the functional scale outlined in Table 11-4.
  - Dyspnea on exertion (DOE): brought on by exercise or activity.
  - Orthopnea: inability to breathe when in a reclining position.
  - Paroxysmal nocturnal dyspnea (PND): inability to breathe occurring during sleep.
- Fatigue: overall feeling of tiredness. If provoked by minimal exertion, it may indicate aortic valve dysfunction, cardiomyopathy, or myocarditis.[18] If cardiac in nature, fatigue is often accompanied by associated symptoms, such as dyspnea, chest pains, palpitations, or headache.[18]

TABLE 11-4. FUNCTIONAL SCALE FOR DYSPNEA

RATING	DESCRIPTION
0	Not troubled with breathlessness except with strenuous exercise
1	Troubled by shortness of breath when hurrying on the level or walking up a slight hill
2	Walks slower than people of the same age on the level because of breathlessness or has to stop for breath when walking at own pace on the level
3	Stops for breath after walking about 100 meters or after a few minutes on the level
4	Too breathless to leave the house or breathless when dressing or undressing

Data from Papiris SA, Daniil ZD, Malagari K, et al: The Medical Research Council dyspnea scale in the estimation of disease severity in idiopathic pulmonary fibrosis. *Respir Med.* 2005;99:755-761. Epub Nov 24, 2004.

- Intermittent claudication: pain, cramping, and fatigue brought on by a consistent amount of exercise or activities, and relieved by rest; associated with PVD.
  - Related to arterial insufficiency: pain is typically in calf; may also be in thigh, hips, or buttocks.
  - Patient may experience pain at rest with severe decrease in arterial blood supply; typically in forefoot, and worse at night.
- Palpitations: has the patient noticed an irregular heartbeat/heart rhythm? Examples include skipped or extra beats, pounding, or fluttering. Rhythm abnormalities may be caused by a relatively benign condition (eg, mitral valve prolapse, athlete's heart, caffeine, anxiety, exercise) or a severe condition (eg, coronary artery disease, cardiomyopathy, complete heart block, ventricular aneurysm, atrioventricular valve disease, mitral or aortic stenosis).[18]
- Dizziness, syncope (mild syncope—lightheadedness, severe syncope: transient loss of consciousness): can be caused by inadequate cerebral blood flow due to arrhythmias, orthostatic hypotension, aortic dissection, hypertrophic cardiomyopathy, CAD, and vertebral artery insufficiency.[18]
- Cough[18]: usually associated with pulmonary condition but may occur as a pulmonary complication of a cardiovascular pathologic condition. Left ventricular dysfunction, including mitral valve dysfunction may result in a cough when aggravated by exercise, metabolic stress, or supine position. A persistent, dry cough can develop as a side effect of some cardiovascular medications.
- Past medical history: comorbidities, previous or related surgeries, current medications.
- Social history: lifestyle, living situation, family/social support, education level, level of employment.

Presence of Risk Factors. Risk factors jointly accepted by the American Heart Association and the American College of Cardiology are divided into major independent risk factors and other risk factors:

Major Independent Risk Factors

- Cigarette smoking
- Hypertension
- Hypercholesterolemia (elevated serum total (and LDL) cholesterol)
- Low serum HDL cholesterol
- Diabetes mellitus
- Advancing age

Other Risk (Predisposing) Factors

- Obesity: body mass index (BMI) of greater than or equal to 30 kg
- Abdominal obesity: waist girth of greater than 100 cm
- Physical inactivity
- Family history of premature coronary heart disease
- Ethnic characteristics

- Psychosocial factors
- Elevated serum triglycerides
- Small LDL particles
- Elevated serum homocysteine
- Impaired fasting glucose: fasting blood glucose of greater than or equal to 110 mg/dL.
- Elevated serum lipoprotein
- Prothrombotic factors (eg, fibrinogen)
- Inflammatory markers (eg, C-reactive protein)

OBSERVATION

The clinician should observe for obvious signs of serious pathology. JACCEL, a mnemonic for **J**aundice, suggestion of **A**naemia (pale color of skin or conjunctiva), **C**yanosis (blue coloration of lips or extremities), **C**lubbing of fingernails, **E**dema of ankles, **L**ymph nodes of neck, armpits, and groin. The patient should be checked for the following signs and symptoms:

- Diaphoresis: excess sweating, which may be associated with decreased cardiac output.
- Neck vein distension (> 2 cm) above the sternal angle: may indicate right-sided heart failure.
- Changes in the eyes
  - Xanthelasma: yellow lipid lesions of the eyes associated with hyperlipidemia.
  - Pale conjunctiva: may indicate anemia.
  - Petechiae on the conjunctiva: may indicate a fat embolus, or bacterial endocarditis.
- Skin changes
  - Cyanosis: bluish color, especially of the lips, fingertips, nail beds that may be related to vasoconstriction or hypoxia, decreased cardiac output, or cold temperatures.
  - Pallor: associated with decreased peripheral blood flow, and with peripheral vascular disease (PVD).
  - Rubor: dependent redness of skin associated with PVD.
  - Clubbing of the nails: associated with chronic oxygen deficiency, heart failure.
  - Splinter-like hemorrhages of the nailbeds: may indicate bacterial endocarditis.
  - Pale, shiny, dry skin, with loss of hair: associated with PVD.
  - Abnormal pigmentation, ulceration, dermatitis, gangrene: associated with PVD.
  - Turgor: the clinician pinches an area of skin. If upon releasing the skin, the skin remains pinched (tenting), may indicate interstitial dehydration.
- Evidence of edema[18]: swelling, especially in dependent body parts/lower extremities. Peripheral, dependent edema is the hallmark of right ventricular failure—it is usually bilateral and dependent and may be accompanied by jugular venous distention. Edema also occurs as a result of cardiac surgery, venous valve incompetence or obstruction, cardiac valve stenosis, CAD, or mitral valve dysfunction. Periorbital edema may indicate renal dysfunction.

- Measurement of girth using a tape, or volumetric measurements using a volumeter (useful with irregular body parts such as hand or foot).
- Pitting edema (indentation): Depression is maintained when finger is pressed firmly; grading scale:
  Mild 1+: < 1/4" depth of depression
  Moderate 2+: 1/4" to 1/2" depth of depression
  Severe 3+: 1/2" to 1 inch of depression

Tests and Measures

Basic Biometrics. Assess height, weight, and body mass index (BMI).

Chest Expansion. The normal chest expansion difference between the resting position and the fully inhaled position is 2 to 4 cm (females > males). The clinician should compare measurements of both the anterior-posterior diameter, and the transverse diameter, during rest and at full inhalation. The ratio is normally 1:2 and 5:7, respectively.

- An increase in these ratios suggests conditions such as senile emphysema, or osteoporosis with kyphosis.
- Bulging of the intercostal spaces during inspiration are signs of asthma, emphysema, or pleural effusion.

Vital Signs. There are four so-called *vital signs* which are standard in most medical settings: temperature, pulse and blood pressure, and respiratory rate. The equipment needed to assess these vital signs is a thermometer, a blood pressure (BP) cuff with a stethoscope (or an automatic BP machine), and a watch or clock. Though a pulse can often be taken by hand, a stethoscope may be required for a patient with a very weak pulse. There is no standard "fifth vital sign", but some proposals include

- Urinary continence.
- Pain.
- Pulse oximetry (an electronic device that measures the degree of saturation of hemoglobin with oxygen [Sao_2]). Normal oxygen saturation levels are between 96% and 100%. In general, saturation levels below 90% are considered significant and warrant additional testing beyond the data provided by pulse oximetry (eg, arterial blood gas analysis—see Chapter 10), as well as mark the potential need for administration of supplemental oxygen.[12]
- End-tidal CO_2.
- Emotional distress.
- Spirometry.
- Military deployment.
- Glucose levels.

Pain. The examination of pain specific to the cardiovascular examination includes

- Chest pain: may be cardiac or noncardiac in origin.
- Ischemic cardiac pain (angina or myocardial infarction): Diffuse retrosternal pain; or sensation of tightness, achiness, in the chest; associated with dyspnea, sweating, indigestion, dizziness, syncope, anxiety.

- Angina: sudden or gradual onset; occurs at rest or with activity; precipitated by physical or emotional factors, hot or cold temperatures; relieved by rest or nitroglycerin.

Anginal scale:

- 1+ light, barely noticeable
- 2+ moderate, bothersome
- 3+ severe, very uncomfortable
- 4+ most severe pain ever experienced

- Myocardial infarction pain: sudden onset; pain lasts for more than a minute; may have no precipitating factors; not relieved by medications.
- Referred pain: Cardiac pain can refer to shoulders, arms, neck, or jaw. Pain referred to the back can occur from dissecting aortic aneurysm.

Temperature. The temperature recording gives an indication of core body temperature which is normally tightly controlled (thermoregulation) as it affects the rate of chemical reactions. The normal core body temperature of a healthy, resting adult human being is 98.6°F or 37.0°C. The body temperature though does vary with time of day and body conditions. For example, the body temperature is lower in the morning, due to the rest the body received and higher at night after a day of muscular activity and after food intake. Body temperature also varies at different parts of the body.

- Axillary temperatures are typically 97.6°F or 36.4°C.
- Rectal temperatures are typically 99.6°F or 37.6°C.

Prolonged significant temperature elevation (hyperthermia—106°F/41.1°C), or depression (hypothermia—85°F/29.4°C), is incompatible with life.

Pulse. The pulse is caused by pressure waves moving through the blood vessels. The pulse rate (or frequency) is the number of pulsations (peripheral pulse waves) per minute. The term pulse is often used, although incorrectly, to denote the frequency of the heart beat, usually measured in beats per minute.

The peripheral pulse is typically taken by palpating the radial artery at the wrist. If the pulse cannot be taken at the wrist, it is taken at the elbow (brachial artery), at the neck against the carotid artery (carotid pulse), in the inguinal region (femoral artery), behind the knee (popliteal artery), or in the foot (dorsalis pedis or posterior tibial arteries).

To take a peripheral pulse, the clinician's fingers must be placed near the artery and then pressed gently against a firm structure, usually a bone. The clinician should avoid using the thumb when taking a pulse as it has its own pulse which can interfere with detecting the patient's pulse. The clinician should palpate for 15 seconds and multiply the total by 4 with regular rhythm (evenly spaced beats), 1 minute with regularly irregular (regular pattern overall with "skipped" beats) or irregularly irregular (chaotic, no real pattern) rhythm (Table 11-5).

Study Pearl

In most people, the pulse is an accurate measure of heart rate. However, in certain cases, including arrhythmias, the heart rate can be much higher than the pulse rate. In these cases, the heart rate should be determined by auscultation of the central, or apex, pulse at the heart apex (located at the fifth interspace, midclavicular vertical line). The pulse deficit (difference between the heart beat and pulsations at the periphery) is determined by simultaneous palpation at the radial artery and auscultation at the heart apex.

Study Pearl

The carotid artery must be palpated gently to avoid stimulating the baroreceptors which can provoke severe bradycardia or even stop the heart in some sensitive persons. Also, the clinician should avoid palpating an individual's two carotid arteries at the same time, to avoid the risk of fainting or brain ischemia.

Study Pearl

The normal adult heart rate is 70 beats/min, with a range of 60 to 80 beats/min.

- A rate of greater than 100 beats/min is referred to as *tachycardia*.
- A rate of less than 60 beats/min is referred to as *bradycardia*. The rate for a newborn is 120 beats/min (normal range 70 to 170 beats/min)

TABLE 11-5. NORMAL AND ABNORMAL PULSES

TYPE	DESCRIPTION
Normal	The pulse is smooth and regular.
Large, bounding	The pulse feels strong and bounding. Causes include: ▶ An increased stroke volume ▶ Decrease peripheral resistance ▶ Complete heart block ▶ Decrease compliance of the aortic walls, as in aging or atherosclerosis
Bisferiens	An increased arterial pulse. Causes include: ▶ Aortic regurgitation ▶ Combined aortic stenosis and regurgitation
Pulsus alterans	The pulse alternates in amplitude from beat to beat even though the rhythm is basically regular. Usually indicates left ventricular failure.
Bigeminal	May masquerade as pulsus alternans. Caused by a normal beat alternating with a premature contraction.
Paradoxical	A palpable decrease in the pulse amplitude on quiet inspiration. Typically associated with pericardial tamponade, constrictive pericarditis, and obstructive lung disease.

Data from Schmitz TJ: Vital signs. In: O'Sullivan SB, Schmitz TJ, eds. *Physical Rehabilitation*. 5th ed. Philadelphia, PA: FA Davis; 2007:81-120.

Study Pearl

The ease of palpability of a pulse is dictated by the patient's blood pressure. If his or her systolic blood pressure is

- ▶ Below 90 mm Hg, the radial pulse will not be palpable.
- ▶ Below 80 mm Hg, the brachial pulse will not be palpable.
- ▶ Below 60 mm Hg, the carotid pulse will not be palpable. Since systolic blood pressure rarely drops that low, the lack of a carotid pulse usually indicates death.

Study Pearl

To grade a peripheral pulse, the following scales may be used:

0-3 Scale

0 Absent
1+ Weak/thready pulse
2+ Normal
3+ Bounding

Pulse Amplitude

0 Absent
1+ Barely palpable
2+ Normal
3+ Moderately increased
4+ Markedly increased, aneurysmal

In addition to noting the pulse rate, the clinician should note the rhythm and quality of the pulse.

- ▶ The pulse rhythm is the pattern of pulsations and the intervals between them.[12] In a healthy individual, the rhythm is regular and indicates that the time intervals between pulse beats are essentially equal. Arrhythmia or dysrhythmia refers to an irregular rhythm in which pulses are not evenly spaced.[12]
- ▶ The quality of the pulse refers to the amount of force created by the ejected blood against the arterial wall during each ventricular contraction.[12] Doppler ultrasound is a noninvasive instrument used to examine pulses which have a poor quality (refer to Diagnostic Tests section).

The pulse quality and rate is influenced by a number of factors including the age of the patient, patient gender, the force of contraction, the volume and viscosity of blood, the diameter and a elasticity of vessels; the patient emotions, the amount of exercise performed prior to testing, medications, systemic or local temperature, and hormones.

Examination of Respiration. Refer to Chapter 10.

Examination of Heart Sounds. To examine heart sounds, the clinician places a stethoscope directly on the chest using recognized auscultation landmarks and notes the intensity and quality of the heart sounds produced by the closing of the AV and semilunar valves ("lub-dub").

- ▶ The lub, or first sound, is produced with the normal closure of the AV valves (mitral and tricuspid valves) during isovolumetric contraction of the ventricles at systole (Figure 11-3).
- ▶ The second sound ("dub") is produced with the normal closure of the semilunar valves (aortic and pulmonary) when the pressure in the ventricles falls below the pressure in the arteries (at the end of systole/beginning of diastole).

Heart Murmurs. A heart murmur is a sound produced as blood flows through the chambers and large blood vessels of the heart during the cardiac cycle of contraction and relaxation. A pathologic heart murmur is one associated with a structural or functional abnormality of the heart, often a defective heart valve. Murmurs also can be caused by conditions such as pregnancy, fever, thyrotoxicosis, or anemia. Some murmurs are benign or harmless and are not associated with any significant underlying abnormality of the heart or its vessels. Murmurs are named as to when they occur:

- A diastolic murmur occurs when the heart muscle relaxes between beats.
- A systolic murmur occurs when the heart muscle contracts. Systolic murmurs are graded by intensity (loudness) from 1 to 6. A grade 1/6 is very faint, heard only with a special effort. A grade 6/6 is extremely loud and can be heard with a stethoscope slightly removed from the chest.

Examination of the Heart Rhythm. The most accurate way to examine heart rhythm is to use an electrocardiogram (ECG).[8] Alterations in rhythm may originate from within the normal conduction pathway, specifically, from normal pacemakers of cardiac depolarization: the SA node or the AV node. Rhythm disturbances may also arise from outside the normal conduction pathway. The ectopic foci consist of areas of irritable myocardium which can spontaneously depolarize. A typical ECG tracing of a normal heartbeat consists of a P-wave, QRS complex, and T-wave (Figure 11-3).

P-Wave. The P-wave is the electrical signature of the current that causes atrial contraction.[9] Both the left and right atria contract simultaneously. The relationship between the P-wave and the QRS complexes determines the presence of a heart block.

- The shape of the P-waves may indicate atrial problems.
- Irregular or absent P-waves may indicate arrhythmia.

QRS Complex. The QRS complex corresponds to the current that causes contraction of the left and right ventricles.[9] All QRS complexes in a sequence should be identical to one another. The normal duration of a QRS complex is 0.6 to 0.10 seconds (1.5 to 2.5 small boxes). Abnormalities in the QRS complex may indicate bundle branch block (when wide), ventricular origin of tachycardia, ventricular hypertrophy or other ventricular abnormalities. Irregularities in ventricular conduction include flutter, fibrillation, and premature contractions (PVCs). Flutters and fibrillation usually develop following ventricular tachycardia and show a progressive degeneration of organized myocardial electrical activity. The complexes are often small in pericarditis or pericardial effusion.

The Q-wave. The Q-wave, when present, represents the small horizontal (left to right) current as the action potential travels through the interventricular septum.[9] Very wide and deep Q-waves do not have a septal origin, but indicate myocardial infarction that involved the full depth of the myocardium and has left a scar.

Study Pearl

The ST segment connects the QRS complex and the T-wave. The ST segment can be depressed in ischemia and elevated in myocardial infarction, and upslopes in digoxin use. T-wave abnormalities may indicate electrolyte disturbance, such as hyperkalemia and hypokalemia.

R- and S-Waves. The R- and S-waves indicate contraction of the myocardium itself.

T-Wave. The T-wave represents the repolarization of the ventricles.[9] The QRS complex usually obscures the atrial repolarization wave so that it is not usually seen. In most leads, the T-wave is positive.

In order to correctly interpret an ECG, the clinician should take the following steps:

- Calculate the rate. This can be done a number of ways.
  - Multiply the number of QRS complexes in a 6-second strip (most ECG papers has markers every 1, 3, or 6 seconds) by 10 (chart speed = 25 mm/s). Estimate the portion of the RR interval when only a portion of one is contained at the end of 6 seconds.
  - Divide 300 by the number of whole or partial large boxes between two consecutive R-waves.
  - Find an R-wave that falls on a large box line and count how many large boxes are in the interval before the next R-wave. Memorize the values for each large box interval. For example, one large box represents a heart rate of 300, two large boxes represent a heart rate of 150.
  - Divide 1500 by the number of small boxes between consecutive R-waves.
- Examine the rhythm and determine whether it is regular or irregular.
  - Identify the P-waves.
  - Assess the duration of the P-R interval and the relationship of the P-wave to the QRS complex.
  - Assess the QRS complex for shape and duration.
  - Determine whether there are any extra waves or complexes.
  - Assess clinical significance of a dysrhythmia.

Study Pearl

- Asystole is an event involving a cardiac standstill with no cardiac output and no ventricular depolarization. Asystole can be primary or secondary.
- Primary asystole occurs when the heart's electrical system fails to generate a ventricular depolarization.
- Secondary asystole occurs when factors external to the heart's electrical conduction system result in a failure to generate any electrical depolarization.

Cardiac Rhythms and Arrhythmias. Cardiac rhythms are generally named by the beat that initiates conduction to the ventricles and the rate (Table 11-6). For example, sinus bradycardia is a slow rate originating in the S-A node, a junctional (or nodal) rhythm is a normal rate originating in the A-V junction, and ventricular tachycardia is a rapid rhythm originating in the ventricles. Extra waves or complexes signify myocardial irritability, with the problem being atrial, junctional, and/or ventricular.

The severity of an arrhythmia is related to the location, frequency, and number of sites where the extra beats are initiated.

- RR interval: a regular rhythm has equally-sized spaces between all intervals. An intermittently irregular rhythm is generally regular with occasional disruptions (for example, extra beats). A regularly irregular rhythm has a cyclical pattern of varying RR intervals. An irregularly irregular rhythm has no recurring pattern; RR intervals vary in an inconsistent manner.
- QT interval: the QT interval is measured from the beginning of the QRS complex to the end of the T-wave. A normal QT interval is usually about 0.40 second.

TABLE 11-6. ECG CHARACTERISTICS OF ABNORMAL CARDIAC RHYTHMS

RHYTHM	DESCRIPTION	ECG CHARACTERISTIC
Sinus bradycardia	A heart rate less than 60 bpm	P-wave rate < 60/min QRS rate < 60/min
Sinus tachycardia	A heart rate greater than 100 bpm	P-wave rate < 100/min QRS rate < 100/min
Premature atrial contraction (PAC)	Originate from areas of irritable, sometimes ischemic, myocardium that form the wall of the atrium. PACs are generally not as important as premature ventricular contractions: the loss of adequate filling and contraction of the atria associated with PACs are not as hemodynamically disruptive as premature contractions within the ventricles.	P-QRS occur earlier P-wave may be abnormal in shape/configuration QRS is normal P-R interval may be altered Incomplete compensatory pause
Paroxysmal atrial tachycardia		P-wave rate: 150-250/min QRS rate: 150-250/min P-waves may be fused on T-waves
Atrial flutter		Characterized by multiple P-waves to every QRS response. P-wave rate: 250-350/min (have a typical "sawtooth" pattern) QRS rate < P-wave rate Regular R-R interval 2:1, 3:1, 4:1 or variable AV block
Atrial fibrillation	Atrial fibrillation is characterized by multiple ectopic foci, or firing at random throughout the cardiac cycle with no single, unified wave of depolarization in the atria, and thus no organized myocardial contraction.	Absence of P-waves—fibrillatory base line Fibrillatory rate > 350/min Irregular R-R interval QRS rate < P-wave rate
Junctional rhythm		P-wave may be inverted and before the QRS/buried in the QRS/after the QRS QRS rate: 40-60/min Regular R-R interval
Accelerated junctional rhythm		Findings as with junctional rhythm QRS rate: 60-100/min
Ventricular tachycardia	A run of three or more PVCs occurring sequentially; very rapid rate (150-200 bpm); may occur paroxysmally (abrupt onset); usually the result of an ischemic ventricle.	QRS rate > 100/min, regular (refer to idioventricular rhythm for other characteristics)
Ventricular fibrillation	Chaotic activity of ventricle originating from multiple foci resulting in a pulseless, emergency situation requiring emergency medical treatment: cardiopulmonary resuscitation (CPR), defibrillation, medications.	Coarse waviness of baseline Fine waviness of baseline No visible QRS complexes
Junctional tachycardia		QRS rate: 100-150/min See Junctional rhythm characteristics
Premature ventricular contraction (PVC)	A premature beat arising from the ventricle; occurs occasionally in the majority of the normal population.	QRS duration > 0.10 s T-wave is opposite polarity of QRS Complete compensatory pause
Idioventricular rhythm		No P-waves QRS rate: 20-40/min QRS duration: > 0.10 s Regular R-R interval T-waves opposite polarity of QRS
Accelerated idioventricular rhythm		QRS rate: 40-100/min Refer to idioventricular rhythm characteristics

Study Pearl

A compensatory pause is the duration of the pause that occurs after an extrasystole (an ectopic beat that is both premature and constantly related to the previous beat):

- A complete compensatory pause occurs when the sum of the coupling interval and the compensatory pause is equal to twice the sinus cycle length. It is characteristic of a ventricular ectopic foci which fails to conduct back to the atria, hence leaving the sinus node undisturbed.
- An incomplete compensatory pause arises if the sinus node is discharged early by the ectopic depolarization.

The pause "compensates" for the prematurity of the extrasystole and the sinus rhythm resumes on schedule.

Study Pearl

- Bigeminy: premature beats alternating regularly with normal beats. Bigeminy can be either atrial or ventricular, depending upon whether the alternating regular premature beats are atrial or ventricular. Bigeminy can be associated with hypoxia, ischemia, acute myocardial infarction, and medication overdose.
- Trigeminy: a type of PVC pattern. The PVC follows very two normal QRS complexes. Possible causes are electrolyte imbalances, hypoxia, ischemia, acute myocardial infarction, and medication toxicity.

- PR interval: the PR interval is measured from the P-wave to the QRS complex. It is usually 0.12 to 0.20 seconds (3-5 small boxes). A prolonged P-R indicates a slowing of conduction from the S-A node into the A-V junction and defines a first degree (atrioventricular) heart block, while a shortening of the P-R indicates increased A-V conduction or an atrial impulse that does not originate in the S-A node.

Heart Blocks. Heart blocks occur when conduction from the SA node to the AV node gets changed, usually at the level of the AV node. Heart blocks are graded by levels of severity, from first-degree, to second-degree, to third-degree. A third-degree block is a complete heart block and usually requires the insertion of an artificial pacemaker.

Dysrthymias. The presence of any of the following dysrhythmias may prove potentially dangerous:[9]

- Sinus rhythm with short episodes of ventricular tachycardia
- Sinus rhythm with short episodes of paroxysmal supraventricular tachycardia
- Accelerated junctional rhythms
- Artificial pacemaker rhythm with premature ventricular contractions that are new, multi-focal, or couplets
- Sinus rhythm with second-degree AV block
- Atrial flutter or fibrillation with tachycardia ventricular rates
- Sinus rhythm with sinus arrest
- Sinus bradycardia with rates below 50 per minute

The following dysrhythmias are associated with significantly altered hemodynamics:[9]

- Ventricular tachycardia (with pulses)
- Sinus rhythm or atrial fibrillation with complete heart block
- Very slow (40 per minute or below) sinus, junctional, or ideoventricular rhythms
- Malfunctioning artificial pacemakers with ideoventricular rhythms

Examination of Blood Pressure. The manual method of measuring blood pressure (BP) is commonly used by the physical therapist. While listening with a stethoscope placed over the brachial artery at the elbow, the clinician slowly inflates the blood pressure cuff until the sound of the artery is completely occluded. At this point, the clinician slowly releases the pressure in the cuff. At the point when the clinician begins to hear a "whooshing" or pounding sound (first Korotkoff sound—see below) the pressure reading (systolic) is noted. The cuff pressure is further released until no sound can be heard (fifth Korotkoff sound). This is the diastolic blood pressure.

Normally, the systolic blood pressure has been taken to be the pressure at which the first Korotkoff sound is first heard and the diastolic blood pressure reading is taken at the point at which the fourth Korotkoff sound is just barely audible. However, there has recently been a move towards the use of the fifth Korotkoff sound (ie, silence) as the diastolic blood pressure, as this has been felt to be more reproducible.[19-24] In pregnancy a fifth phase may not be identifiable, in which case the fourth is used.[25-27]

Relevance of Blood Pressure to Rehabilitation. Under normal conditions, systolic BP rises rapidly and diastolic pressure rises slightly during the first few minutes of aerobic exercise and then both level off.[1,28] With resistance training, systolic BP rises more considerably. High-level resistance training can cause rises in systolic BP that can be harmful for individuals with preexisting hypertension or heart disease and therefore loads should be kept lower in such patients. Aerobic exercise performed with the arms produces a greater rise in systolic and diastolic BP than lower extremity exercise performed at the same intensity (as measured by percent of maximal oxygen uptake).

Although exercise causes an acute increase in BP, regular submaximal aerobic and resistance training do not cause long-term increases in resting BP, but rather result in lowered BP for 2 to 3 hours after exercise, lowered resting BP, and blunting of the BP response to this form of exercise.

Exercise Tolerance Testing. Exercise tolerance testing is an important diagnostic and prognostic tool for assessing the ability of the cardiovascular system to accommodate increasing Vo_2 in patients with suspected or known ischemic heart disease. The patient exercises through stages of increasing workloads, expressed in units of oxygen –L/min, mL O_2/kg/min, kcal, or metabolic equivalents (METs).[2] The two major goals of exercise testing are to detect the presence of ischemia and to determine the functional aerobic capacity of the individual.[2] Indications for this test include:[1]

- Assessment of chest pain in patients with intermediate probability for coronary artery disease
- Arrhythmia provocation
- Assessment of symptoms (eg, presyncope) occurring during or after exercise

Contraindications for exercise tolerance testing include[1]:

- Acute myocardial infarction (within 4-6 days)
- Unstable angina (rest pain in previous 48 hours)
- Uncontrolled heart failure (atrial or ventricular dysrhythmias)
- Acute myocarditis or pericarditis
- Acute systemic infection
- Deep vein thrombosis
- Uncontrolled hypertension (systolic blood pressure > 220 mm Hg, diastolic > 120 mm Hg)
- Severe aortic stenosis
- Severe hypertrophic obstructive cardiomyopathy
- Untreated life threatening arrhythmia
- Dissecting aneurysm
- Recent aortic surgery

Although exercise testing has been shown to have a sensitivity of 78% and a specificity of 70% for detecting coronary artery disease, it cannot be used to rule in or rule out ischemic heart disease unless the probability of coronary artery disease is taken into account.[29-33]

Study Pearl

Korotkoff sounds are the sounds that medical personnel listen for when they are taking blood pressure. Korotkoff actually described five phases of sounds:

- The first clear, clear, rhythmic tapping sound that gradually increases in intensity. This represents the highest pressure in the arterial system during ventricular contraction and is recorded as the systolic pressure (Figure 11-3). An auscultatory gap is the temporary disappearance of sound normally heard over the brachial artery between phase 1 and phase 2 and may cover a range of as much as 40 mm Hg.[12] Failure to identify this gap may lead to an underestimation of systolic pressure and overestimation of diastolic pressure.[12]
- A murmur or swishing sound heard as the artery widens and more blood flows through the artery. This sound is heard for most of the time—between the systolic and diastolic pressures.
- Sounds become crisp, more intense, and louder.
- The sound is distinct, abrupt muffling; soft blowing quality. At pressures within 10 mm Hg above the diastolic blood pressure (in children less than 13 years old, pregnant women, in patients with high cardiac output or peripheral vasodilation) the muffling sound should be used to indicate diastolic pressure, but both muffling (phase 4) and disappearance (phase 5) should be recorded.
- The last sound that is heard, which is traditionally recorded as diastolic blood pressure.

Study Pearl

Normal adult BP: < 120 mm Hg systolic; < 80 mm Hg diastolic.

- Pre-hypertension: 120 to 139 mm Hg systolic; 80 to 89 mm Hg diastolic.
- Hypertension (primary or secondary):
  - Stage one: 140 to 159 mm Hg systolic; 90 to 99 mm Hg diastolic
  - Stage two: greater than or equal to 160 mm Hg systolic; greater than equal to 100 mm Hg diastolic.
- Normal pediatric BP
  - Infants less than two years: 106 to 110 mm Hg systolic; 59 to 63 mm Hg diastolic.
  - Children 3 to 5 years: 113 to 116 mm Hg systolic, 67 to 74 mm Hg diastolic.

In each of the following tests, the patient's pulse is recorded before and after the test to provide an estimate of oxygen consumption, the presence or absence of heart disease, or fitness level.

Throughout the testing procedure the patient should be monitored for

- General appearance, including signs and symptoms of exercise intolerance.
- Unusual changes in heart rate. The heart rate should increase linearly in relation to workload (workload is a reflection of oxygen consumption and hence energy use). During the test an electrocardiogram machine or a halter monitor (Table 11-7) can be used to provide a continuous record of the heart rate, and the 12-lead electrocardiogram is recorded intermittently. The aim of the exercise is for the patient to achieve their maximum predicted heart rate.
- Changes in blood pressure. Blood pressure must be measured before the exercise begins and at the end of each exercise stage. Blood pressure may fall or remain static during the initial stage of exercise. This is the result of an anxious patient relaxing. As the test progresses, however, systolic blood pressure should rise as exercise increases. A level of up to 225 mm Hg is normal in adults, although athletes can have higher levels. Diastolic blood pressure tends to fall slightly.

Numerous protocols for exercise tests, and other tests (Table 11-7) have been devised to assess cardiac responses to increased workloads.

Study Pearl

- The symptoms of exercise intolerance include persistent dyspnea, complaints of vertigo, chest pain, leg cramps (claudication).
- The signs of exercise intolerance include incoordination, ataxia, confusion, pallor, cyanosis, abnormal diaphoresis.

Step Tests. There are three traditional step tests[1]:

- Master's two-step test: a test in which subjects ascend and descend two steps, with specified dimensions for height and width, in synchrony with a metronome.
- One-step test: consists of one step that is ascended and descended in such a way that the subject initially steps onto the step with the right foot and then brings the left foot onto the step. The right foot is then removed from the step and placed on the floor which is followed by the left foot. The stepping sequence begins again, but the left foot is initially placed on the step followed by the right. This reciprocal sequence is performed in synchrony with a metronome.
- Climbing step test: also utilizes standardized step heights in addition to standardized arm heights for climbing.

Cycle Ergometry Tests. A number of standardized cycle ergometry testing, with developed normal values, exist, but the most common appear to be the Astrand-Rhyming protocol,[34-36] the YMCA protocol, and various ramping protocols.

Treadmill Tests. The Bruce exercise testing protocol is the most popular protocol for testing patients with known or suspected heart disease. The protocol has seven stages, each lasting 3 minutes, resulting in 21 minutes of exercise for a complete test. In clinical practice, patients rarely exercise for the full duration. However, completion of 9 to 12 minutes of exercise or reaching 85% of the maximum

TABLE 11-7. CARDIAC DIAGNOSTIC TESTING AND MONITORING

TEST	DESCRIPTION
Holter monitor	A small, portable, battery-powered ECG machine worn by a patient to record heartbeats on tape over a period of 24-48 hours during normal activities. At the end of the time period, the monitor is returned to the physician's office so the tape can be read and evaluated.
Exercise gated blood pool scan, exercise MUGA, or exercise radionuclide angiography	A nuclear scan to see how the heart wall moves and how much blood is expelled with each heartbeat, just after the patient has walked on a treadmill or ridden on a stationary bike. **Resting First Pass** The scan taken while the patient is at rest to measure the percentage of blood going through the heart with each beat. **Exercise First Pass** The scan taken while the patient is exercising to measure the percentage of blood going through the heart with each beat.
Event recorder	A small, portable, battery-powered machine used by a patient to record ECG over a long period of time. Patients may keep the recorder for several weeks. Each time symptoms are experienced, the patient presses a button on the recorder to record the ECG sample. As soon as possible, this sample is transmitted to the physician's office by telephone hookup for evaluation.
Thallium scans or myocardial perfusion scans	**Resting SPECT Thallium Scan or Myocardial Perfusion Scan** A nuclear scan given while the patient is at rest that may reveal areas of the heart muscle that are not getting enough blood. **Exercise Thallium Scan or Myocardial Perfusion Scan** A nuclear scan given while the patient is exercising that may reveal areas of the heart muscle that are not getting enough blood. **Persantine Thallium Scan or Myocardial Perfusion Scan** A nuclear scan given to a patient who is unable to exercise to reveal areas of the heart muscle that are not getting enough blood. Chemicals injected include dipyridamole thallium (thallium-201, a potent vasodilator) and dobutamine.
Positron emission tomography (PET) scan	A nuclear scan that gives information about the flow of blood through the coronary arteries to the heart muscle.
PET F-18 FDG (fluorodeoxyglucose) scan	A glucose scan sometimes done immediately after the PET scan to determine if heart muscle has permanent damage.
Radionuclide angiography[a]	Red blood cells tagged with a radionuclide are injected into the blood; ventricular wall motion can be evaluated and the ejection fraction determined; abnormal blood flow with valve and congenital defects can also be detected; techniques include gated-pool equilibrium studies and first-pass techniques.
Technetium 99m scanning (hotspot imaging)[a]	Technetium 99m injected into the blood is taken up by damaged myocardial tissue; this identifies and localizes acute myocardial infarctions. This radioisotope is readily available, and its short half-life reduces handling problems and patient exposure.
Thallium-201 myocardial perfusion imaging (cold spot imaging)[a]	Thallium-201 injected into the blood at peak exercise; scanning identifies ischemic and infarcted myocardium, which does not take up thallium-201; used to diagnose coronary artery disease and perfusion particularly when ECG is equivocal.
Cardiac catheterization	The passage of a tiny tube into heart via blood vessels with the introduction of a contrast medium into coronary arteries which is then visualized with cinefluoroscopy to evaluate narrowing or occlusion of arteries. ▶ Provides information about anatomy of heart and great vessels, ventricular function, cardiac output, and abnormal wall movement. ▶ Allows determination of intracardiac, transvalve, pulmonary artery pressures, ejection fraction (EF), and blood gas pressures.

[a]Data from Rothstein JM, Roy SH, Wolf SL: Vascular anatomy, cardiology, and cardiac rehabilitation. *The Rehabilitation Specialists Handbook.* Philadelphia, PA: FA Davis. 1991:548-550.

predicted changes in heart rate is usually satisfactory.[29-33] In stage 1 the patient walks at 1.7 mph (2.7 km) up a 10% incline. Energy expenditure is estimated to be 4.8 METs (metabolic equivalents) during this stage. The speed and incline increase with each stage. A modified Bruce protocol (mini-Bruce) is used for exercise testing within one week of myocardial infarction.

Walk Tests. Walk tests have been used extensively in the examination of patients with heart failure. Although the 6-minute walk test is considered submaximal, it appears to provide information about the functional status, exercise tolerance, oxygen consumption, and survival of persons with cardiac pump failure.

Special Tests

Percussion Test. The percussion test is used to determine the competence of the greater saphenous vein. While the patient is standing, the clinician palpates one segment of the vein while percussing the vein at a point approximately 20 cm higher. If a pulse wave is felt by the lower hand, an assumption can be made that the intervening valves are incompetent.

Trendelenburg's Test. The Trendelenburg test (retrograde filling test) can be used to determine the competence of the communicating veins of the saphenous system. The patient is positioned in supine with their legs elevated to 60 degrees. A tourniquet is placed on the proximal thigh and the patient is then asked to stand. The clinician assesses whether the veins fill in a normal pattern. The filling should take approximately 30 seconds.

Rubor of Dependency. The rubor of dependency is a test of peripheral arterial circulation patency. The clinician assesses whether changes in skin occur during elevation of foot followed by placing the limb in a position of dependency (seated, hanging position). With insufficiency, pallor develops in elevated position; relative hyperemia (rubor of dependency) develops in dependent position.

Diagnostic Tests. A number of diagnostic tests are available for the cardiovascular system (Table 11-7).

Laboratory Tests and Values

Enzyme Studies. Cardiac enzyme studies measure the levels of the enzymes troponin (TnI, TnT) and creatine phosphokinase (CPK, CK) in the blood. The values listed in the tables can be used as a general guide (see Tables A4 to A6 in the Appendix).

Lipid Profile. A group of tests often ordered together to help determine coronary risk based on target levels. The lipid profile includes total cholesterol, HDL-cholesterol (often called good cholesterol), LDL-cholesterol (often called bad cholesterol), and triglycerides. An LDL/HDL ratio is sometimes also included. The values listed below can be used as a general guide.

- Cholesterol: desirable: < 200, border line: 200 to 230, high-risk: > 240
- High density lipoprotein (HDL): low risk (negative risk factor): > 60, moderate risk: 35 to 60, high-risk: < 35

- Low density lipoprotein (LDL): < 100 with heart disease or diabetes, > 100 with multiple risk factors, > 160 for low-risk individuals
- Triglycerides: desirable: < 165
- LDL/HDL ratio: low risk: 0.5 to 3.0, moderate risk: 3.0 to 6.0: high risk: > 6.0

CARDIOVASCULAR CONDITIONS

Risk Factors Associated with Cardiovascular Dysfunction

Physical therapists often examine and treat patients with one or more chronic medical condition that is the inherent cause of dependence, dysfunction and disability, and/or increases the risk of other pathologic conditions.

- Comorbidity[37,38]
  - Atherosclerosis: a major contributing factor to coronary heart disease, including angina pectoris and myocardial infarction.[39]
  - Hypertension: causes mechanical damage to vascular endothelium resulting in areas that are stripped of normal endothelial cells. Associated with increased thrombus and plaque formation, intracerebral aneurysms and hemorrhage, and left ventricular hypertrophy.[40,41]
  - Hyperlipidemia (high blood cholesterol).[42]
  - Diabetes: a complex mix of physiological abnormalities which accelerates the development of atherosclerosis and leads to many cardiovascular complications.[43-45]
  - Osteoporosis: can be associated with classic spinal deformities including increased kyphosis with loss of height, thoracic vertebral body fractures, back pain, and decreased vital capacity.
  - Ankylosing spondylitis: pulmonary involvement including nonspecific fibrosis, dilated bronchi, stiffening and straightening of the spine, decreased intestinal compliance, the latter of which increases the potential for pneumothorax, atelectasis, and aspiration.
  - Idiopathic scoliosis: the lateral curve plus the rotation of the involved thoracic vertebrae around a vertical axis causes a decrease in lung function.
  - Pectus deformities: includes pectus excavatum (funnel chest) and pectus carinatum (pigeon breast).
  - Sarcoidosis: a systemic disease that primarily affects the lungs and the lymphatic system.
  - Systemic lupus erythematosus: affects the pulmonary system more frequently than any other collagen vascular disease. Can be associated with pleuritis, pneumonitis, pulmonary interstitial fibrosis, and pulmonary hypertension.
  - Neurologic disease
    - Cerebrovascular accident: cardiovascular disease is the most common cause of death in long-term survivors of stroke.[46-49]

- Spinal cord injury: stimulation of the cardiopulmonary system is impaired due to lack of innervation to the autonomic nervous system, thereby reducing the ability to support higher rates of aerobic metabolism.[50,51]
- Multiple sclerosis: the loss of myelin reduces the speed of nerve conduction, thus interfering with smooth, rapid, and coordinated movement.[52]
- Parkinson disease: associated with bradykinesia, slow and shuffling gait, freezing, kyphotic posture, and overall flexed posture.[53]

- Medications: aspirin resistance may increase the risk of major adverse cardiac events (MACE) more than threefold in patients with stable coronary artery disease (CAD).[54]
- Lifestyle: cigarette smoking substantially increases the risk for cardiovascular disease in addition to other diseases, notably chronic obstructive pulmonary disease and lung cancer.[55]
- Obesity: many of the effects of obesity appear to be mediated through other risk factors including diabetes and hypertension.[56]
- Physical inactivity: physical inactivity may exert much of its influence through other risk factors.[57] However, numerous public health and medical associations have identified physical inactivity as a significant risk factor for cardiovascular and other diseases.[58]
- Race: African-American women have the highest risk of death from heart disease; Native Americans, particularly those living in North Dakota and South Dakota, also have a higher risk.[59]
- Gender: CAD is the number one killer of women, surpassing all forms of cancer, including breast cancer, combined.[60] At the onset of menopause, women's CAD risk begins to approach that of men's.[60,61]
- Family history: family history is considered positive if myocardial infarction or sudden cardiac death occurred in a primary male relative, age 55 or less, or in a primary female relative, age 65 or less.[62]
- Psychosocial factors: an individual's response to stress can be a determinant factor in the development of CAD. Depression, social isolation, and chronic stress have all been shown to be associated with CAD.[63]

Peripheral Arterial and Vascular Disease

Arterial Disease

Arteriosclerosis. Arteriosclerosis is a cluster of diseases characterized by thickening and loss of elasticity (hardening) of the arterial wall. Arteriosclerosis can be divided into three types:

- Atherosclerosis: plaques of fatty deposits form in the inner layer (intima) of the arteries (see Coronary Artery Disease).
- Mönckeberg's arteriosclerosis: involves the middle layer of the arteries with destruction of muscle and elastic fibers and formation of calcium deposits.
- Arteriolosclerosis or arteriolar sclerosis: characterized by thickening of the walls of small arteries (arterioles).

Arteriovenous Malformations. Arteriovenous malformations (AVM) are congenital vascular malformations of the cerebral vasculature—the result of localized poor development of the primitive vascular plexus of the heart. AVMs vary in size and location and therefore in clinical presentation. Early diagnosis can reduce the chance of hemorrhage.

Aneurysm. An aneurysm is an abnormal stretching in the wall of an artery, a vein, or the heart with a diameter that is at least 50% greater than normal.[18] Aneurysms are named according to the specific site of formation. Aortic aneurysms can form a thoracic aneurysm (involving the ascending, transverse, or first half of the descending portion of the aorta), or an abdominal aneurysm (involving the aorta between the renal arteries and iliac branches). The underlying causes of aortic aneurysms are associated with numerous factors, including atherosclerosis, hypertension, medial degeneration and aging, aortitis, congenital abnormalities, trauma, smoking, cellular enzyme dysfunction, and hyperlipidemia.[64]

An acute aortic dissection is characterized by the onset of intense pain, described as sharp, tearing, or stabbing. The pain occurs in the chest and spreads toward the back and into the abdomen. The pain associated with this condition is unaffected by position. The distal pulses are frequently decreased or absent. This is a potentially life-threatening condition requiring immediate transport of the patient to an emergency department. The patient is admitted to the intensive care unit for further evaluation and to temporarily manage the crisis with antihypertensive medications.[64]

Arteritis. Arteritis (giant cell arteritis, cranial or temporal arteritis) is a vasculitis primarily involving multiple sites of temporal and cranial arteries. Early diagnosis is important to prevent blindness.

Thromboangiitis Obliterans. Thromboangiitis obliterans (Buerger's disease), a chronic, inflammatory vasculitis affecting the peripheral blood vessels (small arteries and veins), occurs commonly in young adults, generally males, who smoke heavily. It has a risk of ulceration, gangrene, and amputation if left untreated.

Patients typically exhibit paresthesias or pain, cyanotic cold extremity, diminished temperature sensation, and intermittent claudication, due to occlusion of the arteries.

Intervention includes cessation of smoking and avoidance of any environmental or secondhand smoke inhalation, pharmacological intervention (vasodilators, pain relief) and physical therapy.

Diabetic Angiopathy. Diabetic angiopathy is an inappropriate elevation of blood glucose levels and accelerated atherosclerosis if untreated. Complications include neuropathy and/or neurotrophic ulcers, the latter of which may lead to gangrene and amputation.

Raynaud's Disease. Raynaud's disease or phenomenon results in intermittent spasms of small arteries and arterioles, which cause temporary pallor and cyanosis of the digits, and which is usually exacerbated by exposure to cold or emotional stress.

- Abnormal vasoconstrictor reflex results in pallor, cyanosis, numbness and tingling of digits (fingertips more often than toes).
- Affects largely females.
- Occlusive disease is not usually a factor.

Study Pearl

The differential diagnosis of paresthesias and peripheral neuropathy is difficult. Peripheral neuropathies can be caused by entrapment syndromes, trauma, diabetes, hypothyroidism, vitamin B_{12} deficiency, alcoholism, inflammatory conditions, connective tissue disorders, toxic injury, hereditary conditions, malignancy, infections, and miscellaneous causes.[65] Peripheral neuropathy can also be mimicked by myelopathy, syringomyelia or dorsal column disorders, such as tabes dorsalis.[66] Hysterical symptoms can sometimes mimic a neuropathy. Many medications can cause a peripheral neuropathy (Table 11-8).[66]

TABLE 11-8. MEDICATIONS THAT MAY CAUSE NEUROPATHIES

AXONAL	DEMYELINATING	NEURONOPATHY
Vincristine (Oncovin, Vincosar PFS)	Amiodarone (Cordarone)	Thalidomide (Synovir)
Paclitaxel (Taxol)	Chloroquine	Cisplatin (Platinol)
Nitrous oxide	Suramin (Fourneau 309, Bayer 205, Germanin)	Pyridoxine
Colchicine (Probenecid, Col-Probenecid)	Gold	
Isoniazid (Laniazid)		
Hydralazine (Apresoline)		
Metronidazole (Flagyl)		
Pyridoxine (Nestrex, Beesix)		
Didanosine (Videx)		
Lithium		
Alfa interferon (Roferon-A, Intron A, Alferon N)		
Dapsone		
Phenytoin (Dilantin)		
Cimetidine (Tagamet)		
Disulfiram (Antabuse)		
Chloroquine (Aralen)		
Ethambutol (Myambutol)		
Amitriptyline (Elavil, Endep)		

Hypertension. Hypertension (hypertensive vascular disease) (see Chapter 14) includes, hypertensive heart disease, pulmonary hypertension (see Chapter 10), and pulmonary heart disease.

Hypotension. Blood pressure that is too low is known as hypotension. Low blood pressure may be a sign of severe disease and requires more urgent medical attention. When blood pressure and blood flow is very low, the perfusion of the brain may be critically decreased (ie, the blood supply is not sufficient), causing lightheadedness, dizziness, weakness, and fainting. Sometimes the blood pressure drops significantly when a patient stands up from sitting—orthostatic hypotension (see next). Other causes of low blood pressure include

- Sepsis
- Hemorrhage
- Toxins including toxic doses of blood pressure medicine
- Hormonal abnormalities, such as Addison's disease
- Shock. Shock is a complex condition which leads to critically decreased blood perfusion. The usual mechanisms are loss of blood volume, pooling of blood within the veins reducing adequate return to the heart, and/or low effective heart pumping. Low blood pressure, especially low pulse pressure, is a sign of shock and contributes to/reflects decreased perfusion.

Orthostatic Hypotension. Orthostatic hypotension is associated with an extreme drop in blood pressure—the primary cause is a decreased compensatory vasoconstriction, especially in the large vascular beds in conjunction with venous pooling in the lower extremities, which reduces venous blood return, SV, and BP. Orthostatic hypotension can be classified as neurogenic (dysfunction of the ANS, such as that which can be associated with a spinal cord injury or post cerebrovascular accident), non-neurogenic (low blood volume in patients who

TABLE 11-9. ETIOLOGIES AND DRUGS THAT CAN CAUSE ORTHOSTATIC HYPOTENSION

NON-NEUROGENIC ETIOLOGIES	NEUROGENIC ETIOLOGIES	MEDICATIONS
Cardiac pump failure	Spinal cord problems	Alpha and beta blockers
Aortic stenosis	Syringomyelia	Antihypertensives
Bradyarrhythmia	Tabes dorsalis	Bromocriptine (Parlodel)
Myocardial infarction	Transverse myelitis	Diuretics
Myocarditis	Tumors	Insulin
Pericarditis	Peripheral nervous system problems	MAO inhibitors
Tachyarrhythmia	HIV/AIDS	Marijuana
Reduced intravascular volume	Alcoholic polyneuropathy	Minor tranquilizers
Adrenal insufficiency	Amyloidosis	Narcotics/sedatives
Burns	Diabetes mellitus	Nitrates
Dehydration	Dopamine beta-hydroxylase deficiency	Phenothiazines
Diabetes insipidus	Guillain-Barré syndrome	Sildenafil (Viagra)
Diarrhea	Paraneoplastic syndrome	Sympatholytics
Hemorrhage	Renal failure	Sympathomimetics (with prolonged use)
Salt-losing nephropathy	Vitamin B_{12} or folate deficiency	Tricyclic antidepressants
Straining with heavy lifting, urination, or defecation	Other neurogenic etiologies	Vasodilators
Vomiting	Brain-stem lesions	Vincristine (Oncovin)
Venous pooling	Brain tumors	
Alcohol consumption	Carotid sinus hypersensitivity	
Fever	Cerebral vascular accidents	
Heat (eg, hot environment, hot shower or bath)	Dysautonomias	
Postprandial dilation of splanchnic vessel beds	Multiple sclerosis	
Prolonged recumbency or standing	Neurocardiogenic syncope	
Sepsis	Parkinson disease	
Vigorous exercise with dilation of skeletal vessel beds	Pure autonomic failure	
	Sepsis Syringobulbia	

Data from Engstrom JW, Aminoff MJ: Evaluation and treatment of orthostatic hypotension. *Am Fam Physician.* 1997;56:1379.

are post operative or dehydrated), or iatrogenic (eg, caused by medication, such as antihypertensive medications) (Table 11-9).[14]

Orthostatic hypotension occurs more frequently in the elderly, especially in persons who are sick and frail. In cases of suspected orthostatic hypotension, the clinician should position the patient in the supine position, take a blood pressure measurement and then repeat the blood pressure measurement at one and three minutes after the patient assumes a standing or sitting position.

Intervention strategies to help minimize the potential for an orthostatic hypotensive episode include progressive elevation of the head of the bed, progressive sitting on the edge of the bed, and deep breathing.[67] Elastic stockings should be worn over the lower extremities.[67] Elevating the head of the bed by 5 to 20 degrees during sleep also is recommended.[67]

Study Pearl

Activities that can increase the potential for orthostatic hypotension, such as application of heat modalities, hydrotherapy, moderate to vigorous exercise using the large muscles, and sudden changes of position should be avoided in susceptible patients.[14]

Study Pearl

Instances of orthostatic hypotension should be reported to the patient's physician because of its association with several diagnoses and conditions.

Venous Insufficiency. In venous insufficiency states, venous blood escapes from its normal antegrade path of flow and refluxes backward down the veins into an already congested leg. Venous insufficiency syndromes are caused by valvular incompetence in the high-pressure deep venous system, low-pressure superficial venous system, or both. Physical examination alone is not a reliable means of assessing the venous system—diagnostic testing nearly always is necessary to rule out deep venous obstruction, to assess the paths of reflux, and to guide treatment planning. The Trendelenburg test (see Special Tests) is traditionally part of the physical examination and may be helpful in making the differential diagnosis.

Deep Venous Insufficiency. Deep venous insufficiency occurs when the valves of the deep veins are damaged as a result of deep venous thrombosis (DVT)—see Deep Vein Thrombophlebitis. With no valves to control deep system reflux, the hydrostatic venous pressure in the lower extremity increases dramatically.

Superficial Venous Insufficiency. In superficial venous insufficiency, the deep veins are normal, but venous blood escapes from a normal deep system and flows backwards through dilated superficial veins in which the valves have failed.

Most cases of superficial vein valve failure occur after a single point of high-pressure leakage develops between the deep system and the superficial system. High pressure causes secondary valve failure when otherwise normal superficial veins become so widely dilated that the thin flaps of the venous valves can no longer make contact in the lumen of the vessel. Over time, these ineffectual superficial veins become visibly dilated, at which point they are recognized as varicose veins.

Klippel-Trenaunay-Weber. A less common cause of venous insufficiency is Klippel-Trenaunay-Weber (KTW) syndrome, which involves port-wine stains, varicose veins, and bony or soft-tissue hypertrophy. High pressure can enter the superficial veins as a result of the failure of key valves at any point of communication between the deep system and the superficial system.

Patients with venous insufficiency often report subjective symptoms that are typically bothersome early in the disease, become less severe in the middle phases, and then worsen again with advancing age. Common symptoms include the following:

- Burning
- Swelling
- Throbbing
- Cramping
- Aching
- Heaviness
- Restless legs
- Leg fatigue

Pain caused by venous insufficiency often is improved by walking or by elevating the legs.

Thrombophlebitis. There are two types of venous thrombosis: superficial vein thrombophlebitis and deep vein thrombophlebitis, both of which share the same pathophysiology, pathogenesis, and risk factors.

Superficial Vein Thrombophlebitis. Superficial vein thrombophlebitis may either occur spontaneously or as a complication of medical or surgical interventions. Patients typically report a gradual onset of localized tenderness, followed by the appearance of an area of erythema along the path of a superficial vein. There may be a history of local trauma, prior similar episodes, varicose veins, prolonged travel, or enforced stasis. Swelling may result from acute venous obstruction (as in deep vein thrombosis) or from deep or superficial venous reflux, or it may be caused by an unrelated disease condition such as hepatic insufficiency, renal failure, cardiac decompensation, infection, trauma, or environmental effects. Palpation of a painful or tender area may reveal a firm, thickened, thrombosed vein.

Duplex ultrasound is the initial diagnostic study of choice for most patients with signs and symptoms of phlebitis.

Graduated compression stockings have been proven effective in the prophylaxis of thromboembolism and are also effective in preventing progression of thrombus in patients who already have superficial phlebitis or actual DVT and PE.[68-71]

Study Pearl

Perthes percussive test can be used to test whether venous segments are interconnected. With the patient in a standing position, a vein segment is tapped at one location while an examining hand feels for a pulse wave at another location. Propagation of a palpable pulse wave suggests that a fluid-filled vessel with open or incompetent valves connects the two locations.

Deep Vein Thrombophlebitis. Deep venous thrombosis (DVT) and its sequela, pulmonary embolism, are the leading causes of preventable in-hospital mortality in the United States.[72] The Virchow triad, as first formulated (ie, venous stasis, vessel wall injury, hypercoagulable state), is still the primary mechanism for the development of venous thrombosis.[72] Hypercoagulable states include

- Genetic: includes antithrombin C deficiency, protein C deficiency, and protein S efficiency.
- Acquired: includes postoperative, postpartum, prolonged bed rest or immobilization, severe trauma, cancer, congestive heart failure, obesity, and prior thromboembolism.

Study Pearl

Patients who undergo total hip arthroplasty or total knee arthroplasty are at high risk for DVT. If no prophylaxis is used, DVT occurs in 40% to 80% of these patients, and the proximal DVT occurs in 15% to 50%.[73]

The signs and symptoms of DVT are related to the degree of obstruction to venous outflow and inflammation of the vessel wall. No single physical finding or combination of symptoms and signs is sufficiently accurate to establish the diagnosis of DVT.[72] The following is a list outlining the most sensitive and specific physical findings in DVT[72,74-76]:

- Edema, principally unilateral.
- Tenderness, if present, is usually confined to the calf muscles or over the course of the deep veins in the thigh.
- Pain and/or tenderness away from these areas are not consistent with venous thrombosis and usually indicate another diagnosis.
- Homans' sign. Discomfort in the calf muscles on forced dorsiflexion of the foot with the knee straight has been a time-honored sign of DVT. However, this sign is found in more than 50% of patients without DVT and is present in less than one third of patients with confirmed DVT, making it very nonspecific.
- Venous distension and prominence of the subcutaneous veins.
- Superficial thrombophlebitis is characterized by the finding of a palpable, indurated, cordlike, tender subcutaneous venous

segment. Patients with superficial thrombophlebitis without coexisting varicose veins and with no other obvious etiology (eg, IV catheters, IV drug abuse, soft tissue injury) are at high risk because associated DVT is found in as many as 40% of these patients. Patients with superficial thrombophlebitis extending to the saphenofemoral junction are also at higher risk for associated DVT.

- Fever. Patients may have a fever, usually low grade. High fever is usually indicative of an infectious process such as cellulitis or lymphangitis.

Study Pearl

In the event of a suspected DVT the therapist should hold the therapeutic interventions and inform the physician. The patient should be positioned in non-weight bearing on the affected lower extremity.

Prophylaxic treatment of DVT includes medication (heparin, warfarin, aspirin, and dextran) and the use of mechanical modalities such as external pneumatic compression devices and compression stockings.

Kawasaki Disease

Kawasaki disease is an acute febrile illness associated with systemic vasculitis (see Chapter 16).[77]

Heart Failure

Heart failure is the pathophysiologic state in which the heart fails to pump blood at a rate commensurate with the requirements of the metabolizing tissues.[78]

Congestive Heart Failure. CHF can be categorized as forward or backward ventricular failure:

- Forward ventricular failure is secondary to reduced forward flow into the aorta and systemic circulation.
- Backward failure is secondary to elevated systemic venous pressure.

Heart failure can also be subdivided into systolic and diastolic dysfunction.

- Systolic (left heart) failure: involves a decrease in SV, which leads to activation of peripheral and central baroreflexes and chemoreflexes, which are capable of eliciting marked increases in sympathetic nerve activity. This in turn produces a temporary improvement in systolic BP and tissue perfusion. Signs and symptoms of left sided heart failure include progressive severity of (1) exertional dyspnea, (2) orthopnea, (3) paroxysmal nocturnal dyspnea, (4) dyspnea at rest, and (5) acute pulmonary edema (termed congestive heart failure). Systolic failure can be further categorized as ischemic or nonischemic heart failure:
  - Ischemic: the breakdown of the heart muscle because of lack of blood flow to the coronary vessels that may occur with or without myocardial infarction.
  - Results from any process other than coronary artery disease (CAD).

- Diastolic (right heart) failure: involves a decrease in SV with the same outcome as with systolic failure but through different mechanisms. The altered relaxation of the ventricle (due to delayed calcium uptake and delayed calcium efflux) occurs in response to an increase in ventricular afterload (pressure overload). This impaired relaxation of the ventricle leads to impaired diastolic filling of the left ventricle. Signs and symptoms of left sided heart failure include ascites, congestive hepatomegaly, and anasarca (generalized edema).

Regardless of etiology or classification, heart failure is characterized by an inability of the heart to meet the demands of the body—the finite adaptive mechanisms that may be adequate to maintain the overall contractile performance of the heart at relatively normal levels become maladaptive when trying to sustain adequate cardiac performance at higher levels. This results in the hallmark symptom of heart failure: exercise intolerance. The New York Heart Association uses the following functional classification:

- Class I describes a patient who is not limited with normal physical activity by symptoms.
- Class II occurs when ordinary physical activity results in fatigue, dyspnea, or other symptoms.
- Class III is characterized by a marked limitation in normal physical activity.
- Class IV is defined by symptoms at rest or with any physical activity.

A normal exercise response requires the coordination of multiple systems, including the cardiac, pulmonary, vascular, and musculoskeletal. During exercise, cardiac output should be able to increase to 4 to 6 times its resting level. Patients with heart failure can often only achieve half this normal increase in cardiac output during exercise.[79-81]

The medical intervention for heart failure focuses on improving central hemodynamics through three main goals: (1) preload reduction, (2) reduction of systemic vascular resistance (afterload reduction) through administration of vasodilators and (3) inhibition of both the renin-angiotensin-aldosterone systems and the vasoconstrictor neurohumoral factors (inotropic support) produced by the sympathetic nervous system in patients with heart failure.

Cor Pulmonale

Cor pulmonale is defined as an alteration in the structure and function of the right ventricle caused by a primary disorder of the respiratory system.[82-86] Pulmonary hypertension (see Chapter 10) is the common link between lung dysfunction and the heart in cor pulmonale. Cor pulmonale can develop secondary to a wide variety of cardiopulmonary disease processes. Although cor pulmonale commonly has a chronic and slowly progressive course, acute onset or worsening cor pulmonale with life-threatening complications can occur. Several different pathophysiologic mechanisms can lead to pulmonary hypertension and, subsequently, to cor pulmonale. These pathogenetic mechanisms include

- Pulmonary vasoconstriction due to alveolar hypoxia or blood acidemia
- Anatomic compromise of the pulmonary vascular bed secondary to lung disorders, eg, emphysema, pulmonary thromboembolism, interstitial lung disease
- Increased blood viscosity secondary to blood disorders, eg, polycythemia vera, sickle cell disease, macroglobulinemia
- Idiopathic primary pulmonary hypertension

Clinical manifestations of cor pulmonale are generally nonspecific and subtle, especially in early stages of the disease, and mistakenly may be attributed to the underlying pulmonary pathology. The patient may complain of fatigue, exertional dyspnea, and syncope with exertion as a result of an inability to increase cardiac output during exercise with a subsequent drop in the systemic arterial pressure. Exertional chest pain also can occur and may be due to pulmonary artery stretching and right ventricular ischemia. Other symptoms mainly related to pulmonary artery hypertension are cough, hemoptysis, and, rarely, hoarseness due to compression of the left recurrent laryngeal nerve by a dilated pulmonary artery. In advanced stages, passive hepatic congestion secondary to severe right ventricular failure may lead to anorexia, right upper quadrant abdominal discomfort, and jaundice. Swelling of the legs also can occur, and syncope is a late and ominous occurrence. The most obvious physical findings in cor pulmonale reflect the underlying lung disease, with an increase in chest diameter, labored respiratory efforts with retractions of the chest wall, hyperresonance to percussion, diminished breath sounds, wheezing, distant heart sounds, and, rarely, cyanosis. The medical intervention for cor pulmonale varies according to type:

- Acute cor pulmonale with resultant acute right ventricular failure: fluid loading and vasoconstrictor, eg, epinephrine, administration
- Chronic cor pulmonale: oxygen therapy, diuretics, vasodilators, digitalis, theophylline, and anticoagulation therapy

Phlebotomy is indicated in patients with chronic cor pulmonale and chronic hypoxia causing severe polycythemia.

Congenital Lesions

The incidence of congenital cardiac anomalies is 8 per 1000 live births. The anomalies occur during the first trimester. There are two categories:

- Cyanotic: result from obstruction of blood flow to the lungs, or mixing of desaturated blue venous blood with fully saturated red arterial blood within the chambers of the heart.[18]
- Acyanotic: usually involve left to right shunting through an abnormal opening.

Rubella is the most common infection related to congenital cardiovascular defects.[87] Other possible causes include exposure to x-rays, alcohol, infection or drugs, maternal diabetes, family history, and some hereditary dysplasia such as Down's syndrome.[18]

Cardiomyopathy

Cardiomyopathy is one of a group of conditions affecting the heart muscle so that the fibers involved with contraction and relaxation of the myocardial muscle are impaired. Causes include coronary artery disease CAD (see later), valvular disorders, hypertension, congenital defects, and pulmonary vascular disorders.

Valvular Disease

Impairment of the valves may be caused by infection such as endocarditis, congenital deformity, or disease. Three types of valve deformities may affect aortic, mitral, tricuspid, or pulmonary valves: stenosis, insufficiency, or prolapse.

- Mitral stenosis: a consequence of rheumatic heart disease that primarily affects women.
- Mitral regurgitation: has many causes, but involvement of the mitral valve accounts for approximately 50% of all cases. Other causes include infective endocarditis, dilated cardiomyopathy, rheumatic disease, collagen vascular disease, rupture of the chordae tendineae, and, rarely, cardiac tumors.[18]
- Mitral valve prolapse (Barlow's syndrome): characterized by a slight variation in shape or structure of the mitral valve. Unknown etiology, although there may be a genetic component.
- Aortic stenosis: a disease of aging most commonly caused by progressive valvular calcification.
- Aortic regurgitation (insufficiency): traditionally associated with rheumatic fever but antibiotics have reduced the number of rheumatic-related cases. Nonrheumatic causes include congenital defects, infective endocarditis, hypertension, or secondary to aortic dissection.
- Tricuspid stenosis and regurgitation: usually occurs in people with severe mitral valve disease. Uncommon.

Arrhythmias

Arrhythmias are usually classified according to their origin (ventricular, or supraventricular [atrial]), pattern (fibrillation or flutter), or the speed or rate at which they occur (tachycardia or bradycardia). Causes include hypertrophy of the heart muscle fibers, congenital defects, valvular heart disease, or degeneration of the conductive tissue.

Coronary Artery Disease

Coronary artery disease (CAD), a complex disease involving a narrowing of the lumen of one or more of the arteries that encircle and supply the heart, involves ischemia to the myocardium. Injury to the endothelial lining of arteries, an inflammatory reaction, thrombosis, calcification, and hemorrhage all contribute to arteriosclerosis or scarring of an artery wall.

ATHEROSCLEROSIS

Atherosclerosis, the most common form of arteriosclerosis is a chronic thickening of the arterial wall of medium and large sized vessels, through the accumulation of lipids, macrophages, T-lymphocytes, smooth muscle cells, extracellular matrix, calcium, and necrotic debris. Atherosclerosis primarily affects the lower extremities. When the arteries of the heart are affected it is referred to as coronary artery disease (CAD) or coronary heart disease (CHD); when the arteries to the brain are affected, cerebrovascular disease (CVD) develops.[88] Common symptoms of atherosclerosis include:

- Decreased or absent peripheral pulses.
- Skin color: pale on elevation, dusky red on dependency.
- Intermittent claudication (early stages): pain is described as burning, searing, aching, tightness, or cramping.
- In the later stages, patients exhibit ischemia and rest pain; ulcerations and gangrene, trophic changes.

Risk factors for CAD are classified as modifiable or unmodifiable.

- Modifiable risk factors: smoking, exposure to second-hand smoke, hypertension, hyperlipidemia, high cholesterol (total or LDL-C) levels, low HDL-C) levels, high triglyceride levels, diabetes, abdominal obesity, sedentary lifestyle, high homocysteine levels, and high levels of C-reactive protein (which indicates inflammation).
- Unmodifiable risk factors: age, male sex, race, and family history.

The clinical symptoms of CAD include any symptoms that may represent cardiac ischemia, such as an ache, pressure, pain, other discomfort, or possibly just decreased activity tolerance due to fatigue, shortness of breath or palpitations.

ANGINA PECTORIS

Angina pectoris, caused by an imbalance between myocardial blood supply and oxygen demand, forces the myocardial cells to switch from aerobic to anaerobic metabolism, with a progressive impairment of metabolic, mechanical, and electrical functions.[89]

- Most patients with angina pectoris complain of retrosternal chest discomfort rather than frank pain. The former is usually described as a pressure, heaviness, or squeezing sensation. Anginal pain may be localized primarily in the epigastrium, back, neck, or jaw. Typical locations for radiation of pain are the arms, shoulders, and neck (C8-T4 dermatomes). Exertion, eating, and exposure to cold, or emotional stress are common triggers for angina. Episodes typically last for approximately 1 to 5 minutes and are relieved by rest or by taking nitroglycerin.

- The New York Heart Association classification (see Congestive Heart Failure) may be used to quantify the functional limitation imposed by patients' symptoms. Types of angina include[87]:
  - Chronic stable: classic exertional angina, which occurs in a predictable rate-pressure product, RPP (HR × BP). This type is predictable in appearance; after exercise, eating, or emotional stress and relieved by rest, nitrates, or other coronary artery vasodilators. The discomfort is most often substernal, precordium, epigastrium with radiation to the left arm, jaw, or neck.
  - Unstable (preinfarction, crescendo angina): unstable angina can occur at rest or with activity—doesn't occur at predictable RPP. The pain is similar to that with typical stable angina but may be more intense and may last several hours; ST segment depression or elevation occurs. Pain is difficult to control. New onset angina pectoris, which has developed the first time within the last 60 days is also considered unstable.
  - Prinzmetal (vasospastic, variant): occurs principally at rest and may occur in a circadian manner, at a similar time of day, often in the early morning hours. An ST segment elevation is seen on ECG, and sometimes painless episodes of ST segment elevation occur. A less frequent finding is ST segment depression. It is more common in women (under 50). Coronary artery spasm in normal or obstructed arteries has been found with this type of angina.
- Syndrome X (insulin-resistant syndrome). Chest pain that is seemingly ischemic in origin (microvascular) but with a normal arteriogram and normal ECG. More prevalent among women, particularly those who have undergone hysterectomy.[18] It may be the result of referred pain.

Myocardial Infarction

Myocardial infarction (MI) is the rapid development of myocardial necrosis caused by a critical imbalance between the oxygen supply and demand of the myocardium.[90] This usually results from plaque rupture with thrombus formation in a coronary vessel, resulting in an acute reduction of blood supply to a portion of the myocardium.

- Atherosclerotic causes: the most common cause of MI. Plaque rupture with subsequent exposure of the basement membrane results in platelet aggregation, thrombus formation, fibrin accumulation, hemorrhage into the plaque, and varying degrees of vasospasm. MI occurs most frequently in persons older than 45 years.
- Nonatherosclerotic causes: include coronary vasospasm as seen in Prinzmetal (variant) angina and in patients using cocaine and amphetamines; coronary emboli from sources such as an infected heart valve; occlusion of the coronaries due to vasculitis, or other causes leading to mismatch of oxygen supply and demand, such as acute anemia from GI bleeding.

Signs and symptoms of MI include:

- Chest pain, typically described as tightness, pressure, or squeezing, located across the anterior precordium. Pain may radiate to the jaw, neck, arms, back, and epigastrium. The left arm is affected more frequently; however, pain may be felt in both arms.
- Dyspnea, which may accompany chest pain or occur as an isolated complaint.
- Nausea and/or abdominal pain often are present in infarcts involving the inferior or posterior wall.
- Lightheadedness with or without syncope.
- Nausea with or without vomiting.
- Diaphoresis.

Inflammatory Conditions of the Heart

Myocarditis, pericarditis, and infective endocarditis are all inflammatory conditions of the heart.

- Myocarditis: uncommon inflammatory condition of the muscular walls (myocardium) of the heart, usually as a result of bacterial or viral infection. Other possible causes include chest radiation for treatment of malignancy, sarcoidosis, and drugs such as lithium and cocaine.[18]
- Pericarditis: commonly drug-induced or in association with an autoimmune disease (eg, connective tissue disorders such as SLP, rheumatoid arthritis), postmyocardial infarction, with renal failure, after open-heart surgery, and after radiation therapy.[18]
- Infective endocarditis: an infection (frequently streptococci or staphylococci) of the endocardium, including the heart valves.
- Rheumatic fever: a form of endocarditis caused by streptococcal group A bacteria.

Hematopoietic System Disorders

Sickle Cell Disease. A generic term for a group of inherited, autosomal recessive disorders characterized by the presence of an abnormal form of hemoglobin within the erythrocytes (crescent or sickle shape versus usual biconcave disc shape)—see Chapter 12.

The Thalassemias. A group of inherited, chronic hemolytic anemias predominantly affecting people of Mediterranean or southern Chinese ancestry—see Chapter 12.

Fanconi's Anemia. Fanconi's anemia is an autosomal recessive inherited disease that primarily affects the bone marrow, resulting in decreased production of all types of blood cells. The lack of white blood cells predisposes the patient to infections, while the lack of platelets and red blood cells may result in bleeding, and fatigue (anemia), respectively.

Gaucher Disease. Gaucher disease is an inherited metabolic disorder. All Gaucher patients exhibit a deficiency of an enzyme called *glucocerebrosidase*, which is involved in the breakdown and recycling of glucocerebroside. The buildup of this fatty material within cells prevents the cells and organs from functioning properly, and a fatty substance called *glucocerebroside* accumulates in the spleen, liver, lungs, bone marrow, and sometimes in the brain. There are three types of Gaucher disease:

- **Type 1:** the most common. Patients in this group usually bruise easily, experience fatigue due to anemia and low blood platelets, and have an enlarged liver and spleen, skeletal disorders, and, in some instances, lung and kidney impairment.
- **Type 2:** Gaucher disease—liver and spleen enlargement are apparent by 3 months of age. Patients have extensive and progressive brain damage and usually die by 2 years of age
- **Type 3:** liver and spleen enlargement is variable, and signs of brain involvement such as seizures gradually become apparent.

Hemophilia. Refer to Chapter 16.

Leukemia. Leukemia is divided into four major categories:

- Acute myelogenous: a malignant disease of the bone marrow in which hematopoietic precursors are arrested in an early stage of development.
- Acute lymphocytic (acute lymphoblastic leukemia and acute lymphoid leukemia): most cases of acute lymphocytic leukemia (ALL) occur in children under age 10, but it can appear in all age groups. ALL is an acute leukemia of unknown etiology caused by a change in the cells in the bone marrow.
- Chronic myelogenous: a malignant cancer of the bone marrow, which can occur in adults (usually middle-aged) and children. It is usually associated with a chromosome abnormality called the Philadelphia chromosome.
- Chronic lymphocytic: a disorder of morphologically mature but immunologically less mature lymphocytes that is manifested by progressive accumulation of these cells in the blood, bone marrow, and lymphatic tissues.

Lymphatic Disease

Lymphedema. In a diseased state, the lymphatic transport capacity is compromised, causing the normal volume of interstitial fluid formation to exceed the rate of lymphatic return, which results in the stagnation of high molecular weight proteins in the interstitium. This high oncotic pressure in the interstitium favors the accumulation of additional water. Accumulation of interstitial fluid leads to significant dilatation of the remaining outflow tracts and valvular incompetence resulting in a reversal of flow from subcutaneous tissues into the dermal plexus. The protein and fluid accumulation initiates a marked inflammatory reaction. Macrophage activity is increased, resulting in destruction of elastic fibers and production

Study Pearl

The result of the inflammatory reaction in the interstitium is a change from the initial pitting edema to the brawny non-pitting edema characteristic of lymphedema.

of fibrosclerotic tissue. Fibroblasts migrate into the interstitium and deposit collagen. The lymphatic walls undergo fibrosis, and fibrinoid thrombi accumulate within the lumen, destroying much of the remaining lymph channels. Spontaneous lymphovenous shunts may form. Lymph nodes harden and shrink, losing their normal architecture.

The overlying skin becomes thickened and displays the typical peau d'orange (orange skin) appearance of congested dermal lymphatics. The epidermis forms thick scaly deposits of keratinized debris; cracks and furrows often develop and accommodate debris and bacteria, resulting in the leakage of lymph onto the surface of the skin. Lymphedema may be classified as primary or secondary, based on underlying etiology, although this classification usually has little significance in determining treatment modality.

Primary Lymphedema. Primary lymphedema represents a developmental abnormality of the lymphatic system that is present, but not always clinically evident, at birth. Thus, primary lymphedema has been further subdivided based on age of onset[91-97]:

- Congenital lymphedema: represents all forms that are clinically evident at birth and accounts for 10% to 25% of all primary lymphedema cases. Females are affected twice as often as males, and the lower extremity is involved 3 times more frequently than the upper extremity. Two-thirds of patients have bilateral lymphedema, and this form may improve spontaneously with increasing age.
- Lymphedema praecox: the most common form of primary lymphedema (also known as Meige disease). It becomes clinically evident after birth and before age 35 years, most often arising during puberty. Females are affected 4 times as often as males.
- Lymphedema tarda: does not become clinically evident until age 35 years or older. These conditions are most often sporadic, with no family history, and involve the lower extremity almost exclusively.

Secondary Lymphedema. Secondary lymphedema represents an acquired dysfunction of otherwise normal lymphatics that occurs as a result of obstruction of lymphatic flow by known mechanisms, ie, filariasis (infestation of lymph nodes by the parasite Wuchereria bancrofti), silica, obstruction by a proximal mass, postsurgical mechanisms (eg, mastectomy, peripheral vascular surgery, lipectomy), burns, burn scar excision, insect bites, and fibrosis secondary to chronic infections.

Patients with secondary lymphedema present with varying degrees of severity, from mild swelling to severe disabling enlargement with potentially life-threatening complications. This disease is often first noticed by the patient as an asymmetry or increased circumference of an extremity. The diagnosis is usually made with a thorough history and physical examination. Other causes of edema, such as edema secondary to congestive heart failure, renal insufficiency, hepatic insufficiency, or venous stasis disease, must be excluded. Malignancy must always be considered, particularly when patients report sudden onset, rapid progression, or associated pain.

If lymphedema is not treated it progresses through the following stages:

- Stage 0 (latency/subclinical stage): characterized by reduction of the normal lymph transport capacity, but there will be no measurable increase in volume.
- Stage I (reversible lymphedema): characterized by the presence of protein rich edema and associated with a measurable increase in volume, including pitting edema. Activity, heat, and humidity may cause or increase stage I lymphedema.
- Stage II (spontaneously irreversible lymphedema): presents with increased volume, replacement of some of the protein rich lymphatic fluid with tissue fibrosis, and a positive Stemmer's sign (the inability to lift the thickened cutaneous folds at the dorsum of the toes or fingers).
- Stage III (lymphostatic elephantiasis): characterized by subcutaneous fibrosclerosis and severe skin alterations, including hyperkeratosis and papillomatosis.

Lymphadenopathy. Lymphadenopathy can be caused by an increase in normal lymphocytes and macrophages during a response to an antigen (eg, viral illness), nodal infiltration by inflammatory cells in response to an infection in the nodes themselves (lymphadenitis), proliferation of neoplastic lymphocytes or macrophages (lymphoma), or infiltration of nodes by metabolite-laden macrophages in lipid storage diseases (Gaucher disease, Niemann-Pick disease, Fabry disease).

Generalized lymphadenopathy is defined as enlargement of more than 2 noncontiguous lymph node groups. Causes of generalized lymphadenopathy include infections, autoimmune diseases, malignancies, histiocytoses, storage diseases, benign hyperplasia, and drug reactions.

CARDIOVASCULAR PHYSICAL THERAPY

Physical therapy interventions for cardiovascular conditions can be broadly classified into primary prevention and secondary intervention, although it must be remembered that both of these categories are linked by physiologic, epidemiologic, and clinical elements.

- Primary prevention: the prevention of a cardiovascular disease from developing, even among individuals with risk factors—Preferred Practice Pattern 6A.
- Secondary intervention: aimed at reducing symptoms and/or slowing the progression of a cardiovascular disease. Patients in this category have
  - Impaired aerobic capacity/endurance associated with deconditioning—Preferred Practice Pattern 6B
  - Impaired aerobic capacity/endurance associated with cardiovascular pump dysfunction or failure—Preferred Practice Pattern 6D
  - Impaired circulation and anthropometric dimensions associated with lymphatic system disorders—Preferred Practice Pattern 6H

(Preferred practice patterns 6C, 6E, 6F, and 6G are covered in Chapter 10.)

PHYSICAL THERAPY ASSOCIATED WITH PRIMARY PREVENTION, RISK REDUCTION, AND DECONDITIONING

Patients who have identifiable risk factors should be encouraged to adopt lifestyle behaviors that can modify the risk factors. These include

- Activity recommendations
- Dietary recommendations
- Smoking cessation
- The effects of medications
- Importance of compliance

Exercise Prescription. Any prescribed exercise for this population must be quantified. The quantification can be expressed in a number of ways—total distance walked and time taken; workload expressed in watts when using an ergometer; heart rate (which is proportional to both cardiac output and systemic oxygen consumption) and blood pressure taken at rest, during, and after the activity.[98] A patient's abnormal cardiovascular response to exercise may be categorized as dysrhythmia, ischemia, or congestive heart failure.[99]

Dysrhythmia. Dysrhythmia can occur normally, but may result from premature atrial contractions (PACs), premature ventricular contractions (PVCs), or atrial fibrillation (refer to Examination of the Heart Rhythm). If PVC exists at rest, the clinician must consider the impact that exercise might have.

- PVCs that decrease with exercise is a good sign as it would tend to indicate that the PVCs are suppressed by a higher order pacemaker (overdrive suppression) as physical activity and heart rate increases.
- PVCs that increase with exercise is a less desirable response as it would tend to indicate that the PVCs are ischemic in origin.
- PVCs that do not change with exercise would tend to indicate that the PVCs are unrelated to exercise.

Ischemia. Ischemia occurs when the demand for oxygen by cardiac muscle outstrips the supply of oxygen available to it. This condition frequently arises during exercise with the onset of chest pain, or angina.

Congestive Heart Failure. Shortness of breath with exercise does not necessarily indicate congestive heart failure. A thorough medical history is important.

- In left-sided failure, the pressure builds up in the left ventricle and is reflected backward, up through the left atrium, and into the lungs. The lungs become wet, stiff, soggy, and difficult to move, thus the feeling of shortness of breath.

- In right-sided failure, the cause is often the result of left-sided heart failure. Because of the restriction in forward blood flow, the pressure passes through the lungs and is reflected through the right ventricle and right atrium and into the venous circulatory system. This may result in distension of the jugular vein, organomegaly, or pitting edema in the lower extremities.

Other signs and symptoms of exercise intolerance:

- The appearance of ST-segment elevation at rest with a significant Q-wave (on ECG) may indicate the residual effects of a myocardial infarction (eg, an aneurysm) and should be noted as such.
- Heart murmur: in the setting of myocardial infarction, this murmur usually indicates papillary muscle dysfunction.
- A fall in systolic blood pressure with exercise that occurs beyond the transient drop in BP (usually as a result of regional shunting of blood). Absence of a rise in systolic BP with exercise may signify growing left ventricular dysfunction.
- Chest pain, shortness of breath.
- Reports of skipped beats or "fluttering" of the heart, especially in the presence of dizziness, light-headedness, or syncope.
- Pallor, diaphoresis.
- Unresponsiveness to questions.

Physical Therapy Associated with Impaired Aerobic Capacity/Endurance Associated with Cardiovascular Pump Dysfunction or Failure

According to the APTA Guide to Physical Therapist Practice,[100] the development of specific anticipated goals and expected outcomes is based on the following general goals of physical therapy intervention[2]:

1. Aerobic capacity is increased.
2. Ability to perform physical tasks related to self-care, home management, community and work integration or reintegration, and leisure activities is increased.
3. Physiological response to increased oxygen demand is improved.
4. Strength, power, and endurance are increased.
5. Symptoms associated with increased oxygen demand are decreased.
6. Ability to recognize a recurrence is increased, and intervention is sought in a timely manner.
7. Risk of recurrence is reduced.
8. Behaviors that foster healthy habits, wellness, and prevention are required.
9. Decision-making is enhanced: help a patient, and the use of health care resources by patient/client, family, significant others, and caregivers.

Rehabilitation interventions for patients with heart failure focus primarily on different types of exercise. Appropriate exercise, in combination with optimal medical care, can improve function, symptoms, and quality of life in patients with chronic heart failure.[101-107] In patients with heart failure, exercise tolerance is limited by an inadequate cardiac output response because of a reduction in both stroke volume and heart rate. Alterations in gas exchange also limit exercise tolerance in this patient population.[108] Fluid accumulation in the lungs results in abnormal gas exchange and can cause shortness of breath.[108] Patients with heart failure also have more vasoconstriction at rest because of elevated sympathetic tone, which further limits the delivery of oxygenated blood to the muscles.[108]

Cardiac Rehabilitation. provides many benefits for patients. The most important benefits of cardiac rehabilitation are[109]

- Improved exercise tolerance
- Control of symptoms
- Improvement in the blood levels of lipids
- Beneficial effect on body weight
- Possible improvement with high blood pressure
- Improved psychosocial well being
- Return to work
- Reduced mortality

The goals of a cardiac rehabilitation program can be separated into short and long-term goals:

Short-Term Goals

- "Reconditioning" sufficient enough for resumption of customary activities
- Limiting the physiologic and psychological effects of heart disease
- Decreasing the risk of sudden cardiac arrest or reinfarction
- Controlling the symptoms of cardiac disease

Long-Term Goals

- Identification and treatment of risk factors
- Stabilizing or even reversing the atherosclerotic process
- Enhancing the psychological status of the patients

Phases of Cardiac Rehabilitation. Cardiac rehabilitation programs can be stratified into four phases[110,111]:

Phase 1. This phase occurs in the hospital inpatient (IP) department, starting in the CICU and continuing through the step down phase (approximately 24 days). This program includes a visit by a member of the cardiac rehabilitation team (cardiac nurse, exercise specialist, physical therapist, occupational therapist, dietitian, and social worker), education regarding the disease and its recovery process, personal encouragement, and inclusion of family members in classroom group meetings.

In the coronary care (CCU) unit, assisted range of motion exercises can be initiated within the first 24 to 48 hours. Low-risk patients are encouraged to sit in a bedside chair and begin to perform self-care activities (eg, shaving, oral hygiene, sponge bathing).

Early mobilization programs are designed to progressively increase activity levels in three areas—active exercises, activities of daily living, and educational activities with the goal of early return to independence. On transfer to the step-down unit, patients are encouraged to try to sit up, stand, and walk in their rooms in the beginning. Subsequently, the patients are encouraged to walk in the hallway at least twice daily either for certain specific distances or as tolerated without unduly pushing them or holding them back. Standing heart rates and blood pressures are obtained followed by 5 minutes of warm-up or stretching. Walking, often with assistance, is resumed with target heart rate of < 20 beats above the resting heart rate, and RPE under 14. Starting with 5 to 10 minutes of walking each day, exercise time gradually can be increased to up to 30 minutes daily.

Team members should incorporate in the discharge planning an appropriate emphasis on secondary prevention through risk factor modification and therapeutic lifestyle changes. They must also ensure that phase 1 patients get referred to appropriate local, convenient, and comprehensive phase 2 programs.

Phase 1.5 (Post-Discharge Phase). This phase begins after the patient returns home from the hospital. Team members check the patient's medical status and continuing recovery, and provide education about risk reduction strategies. This phase of recovery includes low-level exercise and physical activity and instruction about changes for resumption of an active lifestyle. After 2 to 6 weeks of recovery at home, the patient is ready to start cardiac rehabilitation phase 2.

Phase 2 (Supervised Exercise). The patients who have completed hospitalization and 2 to 6 weeks of recovery at home generally begin phase 2 of their cardiac rehabilitation program. This phase is designed to allow the heart muscle time to heal and to progress the patient to full resumption of activities of daily living. During this phase, patients are allowed to return to work and are advised to commence a walking or biking program.

Physician and cardiac rehabilitation staff members formulate the level of exercise to meet an individual patient's needs. Exercise treatments usually are scheduled 3 times a week at a rehabilitation facility.

Constant medical supervision is provided, including exercise electrocardiograms (ECGs), as well as supervision by a nurse and exercise specialist. Patients are gradually weaned from continuous monitoring of vital signs to spot checks and then self-monitoring. Risk factor modification, activity pacing, and energy conservation are emphasized. For example, in addition to exercise, counseling, and education about stress management, smoking cessation, nutrition, and weight loss also are incorporated. This phase of rehabilitation may last 3 to 6 months.

Phase 3 (Maintenance Phase). Phase 3 of cardiac rehabilitation is a maintenance program designed to continue for the patient's lifetime.

Activities consist of the type of exercises the patient enjoys, such as walking, bicycling, or jogging. The main goal of phase 3 is to promote habits that lead to a healthy and satisfying lifestyle.

Phase 3 programs do not usually require medical or nursing supervision. In fact, most patients participate in "phase 3" equivalent exercises at the exercise facilities in the community. Entrance into this phase begins with the performance of a maximum, symptom-limited

TABLE 11-10. RATING OF PERCEIVED EXERTION

SCALE	VERBAL RATING
6	
7	Very, very light
8	
9	Very light
10	
11	Fairly light
12	
13	Somewhat hard
14	
15	Hard
16	
17	Very hard
18	
19	Very, very hard
20	

Data from Borg GAV: Psychophysical basis of perceived exertion. *Med Sci Sports Exerc.* 1992;14:377-381.

exercise test, the results of which are used to write an exercise prescription. During this phase, patients exercise at 65% to 85% of their maximum heart rate. Three main components of an exercise-training program are as follows:

- Frequency: the minimum frequency for exercising to improve cardiovascular fitness is 3 times weekly.
- Time: patients usually need to allow 30 to 60 minutes for each session, which includes a warm-up of at least 10 minutes.
- Intensity: the intensity prescribed is in relation to one's target heart rate. Aerobic conditioning is emphasized in the first few weeks of exercise. Strength training is introduced later. The Borg scale of Rate of Perceived Exertion (RPE) is used (Table 11-10). Patients usually should exercise at an RPE of 13-15.

Physical Therapy Associated with Impaired Circulation and Anthropometric Dimensions Associated with Lymphatic System Disorders

Lymphedema. The intervention for lymphedema is multifaceted. Patients should be encouraged to

- Lose weight.
- Avoid even minor trauma. Skin care and avoidance of trauma are important to avoid lymphangitis, cellulitis, and ulceration. The skin should be kept well lubricated and should not be exposed to strong soaps or detergents. Acute lymphangitis, which can either precede or follow chronic lymphedema is usually treated with a combination of rest, elevation, and antibiotics.
- Avoid overheating local body parts or a rise in core body temperature.
- Avoid lifting heavy objects; no heavy handbags with over the shoulder straps.

- Avoid constrictive clothing and jewelry that might have a tourniquet effect.
- Elevate the affected extremity whenever possible, particularly at night. For lower extremity lymphedema, this may be accomplished by elevating the foot of the bed to an appropriate level.

In addition, patients should use compression garments. These are worn continuously during the day, but may be removed at night when the extremity is elevated in bed, and should be replaced promptly each morning. To encourage compliance, the elastic compression garments must be comfortable and fit appropriately—should be custom fit when the extremity is decompressed, have graduated compression, increasing from distal to proximal, on the affected extremity, and should not have a tourniquet effect.

Patients should exercise with compression applied to be involved extremity or area. Simple active exercises should be prescribed that require the joints to maintain range of motion and activate the muscle and joint pump.

Intermittent pneumatic pump compression therapy may also be instituted on an outpatient basis or in the home (refer to Chapter 18). These devices provide sequential active compression from distal to proximal, effectively milking the lymph from the extremity.

Manual lymphatic drainage (MLD) according to the Vodder and/or Leduc techniques may also be prescribed (refer to Chapter 18).[112,113]

Venous Insufficiency. Treatment is aimed at ameliorating the symptoms and, whenever possible, at correcting the underlying abnormality. Deep system disease is often refractory to treatment, but superficial system disease can usually be treated by ablating the refluxing vessels.

Graduated Compression. Graduated compression is the cornerstone of the modern treatment of venous insufficiency. Properly fitted gradient compression stockings provide 30 to 40 or 40 to 50 mm Hg of compression at the ankle, with gradually decreasing compression at more proximal levels of the leg. This amount of gradient compression is sufficient to restore normal venous flow patterns in many or most patients with superficial venous reflux and to improve venous flow, even in patients with severe deep venous incompetence.

The compression gradient is extremely important because nongradient stockings or high-stretch elastic bandages (eg, ACE wraps) may cause a tourniquet effect, with worsening of the venous insufficiency. Antiembolic stockings do not provide sufficient compression to improve the venous return from the legs. No patient with symptoms due to venous insufficiency should be without gradient compression hose, which can be prescribed by a physician. The prescription should specify one pair of gradient compression hose with a 30- to 40-mm Hg gradient that is calf-high (or thigh-high with waist attachment or panty hose style), with refills as needed.

Venoablation. All methods of venoablation are effective. Once the overall volume of venous reflux is reduced below a critical threshold by any mechanism, venous ulcerations heal, and patient symptoms are resolved.

Endovenous Laser Therapy. Endovenous laser therapy (EVLT), a newer procedure, is performed by passing a laser fiber from the knee to the groin and then delivering laser energy along the entire course of the vein.[114-116] Destruction of the vascular wall is followed by fibrosis of the treated vessel. EVLT has demonstrated excellent early (4 years) results and an extremely low rate of complications, but the duration of follow-up is not yet long enough to provide information about mid-term and long-term results.

Radiofrequency Ablation. Radiofrequency ablation (RFA) is a relatively new procedure that has a low rate of complications.[117] It has produced excellent results that have been confirmed after several years of follow-up. RFA is performed by passing a special radiofrequency (RF) catheter from the knee to the groin and by heating the vessel until thermal injury causes shrinkage. The process is repeated every few centimeters along the course of the vein. Initial thermal injury is followed by fibrosis of the treated vessel.

MANAGEMENT OF PERIPHERAL VASCULAR DISORDERS

Patients with peripheral vascular disease (PVD) often have multiple diagnoses and may have socioeconomic constraints. The best intervention for all forms of PVD is prevention—appropriate exercise, healthy diet, and avoidance of smoking.

Arterial Disease. When the metabolic demands of a muscle or group of muscles exceed blood flow, claudication symptoms ensue. A useful tool in assessing a patient with claudication is the ankle-brachial index (ABI), which is calculated as the ratio of systolic blood pressure at the ankle to the arm. A normal ABI is 0.9 to 1.1. However, any patient with an ABI less than 0.9, by definition, has some degree of arterial disease.

The physical therapy intervention for patients with arterial disease depends on the level of severity, a simple four-point functional grading system can be used to help select the appropriate intervention[118]:

- Grade I: no functional limitations.
- Grade II: ambulatory more than four blocks before onset of claudication.
- Grade III: ambulatory less than four blocks before onset of claudication.
- Grade IV: nonambulatory because of ischemic pain at rest.

For those patients in grades I and II, exercise therapy is advised. Exercises can include

- Ambulation at a steady pace up to, but not beyond, the point of pain. A daily walking program of 45 to 60 minutes is recommended. The patient is instructed to walk until claudication pain occurs, rest until the pain subsides, and repeat the cycle. A small heel lift can be used to help reduce the oxygen demand in the gastrocnemius.
- Modified Bueger-Allen exercises (postural exercises, active ankle plantarflexion/dorsiflexion).
- Resistive calf exercises.

Grade III patients, who are not surgical candidates, exercises within pain free limits are advocated.

Since Grade IV patients are ischemic at rest, under no circumstances should they be put on an exercise program.

For all grades, risk factor modification should be encouraged. Medications may be prescribed to decrease blood viscosity and prevent thrombus formation. Patients with limb-threatening ischemia or lifestyle-limiting claudication are referred to a vascular surgeon.

Venous Disease

- Acute thrombophlebitis: requires only rest, elevation, and warm soaks until symptoms subside if limited to a superficial vein.
- Deep vein thrombophlebitis (DVT): associated with long-term venous insufficiency if poorly managed. In acute cases, patients are placed on bed rest and elevation of the involved extremity until signs of inflammation have subsided. Exercise therapy is contraindicated during this phase because of the potential to dislodge the clot, which can result in a pulmonary embolism, a potentially fatal condition. Once the local tenderness and swelling has resolved, passive range of motion and ambulation, while wearing elastic stockings, is permitted. Early exercise is thought to promote fibrinolysis and maintain patency of the deep vein. Patients are advised to not wear high-heeled shoes and to stretch the heel cords regularly to lessen compression of the deep veins.
- Chronic venous insufficiency (CVI): varies by severity. Patients are advised to wear well-fitted support hosiery and to perform frequent muscle pumping (using active and active resistive plantar flexion/dorsiflexion exercises), ambulation as tolerated, and extremity elevation throughout the day. Weight reduction to reduce the strain on the venous system is also indicated if the patient is obese. Patients may also benefit from intermittent pneumatic compression.
- Stasis ulcers: approached in a variety of ways including whirlpool, hyperbaric oxygen, electrical stimulation, and surgery (ligation and vein stripping, vein grafts).

Questions for this chapter and the entire book appear on the included CD-ROM, with additional questions at www.DuttonNPTE.com.

REFERENCES

1. DeTurk WE, Cassady SL: Essentials of exercise physiology. In: DeTurk WE, Cahalin LP, eds. *Cardiovascular and Pulmonary Physical Therapy: An Evidence-Based Approach.* New York, NY: McGraw-Hill. 2004:35-72.
2. Grimes K: Heart disease. In: O'Sullivan SB, Schmitz TJ, eds. *Physical Rehabilitation, 5th ed.* Philadelphia, PA: FA Davis; 2007:589-641.

3. Molloi S, Wong JT: Regional blood flow analysis and its relationship with arterial branch lengths and lumen volume in the coronary arterial tree. *Phys Med Biol.* 2007;52:1495-1503. Epub Feb. 12, 2007.
4. Yildirim A, Soylu O, Dagdeviren B, et al: Cardiac resynchronization improves coronary blood flow. *Tohoku J Exp Med.* 2007; 211:43-47.
5. Carabello BA: Understanding coronary blood flow: the wave of the future. *Circulation.* 2006;113:1721-1722.
6. Tanaka N, Takeda K, Nishi S, et al: A new method for measuring total coronary blood flow using the lithium dilution method. *Osaka City Med J.* 2005;51:11-18.
7. Mittal N, Zhou Y, Linares C, et al: Analysis of blood flow in the entire coronary arterial tree. *Am J Physiol Heart Circ Physiol.* 2005;289:H439-H446. Epub Mar. 25, 2005.
8. DeTurk WE, Cahalin LP: Electrocardiography. In: DeTurk WE, Cahalin LP, eds. *Cardiovascular and Pulmonary Physical Therapy: An Evidence-Based Approach.* New York, NY: McGraw-Hill. 2004:325-359.
9. Cahalin LP: Cardiovascular evaluation. In: DeTurk WE, Cahalin LP, eds. *Cardiovascular and Pulmonary Physical Therapy: An Evidence-Based Approach.* New York, NY: McGraw-Hill. 2004: 273-324.
10. Van de Graaff KM, Fox SI: Circulatory system: cardiac output and blood flow. In: Van de Graaff KM, Fox SI, eds. *Concepts of Human Anatomy and Physiology.* New York, NY: WCB/ McGraw-Hill. 1999:655-691.
11. Di Salvo G, Pergola V, Ratti G, et al: Atrial natriuretic factor and mitral valve prolapse syndrome. *Minerva Cardioangiol.* 2001;49:317-325.
12. Schmitz TJ: Vital signs. In: O'Sullivan SB, Schmitz TJ, eds. *Physical Rehabilitation, 5th ed.* Philadelphia, PA: FA Davis. 2007:81-120.
13. Judge RD, Zuidema GD, Fitzgerald FT: Vital signs. In: Judge RD, Zuidema GD, Fitzgerald FT, eds. *Clinical Diagnosis.* 4th ed. Boston, MA: Little, Brown and Company. 1982:49-58.
14. Bailey MK: Physical examination procedures to screen for serious disorders of the low back and lower quarter. In: Wilmarth MA, ed. *Medical Screening for the Physical Therapist.* Orthopaedic Section Independent Study Course 14.1.1 La Crosse, WI: Orthopaedic Section, APTA, Inc. 2003:1-35.
15. Huber MA, Terezhalmy GT, Moore WS: White coat hypertension. *Quintessence Int.* 2004;35:678-679.
16. Chung I, Lip GY: White coat hypertension: not so benign after all? *J Hum Hypertens.* 2003;17:807-809.
17. Alves LM, Nogueira MS, Veiga EV, et al: White coat hypertension and nursing care. *Can J Cardiovasc Nurs.* 2003;13:29-34.
18. Goodman CC: The cardiovascular system. In: Goodman CC, Boissonnault WG, Fuller KS, eds. *Pathology: Implications for the Physical Therapist, 2nd ed.* Philadelphia, PA: Saunders. 2003: 367-476.
19. O'Sullivan J, Allen J, Murray A: The forgotten Korotkoff phases: how often are phases II and III present, and how do they relate to the other Korotkoff phases? *Am J Hypertens.* 2002;15: 264-268.

20. Venet R, Miric D, Pavie A, et al: Korotkoff sound: the cavitation hypothesis. *Med Hypotheses.* 2000;55:141-146.
21. Weber F, Anlauf M, Hirche H, et al: Differences in blood pressure values by simultaneous auscultation of Korotkoff sounds inside the cuff and in the antecubital fossa. *J Hum Hypertens.* 1999; 13:695-700.
22. Paskalev D, Kircheva A, Krivoshiev S: A centenary of auscultatory blood pressure measurement: a tribute to Nikolai Korotkoff. *Kidney Blood Press Res.* 2005;28:259-263.
23. Perloff D, Grim C, Flack J, et al: Human blood pressure determination by sphygmomanometry. *Circulation.* 1993; 88:2460-2470.
24. Strugo V, Glew FJ, Davis J, et al: Update: Recommendations for human blood pressure determination by sphygmomanometers. *Hypertension.* 1990;16:594.
25. Higgins JR, Walker SP, Brennecke SP: Re: Which Korotkoff sound should be used for diastolic blood pressure in pregnancy? *Aust N Z J Obstet Gynaecol.* 1998;38:480-481.
26. Likeman RK: Re: Which Korotkoff sound should be used for diastolic blood pressure in pregnancy? *Aust N Z J Obstet Gynaecol.* 1998;38:479-480.
27. Franx A, Evers IM, van der Pant KA, et al: The fourth sound of Korotkoff in pregnancy: a myth. *Eur J Obstet Gynecol Reprod Biol.* 1998;76:53-59.
28. Peterson BK: Vital signs. In: Cameron MH, Monroe LG, eds. *Physical Rehabilitation: Evidence-Based Examination, Evaluation, and Intervention.* St Louis, MO: Saunders/Elsevier. 2007:598-624.
29. Fletcher GF, Mills WC, Taylor WC: Update on exercise stress testing. *Am Fam Physician.* 2006;74:1749-1754.
30. Kharabsheh SM, Al-Sugair A, Al-Buraiki J, et al: Overview of exercise stress testing. *Ann Saudi Med.* 2006;26:1-6.
31. Michaelides AP, Aigyprladou MN, Andrikopoulos GK, et al: The prognostic value of a QRS score during exercise testing. *Clin Cardiol.* 2005;28:375-380.
32. Yosefy C, Cantor A, Reisin L, et al: The diagnostic value of QRS changes for prediction of coronary artery disease during exercise testing in women: false-positive rates. *Coron Artery Dis.* 2004;15:147-154.
33. Fowler-Brown A, Pignone M, Pletcher M, et al: Exercise tolerance testing to screen for coronary heart disease: a systematic review for the technical support for the U.S. Preventive Services Task Force. *Ann Intern Med.* 2004;140:W9-W24.
34. Cullinane EM, Siconolfi S, Carleton RA, et al: Modification of the Astrand-Rhyming sub-maximal bicycle test for estimating Vo_2 max of inactive men and women. *Med Sci Sports Exerc.* 1988;20:317-318.
35. Jessup GT, Riggs CE, Lambert J, et al: The effect of pedalling speed on the validity of the Astrand-Rhyming aerobic work capacity test. *J Sports Med Phys Fitness.* 1977;17:367-371.
36. Pollock ML, Linnerud AC: Observations of the Astrand-Rhyming nomogram as related to the evaluation of training. *Am Correct Ther J.* 1971;25:162-165.
37. Cay S, Metin F, Korkmaz S: Association of renal functional impairment and the severity of coronary artery disease. *Anadolu Kardiyol Derg.* 2007;7:44-48.

38. Junnila JL, Runkle GP: Coronary artery disease screening, treatment, and follow-up. *Prim Care.* 2006;33:863-885, vi.
39. Sbarsi I, Falcone C, Boiocchi C, et al: Inflammation and atherosclerosis: the role of TNF and TNF receptors polymorphisms in coronary artery disease. *Int J Immunopathol Pharmacol.* 2007;20: 145-154.
40. Ask the doctors: I recently read that patients with coronary artery disease ought to have their blood pressure reduced to less than 120/80. I thought 120/80 was normal blood pressure, so why would you want blood pressure to be lower than normal? *Heart Advis.* 2007;10:8.
41. Dzielinska Z, Januszewicz A, Demkow M, et al: Cardiovascular risk factors in hypertensive patients with coronary artery disease and coexisting renal artery stenosis. *J Hypertens.* 2007;25:663-670.
42. DeFaria Yeh D, Freeman MW, Meigs JB, et al: Risk factors for coronary artery disease in patients with elevated high-density lipoprotein cholesterol. *Am J Cardiol.* 2007;99:1-4.
43. Carneiro AV: Coronary heart disease in diabetes mellitus: risk factors and epidemiology. *Rev Port Cardiol.* 2004;23:1359-1366.
44. Graner M, Syvanne M, Kahri J, et al: Insulin resistance as predictor of the angiographic severity and extent of coronary artery disease. *Ann Med.* 2007;39:137-144.
45. Orchard TJ, Costacou T, Kretowski A, et al: Type 1 diabetes and coronary artery disease. *Diabetes Care.* 2006;29:2528-2538.
46. Pepine CJ, Kowey PR, Kupfer S, et al: Predictors of adverse outcome among patients with hypertension and coronary artery disease. *J Am Coll Cardiol.* 2006;47:547-551.
47. Hennessey JV, Westrick E: Coronary artery disease and cerebrovascular disease prevention in diabetes mellitus: early identification and aggressive modification of risk factors. *Med Health R I.* 1998;81:350-352.
48. Sukhija R, Aronow WS, Yalamanchili K, et al: Prevalence of coronary artery disease, lower extremity peripheral arterial disease, and cerebrovascular disease in 110 men with an abdominal aortic aneurysm. *Am J Cardiol.* 2004;94:1358-1359.
49. Ness J, Aronow WS: Prevalence of coronary artery disease, ischemic stroke, peripheral arterial disease, and coronary revascularization in older African-Americans, Asians, Hispanics, whites, men, and women. *Am J Cardiol.* 1999;84:932-933, A7.
50. Lee CS, Lu YH, Lee ST, et al: Evaluating the prevalence of silent coronary artery disease in asymptomatic patients with spinal cord injury. *Int Heart J.* 2006;47:325-330.
51. Bauman WA, Spungen AM, Raza M, et al: Coronary artery disease: metabolic risk factors and latent disease in individuals with paraplegia. *Mt Sinai J Med.* 1992;59:163-168.
52. White LJ, McCoy SC, Castellano V, et al: Effect of resistance training on risk of coronary artery disease in women with multiple sclerosis. *Scand J Clin Lab Invest.* 2006;66:351-355.
53. Steffens DC, O'Connor CM, Jiang WJ, et al: The effect of major depression on functional status in patients with coronary artery disease. *J Am Geriatr Soc.* 1999;47:319-322.
54. Pamukcu B, Oflaz H, Onur I, et al: Clinical relevance of aspirin resistance in patients with stable coronary artery disease: a prospective follow-up study (PROSPECTAR). *Blood Coagul Fibrinolysis.* 2007;18:187-192.

55. Ludvig J, Miner B, Eisenberg MJ: Smoking cessation in patients with coronary artery disease. *Am Heart J.* 2005;149:565-572.
56. Schooling CM, Lam TH, Leung GM: Effect of obesity in patients with coronary artery disease. *Lancet.* 2006;368:1645; author reply 1645-1646.
57. Lundberg GD: A new aggressive approach to screening and early intervention to prevent death from coronary artery disease. *MedGenMed.* 2006;8:22.
58. Boekholdt SM, Sandhu MS, Day NE, et al: Physical activity, C-reactive protein levels and the risk of future coronary artery disease in apparently healthy men and women: the EPIC-Norfolk prospective population study. *Eur J Cardiovasc Prev Rehabil.* 2006;13:970-976.
59. Prayaga S: Asian Indians and coronary artery disease risk. *Am J Med.* 2007;120:e15; author reply e19.
60. Chambers TA, Bagai A, Ivascu N: Current trends in coronary artery disease in women. *Curr Opin Anaesthesiol.* 2007;20:75-82.
61. Turhan S, Tulunay C, Gulec S, et al: The association between androgen levels and premature coronary artery disease in men. *Coron Artery Dis.* 2007;18:159-162.
62. Saghafi H, Mahmoodi MJ, Fakhrzadeh H, et al: Cardiovascular risk factors in first-degree relatives of patients with premature coronary artery disease. *Acta Cardiol.* 2006;61:607-613.
63. Ahmed A, Lefante CM, Alam N: Depression and nursing home admission among hospitalized older adults with coronary artery disease: a propensity score analysis. *Am J Geriatr Cardiol.* 2007;16:76-83.
64. Nauer KA: Acute dissection of the aorta: a review for nurses. *Critical Care Nursing Quarterly.* 2000;23:20-27.
65. McKnight JT, Adcock BB: Paresthesias: a practical diagnostic approach. *Am Fam Physician.* 1997;56:2253-2260.
66. Poncelet AN: An algorithm for the evaluation of peripheral neuropathy. *Am Fam Physician.* 1998;57:755-764.
67. Gillette PD: Exercise in aging and disease. In: Placzek JD, Boyce DA, eds. *Orthopaedic Physical Therapy Secrets.* Philadelphia, PA: Hanley & Belfus, Inc. 2001:235-242.
68. Clarke M, Hpewell S, Juszczak E, et al: Compression stockings to prevent deep vein thrombosis in long-haul airline passengers. *Int J Epidemiol.* 2006;35:1410-1411; discussion 1411.
69. Ali A, Caine MP, Snow BG: Graduated compression stockings: physiological and perceptual responses during and after exercise. *J Sports Sci.* 2007;25:413-419.
70. Compression stockings. How hosiery can help circulation and leg swelling. *Mayo Clin Womens Healthsource.* 2006;10:6.
71. Graduated Compression Stockings: Prevention of postoperative venous thromboembolism is crucial. *Am J Nurs.* 2006; 106: 72AA-DD.
72. Motsch J, Walther A, Bock M, et al: Update in the prevention and treatment of deep vein thrombosis and pulmonary embolism. *Curr Opin Anaesthesiol.* 2006;19:52-58.
73. Garmon RG: Pulmonary embolism: incidence, diagnosis, prevention, and treatment. *J Am Osteopath Assoc.* 1985;85:176-185.
74. Bounameaux H, Reber-Wasem MA: Superficial thrombophlebitis and deep vein thrombosis: a controversial association. *Arch Intern Med.* 1997;157:1822-1824.

75. Gorman WP, Davis KR, Donnelly R: ABC of arterial and venous disease. Swollen lower limb-1: general assessment and deep vein thrombosis. *BMJ.* 2000;320:1453-1456.
76. Aschwanden M, Labs KH, Engel H, et al: Acute deep vein thrombosis: early mobilization does not increase the frequency of pulmonary embolism. *Thromb Haemost.* 2001;85:42-46.
77. Fukazawa R, Ikegam E, Watanabe M, et al: Coronary artery aneurysm induced by Kawasaki disease in children show features typical senescence. *Circ J.* 2007;71:709-715.
78. Zevitz ME: Heart Failure, Available at: http://www.emedicine.com/med/topic3552.htm, 2005.
79. Rees K, Taylor RS, Singh S, et al: Exercise based rehabilitation for heart failure. *Cochrane Database Syst Rev.* 2004;3:CD003331.
80. Pina IL, Daoud S: Exercise and heart failure. *Minerva Cardioangiol.* 2004;52:537-546.
81. Pina IL, Apstein CS, Balady GJ, et al: Exercise and heart failure: a statement from the American Heart Association Committee on exercise, rehabilitation, and prevention. *Circulation.* 2003;107:1210-1225.
82. Budev MM, Arroliga AC, Wiedemann HP, et al: Cor pulmonale: an overview. *Semin Respir Crit Care Med.* 2003;24:233-244.
83. Weitzenblum E: Chronic cor pulmonale. *Heart.* 2003;89:225-230.
84. Lehrman S, Romano P, Frishman W, et al: Primary pulmonary hypertension and cor pulmonale. *Cardiol Rev.* 2002;10:265-278.
85. Romano PM, Peterson S: The management of cor pulmonale. *Heart Dis.* 2000;2:431-437.
86. Missov ED, De Marco T: Cor pulmonale. *Curr Treat Options Cardiovasc Med.* 2000;2:149-158.
87. Rothstein JM, Roy SH, Wolf SL: Vascular anatomy, cardiology, and cardiac rehabilitation. *The Rehabilitation Specialists Handbook.* Philadelphia, PA: FA Davis. 1991:548-550.
88. Roffe C: Aging of the heart. *Br J Biomed Sci.* 1998;55:136-148.
89. Alaeddini J, Alimohammadi B: *Angina Pectoris.* Available at: http://www.emedicine.com/med/topic133.htm, 2006.
90. Fenton DE, Stahmer S: Myocardial infarction. Available at: http://www.emedicine.com/EMERG/topic327.htm, 2006.
91. Gragnani SG, Michelotti F, Rocca R, et al: Primary congenital lymphedema. A case report. *Minerva Pediatr.* 1999;51:217-219.
92. Wananukul S, Jittitaworn S: Primary congenital lymphedema involving all limbs and genitalia. *J Med Assoc Thai.* 2005;88:1958-1961.
93. Bauer T, Wechselberger G, Schoeller T, et al: Lymphedema praecox of the lower extremity. *Surgery.* 2002;132:899-900.
94. Lewis JM, Wald ER: Lymphedema praecox. *J Pediatr.* 1984;104:641-648.
95. Wheeler ES, Chan V, Wassman R, et al: Familial lymphedema praecox: Meige's disease. *Plast Reconstr Surg.* 1981;67:362-364.
96. Majeski J: Lymphedema tarda. *Cutis.* 1986;38:105-107.
97. Saab S, Nguyen S, Collins J, et al: Lymphedema tarda after liver transplantation: a case report and review of the literature. *Exp Clin Transplant.* 2006;4:567-570.
98. Mancini MC, Gangahar DM: *Heart Transplantation.* Available at: http://www.emedicine.com/med/topic3187.htm, 2006.
99. DeTurk WE: Exercise and the intolerant heart. *Clin Manage.* 1992;12:67-73.

100. Guide to Physical Therapist Practice. Second Edition. American Physical Therapy Association. *Phys Ther.* 2001;81:1-746.
101. Laethem CV, Van De Veire N, Backer GD, et al: Response of the oxygen uptake efficiency slope to exercise training in patients with chronic heart failure. *Eur J Heart Fail.* 2007;7:7.
102. Klecha A, Kawecka-Jaszcz K, Bacior B, et al: Physical training in patients with chronic heart failure of ischemic origin: effect on exercise capacity and left ventricular remodeling. *Eur J Cardiovasc Prev Rehabil.* 2007;14:85-91.
103. Maria Sarullo F, Gristina T, Brusca I, et al: Effect of physical training on exercise capacity, gas exchange and N-terminal pro-brain natriuretic peptide levels in patients with chronic heart failure. *Eur J Cardiovasc Prev Rehabil.* 2006;13:812-817.
104. van Tol BA, Huijsmans RJ, Kroon DW, et al: Effects of exercise training on cardiac performance, exercise capacity and quality of life in patients with heart failure: a meta-analysis. *Eur J Heart Fail.* 2006;8:841-850. Epub May 18, 2006.
105. Keteyian SJ, Brawner CA, Schairer JR: Exercise testing and training of patients with heart failure due to left ventricular systolic dysfunction. *J Cardiopulm Rehabil.* 1997;17:19-28.
106. Keteyian SJ, Levine AB, Brawner CA, et al: Exercise training in patients with heart failure. A randomized, controlled trial. *Ann Intern Med.* 1996;124:1051-1057.
107. McKelvie RS, Teo KK, McCartney N, et al: Effects of exercise training in patients with congestive heart failure: a critical review. *J Am Coll Cardiol.* 1995;25:789-796.
108. Dekerlegand J: Congestive heart failure. In: Cameron MH, Monroe LG, eds. *Physical Rehabilitation: Evidence-Based Examination, Evaluation, and Intervention.* St Louis, MO: Saunders/Elsevier. 2007:669-688.
109. de Carvalho T, Curi AL, Andrade DF, et al: Cardiovascular rehabilitation of patients with ischemic heart disease undergoing medical treatment, percutaneous transluminal coronary angioplasty, and coronary artery bypass grafting. *Arq Bras Cardiol.* 2007;88:72-78.
110. Certo CM, DeTurk WE, Cahalin LP: History of cardiopulmonary rehabilitation. In: DeTurk WE, Cahalin LP, eds. *Cardiovascular and Pulmonary Physical Therapy.* New York, NY: McGraw-Hill. 2004:3-14.
111. Vibhuti NS, Schocken DD: *Cardiac Rehabilitation.* Available at: http://www.emedicine.com/pmr/topic180.htm, 2006.
112. Kafejian-Haddad AP, Perez JM, Castiglioni ML, et al: Lymphscintigraphic evaluation of manual lymphatic drainage for lower extremity lymphedema. *Lymphology.* 2006;39:41-48.
113. Williams AF, Vadgama A, Franks PJ, et al: A randomized controlled crossover study of manual lymphatic drainage therapy in women with breast cancer-related lymphoedema. *Eur J Cancer Care (Engl).* 2002;11:254-261.
114. Reijnen MM, Disselhoff BC, Zeebregts CJ: Varicose vein surgery and endovenous laser therapy. *Surg Technol Int.* 2007;16:167-174.
115. Schmedt CG, Meissner OA, Hunger K, et al: Evaluation of endovenous radiofrequency ablation and laser therapy with endoluminal optical coherence tomography in an ex vivo model. *J Vasc Surg.* 2007;45:1047–1058.

116. Myers K, Fris R, Jolley D: Treatment of varicose veins by endovenous laser therapy: assessment of results by ultrasound surveillance. *Med J Aust.* 2006;185:199-202.
117. Peden E, Lumsden A: Radiofrequency ablation of incompetent perforator veins. *Perspect Vasc Surg Endovasc Ther.* 2007;19: 73-77.
118. Winsor T, Hyman C: *A Primer of Peripheral Vascular Diseases.* Philadelphia, PA: Lea & Febiger. 1965.

Pathology and Psychology

THE IMMUNE SYSTEM

Together with a series of physical barriers (the skin, mucous membranes, tears, and stomach acid), the immune system helps to defend the body against foreign or harmful substances that attempt to infiltrate it (Table 12-1). Such substances include microorganisms (bacteria, viruses, and fungi), parasites (such as worms), cancer cells, and even transplanted organs and tissues. *Antigens* are entities within or on bacteria, viruses, other microorganisms, or cancer cells that stimulate an immune response in the body. Antigens may also exist independently—eg, as pollen or food molecules. A normal immune response consists of the initial recognition of a foreign antigen, and the mobilization of forces to defend against it.

Dysfunction of the immune system occurs when:

- The body initiates an immune response against itself (an autoimmune disorder).
- The body cannot initiate suitable immune responses against invading microorganisms (an immunodeficiency disorder).
- A normal immune response to foreign antigens results in damage to normal tissues (an allergic reaction).

The body's first line of protection against invaders is through mechanical or physical barriers: the skin; the cornea of the eye; and the membranes lining the respiratory, digestive, urinary, and reproductive tracts. As long as these barriers remain unbroken, many invaders cannot penetrate them. A break in this barrier increases the chance of contamination—eg, an extensive burn damages much of the skin, leaving it prone to contamination. In addition, secretions containing enzymes can destroy bacteria defend the barriers. Examples are tears in the eyes and secretions in the digestive tract and vagina.

The next line of protection includes white blood cells (leukocytes) that travel through the bloodstream and into tissues, seeking

TABLE 12-1. TERMS AND DEFINITIONS OF THE IMMUNE SYSTEM[a]

TERM	DEFINITION
Antibody (immunoglobulin)	A protein that is produced by B lymphocytes and that interacts with a specific antigen
Antigen	Any substance that can stimulate an immune response
Baso phil	A white blood cell that releases histamine (a substance involved in allergic reactions) and produces substances to attract neutrophils and eosinophils to a trouble spot
Cell	The smallest unit of a living organism, composed of a nucleus and cytoplasm surrounded by a membrane
Chemotaxis	The process of attracting cells by means of a chemical substance
Complement system	A group of proteins with various immune functions, such as killing bacteria and other foreign cells, making foreign cells easier for macrophages to identify and ingest, attracting macrophages and neutrophils to a trouble spot, and enhancing the effectiveness of antibodies
Cytokines	The immune system's messengers, which help regulate an immune response
Dendritic cell	A white blood cell that usually resides in tissues and that helps T lymphocytes recognize foreign antigens
Eosinophil	A white blood cell that can ingest bacteria and other foreign cells, that may help immobilize and kill parasites, that participates in allergic reactions, and that helps destroy cancer cells
Helper T cell	A white blood cell that helps B lymphocytes recognize and produce antibodies against foreign antigens
Histocompatibility	Literally, compatibility of tissue; determined by human leukocyte antigens (the major histocompatibility complex) and used to determine whether a transplanted tissue or organ will be accepted by the recipient
Human leukocyte antigens (HLA)	A group of molecules that are located on the surface of cells and that are unique in each organism, enabling the body to distinguish self from nonself; also called the major histocompatibility complex
Immune response	The reaction of the immune system to an antigen
Immunoglobulin	A synonym for antibody
Interleukin	A type of cytokine secreted by some white blood cells to affect other white blood cells
Killer (cytotoxic) T cell	A lymphocyte that attaches to foreign or abnormal cells and kills them
Leukocyte	A white blood cell, such as a monocyte, a neutrophil, an eosinophil, a basophil, or a lymphocyte
Lymphocyte	The white blood cell responsible for specific immunity, including producing antibodies (by B lymphocytes) and distinguishing self from nonself (by T lymphocytes)
Macrophage	A large cell that is derived from a white blood cell called a monocyte, that ingests bacteria and other foreign cells, and that helps white blood cells identify microorganisms and other foreign substances
Major histocompatibility complex (MHC)	A synonym for human leukocyte antigens
Mast cell	A cell in tissues that releases histamine and other substances involved in allergic reactions
Molecule	A group of atoms chemically combined to form a unique chemical substance
Natural killer cell	A type of lymphocyte that, unlike other lymphocytes, is formed ready to kill certain microorganisms and cancer cells
Neutrophil	A white blood cell that ingests and kills bacteria and other foreign cells
Phagocyte	A cell that ingests and kills invading microorganisms, other cells, and cell fragments
Phagocytosis	The process of a cell ingesting an invading microorganism, another cell, or a cell fragment
Receptor	A molecule on a cell's surface or inside the cell that allows only molecules that fit precisely to it—as a key fits in its lock—to attach to it
Suppressor T cell	A white blood cell that helps end an immune response

[a]Merck Manuals on-line library, home edition.

and attacking microorganisms and other invaders. This mode of protection has two parts:

- Nonspecific (innate) immunity: the first step, which involves different types of leukocytes that on most occasions act independently to destroy invaders.
- Specific (adaptive) immunity: the second step, which involves leukocytes combining to destroy invaders. Some of these cells do not destroy invaders themselves but enable other white blood cells to recognize and destroy the invaders.

Nonspecific immunity and specific immunity interact and impact each other either directly or through substances that attract or activate other cells of the immune system. These substances include cytokines (the messengers of the immune system), antibodies, and complement proteins (a part of the complement system). These substances dissolve in a body fluid, such as plasma, the liquid part of blood.

To be effective, the immune system must be able to distinguish what is *nonself* (foreign) from what is *self*. Identification molecules on the exterior of all human cells—human leukocyte antigens (HLA), or the major histocompatibility complex (MHC), allow this to occur. Each individual has unique HLAs, and any cell with molecules on its surface that are not identical with those of the body's own cells provokes an attack from the immune system. T lymphocytes provide the surveillance part of the immune system as they travel through the bloodstream and lymphatic system (see Chapter 11), looking for antigens. However, unless an antigen undergoes processing into antigen fragments by another white blood cell, called an antigen-presenting cell, the T lymphocyte cannot recognize it as foreign. Antigen-presenting cells consist of dendritic cells (which are the most effective), macrophages, and B lymphocytes.

A specialized molecule called a T-cell receptor, found on the exterior of a T lymphocyte, recognizes the antigen fragment when an HLA molecule presents it. The T-cell receptor then attaches to the part of the HLA molecule presenting the antigen fragment, fitting in it as a key fits in a lock.

ORGANS OF THE IMMUNE SYSTEM

The immune system consists of several organs as well as cells scattered throughout the body. Lymphoid organs can be classified as primary or secondary.

- Primary: the thymus gland and bone marrow—the sites of white blood cell (WBC) production.
    - Production and preparation of the T lymphocytes (necessary for specific immunity) occurs in the thymus gland.
    - The bone marrow produces several types of white blood cell, including neutrophils, monocytes, and B lymphocytes.
- Secondary: spleen, tonsils, liver, appendix, and Peyer patches in the small intestine. These organs ensnare microorganisms and other foreign substances and provide a place for mature cells of the immune system to gather, interact with one another and with the foreign substances, and produce a specific immune response.

IMMUNODEFICIENCY

In *immunodeficiency*, the immune response is absent or depressed. Autoimmune diseases manifest as a self-destructive immune system response directed against normal tissue. Autoimmune diseases can develop according to involvement:

- Organ specific: eg, Hashimoto thyroiditis, Addison disease, Crohn disease, and diabetes mellitus
- Nonorgan specific (systemic): eg, systemic lupus erythematosus (SLE), fibromyalgia, ankylosing spondylitis, multiple sclerosis, psoriasis, and Reiter syndrome

The etiology of autoimmune diseases is often unknown. Possible causes include a genetic predisposition, hormonal changes, and environmental factors, viral infection, or stress. Added risk factors include a compromised immune system, poor physiologic and psychological health, advanced age, or a coexistence of other diseases or conditions. The main causes of immunodeficiency can be grouped into primary, secondary, or iatrogenic disorders:

- Primary disorders: a defect involving T cells, B cells, NK (natural killer) cells, phagocytic cells, complement proteins, or lymphoid tissues. Genetically determined immunodeficiency can cause increased susceptibility to infection, autoimmunity, and increased risk of cancer.
- Secondary disorders: result from an underlying disease or cause that depresses or blocks the immune response. These include:
  - Leukemia or Hodgkin disease.
  - Nonspecific deficiencies in the immune system, which occur because of viral and other infections, malnourishment, alcoholism, cancer, chronic disease, chemotherapy, and radiation.
  - Autoimmune disease, diabetes mellitus, renal disease.
  - Acquired immunodeficiency syndrome (AIDS).
  - Organ transplantation—graft versus host disease.
  - Iatrogenic disorders: induced by immunosuppressive drugs, or radiation therapy.

Examples of immunosuppressive drugs include corticosteroids, cyclosporine, cytotoxic drugs.

Study Pearl

Autoimmune disorders certain clinical features and findings in common. These include:

- Synovitis
- Pleuritis
- Myocarditis
- Vasculitis
- Myositis
- Nephritis
- Constitutional symptoms, including fatigue, malaise, myalgias, and arthralgias

PATHOLOGY

INFECTIOUS DISEASE

Infection is a process in which an organism establishes a parasitic relationship with its host.[1] This invasion and multiplication of microorganisms produces an immune response and subsequent signs and symptoms. A great variety of microorganisms are responsible for infectious diseases, including fungi (yeast and molds); helminths (eg, tapeworms); mycobacteria; viruses; mycoplasmas; bacteria; rickettsiae; chlamydiae; protozoa; and prions.

Types of Organisms

Fungus. Certain types of fungi (such as *Candida*) are commonly present on body surfaces or in the intestines. Although generally innocuous, these fungi sometimes cause local infections of the skin and nails, vagina, mouth, or sinuses in immunocompromised individuals, which can prove fatal.

Even in otherwise healthy people, some fungal infections (eg, blastomycosis and coccidioidomycosis) can have serious outcomes.

Although several drugs are effective against fungal infections, the chemical makeup of fungi makes them difficult to treat.

> **Study Pearl**
>
> Fungal diseases in humans are called *mycoses.*

Bacteria. *Bacteria* are microscopic, single-celled organisms, which are encountered in the environment, on the skin, in the airways, in the mouth, and in the digestive and genitourinary tracts.

Gram-positive and gram-negative bacteria differ in the types of infections they produce and in the types of antibiotics that are required to manage them.

> **Study Pearl**
>
> Bacteria can be classified according to:
> - Shape (cocci [spherical], bacilli [rod-like], and spirochetes [spiral or helical])
> - Their use of oxygen (aerobes, those that can live and grow in the presence of oxygen, and anaerobes, those that can tolerate only low levels of oxygen such as those found in the intestine, or in decaying tissue)
> - By color after a particular chemical (Gram) stain is applied (the bacteria that stain blue are called gram positive, whereas those that stain pink are called gram negative)

Gram-Negative Bacteria. This type possesses a unique outer membrane that is rich in molecules called lipopolysaccharides that makes them more resistant to antibiotics than gram-positive bacteria. The lipopolysaccharides, or endotoxins, can potentially cause high fever and a life-threatening drop in blood pressure. Gram-negative bacteria have a great facility for mutation.

Gram-Positive Bacteria. This type is usually slow to develop resistance to antibiotics, but can produce toxins that cause serious illness. Disease-causing anaerobes include clostridia, peptococci, and peptostreptococci, the latter two of which are part of the normal bacterial population (flora) of the mouth, upper respiratory tract, and large intestine.

> **Study Pearl**
>
> *Bacteremia* is the presence of viable bacteria in the circulating blood. If the bacteria become viable, they may establish a focal infection, or the infection may progress to septicemia, multiple organ failure, and death.[2]

Mycoplasmas. Mycoplasmas are self-replicating bacteria that have no cell wall component and possess very small genomes.[1] For this reason, antibiotics that are active against bacterial cell walls have no effect on mycoplasmas.[1]

Clostridia. Clostridia, which normally inhabit the human intestinal tract, the soil, and decaying vegetation, are toxin-producing anaerobes that can cause tetanus, botulism, and tissue infections.[3] Clostridia, particularly *Clostridium perfringens,* also infect wounds. Clostridial wound infections, including skin gangrene, muscle gangrene (clostridial myonecrosis), and tetanus, are rather uncommon but may be fatal.[3]

Rickettsiae. Rickettsiae are small, gram-negative, obligate intracellular organisms that cause several diseases, including Rocky Mountain spotted fever and epidemic typhus.[4-10] Like viruses, rickettsiae require a host for replication and cannot survive on their own in the environment. In humans, rickettsiae infect the cells lining small blood vessels, causing the blood vessels to become inflamed or choked or to bleed into the surrounding tissue. The various types of rickettsial infections produce similar symptoms, which include: fever, severe headache, a characteristic skin rash, and a general feeling of malaise. As rickettsial disease progresses, a person typically experiences confusion and severe weakness—often with cough, dyspnea, and sometimes vomiting and diarrhea. In some people, the liver or spleen enlarges, the kidneys fail, and blood pressure falls dangerously low. Death can occur.

Because ticks, mites, fleas, and lice transmit rickettsiae, a report of a bite from one or more of these vectors is a helpful clue—particularly in geographic areas where rickettsial infection is common.

Ehrlichioses. Ehrlichiae are similar to rickettsiae: they are microorganisms that can live only inside the cells of an animal or person.[11-13] Unlike rickettsiae, however, ehrlichiae inhabit white blood cells (such as granulocytes and monocytes). Ehrlichioses occur in the United States and Europe, but are most common in the midwestern, southeastern, and south-central United States. Ehrlichioses are most likely to develop between spring and late fall, when ticks are most active.

Virus. A *virus* is a subcellular organism consisting of a ribonucleic acid (RNA) or a deoxyribonucleic acid (DNA) nucleus covered with proteins.[1] Viruses cannot replicate unless they invade a host cell and stimulate it to participate in the formation of additional virus particles.[1] Some viruses leave their genetic material in the host cell where it remains dormant for an extended time (latent infection), eg, herpes viruses (see Chapter 13). Viruses are not vulnerable to antibiotics and cannot be destroyed by pharmacologic means.[1] However, antiviral medications can mitigate the course of the viral illness.[1]

Probably the most common viral infections are upper respiratory infections.

Some viruses (eg, rabies, West Nile virus, and several encephalitis viruses) infect the nervous system. Viral infections may also develop in the skin, sometimes resulting in warts or other blemishes.

Prions. Prions are proteinaceous, infectious particles consisting of proteins but without nucleic acids.[1] These particles are transmitted from animals to humans and are characterized by a long, latent interval in the host. Examples include Creutzfeldt-Jakob disease, bovine spongiform encephalopathy or "mad cow disease."[1]

Parasite. A *parasite* is an organism that resides on or inside a host organism and causes harm to the host.[14-16] Some parasites, particularly those that are single celled, reproduce inside the host. Other parasites have complex life cycles, producing larvae that spend time in the environment or as an insect vector before becoming infective.

Parasites enter the body through the mouth or skin. The diagnosis of a parasitic infection can be made from samples of blood, tissue, stool, or urine for laboratory analysis.

If egg-laying parasites live in the digestive tract, their eggs may be found in the person's stool when a sample is examined under a microscope. Antibiotics, laxatives, and antacids can substantially reduce the number of parasites to make their detection in a stool sample more difficult.

Food, drink, and water are often contaminated with parasites in areas of the world with poor sanitation and unhygienic practices.

Infectious Agents

Infectious agents are now suspected in the origins of chronic diseases such as sarcoidosis, various forms of inflammatory bowel disease, scleroderma, rheumatoid arthritis (RA), systemic lupus erythematosus (SLE), diabetes mellitus (DM), Kawasaki disease, Alzheimer disease, and many forms of cancer. All health-care professionals need to have an understanding of the infectious process, the sequence of transmission, and approaches to lessen the spread of infections.

Study Pearl

Nosocomial infections are those that originate or occur in a hospital or hospital-like setting. Clinicians can help prevent transmission of nosocomial infections from themselves to others, from client to client, and from client to self by following standard precautions, infection control procedures, isolation techniques, and proper handwashing techniques (Chapter 5).

Staphylococcal Infections. Most infections caused by staphylococci result from *Staphylococcus aureus.* However, the prevalence of infections because of *S. epidermidis* and other coagulase-negative staphylococci has been steadily increasing in recent years.

Study Pearl

Coagulase-negative staphylococci, particularly *S. epidermidis,* produce an exopolysaccharide (slime) that promotes foreign body adherence and resistance to phagocytosis.

Staphylococcus aureus (S. aureus): *Staphylococcus aureus* is a gram-positive coccus that is catalase positive and coagulase positive. They produce a wide variety of toxins, including enterotoxins, Panton-Valentine leukocidin (PVL)—associated with necrotic skin and lung infections, and toxic shock syndrome toxin-1 (TSST-1).[17-19]

S. aureus occurs with a worldwide distribution. Health-care workers, anyone with diabetes, and patients on dialysis all have higher rates of colonization. The anterior nares are the chief site of colonization in adults; other potential sites of colonization include the axilla, rectum, and perineum.[20]

Common characteristics of staphylococcal infections include skin, wound and soft tissue infections, toxic shock syndrome, endocarditis, osteomyelitis, food poisoning, and infections related to prosthetic devices, including catheters.[20] The clinical manifestations vary enormously according to the site and type of infection.[1]

Many antibiotics are effective against *S. aureus*. Methicillin-resistant *S. aureus* (MRSA) are resistant to most agents other than vancomycin or non–beta-lactam antibiotics. Many coagulase-negative staphylococci are resistant to all antimicrobials other than vancomycin.

Streptococcal Infections. *Streptococcus pyogenes* (group A *Streptococcus*) causes many diseases throughout diverse organ systems ranging from skin infections to infections of the upper respiratory tract.[21-29] Spread is by skin contact, not by the respiratory tract, although impetigo serotypes may colonize the throat. Respiratory droplet spread is the major route for transmission of strains associated with upper respiratory tract infection. Fingernails and the perianal region can harbor streptococci and play a role in spreading impetigo.

Signs and symptoms of streptococcal contamination are varied. Classic acute disease involves the skin and oropharynx, but any organ system may be involved.

Diagnosis is by culturing group A streptococci from pharyngeal secretions, blood, cerebrospinal fluid (CSF), joint aspirate, skin biopsy specimen, sputum, bronchoalveolar lavage fluid, or thoracocentesis fluid. Types include:

- Group A (pyogenes)—responsible for pharyngitis, rheumatic fever, scarlet fever, impetigo, necrotizing fasciitis, cellulitis, myositis

- Group B (agalactiae)—responsible for neonatal and adult infections
- Group C (pneumoniae)—responsible for pneumonia, otitis media, meningitis, endocarditis

The interventions vary depending on the clinical syndrome. In general, penicillin therapy remains the intervention of choice in most situations (except in penicillin-allergic individuals). Remarkably, no penicillin-resistant strains of *S. pyogenes* have yet been encountered in clinical practice.

Hepatitis. *Hepatitis* is defined as an inflammation of the liver. Several different viruses cause viral hepatitis.[30-36] They are named the hepatitis A, B, C, D, and E viruses. Some cases of viral hepatitis cannot be attributed to the hepatitis A, B, C, D, or E viruses. These types are called non A-E hepatitis.

All of the hepatitis viruses can cause acute, or short-term, viral hepatitis. The hepatitis B, C, and D viruses can also cause chronic hepatitis.

Signs and symptoms of viral hepatitis include:

- Low-grade fever.
- Jaundice.
- Elevated lab values (hepatic transaminases and bilirubin)

Acquired Immunodeficiency Syndrome. The primary cause of acquired immunodeficiency syndrome (AIDS) is through transmission of the HIV retrovirus by body fluid exchange (in particular blood and semen), which is associative with high-risk behaviors:

- Unprotected sexual contact
- Contaminated needles.
- Maternal-fetal transmission in utero or at delivery or through contaminated breast milk

Low-risk behaviors for HIV transmission include:

- Occupational transmission: needle sticks
- Casual contact: kissing

The HIV retrovirus chiefly infects human T4 (helper) lymphocytes, the major regulators of the immune response, by destroying or inactivating them.[48] HIV contains reverse transcriptase, an enzyme that allows for successful replication of the virus in reverse fashion, transcribing the RNA code into DNA.[47]

HIV infection manifests itself in many different ways and differs between adult and pediatric populations.[47,48]

The diagnosis is by clinical findings and systemic evidence of HIV infection and nonexistence of other known causes of immunodeficiency.

Physical Therapy Intervention. HIV is now considered as a chronic rather than a terminal illness. The goals of physical therapy will depend on the presenting signs and symptoms. The clinician must remember to follow universal AIDS/HIV precautions. The following interventions are recommended:[49]

- Exercise: moderate aerobic exercise training is recommended to improve cardiopulmonary function while avoiding exhaustive exercise. In addition, strength training should be introduced as tolerated.
- Energy conservation techniques.
- Postural education and instruction with body mechanics.
- Balance and proprioceptive training for patients with neurological deficits.

Influenza. Influenza is one of the most contagious airborne communicable diseases and is associated with significant morbidity and mortality in acute and long-term health-care facilities. The mode of transmission is person-to-person by direct deposition of virus-laden droplets onto the mucosa of the upper respiratory tract of an immunologically liable person.

- Influenza results from contamination with one of three key types of virus, A, B, or C.
- Influenza A is more pathogenic than influenza B.[50-52]

The general appearance among patients who present with influenza varies, with some appearing acutely ill, with some weakness and respiratory findings, while others may seem only mildly sick.

All health-care workers must follow the guidelines for isolation precautions (see later) about prevention of transmission of influenza both for themselves and their patients. This is especially important for the clinician treating aged, immunocompromised, or, chronically ill individuals.

Centers for Disease Control Guidelines for Isolation Precautions

Standard, Airborne, Droplet, and Contact Precautions. Refer to Table 5-37.

Departmental Infection Control.

Sterilization. Sterilization is the killing of all microorganisms in a material or on the surface of an object. There are several common methods of sterilization:

Heat. An autoclave is an instrument used to sterilize equipment and functions by subjecting them to high-pressured steam (103 kPa [15 psi)]) at 121°C (250°F) for around 15–20 minutes depending on the size of the load. Although autoclave treatment inactivates all fungi, bacteria, viruses, and bacterial spores, it does not necessarily eliminate prions.

Boiling in water for 15 minutes kills non-spore forming organisms (bacteria and viruses), but is unsuitable for sterilization as it is ineffective against many bacterial spores and prions. Dry heat can be used to sterilize items. The standard setting for a hot air oven is at least 2 hours at 160°C (320°F). A rapid method can heat air to 190°C (374°F) for 6 to 12 hours.

Chemical. Chemicals are also used for sterilization:

- Phenols: general disinfectant.
- Halogens (chlorine, iodine, bromine).
- Chlorine bleach is a liquid sterilizing agent. Household bleach, also used in hospitals and biological research laboratories, consists of 5.25% sodium hypochlorite. At this concentration it is most stable for storage, but not most active. Bleach will kill many spores, but is ineffectual against certain resistant spores.
- Ethylene oxide gas: commonly used to sterilize objects such as plastics, optics, and electrics. Ethylene oxide can kill all known viruses, bacteria, and fungi, including bacterial spores. However, it is highly flammable, toxic, and carcinogenic.
- Chlorination: used for water disinfection, filtration systems, and cleaning surfaces.
- Iodines: used in hydrotherapy; provide full bactericidal activity when organic matter (skin, feces, urine) is present.
- Bleach: kills many organisms immediately, but for full sterilization it should be allowed to react for 20 minutes. It is also highly corrosive.
- Alcohol.
- Quaternary ammonia salts: powerful disinfectants with extra surfactant (detergent) action. As well as acting against bacteria, their surfactant action removes excess mucus-containing parasites and bacteria, eg, Zephiran.
- Glutaraldehyde and formaldehyde solutions are accepted liquid-sterilizing agents, provided the immersion time is long enough—it can take up to 24 hours for glutaraldehyde to kill all spores, and even longer for formaldehyde.
- Ionizing radiation (x-rays, gamma rays): used to sterilize some medication, plastics, sutures.
- Ultraviolet light: can also be used for irradiation, but only on surfaces and some transparent objects. It also damages many plastics and is harmful to unprotected skin and eyes.

Filtration. Uses forceful air purification.

Physical Cleaning.

- Ultrasonic—disinfects instruments
- Hand washing with an antimicrobial product

Disinfection. Disinfection applies to the process of reducing the number of viable microorganisms present in a sample. Not all disinfectants are capable of sterilizing. An ideal disinfectant should be:

- Fast acting.
- Effective against all types of infectious agents (broadly active) without destroying tissues or being poisonous.
- Able to easily penetrate material to be disinfected without damaging or discoloring the material.
- Easy to prepare and stable even when exposed to light, heat, or other environmental factors.
- Inexpensive and easy to obtain and use.

An *antiseptic* is a chemical agent that is applied to living tissue to kill microbes. *Sanitization* is the cleaning of pathogenic microorganisms from public eating utensils and objects such as that done by the kitchen of a restaurant.

HEMATOLOGIC (BLOOD) DISORDERS

Hematology is the study of the form and structure of blood and blood-forming tissues. Manifestations of hematological system dysfunction are outlined in Table 12-2. Hematologic dysfunctions alter the oxygen-carrying capacity of the blood and the constituents, structure, consistency, and flow of the blood.[49] These changes can contribute to hypo- or hypercoagulopathy, increased work of the heart and breathing, impaired tissue perfusion, and increased risk of thrombus.

Disorders of Iron Absorption

Hemochromatosis. *Hemochromatosis* is an autosomal recessive hereditary disorder that produces excessive iron absorption by the small intestine.[49] Individuals with this condition lack an effective way to remove iron and the iron begins to build up in various organs.[55,56] Symptoms include fatigue, abdominal pain, arthralgia or arthritis, enlarged liver, and darkened skin. Hemochromatosis is characterized by:

- Chronic hemolytic anemia in which hemoglobin is released into plasma with resultant reduced oxygen delivery to the tissues.
- Vaso-occlusion because of the misshapen erythrocytes, which can result in ischemia, occlusion, and infarction of any bordering tissue.

Diagnosis is made by a simple genetic test based on family history.[49]

TABLE 12-2. MANIFESTATIONS OF HEMATOLOGICAL SYSTEM DYSFUNCTION

MANIFESTATION	DESCRIPTION
Edema	Build-up of excessive fluid within the interstitial tissues or within body cavities
Congestion	The build-up of excess blood within the blood vessels of an organ or tissue
Infarction	A localized region of necrosis caused by reduction of arterial perfusion below the level required for cell viability
Thrombosis and embolism	▶ Thrombus: a solid mass of clotted blood within an intact blood vessel or chamber of the heart ▶ Embolus: a mass of solid, liquid, or gas that moves within a blood vessel to lodge at a site distant from its place of origin
Lymphedema	A chronic swelling of an area because of a build-up of interstitial fluid secondary to obstruction of lymphatic vessels or lymph nodes. Although it presents commonly in the limbs, it can develop in other areas as well. Lymphedema is a localized and asymmetrical condition
Hypotension and shock	The result of reduced arterial blood circulation and thus decreased perfusion to an organ or tissue

Data from Goodman CC: The hematologic system. In: Goodman CC, Boissonnault WG, Fuller KS, eds. *Pathology: Implications for the Physical Therapist, 2nd ed.* Philadelphia, PA: Saunders. 2003: 509-552.

Physical Therapy Role. Because arthropathy occurs in 40% to 60% of individuals with hemochromatosis, therapeutic intervention is essential in providing flexibility, strength, and proper alignment to promote function, and prevent the loss of independence in activities of daily living (evaluating the need for assistive devices, orthotics, and splints).[49]

Disorders of Erythrocytes

Anemia. *Anemia* is one of the more common blood disorders and is characterized by an abnormality in the quantity or quality of the blood. Anemia is a symptom of many other disorders including:[49]

- Dietary deficiency (nutritional anemia): iron, vitamin B, folic acid deficiency
- Decreased production of erythrocytes in chronic diseases such as rheumatoid arthritis, tuberculosis, and cancer; bone marrow failure; inborn or acquired metabolic defects
- Acute or chronic blood loss (iron deficiency) which can occur with trauma, bleeding peptic ulcer, excessive menstruation, or bleeding hemorrhoids
- Congenital defects of hemoglobin (sickle cell diseases)
- Destruction of erythrocytes (mechanical or autoimmune hemolysis, enzyme defects, hypersplenism)

Study Pearl

Exercise intolerance can be an adverse side-effect of anemia. Vital signs should be monitored for tachycardia, which is usually accompanied by a sense of generalized weakness, loss of stamina, and exertional dyspnea. Central nervous system (CNS) symptoms can develop in cases of severe pernicious anemia.[49]

Treatment of anemia is directed toward alleviating or controlling the causes, relieving the symptoms, and preventing complications.[49]

Physical Therapy Role. Exercise for any patient with anemia should be approved by the physician. A knowledge of red flag symptoms, indicating the need for alteration of the program or medical referral is essential.[49] Examples include:[49]

- Evidence of easy bruising in response to the slightest trauma.
- Decreased oxygen delivery to the skin results in impaired or delayed healing and loss of the skin's natural elasticity.
- Paresthesias, gait disturbances, and extreme weakness.
- Tachycardia and palpitations.

Hemostasis Disorders

Sickle Cell Disease. This is a cluster of inherited, autosomal recessive disorders in which the erythrocytes, particularly hemoglobin S, are crescent or sickle shaped instead of being biconcave.[57-60] The condition is chronic and can be fatal. The two primary pathophysiologic features of sickle cell disorders are chronic hemolytic anemia and vaso-occlusion resulting in ischemic injury.[49]

Sickle Cell Anemia. *Sickle cell anemia* is a hereditary, chronic form of hemolytic anemia, that is merely a result of the disease and not the disease itself.[49] In sickle cell anemia the erythrocytes rupture releasing hemoglobin prematurely into the plasma, thereby reducing oxygen delivery capacity to the tissues. It is important that the physical therapist be able to recognize the signs and symptoms associated with sickle cell anemia, and a condition called sickle cell crisis (Table 12-2). It also important for the clinician to recognize signs of complications associated with sickle cell anemia, which include cerebrovascular accidents, convulsions, blindness, and avascular necrosis (AVN) of the femoral head.[49]

Hemophilia. *Hemophilia*, a bleeding disorder inherited as a sex-linked autosomal recessive trait (males are affected, females are carriers) is caused by an abnormality of plasma-clotting proteins (clotting factor VIII in hemophilia A; clotting factor IX in hemophilia B or Christmas disease) necessary for blood coagulation. This abnormality produces a prolonged but not faster bleeding than occurred in a normal person with the same injury.[61-65] Complications include:

- Joint contracture(s) and deformities, especially at the hip, knee, elbow, and ankle joints
- Hemophiliac arthropathy—the articular cartilage becomes pitted and fragmented[49]
- Muscle weakness and atrophy
- Decreased aerobic fitness

Currently, no known cure or prenatal treatment for hemophilia exists.[49]

The Thalassemias. *The Thalassemias*, a group of inherited, chronic hemolytic anemias commonly affecting people of Mediterranean or southern Chinese ancestry, are characterized by production of extremely thin, fragile erythrocytes, called target cells.[49,74] The onset of thalassemia is usually insidious and the symptoms resemble those of other hemolytic anemias (jaundice, leg ulcers, splenomegaly), and bony changes in older children if untreated.[49]

Histiocytosis X. *Histiocytosis* is the name given for a group of syndromes characterized by an abnormal increase in the number of specific immune cells called histiocyte cells, including monocytes, macrophages, and dendritic cells.[75-77] Most cases of histiocytosis X affect children between ages 1 and 15 years old. The extra immune cells may form tumors, which can affect various parts of the body. The skull is frequently affected.

Physical Therapy Intervention for Hematologic Disorders. Physical therapy intervention should be geared toward enhancing flexibility, strength, and appropriate trunk and extremity alignment to promote function, preventing contracture formation, preventing falls, and preventing the reduction of independence with ADLs.[49] The physical therapist needs to be able to recognize any signs of early (first 24-48 hours) bleeding episodes (warm, swollen, and painful joints with decreased range of motion, paresthesias, protective muscle spasm) and sickle cell crisis in those patients with hemostasis disorders (Table 12-3).[49]

> **Study Pearl**
>
> Patients with sickle cell disease must be closely monitored for cardiorespiratory and adverse metabolic responses during exercise.

ONCOLOGY

Cancer refers to a large group of diseases characterized by uncontrolled cell growth and the dispersion of abnormal cells (Table 12-4).

TABLE 12-3. SIGNS AND SYMPTOMS OF SICKLE CELL ANEMIA AND SICKLE CELL CRISIS

SICKLE CELL ANEMIA	SICKLE CELL CRISIS
Pain (abdominal, chest, headache)	Acute and severe pain because of ischemia
Fatigue	Recurrent joint, extremity, and back pain
Weakness	Neurologic manifestations: dizziness, paresthesias, blindness, and cranial nerve palsies
Dyspnea on effort	Renal compensations
Tachycardia	
Pallor or yellow skin	

Data from Goodman CC: The hematologic system. In: Goodman CC, Boissonnault WG, Fuller KS, eds. *Pathology: Implications for the Physical Therapist, 2nd ed.* Philadelphia, PA: Saunders. 2003: 509-552.

The cause of cancer varies, and the causative agents are subdivided into two categories:

- Endogenous (genetic)
- Exogenous (environmental or external): viruses (HIV), chemical agents (hydrocarbons, nickel, arsenic), physical agents (radiation, asbestos), drugs (cytotoxic drugs including steroids), tobacco use

Staging and Grading. Cancer is graded using stages according to the degree of malignancy and differentiation of malignant cells.

- Stage 0 (carcinoma in situ): the abnormal cells are found only in the first layer of cells of the primary site and have not invaded the deeper tissues.
- Stage I: cancer involves the primary site, and has not spread to nearby tissues.
- Stage IA: a very small amount of cancer—visible under a microscope—is found deeper in the tissues.
- Stage IB: a larger amount of cancer is found in the tissues.
- Stage II: cancer has metastasized to nearby areas but is still inside the primary site.

TABLE 12-4. ONCOLOGIC DEFINITIONS

TERM	DEFINITION
Tumor/neoplasm	Abnormal growths of new tissues that serve no useful purpose and may harm the host organism by competing for blood supply and nutrients. These new growths may be benign or malignant
Benign tumor	Localized, slow growing, usually encapsulated; not invasive, however, can become large enough to disband, compress, or obstruct normal tissues and to impair normal body functions
Malignant tumor	Invasive, rapid growth giving rise to metastasis; can be life threatening
Lymphoma	Malignancy originating in the lymphoid tissues, eg, Hodgkin disease, lymphatic leukemia
Carcinoma	Originating in epithelial tissues, eg, skin, stomach, colon, breast, and rectum
Sarcoma	Originating in connective and mesodermal tissues, eg, muscle, bone, fat
Leukemias and myelomas	Involve the blood (unrestrained growth of leukocytes) and blood-forming organs (bone marrow)
Dysplasia	A general category that suggests a disorganization of cells in which an adult cell varies from its normal size, shape, or organization
Differentiation	The process by which normal cells undergo physical and structural changes, as they develop to form different tissues of the body
Metaplasia	The first level of dysplasia. A reversible and benign but abnormal change in which one adult cell changes from one type to another
Hyperplasia	An increase in the number of cells in tissue, resulting in increased tissue mass
Metastasis	Movement of cancer cells from one body part to another; spread is by lymphatic system or bloodstream

- Stage IIA: cancer has metastasized beyond the primary site.
- Stage IIB: cancer has metastasized to other tissue around the primary site.
- Stage III: cancer has metastasized throughout the nearby area.
- Stage IV: cancer has metastasized to other parts of the body.
- Stage IVA: cancer has metastasized to organs close to the pelvic area.
- Stage IVB: cancer has metastasized to distant organs, such as the lungs.

The most common clinical manifestations of cancer include:

- Unusual bleeding or discharge
- A lump or thickening of any area, eg, breast
- A change in bladder or bowel habits
- Unexplained weight loss
- Night pain not related to movement
- Change in the size or appearance of a wart or mole

Physical Therapy Intervention. The physical therapy intervention varies according to the physical condition of the patient, the stage of cancer, and the cancer treatment the patient is undergoing. Common side effects while undergoing treatment for cancer can include limited motion, soreness, disuse atrophy, pain, fatigue, sensory loss, weakness, sleep disturbance, and lymphedema. Table 12-5 outlines the side effects of various cancer treatments.[82]

Study Pearl

Cancer can also be staged using the TNM classification. This records:

- Size of the primary tumor (T)
- Regional lymph node involvement (N)
- Distant metastasis (M)

Numbers are used to denote the extent of involvement from one to four (least to most).

Other parameters can be used, including:

G: the grade of the cancer cells. Low-grade cancer cells appear similar to normal cells, while high grade cancer cells appear poorly differentiated.

R: the completeness of the surgical operation (resection-boundaries free of cancer cells or not)

L: invasion into lymphatic vessels

V: invasion into a vein

TABLE 12-5. THE VARIOUS SIDE EFFECTS OF CANCER TREATMENTS

SURGERY	RADIATION	CHEMOTHERAPY	BIOTHERAPY	HORMONAL THERAPY
Fatigue	Fatigue	Fatigue	Fever	Hypertension
Disfigurement	Radiation sickness	Gastrointestinal effects	Chills	Steroid-induced diabetes
Loss of function	Immunosuppression	▶ Anorexia	Nausea	Myopathy (steroid induced)
Infection	Decreased platelets	▶ Nausea	Vomiting	Weight gain
Increased pain	Decreased white blood cells	▶ Vomiting	Anorexia	Hot flashes
Deformity	Infection	▶ Diarrhea	Fluid retention	Impotence
Bleeding	Fibrosis	▶ Constipation	Fatigue	Decreased libido
Scar tissue	Burns	Fluid/electrolyte imbalance from GI effects	CNS effects	Vaginal dryness
Fibrosis	Mucositis	Hepatotoxicity	Inflammatory reactions at injection sites	
	Diarrhea	Hemorrhage	Anemia	
	Edema	Bone marrow suppression	Leukopenia	
	Hair loss	Anemia	Altered taste sensation	
	Ulceration, delayed wound healing	Leukopenia (infection)		
	CNS/PNS effects	Thrombocytopenia		
	Malignancy	Decreased bone density with ovarian failure		
		Muscle weakness		
		Skin rashes		
		Neuropathies		
		Hair loss		
		Sterilization		
		Stomatitis, mucositis		
		Sexual dysfunction		

Reproduced, with permission, from Goodman CC, Snyder TK: Oncology. In: Goodman CC, Boissonnault WG, Fuller KS, eds. *Pathology: Implications for the Physical Therapist, 2nd ed.* Philadelphia, PA: Saunders. 2003: 236-263.

GENITOURINARY

The genitourinary system includes the male and female reproductive organs and the urinary system (the kidneys, the bladder, and the ureters). This section will focus on the renal urologic systems.

Water Balance. Fluid found inside the cells, called the intracellular fluid (ICF), accounts for two-thirds of the total body fluid. The fluid in the interstitial and intravascular compartment, called the extracellular fluid (ECF), comprises the remaining one-third of the body fluid. The ICF and ECF contain electrolytes (sodium, calcium, potassium, magnesium, chloride, and bicarbonate) that are essential to human life. When dissolved in water, electrolytes separate into electrically charged particles called ions, allowing them to conduct an electrical charge. This electrical charge is necessary for metabolic activities and is essential for the normal function of all cells.

The kidneys regulate body water balance through a combination of intrinsic and extrinsic mechanisms. The 1 to 2 L of water normally taken in each day join the body's fluid volume, and a similar amount is normally excreted in urine. The two intrinsic mechanisms that help maintain the water balance are the glomerular tubular balance (GTB) and the countercurrent mechanism:

- GTB: the fluid the tubules receive by glomerular filtration determines the amount they reabsorb or excrete.
- Countercurrent mechanism: a continuous process of concentrating urine as needed.

The extrinsic factors for regulating body water include the thirst mechanism and the antidiuretic hormone (ADH), both of which work together.

Study Pearl

As a general guideline, cancer patients should not be treated with electric or deep-heating thermal physical agents (ultrasound in particular), even if the site is distant from the neoplasm. However, the effect of ultrasound on micrometastasis is not known (refer to Chapter 18).

Study Pearl

An increase in intravascular fluid may result in congestive heart failure (CHF), increased pulse, and increased respiration. A decrease in intravascular fluid may result in decreased blood pressure, an increased pulse, and increased respiration. Conversely, an increase in extravascular fluid may cause edema, ascites, or pleural effusion, while a decrease in extravascular fluid may result in decreased skin turgor and fatigue.

Regulation of Fluids and Electrolytes.[83] Elevation or depression of electrolytes is diagnostically and clinically significant in a number of metabolic disorders (see next section). The following five types of fluid imbalances may occur:

- ECF volume deficit
- ECF volume excess
- ECF volume shift
- ICF volume excess
- ICF volume deficit

The most common causes and manifestations of fluid and electrolyte imbalances are seen in burns, diabetes mellitus, malignancy, acute alcoholism, dehydration (Table 12-6), edema, and congestive heart failure. An excess of body fluids can occur because of excessive intake; disturbances of output including acute renal failure, congestive heart failure, and cirrhosis.

The normal levels of the various electrolytes and the potential causes of their imbalances are listed in Table 12-7. The clinical features of various electrolyte imbalances are listed in Table 12-8.

TABLE 12-6. CLINICAL MANIFESTATIONS OF DEHYDRATION

Absent perspiration, tearing, and salivation
Abnormal body temperature
Confusion
Disorientation; comatose; convulsions
Dizziness when standing
Dry, brittle hair
Dry mucous membranes, furrowed tongue
Headache
Incoordination
Irritability
Lethargy
Postural hypotension
Rapid pulse
Rapid respiration
Skin changes:
▶ Color: gray
▶ Temperature: cold
▶ Turgor: poor
▶ Feel: warm, dry if mild; cool, clammy if severe
Sunken eyeballs
Sunken fontanel (children)

Reproduced, with permission, from Goodman CC, Snyder TK: Problems affecting multiple systems. In: Goodman CC, Boissonnault WG, Fuller KS, eds. *Pathology: Implications for the Physical Therapist, 2nd ed.* Philadelphia, PA: Saunders. 2003:85-119.

Acid–Base Imbalances. Acid–base imbalances are recognized clinically as abnormalities of serum pH. Normal serum pH is 7.35 to 7.45 (slightly alkaline).[83] Cell function is seriously compromised when the pH falls to 7.2 or lower or rises to 7.55 or higher. Three physiologic systems act interdependently to preserve normal serum pH:

- Blood buffer systems that provide an immediate buffering of excess acid or base.
- Excretion of acid by the lungs that occurs within hours.
- Excretion of acid or reclamation of base by the kidneys that occurs within days.

The four general classes of acid–base imbalance are respiratory acidosis, respiratory alkalosis, metabolic acidosis, and metabolic alkalosis (refer to Chapter 10).

Urinary Tract Disorders. An infection anywhere along the urinary tract is referred to as a urinary tract infection (UTI).[84]

Urinary Tract Infections. UTIs are usually classified as upper or lower according to where they occur along the urinary tract.

- Lower UTIs: infections of the urethra (urethritis) or bladder (cystitis).
- Upper UTIs: infections of the kidneys (pyelonephritis) or ureters (ureteritis).[84]

Study Pearl

The genitourinary structures involved with urine excretion are:
- Upper urinary tract: kidney and ureters
- Lower urinary tract: bladder and urethra

TABLE 12-7. NORMAL LEVELS AND CAUSES OF ELECTROLYTE IMBALANCES

ELECTROLYTE	NORMAL LEVELS (FOR ADULTS) AND RISK FACTORS FOR IMBALANCE
Potassium	Normal serum level is 3.5-5.5 mEq/L
Hypokalemia	Dietary deficiency (rare)
	Intestinal or urinary losses as a result of diarrhea or vomiting (anorexia, dehydration), drainage from fistulas, overuse of gastric suction
	Trauma (injury, burns, surgery): damaged cells release potassium, are excreted in urine
	Chronic renal disease
	Medications such as potassium-wasting diuretics, steroids, sodium-containing antibiotics
	Alkalosis
	Hyperglycemia
	Cushing syndrome, primary aldosteronism, severe magnesium deficiency
Hyperkalemia	Conditions that alter kidney function or decrease its ability to excrete potassium
	Intestinal obstruction that prevents elimination of potassium in the feces
	Addison disease
	Chronic heparin therapy, lead poisoning, insulin deficit
	Trauma: crush injuries, burns
	Acidosis
Sodium	Normal serum level is 134-145 mEq/L
Hyponatremia	Inadequate sodium intake (low-sodium diets)
	Excessive intake or retention of water (kidney failure and heart failure)
	Excessive water loss and electrolytes (vomiting, excessive perspiration, tap-water enemas, suctioning, use of diuretics)
	Loss of bile (high in sodium) as a result of fistulas, drainage, CI surgery, and suction
	Trauma (loss of sodium through burn wounds, wound drainage from surgery)
	IV fluids that do not contain electrolytes
	Adrenal gland insufficiency (Addison disease) or hyperaldosteronism
	Cirrhosis of the liver with ascites
	SIADH: brain tumor, cerebrovascular accident, pulmonary disease, neoplasm with ADH production, medications
Hypernatremia	Decreased water intake (comatose, mentally confused, or debilitated client)
	Water loss (excessive sweating, diarrhea, failure of kidney to reabsorb water from urine)
	ADH deficiency (diabetes insipidus)
	Excess adrenocortical hormones (Cushing syndrome)
	IV administration of high-protein, hyperosmotic tube feedings and diuretics
Calcium	Normal serum level is 9-11 mg/dL
Hypocalcemia	Inadequate dietary intake of calcium and inadequate exposure to sunlight (vitamin D) necessary for calcium use
	Impaired absorption of calcium from intestinal tract (severe diarrhea, overuse of laxative, and enemas containing phosphates; phosphorus tends to be more readily absorbed from the intestinal tract than calcium and suppresses calcium retention in the body)
	Hypoparathyroidism (injury, disease, surgery)
	Severe infections or burns
	Overcorrection of acidosis
	Pancreatic insufficiency
	Renal failure
	Hypomagnesemia
Hypercalcemia	Hyperparathyroidism, hyperthyroidism, adrenal insufficiency
	Tumors (bone, lung, stomach, and kidney)
	Multiple fractures
	Excess intake of calcium (excessive antacids), excess intake of vitamin D, milk alkali syndrome
	Osteoporosis, immobility, multiple myeloma
	Thiazide diuretics
	Sarcoidosis

(*Continued*)

TABLE 12-7. NORMAL LEVELS AND CAUSES OF ELECTROLYTE IMBALANCES (*continued*)

ELECTROLYTE	NORMAL LEVELS (FOR ADULTS) AND RISK FACTORS FOR IMBALANCE
Magnesium	Normal serum level is 1.5-2.5 mEq/L
Hypomagnesemia	Decreased magnesium intake or absorption (chronic malnutrition, chronic diarrhea, bowel resection with ileostomy or colostomy, chronic alcoholism, prolonged gastric suction, acute pancreatitis, biliary or intestinal fistula, diuretic therapy)
	Excessive loss of magnesium (diabetic ketoacidosis, severe dehydration, hyperaldosteronism and hypoparathyroidism, diuretic therapy)
Hypermagnesemia	Chronic renal and adrenal insufficiency
	Overuse of antacids and laxatives containing magnesium
	Severe dehydration (resulting oliguria can cause magnesium retention)
	Overcorrection of hypomagnesemia
	Near-drowning (aspiration of sea water)

Data from Goodman CC, Snyder TK: Problems affecting multiple systems. In: Goodman CC, Boissonnault WG, Fuller KS, eds. *Pathology: Implications for the Physical Therapist, 2nd ed.* Philadelphia, PA: Saunders. 2003: 85-119. Home M, Bond E: Fluid, electrolyte, and acid-base imbalances. In: Lewis S, Heitkempcr M, Dirksen S, eds. Medical-Surgical Nursing: Assessment and Management of Clinical problems, *5th ed.* St Louis: Mosby. 2000: 67-98.

Symptoms of UTIs often include:[84]

- A frequent urge to urinate. Despite the urge to urinate, only a small amount of urine is passed.
- A painful, burning feeling around the bladder or urethra during urination (dysuria).
- Complaints of pain, unrelated to urinating.
  - Women may feel an uncomfortable pressure above the pubic bone.
  - Men may experience fullness in the rectum.
- Urine may look milky or cloudy, or reddish if blood (hematuria) is present.
- Fever.
- Pain in the back or side, below the ribs, particularly if the kidneys become involved.
- Nausea.
- Vomiting.

Early detection and treatment of this disorder are vital to reduce the potential for permanent structural damage. In the case of insidious onset of back or shoulder pain, especially when accompanied by a recent history of any infection, warrants a medical screening examination.[84]

Interstitial Cystitis. Interstitial cystitis (IC) is a chronic disorder characterized by an inflamed, or irritated, bladder wall that can lead to scarring and stiffening of the bladder, decreased bladder capacity, glomerulations (pinpoint bleeding) and, rarely, ulcers in the bladder lining. IC may also be known as:[85]

- Painful bladder syndrome
- Frequency-urgency-dysuria syndrome

The symptoms of IC vary but often resemble the symptoms of a UTI.

TABLE 12-8. THE CLINICAL FEATURES OF VARIOUS ELECTROLYTE IMBALANCES

POTASSIUM IMBALANCE	HYPOKALEMIA	HYPERKALEMIA
Cardiovascular	Dizziness, hypotension, arrhythmias, ECG changes, cardiac arrest (with serum potassium levels 2.5 mEq/L)	Tachycardia and later bradycardia, ECG changes, cardiac arrest (with levels > 7.0 mEq/L)
Gastrointestinal	Nausea and vomiting, anorexia, diarrhea, abdominal distention, paralytic ileus, or decreased peristalsis	Nausea, diarrhea, abdominal cramps
Musculoskeletal	Muscle weakness and fatigue, leg cramps	Muscle weakness, flaccid paralysis
Central nervous system	Malaise, irritability, confusion, mental depression, speech changes, decreased reflexes, respiratory paralysis	Hyperreflexia progressing to weakness, numbness, tingling, and flaccid paralysis
Genitourinary	Polyuria	Oliguria, anuria
Acid-base balance	Metabolic alkalosis	Metabolic acidosis
CALCIUM IMBALANCE	**HYPOCALCEMIA**	**HYPERCALCEMIA**
Central nervous system	Anxiety, irritability, twitching around mouth, laryngospasm, convulsions, Chvostek sign, Trousseau sign	Drowsiness, lethargy, headaches, depression or apathy, irritability, confusion
Musculoskeletal	Paresthesia (tingling and numbness of the fingers), tetany or painful tonic muscle spasms, facial spasms, abdominal cramps, muscle cramps, spasmodic contractions	Weakness, muscle flaccidity, bone pain, pathologic fractures
Cardiovascular	Arrhythmias, hypotension	Signs of heart block, cardiac arrest in systole, hypertension
Gastrointestinal	Increased GI motility, diarrhea	Anorexia, nausea, vomiting, constipation, dehydration, polydipsia
Other	Blood-clotting abnormalities	Renal polyuria, flank pain, and, eventually, azotemia
SODIUM IMBALANCE	**HYPONATREMIA**	**HYPERNATREMIA**
Central nervous system	Anxiety, headaches, muscle twitching and weakness, convulsions	Fever, agitation, restlessness, convulsions
Cardiovascular	Hypotension; tachycardia; with severe deficit, vasomotor collapse, thready pulse	Hypertension, tachycardia, pitting edema, excessive weight gain
Gastrointestinal	Nausea, vomiting, abdominal cramps	Rough, dry tongue; intense thirst
Genitourinary	Oliguria or anuria	Oliguria
Respiratory	Cyanosis with severe deficiency	Dyspnea, respiratory arrest, and death (from dramatic rise in osmotic pressure)
Cutaneous	Cold clammy skin, decreased skin turgor	Flushed skin; dry, sticky mucous membranes

Reproduced, with permission, from Goodman CC, Snyder TK: Problems affecting multiple systems. In: Goodman CC, Boissonnault WG, Fuller KS, eds. *Pathology: Implications for the Physical Therapist, 2nd ed.* Philadelphia, PA: Saunders. 2003:85-119.

Urinary Incontinence. Urinary incontinence is an involuntary loss of urine that is sufficient to be a problem and which occurs most often when bladder pressure exceeds sphincter resistance. The following four categories can be used to classify urinary incontinence:[84]

- Functional incontinence: includes those individuals who have normal urine control but are unwilling (impaired cognition), or who have difficulty reaching a toilet in time (muscle or joint dysfunction or environmental barriers).
- Stress incontinence: the loss of urine during activities that increase intraabdominal pressure such as coughing, lifting, or laughing.
- Overflow incontinence: the constant leaking of urine from a bladder that is full but unable to empty:
  - Anatomic obstruction, eg, prostate enlargement.
  - Neurogenic bladder, eg, spinal cord injury (see Chapter 9).
- Urge incontinence: the sudden unexpected urge to urinate and the uncontrolled loss of urine; often related to reduced bladder capacity, detrusor instability, or hypersensitive bladder.

Medical management of urinary incontinence is aimed at prevention, and may include:

- Nutritional counseling to help prevent constipation and to encourage adequate hydration.
- Medications to relieve urge incontinence such as estrogen replacement therapy (ERT); anticholinergics; alpha-adrenergic blockers to increase bladder outlet/sphincter tone; antispasmodics, and combination therapy with tricyclic antidepressant agents and antidiuretic hormone.[88-92]
- Surgical intervention can include catheterization, penile clamps, and surgically implanted artificial sphincters and bladder generators, the latter of which sends impulses to the nerves that control the bladder function.

Physical Therapy Role. Physical therapists have an important direct role in the assessment and treatment intervention of urge and stress urinary incontinence:

- Patient education:
  - To avoid the Valsalva maneuver.
  - To avoid activities that strains the pelvic floor and abdominal muscles.
  - Exercise to improve control of pelvic floor and to maintain abdominal function, which are referred to as pelvic floor muscle (pubococcygeal muscle) exercises:[93-95] The most commonly prescribed exercises for this condition are Kegal exercises:
- Type 1—works on holding contractions, progressing to 10-second holds, rest 10 seconds between contractions.
- Type 2—works on quick contractions to shut off urine flow; 10 to 80 repetitions per day, while avoiding buttock squeezing, or contracting abdominals.

The patient is encouraged to incorporate Kegal exercises into everyday life, especially with lifting, coughing, laughing, changing positions, etc.

- Progressive strengthening of pelvic floor musculature:
  - Weighted vaginal cones.
  - Pelvic floor exercises.
- Biofeedback to reinforce active contraction-relaxation of bladder.[96]
- Functional electric stimulation for muscle reeducation of the bladder and pelvic floor muscles.[96]
- Noninvasive pulsed magnetic fields (extracorporeal magnetic innervation), which are used for pelvic floor muscle strengthening.[97]
- Education to preserve acceptable skin condition:[97]
  - Adequate protection—adult diapers, under pads.
- Maintenance of toileting schedule.
- Providing psychological and emotional support.

Study Pearl

- *Nephritis:* inflammation of the kidney tissue.
- *Glomerulonephritis:* inflammation of the glomeruli.
- *Pyelonephritis:* inflammation of the renal pelvis, the calycis, and the tubules from within one or both kidneys.

Renal Disorders

Pyelonephritis. Pyelonephritis, which is more common in women than in men, is an infectious, inflammatory disease involving the kidney, parenchyma, and renal pelvis.[84] *Escherichia coli* causes about 90% of cases of pyelonephritis.[98,99]

Although urine is typically sterile, the distal end of the urethra is commonly colonized by bacterial flora.[84] In a person with a healthy urinary tract, an infection is prevented from moving up the ureters into the kidneys by the regular flow of urine washing organisms out and by closure of the ureters at their entrance to the bladder.[98,99]

However, any physical obstruction to the flow of urine, such as a structural abnormality, kidney stone, or an enlarged prostate, or the backflow (reflux) of urine from the bladder into the ureters increases the likelihood of pyelonephritis.[98]

Study Pearl

During pregnancy, the enlarging uterus puts pressure on the ureters, which partially obstructs the normal downward flow of urine. Pregnancy also increases the risk of reflux of urine up the ureters by causing the ureters to dilate and reducing the muscle contractions that propel urine down the ureters into the bladder.[98,100]

The signs and symptoms of pyelonephritis often begin unexpectedly with chills, fever, pain in the lower part of the back (on either side), nausea, and vomiting.[98,99] In a long-standing infection (chronic pyelonephritis), the pain may be vague, and fever may fluctuate. Chronic pyelonephritis occurs only in people who have major underlying abnormalities, such as a urinary tract obstruction, large kidney stones that persist.[101]

Renal Cell Carcinoma. Adult kidney neoplasms account for approximately 2% of all adult cancers, with smoking and obesity being established risk factors for renal cell carcinomas.[84] Other risk factors include hypertension, reduced consumption of fruits and vegetables, and occupational exposure to substances such as solvents and asbestos.

The initial stages of this condition are generally insidious with symptoms associated with metastasis. The classic triad associated with renal cancer consists of hematuria, abdominal or flank pain, and a palpable abdominal mass.

Surgical intervention, including radical nephrectomy and regional lymph node dissection is the intervention of choice for all resectable tumors.

Physical therapists working primarily with the geriatric population need to be aware of the symptoms and signs of this disease. Questions and history related to hematuria, unexplained weight loss, fatigue, fever, and malaise are important with this population.

Renal Cystic Disease. A renal cyst is a cavity filled with fluid or renal tubular elements making up a semisolid material.[84] The four types of renal cystic disease are:[84]

- Polycystic kidney disease
- Medullary sponge kidney
- Acquired cystic disease
- Single or multiple cysts

Renal cysts are usually asymptomatic but may include pain, hematuria, fever, and hypertension. Physical therapists working with a patient with a history of renal cystic disease should be aware of symptoms and signs suggesting that the condition is worsening.[84]

Renal Calculi. Urinary stone disease is the third most common urinary tract disorder, exceeded only by infections and prostate disease.[84] Clinical manifestations include pain associated with urinary tract obstruction (renal colic), which usually occurs once the stone has moved out of the kidney into the ureter. The pain is usually acute and intolerable, located on the flank and upper outer abdominal quadrant.[84] Nausea and vomiting; urinary urgency and frequency; blood in the urine; and cool, clammy skin may also be present.[84]

Physical therapists need to be aware that depending on where the urinary collecting system is obstructed, the condition may only be manifested solely by unilateral back pain ranging from the thoracolumbar junction to the iliac crest.[84]

Acute Renal Failure. In acute renal failure, the ability of the kidneys to excrete waste and regulate the homeostasis of blood volume, pH, and electrolytes worsens over a short period of time (hours to days). There is a rise in serum urea and blood creatinine concentration, and a decrease in the renal plasma clearance of creatinine.

Chronic Renal Failure. Chronic renal failure (renal insufficiency or kidney failure) can be attributed to various conditions that result in permanent loss of nephrons, which in turn results in a progressive decline of glomerular filtration, tubular reabsorption, and the endocrine functions of the kidneys.[84] Diabetes mellitus and controlled or poorly controlled high blood pressure are the two leading causes of chronic renal failure.[84] Uremia is the term used to describe the clinical manifestations of the end-stage of renal disease—almost all body systems are involved, with a multitude of symptoms and signs being present (Table 12-9).

Dialysis. Dialysis is the mechanical process of diffusing blood across a semi-permeable membrane for the removal of toxic substances; fluid

TABLE 12-9. CHRONIC RENAL FAILURE: SUMMARY OF CLINICAL MANIFESTATIONS

SYSTEM	MANIFESTATIONS
General	Fatigue, weakness, decreased alertness, inability to concentrate
Skin	Pallor, ecchymosis, pruritis, dry skin and mucous membranes, thin/brittle fingernails, urine odor on skin
Hematologic	Anemia, tendency to bleed easily
Body fluids	Polyuria, nocturia, dehydration, hyperkalemia, metabolic acidosis, hypocalcemia, hyperphosphatemia
Ear, eye, nose, throat	Metallic taste in mouth, nosebleeds, urinous breath, pale conjunctiva
Pulmonary	Dyspnea, rales, pleural effusion
Cardiovascular	Dyspnea on exertion, hypertension, friction rub, retrosternal pain on inspiration
Gastrointestinal	Anorexia, nausea, vomiting, hiccups, gastrointestinal bleeding
Genitourinary	Impotence, amenorrhea, loss of libido
Skeletal	Osteomalacia, osteoporosis, bone pain, fracture, metastatic calcification of soft tissues, edema
Neurologic	Recent memory loss, coma, seizures, muscle tremors, paresthesias, muscle weakness, restless legs, cramping

Reproduced, with permission, from Boissonnault WG, Goodman CC: The renal and urologic systems. In: Goodman CC, Boissonnault WG, Fuller KS, eds. *Pathology: Implications for the Physical Therapist, 2nd ed.* Philadelphia, PA: Saunders. 2003:704-728.

maintenance, electrolyte, and acid–base balance in the presence of renal failure. The complications of dialysis are multiple and varied:[84]

- Dialysis disequilibrium: the result of drastic changes at the beginning of dialysis; manifested by symptoms of nausea, vomiting, drowsiness, headache, and seizures.
- Dialysis dementia: the result of chronic dialysis treatment; manifested by signs and symptoms of cerebral dysfunction including speech difficulties, mental confusion, seizures, and occasionally death.
- Loss of lean body mass: the result of the catabolism and anorexia associated with progressive renal failure. However, weight gain because of fluid retention can mask this loss of body mass.
- Increased susceptibility to infection: patients on dialysis are immunosuppressed, and the dialysis process requires vascular access for prolonged periods of time.
- Myopathy.
- Neuropathy.

Physical Therapy Role With Dialysis. Given the multiple and varied complications that can be associated with dialysis, the physical therapist must record vital signs regularly while the patient is exercising. Care must be taken when taking blood pressure to avoid the dialysis shunts (taking blood pressure at the shunt site is contraindicated) and to avoid trauma to the peritoneal catheters.

ENDOCRINE DISORDERS

The clinical manifestations of endocrine and metabolic disorders are fatigue, muscle weakness, and occasionally pain. These complaints may be early manifestations of diabetes, thyroid or parathyroid disease, acromegaly, Cushing syndrome (adrenal hyperfunction), or osteomalacia.

Diabetes Mellitus. Diabetes mellitus (DM) is a chronic disorder of carbohydrates, fats, and protein metabolism that is caused by a deficiency or absence of the insulin secreting beta cells of the pancreas, or by defects of the insulin receptors. Patients diagnosed with diabetes accounted for 6.2% of the US population in 2002.[102-104] The two basic types of diabetes mellitus are type 1 and type 2.

Type 1 (Insulin-Dependent Diabetes Mellitus). Type 1 DM or insulin-dependent diabetes mellitus (IDDM) is caused by a decrease in size and number of islet cells resulting in inadequate production of insulin.[105] Type 1 DM can occur at any age and is characterized by the marked inability of the pancreas to secrete insulin because of autoimmune destruction of the beta cells.

The distinguishing characteristic of a patient with type 1 DM, versus the type 2 is that, if the patient's insulin is withdrawn, ketosis and eventually ketoacidosis develop.[105] Therefore, these patients are dependent on exogenous insulin.

Type 2 (Formerly Called Adult-Onset Diabetes)/Non-Insulin-Dependent Diabetes Mellitus. Type 2 diabetes or non-insulin-dependent diabetes mellitus (NIDDM) is characterized by a gradual increase in peripheral insulin resistance with an insulin-secretory defect that varies in severity.[106] For type 2 diabetes to develop, both defects must exist: All overweight individuals have insulin resistance, but only those with an inability to increase beta-cell production of insulin develop diabetes.[106] About 90% of patients who develop type 2 diabetes are obese.[107] Type 2 DM is more prevalent among Hispanics, Native Americans, African Americans, and Asians/Pacific Islanders than in non-Hispanic whites.[107] The incidence is essentially equal in women and men in all populations.

Because patients with type 2 diabetes retain the ability to secrete some endogenous insulin, those who are taking insulin do not develop diabetic ketoacidosis (DKA) if they stop taking it for some reason. Therefore, they are considered to require insulin but not to be dependent on insulin.[107] Besides, patients with type 2 diabetes often do not need treatment with oral antidiabetic medication or insulin if they lose weight.[108] Patients with type 2 diabetes are often asymptomatic, and their disease remains undiagnosed for many years.

Subtypes of DM

- Maturity-onset diabetes of the young (MODY): a heterogeneous group of autosomal dominantly inherited, young-onset beta-cell disorders with an onset in individuals younger than 25 years.[109]
- Impaired glucose tolerance (IGT): asymptomatic or borderline diabetes with abnormal response to oral glucose test.[110,111] From 10% to 15% of individuals will convert to type 2 diabetes within 10 years.[110,111]
- Gestational diabetes mellitus (GDM) is defined as any degree of glucose intolerance with onset or first recognition during pregnancy.[112,113] GDM is a complication in about 4% of all pregnancies in the United States.[112,113]
- Prediabetes: the circumstances of having chronically high blood sugars but not meeting diagnostic criteria for diabetes.[114]

Prediabetes often precedes overt type 2 diabetes.[114] Prediabetes is defined by a fasting blood glucose level of 100-125 mg/dL.[114,115] Patients who have prediabetes have an increased risk for macrovascular disease, as well as diabetes.[114,115] Metabolic syndrome (also called syndrome X or the insulin-resistance syndrome) is often confused with prediabetes. Metabolic syndrome, thought to be because of insulin resistance, can occur in patients with overtly normal glucose tolerance, prediabetes, or diabetes.[116] It is characterized by central obesity, then by dyslipidemia.[116] Hypertension is a common feature.[116] Eventually, clinically obvious insulin resistance develops.[116]

Signs and Symptoms of DM. The classic signs and symptoms of DM include:

- Hyperglycemia (raised blood sugar)
- Glycosuria (raised sugar in the urine)
- Polyuria (excessive excretion of urine)
- Polydipsia (excessive thirst)
- Excessive hunger (polyphagia) and weight loss
- Fatigue

The morbidity and mortality associated with diabetes are related to the short- and long-term complications. Complications of DM include:

- Hypoglycemia:
  - Low blood sugar.
  - Usually has a rapid onset (within minutes).
  - Results from failure to eat after taking insulin, excessive insulin.
  - Can be precipitated by exercise.
  - Results in CNS changes (irritability, headache, blurred vision, slurred speech, difficulty concentrating, confusion, incoordination) and sympathetic changes (diaphoresis, pallor, piloerection, tachycardia, shakiness, hunger).
  - Hypoglycemic coma: a loss of consciousness that results from an abnormally low blood sugar level. If the patient is awake, give him or her some form of sugar (fruit juice, candy bar); if the patient is unresponsive, medical intervention is necessary.
- Hyperglycemia:
  - Abnormally high blood sugar.
  - Gradual onset (within days).
  - CNS changes: confused, diminished reflexes, paresthesia.
  - Fruity odor to the breath.
  - Weakness.
  - Complaints of thirst.
  - Rapid and weak pulse.
  - Rapid and deep respirations.
  - May lapse into hypoglycemic coma, which can lead to death.
  - Increased risk of infections and skin ulcerations.
  - Microvascular disease and complications (eg, retinopathy, nephropathy, myocardial infarction, stroke).[117,118]
  - Neuropathic complications (polyneuropathy) associated with long-term diabetes and poor glucose control.
  - Blindness.

Physical Therapy Role

Examination. A diabetes-focused examination includes vital signs, limited vascular and neurologic examinations, and a foot assessment. Other organ systems should be examined as indicated by the patient's clinical findings.

- Assessment of vital signs.
- Is the patient hypertensive or hypotensive?
- If the respiratory rate and pattern suggest Kussmaul respiration, diabetic ketoacidosis must be considered immediately, and an appropriate referral made.
- Foot examination.
- The dorsalis pedis and posterior tibialis pulses should be palpated and their presence or absence noted.
- Documenting lower extremity sensory neuropathy is useful in patients who present with foot ulcers.

Although physical therapists do not prescribe medications, being acquainted with the drugs used and their adverse effects and contraindications is useful (refer to Chapter 19).

Intervention

- Patient education: Education of the patient/family member should include:
  - Emphasis on proper diabetic foot care—good footwear, hygiene
  - Control of risk factors—obesity, physical inactivity, prolonged stress, smoking
  - Injury prevention strategies
  - Self-management strategies
- Exercise[102,103,119-123]: Exercise is another ingredient in the overall intervention plan as it has been shown to delay disease onset, improve blood glucose levels and circulation, reduce cardiovascular risk, and to aid in weight control and strength gains. The patient's exercise tolerance is dependent on the adequacy of disease control. As exercise can produce hypoglycemia, the following precautions must be taken:
  - The patient's glucose levels should be taken before and following exercise.
  - The patient should not exercise without eating at least 2 hours before exercise; as a precaution the physical therapist or patient should have a carbohydrate snack readily available during exercise.
  - Adequate hydration needs to be maintained both during and after the exercise session.
- The patient should not exercise when:
  - Blood glucose levels are high (at or near 250 mg/dL) or if their blood glucose levels are poorly controlled.
  - If the urine test is positive for ketones.
  - The exercise environment is not at a comfortable temperature.

Thyroid Disorders

The thyroid gland is located in the base of the neck on both sides of the lower part of the larynx and upper part of the trachea. Thyroid diseases can be broadly divided into hyperthyroidism and hypothyroidism.

Hyperthyroidism. *Hyperthyroidism* occurs because of an imbalance of metabolism caused by overproduction of thyroid hormone (hyperthyroidism).[124-126] Hyperthyroidism or thyrotoxicosis occurs when the thyroid releases too many of its hormones over a short (acute) or long (chronic) period of time. Many diseases and conditions can cause this problem, including:

- Grave disease (accounts for 85% of all cases of hyperthyroidism)
- Noncancerous growths of the thyroid gland
- Tumors of the testes or ovaries
- Inflammation (irritation and swelling) of the thyroid because of viral infections or other causes
- Ingestion of excessive amounts of iodine, or excessive amounts of thyroid hormone
- Underproduction of thyroid hormone (hypothyroidism)
- Benign (noncancerous) thyroid disease
- Thyroid cancer

Symptoms associated with hyperthyroidism include:

- Nervousness
- Hyperreflexia
- Weight loss
- Hunger
- Heat intolerance
- Palpitations
- Bounding pulse/tachycardia
- Diarrhea
- Increase in metabolic processes
- Possible exercise intolerance

Hyperthyroidism is usually treated with antithyroid medications, radioactive iodine (which destroys the thyroid and thus stops the excess production of hormones), or surgery to remove the thyroid.

Hypothyroidism. *Hypothyroidism*, the most common pathologic hormone deficiency, is usually a primary process resulting from failure of the gland to produce adequate amounts of hormone.[127-130] It may also be caused by a lack of thyroid hormone secretion secondary to the failure of adequate thyrotropin (ie, thyroid-stimulating hormone [TSH]) secretion from the pituitary gland or thyrotropin-releasing hormone (TRH) from the hypothalamus (secondary or tertiary hypothyroidism). Cretinism refers to congenital hypothyroidism. The signs and symptoms associated with a hypothyroidism include:

- Weight gain
- Increased appetite
- Lethargy and fatigue
- Low blood pressure
- Cold intolerance
- Dry skin and hair
- Possible presence of goiter (visibly enlarged thyroid)
- Possible exercise intolerance and exercise-induced myalgia
- Reduced cardiac output

Hypothyroidism is usually treated with lifelong thyroid replacement therapy.

Parathyroid Disorders

Hyperparathyroidism.[127]

- *Primary hyperparathyroidism (HPT)* is defined as an abnormal hypersecretion of parathyroid hormone (PTH), producing hypercalcemia and hyperphosphatemia.[131-134] Primary HPT is the most common cause of elevated PTH and calcium levels. Approximately 85% of cases are found to be caused by an isolated adenoma, 15% caused by diffuse hyperplasia, and less than 1% by parathyroid carcinoma.
- Secondary HPT is a compensatory hyperfunctioning of the parathyroid glands caused by hypocalcemia or peripheral resistance to PTH. As opposed to primary HPT, treating the underlying cause can reverse secondary HPT. Secondary HPT is often associated with a patient with end-organ failure from chronic renal insufficiency, with hypocalcemia and hyperphosphatemia. Less commonly, it may be caused by calcium malabsorption, osteomalacia, vitamin D deficiency, or deranged vitamin D metabolism.
- Tertiary HPT occurs in a setting of previous secondary HPT in which the glandular hyperfunction and hypersecretion continue despite correction of the underlying abnormality, as in renal transplantation.
- Familial hypocalciuric hypercalcemia (FHH) is a disease with an autosomal dominant mode of inheritance. The exact mechanism of the disease is not known, but it appears that affected individuals have an abnormal calcium sensor.

Hypoparathyroidism.[127] *Hypoparathyroidism* is an uncommon congenital or acquired condition in which PTH secretion is deficient or absent.[135-137] Hypocalcemia and hyperphosphatemia are usually present. By far, hypoparathyroidism most commonly results from an iatrogenic cause; it usually follows parathyroid surgery or total thyroidectomy. Some cases of hypoparathyroidism categorized as idiopathic may have an autoimmune basis and other endocrine deficiencies; T-cell dysfunction also may be involved.

Acromegaly. *Acromegaly* is the result of increased and unregulated growth hormone (GH) production, usually caused by a GH-secreting pituitary tumor (somatotroph tumor).[138-146] More than 95% of acromegaly cases are caused by a pituitary adenoma. The pathologic effects of GH excess include acral overgrowth (ie, macrognathia; enlargement of the facial bone structure; enlarged hands and feet; visceral overgrowth, including macroglossia and enlarged heart muscle, thyroid, liver, kidney), insulin antagonism, nitrogen retention, and increased risk of colon polyps/tumors.

Symptoms develop insidiously, taking from years to decades to become apparent, with a mean duration of symptom onset to diagnosis of 12 years. Excess GH produces a myriad of signs and symptoms and significantly increases morbidity and mortality rates.

Study Pearl

The principal hormones produced by the adrenal cortex are cortisol (hydrocortisone), aldosterone, and dehydroepiandrosterone (DHEA). The adrenal cortex also secretes male sex hormones, glucocorticoids, and mineralocorticoids.

ADRENAL DISORDERS

Located on top of both kidneys, the adrenal glands are triangular shaped and measure approximately ½ in. in height and 3 in. in length. The inner part is called the adrenal medulla, while the outer portion is called the adrenal cortex.

Dysfunction of the adrenal cortex can be classified according to hypofunction or hyperfunction:

Hypofunction (Addison Disease). Addison disease occurs when the adrenal glands do not produce enough of the cortisol hormone and in some cases, the aldosterone hormone.[147-150] For this reason, the disease is sometimes called *chronic adrenal insufficiency*, or *hypocortisolism*.

Addison disease is characterized by an increased excretion of sodium and decreased excretion of potassium, chiefly in the urine, which is isotonic, and also in the sweat, saliva, and GI tract. Low blood concentrations of sodium and chloride and a high concentration of serum potassium result. Inability to concentrate the urine, combined with changes in electrolyte balance, produces severe dehydration, plasma hypertonicity, acidosis, decreased circulatory volume, hypotension, and eventual circulatory collapse.

Common signs and symptoms associated with Addison's disease include weight loss, muscle weakness, fatigue, low blood pressure (dizziness and syncope), and sometimes darkening of the skin. Adrenal crisis, a medical emergency, is characterized by profound asthenia; severe pains in the abdomen, lower back, or legs; peripheral vascular collapse; and, finally, renal shutdown.

Other causes of adrenal hypofunction include destruction of the adrenal gland by granuloma (eg, tuberculosis, which has become increasingly common recently, especially in developing countries), tumor, amyloidosis, or inflammatory necrosis.

Hyperfunction. Hypersecretion of one or more adrenocortical hormones produces distinct clinical syndromes:

- Excessive production of androgens results in adrenal virilism[151,152]: In adult women, adrenal virilism is caused by adrenal hyperplasia or an adrenal tumor. Whether involving a male or female, the symptoms and signs include hirsutism, baldness, acne, deepening of the voice, amenorrhea, atrophy of the uterus, clitoral hypertrophy, decreased breast size, and increased muscularity.
- Hypersecretion of glucocorticoids produces Cushing syndrome[153-159]:
  - Cushing syndrome has been applied to the clinical picture resulting from cortisol excess regardless of the cause, hyperfunction of the adrenal cortex resulting from pituitary ACTH excess has frequently been referred to as Cushing disease, implying a particular physiologic abnormality.
- Patients with Cushing disease may have a basophilic or a chromophobe adenoma of the pituitary gland.
- Clinical manifestations of Cushing disease include rounded "moon" facies with a plethoric appearance. There is truncal obesity with prominent supraclavicular and dorsal cervical fat

pads (buffalo hump); the distal extremities and fingers are usually quite slender. Muscle wasting and weakness are commonly present. The skin is thin and atrophic, with poor wound healing and easy bruising. Purple striae may appear on the abdomen. Hypertension, renal calculi, osteoporosis, glucose intolerance, reduced resistance to infection, and psychiatric disturbances are common. Cessation of linear growth is characteristic in children. Females usually have menstrual irregularities. In adrenal tumors, an increased production of androgens, in addition to cortisol, may lead to hypertrichosis, temporal balding, and other signs of virilism in the female.

- Excess aldosterone output results in hyperaldosteronism (aldosteronism).[160-164] Aldosterone secretion is regulated by the renin-angiotensin mechanism and to a lesser extent by ACTH.
- Primary aldosteronism (Conn syndrome) is due to an adenoma, usually unilateral, of the glomerulosa cells of the adrenal cortex or, more rarely, to an adrenal carcinoma or hyperplasia.
- Hypersecretion of aldosterone may result in hypernatremia, hyperchlorhydria, hypervolemia, and a hypokalemic alkalosis manifested by episodic weakness, paresthesias, transient paralysis, and tetany. Diastolic hypertension and a hypokalemic nephropathy with polyuria and polydipsia are common.
- Secondary aldosteronism, an increased production of aldosterone by the adrenal cortex caused by stimuli originating outside the adrenal, mimics the primary condition and is related to hypertension and edematous disorders (eg, cardiac failure, cirrhosis with ascites, the nephrotic syndrome).

Metabolic Disorders

Osteoporosis. Refer to Chapter 8.

Osteomalacia. Refer to Chapter 8

Paget Disease. Refer to Chapter 8.

OBSTETRICS AND GYNECOLOGY

An obstetrician is a physician who specializes in the management of pregnancy, labor, and postpartum care.[165] Many terms are used in obstetrics to describe the number of pregnancies and deliveries and the stages of pregnancy, labor, and postpartum phase (Table 12-10).

Physiologic Changes That Occur During Pregnancy

A number of physiologic changes occur during pregnancy and the postpartum period within the various body systems.

Endocrine System. Changes that occur in the endocrine system include, but are not limited to the following:

TABLE 12-10. CLASSIFICATION OF MATERNAL CIRCUMSTANCE BY NUMBER OF PREGNANCIES, LIVE BIRTH, AND PERIOD DURING THE CHILDBEARING YEAR

TERM	DEFINITION
Nullipara	A woman who has not been pregnant or has never completed a pregnancy beyond 20 weeks of gestation
Primipara	A woman who has had one delivery beyond 20 weeks of gestation
Multipara	A woman who has delivered two or more pregnancies beyond 20 weeks of gestation regardless of whether the fetuses were born alive or stillborn (not the number of fetuses delivered)
Nulligravida	A woman who is not now or who never has been pregnant
Primigravida	A woman who has been pregnant once, regardless of outcome
Multigravida	A woman who has had more than one pregnancy, regardless of the outcome. The number represents the number of pregnancies
Postpartum	The period after childbirth
Puerperal	The period from the end of labor until the uterus return to prepregnancy size, generally from 3-6 weeks postpartum. Puerpera refers to woman who has just delivered
Gestation	Duration of the pregnancy, usually 280 days, or 40 weeks, marked from the first day of the last menstrual period
Trimesters	Division of weeks of pregnancy: first, 1-13 weeks; second, 14-17 weeks; third, 28-40 weeks
EDC/EDD	"Expected date of confinement" (EDC) is an old-fashioned term indicating the date a woman was expected to deliver and be confined. A more modern term, estimated date of delivery (EDD) is now commonly used
Parturient	A woman in labor
Preterm labor	Labor that starts after the 20th but before the 37th week
Term labor	Labor initiated after the 37th week of pregnancy but before the 42nd week
Postterm/postdates	Labor initiated after the 37th week of pregnancy but before the 42nd week

Reproduced, with permission, from Boissonnault J, Stephenson R: The obstetric patient. In: Boissonnault WG, ed. *Primary Care for the Physical Therapist: Examination and Triage*. St Louis: Elsevier Saunders. 2005:239-270.

- The adrenal, thyroid, parathyroid, and pituitary glands enlarge.
- Increase in hormone levels to support the pregnancy and the placenta, and to prepare the mother's body for labor. For example, a female hormone (relaxin) is released that assists in the softening of the pubic symphysis so that during delivery, the female pelvis can stretch enough to allow birth. However, these hormonal changes are also thought to induce a greater laxity in all joints.[166,167] This can result in:
  - Joint hypermobility, especially throughout the pelvic ring as it relies heavily on ligamentous support[168]
  - Symphysis pubic dysfunction (SPD) (see Complications Associated with Pregnancy)
  - SIJ dysfunction (see Complications Associated with Pregnancy)
  - Increased susceptibility to injury

Musculoskeletal System. The average pregnancy weight gain is 20 to 30 lb.[169] This weight change can produce a number of changes within the musculoskeletal system:

- The abdominal muscles are stretched and weakened as pregnancy develops (see Complications Associated with Pregnancy).
- The rib cage circumference increases, increasing the subcostal angle and the transverse diameter.
- Pelvic floor weakness can develop with advanced pregnancy and childbirth. This can result in stress incontinence (refer to Urinary Incontinence in Genitourinary section).

- Postural changes related to the weight of growing breasts, and the uterus and fetus, which can result in a shift in the woman's center of gravity in an anterior and superior direction. In advanced pregnancy, the patient develops a wider base of support and has increased difficulty with walking, stair climbing, and rapid changes in position. Specific postural changes include:[170]
  - Thoracic kyphosis with scapular retraction
  - Increased cervical lordosis and forward head
  - Increased lumbar lordosis

Study Pearl

Pregnant females should be taught correct body mechanics, and postural exercises to stretch, strengthen, and train postural muscles.

Due to the alterations in ligament extensibility, postural changes become more significant.

Table 12-11 contains a partial list of symptoms during pregnancy that may result from musculoskeletal dysfunction or from medical conditions.[165]

TABLE 12-11. SYMPTOMS THAT CAN MIMIC MUSCULOSKELETAL CONDITIONS IN PREGNANCY

SYMPTOMS	POSSIBLE MEDICAL CONDITION	POSSIBLE MUSCULOSKELETAL DYSFUNCTION	DIFFERENTIATING TESTS OR MEASURES
Calf, proximal thigh, or inguinal pain	Deep vein thrombosis	Gastrosoleus sprain; radicular symptoms from nerve root impingement; compartment syndrome; pubic symphysis dysfunction	Duplex ultrasonography; positive Homan sign; assessment of response to treatment and provocation of pain by musculoskeletal examination of the pelvis and lower quadrant
Urinary incontinence	Urinary tract infection	Pelvic floor muscle dysfunction; cauda equina syndrome	Urinalysis; assessment of onset (acute or gradual) and aggravating factors
Lower abdominal pain	Abruption of the placenta; ectopic pregnancy	Pubic symphysis dysfunction (shear or separation)	Assessment of nature of pain (constant or intermittent) and aggravating factors; provocation of pain by musculoskeletal assessment of the pelvis; diagnostic ultrasound
Lower back pain or hip pain	Osteoporosis of pregnancy with or without fracture	Mechanical dysfunction of the lower back or pelvic ring; disk disease; spondylolisthesis	Height assessment; pain pattern assessment; objective findings (provocation tests, palpatory findings, neurologic findings, end-feels)
Flank pain	Upper urinary tract infection (kidney)	Rib or thoracic spine dysfunction	Percussion over the ribs; assessment of response to treatment and provocation of pain by musculoskeletal examination of the thorax; fever assessment; urinalysis
Right upper quadrant/ scapular pain	Gallstones	Shoulder girdle or thoracic spine/rib dysfunction	Diagnostic ultrasound; assessment of response to treatment and nature of symptoms (whether pain is constant or provoked by activity)
Headache	Pregnancy-induced hypertension or preeclampsia	Upper cervical dysfunction or tension-type headache	Blood-pressure assessment for hypertension; signs of recent onset of edema; provocation of headache by musculoskeletal assessment of the upper cervical spine

Reproduced, with permission, from Boissonnault JS, Stephenson R: The obstetric patient. In: Boissonnault WG, ed. *Primary Care for the Physical Therapist: Examination and Triage.* St Louis, MO: Elsevier Saunders. 2005:239-270.

Neurologic System. Swelling and increased fluid volume can cause nerve compression of the thoracic outlet, wrists, or groin (brachial plexus, median nerve, and lateral [femoral] cutaneous nerve of the thigh, respectively).[171-173]

Gastrointestinal System. Nausea and vomiting may occur in early pregnancy, and are generally confined to the first 16 weeks of pregnancy but occasionally remain throughout the entire 10 lunar months (see Complications Associated with Pregnancy).[165,174-177] Other changes related to the gastrointestinal system include:[174-177]

- A slowing of intestinal motility.
- The development of constipation, abdominal bloating, and hemorrhoids.
- Esophageal reflux.
- Heartburn (pyrosis). About 50% to 80% of women report heartburn during pregnancy, with its incidence peaking in the third trimester.[165]
- An increase in the incident and symptoms of gallbladder disease.

Respiratory System. Adaptive changes that occur in the pulmonary system during pregnancy include:

- The diaphragm elevates with a widening of the thoracic cage. This results in a predominance of costal versus abdominal breathing.
- Mild increases in tidal volume and oxygen consumption, which is caused by increased respiratory center sensitivity (see Chapter 10) and drive due to the increased oxygen requirement of the fetus.[178] With mild exercise, pregnant women have a greater increase in respiratory frequency and oxygen consumption to meet their greater oxygen demand.[178] As exercise increases to moderate and then maximal levels, however, pregnant women demonstrate decreased respiratory frequency, lower tidal volume, and maximal oxygen consumption.[178]
- A compensated respiratory alkalosis (see Chapter 10).[179]
- A low expiratory reserve volume (see Chapter 11). The vital capacity and measures of forced expiration are well preserved.[178,180]

Cardiovascular System. The pregnancy-induced changes in the cardiovascular system develop primarily to meet the increased metabolic demands of the mother and fetus. These include:

- Increased blood volume: increases progressively from 6- to 8-week gestation (pregnancy) and reaches a maximum at approximately 32 to 34 weeks with little change thereafter.[181] The increased blood volume serves two purposes:[182,183]
  - It facilitates maternal and fetal exchanges of respiratory gases, nutrients, and metabolites.
  - It reduces the impact of maternal blood loss at delivery. Typical losses of 300 to 500 mL for vaginal births and 750 to 1000 mL for caesarean sections are thus compensated with

the so-called "autotransfusion" of blood from the contracting uterus.

- Increased plasma volume (40%-50%) is relatively greater than that of red cell mass (20%-30%) resulting in hemodilution and a decrease in hemoglobin concentration (intake of supplemental iron and folic acid is necessary to restore hemoglobin levels to normal, ie, 12 g/dL).[182,184,185]
- Increased cardiac output: increases to a similar degree as the blood volume.[182,183] During the first trimester cardiac output is 30% to 40% higher than in the nonpregnant state.[184] During labor, further increases are seen. The heart is enlarged by both chamber dilation and hypertrophy.

Metabolic System. Because of the increased demand for tissue growth, insulin is elevated from plasma expansion, and blood glucose is reduced for a given insulin load. The metabolic rate increases during both exercise and pregnancy, resulting in greater heat production. Fetoplacental metabolism generates additional heat, which maintains fetal temperature at 0.5°C to 1.0°C (0.9°F to 1.8°F) above maternal levels.[186-188]

Renal and Urologic Systems. During pregnancy, the renal threshold for glucose drops because of an increase in the glomerular filtration rate (GFR) and there is an increase in sodium and water retention.[165] Anatomic and hormonal changes during pregnancy place the pregnant woman at risk for both lower and upper UTIs and for urinary incontinence.[165] As the fetus grows, stress on the mother's bladder can occur. This can result in urinary incontinence (refer to Urinary Incontinence under the Genitourinary section in this chapter).

COMPLICATIONS ASSOCIATED WITH PREGNANCY

Hypertension. Hypertensive disorders complicating pregnancy are the most common medical risk factor responsible for maternal morbidity and death related to pregnancy.[165] Hypertensive disorders complicating pregnancy have been divided into five types (Table 12-12).

Symphysis Pubis Dysfunction (SPD) and Diastasis Symphysis Pubis (DSP).[189-192]. The symptoms of SPD and DSP vary from person to person. On examination, the patient typically demonstrates an antalgic, waddling gait. Subjectively the patient reports pelvic pain with any activity that involves lifting one leg at a time or parting the legs. Lifting the leg to put on clothes, getting out of a car, turning over in bed, sitting down or getting up, walking up stairs, and standing on one leg are all painful. Patients may also report that the hip joint seems stuck in place or they describe having to wait for it to "pop into place" before being able to walk. Palpation reveals anterior pubic symphyseal tenderness. Occasional clicking can be felt or heard. The findings on the physical examination include positive sacroiliac joint stress tests (compression, distraction, and FABER tests). The range of hip movements will be limited by pain, and there is an inability to stand on one leg. Characteristic pain can often be evoked by bilateral pressure on the trochanters or by hip flexion with the knees in extension. However, such maneuvers may result in severe pain or muscle spasm and are not necessary for diagnosis. Radiological

Study Pearl

Changes in blood pressure during pregnancy include:

- Systemic arterial pressure is never increased during normal gestation.
- Pulmonary arterial pressure also maintains a constant level.
- Vascular tone is more dependent upon sympathetic control than in the nonpregnant state, so that hypotension develops more readily and more markedly.
- Central venous and brachial venous pressures remain unchanged during pregnancy, but femoral venous pressure is progressively increased due to mechanical factors.

TABLE 12-12. SUMMARY OF TYPES OF HYPERTENSION DURING PREGNANCY

DISORDER/INCIDENCE	DEFINITION	DIAGNOSTIC CRITERIA	SIGNS/SYMPTOMS
Gestational hypertension: affects nulliparous women most often	Diagnoses made retrospectively when preeclampsia does not develop and blood pressure returns to normal by the 12th week postpartum	Blood pressure 140/90 mm Hg or greater for the first time during pregnancy; no proteinuria; blood pressure returns to normal by 12 weeks postpartum	Epigastric pain, thrombocytopenia, headache
Preeclampsia: 5% incidence influenced by parity, race, ethnicity, and environmental factors	A life-threatening disorder that occurs only during pregnancy and the postpartum period (in at least 5% of all pregnancies) and affects both the mother and the unborn baby. The syndrome involves reduced organ perfusion from vasospasm and endothelial activation	Blood pressure 140/90 mm Hg or greater after 20-weeks gestation; proteinuria: 300 mg or more of urinary protein in a 24-hour period or persistent 30 mg/dL in random urine samples	The more severe the hypertension or proteinuria, the more certain is the severity of preeclampsia; symptoms of eclampsia, such as headache, cerebral visual disturbance, and epigastric pain can occur
Eclampsia: 1 in 3250 in United States (1998)	Seizures in a pregnant woman with preeclampsia not assigned to other causes	Grand mal seizures appearing before, during, or after labor; in nulliparas, seizures may develop 48 hours to 10 days after delivery	Mother may develop abruptio placentae, neurological deficits, aspiration pneumonia, pulmonary edema, cardiopulmonary arrest, acute renal failure; maternal death
Superimposed preeclampsia on chronic hypertension	Chronic hypertensive disorders predispose the development of superimposed preeclampsia or eclampsia	New-onset proteinuria of 300 mg or more in 24 hours in hypertensive women; no proteinuria before 20-weeks gestation	The risk of abruptio placentae; fetus at risk for growth restriction and death
Chronic hypertension: strong familial history of essential hypertension and/or multiparous women with hypertension complicated by a previous pregnancy beyond the first one	Hypertension that persists longer than 12 weeks after delivery	Blood pressure 140/90 mm Hg or greater before pregnancy; hypertension 140/90 mm Hg or greater detected before 20- weeks, gestation; persistent hypertension long after delivery	Risk of abruptio placentae; fetus at risk for growth restriction and death; pulmonary edema; hypertensive encephalopathy; renal failure

Data from Boissonnault JS, Stephenson R: The obstetric patient. In: Boissonnault WG, ed. *Primary Care for the Physical Therapist: Examination and Triage.* St Louis: Elsevier Saunders. 2005: 239-270. American College of Obstetrics and Gynecology. Practice bulletin 29: chronic hypertension in pregnancy. *Obstet Gynecol.* 2001;98:177-185. Cunningham FG, Gant NF, Leveno KJ, et al. *Williams Obstetrics,* 21st ed. New York: McGraw-Hill; 2001:1210-1220. Livingston JC, Baha MS: Chronic hypertension in pregnancy. *Obstet Gynecol Clin North Am.* 2001;28:447-463. Terry MB, Perrin M, Salafia CM, et al. Preeclampsia, pregnancy-related hypertension, and breast cancer risk. *Am J Epidemiol.* 2007 May 1;165(9):1007-1014. Anderson CM: Preeclampsia: exposing future cardiovascular risk in mothers and their children. *J Obstet Gynecol Neonatal Nurs.* 2007;36:3-8. Barton JR, Sibai BM: Life-threatening emergencies in preeclampsia-eclampsia. *J Ky Med Assoc.* 2006;104:410-418. Lindheimer MD, Umans JG: Explaining and predicting preeclampsia. *N Engl J Med.* 2006;355:1056-1058. Arafeh JM: Preeclampsia: pieces of the puzzle revealed. *J Perinat Neonatal Nurs.* 2006;20:85-87.

evaluation may occasionally be useful in confirming the diagnosis.[193] The amount of symphyseal separation does not always correlate with the severity of symptoms or the degree of disability. Therefore, the intervention is based on the severity of symptoms rather than the degree of separation as measured by imaging studies.[193]

A conservative management approach is often effective in cases of SPD. In more severe cases, the interventions can include bed rest in the lateral decubitus position, pelvic support with a brace or girdle, ambulation with assistance or devices such as walkers and graded exercise protocols.[193] In all cases, patient education is extremely important in terms of providing advice on how to avoid stress to the area. Many of the suggestions to give include:

- Use a pillow between the legs when sleeping.
- Move slowly and without sudden movements. Keep the legs and hips parallel and as symmetrical as possible when moving or turning in standing. Silk/satin sheets and night garments may make it easier to turn over in bed.
- A waterbed mattress may be helpful.
- When standing, stand symmetrically, with the weight evenly distributed through both legs. Avoid "straddle" movements.
- Sit down to get dressed, especially when putting on underwear or pants.
- An ice pack may feel soothing and help reduce inflammation in the pubic area.

> **Study Pearl**
>
> Symphysis pubic dysfunction (SPD) should always be considered when examining patients in the postpartum period who are experiencing suprapubic, sacroiliac, or thigh pain.

Swimming may help relieve pressure on the joint (the breaststroke may prove aggravating). Deep-water aerobics or deep-water running using floatation devices may also be helpful.

The most common outcome in SDP and DSP is the resolution of symptoms in approximately 6 to 8 weeks with no lasting sequela.[193] Occasionally, patients report residual pain requiring several months of physical therapy but long-term impairment is unusual. Surgical intervention is rarely required but may be utilized in cases of inadequate reduction, recurrent diastasis, or persistent symptoms.

Low Back Pain. Low back pain is said to occur in 50% to 90% of pregnant women.[170,194-201] However, it is not clear whether the low back pain is the result of the shift in the center of gravity and concomitant changes in the spinal curvature.

> **Study Pearl**
>
> It is worth remembering that complaints of low back pain in this population may be because of a kidney or urinary tract infection.

Coccydynia. *Coccygeal pain*, pain in and around the region of the coccyx, is relatively common postpartum.[202-206] Symptoms include pain with sitting. The patient should be provided with seating adaptation (donut cushion) to lessen the weight on the coccyx and to support the lumbar lordosis.

If symptoms persist for more than a few weeks, the displaced coccyx can often be corrected manually by grasping the coccyx after inserting the index finger in the anal canal. The coccyx is distracted and pulled posteriorly, while pulling laterally on the medial surface of the ischial tuberosity.

Gestational Diabetes. *Gestational diabetes* is defined as carbohydrate intolerance of variable severity, with onset or first recognition during pregnancy. After the birth, blood sugars usually return to normal levels; however, frank diabetes often develops later in life. Typical causes include:

- Genetic predisposition.
- High-risk populations include Aboriginal people, people of Hispanic, Asian, or African descent.
- Family history of diabetes, gestational diabetes, or glucose intolerance.

- Increased tissue resistance to insulin during pregnancy, caused by increased levels of estrogen and progesterone.

Current risk factors include:

- Maternal obesity (> 20% above ideal weight)
- Excessive weight gain during pregnancy
- Low level of high-density-lipoprotein (HDL) cholesterol (< 0.9 mmol/L) or elevated fasting level of triglycerides (> 2.8 mmol/L)
- Hypertension or preeclampsia (risk for gestational diabetes is increased to 10%-15% when hypertension is diagnosed)
- Maternal age > 25 years

Most individuals with gestational diabetes are asymptomatic. However, subjectively the patient may complain of:

- Polydipsia
- Polyuria
- Polyphagia
- Weight loss

Diastasis Recti Abdominis. *Diastasis recti abdominis* is defined as a lateral separation of greater than two fingertip widths of the two bellies of the rectus abdominis at the linea alba (or linea nigra, in pregnancy).

If diastasis recti abdominis is confirmed, corrective exercises need to be performed to prevent further muscle trauma. The patient can perform any exercise that does not increase intra-abdominal pressure including partial sit-ups, posterior pelvic tilts while using hands to support the abdominal wall and transverses abdominis exercises. Traditional abdominal exercises, such as full sit-ups or bilateral straight leg raises can be resumed when the separation is less than 2 cm.

Cesarean Childbirth. Cesarean delivery, also known as cesarean section, is a major abdominal surgery involving two incisions:

- An incision through the abdominal wall
- An incision involving the uterus to deliver the baby

Although the physical therapist is not involved in the surgical procedure, they can play an important role postoperatively:

- TENS can be prescribed to decrease incisional pain (electrodes are placed parallel to the incision).
- Patient education:
  - Correct breathing and coughing to prevent postsurgical pulmonary complications
  - Heavy lifting precautions (4-6 weeks), use of pillow for incisional support
  - Instruction on transverse fictional massage to prevent incisional adhesions
  - Ambulation

- Exercise:
  - Postural exercises
  - Pelvic floor exercises
  - Gentle abdominal exercises

Hyperemesis Gravidarum. The causes of this condition are largely unknown. Indications that the patient may have this condition include persistent and excessive nausea and vomiting throughout the day and an inability to keep down any solids or liquids. If the condition is prolonged, the patient may also report:[174,177]

- Fatigue, lethargy
- Headache
- Faintness

Various degrees of dehydration may be present: skin may be pale, there may be dark circles under eyes, eyes may appear sunken, mucous membranes may be dry, skin turgor may be poor.[174,177]

Supine Hypotension. Supine hypotension (also known as inferior vena cava syndrome) may develop in the supine position, especially after the first trimester. The decrease in blood pressure is thought to be caused by the occlusion of the aorta and inferior vena cava by the increased weight and size of the uterus. Spontaneous recovery usually occurs upon a change in maternal position. However, patients should not be allowed to stand up quickly to decrease the potential for hypotension. Signs and symptoms of this condition include:

- Bradycardia
- Shortness of breath
- Syncope (fainting)
- Dizziness
- Nausea and vomiting
- Sweating or cold, clammy skin
- Headache
- Numbness in extremities
- Weakness
- Restlessness

Psychiatric Changes. Pregnancy-related depression and postpartum depression may occur. Postnatal depression has been documented to occur in 5% to 20% of all postpartum mothers,[207-209] but can also occur in fathers.[210] Depressive postpartum disorders range from "postpartum blues," which occurs from 1 to 5 days after birth and lasts for only a few days, to postpartum depression and postpartum psychosis, the latter two of which are more serious conditions and require medical or social intervention to avoid serious ramifications of the family unit.[165,211,212]

PHYSICAL THERAPY EXAMINATION

Special questions for the pregnant patients should include the following:[165]

- Have you had any complications with the pregnancy? Complications include those previously mentioned. A positive response to this question may alter the rigor of the physical examination and any exercise prescribed. It may also necessitate monitoring of vital signs and other signs and symptoms with each visit.

- Have you had any complications with a previous pregnancy or delivery that is placing you at high risk now? For example, preterm labor in one pregnancy places a woman at risk for similar outcome in subsequent pregnancies.
- Did you have any of your current musculoskeletal symptoms during a previous pregnancy, and, if so, what was done for them, and was the treatment successful?
- Which medications are you currently taking and what medications did you stop taking because of the pregnancy? Many prescription and some over-the-counter medications and herbal remedies are contraindicated in pregnancy because of the risk to the fetus or the mother. Medications such as nonsteroidal anti-inflammatories, antidepressants, and migraine prescriptions are contraindicated in pregnancy. Herbal remedies containing aloe, cascara, anthraquinone, or phenolphthalein should be avoided.
- Do you currently have any urinary stress incontinence? Recognition of this condition will help a physical therapist and patient with the intervention before and after delivery.

PHYSICAL THERAPY INTERVENTION

Given the number of physiologic changes that occur during pregnancy and the postpartum period within the various body systems, the extent of the physical therapy intervention will depend on the findings of the examination. Therapeutic exercise seems to play a key role with this patient population.

Both exercise and pregnancy are associated with a high demand for energy. Caloric demands with exercise are even higher. The competing energy demands of the exercising mother and the growing fetus raise the theoretic concern that excessive exercise might adversely affect fetal development.[165] Theoretically, because of the physiologic changes associated with pregnancy, as well as the hemodynamic response to exercise, some precautions should be observed during exercise:[213-220]

- Exercise activity should occur at a moderate rate during a low-risk pregnancy. Guidelines permit women to remain at 50% to 60% of their maximal heart rate (monitored intermittently) for approximately 30 minutes per session.
- Increases in joint laxity due to changes in hormonal levels may lead to a higher risk of strains or sprains, so weight-bearing exercises should be prescribed judiciously.
- Women should avoid becoming overtired and should not exercise in the supine position for more than a few minutes after the first trimester (see Supine Hypotension).
- Positions that involve abdominal compression (flat prone lying) should be avoided in mid-to-late pregnancy.
- Adequate hydration and appropriate ventilation are important in preventing the possible teratogenic effects of overheating.

Study Pearl

Warning signs associated with exercise during pregnancy include:

- Pain
- Vaginal bleeding
- Dizziness, feeling faint
- Tachycardia
- Dyspnea
- Chest pain
- Uterine contractions

COMPLEX DISORDERS

Complex disorders include those poorly understood syndromes that do not fit the traditional allopathic model of illness with specific etiology and pathogenesis.

Chronic Fatigue Syndrome.[221-226] *Chronic fatigue syndrome* (CFS) is characterized by debilitating fatigue, neurological problems, and a variety of flu-like symptoms. In the past the syndrome has been known as chronic Epstein-Barr virus (CEBV).

In addition to the eight core symptoms of CFS, other signs and symptoms include, but are not limited to:

- Jaw pain
- Morning stiffness
- Psychological problems, such as depression, irritability, anxiety disorders, and panic attacks
- Tingling sensations

The severity of CFS can differ widely among patients, and can also vary over time for the same patient, which makes CFS difficult to diagnose. The etiology of CFS is not yet known, but it can occur after an infection (cold, flu) or shortly after a period of high stress and can sometimes last for years. Possible causes include:

- Neuro-endocrine dysfunction
- Viral (Epstein-Barr virus or human herpes virus 6)
- Environmental toxins
- Genetic predisposition
- Iron deficiency anemia
- Low blood sugar (hypoglycemia)
- History of allergies
- Dysfunction in the immune system
- Changes in the levels of hormones produced in the hypothalamus, pituitary glands, or adrenal glands
- Mild, chronic low blood pressure (hypotension)

As no single test confirms its presence, the diagnosis of CFS is based on exclusion. Women are diagnosed with CFS two to four times as often as men are. According to the International Chronic Fatigue Syndrome Study Group, a person meets the diagnostic criteria of CFS when unexplained persistent fatigue occurs for 6 months or more with at least four of the eight primary signs and symptoms also present.

Fibromyalgia Syndrome. *Fibromyalgia syndrome* (FMS) is a chronic muscular endurance disorder, with substantial overlap into a major depressive disorder, various anxiety disorders, CFS, and in multiple regional pain syndromes.[227-230] FMS affects more women than men (9:1) and occurs in people of all ages.[231-233] The exact cause of fibromyalgia is unknown, although it is associated with any condition that diminishes the endurance of the muscles. Recent studies suggest that FMS may best be characterized as a biologic disorder associated with neurohormonal dysfunction of the ANS. Pain is the primary symptom of fibromyalgia, often described as aching or burning.

Study Pearl

The eight core symptoms of CFS include:

- Postexertional malaise lasting more than 24 hours
- Tender lymph nodes
- Muscle pain
- Multiple arthralgias without swelling or redness
- Substantial impairment in short-term memory or concentration
- Headaches of a new type, pattern, or severity
- Sore throat
- Unrefreshing sleep

Study Pearl

Other conditions associated with fibromyalgia include:

- Allergies and infections
- Irritable bowel syndrome
- Dysmenorrhea
- Depression
- Raynaud phenomenon
- Loss of stage IV sleep
- Arthralgias

The apparent pain in patients with FM derives partly from a generalized decrease in the pain perception threshold, reflecting discrimination of a nociceptive quality from a nonnociceptive quality (eg, tactile, thermal), and in the threshold for pain tolerance, reflecting a reluctance to receive more intense stimulation.[234,235] Underlying these threshold changes is altered processing of nociceptive stimuli in the CNS (central sensitization).[234,235]

One characteristic of FMS is the presence of multiple tender points. This refers to specific points in the neck, spine, shoulders, and hips that feel tender. Other symptoms include:

- Fatigue and poor sleep.
- Depression.
- Headaches.
- Alternating diarrhea and constipation.
- Numbness and tingling in the hands and feet.
- Feelings of weakness.
- Short-term memory and cognitive difficulties.
- Dizziness.
- Difficulty breathing—the diaphragm can be so significantly affected in fibromyalgia to the point that it ceases to function as the major breathing muscle and the accessory muscles of the neck and upper chest take over.[48]

Study Pearl

The 1990 American College of Rheumatology classification criteria for FM include:[233]

- The presence of widespread pain for more than 3 months, located on the right and left sides of the body as well as above and below the waist
- Pain, not just tenderness, that can be elicited by manual pressure of approximately 4 kg/cm^2 at 11 or more defined tender points. The number of painful tender points is correlated strongly with psychologic distress, not only in patients with FM but also in the general population.

These criteria are classification criteria for the selection of subjects for research studies, not diagnostic criteria and should not be used for clinic diagnosis.[233]

The diagnosis of FMS is based on the history and physical examination.

The approach with FMS usually involves:

- Empathetic listening and acknowledgment
- Medications:
  - Serotonin: to modulate or dampen the pain response.
  - Low doses of antidepressant drugs taken before bed to improve sleep.
  - Nonsteroidal anti-inflammatory drugs may help decrease pain.
  - Administration of thyroid hormone (metabolic rehabilitation).[236,237]
  - Dehydroepiandrosterone (DHEA): responsible for initiating the cascade of events that result in muscle tissue repair.
  - Psychologic and behavioral approaches. Often if stressful situations are resolved, fibromyalgia may improve and medications may not be necessary.
  - Chronic pain program.
  - Nutritional consult: higher levels of protein in diet is recommended.
  - Physical therapy (see Physical Therapy Role in Complex Disorders).

Myofascial Pain Syndrome. *Myofascial pain syndrome* (MPS) is a common painful disorder that can affect any skeletal muscle in the body. MPS is characterized by the presence of myofascial trigger points (MTrPs).[238-242] An *MTrP* is a hyperirritable location, approximately 2 to 5 cm in diameter,[243] within a taut band of muscle fibers that is painful when compressed and that can give rise to characteristic referred pain, tenderness, and tightness.[244] The patient's reaction to firm palpation of the MTrP is a distinguishing characteristic of MPS and is termed a *positive jump sign.*[245] This hyperirritability appears to be a result of sensitization of the chemonociceptors and mechanonociceptors located within the muscle, which can be triggered following a microtrauma or macrotrauma, or a sustained muscle contraction from a postural dysfunction.[246] Thus, MTrPs are typically located in areas that are prone to increased mechanical strain or impaired circulation (eg, upper trapezius, levator scapulae, infraspinatus, quadratus lumborum, and gluteus minimus).

Stimulation of these receptors can cause:[239,248]

- *Localized ischemia:* Ischemia to the nerves and muscles results in a bombardment of the nervous system with abnormal impulses, creating hyperalgesia in the segmentally related muscles and referral zones.[248-250]
- Edema.
- Fibrosis.
- Temperature changes.
- *Focal or regional autonomic dysfunction:* This can include localized vasoconstriction, persistent hyperemia after palpation, diaphoresis, lacrimation, salivation, and pilomotor activity.

MTrPs, which can give rise to both referred pain and autonomic phenomena, are classified as either active or latent. Active MTrPs are believed to cause pain, whereas latent trigger points are said to restrict range of motion and produce weakness of the affected muscle, with the patient unaware of the tender area until the examination.[246] Latent trigger points can persist for years after a patient recovers from an injury and may become active and create acute pain in response to minor overstretching, overuse, or chilling of the muscle.[239,253]

According to Simons,[254] the diagnosis of MPS can be made if five major criteria and at least one out of three minor criteria are met. The major criteria are:

1. Localized spontaneous pain
2. Spontaneous pain or altered sensations in the expected referred pain area for a given trigger point
3. Presence of a taut palpable band in an accessible muscle
4. Exquisite localized tenderness in a precise point along the taut band
5. Some degree of reduced range of movement when measurable

Minor criteria include:

1. Reproduction of spontaneously perceived pain and altered sensations by pressure on the trigger point
2. Elicitation of a local twitch response of muscular fibers by "transverse" snapping palpation, or by needle insertion into the trigger point
3. Pain relieved by muscle stretching or injection of the trigger point

Complex Regional Pain Syndrome. *Complex regional pain syndrome (CRPS)* is an incompletely understood response of the body

Study Pearl

Some confusion exists as to the difference between trigger points and tender points. Although MTrPs can occur in the same sites as the tender points of fibromyalgia, they can cause referral of pain in a distinct and characteristic area, remote from the trigger point site, not necessarily in a dermatomal distribution.[238] Referred pain is, by definition, absent in the tender points of fibromyalgia.[241,247]

Study Pearl

As with all chronic pain conditions, concomitant social, behavioral, and psychological disturbances often precede or follow their development.[251,252]

Study Pearl

Some of the precipitating events that can cause CRPS I include:

- Fractures
- Soft tissue trauma
- Frostbite
- Myocardial infarction
- Crushing injury
- Surgical procedures
- Amputations

Study Pearl

Some of the sensory abnormalities seen with CRPS I and II include hyperpathia (abnormal response to a repetitious stimuli), dysesthesia (change in sensitivity), hypoesthesia, hyperesthesia, allodynia (painful response to nonpainful stimuli), and paresthesia.

Study Pearl

Diseases associated with CRPS include:

- Spinal cord injuries
- Syringomyelia
- Vascular diseases

to an external stimulus, resulting in pain that usually is nonanatomic and disproportionate to the inciting event or expected healing response. Two types are recognized (I and II). A number of terms were previously used to describe CRPS including reflex sympathetic dystrophy (RSD), causalgia, neurodystrophy, shoulder hand syndrome, Sudeck atrophy, and sympathalgia.

Efferent sympathetic nervous system overactivity and/or abnormal activity involving spinal internuncial neurons, peripheral nociceptors, and/or mechanoreceptors have been postulated as an etiology for, or at least as a significant component of CRPS.

CRPS I affects both men and women, but is more common in women, and while it can occur at any age, it usually affects people between 40 and 60.

Various attempts have been made to relate the various stages of disease to signs and symptoms, but because the course of the disease is so unpredictable, and because overlap is common, staging has been difficult. Nevertheless, understanding the stages provides some insight as to the nature and progression of the disease:

- Stage 1: Lasting about 1 to 2 months and involving nonfocal pain, burning, swelling with associated joint stiffness, decreased range of motion, and increased skin temperature.
- Stage 2: Lasting about 3 to 6 months. Pain continues but decreases over time. Swelling evolves into thickening of the dermis and fascia. Joint stiffness worsens. Early signs of atrophy and osteoporosis become evident, and the extremity becomes cooler. The nails may begin to deteriorate.
- Stage 3 is the atrophic stage. Pain continues and atrophy is exacerbated by continued decreased range of motion, increased joint stiffness, and joint deterioration. The extremity is cooler with decreased vascularity.

Unfortunately, a diagnosis of CRPS is often delayed as no specific test for CRPS exists. Radionuclide bone imaging (RNBI) is the only generally accepted imaging technique to provide objective and relatively specific evidence of RSD in the upper and lower extremities, predominantly the hands and feet.

If conservative methods fail, a continuum involving sympathetic nerve blocks, sympathectomy, spinal cord stimulation, and morphine pumps are available.

Physical Therapy Role in Complex Disorders.[255-259]

- Increase function:
  - Improve sleep through relaxation techniques
  - Energy conservation techniques
  - Ergonomic education
- Decrease pain and fatigue.
  - Soft tissue techniques and joint mobilizations
  - Carefully controlled and graded exercises
  - Cardiovascular fitness training (eg, low-impact aerobics, walking, water aerobics, stationary bicycle)
  - Flexibility exercises—stretching tight, sore muscles
- Recommend lifestyle changes, such as stress reduction and using relaxation techniques. In particular, anxiety and depression need to be treated to reduce stress.

- Heat, massage, and myofascial release provide anecdotal benefit, but are passive modalities of questionable long-term benefit that do not promote self-efficacy.

PSYCHOLOGY

Psychosocial factors pertain to the psychological development of an individual in relation to his or her social environment. A number of the psychosocial factors can influence the direction of physical therapy intervention. Mental health status has been shown to be one of the most important predictors of physical health.[260-262]

ANXIETY

Anxiety disorders are illnesses related to overwhelming anxiety and fear. The following definitions may help the physical therapist understand these conditions:

- Panic attack—repeated episodes of intense fear that strike often and without warning. Physical symptoms include heart palpitations, shortness of breath, dizziness, abdominal distress, and feelings of unreality.
- Obsessive-compulsive disorder—repeated, unwanted thoughts or compulsive behaviors that seem impossible to stop or control.
- Phobias—two major types:
  - Social phobia, which involves an overwhelming and disabling fear of scrutiny, embarrassment, or humiliation in social situations, and which can lead to the avoidance of many potentially pleasurable and meaningful activities.
  - Specific phobia, which involves an extreme, disabling, and irrational fear of something that poses little or no actual danger, which can lead to avoidance of objects or situations.
- Generalized anxiety disorder—constant, exaggerated worrisome thoughts and tension about everyday routine life events and activities, lasting at least 6 months.

ACUTE STRESS DISORDER AND POSTTRAUMATIC STRESS DISORDER

Both acute stress disorder (ASD) and posttraumatic stress disorder (PTSD) are specific forms or subsets of anxiety that occur after experiencing or witnessing a traumatic event. Such traumatic events can include rape or other criminal assault, war, child abuse, and natural or human-caused disasters. The symptoms can comprise of nightmares, flashbacks, numbing of emotions, depression, hostile behavior, and increased irritability. According to the triple vulnerability model, three vulnerabilities need to be present to develop an anxiety disorder:[263,264]

- A biological vulnerability
- A generalized psychological vulnerability (existing experiences of loss control over unpredictable events)
- A specific psychological vulnerability that links anxiety to specific situations

Chronic pain frequently occurs concurrently with PTSD, and the occurrence of both disorders tend to negatively affect the treatment outcome for each.[264,265] The main design outcome of treatment for PTSD should be engagement in healthy, satisfying, necessary, activities.[264]

Coping/Defense Mechanisms

These are typically unconscious behaviors by which the individual resolves or conceals complex anxieties. Table 12-13 lists some of the more common coping/defense mechanisms.

TABLE 12-13. COPING/DEFENSE MECHANISMS

MECHANISM	DEFINITION
Acting out	Instead of expressing feelings verbally, the patient uses actions to release stress. Acting out occurs because certain feeling such as anger and hurt are too difficult to express verbally.
Aim inhibition	Lowering sights to what seems more achievable.
Altruism	The patient becomes dedicated to helping others in order to manage his or her own stress.
Attacking	Trying to beat down something which is threatening.
Autistic fantasy	The patient engages in excessive daydreaming instead of pursuing human relationships in order to decrease stress.
Avoidance	Mentally or physically avoiding something that causes distress.
Compartmentalization	Separating conflicting thoughts into separated compartments.
Compensation	Making up for a weakness in one area by gaining strength in another.
Conversion	Subconsciously converting stress into physical symptoms.
Denial	Denial protects the ego from being overwhelmed by pain through an unrelenting process of disbelief. The patient refuses to acknowledge that an event has occurred.
Devaluation	The patient is overly critical of others and of him or herself and may insult therapists and other personnel.
Displacement	The patient shifts an intended action or response onto a less threatening object to minimize stress.
Dissociation	Separating oneself from parts of his/her life.
Humor	Humor can be used to minimize stress by highlighting the ironic or amusing aspects of a stressful situation.
Idealization	Playing up the good points and ignoring limitations of things desired.
Identification	Copying others to take on their characteristics.
Intellectualization	A patient uses intellectual reasoning rather than expressing emotions in order to avoid painful feelings.
Introjection	Bringing things from the outer world into the inner world.
Omnipotence	A patient feels or acts as if he or she is better than others to guard against feelings of inadequacy.
Passive aggression	Avoiding refusal by passive avoidance.
Projection	A patient transfers his or her own unacceptable feelings, thoughts, and beliefs onto another person and becomes certain that the other person really feels, thinks, and believes that way.
Rationalization	A patient uses elaborate explanations to reassure him/her that his/her actions are driven by sound motives, when he/she may truly be unsure.
Regression	Returning to a child state to avoid problems.
Repression	Subconsciously hiding uncomfortable thoughts.
Somatization	Psychological problems turned into physical symptoms.
Sublimation	Occurs when patients transform unacceptable emotions or desires into socially acceptable actions.
Suppression	A patient intentionally avoids thoughts of disturbing feelings, situations, experiences, or problems in order to reduce stress.
Trivializing	Making small what is really something big.

Data from Precin P: Influence of psychosocial factors on rehabilitation. In: O'Sullivan SB, Schmitz TJ, eds. *Physical Rehabilitation, 5th ed.* Philadelphia, PA: FA Davis. 2007:27-63.

DEPRESSION

Depression is due to an inappropriate environmental responsiveness, and defective habituation (ie, a slower return to baseline functioning following a perturbation). The underlying pathophysiology of depression has not been clearly defined, although clinical and preclinical trials suggest a disturbance in CNS serotonin activity as an important factor. The various conditions associated with depression include:

- Learned helplessness. Humans who are exposed to a major stressor are subsequently unable to learn to escape that stressor.
- Desynchronization of circadian rhythms:
  - Decreased total sleep time
  - Increased sleep onset latency
  - Decreased sleep arousal threshold
  - Increased wakefulness
  - More frequent changes between sleep stages, and terminal insomnia
  - Behavioral sensitization. Behavior becomes more severe and occurs more rapidly in response to the same dose of a given psychomotor stimulant.

No physical findings have been found to be specific to depression, making the history and the mental status examination of paramount importance. In more severe cases, a flat affect, and an overall decline in grooming and hygiene can be observed, as well as a change in weight.

If untreated, depression can spiral into greater severity and may result in suicide; 15% of people who are depressed commit suicide each year.[266] Fortunately a number of medical interventions are available including psychotherapy, medications, electroconvulsive therapy (ECT), light therapy (for seasonal affective disorder), transcranial magnetic stimulation, and vagus nerve stimulation.

From a physical therapy perspective, depression usually affects performance negatively. Depressed patients may not want to make gains in rehabilitation because of decreased motivation and lack of pleasure in life.[264] Physical therapists can facilitate motivation by providing encouragement, emphasizing strength, offering positive feedback, addressing values, and mobilizing guilt into goal acquisition.[264]

Study Pearl

Factors that can hinder the grieving process include:

- Avoidance or minimization of one's emotions
- Use of alcohol or drugs to self-medicate
- Use of work (overfunction at workplace) to avoid feelings

Healthy responses to grief include:

- Allowing sufficient time to experience thoughts and feelings openly to self
- Acknowledging and accepting all feelings, both positive and negative
- Using a journal to document the healing process
- Confiding in a trusted individual
- Expressing feelings openly; crying offers a release
- Identifying any unfinished business and attempting to come to a resolution
- Attending bereavement groups—can provide an opportunity to share grief with others who have experienced similar loss

THE GRIEF PROCESS

Grief is a normal and natural response to the loss of someone or something (loved one, a job, or possibly a role—entering retirement). It is important to realize that acknowledging the grief promotes the healing process. There are a variety of ways that individuals respond to loss, some healthy and some that may hinder the grieving process.

The grieving process invariably consists of a series of stages unique to each individual. These stages of grief reflect a variety of reactions that may surface as an individual makes sense of how a loss impacts them. Experiencing and accepting all feelings remains an important part of the healing process.

Shock, Numbness, Denial, and Disbelief. Shock usually occurs as the initial reaction to a psychological trauma or severe and sudden physical injury.[264] During stressful situations, individuals express themselves through physiological and emotional responses. These reactions serve to protect the individual from an overwhelming experience.

- Numbness is a normal reaction to an immediate loss and should not be confused with "lack of caring."
- Denial is often used as a defense mechanism to alleviate anxiety and pain associated with a disability or illness.[264] Denial, and feelings of disbelief, occur as a specific phase early in the adaptation process and serve to protect the person from having to confront the overwhelming implications of illness or injury at once.[264] Denial and disbelief will diminish as the individual slowly acknowledges the impact of this loss and accompanying feelings.

Bargaining. At times, individuals may ruminate about what could have been done to prevent the loss. Individuals can become preoccupied about ways that things could have been better, imagining all the things that will never be. This reaction can provide insight into the impact of the loss; however, if not properly resolved, intense feelings of remorse or guilt may hinder the healing process. This phase may be marked by externalized hostility toward other people or objects in the environment.

Depression. After recognizing the true extent of the loss, some individuals may experience depressive symptoms. Sleep and appetite disturbance, lack of energy and concentration, and crying spells are some typical symptoms. Feelings of loneliness, emptiness, isolation, and self-pity can also surface during this phase, contributing to this reactive depression. For many, this phase must be experienced in order to begin reorganizing one's life.

Anger. This reaction usually occurs when an individual feels helpless and powerless. Anger may result from feeling abandoned, occurring in cases of loss through death. Feelings of resentment may occur toward one's higher power or toward life in general for the injustice of this loss. After an individual acknowledges anger, guilt may surface due to expressing these negative feelings.

Acknowledgment. Acknowledgment is the first sign that the patient has accepted or recognized the permanency of the condition and its future implications.[264]

Acceptance. Time allows the individual an opportunity to resolve the range of feelings that surface.

Adjustment. Adjustment is the final phase in adaptation and involves the development of new ways of interacting successfully with others and one's environment.[264]

Elizabeth Kubler Ross' Model of Grief Stages.[267]

- Stage 1: Shock and denial. It is common for people to avoid making decisions or taking action at this point.
- Stage 2: Anger. Making decisions at this point is difficult because all one's energy gets put into the emotion rather than problem solving.
- Stage 3: Depression and detachment. Because it is hard to make decisions at this stage, consider asking a family member, friend, or professional for help if important decisions need to be made.
- Stage 4: Dialogue and bargaining. People become more willing to explore alternatives after expressing their feelings.
- Stage 5: Acceptance. Decisions are much easier to make because people have found new purpose and meaning as they have begun to accept the loss.

Physical Therapy Approach During the Grieving Process

- Discuss quality-of-life issues with patient/family and help them realize that the phases of terminality are being redefined.
- Make time for grief work.
- Focus on the positive: realize and maximize all clinical opportunities.
- Learn to deal with the patient's or family's anger during the discharge crisis.
- Realize the importance of comfort measures and pain management to patient/family.
- Work with appropriate pastoral supports.
- Try to engage patient's interest in things.
- Respect the needs of privacy, independence, and decathexis (the gradual weakening and separating of emotional ties) on the part of the patient.

Psychosocial Pathologies

Affective Disorders. Affective disorders (Table 12-14) refer to disorders of mood.

TABLE 12-14. AFFECTIVE DISORDERS

Psychosis	A nonspecific cluster of signs and symptoms that may occur in a broad array of medical, neurologic, and surgical disorders, or as a consequence of pharmacologic treatment, substance abuse, or the withdrawal of drugs and alcohol. There are three major categories of this syndrome: ▶ Schizophrenia ▶ Paranoia ▶ Depression
Anxiety disorders	Apprehension of danger and dread accompanied by restlessness, tension, tachycardia, and dyspnea secondary to an unidentifiable reason. Characterized by an adherence either to fixed, false beliefs outside the normal range of a person's subculture, or by a hallucinatory experience, and by a formally defined disorder of thought.
Behavioral disturbances	Manifested in a variety of abnormal actions
Neurosis	A disorder with anxiety as its primary characteristic. Includes depression, obsessive-compulsive states, and hysteria (refer to Neuroses Disorders)
Delusions	Commonly defined as a fixed false belief and is used in everyday language to describe a belief that is either false, fanciful, or derived from deception. In psychiatry, the definition is necessarily more precise and implies that the belief is pathological (the result of an illness or illness process).

Bipolar Disorder. *Bipolar disorder*, also known as manic-depressive illness, is one of the most common, severe, and persistent mental illnesses. The condition is characterized by periods of deep, prolonged, and profound depression that alternate with periods of excessively elevated and/or irritable mood known as mania. Between these highs and lows, patients usually experience periods of higher functionality and can lead a productive life.

The etiology and pathophysiology of bipolar disorder have not been determined. However, twin, family, and adoption studies all indicate strongly that bipolar disorder has a genetic component. There are a wide range of medications that are utilized to treat affective disorders (refer to Chapter 19).

Neuroses Disorders. The term *neurosis*, also known as psychoneurosis or neurotic disorder, is a general term that refers to any mental imbalance that causes distress, but does not interfere with rational thought, or an individual's ability to function in daily life.

There are many different specific forms of neuroses: pyromania, obsessive-compulsive disorder, anxiety neurosis, hysteria (in which anxiety may be discharged through a physical symptom).

Dissociative Disorders. A dissociative disorder occurs when there is a breakdown of one's perception of his/her surroundings, memory, identity, or consciousness. There are four main kinds of dissociative disorders:

- Dissociative amnesia: the essential feature is an inability to recall important personal information that is more extensive than can be explained by normal forgetfulness. Remembering such information is usually traumatic or produces stress.
- Dissociative fugue: characterized by sudden, unexpected travels from the home or workplace with an inability to recall some or all of one's past. Some of these patients assume a new identity or are confused about their own identity.
- Dissociative identity disorder: formerly referred to as multiple personality disorder, this is characterized by the existence of two or more identities or personality traits within a single individual. Patients with this disorder demonstrate transfer of behavioral control among other identities either by state transitions or by inference and overlap of others who manifest themselves simultaneously. It is observed in 1% to 3% of the general population.
- Depersonalization disorder: Derealization or depersonalization is characterized by feelings that the objects of the external environment are changing shape and size, or that people are automated and inhuman, and features detachment as a major defense. Depersonalization disorder usually begins in adolescence; typically, patients have continuous symptoms. Onset can be sudden or gradual.

Somatoform Disorders. *Somatoform disorders* represent a group of disorders characterized by physical symptoms that cannot be fully explained by a medical disorder, substance use, or another mental disorder. These somatoform disorders can challenge medical providers who must distinguish between a physical and psychiatric source for the patient's complaints. Somatosensory amplification refers to the tendency to experience somatic sensation as intense, noxious, and disturbing. Barsky and colleagues[268] introduced the concept of somatosensory amplification as an important feature of hypochondriasis. Somatosensory amplification is observed in patients whose extreme anxiety leads to an increase in their perception of pain.

The term *nonorganic* was proposed by Waddell[269] to define the abnormal illness behaviors exhibited by patients suffering from depression, emotional disturbance, or anxiety states. The presence of three of five of the following Waddell signs has been correlated significantly with disability.[270]

- Superficial or nonanatomic tenderness to light touch that is widespread and refers pain to other areas.
- Simulation tests. These are a series of tests that should be comfortable to perform. Examples include axial loading of the spine through the patient's head with light pressure to the skull and passive hip and shoulder rotation with the patient positioned standing. Neither of these tests should produce low back pain. If pain is reported with these tests, a nonorganic origin should be suspected.
- Distraction test.[271] This test involves checking a positive finding elicited during the examination on the distracted patient. For example, if a patient is unable to perform a seated trunk flexion maneuver, the same patient can be observed when asked to remove his or her shoes. A difference of 40 to 45 degrees is significant for inconsistency.
- Regional disturbances. These signs include sensory or motor disturbances that have no neurologic basis.
- Overreaction. This includes disproportionate verbalization, muscle tension, tremors, and grimacing during the examination.

The Somatosensory Amplification Rating Scale is a version of Waddell's nonorganic physical signs that has been modified to allow for a more accurate appraisal of the patient with exaggerated illness behavior.[268]

Study Pearl

It is important to remember that the Waddell and SARS assessment tools are designed not to detect whether patients are malingering, but only to indicate whether they have symptoms of a nonorganic origin (symptom magnification syndrome).

Schizophrenia Disorders. Schizophrenia is characterized by hallucinations (visual—see images, and auditory—hear voices) and delusions (altered beliefs, persecutory or grandiose, etc). There are three subtypes of schizophrenia:[272-276]

- Paranoid: the most common type of schizophrenia in most parts of the world. The clinical picture is dominated by relatively stable, often paranoid, delusions, usually accompanied by hallucinations, particularly of the auditory variety, and perceptual disturbances. Disturbances of affect, volition, and speech, and catatonic symptoms, are not prominent.
- Disorganized: characterized by early age of onset and the presence of pronounced thought and speech disorder, altered affect, and strange behavior.
- Catatonic: characterized by auditory and visual hallucinations and most typically the presence of bizarre motor activity. Immobility, bizarre postures, excessive purposeless movements,

TABLE 12-15. THE 10 RECOGNIZED PERSONALITY DISORDERS

DISORDER	DESCRIPTION
Antisocial personality	Lack of regard for the moral or legal standards in the local culture, marked inability to get along with others or abide by societal rules; sometimes called psychopaths or sociopaths
Avoidant personality	Marked social inhibition, feelings of inadequacy, and extremely sensitive to criticism
Borderline personality	Lack of one's own identity, with rapid changes in mood, intense unstable interpersonal relationships, marked impulsiveness, instability in affect and in self-image
Dependent personality	Extreme need of other people, to a point where the person is unable to make any decisions or take an independent stand on his or her own; fear of separation and submissive behavior; marked lack of decisiveness and self-confidence
Histrionic personality	Exaggerated and often inappropriate displays of emotional reactions, approaching theatricality, in everyday behavior; sudden and rapidly shifting expressions of emotion
Narcissistic personality	Behavior or a fantasy of grandiosity, a lack of empathy, a need to be admired by others, an inability to see the viewpoints of others, and hypersensitive to the opinions of others
Obsessive-compulsive personality	Characterized by perfectionism and inflexibility; preoccupation with uncontrollable patterns of thought and action
Paranoid personality	Marked distrust of others, including the belief, without reason, that others are exploiting, harming, or trying to deceive him or her; lack of trust; belief of others' betrayal; belief in hidden meanings; unforgiving and grudge holding
Schizoid personality	Primarily characterized by a very limited range of emotion, both in expression and experiencing; indifferent to social relationships
Schizotypal personality	Peculiarities of thinking, odd beliefs, and eccentricities of appearance, behavior, interpersonal style, and thought (eg, belief in psychic phenomena and having magical powers)

and mutism characterize the disease. Other symptoms include: prolonged maintenance of a fixed posture (catalepsy), grimacing, parrot-like repetition of a word or phrase just spoken by someone else (echolalia), repetitive imitation of the movements of another person (echopraxia), stupor, or excitement.

Personality Disorders. Personality disorders are not illnesses in a strict sense as they do not disrupt emotional, intellectual, or perceptual functioning. However, those with personality disorders suffer a life that is not positive, proactive, or fulfilling.

Currently, there are 10 distinct personality disorders identified in the *DSM-IV*[277-282] (Table 12-15).

PHYSICAL THERAPY INTERVENTION

Although the treatment for psychological and psychiatric disorders is mainly pharmacologic, the physical therapist can encounter this patient population as they may have been prescribed physical therapy for another condition. As with any other patient, but particularly with those patients who have an affective disorder, the following guidelines are recommended:

- Maintain a positive attitude, but avoid excessive cheerfulness.
- Consistently demonstrate warmth and interest.
- Use positive reinforcement, building on successful treatment experiences.
- Involve the patient in the treatment decisions.
- Take all suicide ideations seriously.

Empathy vs Sympathy. Empathy is a communication skill that is often misunderstood and underused. Empathy refers to the capacity to recognize and, to some extent, share feelings that are being experienced by another individual. Sympathy on the other hand is rarely helpful or therapeutic. Appropriate use of empathy as a communication tool facilitates the clinical interview, increases the efficiency of gathering information, and honors the patient's feelings. The key steps to effective empathy include:

- Establishing the boundaries of the professional relationship while recognizing the potential for strong emotions in the clinical setting (ie, fear, anger, grief, disappointment)
- Providing an environment conducive to the patient's emotional state, learning, and optimal function
- Setting realistic, meaningful goals and involving the patient and family in the goal setting process
- Legitimizing the patient's feelings by using statements such as "I can imagine that must be ..." or "It sounds like you're upset about ...."
- Respecting the patient's effort to cope with the predicament, while recognizing secondary gains or unacceptable behavior
- By not reinforcing unacceptable behaviors
- Helping the patient to identify feelings, successful coping strategies, and successful conflict resolutions

Questions for this chapter and the entire book appear on the included CD-ROM, with additional questions at www.DuttonNPTE.com.

REFERENCES

1. Goodman CC, Kelly Snyder TE: Infectious disease. In: Goodman CC, Boissonnault WG, Fuller KS, eds. *Pathology: Implications for the Physical Therapist, 2nd ed.* Philadelphia, PA: Saunders; 2003: 194-235.
2. Bass JW, Wittler RR, Weisse ME: Social smile and occult bacteremia. *Pediatr Infect Dis J.* 1996;15:541.
3. Bohnel H, Gessler F: Clostridia and clostridioses. *FEMS Immunol Med Microbiol.* 1999;24:v.
4. Esiri MM: Viruses and rickettsiae. *Brain Pathol.* 1997;7:695-709.
5. Ormsbee RA: Rickettsiae as organisms. *Acta Virol.* 1985; 29:432-448.
6. Osterman JV: Rickettsiae and hosts. *Acta Virol.* 1985;29:166-173.
7. Raoult D, Fournier PE, Eremeeva M, et al. Naming of Rickettsiae and rickettsial diseases. *Ann N Y Acad Sci.* 2005;1063:1-12.
8. Vitorino L, Chelo IM, Bacellar F, Ze-Ze L. Rickettsiae phylogeny: a multigenic approach. *Microbiology.* 2007;153:160-168.
9. Weisburg WG, Dobson ME, Samuel JE, Dasch GA, Mallavia LP: Phylogenetic diversity of the Rickettsiae. *J Bacteriol.* 1989;171: 4202-4206.
10. Wood DO, Azad AF: Genetic manipulation of rickettsiae: a preview. *Infect Immun.* 2000;68:6091-6093.
11. Dumler JS: Ehrlichioses: emerging infections. *Curr Opin Infect Dis.* 1998;11:183-187.

12. McQuiston JH, Paddock CD, Holman RC, et al: The human ehrlichioses in the United States. *Emerg Infect Dis.* 1999;5: 635-642.
13. Olano JP, Walker DH: Human ehrlichioses. *Med Clin North Am.* 2002;86:375-392.
14. Crompton, DWT: Human nutrition and parasitic infection. *Parasitology.* 1993;107(suppl):S1-S203.
15. Protection and pathology in parasitic infection. *Parasite Immunol.* 2000;22:595.
16. Stear MJ, Wakelin D: Genetic resistance to parasitic infection. *Rev Sci Tech.* 1998;17:143-153.
17. Fitzgerald JR, Reid SD, Ruotsalainen E, et al: Genome diversification in *Staphylococcus aureus*: molecular evolution of a highly variable chromosomal region encoding the staphylococcal exotoxin-like family of proteins. *Infect Immun.* 2003;71:2827-2838.
18. O'Kane GM, Gottlieb T, Bradbury R: Staphylococcal bacteraemia: the hospital or the home? A review of *Staphylococcus aureus* bacteraemia at Concord Hospital in 1993. *Aust N Z J Med.* 1998;28:23-27.
19. Szczepanik A, Koziol-Montewka M, Al-Doori Z, et al. Spread of a single multiresistant methicillin-resistant *Staphylococcus aureus* clone carrying a variant of staphylococcal cassette chromosome mec type III isolated in a university hospital. *Eur J Clin Microbiol Infect Dis.* 2007;26:29-35.
20. Eady EA, Cove JH: Staphylococcal resistance revisited: community-acquired methicillin resistant *Staphylococcus aureus*—an emerging problem for the management of skin and soft tissue infections. *Curr Opin Infect Dis.* 2003;16:103-124.
21. Brogan TV, Nizet V, Waldhausen JH: Streptococcal skin infections. *N Engl J Med.* 1996;334:1478.
22. Duggan JM, Georgiadis G, VanGorp C, Kleshinski J: Group B streptococcal prosthetic joint infections. *J South Orthop Assoc.* 2001;10:209-214; discussion 214.
23. Edwards MS, Baker CJ: Group B streptococcal infections in elderly adults. *Clin Infect Dis.* 2005;41:839-847.
24. Ekelund K, Skinhoj P, Madsen J, et al: Invasive group A, B, C and G streptococcal infections in Denmark 1999-2002: epidemiological and clinical aspects. *Clin Microbiol Infect.* 2005;11:569-576.
25. Gotoff SP: Group B streptococcal infections. *Pediatr Rev.* 2002;23:381-386.
26. Jaggi P, Shulman ST: Group A streptococcal infections. *Pediatr Rev.* 2006;27:99-105.
27. Lee NY, Yan JJ, Wu JJ, et al: Group B streptococcal soft tissue infections in non-pregnant adults. *Clin Microbiol Infect.* 2005;11:577-579.
28. Mulla ZD: Group A streptococcal infections in long-term care facilities. *Am J Infect Control.* 2005;33:375-376.
29. Weir E, Main C: Invasive group A streptococcal infections. *CMAJ.* 2006;175:32.
30. Amaro R, Schiff ER: Viral hepatitis. *Curr Opin Gastroenterol.* 2001;17:262-267.
31. Gonzalez-Aseguinolaza G, Crettaz J, Ochoa L, Otano I, Aldabe. R, Paneda A: Gene therapy for viral hepatitis. *Expert Opin Biol Ther.* 2006;6:1263-1278.
32. Mallat D, Schiff E: Viral hepatitis. *Curr Opin Gastroenterol.* 2000;16:255-261.

33. Marrero R, Schiff E: Viral hepatitis. *Curr Opin Gastroenterol.* 2002;18:330-333.
34. Regev A, Schiff ER: Viral hepatitis. *Curr Opin Gastroenterol.* 1999; 15:234-239.
35. Rehermann B, Naoumov NV: Immunological techniques in viral hepatitis. *J Hepatol.* 2007;46:508-520.
36. Trepo C, Zoulim F, Pradat P: Viral hepatitis. *Curr Opin Infect Dis.* 1999;12:481-490.
37. Achord JL: Acute pancreatitis with infectious hepatitis. *JAMA.* 1968;205:837-840.
38. Canosa CA, Gosalvez JA, Abeledo G, Dalmau J: Acute infectious hepatitis. Clinical and epidemiological study. *Helv Paediatr Acta.* 1977;32:21-28.
39. Parana R, Codes L, Andrade Z, et al. Clinical, histologic and serologic evaluation of patients with acute non-A-E hepatitis in north-eastern Brazil: is it an infectious disease? *Int J Infect Dis.* 2003;7:222-230.
40. Tabor E, April M, Seeff LB, Gerety RJ: Acute non-A, non-B hepatitis. Prolonged presence of the infectious agent in blood. *Gastroenterology.* 1979;76:680-684.
41. Liu CJ, Kao JH: Hepatitis B virus-related hepatocellular carcinoma: epidemiology and pathogenic role of viral factors. *J Chin Med Assoc.* 2007;70:141-145.
42. Modi AA, Feld JJ: Viral hepatitis and HIV in Africa. *AIDS Rev.* 2007;9:25-39.
43. Wu CA, Lin SY, So SK, Chang ET: Hepatitis B and liver cancer knowledge and preventive practices among Asian Americans in the San Francisco Bay Area, California. *Asian Pac J Cancer Prev.* 2007;8:127-134.
44. Camarero C, Ramos N, Moreno A, et al: Hepatitis C virus infection acquired in childhood. Eur J Pediatr, 2007;150:168-174.
45. Hahn JA: Sex, drugs, and hepatitis C virus. *J Infect Dis.* 2007; 195:1556-1559.
46. Dalton HR, Fellows HJ, Gane EJ, et al: Hepatitis E in New Zealand. *J Gastroenterol Hepatol.* 2007;22:1236-1240.
47. Wong KH, Lee SS, Chan KC: Twenty years of clinical human immunodeficiency virus (HIV) and acquired immunodeficiency syndrome (AIDS) in Hong Kong. *Hong Kong Med J.* 2006;12:133-140.
48. Goodman CC: The immune system. In: Goodman CC, Boissonnault WG, Fuller KS, eds. *Pathology: Implications for the Physical Therapist, 2nd ed.* Philadelphia, PA: Saunders; 2003: 153-193.
49. Goodman CC: The hematologic system. In: Goodman CC, Boissonnault WG, Fuller KS, eds. *Pathology: Implications for the Physical Therapist, 2nd ed.* Philadelphia, PA: Saunders; 2003: 509-552.
50. Thomas JK, Noppenberger J: Avian influenza: a review. *Am J Health Syst Pharm.* 2007;64:149-165.
51. Lamabadusuriya SP: Avian influenza. *Ceylon Med J.* 2006;51:77.
52. Influenza. *Wkly Epidemiol Rec.* 2006;81:480.
53. La Gruta NL, Kedzierska K, Stambas J, Doherty PC: A question of self-preservation: immunopathology in influenza virus infection. *Immunol Cell Biol.* 2007;9:9.

54. Langley JM: Review: Antiviral agents reduce the risk of influenza in healthy adults and alleviate symptoms faster than placebo. *Evid Based Med.* 2006;11:141.
55. Beaton MD, Adams PC: The myths and realities of hemochromatosis. *Can J Gastroenterol.* 2007;21:101-104.
56. Davies MB, Saxby T: Ankle arthropathy of hemochromatosis: a case series and review of the literature. *Foot Ankle Int.* 2006;27:902-906.
57. de Gheldere A, Ndjoko R, Docquier PL, Mousny M, Rombouts JJ: Orthopaedic complications associated with sickle-cell disease. *Acta Orthop Belg.* 2006;72:741-747.
58. Sarrai M, Duroseau H, D'Augustine J, et al: Bone mass density in adults with sickle cell disease. *Br J Haematol.* 2007;11:11.
59. Yoon SL, Black S: Comprehensive, integrative management of pain for patients with sickle-cell disease. *J Altern Complement Med.* 2006;12:995-1001.
60. Sathappan SS, Ginat D, Di Cesare PE: Multidisciplinary management of orthopedic patients with sickle cell disease. *Orthopedics.* 2006;29:1094-1101; quiz 1102-1103.
61. Williams V, Griffiths A, Tapp H, Mangos H, Casey G: A hemophilic son of a hemophiliac: did my son inherit my hemophilia? *J Thromb Haemost.* 2007;5:210-211.
62. Lusher JM, Brownstein AP: Hemophilia and HIV. *J Thromb Haemost.* 2007;12:12.
63. Hoots WK, Nugent DJ: Evidence for the benefits of prophylaxis in the management of hemophilia A. *Thromb Haemost.* 2006;96:433-440.
64. Evatt BL: The tragic history of AIDS in the hemophilia population, 1982-1984. *J Thromb Haemost.* 2006;4:2295-2301; Epub 2006 Sep 14.
65. Hilliard P, Funk S, Zourikian N, et al. Hemophilia joint health score reliability study. *Haemophilia.* 2006;12:518-525.
66. Schafer AI: Thrombocytosis: when is an incidental finding serious? *Cleve Clin J Med.* 2006;73:767-774.
67. Vlacha V, Feketea G: Thrombocytosis in pediatric patients is associated with severe lower respiratory tract inflammation. *Arch Med Res.* 2006;37:755-759.
68. Papageorgiou T, Theodoridou A, Kourti M, et al: Childhood essential thrombocytosis. *Pediatr Blood Cancer.* 2006;47:970-971.
69. Dan K: Thrombocytosis in iron deficiency anemia. *Intern Med.* 2005;44:1025-1026.
70. Salacz ME, Lankiewicz MW, Weissman DE: Management of thrombocytopenia in bone marrow failure: a review. *J Palliat Med.* 2007;10:236-244.
71. Li X, Swisher KK, Vesely SK, George JN: Drug-induced thrombocytopenia: an updated systematic review, 2006. *Drug Saf.* 2007;30:185-186.
72. Murphy MF, Bussel JB: Advances in the management of alloimmune thrombocytopenia. *Br J Haematol.* 2007;136:366-378.
73. Girolami B, Girolami A: Heparin-induced thrombocytopenia: a review. *Semin Thromb Hemost.* 2006;32:803-809.
74. Marengo-Rowe AJ: The thalassemias and related disorders. *Proc (Bayl Univ Med Cent).* 2007;20:27-31.
75. Al-Jahdali H, Al-Shimemeri A, Bamefleh H, et al: Pulmonary histiocytosis X. *Ann Saudi Med.* 1998;18:437-439.

76. de Brito Macedo Ferreira LM, de Carvalho JD, Pereira ST, et al: Histiocytosis X of the temporal bone. *Rev Bras Otorrinolaringol (Engl Ed).* 2006;72:575.
77. Rizvi RM, Nasreen C, Jafri N: Histiocytosis X of the vulva. *J Pak Med Assoc.* 2002;52:430.
78. Flenaugh EL, Henriques-Forsythe MN: Lung cancer disparities in African Americans: health versus health care. *Clin Chest Med.* 2006;27:431-439, vi.
79. Kendall J, Catts ZA, Kendall C, Jones L: African Americans' knowledge of cancer genetic counseling: an examination of information delivery. *Del Med J.* 2006;78:453-458.
80. O'Keefe SJ, Chung D, Mahmoud N, Sepulveda AR, Manafe M: Why do African Americans get more colon cancer than Native Africans? *J Nutr.* 2007;137:175S-182S.
81. Overmyer M: Search narrows for gene tied to prostate cancer in African-Americans. *RN.* 2007;70(2):suppl 2.
82. Goodman CC, Snyder TK: Oncology. In: Goodman CC, Boissonnault WG, Fuller KS, eds. *Pathology: Implications for the Physical Therapist, 2nd ed.* Philadelphia, PA: Saunders. 2003: 236-263.
83. Goodman CC, Snyder TK: Problems affecting multiple systems. In Goodman CC, Boissonnault WG, Fuller KS, eds. *Pathology: Implications for the Physical Therapist, 2nd ed.* Philadelphia, PA: Saunders. 2003: 85-119.
84. Boissonnault WG, Goodman CC, The renal and urologic systems. In: Goodman CC, Boissonnault WG, Fuller KS, eds. *Pathology: Implications for the Physical Therapist, 2nd ed.* Philadelphia, PA: Saunders. 2003: 704-728.
85. Mayer R: Interstitial cystitis pathogenesis and treatment. *Curr Opin Infect Dis.* 2007;20:77-82.
86. Kelada E, Jones A. Interstitial cystitis. *Arch Gynecol Obstet.* 2006;22:22.
87. Sant GR: Etiology, pathogenesis, and diagnosis of interstitial cystitis. *Rev Urol.* 2002;4:S9-S15.
88. Urinary incontinence. Know your drug options. *Mayo Clin Health Lett.* 2005;23:6.
89. Blackwell RE: Estrogen, progestin, and urinary incontinence. *JAMA.* 2005;294:2696-2698.
90. Bren L: Controlling urinary incontinence. *FDA Consum.* 2005;39:10-15.
91. Castro-Diaz D, Amoros MA: Pharmacotherapy for stress urinary incontinence. *Curr Opin Urol.* 2005;15:227-230.
92. Kelleher C, Cardozo L, Kobashi K, et al. Solifenacin: as effective in mixed urinary incontinence as in urge urinary incontinence. *Int Urogynecol J Pelvic Floor Dysfunct.* 2006;17:382-388.
93. Borello-France DF, Zyczynski HM, Downey PA, et al. Effect of pelvic-floor muscle exercise position on continence and quality-of-life outcomes in women with stress urinary incontinence. *Phys Ther.* 2006;86:974-986.
94. Neumann PB, Grimmer KA, Deenadayalan Y: Pelvic floor muscle training and adjunctive therapies for the treatment of stress urinary incontinence in women: a systematic review. *BMC Womens Health.* 2006;6:11.
95. Hay-Smith EJ, Dumoulin C: Pelvic floor muscle training versus no treatment, or inactive control treatments, for urinary incontinence in women. *Cochrane Database Syst Rev.* 2006;CD005654.

96. Anders K: Treatments for stress urinary incontinence. *Nurs Times.* 2006;102:55-57.
97. Wilson MM: Urinary in continence: selected current concepts. *Med Clin North Am.* 2006;90:825-836.
98. Berger RE: Risk factors associated with acute pyelonephritis in healthy women. *J Urol.* 2005;174:1841.
99. Ramakrishnan K, Scheid DC: Diagnosis and management of acute pyelonephritis in adults. *Am Fam Physician.* 2005;71:933-942.
100. Hill JB, Sheffield JS, McIntire DD, et al. Acute pyelonephritis in pregnancy. *Obstet Gynecol.* 2005;105:18-23.
101. Rollino C, Boero R, Ferro M, et al: Acute pyelonephritis: analysis of 52 cases. *Ren Fail.* 2002;24:601-608.
102. Gaesser GA: Exercise for prevention and treatment of cardiovascular disease, type 2 diabetes, and metabolic syndrome. *Curr Diab Rep.* 2007;7:14-19.
103. Cayley WE: The role of exercise in patients with type 2 diabetes. *Am Fam Physician.* 2007;75:335-336.
104. Orchard TJ, Costacou T, Kretowski A, et al: Type 1 diabetes and coronary artery disease. *Diabetes Care.* 2006;29:2528-2538.
105. Toni S, Reali MF, Barni F, Lenzi L, Festini F: Managing insulin therapy during exercise in type 1 diabetes mellitus. *Acta Biomed.* 2006;77(suppl 1):34-40.
106. Davies MJ: The prevention of type 2 diabetes mellitus. *Clin Med.* 2003;3:470-474.
107. Bhaskarabhatla KV, Birrer R: Physical activity and diabetes mellitus. *Compr Ther.* 2005;31:291-298.
108. Choudhary P: Review of dietary recommendations for diabetes mellitus. *Diabetes Res Clin Pract.* 2004;65(suppl 1):S9-S15.
109. Owen K, Hattersley AT: Maturity-onset diabetes of the young: from clinical description to molecular genetic characterization. *Best Pract Res Clin Endocrinol Metab.* 2001;15:309-323.
110. Kaarisalo MM, Raiha I, Arve S, et al: Impaired glucose tolerance as a risk factor for stroke in a cohort of non-institutionalised people aged 70 years. *Age Ageing.* 2006;35:592-596.
111. Fujita M, Asanuma H, Kim J, et al: Impaired glucose tolerance: a possible contributor to left ventricular hypertrophy and diastolic dysfunction. *Int J Cardiol.* 2007;118(1):76-80.
112. Oztekin O: Screening for gestational diabetes mellitus. *Acta Obstet Gynecol Scand.* 2006;85:763.
113. Ross G: Gestational diabetes. *Aust Fam Physician.* 2006;35:392-396.
114. Files D: Pre-diabetes. *Aviat Space Environ Med.* 2006;77:658-689.
115. Ryden L, Standl E, Bartnik M, et al: Guidelines on diabetes, pre-diabetes, and cardiovascular diseases: executive summary. The Task Force on Diabetes and Cardiovascular Diseases of the European Society of Cardiology (ESC) and of the European Association for the Study of Diabetes (EASD). *Eur Heart J.* 2007;28:88-136.
116. Vitale C, Marazzi G, Volterrani M, et al: Metabolic syndrome. *Minerva Med.* 2006;97:219-229.
117. Maier B, Thimme W, Kallischnigg G, et al: Does diabetes mellitus explain the higher hospital mortality of women with acute myocardial infarction? Results from the Berlin Myocardial Infarction Registry. *J Investig Med.* 2006;54:143-151.
118. Toyoda K, Nakano A, Fujibayashi Y, et al: Diabetes mellitus impairs myocardial oxygen metabolism even in non-infarct-related

areas in patients with acute myocardial infarction. *Int J Cardiol.* 2007;115:297-304.

119. Carrier J: Review: exercise improves glycaemic control and reduces plasma triglycerides and visceral adipose tissue in type 2 diabetes. *Evid Based Nurs.* 2007;10:11.
120. Follow these exercise guidelines to manage type 2 diabetes. *Health News.* 2006;12:12.
121. Feher M: Exercise and sport in diabetes. *J Hum Hypertens.* 2006;20:907.
122. Cauza E, Hanusch-Enserer U, Strasser B, et al: The metabolic effects of long term exercise in type 2 diabetes patients. *Wien Med Wochenschr.* 2006;156:515-519.
123. Chipkin SR, Klugh SA, Chasan-Taber L: Exercise and diabetes. *Cardiol Clin.* 2001; 19:489-505.
124. Welch TR: Hyperthyroidism: impact on bone. *J Pediatr.* 2007;150:a3.
125. Maji D: Hyperthyroidism. *J Indian Med Assoc.* 2006;104:563-564, 566-567.
126. Cooper DS: Approach to the patient with subclinical hyperthyroidism. *J Clin Endocrinol Metab.* 2007;92:3-9.
127. Sutandar M, Garcia-Bournissen F, Koren G: Hypothyroidism in pregnancy. *J Obstet Gynaecol Can.* 2007;29:354-356.
128. Lazarus JH: Aspects of treatment of subclinical hypothyroidism. *Thyroid.* 2007;17:313-316.
129. Bungard TJ, Hurlburt M: Management of hypothyroidism during pregnancy. *CMAJ.* 2007;176:1077-1078.
130. Jayakumar RV: Hypothyroidism. *J Indian Med Assoc.* 2006;104: 557-560, 562.
131. Hamidi S, Soltani A, Hedayat A, et al: Primary hyperparathyroidism: a review of 177 cases. *Med Sci Monit.* 2006;12:CR86-CR89.
132. Mikhail N, Cope D: Evaluation and treatment of primary hyperparathyroidism. *JAMA.* 2005;294:2700.
133. Grey A, Bolland M, Reid IR: Evaluation and treatment of primary hyperparathyroidism. *JAMA.* 2005;294:2699-2700.
134. Thaunat M, Gaudin P, Naret C, et al: Role of secondary hyperparathyroidism in spontaneous rupture of the quadriceps tendon complicating chronic renal failure. *Rheumatology (Oxford).* 2006;45:234-235.
135. Maeda SS, Fortes EM, Oliveira UM, et al: Hypoparathyroidism and pseudohypoparathyroidism. *Arq Bras Endocrinol Metabol.* 2006;50:664-673.
136. Korkmaz C, Yasar S, Binboga A: Hypoparathyroidism simulating ankylosing spondylitis. *Joint Bone Spine.* 2005;72:89-91.
137. De Sanctis C, De Sanctis V, Radetti G, et al: Hypoparathyroidism and pseudohypoparathyroidism. *Minerva Pediatr.* 2002; 54:271-278.
138. Pantanetti P, Sonino N, Arnaldi G, et al: The quality of life in acromegaly. *J Endocrinol Invest.* 2003;26:35-38.
139. Terzolo M, Daffara F, Reimondo G, et al: The neoplastic complications of acromegaly. *J Endocrinol Invest.* 2003;26:32-34.
140. Bondanelli M, Zatelli MC, Ambrosio MR, et al: The vascular complications of acromegaly. *J Endocrinol Invest.* 2003;26:28-31.
141. Maffei P, Martini C, Mioni R, et al: The cardiac complications of acromegaly. *J Endocrinol Invest.* 2003;26:20-27.
142. Angeletti G: The metabolic complications of acromegaly. *J Endocrinol Invest.* 2003;26:18-19.

143. Ezzat S: Pharmacological approach to the treatment of acromegaly. *Neurosurg Focus.* 2004;16:E3.
144. Giustina A, Casanueva FF, Cavagnini F, et al: Diagnosis and treatment of acromegaly complications. *J Endocrinol Invest.* 2003;26:1242-1247.
145. Sacca L, Napoli R, Cittadini A: Growth hormone, acromegaly, and heart failure: an intricate triangulation. *Clin Endocrinol (Oxf).* 2003;59:660-671.
146. Paisley AN, Trainer PJ: Medical treatment in acromegaly. *Curr Opin Pharmacol.* 2003;3:672-677.
147. Nieman LK, Chanco Turner ML: Addison's disease. *Clin Dermatol.* 2006;24:276-280.
148. Lovas K, Husebye ES: Addison's disease. *Lancet.* 2005;365:2058-2061.
149. Marzotti S, Falorni A: Addison's disease. *Autoimmunity.* 2004;37:333-336.
150. Chhangani NP, Sharma P: Addison's disease. *Indian Pediatr.* 2003;40:904-905.
151. Riddick DH, Hammond CB: Adrenal virilism due to 21-hydroxylase deficiency in the postmenarchial female. *Obstet Gynecol.* 1975; 45:21-24.
152. David RR: Adrenal virilism in childhood. *Ann N Y Acad Sci.* 1967;142:787-793.
153. Storr HL, Chan LF, Grossman AB, et al: Paediatric Cushing's syndrome: epidemiology, investigation and therapeutic advances. *Trends Endocrinol Metab.* 2007;18:167-174.
154. Makras P, Toloumis G, Papadogias D, et al: The diagnosis and differential diagnosis of endogenous Cushing's syndrome. *Hormones (Athens)* 2006;5:231-250.
155. Magiakou MA, Smyrnaki P, Chrousos GP: Hypertension in Cushing's syndrome. *Best Pract Res Clin Endocrinol Metab.* 2006;20:467-482.
156. Elte JW: Diagnosis of Cushing's syndrome. *Eur J Intern Med.* 2006;17:311-312.
157. Shibli-Rahhal A, Van Beek M, Schlechte JA: Cushing's syndrome. *Clin Dermatol.* 2006;24:260-265.
158. Newell-Price J, Bertagna X, Grossman AB, et al: Cushing's syndrome. *Lancet.* 2006;367:1605-1617.
159. Miyachi Y: Pathophysiology and diagnosis of Cushing's syndrome. *Biomed Pharmacother.* 2000;54(suppl 1):113s-117s.
160. Nadar S, Lip GY, Beevers DG: Primary hyperaldosteronism. *Ann Clin Biochem.* 2003;40:439-452.
161. Quinkler M, Lepenies J, Diederich S: Primary hyperaldosteronism. *Exp Clin Endocrinol Diabetes.* 2002;110:263-271.
162. Stowasser M: Hyperaldosteronism: primary versus tertiary. *J Hypertens.* 2002;20:17-19.
163. Stowasser M, Gordon RD: Familial hyperaldosteronism. *J Steroid Biochem Mol Biol.* 2001;78:215-229.
164. Soule S, Davidson JS, Rayner BL: The evaluation of primary hyperaldosteronism. *S Afr Med J.* 2000;90:387-394.
165. Boissonnault JS, Stephenson R: The obstetric patient. In Boissonnault WG, ed. *Primary Care for the Physical Therapist: Examination and Triage.* St Louis: Elsevier Saunders; 2005:239-270.
166. Lee HY, Zhao S, Fields PA, et al: Clinical use of relaxin to facilitate birth: reasons for investigating the premise. *Ann N Y Acad Sci.* 2005;1041:351-366.

167. Lubahn J, Ivance D, Konieczko E, et al: Immunohistochemical detection of relaxin binding to the volar oblique ligament. *J Hand Surg [Am].* 2006;31:80-84.
168. Goldsmith LT, Weiss G, Steinetz BG: Relaxin and its role in pregnancy. *Endocrinol Metab Clin North Am.* 1995;24:171-186.
169. Wiles R: The views of women of above average weight about appropriate weight gain in pregnancy. *Midwifery.* 1998;14: 254-260.
170. Moore K, Dumas GA, Reid JG: Postural changes associated with pregnancy and their relationship with low back pain. *Clin Biomech (Bristol, Avon).* 1990;5:169-174.
171. Noronha A: Neurologic disorders during pregnancy and the puerperium. *Clin Perinatol.* 1985;12:695-713.
172. Godfrey CM: Carpal tunnel syndrome in pregnancy. *Can Med Assoc J.* 1983;129:928.
173. Graham JG: Neurological complications of pregnancy and anaesthesia. *Clin Obstet Gynaecol.* 1982;9:333-350.
174. Lamondy AM: Managing hyperemesis gravidarum. *Nursing.* 2007;37:66-68.
175. Dodds L, Fell DB, Joseph KS, et al: Outcomes of pregnancies complicated by hyperemesis gravidarum. *Obstet Gynecol.* 2006;107:285-292.
176. Fell DB, Dodds L, Joseph KS, et al: Risk factors for hyperemesis gravidarum requiring hospital admission during pregnancy. *Obstet Gynecol.* 2006;107:277-284.
177. Loh KY, Sivalingam N: Understanding hyperemesis gravidarum. *Med J Malaysia.* 2005;60:394-349; quiz 400.
178. Wise RA, Polito AJ, Krishnan V: Respiratory physiologic changes in pregnancy. *Immunol Allergy Clin North Am.* 2006;26:1-12.
179. Prowse CM, Gaensler EA: Respiratory and acid-base changes during pregnancy. *Anesthesiology.* 1965;26:381-392.
180. Bonica JJ: Maternal respiratory changes during pregnancy and parturition. *Clin Anesth.* 1974;10:1-19.
181. Sadaniantz A, Kocheril AG, Emaus SP, et al: Cardiovascular changes in pregnancy evaluated by two-dimensional and Doppler echocardiography. *J Am Soc Echocardiogr.* 1992;5:253-258.
182. Atkins AF, Watt JM, Milan P, et al: A longitudinal study of cardiovascular dynamic changes throughout pregnancy. *Eur J Obstet Gynecol Reprod Biol.* 1981;12:215-224.
183. Chesley LC: Cardiovascular changes in pregnancy. *Obstet Gynecol Annu.* 1975;4:71-97.
184. Capeless EL, Clapp JF: Cardiovascular changes in early phase of pregnancy. *Am J Obstet Gynecol.* 1989;161:1449-1453.
185. Walters WA, Lim YL: Changes in the materal cardiovascular system during human pregnancy. *Surg Gynecol Obstet.* 1970;131: 765-784.
186. Urman BC, McComb PF: A biphasic basal body temperature record during pregnancy. *Acta Eur Fertil.* 1989;20:371-372.
187. Grant A, Mc BW: The 100 day basal body temperature graph in early pregnancy. *Med J Aust.* 1959;46:458-460.
188. Siegler AM: Basal body temperature in pregnancy. *Obstet Gynecol.* 1955;5:830-832.
189. Depledge J, McNair PJ, Keal-Smith C, et al: Management of symphysis pubis dysfunction during pregnancy using exercise and pelvic support belts. *Phys Ther.* 2005;85:1290-1300.

190. Leadbetter RE, Mawer D, Lindow SW: Symphysis pubis dysfunction: a review of the literature. *J Matern Fetal Neonatal Med.* 2004;16:349-354.
191. Owens K, Pearson A, Mason G: Symphysis pubis dysfunction—a cause of significant obstetric morbidity. *Eur J Obstet Gynecol Reprod Biol.* 2002;105:143-146.
192. Allsop JR: Symphysis pubis dysfunction. *Br J Gen Pract.* 1997;47:256.
193. Snow RE, Neubert AG: Peripartum pubic symphysis separation: a case series and review of the literature. *Obstet Gynecol Survey.* 1997;52:438-443.
194. Whitman JM: Pregnancy, low back pain, and manual physical therapy interventions. *J Orthop Sports Phys Ther.* 2002;32: 314-317.
195. Mogren IM, Pohjanen AI: Low back pain and pelvic pain during pregnancy: prevalence and risk factors. *Spine.* 2005;30:983-991.
196. Pool-Goudzwaard AL, Slieker ten Hove MC, Vierhout ME, et al: Relations between pregnancy-related low back pain, pelvic floor activity and pelvic floor dysfunction. *Int Urogynecol J Pelvic Floor Dysfunct.* 2005;16:468-474; Epub 2005 Apr 1.
197. Wang SM, Dezinno P, Maranets I, et al: Low back pain during pregnancy: prevalence, risk factors, and outcomes. *Obstet Gynecol.* 2004;104:65-70.
198. Fast A, Weiss L, Ducommun EJ, et al: Low back pain in pregnancy. Abdominal muscles, sit-up performance and back pain. *Spine.* 1990;15:28-30.
199. Berg G, Hammar M, Moller-Nielsen J, et al: Low back pain during pregnancy. *Obstet Gynecol.* 1988;71:71-75.
200. Bullock JE, Jull GA, Bullock MI: The relationship of low back pain to postural changes during pregnancy. *Aust J Physiother.* 1987;33:10-17.
201. Ostgaard HC, Andersson GBJ, Schultz AB, et al: Influence of some biomechanical factors on low back pain in pregnancy. *Spine.* 1993;18:61-65.
202. Hodges SD, Eck JC, Humphreys SC: A treatment and outcomes analysis of patients with coccydynia. *Spine J.* 2004;4:138-140.
203. Ryder I, Alexander J: Coccydynia: a woman's tail. *Midwifery.* 2000;16:155-160.
204. Maigne JY, Lagauche D, Doursounian L: Instability of the coccyx in coccydynia. *J Bone Joint Surg Br.* 2000;82:1038-1041.
205. Boeglin ER, Jr: Coccydynia. *J Bone Joint Surg Br.* 1991;73:1009.
206. Wray CC, Easom S, Hoskinson J: Coccydynia. Aetiology and treatment. *J Bone Joint Surg Br.* 1991;73:335-338.
207. Lee DT, Chung TK: Postnatal depression: an update. *Best Pract Res Clin Obstet Gynaecol.* 2006;21:183-189.
208. Howard L: Postnatal depression. *Clin Evid.* 2006;1919-1931.
209. Howard L: Postnatal depression. *Clin Evid.* 2005;1764-1775.
210. Cox J: Postnatal depression in fathers. *Lancet.* 2005;366:982.
211. Hanley J: The assessment and treatment of postnatal depression. *Nurs Times.* 2006;102:24-26.
212. Mallikarjun PK, Oyebode F: Prevention of postnatal depression. *J R Soc Health.* 2005;125:221-226.
213. Snyder S, Pendergraph B: Exercise during pregnancy: what do we really know? *Am Fam Physician.* 2004;69:1053, 1056.

214. Parker KM, Smith SA: Aquatic-aerobic exercise as a means of stress reduction during pregnancy. *J Perinat Educ.* 2003;12:6-17.
215. Kramer MS, McDonald SW: Aerobic exercise for women during pregnancy. *Cochrane Database Syst Rev.* 2006;3:CD000180.
216. Morris SN, Johnson NR: Exercise during pregnancy: a critical appraisal of the literature. *J Reprod Med.* 2005;50:181-188.
217. Larsson L, Lindqvist PG: Low-impact exercise during pregnancy—a study of safety. *Acta Obstet Gynecol Scand.* 2005;84:34-38.
218. Fazlani SA: Protocols for exercise during pregnancy. *J Pak Med Assoc.* 2004;54:226-229.
219. Paisley TS, Joy EA, Price RJ, Jr: Exercise during pregnancy: a practical approach. *Curr Sports Med Rep.* 2003;2:325-330.
220. Information from your family doctor. Pregnancy and exercise. *Am Fam Physician.* 2003;68:1168.
221. The Centers for Disease Control and Prevention. Inability of retroviral tests to identify persons with chronic fatigue syndrome, 1992. *JAMA.* 1993;269:1779,1782.
222. Albrecht F: Chronic fatigue syndrome. *J Am Acad Child Adolesc Psychiatry.* 2000;39:808-809.
223. Darbishire L, Ridsdale L, Seed PT: Distinguishing patients with chronic fatigue from those with chronic fatigue syndrome: a diagnostic study in UK primary care. *Br J Gen Pract.* 2003;53:441-445.
224. Lee P: Recent developments in chronic fatigue syndrome. *Am J Med.* 1998;105:1S.
225. Mawle AC: Chronic fatigue syndrome. *Immunol Invest.* 1997; 26:269-273.
226. Tan EM, Sugiura K, Gupta S: The case definition of chronic fatigue syndrome. *J Clin Immunol.* 2002;22:8-12.
227. Amital D, Fostick L, Polliack ML, et al. Posttraumatic stress disorder, tenderness, and fibromyalgia syndrome: are they different entities? *J Psychosom Res.* 2006;61:663-669.
228. Glass JM: Cognitive dysfunction in fibromyalgia and chronic fatigue syndrome: new trends and future directions. *Curr Rheumatol Rep.* 2006;8:425-429.
229. Mehendale AW, Goldman MP: Fibromyalgia syndrome, idiopathic widespread persistent pain or syndrome of myalgic encephalomyelopathy (SME): what is its nature? *Pain Pract.* 2002;2:35-46.
230. Thieme K, Rose U, Pinkpank T, et al: Psychophysiological responses in patients with fibromyalgia syndrome. *J Psychosom Res.* 2006;61:671-679.
231. Cramer CR: Fibromyalgia and chronic fatigue syndrome: an update for athletic trainers. *J Athl Train.* 1998;33:359-361.
232. Goldenberg DL, Burckhardt C, Crofford L: Management of fibromyalgia syndrome. *JAMA* 2004;292:2388-2395.
233. Mease PJ, Clauw DJ, Arnold LM, et al: Fibromyalgia syndrome. *J Rheumatol.* 2005;32:2270-2277.
234. Staud R, Rodriguez ME: Mechanisms of disease: pain in fibromyalgia syndrome. *Nat Clin Pract Rheumatol.* 2006;2:90-98.
235. Wood PB, Patterson JC, II, Sunderland JJ, et al: Reduced presynaptic dopamine activity in fibromyalgia syndrome demonstrated with positron emission tomography: a pilot study. *J Pain.* 2007;8:51-58.
236. Joffe RT, Sokolov ST, Levitt AJ: Lithium and triiodothyronine augmentation of antidepressants. *Can J Psychiatry.* 2006;51:791-793.

237. Agid O, Shalev AY, Lerer B: Triiodothyronine augmentation of selective serotonin reuptake inhibitors in posttraumatic stress disorder. *J Clin Psychiatry.* 2001;62:169-173.
238. McClaflin RR: Myofascial pain syndrome: primary care strategies for early intervention. *Postgrad Med.* 1994;96:56-73.
239. Travell JG, Simons DG: *Myofascial Pain and Dysfunction—The Trigger Point Manual.* Baltimore, MD: Williams & Wilkins. 1983.
240. Fricton JR: Myofascial pain. *Baillieres Clin Rheumatol.* 1994;8: 857-880.
241. Vecchiet L, Giamberardino MA, Saggini R: Myofascial pain syndromes: clinical and pathophysiological aspects. *Clin J Pain.* 7(suppl):16-22.
242. Grodin AJ, Cantu RI: Soft tissue mobilization. In: Basmajian JV, Nyberg R, eds. *Rational Manual Therapies.* Baltimore, MD: Williams & Wilkins. 1993:199-221.
243. Fricton JR: Management of masticatory myofascial pain. *Seminars Orthodontics.* 1995;1:229-243.
244. Esenyel M, Caglar N, Aldemir T: Treatment of myofascial pain. *Am J Phys Med Rehabil.* 2000;79:48-52.
245. Fricton JR: Clinical care for myofascial pain. *Dent Clin N Am.* 1991;35:1-29.
246. Dreyer SJ, Boden SD: Nonoperative treatment of neck and arm pain. *Spine.* 1998;23:2746-2754.
247. Wolfe F, Smythe HA, Yunus MB, et al: The American College of Rheumatology 1990 criteria for the classification of fibromyalgia. *Arthr Rheum.* 1990;33:160-172.
248. Keller K, Corbett J, Nichols D: Repetitive strain injury in computer keyboard users: pathomechanics and treatment principles in individual and group intervention. *J Hand Ther.* 1998;11:9-26.
249. Quinter J, Elvey R: Understanding "RSI": a review of the role of peripheral neural pain and hyperalgesia. *J Man & Manip Ther.* 1993;1:99-105.
250. Goldman LB, Rosenberg NL: Myofascial pain syndrome and fibromyalgia. *Seminars Neurol.* 1991;11:274-280.
251. Fricton JR, Kroening R, Haley D, et al: Myofascial pain syndrome of the head and neck: a review of clinical characteristics of 164 patients. *Oral Surg Oral Med Oral Pathol.* 1985;60:615-623.
252. Fricton JR: Behavioral and psychosocial factors in chronic craniofacial pain. *Anesth Prog.* 1985;32:7-12.
253. Stratton SA, Bryan JM: Dysfunction, evaluation, and treatment of the cervical spine and thoracic inlet. In: Donatelli R, Wooden M, eds. *Orthopaedic Physical Therapy, 2nd ed.* New York: Churchill Livingstone; 1993:77-122.
254. Simons DG: Muscular pain syndromes. In: Fricton JR, Awad E, eds. *Advances in Pain Research and Therapy.* New York: Raven Press; 1990:1-41.
255. Cook DB, Nagelkirk PR, Poluri A, et al: The influence of aerobic fitness and fibromyalgia on cardiorespiratory and perceptual responses to exercise in patients with chronic fatigue syndrome. *Arthritis Rheum.* 2006;54:3351-3362.
256. Havermark AM, Langius-Eklof A: Long-term follow up of a physical therapy programme for patients with fibromyalgia syndrome. *Scand J Caring Sci.* 2006;20:315-322.
257. Karper WB, Jannes CR, Hampton JL: Fibromyalgia syndrome: the beneficial effects of exercise. *Rehabil Nurs.* 2006;31:193-198.

258. Kurtais Y, Kutlay S, Ergin S: Exercise and cognitive-behavioural treatment in fibromyalgia syndrome. *Curr Pharm Des.* 2006;12:37-45.
259. Salek AK, Khan MM, Ahmed SM, et al: Effect of aerobic exercise on patients with primary fibromyalgia syndrome. *Mymensingh Med J.* 2005;14:141-144.
260. Extremera N, Fernandez-Berrocal P: Emotional intelligence as predictor of mental, social, and physical health in university students. *Span J Psychol.* 2006;9:45-51.
261. Penedo FJ, Dahn JR: Exercise and well-being: a review of mental and physical health benefits associated with physical activity. *Curr Opin Psychiatry.* 2005;18:189-193.
262. Scott KM, Bruffaerts R, Tsang A, et al: Depression-anxiety relationships with chronic physical conditions: results from the World Mental Health surveys. *J Affect Disord.* 2007;8:8.
263. Barlow DH: Unraveling the mysteries of anxiety and its disorders from the perspective of emotion theory. *Am Psychol.* 2000;55:1247-1263.
264. Precin P: Influence of psychosocial factors on rehabilitation. In: O'Sullivan SB, Schmitz TJ, eds. *Physical Rehabilitation*, 5th ed. Philadelphia, PA: FA Davis. 2007:27-63.
265. Geisser ME, Roth RS, Bachman JE, et al: The relationship between symptoms of post-traumatic stress disorder and pain, affective disturbance and disability among patients with accident and non-accident related pain. *Pain.* 1996;66:207-214.
266. Nemeroff CB: The neurobiology of depression. *Sci Am.* 1998;278:42-49.
267. Kübler-Ross E: *On Death and Dying.* New York: Macmillan; 1969.
268. Barsky AJ, Goodson JD, Lane RS, et al: The amplification of somatic symptoms. *Psychosom Med.* 1988;50:510-519.
269. Waddell G, Main CJ, Morris EW, et al: Chronic low back pain, psychological distress and illness behavior. *Spine.* 1984;9:209-213.
270. Werneke MW, Harris DE, Lichter RL: Clinical effectiveness of behavioral signs for screening low-back pain patients in a work oriented physical rehabilitation program. *Spine.* 1993;18:2412.
271. Kenna O, Murtagh A: The physical examination of the back. *Aust Fam Physician.* 1985;14:1244-1256.
272. Eack SM, Newhill CE, Anderson CM, et al: Quality of life for persons living with schizophrenia: more than just symptoms. *Psychiatr Rehabil J.* 2007;30:219-222.
273. Howard L, Kirkwood G, Leese M: Risk of hip fracture in patients with a history of schizophrenia. *Br J Psychiatry.* 2007;190:129-134.
274. Mettner J: Inside schizophrenia. *Minn Med.* 2007;90:14-15.
275. Rabinowitz J, Levine SZ, Haim R, Hafner H: The course of schizophrenia: progressive deterioration, amelioration or both? *Schizophr Res.* 2007;91:254-258.
276. Seeman MV: Symptoms of schizophrenia: normal adaptations to inability. *Med Hypotheses.* 2007;69(2):253-237.
277. Bower H: The gender identity disorder in the DSM-IV classification: a critical evaluation. *Aust N Z J Psychiatry.* 2001;35:1-8.
278. Brown TA, Di Nardo PA, Lehman CL, et al: Reliability of DSM-IV anxiety and mood disorders: implications for the classification of emotional disorders. *J Abnorm Psychol.* 2001;110:49-58.
279. Hartman CA, Hox J, Mellenbergh GJ, et al: DSM-IV internal construct validity: when a taxonomy meets data. *J Child Psychol Psychiatry.* 2001;42:817-836.

280. Slade T, Andrews G: DSM-IV and ICD-10 generalized anxiety disorder: discrepant diagnoses and associated disability. Soc *Psychiatry Psychiatr Epidemiol.* 2001;36:45-51.
281. Suneja S: Memorizing and recalling DSM-IV diagnostic criteria. *Psychiatr Serv.* 2001;52:976.
282. Syed EU, Atiq R, Effendi S, et al: Conversion disorder: difficulties in diagnosis using DSM-IV/ICD-10. *J Pak Med Assoc.* 2001; 51:143-145.
283. Dutton M: Pathology. In Dutton M, ed: *Physical Therapist Assistant Exam Review Guide & JB Test Prep: PTA Exam Review.* Sudbury, MA:Jones & Bartlett Learning. 2011:315-362.

Integumentary Physical Therapy

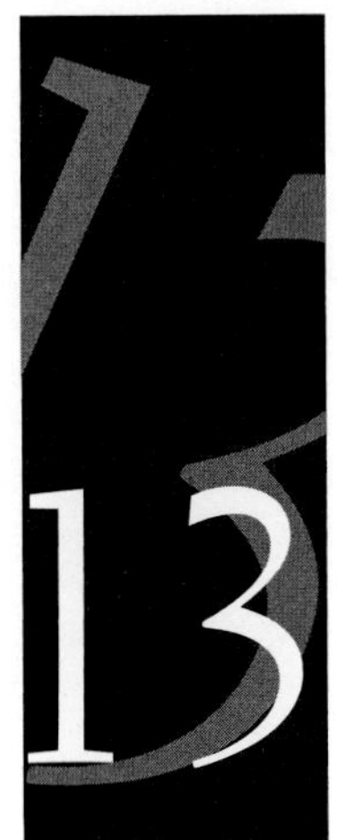

The integumentary system comprises the skin and its appendages (hair follicles, nails, sebaceous glands, and sweat glands). The integument or skin, which is the largest organ system of the body, constitutes 15% to 20% of the body weight.[1]

> **Study Pearl**
>
> Key functions of the skin include
> - Cushioning and protecting against injury or invasion
> - Lubrication through secretion of oils
> - Insulation
> - Maintenance of homeostasis: fluid balance, regulation of body temperature
> - Excretion of excess water, urea, and salt via sweat
> - Maintenance of body shape—provides cosmetic appearance and identity
> - Vitamin D synthesis
> - Storage of nutrients
> - Provision of sensory information via receptors in the dermis

SKIN OR INTEGUMENT

Anatomically, the skin consists of three distinct layers of tissue: the epidermis, the dermis, and the hypodermis, a subcutaneous fat cell layer that is located directly under the dermis and above the muscle fascial layers.[1]

EPIDERMIS

The epidermis is the most superficial layer and is made up of epithelial cells and no blood vessels. Its main function is protection, absorption of nutrients, and homeostasis. In structure, it consists of a keratinized stratified squamous epithelium comprising four types of cells:

- keratinocytes: produce keratin cells that toughen and waterproof the skin. The only portion of skin that is non-keratinized is the lining of skin on the inside of the mouth.
- melanocytes: provide a protective barrier to the ultraviolet radiation in the sunlight; produce melanin and are responsible for skin color.
- Merkel cells
- Langerhans' cells

> **Study Pearl**
>
> Keratin is a fibrous protein that aids in the protection and water-proofing of the skin.

DERMIS

The dermis, the middle layer of the skin, is considered the "true" skin because it contains blood vessels, lymphatics, nerves, collagen, sebaceous and sweat glands, and elastic fibers.[1] The dermis is composed primarily of collagen and elastin fibrous connective tissue.

Study Pearl

The interface between the epidermis and the dermis is termed the *rete peg region*. Rete pegs are the epithelial extensions that project into the underlying connective tissue and which act to overcome the frictional forces that skin is exposed to during daily activity.[1]

The amount of elastin decreases with age. The dermis can be subdivided into two layers, a superficial papillary layer and the deeper reticular layer[1]:

ACCESSORY STRUCTURES OF THE SKIN

HAIR

Hair is formed by epidermal cells that invaginate into the dermal layers. The distribution, function, intensity, and texture of the hair vary according to the region of the body. Certain regions, such as the palms, soles, lips, and nipples are hairless. The primary function of hair is protection, even though its effectiveness is limited. Humans have a number of distinct kinds of hair:

- Lanugo: a fine, silky fetal hair that appears during the last trimester of development.
- Vellus: short, fine, soft, and nonpigmented.
- Angora: grows continuously and is found on the scalp and on the male face.
- Definitive: grows to a certain length and then stops. It is the most common type of hair. Examples include eyelashes, eyebrows, and axillary hair.

NAILS

The nails on the ends of the fingers and toes are formed from the compressed outer layer (stratum corneum) of the epidermis. The hardness of the nails is due to the dense keratin fibrils. Each nail consists of a body, free border, and hidden border. The platelike body of the nail rests on the nail bed, which is actually the stratum spinosum of the epidermis. The sides of the nail body are protected by a nailfold, and the furrow between the sides and body is the nail groove. The stratum corneum layer of the skin covering the nail root is the cuticle (eponychium). The paronychium is the soft tissue surrounding the nail border.

GLANDS

Although they originate in the epidermal layer, all of the glands of the skin are located in the dermis. The glands of the skin are of three basic types:

- Sebaceous glands: commonly called oil glands, sebaceous glands secrete sebum (a fatty substance) onto and along the hair follicles, where it is dispersed to the surface of the skin to provide lubrication and waterproofing of the stratum corneum.
- Sudoriferous (sweat) glands: secrete perspiration (composed of water, salts, urea, and uric acid) onto the surface of the skin to provide evaporative cooling, but also to excrete certain wastes. Two types exist:
  - Eccrine glands: widely distributed, especially on the forehand, back, palms, and soles. These glands are formed before birth and function to help control body temperature.

  - Apocrine glands: these are much larger than eccrine glands and are located in axillary and pubic areas, where they secrete into hair follicles. These glands are not functional until puberty, when they enlarge and become active, producing a characteristically adult odor.
- Ceruminous glands: highly specialized glands that are found only in the external acoustic canal. The glands secrete cerumen (earwax), which is both a water and insect repellent.

Study Pearl

Mammary glands, found within the breast, are specialized sudoriferous glands that secrete milk during lactation.

Vascular Supply

Blood flows through the arteries to get to capillaries of the skin. Dermal blood vessels play an important role in regulating body temperature and blood pressure. Autonomic vasoconstriction or vasodilation responses can either shunt the blood away from the superficial dermal arterioles or allow it to flow freely throughout dermal vessels:

- An increase in blood flow produces an increase in oxyhemoglobin to skin capillaries causing reddening of the skin.
- A decrease in blood flow and a decrease in oxyhemoglobin cause a somewhat blue color appearance to the skin (peripheral cyanosis).

Study Pearl

A condition called central cyanosis occurs when there is a reduced oxygen level in the blood. Some of the causes for this condition include advanced lung disease, congenital heart disease, and abnormal hemoglobin levels.

EXAMINATION OF THE INTEGUMENTARY SYSTEM

Patient/Client History and Systems Review Related to the Integumentary System

- Age, sex, race/ethnicity
- Health habits
  - Skin, hair and nail care habits
  - Alcohol, tobacco, or caffeine use
  - Work, living, environment (exposure to environmental or occupational hazards, dyes, chemicals, sunlight etc)
- General health status
- Body composition
- Body mass index, skinfold thickness
- Height, weight
- Metabolic comorbidity (diabetes mellitus, vascular disorders)
- Nutritional status
- Medical/surgical history
- Functional status/activity level
- Current medications (topical and systemic), eg, corticosteroids, anticoagulants
- Changes in skin: dryness, sores, rashes, lumps, texture, amount of perspiration, changes in wart or mole, changes in color
- Symptoms: pain, itching, bleeding, exudate
- Presence of paresthesias or sensory loss
- Associated symptoms: systemic disease, fever
- Travel history: exposure to diseases and/or bites
- Previous skin problems: sensitivities, skin allergies, hair loss, skin cancer, fungal infections of the nails.

TABLE 13-1. HISTOLOGIC TERMS FOR SKIN LESIONS

TERM	DEFINITION
Acantholysis	Dissolution of intercellular integrity with fragmentation of epidermis
Acanthosis	Hyperplasia of epidermal layer
Dyskeratosis	Abnormal keratinization occurring prematurely in cells below the stratum granulosum
Erosion	Loss of epidermis
Exocytosis	Infiltration of epidermis by inflammatory cells
Hyperkeratosis	Thickening of the stratum corneum with excess abnormal keratin
Papillomatosis	Hyperplasia of the papillary dermis and lengthening and/or widening of the dermal papillae
Spongiosis	Edema limited to the epidermis
Ulceration	Loss of epidermis with variable partial-to-complete loss of dermis

Observation

Examination of the integumentary system is chiefly performed by observation and palpation (Table 13-1). The skin should be palpated for the following:

- Moisture
- Temperature
- Texture
- Turgor
- Mobility

Signs and Symptoms of Skin Disorders

Pruritis. Pruritis (itching), a symptom of underlying systemic disease in the 50% of people with generalized itching, is one of the most common manifestations of dermatologic disease.[2]

- Can lead to damage as scratching injures the skin's protected area.
- Associated with many systemic disorders including diabetes mellitus, drug hypersensitivity, and hyperthyroidism.

Urticaria. Urticaria (hives) is a vascular reaction of the skin marked by the appearance of smooth, slightly elevated patches.

Rash. A generalized term for eruption of the skin, most often on the face, trunk, axilla, and groin.

Blister. Nonspecific term for a fluid-filled lesion. Manifestation of a wide variety of causes including autoimmune origin or secondary to viral or bacterial infections of the skin (eg, herpes simplex, impetigo), local injury to the skin (eg, burns, ischemia, dermatitis), or drug-induced (eg, penicillamine, captopril).

Bulla. Fluid-filled lesion greater than 5 mm in greatest dimension.

Vesicle. Fluid-filled lesion of 5 mm or less.

Xeroderma. Mild form of ichthyosis or excessive dryness of the skin. Characterized by a dry, rough, discolored skin with the formation of scaly desquamation.

DOCUMENTATION OF SKIN LESIONS

Skin lesions should be described according to characteristics, type, exudate, pattern of arrangement, location, and distribution (Table 13-2).

Hair should be examined for the following:

- Color
- Distribution
- Quantity
- Texture

The nails should be inspected for the following:

- Color
- Length
- Configuration
- Symmetry
- Cleanliness
- Ridging and beading

TABLE 13-2. SKIN LESION DESCRIPTIONS

DESCRIPTION	EXAMPLES
Characteristics	▶ Size ▶ Shape ▶ Color ▶ Texture ▶ Elevation or depression
Type	▶ Abrasion: an abrasion or is a wearing away of the upper layer of skin as a result of applied friction force. ▶ Contusion: a contusion (bruise) is caused when blood vessels are damaged or broken as the result of a direct blow to the skin. ▶ Ecchymosis: the skin discoloration caused by the escape of blood into the tissues from ruptured blood vessels. ▶ Hematoma: a localized collection of blood, usually clotted, in a tissue or organ. ▶ Excoriation: lesion of traumatic nature with epidermal loss in a generally linear shape. ▶ Laceration: describes an injury involving penetration of the skin, in which the wound is deeper than the superficial skin level. ▶ Penetrating wound: a wound accompanied by disruption of the body surface that extends into the underlying tissue or into a body cavity ▶ Petechiae: tiny red spots in the skin which do not blanch when pressed upon. Petechiae result from red blood leaking from capillaries into the skin (intradermal hemorrhages). Petechiae are less than 3 mm in diameter. ▶ Puncture: a wound made by a pointed object (like a nail). ▶ Ulcer: a lesion on the surface of the skin or the surface of the mucous membrane, produced by the sloughing of inflammatory, necrotic tissue.
Exudates (see Table 13-3)	▶ Color ▶ Odor ▶ Amount ▶ Consistency
Pattern of arrangement	▶ Annular ▶ Grouped ▶ Linear ▶ Diffuse
Location and distribution	▶ Generalized or localized ▶ Region of the body ▶ Discrete or confluent

EXAMINATION OF A SKIN WOUND

The following outline should provide the clinician with the necessary guidelines to perform a detailed wound assessment[3]:

- Wound history: mechanism, force, and duration of injury, and the time interval between injury and onset of intervention: acute versus chronic.
- Wound examination
  - Photographic records of wound appearance aid narrative descriptions. A marker pen should be used over outlying wound edges on a transparent dressing with a calibrated grid to provide a measuring scale.
  - General inspection of extremity.
  - Location of wound: use anatomic landmarks.
  - Assess size: length, width, depth, wound area.
    - Insert sterile cotton tip applicator into deepest part of wound for depth measurement; indicate gradations of depth from shallow to deep.
    - Examine for tunneling (rimming or undermining): underlying tissue destruction beneath intact skin.
    - Evaluate for sinus tracts (communication with deeper structures): associated with unusual or irregular borders.
  - Presence of edema (pitting, brawny, hard, or mobile) and measurement (circumferential or volumetric).
  - Skin color and temperature.
    - Reddened areas may indicate inflammation or cellulitis.
    - Cyanosis may indicate arterial insufficiency.
    - Use temperature probe (thermistor) to detect surface temperature. Changes in skin temperature correlate with the internal temperature unless skin is exposed to local heat or cold.
    - Examine with backs of fingers for generalized warmth or coolness.
    - Abnormal heat can indicate febrile condition, hyperthyroidism, mental excitement, and excessive salt intake.
    - Abnormal cold can indicate poor circulation or obstruction, eg, vasomotor spasm, venous or arterial thrombosis, and hypothyroidism.
  - Wound color—see Wound bed.
- Wound type[4]
  - Tidy: clean laceration, minimal tissue damage, and minimal contamination.
  - Untidy: significant amount of tissue damage, uncertainty regarding viability of deeper structures, higher degree of contamination.
  - Wound with tissue loss: deeper structures involved (vessels, tendons, nerve, or bone). May require soft tissue coverage:
    - Split thickness graft (epidermis and part of dermis) or full thickness (epidermis and entire underlying dermis).
    - Flap coverage necessary: a flap is a portion of tissue *partly* severed from its place of origin to correct a defect in the body.
  - Infected wound (presently or potentially).
- Type of closure
  - Primary closure
  - Delayed primary closure

TABLE 13-3. EXUDATE CLASSIFICATIONS

TYPE OF EXUDATE	DESCRIPTION
Serous	Presents as clear, light color with a thin, watery consistency. Serous exudate is considered to be normal in a healthy healing wound.
Sanguinous	Presents as red with a thin, watery consistency. Sanguinous exudate appears to be red due to the presence of blood or may be brown if allowed to dehydrate. This type of exudate may be indicative of new blood vessel growth or the disruption of blood vessels.
Serosanguinous	Presents as light red or pink, with a thin, watery consistency. Serosanguinous exudate can be normal in a healthy healing wound.
Seropurulent	Presents as an opaque, yellow or tan color, with a thin, watery consistency. Seropurulent exudate may be an early warning sign of an impending infection.
Purulent	Presents as a yellow or green color with a thick, viscous consistency. This type of exudate is generally an indicator of wound infection.

  - Secondary intention
  - Closure method (sutures, staples, Steri-strips, graft, or flap)
  - Fixation (K-wire, pull-out wire, external fixator)
- ▶ Wound configuration
  - Size, shape, depth
  - Integrity of tissue[5]
  - Viability of wound edges
  - Maceration (softened tissues, due to high fluid environment): moist and white appearance of skin
  - Hematoma/seroma: collection of blood and/or serum; a bleb is a blood- or serum filled blister
- ▶ Exudate (Table 13-3).
  - Color consistency: bloody, serous (watery-like serum), serosanguinous (containing blood), pus (purulent), or dark red.
  - Amount: dry, slight, minimal, moderate, severe.
  - Odor: presence or absence of foul odor.
- ▶ Wound bed
  - Color and extent of granulation tissue (Table 13-4). Granulation tissue consists of a gel-like matrix of collagen, hyaluronic acid, and fibronectin in a newly formed avascular network. Granulation tissue nourishes the macrophages and fibroblasts that have migrated into the wound and, as healing continues, provides a substrate for the migration of epidermal cells.
  - Indolent ulcer: ulcer that is slow to heal; is not painful.
  - Check to see if fascia, muscle, tendons, or bone involved.

TABLE 13-4. RED-YELLOW-BLACK SYSTEM

COLOR	WOUND DESCRIPTION	INTERVENTION GOALS
Red	Healthy, pink granular tissue with absence of necrotic tissue	Protect wound; maintain moist environment
Yellow	Presence of adherent fibrinous exudates and debris (moist yellow slough)	Debride necrotic tissue; absorb drainage
Black	Presence of black, thick eschar (dried necrotic tissue), firmly adhered	Debride necrotic tissue

Data from Cozzell J: The new red, yellow, black color code. *Am J Nurs*. 1989;10:1014.

- Examine viability of periwound tissue.
  - Halo of erythema, warmth, swelling may indicate infection (cellulitis).
  - Maceration of surrounding tissues due to moisture (urine, feces) or wound drainage increases risk for wound deterioration and enlargement.
  - Trophic changes may indicate poor arterial nutrition.

COMMON SKIN DISORDERS OR CONDITIONS

Skin disorders can occur as a result of a wide variety of ecological factors, and can be classified as primary or secondary.

PRIMARY SKIN DISORDERS

Primary skin disorders are the first lesion to appear on the skin as a visually recognizable manifestation of an underlying pathologic process. They can be described a number of ways depending on characteristics.

Macule. A macule is a change in the color of the skin. It is a flat spot, up to 1 cm, undetectable with palpation. A macule greater than 1 cm may be referred to as a patch.

Papule. A papule is a solid raised lesion that has distinct borders and is less than 1 cm in diameter. Papules may have a variety of shapes in profile (domed, flat-topped, umbilicated) and may be associated with secondary features such as crusts or scales.

Plaque. A plaque is a solid, raised, flat-topped lesion greater than 1 cm. in diameter. It is analogous to the geological formation, the plateau.

Nodule. A nodule is a raised solid lesion more than 1 cm and may be in the epidermis, dermis, or subcutaneous tissue.

Wheal. A wheal is an area of edema in the upper epidermis.

Pustule. Pustules are circumscribed elevated lesions that contain pus. They are most commonly infected (as in folliculitis) but may be sterile (as in pustular psoriasis).

Cyst. A cyst is a closed sac having a distinct membrane and developing abnormally in a cavity or structure of the body. Cysts may occur spontaneously, as a result of a developmental error in the embryo during pregnancy, or they may be caused by infections.

SECONDARY SKIN DISORDERS

Secondary skin disorders are the result of changes in the primary lesion or external trauma to the primary lesion:

- Scale.
- Crust.
- Thickening.

- Scar.
- Keloid: a keloid is an overgrowth of dense fibrous tissue that usually develops after healing of a skin injury. The tissue extends beyond the borders of the original wound, does not usually regress spontaneously, and tends to recur after excision.
- Excoriation: a hollowed-out or linear area of the skin covered by a crust.
- Fissure: a groove, natural division, deep furrow, or cleft.
- Ulcer.
- Erosion.
- Atrophy.

VASCULAR SKIN LESIONS

- Purpura: the appearance of red or purple discolorations on the skin, caused by bleeding underneath the skin. Small spots are called petechiae, while large spots are called ecchymoses.
- Spider angioma: an abnormal collection of blood vessels near the surface of the skin. The appearance is often similar to that of a small spider web.
- Venous star (telangiectasia): a small red nodule formed by a dilated vein in the skin caused by increased venous pressure.
- Capillary hemangioma: a unilateral, superonasal, eyelid, or brow lesion. It typically blanches with pressure, unlike the lesions seen with port-wine stains. The mass lesion may be sufficient to cause a ptosis of the involved eyelid. Alternatively, if the lesion extends posteriorly in the orbit, proptosis and visual loss may be present.

ECZEMA AND DERMATITIS

Eczema and dermatitis are terms that describe a superficial inflammation of the skin caused by exposure, allergic sensitization, or generally undetermined idiopathic factors. These conditions may be classified as either acute, subacute, or chronic:

- Acute: characterized by erythema, edema, vesiculation
- Subacute
- Chronic: characterized by mild erythema, scaliness, lichenification (thickening of the epidermis with exaggeration of normal skin lines), with or without hyperpigmentation

Exogenous (Contact) Dermatitis. Dermatitis typically follows some form of contact. Various types exist:

- Irritant contact dermatitis: exposure to direct chemical contact (acids or alkalis) or physical agent on the skin.
- Allergic contact dermatitis: this is a form of cell-mediated response, with the hypersensitivity based on a specific immunologic alteration.

Endogenous (Constitutional) Dermatitis. Various subtypes of endogenous dermatitis exist:

- Atopic: involves increased susceptibility to atopic diseases, (eg, asthma, hay fever, and systemic drug allergy), and an increased production of IgE antibodies. The skin becomes inherently sensitive and dry with a low threshold for itching.

- Seborrheic dermatitis: this type, usually localized in the areas of greatest sebaceous activity, is associated with excessive sebaceous secretion (seborrhea). The skin lesions consist of subacute dermatitis covered by greasy scales (eg, Dandruff), and is frequently associated with acne.
- Rosacea: this is a chronic, benign, but obvious facial disorder of middle-aged and older people of unknown etiology, but has a causal relationship with *Helicobacter pylori.* The characteristic signs of this condition include a rosy appearance of the cheeks, nose, and chin.

Bacterial Infections

A variety of bacterial flora can be found on normal skin, including the major pathogenic varieties of staphylococci and streptococci. These bacteria remain harmless depending on the invasiveness and toxicity of the specific organisms, the integrity of the skin and the immune and cellular defenses of the host. Bacterial infections typically enter through breaks in the skin, eg, abrasions or puncture wounds, or through the respiratory tract.

Bacterial Infections Localized to Hair. All of these infections are caused by *Staphylococcus aureus*, coagulase positive.

- Folliculitis: infection of most superficial part of hair follicle—a pustule pierced by hair.
- Furuncle: painful infection of whole length of hair follicle.
- Carbuncle: infection of a group of follicles.

Generalized Bacterial Skin Infections

- Impetigo contagiosum: an epidermal reaction caused by beta-hemolytic streptococci (*Streptococcuspyogenes*), *Staphylococcus aureus*, or both.
- Ecthyma: affects epidermis and dermis and is bacteriologically similar to impetigo.
- Cellulitis: caused mainly by beta-hemolytic streptococcus.

Viral Infections

These infections are contagious: the clinician must observe *standard precautions*.

Herpes Simplex. Herpes simplex viruses (HSVs), of which to types exist (type 1 [HSV-1] and type 2 [HSV-2], are two members of the herpes virus family, Herpesviridae. HSV-1 is transmitted chiefly by contact with infected saliva, whereas HSV-2 is transmitted sexually or from a mother to her newborn. Both HSV-1 and HSV-2 can cause similar watery blisters in the skin or mucous membranes of the mouth, lips or genitals after contact with infectious secretions.

Herpes Zoster (Shingles). More details on herpes zoster can be found in Chapter 9.

Plantar Wart. A plantar wart (verruca plantaris) is a hyperkeratotic lesion typically found on the plantar surface of the foot (over areas of pressure such as the heel and ball of the foot), caused by the human papillomavirus (HPV), usually of type 1, 2, or 4. Plantar warts are often endophytic (ie, they grow into the deeper layers of skin because of pressure). Although plantar warts are generally self-limiting, they should be treated to lessen symptoms, decrease duration, and reduce transmission.

FUNGAL INFECTIONS

Transmission of fungal infections is person-to-person or animal to person: the clinician must observe *standard precautions*.

Dermatophytes. The dermatophytes are a group of fungi that invade the dead keratin of skin, hair, and nails. Dermatophytosis (tinea) is a fungal infection caused by dermatophytes.

Clinically, tinea infections are classified according to the body region involved (Table 13-5).

Fungal infections may be treated with topical agents (except when treating tinea of the hair and nails) or, in extensive or recalcitrant disease, with oral antifungals.

PARASITIC INFECTIONS

Parasitic infections are caused through insect and animal contacts. Transmission can be either person to person or sexually transmitted so the clinician must observe *standard precautions*. A number of common parasitic infections exist:

- Scabies (mites). This is a highly contagious skin eruption caused by a female parasite that burrows into the skin causing inflammation, itching, and intense pruritus. Treatment involves excavation of the parasite using a needle or scalpel blade, or with a scabicide.
- Pediculosis. This is an infestation of a common parasite that can affect head, body, genital area, that is transmitted from person-to-person usually on shared personal items such as combs, clothes, or furniture. Treatment involves using a special soap or shampoo containing permethrin.

TABLE 13-5. CLASSIFICATIONS OF TINEA INFECTIONS

TINEA	DESCRIPTION
Capitis	Infection of scalp hair
Corporis	Infection of the trunk and extremities
Manuum	Infection of palms and interdigital webs
Pedis	Infection of the soles, and interdigital webs (Athlete's foot)
Cruris	Infection of the groin
Barbae	Infection of the beard area and neck
Faciale	Infection of the face
Unguium	Infection of the nail (onychomycosis)

Melanin Pigment Disorders

Hypopigmentation and Depigmentation

Pityriasis Alba. This condition is common in young children with the lesions consisting of hypopigmented macules with powdery scales. The face is commonly affected. However, patients are usually asymptomatic and the condition gradually disappears with age.

Vitiligo. This is a genetic disease that may be associated with autoimmune disorders such as thyroid diseases, pernicious anemia, Addison's disease, diabetes mellitus, and alopecia areata. Histologic examination shows a marked absence of melanocytes. Vitiligo is associated with localized scattered or confluent depigmented macules, that occur more frequently over friction areas. This disease may have a protracted course and may become generalized,

Hyperpigmentation

Freckles (Ephilides). Freckles occur frequently on light-exposed skin in individuals with red or blonde hair and blue eyes during the summer months.

Neurofibromatosis (von-Recklinghausen's Disease). Neurofibromatosis is characterized by macular hyperpigmentation (cafe-au-lait patches) and neurofibromata (neural tumors) anywhere on the body. The condition may be associated with bone lesions and intracranial and GI lesions and symptoms.

Melasma (Chloasma). Melasma, a blotchy hypermelanosis that occurs most often on the cheeks, forehead, and moustache area (usually in women) is commonly seen in pregnancy. Although the condition causes no other symptoms, there may be cosmetic concerns.

Benign Dermatoses

Psoriasis. Psoriasis, one of the most common dermatoses, appears as a chronic, bilaterally symmetric, erythematous plaquelike lesion with a silvery scale covering. The lesions classically are located over the extensor surfaces of the body, including the elbows, knees, back, and scalp. Psoriasis occasionally is associated with other systemic illnesses, particularly psoriatic arthritis (see Chapter 8), which occurs in approximately 5% to 10% of patients with psoriasis.

Systemic Sclerosis. Systemic sclerosis is a diffuse and chronic connective tissue disease of unknown etiology that causes fibrosis of the skin, joints, blood vessels, and internal organs. The disease is classified according to the degree and extent of skin thickening. The altered vascular function associated with the disease includes increased vasospasm, reduced vasodilatory capacity, and increased adhesiveness of the blood vessels to platelets and lymphocytes. There are three recognized stages of the disease (edematous; sclerotic; atrophic), although not every patient passes through all of the stages.

Discoid Lupus Erythematosus. Discoid lupus is a chronic, relatively common dermatitis that is more common in women than in men. The condition is characterized by erythematous plaques that vary from an atrophic to hyperkeratotic appearance in the region of the face, scalp, neck, extremities, and trunk.

AUTOIMMUNE SKIN DISORDERS

Scleroderma. Scleroderma, also known as progressive systemic scleroderma, describes two distinct diseases, both of unknown etiology: localized scleroderma and systemic scleroderma.[6-13] Localized scleroderma is primarily a cutaneous disease whereas the systemic variety is a multisystem connective tissue disease. There are two main subsets of systemic sclerosis, limited scleroderma (formerly known as CREST syndrome), and diffuse scleroderma:

- ***Limited scleroderma.*** Patients typically have a long history of Raynaud's phenomenon, and mildly puffy or swollen fingers before they present to their physicians with a digital ulcer, heartburn, or shortness of breath.
- ***Diffuse scleroderma.*** Patients have an acute onset of arthralgias, carpal tunnel syndrome, drawn, pursed lips, swollen hands, swollen legs, and crepitus-like friction rubs over the tendon areas of the hands, wrists, and ankles. These patients can have severe problems not only from skin thickening and contractures but also from dysfunction of other organ systems, including gastrointestinal (decreased esophageal motility, esophageal reflux), pulmonary (exertional dyspnea, fibrosis of the lungs, pulmonary hypertension), cardiovascular (myocardial fibrosis, arrhythmias), and renal (renal insufficiency and failure).

Raynaud's phenomenon is present in almost all patients with scleroderma. As there is no cure for scleroderma, the condition is managed with medications (antihypertensives, corticosteroids). The physical therapy intervention emphasizes preventing any loss of range of motion and enhancement of function (bed mobility, transfers, and walking). Modalities such as moist heat or paraffin may prove therapeutic.

Polymyositis. Polymyositis (PM), dermatomyositis (DM), and inclusion body myositis (IBM) are the major members of a group of skeletal muscle diseases called the idiopathic inflammatory myopathies.[14-19] Both PM and DM present with symmetric muscle weakness that develops over weeks to months. The characteristic rash (confluent, purple-red, macular eruption) over the face, trunk, and hands is seen in DM only. Other rashes seen with DM include erythematous nail beds and a scaly, purple erythematous papular eruption over the posterior (dorsal) aspect of the metacarpophalangeal and interphalangeal joints (Gottron sign).

ULCERS

The clinical features of the various types of ulcers are listed in Table 13-6.

Pressure Ulcers. Although the terms pressure ulcer and decubitus ulcer often are used interchangeably, pressure ulcer is the better term to describe this condition because the common denominator

TABLE 13-6. CLINICAL FEATURES OF ULCERS

CLINICAL FEATURES	VENOUS ULCER	ARTERIAL ULCER	DIABETIC ULCER	PRESSURE ULCER
Pulses	Normal	Poor or absent	Maybe present or diminished	
Pain	None to aching (in dependent position)	Often severe, intermittent claudication, progressing to pain at rest	Typically not painful; sensory loss usually present	Can be painful if sensation is intact
Color	Normal or cyanotic. May see dark pigmentation (thick, tender, indurated, fibroused tissue)	Pale on elevation; dusky rubor on dependency		Red, brown/black, or yellow
Temperature	Normal	Cool		May be warm if localized infection present (associated fever)
Edema	Often marked	Usually absent		
Skin changes	Pigmentation, stasis dermatitis, thickening of skin as scarring develops	Trophic changes (thin, shiny, atrophic skin); loss of hair on foot and toes; nails thickens		Inflammatory response with necrotic tissue
Ulceration	May develop, especially on the medial ankle; wet, with large amount of exudate	On toes or feet; can be deep	May develop due to trauma to insensitive skin	Typically occurs over bony prominences ie, sacrum, heels, trochanter, lateral malleolus, ischial areas, elbows
Gangrene	Absent	Black gangrenous skin adjacent to ulcer can develop	May develop	If left untreated

of all such ulcerations is pressure. Pressure ulcers result from sustained or prolonged pressure at levels greater than the level of the tissue's capillary filling pressure resulting in localized ischemia and/or tissue necrosis.[20-32] Most pressure ulcers are avoidable through anticipation and avoidance of the conditions that promote them by the multiple members of the health care team (Table 13-7). The

TABLE 13-7. PRESSURE ULCER PREVENTION

PREVENTION TECHNIQUE	SUGGESTED STRATEGIES
Proper positioning in bed and in wheelchair	Bony prominences protected and pressure distributed equally over large surface areas. Use of pressure distribution equipment such as wheelchair cushions, custom mattresses, and alternating pressure mattress pads.
Frequent changes in position	Every 2 hour when in bed Every 15-20 minutes when seated
Keep skin clean and dry	Good bowel and bladder care with immediate cleansing after episode of incontinence. Current cleansing and drying of skin at least once daily. Inspect skin for areas of redness in a.m. and p.m.
Nutrition	Diet with adequate calories, protein, vitamins, and minerals. Sufficient water intake.
Clothing	Avoid clothes that are either too tight or too loose fitting. Avoid clothes with thick seams, buttons, or zippers in areas of pressure.
Activity	Regular cardiovascular exercise. Gradual buildup of skin tolerance for new activities, equipment, and positions. Avoid movements that rub, drag, or scratch the skin.

Data from Spangler LL: Nonprogressive spinal cord disorders. In: Cameron MH, Monroe LG, eds. *Physical Rehabilitation: Evidence-Based Examination, Evaluation, and Intervention.* St Louis, MO: Saunders/Elsevier. 2007: 538-579.

TABLE 13-8. THE NORTON SCORE FOR ANTICIPATING PRESSURE ULCERS

General physical condition	1. Poor 2. Fair 3. Good 4. Excellent	Score:________
Mobility	1. Immobilized 2. Tubes and restraints 3. Tubes or restraints 4. No impairment	Score:________
Activity	1. Bed rest 2. Bed to chair 3. Bed rest with BRP 4. Up at liberty	Score:________
Mental status	1. Stuporous 2. Withdrawn 3. Confused 4. Alert and oriented	Score:________
Continence	1. Doubly incontinent 2. Frequently incontinent of urine 3. Occasionally incontinent 4. Fully continent	Score:________
Grading	Add the scores for all five categories. If cumulative score is greater than 15, there is little risk for pressure sore development; if cumulative score is less than 15, then there is a significant risk for pressure sore development.	

groups of patients most susceptible include elderly individuals, those who are neurologically impaired, and those who are acutely hospitalized (Tables 13-8 and 13-9). Pressure against the skin over a bony prominence increases the risk for the development of necrosis and ulceration (Table 13-10). Bacterial contamination from improper skin care or urinary or fecal incontinence, while not truly an etiological factor, is important to consider in the treatment of pressure sores as it can delay wound healing. Other contributing factors to pressure ulcers include shear, friction, heat, maceration (softening associated with excessive moisture) medication, malnutrition, and muscle atrophy (Table 13-11). Pressure ulcers can be graded using a four-stage system (Table 13-12).

Study Pearl

The term Marjolin's ulcer is used to describe a type of cancer that arises from any site of chronic inflammation. Ninety percent of Marjolin's ulcers develop from burn scars.[33,34] Other sites include stasis ulcers and decubitus ulcers. Marjolin's ulcers occur most often on the extremities and in wounds that have been present for 30 years or more.[33,34] Clinically, they exhibit exuberant granulation tissue that spills over their well-defined margins onto the surrounding tissue. The differential diagnosis is broad and may include any nonhealing ulcer such as venous stasis ulcers, diabetic ulcers, and arterial ulcers.[33,34]

Arterial Insufficiency (Ischemic) Ulcers. This type of ulcer develops secondary to arterial ischemia usually as a result of atherosclerotic disease of large-sized and medium-sized arteries, such as aortoiliac and femoropopliteal atherosclerosis.[35,36] Arterial insufficiency ulcers are common in the diabetic population due to a number of metabolic abnormalities, including high low-density lipoprotein (LDL) and very-low-density lipoprotein (VLDL) levels, elevated plasma fibrinogen levels, and increased platelet adhesiveness. In addition, individuals with diabetes have a higher incidence of atherosclerosis, thickening of capillary basement membranes, arteriolar hyalinosis, and endothelial proliferation. Mönckeberg sclerosis (calcification and thickening of the arterial media) is also noted with higher frequency in the diabetic population. Complicating matters further is the peripheral neuropathy associated with diabetes. Arterial ulcers occur more frequently on the distal aspects of the foot but may occur more proximally, depending on the location of the occluded artery.

TABLE 13-9. BRADEN SCALE FOR PREDICTING PRESSURE SORE RISK

Patient's Name ______________ Evaluator's Name ______________ Date of Assessmant

SENSORY PERCEPTION ability to respond meaning-fully to pressure-related discomfort	**1. Completely Limited** Unresponsive (does not moan, flinch, or grasp) to painful stimuli, due to diminished level of consciousness or sedation. OR limited ability to feel pain over most of body	**2. Very Limited** Responds only to painful stimuli. Cannot communicate discomfort except by moaning or restlessness OR has a sensory impairment which limits the ability to feel pain or discomfort over ½ of body.	**3. Slightly Limited** Responds to verbal commands, but cannot always communicate discomfort or the need to be turned. OR has some sensory impairment which limits ability to feel pain or discomfort in 1 or 2 extremities.	**4. No Impairment** Responds to verbal commands. Has no sensory deficit which would limit ability to feel or voice pain or discomfort.				
MOISTURE degree to which skin is exposed to moisture	**1. Constantly Moist** Skin is kept moist almost constantly by perspiration, urine, etc. Dampness is detected every time patient is moved or turned.	**2. Very Moist** Skin is often, but not always moist. Linen must be changed at least once a shift.	**3. Occasionally Moist:** Skin is occasionally moist, requiring an extra linen change approximately once a day.	**4. Rarely Moist** Skin is usually dry, linen only requires changing at routine intervals.				
ACTIVITY degree of physical activity	**1. Bedfast** Confined to bed.	**2. Chairfast** Ability to walk severely limited or non-existent. Cannot bear own weight and/or must be assisted into chair or wheelchair.	**3. Walks Occasionally** Walks occasionally during day, but for very short distances, with or without assistance. Spends majority of each shift in bed or chair	**4. Walks Frequently** Walks outside room at least twice a day and inside room at least once every two hours during waking hours				
MOBILITY ability to change and control body position	**1. Completely Immobile** Does not make even slight changes in body or extremity position without assistance	**2. Very Limited** Makes occasional slight changes in body or extremity position but unable to make frequent or significant changes independently.	**3. Slightly Limited** Makes frequent though slight changes in body or extremity position independently.	**4. No Limitation** Makes major and frequent changes in position without assistance.				
NUTRITION usual food intake pattern	**1. Very Poor** Never eats a complete meal. Rarely eats more than of any food offered. Eats 2 servings or less of protein (meat or dairy products) per day. Takes fluids poorly. Does not take a liquid dietary supplement OR is NPO and/or maintained on clear liquids or IV's for more than 5 days.	**2. Probably Inadequate** Rarely eats a complete meal and generally eats only about ½ of any food offered. Protein intake includes only 3 servings of meat or dairy products per day. Occasionally will take a dietary supplement. OR receives less than optimum amount of liquid diet or tube feeding	**3. Adequate** Eats over half of most meals. Eats a total of 4 servings of protein (meat, dairy products per day). Occasionally will refuse a meal, but will usually take a supplement when offered OR is on a tube feeding or TPN regimen which probably meets most of nutritional needs	**4. Excellent** Eats most of every meal. Never refuses a meal. Usually eats a total of 4 or more servings of meat and dairy products. Occasionally eats between meals. Does not require supplementation.				
FRICTION & SHEAR	**1. Problem** Requires moderate to maximum assistance in moving. Complete lifting without sliding against sheets is impossible. Frequently slides down in bed or chair, requiring frequent repositioning with maximum assistance. Spasticity, contractures or agitation leads to almost constant friction	**2. Potential Problem** Moves feebly or requires minimum assistance. During a move skin probably slides to some extent against sheets, chair, restraints or other devices. Maintains relatively good position in chair or bed most of the time but occasionally slides down.	**3. No Apparent Problem** Moves in bed and in chair independently and has sufficient muscle strength to lift up completely during move. Maintains good position in bed or chair.					
				Total Score				

TABLE 13-10. BONY PROMINENCES ASSOCIATED WITH PRESSURE ULCERS

SUPINE	PRONE	SIDELYING	SEATED
Occiput	Forehead	Ears	Spine of scapula
Spine of scapula	Anterior portion of the acromion process	Lateral portion of acromion process	Vertebral spinous processes
Inferior angle of scapula	Anterior head of humerus	Lateral head of humerus	Ischial tuberosities
Vertebral spinous processes	Sternum	Lateral epicondyle of humerus	
Medial epicondyle of humerus	Anterior superior iliac spine	Greater trochanter	
Posterior iliac crest	Patella	Head of fibula	
Sacrum	Dorsum of foot	Lateral malleolus	
Coccyx		Medial malleolus	

Symptomatic patients may present with intermittent claudication, ischemic pain at rest, nonhealing ulceration of the foot, or frank ischemia of the foot. Signs frequently associated with arterial ulcers include a loss of hair on the extremity, poor capillary refill in the toes, and brittle nails.

The typical intervention for an arterial insufficiency ulcer focuses on cleansing the ulcer, rest, reducing risk factors, and limb protection. Patient education emphasizes

- Washing and thorough drying of the feet
- Avoiding unnecessary leg elevation
- Daily inspections of the legs and feet
- The wearing of appropriately sized shoes together with clean, seamless socks
- Using bandages as necessary while avoiding any unnecessary pressure
- Avoiding using heating pads or soaking feet in hot water (to avoid maceration and possible burning)

TABLE 13-11. RISK FACTORS ASSOCIATED WITH PRESSURE ULCERS

Emaciation
Obesity
Elderly
Immobilization
Decrease in activity level
Diabetes
Circulatory disorders
Incontinence
Decreased mental status

TABLE 13-12. NATIONAL PRESSURE ULCER ADVISORY PANEL (NPUAP) PRESSURE ULCERS STAGES

STAGE	CHARACTERISTICS	PREFERRED PRACTICE PATTERN ACCORDING TO THE GUIDE[a]
Stage I	An observable pressure related alteration of intact skin whose indicators as compared to an adjacent or opposite area of the body may include changes in skin color, skin temperature (warm or cool), tissue consistency (firm or boggy), and/or sensation (pain, itching).	7B: Impaired integumentary integrity associated with superficial skin involvement
Stage II	A partial thickness skin loss that involves the epidermis and/or dermis. The ulcer is superficial and presents clinically as an abrasion, a blister, or shallow crater.	7C: Impaired integumentary integrity associated with partial thickness skin involvement and scar formation
Stage III	A full thickness skin loss that involves damage or necrosis of subcutaneous tissue that may extend down to, but not through, underlying fascia. The ulcer presents clinically as a deep crater with or without undermining adjacent tissue.	7D: Impaired integumentary integrity associated with full-thickness skin involvement and scar formation
Stage IV	A full thickness skin loss with extensive destruction, tissue necrosis or damage to muscle, bone or supporting structures (eg, tendon, joint capsule). Undermining or sinus tracts may be present.	7E: Impaired integumentary integrity associated with skin involvement extending into fascia, muscle, or bone and scar formation

[a]Guide to Physical Therapist Practice, 2nd ed. American Physical Therapy Association. *Phys Ther.* 2001;81:1-746.
Data from Pressure ulcer prevention and treatment following spinal cord injury: a clinical practice guideline for health-care professionals. *J Spinal Cord Med.* 2001;24(suppl 1):S40-S101.

Neuropathic Ulcers. A neuropathic ulcer is a secondary complication associated with a combination of ischemia and neuropathy, such as that which occurs with diabetic peripheral neuropathy.[37-44] Because of the decreased sensitization, unnoticed excessive heat or cold, pressure from a poorly fitting shoe, or damage from a blunt or sharp object inadvertently left in the shoe may cause blistering and ulceration before the patient is aware. These factors, combined with a poor arterial inflow, confer a high risk of limb loss on the patient with diabetes. Neuropathic ulcers are frequently found in those areas that are most subjected to weight bearing, such as the malleoli, heel, plantar metatarsal head areas, the tips of the most prominent toes (usually the first or second), and the tips of hammer toes.

Study Pearl

Charcot deformity is seen commonly in patients with advanced stages of diabetic neuropathy. Initial signs often mimic cellulitis. A common finding in diabetic patients with early Charcot changes is a strong pulse with associated diffuse erythema.

Neuropathic ulcers have certain characteristics:

- They are typically well defined by a prominent callus rim and the wound has good granulation tissue with little or no drainage.
- The wound skin often appears to be dry or cracked.
- The distal limb may appear to be shiny and appear somewhat cool to touch.

Patients rarely report pain with neuropathic ulcers in part due to diminished sensation. Pedal pulses are most often diminished or absent. The Wagner Ulcer Grade Classification Scale is commonly used as an assessment instrument for diabetic foot ulcers (Table 13-13).[45,46]

Venous Insufficiency Ulcers. Venous insufficiency ulcers are caused by valvular incompetence in the high-pressure deep venous system, low-pressure superficial venous system, or both.[47-51] Untreated venous insufficiency in the deep or superficial system can cause a progressive syndrome involving pain, swelling, skin changes, and eventual tissue breakdown. Venous ulcers typically are located over the medial malleolus area. They tend to be irregular in shape and possess a good granulation base. The most common subjective symptoms include leg aching, swelling, cramping, heaviness, and soreness, which are improved by walking or by elevating the legs.

Intervention focuses on cleansing the ulcer and applying compression to control the edema. Patient education emphasizes

- Elevating the ulcer above the heart when resting or sleeping
- Attempting frequent active exercise
- Daily inspections of the legs and feet

TABLE 13-13. THE WAGNER ULCER GRADE CLASSIFICATION SCALE

GRADE	DESCRIPTION
0	No open lesion but may possess pre-ulcerative lesions; healed ulcers; presence of bony deformity
1	Superficial ulcer not involving subcutaneous tissue
2	Deep ulcer with penetration through the subcutaneous tissue; potentially exposing bone, tendon, ligament or joint capsule
3	Deep ulcer with osteitis, abscess or osteomyelitis
4	Gangrene of digit
5	Gangrene of foot requiring disarticulation

Data from Gul A, Basit A, Ali SM, et al: Role of wound classification in predicting the outcome of diabetic foot ulcer. *J Pak Med Assoc*. 2006;56:444-447; and Oyibo SO, Jude EB, Tarawneh I, et al: A comparison of two diabetic foot ulcer classification systems: the Wagner and the University of Texas wound classification systems. *Diabetes Care*. 2001;24:84-88.

- Wearing appropriately sized shoes together with clean, seamless socks
- Using bandages as necessary and avoiding scratching or other forms of direct contact

Skin Cancer

Skin cancers are the most prevalent form of cancer.[52-61] Skin cancer can be categorized using three broad categories: benign, premalignant, and malignant.

Benign Tumors.

- Seborrheic keratosis (SK) is a common benign tumor that occurs in advanced and middle-aged persons. It is typically a raised papular lesion of variable color from light to dark brown. SKs may be smooth or wartlike with visible pitting. Common sites include the face, trunk, and extremities.
- Acrochordon, also known as skin tag, fibroepithelial polyp, fibroma molle, and fibroepithelial papilloma, have been observed to follow warts, SKs, inflammatory skin conditions, and are occasionally associated with pregnancy, diabetes mellitus, and intestinal polyposis syndromes. Acrochordons tend to be located in the intertriginous areas of the axilla, groin, and infra mammary regions as well as in the low cervical area along the collar line. They are soft fleshy papules that vary in size from 1 to 6 mm and are usually, although not necessarily, pedunculated.
- Keratinous cyst, also known as a sebaceous cyst, wen, atheroma, or steatoma.
- Nevus. The definition of a nevus can be expanded to include any congenital lesion that is circumscribed to well-defined, including moles. Most nevi appear when individuals are aged 2 to 60 years and have a predictable evolution. They rarely undergo activation or malignant degeneration. Nevi tend to be more common on the head, neck, and trunk. However, a great deal of variability exists with regard to size, shape, and even amount of hair present.

Premalignant Tumors. Actinic keratosis, also known as solar keratosis and senile keratosis, are rough appearing, scaly, erythematous papules or plaques that occur on exposed surfaces (eg, face, hands, ears, neck, legs, thorax) of blue or green-eyed middle-aged persons with fair skin and a history of chronic sun exposure. The most important attribute is its premalignant potential—almost 50% of skin cancer cases begin as actinic keratosis lesions.

Malignant Tumors.

Malignant tumors of the skin include the following:

- Basal cell carcinoma: the most common cutaneous malignancy in humans. These tumors typically appear on sun-exposed skin, are slow growing, and rarely metastasize. The classic description is of a small, well-defined nodule with a translucent, pearly border with overlying telangiectasias. Coloration varies with melanin content and the presence of areas of necrosis. Neglected tumors can lead to significant local destruction and even disfigurement.

- Bowen's disease: also known as carcinoma in situ and squamous intraepidermal neoplasia. These lesions involve predominantly skin unexposed to the sun (ie, protected skin). The lesions are scaly, crusted, erythematous plaques—a persistent, ground to reddish brown, scaly plaque with well-defined margins.
- Squamous cell carcinoma: the second most common form of skin cancer. Frequently arises on the sun-exposed skin of middle-aged and elderly individuals. General risk factors include age older than 50 years, male sex, fair skin, geography (closer to the equator), exposure to UV light (high cumulative dose), exposure to chemical carcinogens (eg, arsenic, tar), exposure to ionizing radiation, and chronic immunosuppression. The tumors often manifest as small, firm nodules with indistinct margins or plaques. The surface may have various irregularities ranging from smooth to verruciform to ulcerated. Skin coloration is often brown to tan. Scaling, bleeding, and crusting also may occur. Typically, squamous cell carcinoma is locally invasive.
- Dermatofibroma protuberans: a low-grade dermal sarcoma. Typically, the lesion occurs as a painless subcutaneous mass after a history of trauma. The lesion grows slowly; however, if left unattended, it can become quite large and have multiple nodules. This malignancy typically has lateral spread, but it can also invade deeper structures and may ulcerate. It is generally reddish blue. Metastasis is unlikely but has been reported.
- Merkel cell carcinoma: an aggressive cutaneous neoplasm observed in sun-exposed areas. The tumor originates in the dermis and appears as a pinkish nodule that enlarges by invading deeper structures.
- Kaposi's sarcoma: a spindle-cell tumor thought to be derived from endothelial cell lineage. Kaposi's sarcoma (KS) can occur in several different clinical settings:
  - Epidemic AIDS-related KS: this type occurs in patients with advanced HIV infection, and is the most common presentation of KS.
  - Immunocompromised KS: this type can occur following solid-organ transplantation or in patients receiving immunosuppressive therapy.
  - Classic KS: this type typically occurs in elderly men of Mediterranean and Eastern European background. Classic KS usually carries a protracted and indolent course.
  - Endemic African KS: this type occurs in men who are HIV seronegative in Africa and may carry an indolent or aggressive course.
- Melanoma: melanoma is a malignancy of pigment-producing cells (melanocytes) located predominantly in the skin, but which can also be found in the eyes, ears, GI tract, leptomeninges, and oral and genital mucous membranes. A changing mole is the most common warning sign for melanoma. Variation in color and/or an increase in diameter, height, or asymmetry of borders of a pigmented lesion are noted by more than 80% of patients with melanoma at the time of diagnosis.

Study Pearl

The pneumonic ABCDE (**A**symmetry, **B**order irregularity, **C**olor variegation, **D**iameter, **E**volving) is an easy way to remember those factors associated with skin cancer. Symptoms such as bleeding, itching, ulceration, and pain in a pigmented lesion are less common but warrant an evaluation.

Four major clinicopathologic (or histogenetic) subtypes of primary cutaneous melanoma, distinguished largely by anatomic site have been identified. These include

- Superficial spreading melanoma: the most common subtype, manifested as a flat or slightly elevated brown lesion with variegate pigmentation (ie, black, blue, pink, or white discoloration).
- Nodular melanoma: most commonly found on the legs and trunk.
- Lentigo maligna melanoma: typically located on the head, neck, and arms (sun-damaged skin) of fair-skinned older individuals.
- Acral lentiginous melanoma: characterized by the development of macular pigmentation ranging from dark brown to black or by raised blue-black nodules.

BURNS

Burn injuries are classified by the depth of skin tissue involved, with the amount of skin destruction being based on temperature and length of time the tissue is exposed to heat.

Superficial Burn. This type of burn, also referred to as an epidermal burn, causes cell damage only to the epidermis. Characteristics include

- Tissue is red, erythematous, often painful, and blanches with pressure.
- Tissue damage is minimal and healing is spontaneous.

Superficial Partial-Thickness Burn. This type of burn involves damage down through the epidermis and into the papillary layer of the dermis. Characteristics include

- Adnexal structures (eg, sweat glands, hair follicles) are often involved, but enough of these structures are preserved for function, and the epithelium lining then can proliferate and allow for regrowth of skin.
- The burned area characteristically has blisters over it and is very painful.

Deep Partial-Thickness Burn. This type of burn involves destruction of the entire epidermis and damage of the dermis down into the reticular layer. Characteristics include[1]

- A mixed red or waxy white color (the deeper the injury, the more white) in appearance.
- Wet surface from broken blisters and leakage of plasma fluid due to alteration of the dermal vascular network.
- Marked edema.
- Involved area has diminished sensation to light touch or soft pinprick, but deep pressure sense is retained.
- Healing occurs through scar formation and re-epithelialization.

- May be associated with the development of hypertrophic and keloid scars.

Full-Thickness Burn. This type of burn involves destruction of all the epidermal and dermal layers. In addition the hypodermis may be damaged to some extent. Characteristics include

- Charring of skin or a translucent white color, with coagulated vessels visible below.
- The area is insensate (without feeling), but the patient complains of pain, which is usually a result of surrounding partial thickness burns.
- As all of the skin tissue and structures are destroyed, there are no sites available for epithelialization of the wound, and skin grafting of tissue over the wound is necessary.

Subdermal Burn. This type of burn involves complete destruction of all tissue from the epidermis down to and through the hypodermis.

Electrical Burn. Electrical burns can occur when an electric current passes through the body after the skin has made contact with an electrical source.

As the body is essentially an electrical system, complications associated with electrical burns include cardiac arrhythmias, ventricular fibrillation, renal failure, spinal cord damage, and respiratory arrest.[1]

Study Pearl

Electric current follows the course of least resistance offered by various tissue:
- Nerves, followed by blood vessels, offer the least resistance.
- Bone offers the most resistance.

Burn Extent. The more body surface area (BSA) involved in a burn, the greater the morbidity and mortality rates. An individual's palmar surface represents 1% of the BSA. A simple method to estimate burn extent is to use the patient's palmar surface to measure the burned area. Burn extent is calculated only on individuals with second-degree or third-degree burns. Classification by a percentage of body area burned:

- Critical: 10% of body with third-degree burns and 30% or more with second-degree; complications, and, eg, respiratory involvement, smoke inhalation.
- Moderate: less than 10% with third-degree burns and 15% to 30% with second-degree.
- Minor: less than 2% with third-degree burns and 15% with second-degree burns.
- Another quick method is to use the Rule of Nines to estimate the extent of burn injury (Table 13-14).

Study Pearl

Burns cause an increased metabolic rate and energy metabolism. How the individual responds to the increased energy demands will dictate recovery.

TABLE 13-14. RULE OF NINES

BODY AREA	ADULTS (%)	CHILDREN (%)
Head: anterior	4.5	18
Head: posterior	4.5	
Arm: anterior	4.5	9
Arm: posterior	4.5	
Leg: anterior	9	14
Leg: posterior	9	
Chest	18	18
Back	18	18
Genitals	1	1

The Lund-Browder charts, which are designed specifically for use with children, are often used for estimating body areas (Figure 13-1).

Complications of Burn Injury. Integument trauma often affects the function of the cardiovascular, pulmonary, renal, metabolic, muscular, nervous and skeletal systems.

Pain. Superficial skin damage generally results in more pain than deeper injuries because the free endings are not destroyed in the

Print a copy of of this page for patients with burns covering large areas or multiple areas.

Complete the table to calculate the total area of burn involved.

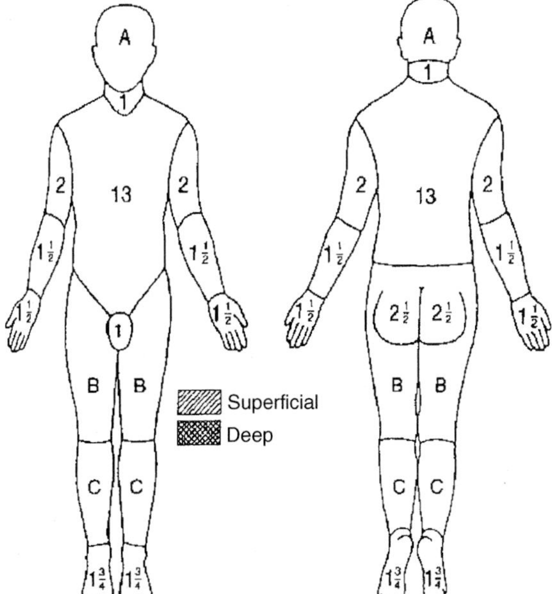

Region	%
Head	
Neck	
Ant. Trunk	
Post. Trunk	
Right arm	
Left arm	
Buttocks	
Genitalia	
Right leg	
Left leg	
Total burn	

Relative percentage of areas affected by growth

Age (years)	0	1	5	10	15	Adult
A - 1/2 of head	9 1/2	8 1/2	6 1/2	5 1/2	4 1/2	3 1/2
B - 1/2 of one thigh	2 3/4	3 1/4	4	4 1/4	4 1/2	4 3/4
C - 1/2 of one leg	2 1/2	2 1/2	2 3/4	3	3 1/4	3

Figure 13-1. Burn diagram.

former. However, as the nerve endings regenerate following a full thickness burn, intense pain may result. Pain is the major deterrent in preventing burn patients from participating in exercises and positioning following a burn injury.

Infection. In addition to the tissue damage, infection is a major source of mortality and the most significant cause of loss of function and cosmetic appearance. A number of factors play a role:

- Vasoconstriction leading to peripheral hypoperfusion, particularly in the burned areas, creates a major defect in immunity, enhancing bacterial invasion.
- Dead tissue, warmth, and moisture are ideal for bacterial growth.

Infection can be reduced or controlled with the following:

- Culturing of wounds and appropriate antibiotic treatment regimen prescribed.

- The application of topical antimicrobial agents.
- Anti-inflammatory agents.
- Standard and transmission-based precautions by healthcare workers.

Cardiac Complications. These include arrhythmias caused by hypovolemia, hypoxia, acidosis, or hyperkalemia.

Pulmonary Complications. An individual who has been burned in a closed space should be suspected of having an inhalation injury. Signs of an inhalation injury include facial burns, singed nasal hairs, harsh cough, hoarseness, abnormal breath sounds, respiratory distress, and carbonaceous sputum and/or hypoxemia.[1,63] The primary complications associated with this injury are carbon monoxide poisoning, tracheal damage, upper airway obstruction, pulmonary edema, and pneumonia.[1] Thermal damage to the lower respiratory tract can be caused by steam inhalation or by the inhalation of hot gases.

- Airway edema can produce upper airway obstruction that develops more slowly.
- Chemical injury to small airway alveolar capillaries can cause delayed progressive respiratory failure.
- Inhaling toxic products (eg, cyanide, carbon monoxide) generated by burning material may result in thermal injuries to the pharynx and upper airway as well as in ventilation injuries.

Study Pearl

- Inhaled carbon monoxide binds to hemoglobin, greatly reducing O_2 transport.

Metabolic Complications. Because thermal injury results in more loss of body mass than any other disease, continued demands are placed on the metabolic system for the significant healing process. Metabolic acidosis may result from poor tissue perfusion due to hypovolemia (monitored through urine output) or to heart failure. The clinician must consider the catabolic state of the patient when designing exercise programs so that the metabolic stress is not increased.

Myoglobinuria. Hemoglobinuria may result from erythrocyte destruction after burns. Myoglobinuria can also result from ischemic constrictions of muscle, crush injuries, or deep thermal or electrical burns of muscle. Initially, osmotic diuresis is needed until the myoglobinuria clears. Without prompt, accurate management, myoglobinuria may result in renal tubular necrosis.

Study Pearl

Types of scarring include

- Hypertrophic scar: a raised scar that stays within the boundaries of the burn wound; characteristically red, raised, firm.
- Keloid scar: a raised scar that extends beyond the boundaries of the original burn wound; red, raised, firm.

Hypertrophic Scarring and Wound Contracture. Contractures are especially likely to develop if wounds are not closed promptly. If a body part is left immobile for a protracted period of time, capsular contraction and shortening of tendon and muscle groups (which cross the joints) occur. This rapid process can be prevented by a program of passive ROM, correct positioning, and splinting. The general rule for splinting is to position the affected joint in the opposite direction from which it will contract.

Upper Extremity. Flexion deformities of the neck can be minimized with thermoplastic neck splints, conformers, and split mattresses. In critically ill patients, positioning the neck in slight extension is often all that can be done. The clinician should ensure that the ventilator tubing does not pull the head so that a contracture develops.

- An axillary contracture can interfere with important upper extremity functions. Axillary adduction contractures can be prevented by positioning the shoulders widely abducted with axillary splints, or a variety of support devices mounted to the bed.
- Elbow contractures, which restrict extension is a common anterior soft tissue complication. Elbow flexion contractures are minimized by statically splinting the elbow in extension using a gutter splint, conforming splint, palmar or dorsal extension splint. Elbow splints can be alternated with flexion splints to help retain a full ROM.

Perhaps the most common upper extremity deformities are posterior (dorsal) hand and web space contractures:

- Dorsal hand contractures are prevented ideally by attention to proper positioning presurgically and postsurgically using wrist splints, thumb spica, and palmar or dorsal extension splints.
- In the normal web space, the leading edge of the anterior aspect of the web is distal to the dorsal aspect, whereas in the typical dorsal web space contracture, this pattern is reversed. Web space contractures can be minimized by proper early surgery and compressive gloves supplemented with web space conformers.

Lower Extremity. Patients who have been supine for extended periods often tolerate immediate upright positioning poorly. Prior to initial efforts at assisted standing, such patients benefit from tilt table training and graduated sitting. Using gentle elastic wraps around the lower extremities prior to placing the patient in an upright position helps to prevent lower extremity edema, which can hinder recovery.

- Flexion contractures of the hips and knees, which are particularly common in infants and very young children who spend little time with the hips in extension, can be prevented by careful positioning and ROM. Prone positioning, although poorly tolerated by some, can assist in minimizing hip flexion contractures. Knee immobilizers can minimize knee flexion contractures. Correction generally requires incisional release and grafting with directed postoperative efforts to maintain knee extension.
- The equinus deformity, in which the ankle is plantar flexed and the foot is in a varus position, is a serious problem that can occur even if the ankles are not burned. This position can be prevented, however, with static splinting of the ankles in the neutral position and performing ROM twice daily. Splints designed for this purpose can cause pressure injury over the metatarsal heads or calcaneus if improperly designed. These injuries can be prevented by using padding to distribute pressure evenly across the metatarsal heads and by extending the footplate of the splint beyond the heel and cutting out the area around the calcaneus.
- A deep dorsal foot burn may result in a contracture of the metatarsophalangeal joints, so that the toes are brought off the ground, causing the patient to have an abnormal gait.

- The role of physical therapy in burn management is described in the Burn Healing and Management section.

PHYSICAL THERAPY INTERVENTION FOR IMPAIRED INTEGUMENTARY INTEGRITY

Patient/Client-Related Instruction

Patient education plays a critical role in the intervention of integumentary disorders. The clinician should determine those activities, positions, and postures that produce or reduce trauma to skin and the level of safety awareness that the patient demonstrates during functional activities. In addition, the following should be addressed:

- The likelihood of future trauma to skin.
- Enhanced disease awareness, healthy behaviors.
- Mechanisms of pressure ulcer development. These include assistive, adaptive, protective, orthotic, or prosthetic devices that produce or reduce skin trauma.
- Avoidance of prolonged positions.
- Safety awareness during self-care and during use of devices and equipment.
- Importance of ongoing activities/exercise program.
- Daily, comprehensive skin inspection, paying particular attention to bony prominences.
- Avoidance of harsh soaps, known irritants, temperature extremes, and exacerbating factors or triggers.
- Avoidance of restrictive clothing, and tight fitting shoes, socks.
- Incontinence management strategies.
- Enhance activities of daily living, functional mobility and safety.
- Pressure relieving devices.
- Enhance self-management of symptoms.
- Edema management through leg/arm elevation and muscle pumping exercises, and compression therapy to facilitate the movement of excess fluid from the extremity.
  - Compression wraps: elastic or tubular bandages.
  - Paste bandages, eg, Unna boot.
  - Compression stockings, eg, Jobst.
  - Compression pump therapy.
- Review of medications. The following medications can have a negative effect on wound repair: nonsteroidal anti-inflammatories, corticosteroids, immunosuppressives, anticoagulants, and prostaglandins.

Burn Healing and Management

Management of burn injuries may be divided into four general phases. The physical therapist is typically not involved until the fourth phase.[64-76]

Initial Evaluation and Resuscitation. Occurs on days 1 to 3 and requires an accurate fluid resuscitation and thorough evaluation for other injuries and comorbidity. At the rescue site, the victim of an acute thermal, chemical, or electrical injury must be immediately removed from the burning process, including removing all clothing, especially smoldering material (eg, melted synthetic shirts, hot tar-laden material). All chemical agents should be flushed off the skin, and burns caused by acids, alkalis, or organic compounds (eg, phenols, cresols) should be flushed with copious amounts of water continuously over an extended time. Immediate care also includes establishing an adequate airway, replacing lost fluid (plasma), and recognizing and managing associated life-threatening major trauma. Aggressive nutritional support is indicated for patients with a burn of > 20% BSA.

Initial Wound Excision and Biologic Closure. This is accomplished typically by a series of staged operations that are completed during the first few days after injury.

Definitive Wound Closure. Involves replacement of temporary wound covers with a definitive cover; there is also closure and acute reconstruction of areas with small surface area but high complexity, such as the face and hands. Restoration of an intact barrier is of critical importance following wounding and may be achieved in numerous ways, including grafting. A skin graft is a surgical procedure in which a piece of skin is taken from a suitable donor area and transplanted to the affected area. There are a variety of skin grafts, some of which provide temporary cover, and others that are for permanent wound coverage:

- Autogenous graft, or autograft: skin transplanted from one location to another on the same individual. If the entire thickness of the dermis is included, the appropriate term is full-thickness skin graft. If less than the entire thickness of the dermis is included, appropriate terms are partial or split-thickness skin graft. Split-thickness skin grafts are further categorized as thin (0.005-0.012 in), intermediate (0.012-0.018 in), or thick (0.018-0.030 in) based on the thickness of graft harvested. An appropriate donor site is selected, typically the anterior, lateral, or medial part of the thigh; the buttock; or the medial aspect of the arm. For larger defects, a large, flat donor surface is ideal.
- Xenograft or heterograft is skin taken from a variety of animals, usually a pig. Heterograft skin became popular because of the limited availability and high expense of human skin tissue. In some cases religious, financial, or cultural objections to the use of human cadaver skin may also be factors. Wound coverage using xenograft or heterograft is a temporary covering used until autograft.
- Allograft, cadaver skin, or homograft is human cadaver skin donated for medical use. Cadaver skin is used as a temporary covering for excised (cleaned) wound surfaces before autograft (permanent) placement. Unmeshed cadaver skin is put over the excised wound and stapled in place. Postoperatively, the cadaver skin may be covered with a dressing. Wound coverage using cadaveric allograft is removed prior to permanent autografting.

Rehabilitation, Reconstruction, and Reintegration.

Although this phase begins during the resuscitation period, it becomes time consuming and involved toward the end of the acute hospital stay. To attain the objective of optimal long-term function, rehabilitation efforts must begin at the outset of burn care.

Based on evaluation, the extent and depth of burn, and the patient's current health status, age, and physical and mental condition, the patient's prognosis can be estimated by the burn care team. The development of specific anticipated goals and expected outcomes is based on the following general goals from the *Guide to Physical Therapist Practice*, and include

- Enhancement of wound and soft tissue healing
- A reduction in the risk of infection and complications
- A reduction in the risk of secondary impairments
- Achievement of maximal range of motion
- Restoration of preinjury level of cardiovascular endurance
- Achievement of good to normal strength
- Achievement of independent ambulation
- Increased independent function in ADLs
- Minimization of scar formation
- Increased patient, family, and caregiver understanding of expectations and goals and outcomes
- Increased aerobic capacity
- Improved self-management of symptoms

Study Pearl

Attention to the security of endotracheal tubes, nasogastric tubes, and arterial and central venous catheters is paramount, as unexpected loss of these devices can contribute to morbidity and mortality.

The principal components of burn therapy include the following:

- Passive ROM and gentle stretching. Passive ROM is best performed twice daily, with the clinician taking all joints through a full ROM. The clinician must be sensitive to the patient's pain, anxiety, wound status, extremity perfusion, and security of the patient's airway and vascular access devices. These procedures should be performed in coordination with the ICU staff.

Other maneuvers that can be used to increase the patient's tolerance for passive ROM include the following:

- Timing of the ROM session with medication, wound cleansing, or dressing changes.
- Administration of opiates or benzodiazepines.
- Gentle conversation, encouragement, and an unhurried approach to therapy sessions.
- Increasing active ROM and progressing to strengthening with resistive exercises. Resisted ROM, isometric exercises, active strengthening, and gait training are important objectives.
- Minimizing dependent edema formation and promoting venous return. Burned and grafted extremities commonly have lingering edema that can contribute to joint stiffness. Reducing this edema facilitates rehabilitation efforts.
- Tubular elastic dressings, elastic wrap dressings, elevation, and retrograde massage help reduce extremity edema.
- ADL training. Performance of ADL tasks and the impending return to play/school/work are important considerations.

- Initial scar management. Topical silicone may have a favorable influence on selected evolving hypertrophic scars.
- Proprioceptive and sensation training.
- Positioning and splinting. Proper antideformity positioning minimizes shortening of tendons, collateral ligaments, and joint capsules; it reduces extremity and facial edema.

Although splints are used less frequently, there are several predictable contractures that occur in patients with burns that can be prevented by a proper ROM, positioning, and splinting program.

The most important therapeutic maneuver is elevation of the extremity, especially for patients with a leg or hand burn. Positioning affected extremities just above the level of the heart reduces edema, which is another important aspect of antideformity positioning. The extremity should be placed above heart level at all times except for periods of ≤20 minutes during the day. Because bed rest with elevation is difficult for an outpatient, hospitalization is often required when the legs are burned.

Postdischarge. Planning appropriate postoperative rehabilitation activities helps patients optimize surgical outcome.

For many burn patients, the first 18 months after discharge are more difficult than the acute stay. The principal rehabilitation goals at this time include the following:

- Providing a home exercise program of progressive ROM and strengthening
- Evaluation of evolving problem areas
- Specific postoperative therapy after reconstructive operations
- Scar management

Ideally, the same clinician who worked with the patient during the acute inpatient hospitalization continues through the outpatient setting. Not only does this continuity enhance the patient's experience, but also it helps the clinician monitor burn recovery. If, for reasons of distance or managed care, it is not possible to maintain this relationship, regular contact at each clinic visit back at the burn unit can achieve this goal indirectly.

Scar Management. Hypertrophic scarring is a difficult problem for burn patients, and scar management is an essential aspect of burn therapy. Scars can form in an organized manner termed *normotrophic* scarring, or in a disorganized manner such as that seen with hypertrophic or keloid scars.

The wound hyperemia seen universally following burn wound healing should begin to resolve about 9 weeks after epithelialization. In wounds destined to become hypertrophic, increased neovascularization occurs with increasing (rather than decreasing) erythema after 9 weeks.

Available tools to modify the progression of hypertrophic scar formation include scar massage, compression garments, topical silicone, steroid injections, and surgery. In some contractures over major joints, serial casting (refer to Chapter 9) may be useful.

Surgical Intervention. Surgical excision or incision and autografting are useful maneuvers when other scar management tools are

> **Study Pearl**
>
> All splints should be inspected at least twice daily for evidence of poor fit or pressure injury; improperly used splints can cause injury. A nursing staff in-service minimizes splint-related skin injury.

> **Study Pearl**
>
> When treating children, it is important to use developmentally appropriate play to facilitate rehabilitation goals. For example, children with serious hand burns are ideally engaged in play that requires the use of their hands at a motor level that is consistent with their development.

> **Study Pearl**
>
> Perhaps the most virulent hypertrophic scarring is seen in deep dermal burns that heal spontaneously in 3 or more weeks; this seems especially true in areas of highly elastic skin (eg, the lower face, submental triangle, anterior chest and neck).

> **Study Pearl**
>
> Extreme pruritus is a frequent part of burn wound healing. Pruritus typically begins shortly after the wound has healed, peaks in intensity 4 to 6 months after injury, and then gradually subsides in most patients. It can be especially troubling at night. In most patients, it is adequately treated with massage, moisturizers, and oral antihistamines at night. Alternative approaches are available, although none works reliably for everyone. In patients particularly troubled by pruritus, a sequential therapeutic trial of each maneuver often identifies one particularly helpful method: topical creams containing vitamin E, topical antihistamine creams, topical cold compresses, frequent application of moisturizing creams, or colloidal baths.

ineffective. Most burn reconstructive procedures can be performed using a combination of some basic techniques: incisional release and grafting, excisional release and grafting, Z-plasty, and random flaps. Tissue expansion and free flaps are needed less commonly.

WOUND CARE

The four primary principles of wound care are

- Wound cleansing, which involves the removal of loose cellular debris, devitalized tissue, metabolic wastes, bacteria, and topical agents that retard wound healing. The wound is cleansed initially and then at each dressing change (Table 13-15).
- Management of edema, which involves monitoring the moisture levels in the wound to optimize healing and prevent the excessive accumulation of fluid.
- Reduction of necrosis, which harnesses enzymes to remove necrotic tissue in conjunction with dressings and debridement technologies. Harsh soaps, alcohol based products, or harsh antiseptic agents should be avoided as they may erode the skin and create an imbalance in the hydration of the wound.
- Control of microorganism level (bioburden management), which is aimed at reducing wound-bed microorganism levels by facilitating the body's normal immune response and using cleansing/debridement technologies and appropriate topical or systemic antimicrobials.

Study Pearl

Proper hydration and adequate perfusion facilitate the formation of granulation tissue and epithelial cell migration.

Study Pearl

Wound debridement can be accomplished in a number of ways:

- Mechanically: whirlpool, pulsatile lavage, other forms of spray irrigation, and the traditional wet-to-dry dressing.
- Surgically: performed by a physician with the patient anesthetized. Sharp debridement removes necrotic tissue by means of a scalpel or other sharp instrument with the patient alert.
- Chemically: the use of enzymes or other topical agents, such as Dakin's solution (weak bleach).
- Autolytically: the body does its own cleaning. This type of debridement is the least traumatic to healthy tissue but may take longer than enzymes or more invasive forms of debridement.

Wound Dressings. Ideally, a dressing creates a moist environment without permitting maceration or desiccation. Two terms are used when describing dressings[77-87]:

- Occlusion: refers to the ability of a dressing to transmit moisture, vapor or gases from the wound bed to the atmosphere. Occlusive dressings are completely impermeable, while non-occlusive dressings are completely permeable. The following dressings are arranged from most occlusive to nonocclusive:
    - Hydrocolloids, hydrogels, semipermeable foam, semipermeable film, impregnated gauze, alginates, and traditional gauze
- Moisture: dressings can be classified according to the ability to retain moisture. The following list of dressings is arranged from most moisture retentive to least moisture retentive:
    - Alginates, semipermeable foam, hydrocolloids, hydrogels, and semipermeable films

The following list describes the most common types of dressing, their indications, advantages, and disadvantages.

Hydrocolloids. These dressings contain gel-forming polymers such as gelatin, pectin, and carboxymethylcellulose with a strong film or foam adhesive backing. These dressings, which are generally designed to be left in place for several days to a week, vary in permeability, thickness, and transparency, and from occlusive to semipermeable. Hydrocolloids absorb exudate (Table 13-3) by swelling into a gel-like mass and by anchoring to intact skin surrounding the wound.

TABLE 13-15. WOUND CARE TERMINOLOGY

TERM	DESCRIPTION
Blanching	Paleness of the skin, usually in response to digital pressure
Clammy	Damp, soft, unusually cool skin
Cyanosis	Bluish discoloration of skin
Debridement	Removal of foreign material, contaminated and devitalized tissues from or adjacent to traumatized or infected lesions until healthy tissue is exposed
Dehiscence	Separation of previously joined edges
Denuded	Stripped or laid bare
Desiccated	Thoroughly dried
Diaphoresis	Profuse perspiration
Ecchymosis	A bruise
Edema	Abnormal accumulation of fluid in tissues
Erythema	Redness of the skin caused by congestion of the capillaries
Eschar	Scab-like structure overlying an open wound, when mature it is black and hard
Exfoliation	Falling off in scales
Exudate	Fluid which has escaped from blood vessels and is deposited in tissues, and which contains cells and proteins
Friability	Easily pulverized, crumbled
Granulation	The process of forming new tissue in response to an injury or wound
Indurated	Hardened tissue
Infection	Invasion and multiplication of microorganisms in body tissues (inflammation plus purulent drainage plus odor)
Inflammation	Body's reaction to injury which results in four classic symptoms: heat, redness, swelling, and pain
Irrigation	Washing cavity or wound with a stream of water or fluid
Ischemia	Inadequate blood supply to a body part, which may result in cell death if allowed to persist
Maceration	Softening of a solid via contact with a liquid
Mottling	Irregular coloration/discoloration of skin
Necrosis	Morphologic changes indicative of cell death
Purulent	Containing or forming pus
Serous drainage	Fluid that is thin and watery like serum
Stasis	A stoppage or diminution of fluid
Turgor	Fullness of the skin, reduced turgor indicates dehydration
Ulcer	A local defect or excavation of the surface of an organ or tissue
Undermining	Excavation beneath the skin surface

- Indications for this type of dressing include partial and full thickness wounds. The dressings can also be used effectively with granular or necrotic wounds.
- Advantages include
  - Provides a moist environment for wound healing, while also providing moderate absorption
  - Enables autolytic debridement
  - Offers protection from microbial contamination
  - Does not require a secondary dressing
  - Provides a waterproof surface
- Disadvantages include
  - May traumatize surrounding intact skin upon removal
  - May tend to roll in areas of excessive friction
  - Cannot be used on infected wounds

Study Pearl

A primary dressing comes into direct contact with the wound, whilst a secondary dressing is placed directly over the primary dressing to provide protection, absorption, and/or occlusion.

Hydrogels. These dressings consist of varying amounts of water and varying amounts of gel-forming materials such as glycerin. The dressings are available in sheet form or amorphous gel form.

- Indications for this type of dressing include superficial and partial thickness wounds (eg, abrasions, blisters, pressure ulcers) that have minimal drainage, and wounds that are prone to desiccation and in dry climates where dehydration is more of a problem Hydrogel dressings also help to soften hard eschar and promote autolytic or mechanical debridement. Rather than absorb drainage, hydrogels are moisture retentive.

- Advantages include
  - Provides a moist environment for wound healing
  - Enables autolytic debridement
  - May reduce pressure and diminish pain
  - Can be used as a coupling agent for ultrasound
  - Minimally adheres to wound
- Disadvantages include
  - Potential for dressings to dehydrate
  - Cannot be used on wounds with significant drainage
  - Typically requires a second dressing

Fiber Dressings. Fiber dressings are composed of carboxymethylcellulose and draw fluid directly into the cellulose fibers. The gelling action is both immediate and nonreversible and the fluid remains in a gel state, which minimizes chances of periwound maceration.[88] Fiber dressings are excellent for highly exudative wound such as venous insufficiency ulcers.[88]

Foam Dressings. These dressings are composed from a hydrophilic (highly absorbent) polyurethane base. The dressings are hydrophilic at the wound contact surface, but hydrophobic on the outer surface. The dressings allow exudate to be absorbed into the foam through the hydrophilic layer. The dressings are most commonly available in sheets or pads with varying degrees of thickness. Semipermeable foam dressings are produced in adhesive and nonadhesive foams. Nonadhesive foams require a second dressing.

- Indications for this type of dressing include partial and full thickness wounds with varying levels of exudate. They can also be used as secondary dressings over amorphous hydrogels.
- Advantages include
  - Provides a moist environment for wound healing
  - Available in adhesive and nonadhesive forms
  - Provides prophylactic protection and cushioning
  - Encourages autolytic debridement
  - Provides moderate absorption
- Disadvantages include
  - May tend to roll in areas of excessive friction
  - Adhesive form may traumatize periwound area upon removal
  - Lack of transparency makes inspection of wound difficult

Semipermeable Film. These dressings are thin membranes made from transparent polyurethane coated with water resistant adhesives. The dressings are permeable to vapor and oxygen, but are mostly impermeable to large molecule bacteria. They are highly elastic, form to a variety of body contours, and allow easy visual inspection of the wound since they are transparent.

- Indications for this type of dressing include superficial wounds (scalds, abrasions, lacerations) or partial thickness wounds with minimal drainage.
- Advantages include
  - Provides a moist environment for wound healing
  - Enables autolytic debridement
  - Allows visualization of the wound
  - Resistant to shearing and frictional forces
  - Cost effective
- Disadvantages include
  - Excessive accumulation of exudate can result in periwound maceration.
  - Adhesive may traumatize periwound area upon removal.
  - Cannot be used on infected wounds.

Gauze. These dressings are manufactured from yarn or thread and are the most readily available dressings used in an inpatient environment. Gauze dressings come in many shapes and sizes (eg, sheets, squares, rolls, packing strips). Impregnated gauze is a variation of woven gauze in which various materials such as Petrolatum, and zinc or antimicrobials have been added.

- Indications for this type of dressing include infected or noninfected wounds of any size. The dressings can be used for wet to wet, wet to moist, or wet to dry debridement.
- Advantages include
  - Readily available, cost effective dressings
  - Can be used alone or in combination with other dressings or topical agents
  - Can modify number of layers to accommodate for changing wound status
  - Can be used on infected or uninfected wounds
- Disadvantages include
  - Has tendency to adhere to wound bed
  - Highly permeable and therefore requires frequent dressing changes (prolonged use decreases cost effectiveness)
  - Increased infection rate compared to occlusive dressings

Alginates. These dressings consist of calcium salt of alganic acid that is extracted from brown algae and kelp. Alginates, which interact with wound exudate to create a gel-like substance that aid in moist wound healing, are highly permeable and nonocclusive. Because alginates dressings provide an excellent avenue for exudate absorption, they require a secondary dressing. Allogeneic dressings are based on the interaction of calcium ions in the dressing and the sodium ions in the wound exudate.

- Indications for the dressings include partial and full thickness draining wounds, such as pressure wounds or venous insufficiency ulcers. Alginates are often used on infected wounds due to the likelihood of excessive drainage.
- Advantages include
  - High absorptive capacity
  - Enables autolytic debridement
  - Offers protection from microbial contamination

- Can be used on infected or uninfected wounds
- Nonadhering to wound

- ▶ Disadvantages include
  - May require frequent dressing changes based on level of exudates
  - Requires a secondary dressing
  - Cannot be used on wounds with an exposed tendon, joint capsule, or bone

Other categories of dressings have evolved to deal with the unique characteristics of the complicated/infected acute wound and the biochemical changes inherent in the chronic wound:

- ▶ Silver dressings: the evolution of silver dressings appears to be related to the increasing prevalence of antibiotic-resistant organisms and that lower concentrations of silver are required for microbial control. Occlusive to semiocclusive technologies, and absorptive materials can be combined with silver to provide a dressing with multiple functions. Silver dressings may be broadly categorized according to silver levels:
  - High-content silver dressings: may provide enhanced microbial control, but they appear to inhibit epithelialization.
  - Lower-content silver dressings: may not provide the same level of microbial control but do not inhibit epithelialization.
- ▶ All silver dressings or preparations release ionic silver that is thought to interfere with microbial respiratory enzymes, protein synthesis, and DNA replication. There is some concern about the possibility of microbes developing silver resistance, since such low levels of silver are utilized by these dressings. These low levels are quite close to the minimum inhibitory concentration for microbes and may allow organisms to survive and mutate.
- ▶ Cadexomer iodine dressings: provide a slow, time release of active iodine to the wound bed as wound fluid is absorbed by the iodine-polymer complex. Sustained release of iodine from this polymer optimizes its antimicrobial effects while preventing the accumulation of active iodine in tissues at levels toxic to wound-bed cells. Toxicity studies have not demonstrated any local or systemic adverse effects. Because of its slow release formulation and rapid excretion by the kidneys, cadexomer iodine is not thought to pose a threat to healing tissues or the central nervous system. Other benefits include no evidence of microbial resistance, good fluid-handling capabilities, an immune-stimulating effect, and facilitation of the wound-healing process.
- ▶ Polyhexamethylene biguanide (PHMB): has bidirectional fluid-handling properties (can absorb or hydrate the wound bed) and uses 0.3% PHMB as the antimicrobial constituent. PHMB is a broad-spectrum antimicrobial dressing that donates fluid to dry areas of the wound, as well as absorbs fluid from overly hydrated areas.
- ▶ Wound-matrix dressings: enhances the function of the extracellular tissue matrix and the cells that reside there. Collagen-based dressings in powder, dried matrices, alginate, hydrogel, and hydrocolloid formulations have evolved to provide support for fibroblast migration and function and growth-factor binding.

These collagen-based dressings act as temporary scaffolding for cells and are reabsorbed or removed as the wound heals. Newer technology includes a collagen (55%) and chemically processed cellulose (45%) blend that works to bind growth factors and bind/disable tissue enzymes (metallomatrix proteinases) that destroy the extracellular matrix in chronic wounds and provides fluid-handling capabilities to control wound exudates.

Negative Pressure Wound Therapy. Negative pressure wound therapy (NPWT), a topical treatment used as an adjunct to wound healing to facilitate wound closure, involves the application of negative pressure to the wound bed.[89-93] NPWT consists of a wound dressing (changed every 12 hours for infected wounds; 48 hours or longer for clean wounds), a drainage tube inserted into the dressing, occlusive transparent film, and a connection to a vacuum source, which supplies the negative pressure.

Selective Debridement. Selective debridement involves the removal of necrotic or infected tissues from the wound as these can interfere with wound healing. The goals of wound debridement include

- Allow for the examination of the ulcer, and determination of the extent of wound
- Decrease the bacterial concentration in a wound; improve wound healing
- Decrease spreading infection, ie, cellulitis or sepsis

Selective debridement is most often performed by sharp debridement, enzymatic debridement, and autolytic debridement:

- Sharp debridement: requires the use of the scalpel, scissors, and forceps to selectively remove devitalized tissues, foreign materials, or debris from the wound. Sharp debridement is most often useful on wounds with large amounts of thick, adherent, necrotic tissue; however, it is also used in the presence of cellulitis or sepsis. Sharp debridement is the most expedient form of removing necrotic tissue.
- Enzymatic debridement: refers to the topical application of enzymes to the surface of necrotic tissue. Enzymatic debridement can be used on infected and uninfected wounds with necrotic tissue. This type of debridement may be used on wounds that have not responded to autolytic debridement or in conjunction with other debridement techniques. Enzyme debridement can be slow to establish a clean wound bed and should be discontinued after removal of devitalized tissues in order to avoid damage.
- Autolytic debridement: refers to using the body's own mechanisms to remove nonviable tissue. Common methods of autolytic debridement include transparent films, hydrocolloids, hydrogels, and alginates. Autolytic debridement results in a moist wound environment that permits rehydration of the necrotic tissue and eschar and allows enzymes to digest the nonviable tissue. Autolytic debridement can be used with any amount of necrotic tissue and is noninvasive and painfree. Patients and caregivers can be instructed to perform autolytic debridement with relative ease; however, this type

Study Pearl

Physical therapists are permitted to perform sharp debridement in the majority of states.

of debridement requires a longer period of time for overall wound healing to occur. Autolytic debridement should not be performed on infected wounds.

Nonselective Debridement. Nonselective debridement, or mechanical debridement, involves removing both viable and nonviable tissues from the wound. Nonselective debridement is most commonly performed by wet to dry dressings, wound irrigation, and hydrotherapy (whirlpool):

- Wet to dry dressings: refers to the application of a moistened gauze dressing placed in an area of necrotic tissue. The dressing is then allowed to dry completely and is later removed along with the necrotic tissue that has adhered to the gauze. Wet to dry dressings are most often used to debride wounds with moderate amounts of exudate and necrotic tissue. This type of debridement should be used sparingly on wounds with both necrotic tissue and viable tissue, as granulation tissue will be traumatized in the process. Removal of dry dressings from granulation tissue may cause bleeding and be extremely painful.
- Wound irrigation: removes necrotic tissue from the wound bed using pressurized fluid. Normal saline (0.9% NaCl) is recommended for most ulcers; nontoxic effect in the wound.
- Cleansing topical agents (povidone-iodine solution, sodium hydrochlorite solution, Dakin's solution, acetic acid solution, hydrogen peroxide), which contain surfactants that level off surface tension, should only be used sparingly as they can be toxic to healing tissues.

Delivery systems include

- Minimal mechanical force: cleansing with coarse cloth or sponge.
- Irrigation: using a syringe, or a squeezable bottle with typical battery-powered irrigation device (pulsatile lavage). Most of these devices permit varying pressure settings (to loosen wound debris) and provide suction for removal of the exudate and debris. Safe and effective irrigation pressures range from 4 to 15 psi.
- Hydrotherapy: the most commonly employed using a whirlpool tank with agitation directed toward a wound that requires debridement. This process results in softening and loosening of adherent necrotic tissue. The physical therapist must be aware of the side effects of hydrotherapy such as dependent position of the lower extremities, systemic effects such as a drop in blood pressure, and maceration of surrounding skin.

Factors Influencing Wound Healing[77]

A number of factors can contribute to the rate and degree of wound healing:

- Age: a decreased metabolism in older adults tends to decrease the overall rate of wound healing.
- Illness: compromised medical status such as cardiovascular disease may significantly delay healing. This often results secondary to diminished oxygen and nutrients at the cellular level.

- Infection: and infected wound will impact essential activity associated with wound healing including fibroblast activity, collagen synthesis, and phagocytosis.
- Lifestyle: regular physical activity results in increased circulation that enhances wound healing. Lifestyle choices such as smoking negatively impact wound healing by limiting the blood's oxygen carrying capability.
- Medication: there are a variety of pharmacological agents that can negatively impact wound healing. Medications falling into this category include steroids, anti-inflammatory drugs, heparin, antineoplastic agents, and oral contraceptives. Undesirable physiological effects include delayed collagen synthesis, reduced blood supply, and decreased tensile strength of connective tissues.

SCAR MANAGEMENT

Intervention guidelines for scar management include

- Massage of the area using cream twice per day (once the wound is completely healed)
- Use of sun block and vitamin E cream on the scar
- Use of silicone gel (softens scar)
- Pressure garments
- Consider ultrasound treatment
- Consider electrical stimulation treatment

THERAPEUTIC EXERCISE

- Strengthening and range of motion exercises
- Aerobic conditioning
- Body mechanics, postural awareness training
- Gait, locomotion, and balance training
- Aquatic therapy

FUNCTIONAL TRAINING

- Activity of daily living training (basic and instrumental)
- Activity pacing and energy conservation; stress management
- Skin and joint protection techniques
- Instruction in safe use of assistive and adaptive devices
- Prescription, application, and training in use of orthotic, protective, or supportive devices

HIGH-VOLTAGE PULSED CURRENT

- Numerous controlled studies have demonstrated the benefits of high-voltage galvanic stimulation in augmenting wound healing, particularly in the management of pressure sores.[88] The standard treatment is 45 minutes to 1 hour in length, with the stimulus being delivered at a frequency of 100 pulses per second at a sufficient intensity to produce a tingling paresthesia. The positive electrode (anode) should be placed over the wound when debridement or epithelialization is the objective.[88] The negative pole (cathode) is used to stimulate production of granulation tissue or to promote antimicrobial or anti-inflammatory effects.[88] Typically the wound is filled loosely with saline-moistened gauze, and an aluminum foil electrode (smaller than the moistened gauze so that no portion of the foil comes in contact with intact skin), connected to an alligator clip lead wire, is used for conductivity.

Questions for this chapter and the entire book appear on the included CD-ROM, with additional questions at www.DuttonNPTE.com.

REFERENCES

1. Richard RL, Ward RS: Burns. In: O'Sullivan SB, Schmitz TJ, eds. *Physical Rehabilitation, 5th ed.* Philadelphia, PA: FA Davis. 2007:1091-1115.
2. Unger P, Goodman CC: The integumentary system. In: Goodman CC, Boissonnault WG, Fuller KS, eds. *Pathology: Implications for the Physical Therapist,* 2nd ed. Philadelphia, PA: Saunders. 2003:264-316.
3. Anthony MS: Wounds. In: Clark GL, Shaw Wilgis EF, Aiello B, et al, eds. *Hand Rehabilitation: A Practical Guide, 2nd ed.* Philadelphia, PA: Churchill Livingstone. 1998:1-15.
4. Noe JM: *Wound Care, 2nd ed.* Greenwich, London: Chesebrough-Pond's Inc; 1985.
5. Baldwin JE, Weber LJ, Simon CLS: *Clinical Assessment Recommendations.* 2nd ed. Chicago, IL: American Society of Hand Therapists; 1992.
6. Eckes B, Hunzelmann N, Moinzadeh P, et al: Scleroderma—news to tell. *Arch Dermatol Res.* 2007;299:139–144.
7. Kreuter A, Altmeyer P, Gambichler T: Treatment of localized scleroderma depends on the clinical subtype. *Br J Dermatol.* 2007;156:1363–1365.
8. Chizzolini C: Update on pathophysiology of scleroderma with special reference to immunoinflammatory events. *Ann Med.* 2007;39:42-53
9. Zivkovic SA, Medsger TA, Jr: Myasthenia gravis and scleroderma: two cases and a review of the literature. *Clin Neurol Neurosurg.* 2007;109:388-391.
10. Verrecchia F, Laboureau J, Verola O, et al: Skin involvement in scleroderma—where histological and clinical scores meet. *Rheumatology (Oxford).* 2007;46:833-841.
11. Ashida R, Ihn H, Mimura Y, et al: Clinical features of scleroderma patients with contracture of phalanges. Clin Rheumatol, 2006;26:1275–1277.
12. Karnen FP, Kongko HR, Kasjmir YI: Scleroderma in a young man. *Acta Med Indones.* 2006;38:213-216.
13. Jablonska S, Blaszczyk M: New treatments in scleroderma: dermatologic perspective. *J Eur Acad Dermatol Venereol.* 2002;16:433-435.
14. Chen YJ, Wu CY, Shen JL: Predicting factors of interstitial lung disease in dermatomyositis and polymyositis. *Acta Derm Venereol.* 2007;87:33-38.

15. Yoshidome Y, Morimoto S, Tamura N, et al: A case of polymyositis complicated with myasthenic crisis. *Clin Rheumatol.* 2006;26:1569–1570.
16. Pongratz D: Therapeutic options in autoimmune inflammatory myopathies (dermatomyositis, polymyositis, inclusion body myositis). *J Neurol.* 2006;253:v64-v65.
17. Ytterberg SR: Treatment of refractory polymyositis and dermatomyositis. *Curr Rheumatol Rep.* 2006;8:167-173.
18. Zampieri S, Ghirardello A, Iaccarino L, et al: Polymyositis-dermatomyositis and infections. *Autoimmunity.* 2006;39:191-196.
19. Bronner IM, Linssen WH, van der Meulen MF, et al: Polymyositis: an ongoing discussion about a disease entity. *Arch Neurol.* 2004;61:132-135.
20. Thomas DR: Prevention and management of pressure ulcers. *Mo Med.* 2007;104:52-57.
21. Evans J, Stephen-Haynes J: Identification of superficial pressure ulcers. *J Wound Care.* 2007;16:54-56.
22. McNees P, Meneses KD: Pressure ulcers and other chronic wounds in patients with and patients without cancer: a retrospective, comparative analysis of healing patterns. *Ostomy Wound Manage.* 2007;53:70-78.
23. Stewart TP, Magnano SJ: Burns or pressure ulcers in the surgical patient? *Adv Skin Wound Care.* 2007;20:74, 77-78, 80.
24. Spilsbury K, Nelson A, Cullum N, et al: Pressure ulcers and their treatment and effects on quality of life: hospital inpatient perspectives. *J Adv Nurs.* 2007;57:494–504.
25. Whitney J, Phillips L, Aslam R, et al: Guidelines for the treatment of pressure ulcers. *Wound Repair Regen.* 2006;14:663-679.
26. Dini V, Bertone M, Romanelli M: Prevention and management of pressure ulcers. *Dermatol Ther.* 2006;19:356-364.
27. Rycroft-Malone J, McInnes L: The prevention of pressure ulcers. *Worldviews Evid Based Nurs.* 2004;1:146-149.
28. Effective methods for preventing pressure ulcers. *J Fam Pract.* 2006;55:942.
29. Benbow M: Guidelines for the prevention and treatment of pressure ulcers. *Nurs Stand.* 2006;20:42-44.
30. Cullum N, Nelson EA, Nixon J: Pressure ulcers. *Clin Evid.* 2006;15:2592-2606.
31. Reddy M, Gill SS, Rochon PA: Preventing pressure ulcers: a systematic review. *JAMA.* 2006;296:974-984.
32. Baranoski S: Pressure ulcers: a renewed awareness. *Nursing.* 2006;36:36-41,quiz.
33. Ratliff CR: Two case studies of Marjolin's ulcers in patients referred for management of chronic pressure ulcers. *J Wound Ostomy Continence Nurs.* 2002;29:266-268.
34. Ozek C, Cankayali R, Bilkay U, et al: Marjolin's ulcers arising in burn scars. *J Burn Care Rehabil.* 2001;22:384-389.
35. Gschwandtner ME, Ambrozy E, Maric S, et al: Microcirculation is similar in ischemic and venous ulcers. *Microvasc Res.* 2001;62:226-235.
36. Jeter KF, Tintle TE: Rethinking ischemic ulcers: from etiology to treatment outcome. Prog Clin Biol Res. 1991;365:45-54.
37. Worley CA: Neuropathic ulcers: diabetes and wounds, part II. Differential diagnosis and treatment. *Dermatol Nurs.* 2006;18: 163-164.

38. Worley CA: Neuropathic ulcers: diabetes and wounds, part I. Etiology and assessment. *Dermatol Nurs.* 2006;18:52, 59.
39. Margolis DJ, Allen-Taylor L, Hoffstad O, et al: Diabetic neuropathic foot ulcers and amputation. *Wound Repair Regen.* 2005;13:230-2306.
40. Steeper R: A critical review of the aetiology of diabetic neuropathic ulcers. *J Wound Care.* 2005;14:101-103.
41. Aksenov IV: Neuropathic diabetic foot ulcers. N Engl J Med. 2004;351:1694-1695.
42. Chang HR: Neuropathic diabetic foot ulcers. *N Engl J Med.* 2004;351:1694-1695; author reply 1694-1695.
43. Zulkowski K, Ratliff CR: Managing venous and neuropathic ulcers. *Nursing.* 2004;34:68.
44. Boulton AJ, Kirsner RS, Vileikyte L: Clinical practice. Neuropathic diabetic foot ulcers. *N Engl J Med.* 2004;351:48-55.
45. Gul A, Basit A, Ali SM, et al: Role of wound classification in predicting the outcome of diabetic foot ulcer. *J Pak Med Assoc.* 2006;56:444-447.
46. Oyibo SO, Jude EB, Tarawneh I, et al: A comparison of two diabetic foot ulcer classification systems: the Wagner and the University of Texas wound classification systems. *Diabetes Care.* 2001;24:84-88.
47. Cunningham D: Treating venous insufficiency ulcers with soft silicone dressing. *Ostomy Wound Manage.* 2005;51:19-20.
48. Galvan L: Assessing venous ulcers and venous insufficiency. *Nursing.* 2005;35:70.
49. Kelechi TJ, Edlund B: Chronic venous insufficiency. Preventing leg ulcers is primary goal. *Adv Nurse Pract.* 2005;13:31-34.
50. Berliner E, Ozbilgin B, Zarin DA: A systematic review of pneumatic compression for treatment of chronic venous insufficiency and venous ulcers. *J Vasc Surg.* 2003;37:539-544.
51. Ruckley CV: Socioeconomic impact of chronic venous insufficiency and leg ulcers. *Angiology.* 1997;48:67-69.
52. Ullrich SE: Sunlight and skin cancer: Lessons from the immune system. *Mol Carcinog.* 2007;46:629–633.
53. Ansems TM, van der Pols JC, Hughes MC, et al: Alcohol intake and risk of skin cancer: a prospective study. *Eur J Clin Nutr.* 2007;8:300–307.
54. Rhee JS, Matthews BA, Neuburg M, et al: The skin cancer index: clinical responsiveness and predictors of quality of life. *Laryngoscope.* 2007;117:399-405.
55. Telfer NR: Skin cancer: prevalence, prevention and treatment. *Clin Med.* 2006;6:622,623.
56. Gloster HM, Jr, Neal K: Skin cancer in skin of color. *J Am Acad Dermatol.* 2006;55:741-760, quiz 761-764.
57. Honda KS: HIV and skin cancer. *Dermatol Clin.* 2006;24:521-530, vii.
58. Information from your family doctor. Checking yourself for signs of skin cancer. *Am Fam Physician.* 2006;74:819-820.
59. Information from your family doctor. Melanoma: a type of skin cancer. *Am Fam Physician.* 2006;74:813-814.
60. Dixon A: Skin cancer in patients with multiple health problems. *Aust Fam Physician.* 2006;35:717-718.
61. Sharpe G: Skin cancer: prevalence, prevention and treatment. *Clin Med.* 2006;6:333-334.

62. Guide to physical therapist practice. *Phys Ther.* 2001;81:S13-S95.
63. Cioffi WG: Inhalation injury. In: Carrougher GJ, ed. *Burn Care and Therapy.* St. Louis, MO: CV Mosby. 1998:35.
64. Sheridan RL: Burn Rehabilitation, Available at: http://www.emedicine.com/pmr/topic163.htm, 2004.
65. Gomez R, Cancio LC: Management of burn wounds in the emergency department. *Emerg Med Clin North Am.* 2007;25:135-146.
66. Prelack K, Dylewski M, Sheridan RL: Practical guidelines for nutritional management of burn injury and recovery. *Burns.* 2007;33:14-24.
67. Khan N, Malik MA: Presentation of burn injuries and their management outcome. *J Pak Med Assoc.* 2006;56:394-397.
68. Abdi S, Zhou Y: Management of pain after burn injury. *Curr Opin Anaesthesiol.* 2002;15:563-7.
69. DeSanti L: Pathophysiology and current management of burn injury. *Adv Skin Wound Care.* 2005;18:323-332; quiz 332-334.
70. Papini R: Management of burn injuries of various depths. *BMJ.* 2004;329:158-160.
71. Hettiaratchy S, Papini R: Initial management of a major burn: II—assessment and resuscitation. *BMJ.* 2004;329:101-103.
72. Hettiaratchy S, Papini R: Initial management of a major burn: I—overview. *BMJ.* 2004;328:1555-1557.
73. Bishop JF: Burn wound assessment and surgical management. *Crit Care Nurs Clin North Am.* 2004;16:145-177.
74. Montgomery RK: Pain management in burn injury. *Crit Care Nurs Clin North Am.* 2004;16:39-49.
75. Danks RR: Burn management. A comprehensive review of the epidemiology and treatment of burn victims. *JEMS.* 2003;28: 118-139; quiz 140-141.
76. Sheridan RL: Airway management and respiratory care of the burn patient. *Int Anesthesiol Clin.* 2000;38:129-145.
77. Dutton M: Integumentary Physical Therapy. In: Dutton M, ed, *Physical Therapist Assistant Exam Review Guide & JB Test Prep: PTA Exam Review.* Sudbury, MA: Jones & Bartlett Learning. 2011:291-314.]
78. Fonder MA, Mamelak AJ, Lazarus GS, et al: Occlusive wound dressings in emergency medicine and acute care. *Emerg Med Clin North Am.* 2007;25:235-242.
79. Burd A: Evaluating the use of hydrogel sheet dressings in comprehensive burn wound care. *Ostomy Wound Manage.* 2007;53:52-62.
80. Fleck CA: Innovative dressings improve wound care management. *Mater Manag Health Care.* 2007;16:24-26, 28.
81. Ovington LG: Advances in wound dressings. *Clin Dermatol.* 2007;25:33-38.
82. Leaper DJ: Silver dressings: their role in wound management. *Int Wound J.* 2006;3:282-294.
83. O'Donnell TF, Jr, Lau J: A systematic review of randomized controlled trials of wound dressings for chronic venous ulcer. *J Vasc Surg.* 2006;44:1118-1125.
84. Shreenivas S, Magnuson JS, Rosenthal EL: Use of negative-pressure dressings to manage a difficult surgical neck wound. *Ear Nose Throat J.* 2006;85:390-391.
85. Attinger CE, Janis JE, Steinberg J, et al: Clinical approach to wounds: debridement and wound bed preparation including the

use of dressings and wound-healing adjuvants. *Plast Reconstr Surg.* 2006;117:72S-109S.

86. Jones V, Grey JE, Harding KG: Wound dressings. *BMJ.* 2006;332:777-780.
87. Wicker P: Wound dressings. *Br J Theatre Nurs.* 1992;2:22-25.
88. Willey T: Use a decision tree to choose wound dressings. *Am J Nurs.* 1992;92:43.
89. McCulloch JM: Wound healing and management. In: Placzek JD, Boyce DA, eds. *Orthopaedic Physical Therapy Secrets.* Philadelphia, PA: Hanley & Belfus, Inc. 2001:171-176.
90. Morris GS, Brueilly KE, Hanzelka H: Negative pressure wound therapy achieved by vacuum-assisted closure: evaluating the assumptions. *Ostomy Wound Manage.* 2007;53:52-57.
91. Vuerstaek JD, Vainas T, Wuite J, et al: State-of-the-art treatment of chronic leg ulcers: a randomized controlled trial comparing vacuum-assisted closure (V.A.C.) with modern wound dressings. *J Vasc Surg.* 2006;44:1029-37; discussion 1038. Epub Sep 26, 2006.
92. Timmers MS, Le Cessie S, Banwell P, et al: The effects of varying degrees of pressure delivered by negative-pressure wound therapy on skin perfusion. *Ann Plast Surg.* 2005;55:665-671.
93. Eginton MT, Brown KR, Seabrook GR, et al: A prospective randomized evaluation of negative-pressure wound dressings for diabetic foot wounds. *Ann Vasc Surg.* 2003;17:645-649. Epub Oct 13, 2003.
94. Wanner MB, Schwarzl F, Strub B, et al: Vacuum-assisted wound closure for cheaper and more comfortable healing of pressure sores: a prospective study. *Scand J Plast Reconstr Surg Hand Surg.* 2003;37:28-33.
95. Horwitz LR, Burke TJ, Carnegie D: Augmentation of wound healing using monochromatic infrared energy. Exploration of a new technology for wound management. *Adv Wound Care.* 1999;12:35-40.
96. Burke TJ: The effect of monochromatic infrared energy on sensation in subjects with diabetic peripheral neuropathy: a double-blind, placebo-controlled study. Response to Clifft et al. *Diabetes Care.* 2006;29:1186-1187.
97. Harkless LB, DeLellis S, Carnegie DH, et al: Improved foot sensitivity and pain reduction in patients with peripheral neuropathy after treatment with monochromatic infrared photo energy—MIRE. *J Diabetes Complications.* 2006;20:81-87.
98. Clifft JK, Kasser RJ, Newton TS, et al: The effect of monochromatic infrared energy on sensation in patients with diabetic peripheral neuropathy: a double-blind, placebo-controlled study. *Diabetes Care.* 2005;28:2896-2900.
99. Londahl M, Katzman P, Nilsson A, et al: A prospective study: hyperbaric oxygen therapy in diabetics with chronic foot ulcers. *J Wound Care.* 2006;15:457-459.
100. Mathieu D: Role of hyperbaric oxygen therapy in the management of lower extremity wounds. *Int J Low Extrem Wounds.* 2006;5:233-235.
101. Koetters KT: Hyperbaric oxygen therapy. *J Emerg Nurs.* 2006;32:417-419.
102. Lin LC, Yau G, Lin TF, et al: The efficacy of hyperbaric oxygen therapy in improving the quality of life in patients with problem wounds. *J Nurs Res.* 2006;14:219-227.

Geriatric Physical Therapy

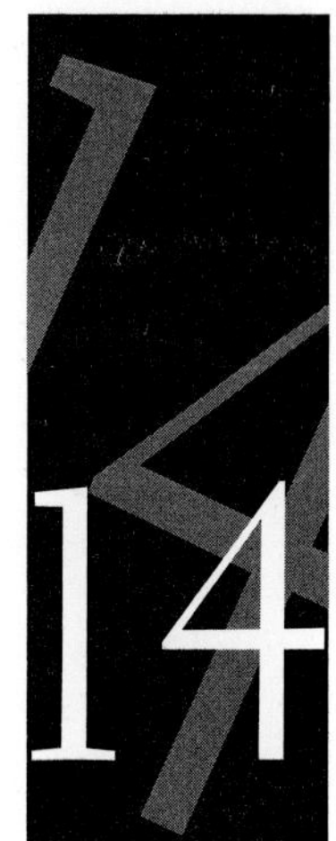

Aging can be defined as the accumulation of diverse adverse changes that increase the risk of death.[1] These aging changes are responsible for both the commonly recognized sequential alterations that accompany advancing age beyond the early period of life, and the progressive increases in the chance of disease and death associated with them.[1]

Study Pearl

- Geriatrics is the branch of medicine that focuses on health promotion and the prevention and treatment of disease and disability in later life.
- Gerontology is the study of the aging process and the science related to the care of the elderly.

THEORIES OF AGING

The changes associated with aging can be attributed to a combination of development, genetic defects, the environment, disease, and an innate factor, the aging process. The rate of aging, that is, the rate of production of aging changes, normally varies from individual to individual, due to differences in genetic and environmental factors that modulate production of aging changes, and thus contribute to differences in the age of death and of the onset of disease.[1] A wide array of theories exist as to why aging occurs, why species have the life spans they do, and what kinds of factors are likely to influence the aging process. For example, the aging process has been attributed to the following:

- Molecular cross-linking (Glycosylation).[2-4] Glycosylation involves the abnormal process of the binding of glucose (simple sugar) to protein, a process that requires oxygen. Once this binding has occurred, the protein becomes impaired and is unable to perform as efficiently. Examples of known cross-linking disorders include senile cataract and the appearance of tough, leathery and yellow skin.
- Changes in immunologic function (neuroendocrine-immuno theory).[5-8] The immune system is the most important line of defense against foreign substances that enter the body. With age the system's ability to produce necessary antibodies that fight disease declines, as does its ability to distinguish between antibodies and proteins. In a sense the immune system itself becomes

self-destructive and reacts against itself. Examples of autoimmune disease are lupus, scleroderma and adult-onset diabetes.

- Damage by free-radical reactions.[9] The term free radical describes any molecule that has a free electron. Theoretically, this free electron reacts with healthy molecules in a destructive way by creating an extra negative charge. This unbalanced energy makes the free radical bind itself to another balanced molecule as it tries to steal electrons. In so doing, the balanced molecule becomes unbalanced and transforms into a free radical itself. It is known that diet, lifestyle, drugs (eg, tobacco and alcohol) and radiation etc, are all accelerators of free radical production within the body. However, there is also natural production of free radicals within the body as a byproduct of energy production, particularly from the mitochondria.
- Senescence genes in the DNA (planned obsolescence).[1] The planned-obsolescence theory focuses on the genetic programming encoded within the DNA, the blueprint of individual life obtained from parents. Individuals are born with a unique code and a predetermined tendency to certain types of physical and mental functioning that regulate the rate at which we age (graying of hair, wrinkles etc). Many genes show changes in expression with age and these premature aging syndromes provide evidence of defective genetic programming: Hutchinson-Gilford syndrome, Werner's syndrome.
- Telomere shortening. This theory was born from the surge of technological breakthroughs in genetics and genetic engineering. Telomeres are DNA-protein complexes that cap the ends of chromosomes and promote genetic stability. Each time a cell divides, a portion of telomeric DNA dwindles away, and after many rounds of cell division, so much telomeric DNA has diminished that the aged cell stops dividing. Thus, telomeres play a critical role in determining the number of times a cell divides, its health, and its life span.
- Caloric restriction. Calorie restriction or energy restriction is a theory proposed after years of animal experiments and research on longevity that demonstrated how, a high nutrient low-calorie diet can dramatically retard the functional, if not the chronological aging process.
- Mutation accumulation (evolutionary theory). Aging is an inevitable result of declining force of natural selection with age. Because evolution acts primarily to maximize reproductive fitness in an individual, longevity is a trait to be selected only if it is beneficial for fitness. Over successive generations, late acting deleterious mutations will accumulate in the population and ultimately lead to pathology and senescence.

DEFINITIONS

AGEISM

Webster defines ageism as "any attitude, action, or institutional structure which subordinates a person, group or perception purely on the basis of age." Age discrimination occurs when that bias is the primary motivation behind acts against a person or group.

LIFESPAN

There are two kinds of life span:

- Maximum life span: the greatest age attainable by any member of a species.
- Average life span: the average age reached by members of a population. This figure has shown changes over time—due to a large extent to medical advances. The average lifespan was 47 years in 1900, and 75 years in 1990. As of the year 2000, in the United States the life expectancy for females is 80 years. For males the comparable figure is 74.

LIFE EXPECTANCY

Life expectancy, the number of years an individual can expect to live, is based on average life spans. Men generally have lower life expectancy rates than women at every age.

SENESCENCE

Senescence is the combination of processes of deterioration that follow the period of development of an organism.

COMPONENT AGE GROUPS

Chronological age is defined as age in years and is, therefore, easily determined. For convenience and simplicity, the following terms are used for the component age groups:

- Middle-age: 45 to 64 years
- Young-old: 65 to 74 years
- Old: 75 to 84 years
- Old-old: 85 to 99 years
- Oldest-old: 100+ years

MORTALITY

Mortality refers to the number of deaths (from a disease or in general) per 1000 people and is typically reported on an annual basis. Reductions in mortality have resulted in impressive increases in life expectancy that have contributed to the growth of the older population, especially at the oldest ages.

MORBIDITY

Morbidity (from Latin morbidus: sick, unhealthy) refers to the number of people who have a disease (prevalence) as compared to the total number of people in a population at a particular point in time. The term morbidity can also refer to

- The state of being diseased
- The degree or severity of a disease
- The incidence of a disease: the number of new cases in a particular population during a particular time interval

PHYSIOLOGICAL CHANGES AND ADAPTATIONS IN THE OLD ADULT

Many changes are associated with aging throughout adulthood and into old age. Table 14-1 summarizes these system changes. Some of these changes are discussed below.

> **Study Pearl**
>
> Resistive exercise prescriptions for the elderly should be directed toward the muscles most susceptible to atrophic changes.[11,12] Additionally, exercises should be geared towards increasing power, not just strength.

IMPAIRED STRENGTH

The decline in strength in elderly individuals has been associated with increases in falls, functional decline, and impaired mobility. However, much of the muscle atrophy that occurs reflects the effects of disuse, and not merely age-related changes.[10] Women experience a less steep absolute decline in strength than men with aging.

IMPAIRED BALANCE

Age-related balance dysfunctions can occur through a loss of sensory elements related to balance (vestibular, vision, and somatosensory), the ability to integrate information, and muscle weakness. Diseases

TABLE 14-1. SUMMARY OF MULTI-SYSTEM CHANGES IN THE ELDERLY

SYSTEM	CHANGES
Musculoskeletal	Muscle mass and strength decrease at a rate of about 30% between the age of 60 and 90.
	Change in muscle fiber type, white and red. Type II fibers (fast twitch) decrease by about 50%.
	Changing differentiation of fiber type, with the red increasing in speed of contraction and white fibers decreasing in the speed of contraction.
	Decrease in recruitment of motor units.
	Decrease in the speed of movement.
	Decreased tensile strength of bone (more than 30% of women over the age of 65 have osteoporosis).
	Females lose about 30% of bone mass by age of 70; males lose about 15% by age of 70.
	Joint flexibility reduced by 25%-30% over the age of 70.
	Decreasing enzymatic activity, cell count, and metabolic substrates in cartilage (collagen fibers increased their cross-linking, resulting in an increase in soft tissue density).
Neuromuscular	Atrophy of neurons; nerve fibers decrease and change in structure.
	Myoneural junction decreases in transmission speed.
	Mitochondrial activity decreases.
	Dopamine level depletion.
	Decrease in nerve conduction velocity by about 0.4% a year after age 70.
	Slowing of motor neuron conduction, which contributes to alterations in the autonomic system.
	Decreasing reflexes result from decrease in nerve conduction. In a population of those 70-80 years old: ankle jerk is absent in about 70%, and knee and biceps jerk are absent in about 15%.
	Overall slow and decreased responsiveness in reaction time (simple reflexes less than complex).
	Increased postural sway (less in women than in men with linear increase with age).
	Changes in sleep patterns that affect neuromuscular functioning.
Neurosensory	Decrease in sweating (implications for modalities and exercise).
	10%-20% decrease in brain weight by age 90.
	Decrease in mechanoreceptors.
	Decrease in efficiency of the neuroendocrine system (ie, decrease in calcium control, affecting heart contraction and causing osteoporosis; thymus function decreases 90% between ages 20 and 80).
	Decrease in visual acuity and ability to accommodate to lighting changes resulting from increased density of lens.
	Decrease in hearing capabilities.
	Decreases in the senses of smell and taste.

(*Continued*)

TABLE 14-1. SUMMARY OF MULTI-SYSTEM CHANGES IN THE ELDERLY (*Continued*)

SYSTEM	CHANGES
Cardiovascular and pulmonary	Decrease in cardiac output by about 0.7% a year after 20 years of age. Increased vascular resistance. Decreased arterial elasticity. Decreased cardiac reserve, decreased physical and psychological response to stress. Decrease in lipid catabolism, which may increase risk for heart disease; about 50% of adults between ages 65 and 74 have evidence of heart disease, and about 30% in this age range have sustained myocardial infarction even in the absence of symptoms of ischemia (in CHF, MIs exceed 50%). Increased irritation of myocardium contributes to increased risk of atrial fibrillation and arrhythmias. Decrease in lung function (from age 25 to age 85 as much as 50% decrease in maximal voluntary ventilation due to an increase in air resistance; get about 40% decrease in vital capacity). Respiratory gas exchange surface decreases at a rate of about 0.27 m^2 a year (maximum oxygen consumption for sedentary individuals of any age is 0.62-0.7 mL/min). Decrease in elastin in the lungs (increased rigidity) and chest wall soft tissues results in decrease in chest wall compliance. Decrease in vital capacity and decrease in pulmonary blood flow contribute to lower oxygen saturation levels. Residual volume doubles. Decreased cough reflex. Decreased ciliary response. Work capacity declines about 30% between the ages of 40 and 70.
Urogenital/renal	Gradual overall structure changes in all renal components. Decreased glomerular filtration rate and creatinine clearance. Change in response to sodium intake. Muscle hypertrophy in the urethra and bladder. Decreased ability to concentrate urine.
Gastrointestinal	Decreasing number of taste buds and ability to taste. Decreased peristalsis. Diminished secretions of pepsin and acid in the stomach. Decreasing hepatic and pancreatic enzymes.
Immunologic	Decrease in overall function with respect to infection. Decreased temperature regulation. Decrease in T cells. Decrease in neuroendocrine system efficiency, diminishing responsiveness.

Data from Bottomley JM: The geriatric population. In: Boissonnault WG, ed. *Primary Care for the Physical Therapist: Examination and Triage.* St Louis, MO: Elsevier Saunders. 2005:288-306; and Bottomley JM: Summary of system changes. Comparing and contrasting age-related changes. In: Bottomley JM, Lewis CB, eds. *Geriatric Rehabilitation: A Clinical Approach, 2nd ed.* Upper Saddleback, NJ: Prentice-Hall. 2003:50-75.

common in aging populations, such as cerebrovascular disease, cerebellar dysfunction, and cardiac disease lead to further deterioration in balance function in some patients.

In addition, elderly patients are more susceptible to dizziness, which can also cause a loss of balance. Dizziness can have a multitude of different causes including

- Cardiac abnormalities
- Medications: certain classes of medications may predispose a person to vestibular dysfunction, including tricyclic antidepressants, antihypertensives, and sedatives (Table 14-6).

The clinical implications of impaired balance include

- Diminished visual acuity, and disorganized postural response patterns (diminished ankle torque, increased hip torque, and increased postural sway) both of which increase the likelihood of falls.

- Delayed reaction times and longer response times by the patient, which increases the likelihood of injury.
- Altered sensory organization: higher dependence upon somatosensory inputs, which makes it difficult for patients to function in low light.

Intervention Strategies for Impaired Balance

- Determine the presence of any disease states that may be contributing to the balance disorder.
- Assess the static and dynamic balance ability of the patient.
- Use fall-risk questionnaires to help identify fall risk.
- Assess the need for appropriate and safe assistive device/adaptive equipment as necessary.
- Strengthening and flexibility exercises to increase stability.
- Weight-bearing exercises to help prevent osteoporosis.
- Balance and gait exercises based on the balance deficits determined in the examination.
- Transfer training: sit to stand transitions.
- Pharmacological reevaluation as appropriate.
- Modify living environment (Table 14-2).
- Safety education.

Impaired Coordination

The most prominent age-related changes impacting coordinated movement include

- Decreased strength
- Slowed reaction time
- Decreased range of motion and flexibility
- Postural changes
- Impaired balance

These changes may be accentuated further by alterations in sensation, perceptual impairments, and diminished vision and hearing acuity.

TABLE 14-2. HOME SAFETY CHECKLIST

ALL LIVING SPACES	BATHROOMS	OUTDOORS
Remove throw rugs.	Install grab bars in the bathtub or shower and by the toilet.	Repair cracked sidewalks.
Secure carpet edges.	Use rubber mats in the bathtub or shower.	Install handrails on stairs and steps.
Remove low furniture and objects on the floor.	Take up floor mats when the bathtub or shower is not in use.	Trim shrubbery along the pathway to the home.
Reduce clutter.	Install a raised toilet seat.	Install adequate lighting by doorways and along walkways leading to doors.
Remove cords and wires on the floor.		
Check lighting for adequate illumination at night (especially in the pathway to the bathroom).		
Secure carpet or treads on stairs.		
Install handrails on staircases.		
Eliminate chairs that are too low to sit in and get out of easily.		
Avoid floor wax (or use nonskid wax).		
Ensure that the telephone can be reached from the floor.		

Data from Rubenstein LZ: Falls. In: Yoshikawa TT, Cobbs EL, Brummel-Smith K, eds. *Ambulatory Geriatric Care.* St. Louis: MO. 1993:296-304.

Impaired Cognition

Age-related changes in the brain typically start at around age 60. However, normal nonprogressive, and negligible declines among the aged do not dramatically impact daily functioning (until the early 80s), but some serious disorders/diseases can significantly affect cognitive function in old age. Not all cognitive disorders are irreversible, but many require timely identification and intervention to minimize permanent dysfunction.

Dementia. Dementia is primarily a disease of the elderly, and is typically associated with neuropsychological problems—a progressive, persistent loss of cognitive and intellectual functions. This loss of cognitive and intellectual functions can include[13-21]:

- Loss of memory, especially short-term memory; long-term memory is usually retained. Impairments tend to be task dependent and occur more frequently with novel conditions.
- Language impairment, including reduction in, or inappropriate use of, vocabulary.
- A decrease in visuospatial skills (see Balance).
- Emotional instability, which manifests as excessive emotional reactions and frequent mood changes.

Dementia is often confused with delirium (also known as acute confusional state). Delirium presents with

- A rapid onset and fluctuating course, which is potentially reversible
- Attention and focal cognitive deficits.

In contrast, dementia progresses slowly, is irreversible, causes profound memory deficits, and it associated with global cognitive deficits.

Intervention Strategies for Impaired Cognition. The intervention for impaired cognition is based on the findings from the examination:

- Cognitive assessment, which may focus either on a patient's current cognitive functioning or any decline in functioning from a previous level. An advantage of assessing the degree of cognitive decline, rather than current functioning, is that the influences of education, premorbid intelligence and cultural differences are discounted in the assessment.
- Determination of any medical problems associated with the cognitive deficits (cardiovascular disease, hypertension, diabetes, or hypothyroidism).
- Pharmacological questioning if drug toxicity suspected.

The mainstays of treatment for cognitive dysfunction include:

- Cognitive training activities (chess, crossword puzzles etc)
- Providing a stimulating and enriching environment.
- The use of context-based tasks versus memorization.

PATHOLOGICAL CONDITIONS ASSOCIATED WITH THE ELDERLY

MUSCULOSKELETAL DISORDERS AND DISEASES

Fractures. Fractures commonly occur among the elderly and can have a significant impact on the morbidity, mortality and functional dependence of this population. Fractures in the elderly have their own set of problems:

- The fractures heal more slowly.
- Older adults are prone to complications
  - Pneumonia
  - Changes in mental status
  - Decubiti
  - Comorbidity

The following are deemed to be the most common fractures to occur in the elderly population:

- Pathological fractures. Pathological fractures are those that occur from low energy injuries to an area of bone weakness with a preexisting abnormality or disease.
- Stress fractures.[22] Stress fractures, including fatigue and insufficiency fractures, are fractures that occur in the absence of a specific traumatic event.
- Proximal humerus fractures. Proximal humerus fractures have been conservatively estimated to account for 5% of all fractures in the elderly, particularly in those who primarily are osteoporotic. Like hip fractures, proximal humerus fractures represent a major morbidity in the elderly population.
- Distal radius fracture.[23] The distal radial fracture is the most common forearm fracture. It is usually caused by a fall onto an outstretched hand (FOOSH), but can also result from direct impact or axial forces. The classification of these fractures is based on distal radial angulation and displacement, intra-articular or extra-articular involvement, and associated anomalies of the ulnar or carpal bones. The most common complication of this type of fracture is peripheral nerve dysfunction, with the median nerve being the most commonly affected, although the ulnar nerve may also be injured.
- Proximal femur/hip fracture. Fracture of the hip can have devastating consequences—the mortality rate is 20%. About 50% of patients who sustain this type of fracture will not resume their premorbid level of function. The various types of proximal femur/hip fracture include
  - Femoral head fracture: most often, this occurs as a result of hip dislocation.
  - Femoral neck fracture: together with intertrochanteric fractures, these constitute the vast majority of all hip fractures.
  - Intertrochanteric fracture: extremity is held in a markedly shortened and externally rotated position.
  - Subtrochanteric fracture: proximal femur usually is held in a flexed and externally rotated position.

- Fractures of the spine. Compression fractures of the vertebral body are common in the elderly and range from mild to severe. While the diagnosis can be suspected from the history and physical examination, plain radiographs, as well as occasional computed tomography or magnetic resonance imaging, are often helpful in accurate diagnosis and prognosis.

NEUROLOGIC DISORDERS AND DISEASES

Cerebrovascular Accident (Stroke). A cerebrovascular accident (CVA) or stroke syndrome results in a sudden loss of circulation to an area of the brain, resulting in a corresponding loss of neurologic function.

CVAs are currently classified as either hemorrhagic or ischemic, although the two can coexist.

- *Hemorrhagic:* results from abnormal bleeding into the extravascular areas of the brain. Causes include, but are not limited to, intracranial aneurysm, hypertension, arteriovenous malformation (AVM), and anticoagulant therapy.
- *Ischemic:* results when a clot blocks or impairs blood flow. Risk factors for ischemic stroke include advanced age, hypertension, smoking, heart disease, and hypercholesterolemia.

Common signs and symptoms of a CVA include abrupt onset of hemiparesis, monoparesis, or quadriparesis; monocular or binocular visual loss; visual field deficits; diplopia; dysarthria; ataxia; vertigo; aphasia; or sudden decrease in the level of consciousness.

The patient's neurologic deficits are often determined by the site of arterial compromise:[24]

- *Anterior cerebral artery (ACA) occlusion:* Primarily produces altered mental status, impaired judgment, neglect, contralateral hemiplegia/hemiparesis and hypesthesia, bowel and bladder incontinence, behavioral changes, apraxia (if located in the nondominant hemisphere), or aphasia (if located in the dominant hemisphere).
- *Middle cerebral artery (MCA):* Occlusions commonly produce contralateral hemiparesis, contralateral hypesthesia, ipsilateral hemianopsia (blindness in one half of the visual field), and gaze preference toward the side of the lesion. Agnosia is common, and receptive or expressive aphasia may result if the lesion occurs in the dominant hemisphere. Since the MCA supplies the upper extremity motor strip, weakness of the arm and face is usually worse than that of the lower limb.
- *Posterior cerebral artery occlusions:* These affect vision and thought, producing homonymous hemianopsia, pain and temperature sensory loss, contralateral hemiplegia (central area), cortical blindness, visual agnosia, altered mental status, and impaired memory.

The neuroanatomic stroke syndrome subtypes include:[24]

- *Anterior communicating artery:* Produces incontinence, impairment of intellect, loss of innovative abilities, and paraparesis.

Study Pearl

Any process that disrupts blood flow to a portion of the brain unleashes an ischemic cascade, leading to the death of neurons and cerebral infarction.

Key Point

Any process that causes dissection of the cerebral arteries also can cause thrombotic stroke (eg, trauma, thoracic aortic dissection, arteritis).

Key Point

A CVA should be considered as a diagnosis in any patient presenting with an acute neurologic deficit (focal or global) or altered level of consciousness.

Key Point

Vertebrobasilar artery occlusions (Table 14-3) are notoriously difficult to detect because they cause a wide variety of cranial nerve, cerebellar, and brainstem deficits. These include vertigo, nystagmus, diplopia, visual field deficits, dysphagia, dysarthria, facial hypesthesia, syncope, and ataxia. Loss of pain and temperature sensation occurs on the ipsilateral face and contralateral body. In contrast, anterior strokes produce findings on one side of the body only.

TABLE 14-3. VERTEBROBASILAR STROKE SYNDROMES

TYPE	SYNDROME	DESCRIPTION
Vertebral artery	Medial medullary syndrome (Dejerine syndrome)	Rare stroke syndrome associated with clinical triad of ipsilateral hypoglossal palsy, contralateral hemiparesis, and contralateral lemniscal sensory loss.
	Lateral medullary syndrome (Wallenberg syndrome)	Result of occlusion to distal branches of the vertebral artery, superior lateral medullary artery or posterior inferior cerebellar artery. Characterized by selective involvement of the spinothalamic sensory modalities with dissociated distribution (ipsilateral trigeminal and contralateral hemibody/limbs), contralateral or bilateral trigeminal sensory impairment, restricted sensory involvement, ipsilateral cerebellar symptoms (ataxia; vertigo, nausea and vomiting; nystagmus), Horner's syndrome (miosis, ptosis, decreased sweating).
Basilar artery	Medial medullary syndrome (Dejerine syndrome)	See above.
	Locked-in syndrome	Due to bilateral ischemic or hemorrhagic ventral pons lesions. Results in preserved consciousness and sensation, but paralysis of all movements except vertical gaze and eyelid opening.
	Lateral pontine syndrome (Marie-Foix syndrome)	Lesion in the lateral pons, including the middle cerebellar peduncle. Results in ipsilateral cerebellar ataxia due to involvement of cerebellar tracts, contralateral hemiparesis due to corticospinal tract involvement, and variable contralateral hemihypesthesia for pain and temperature due to spinothalamic tract involvement.
	Ventral pontine syndrome (Raymond syndrome)	Occlusion of the paramedian branches, resulting in ipsilateral lateral gaze weakness, and weakness of the contralateral upper and lower extremities.
	Inferior medial pontine syndrome (Foville syndrome)	Unilateral lesion in the dorsal pontine tegmentum in the caudal third of the pons. Associated with contralateral hemiplegia (with facial sparing) due to corticospinal tract involvement, ipsilateral peripheral-type facial palsy, due to cranial nerve VII nucleus/fascicle involvement, and inability to move the eyes conjugately to the ipsilateral side (patient unable to look toward the side of the lesion—also called Millard-Gubler syndrome).
		Cortical blindness (Anton syndrome): occlusion of both posterior cerebral arteries, which is associated with bilateral visual loss and unawareness or denial of blindness.

- *Anterior inferior cerebellar artery:* Produces ipsilateral ataxia, loss of contralateral pain and temperature, ipsilateral deafness, ipsilateral facial paralysis, and ipsilateral sensory loss to the face.
- *Paramedian area:* Produces paralysis of one or more cranial nerves on the same side of the body as the lesion, and varying degrees of impairment of sensation and loss of motor function of the arm and leg on the contralateral side.
- *Lateral area:* Produces symptoms of dysfunction of the cerebellum and of the nuclei and tracts in the lateral portion of the brainstem, in particular the motor nuclei of the fifth, seventh, and tenth cranial nerves; the sensory nuclei of the fifth and eighth cranial nerves; the descending sympathetic pathways; and the spinothalamic tract.
- *Internal carotid artery:* Produces aphasia (when in the dominant hemisphere), contralateral hemiplegia, hemianesthesia, hemianopia, and unilateral loss of vision.
- *Posterior inferior cerebral artery:* Produces ataxia, contralateral hemianalgesia, difficulty swallowing, ipsilateral weakness of the tongue and vocal cords, and nystagmus.

- *Superior cerebral artery:* Produces contralateral hemianesthesia/hemianalgesia, contralateral facial weakness, and ipsilateral ataxia.

The medical examination for stroke also includes a number of routine laboratory and diagnostic tests, including:

- Urinalysis
- Blood analysis
- Fasting blood glucose levels
- Blood chemistry profile, including creatinine phosphokinase isoenzyme (CPK-MB), which is elevated with cardiac infarction
- Thyroid function tests
- Full cardiac workup (radiograph of chest, ECG, and echocardiography; see Chapter 11)
- Pertinent imaging studies, including CT scan, MRI, PET scan, transcranial and carotid Doppler, and cerebral angiography

Physical Therapy Intervention. The primary impairments associated with stroke include:

- Loss of or impaired sensation
- Pain—headache, neck and face pain
- Visual changes, including neglect and visual field deficits
- Alterations in motor function, including weakness, alterations in tone, abnormal synergy patterns, abnormal reflexes, altered coordination, bowel and bladder changes, and altered motor programming
- Impairments in postural control and balance
- Impairments of speech, language, and swallowing
- Impairments of perception and cognition
- Changes in emotional status

In many instances, the recovery from a stroke occurs in the sequential manner described by Brunnstrom (Table 14-4) or by Fugl-Meyer and colleagues (Table 14-5):[37]

The goals for the physical therapy intervention should include:[24]

- To maintain or improve range of motion:
  - Positioning techniques
  - Passive ROM/Self ROM
  - Soft tissue/joint mobilizations

TABLE 14-4. BRUNNSTROM'S SEVEN STAGES OF RECOVERY FROM STROKE

STAGE	DESCRIPTION
1	No volitional movement initiated.
2	The appearance of basic limb synergies. The beginning of spasticity.
3	The synergies are performed voluntarily; spasticity increases.
4	Spasticity begins to decrease. Movement patterns are not dictated solely by limb synergies.
5	A further decrease in spasticity is noted with independence from limb synergy patterns.
6	Isolated joint movements are performed with coordination.
7	Normal motor function is restored.

Data from Brunnstrom S: Motor testing procedures in hemiplegia: based on sequential recovery stages. *Phys Ther.* 1966;46:357-375.

TABLE 14-5. THE FUGL-MEYER AND COLLEAGUES STAGES OF STROKE RECOVERY

STAGE	DESCRIPTION
1	Reflexes recur, a period of initial flaccidity with no voluntary movement.
2	Voluntary movement is only possible within the dynamic flexion and extension synergies.
3	Voluntary control in isolated joint movements emerging with a mixing of synergies.
4	Increasing voluntary control out of synergy; coordination deficits present.
5	The patient has maximum scores in stages 1 through 4—control and coordination of movement near normal.

Data from Fugl-Meyer AR, Jaasko L, Leyman I, et al: The post-stroke hemiplegic patient. 1. A method for evaluation of physical performance. *Scand J Rehabil Med.* 1975;7:13-31.

- To maintain or improve strength:
  - Graded strength training combined with careful monitoring of blood pressure, heart rate, and ratings of perceived exertion (RPE)
- Improve postural control and functional mobility:
  - Rolling activities
- Transfer training (supine to sit; sit to supine; sit to stand; sit down transfers).
- Sitting exercises focusing on correct alignment, control, weight shifts, and reaching.
- Bridging.
- Standing activities (modified plantigrade, upright standing, and weight shifts).
- Locomotor and gait training as appropriate.
- Improve manipulation and dexterity skills.
- Assess the need for environmental modifications and/or assistive devices (orthotics, foot and ankle controls [AFO], knee controls, and wheelchairs).
- Minimize secondary complications:
  - Spasticity (refer to Chapter 9)
  - Contracture and deformity prevention
  - Decubiti
  - Confusion
  - Decreased sensorimotor function
- Improve feeding and swallowing deficits using a multidisciplinary approach.

Degenerative Diseases

Parkinson Disease. Parkinson disease (PD), a progressive neurodegenerative disorder, is a pathology associated with a loss of pigmented dopaminergic nigrostriatal neurons in the substantia nigra and the presence of Lewy bodies.[24-36]

- Dopaminergic nigrostriatal neurons: the loss occurs most prominently in the ventral lateral substantia nigra. Approximately 60% to 80% of dopaminergic neurons are lost before clinical symptoms of PD emerge.
- Lewy bodies: the presence of Lewy bodies within pigmented neurons of the substantia nigra is characteristic, but not pathognomonic, of idiopathic PD.

Most cases of idiopathic PD are due to a combination of genetic and environmental factors (exposure to herbicides/pesticides, and proximity to industrial plants or quarries).

The onset of PD is typically asymmetric, with the most common initial finding being an asymmetric resting tremor in an upper extremity, the amplitude of which increases with stress and resolves during sleep. After several months or as much as a few years, the tremor may begin to affect the extremity on the other side, but asymmetry often is maintained. Other signs and symptoms include

- The axial posture becomes progressively flexed and the walking strides become shorter.
- A decreased ability to swallow, which may lead to excess saliva and ultimately drooling.
- Sleep disturbances.

Symptoms of autonomic dysfunction, including constipation, sweating abnormalities, sexual dysfunction, and seborrheic dermatitis are common.

Examination. The three cardinal signs of PD are resting tremor, rigidity, and bradykinesia. Postural instability, which emerges late in the disease (usually after 8 years or more), is the fourth cardinal sign. Parkinson disease can be staged for examination and intervention purposes using the Hoehn and Yahr classification[37]:

I. Minimal or absent disability, unilateral symptoms.
II. Minimal bilateral or midline involvement, no balance involvement.
III. Impaired balance, some restrictions in activity.
IV. All symptoms present and severe. Stands and walks only with assistance.
V. Confinement to bed or wheelchair.

Physical Therapy Intervention. The goal of the physical therapy intervention is for the patient to maintain control of the signs and symptoms for as long as possible while attempting to prevent or minimize the secondary impairments associated with disuse and inactivity. It is important that the clinician continues to monitor changes associated with the disease progression and any side effects that may be caused by the pharmacological interventions.

Alzheimer Disease. Alzheimer disease (AD) is an acquired cognitive and behavioral impairment of sufficient severity to markedly interfere with social and occupational functioning. The cause of AD is unknown.

Patients with AD most commonly present with an insidious and progressive memory loss. This loss can be associated with slowly progressive behavioral changes. Although other neurologic systems (eg, extrapyramidal, cerebellar systems) can also be affected, the most prominent finding as the disease progresses to its moderate and severe stages is progressive memory impairment. In addition to behavioral changes, patients may also develop language disorders (eg, anomia, progressive aphasia) and impairment in their visuospatial skills and executive functions.

Examination. Examination in the clinic or at the patient's bedside should include a discussion with the patient. Any cognitive impairment or language dysfunction should ideally be verified and discussed with the patient's spouse and/or caregivers. Memory dysfunction and problems with activities of daily living (eg, cooking, cleaning, money management, getting lost, confusion, self-care) should also be addressed. A screening language examination and Mini-Mental Status Testing may be warranted (see Table 9-19).

Imaging Studies

- Brain MRI or CT: in assessing AD, brain MRIs or CT scans show diffuse cortical and/or cerebral atrophy. These studies are also used to rule out other CNS disease.
- SPECT: under most circumstances, SPECT is an optional study and not considered mandatory for the routine workup of patients with typical presentations of AD. SPECT is used in qualified cases, usually those involving atypical presentations, such as language disorders (eg, progressive aphasia), visuospatial dysfunction syndromes, or other conditions that may be confused with cerebrovascular disease or other neurodegenerative conditions.

Other Diagnostic Tests

- EEG: EEG can help in ruling out other diseases that cause dementia, such as prion-related diseases (eg, Creutzfeldt-Jakob disease).
- Tau protein test: tau is a constituent of NFTs and amyloid protein (found in senile plaques among other lesions) in the CSF to diagnose AD. However, as levels of tau protein overlap considerably in healthy elderly individuals, in patients with a variety of neurodegenerative disorders, and in those with AD, these levels are not useful as an unequivocal biologic marker of AD.
- Genotyping for apolipoproteins: This test is a research tool that is helpful in determining the risk of AD in populations, but it is of little if any value in making a clinical diagnosis and developing a management plan in individual patients.

Medical Intervention. Medical treatments for AD include psychotropic medications and behavioral interventions. To date, no interventions have been shown to convincingly prevent AD or slow its progression.

Physical Therapy Intervention. Patients with AD appear to benefit from both physical and mental activities, both to prevent deterioration and to slow its rate. However, the mental activities should be kept within a reasonable level of difficulty for the patient so that excessive frustration can be avoided and that they ideally motivate the patient to engage in them frequently.

Cognitive Disorders

Delirium, Dementia. Acute alterations in brain function are commonly referred to as mental status change (MSC) or acute confusional state (ACS), while chronic alterations and any MSC specifically due to nonpsychiatric causes are generally referred to as organic brain syndrome (OBS).

Physical Therapy Examination. Any patient who presents with altered mental status needs a complete physical examination, with particular attention to mental status (orientation, attention, calculation, recall, language) general appearance, vital signs, hydration status, evidence of physical trauma, behavioral changes (restless, agitated, distracted, paranoid, wandering, inappropriate social behavior, repetitive behavior), and neurologic signs.

The Mini-Mental Status Examination (MMSE) (Table 9-19) is a formalized way of documenting the severity and nature of mental status changes. In addition, or as an alternative to the MMSE, the patient can be asked to correctly draw the face of a clock (to include the circle, numbers, and hands). Other simple screening tests include asking the patient to spell "world" backwards or performing "serial 7s," which involves starting at the number 100 and subtracting 7 repeatedly in series (ie, 100...93...86...79...).

Physical Therapy Intervention. The physical therapy intervention will depend on the extent of the disease. The goals typically include

- Improvement of self-care abilities to help the patient carry out activities of daily living (grooming, hygiene, continence).
- The provision of a safe and soothing environment to help decrease agitation, increase attention, prevent falls, injury or further dysfunction.
- Improvement of motor function, gait, and balance.
- The provision of reorienting cues: calendars, memory aids.

Cardiovascular Disorders and Diseases

Hypertension.

As described in Chapter 11, the regulation of normal blood pressure, which is a function of cardiac output and peripheral vascular resistance, is a complex process. Hypertension may be either essential or secondary.

Essential Hypertension. Essential hypertension has been linked to the interaction of multiple factors, including genetic predisposition, excess dietary salt intake, and adrenergic tone.[38-47] Although genetics appears to contribute to essential hypertension, the exact mechanism has not been established. The progression of hypertension begins with an asymmetric period of prehypertension in persons aged 10 to 30 years (due to increased cardiac output) to early hypertension in persons aged 20 to 40 years (in which increased peripheral resistance is prominent) to established hypertension in persons aged 30 to 50 years, and, finally, to complicated hypertension in persons aged 40 to 60 years.

Secondary Hypertension. The historical and physical findings that have been associated with secondary hypertension are a history of known renal disease, abdominal masses, anemia, and urochrome pigmentation.

An accurate measurement of blood pressure is the key to diagnosis (see Chapter 11).

Intervention. In addition to pharmacotherapy, most intervention approaches address lifestyle modifications:

- Lose weight if overweight.
- Limit alcohol intake.

- Increase aerobic activity.
- Reduce sodium intake.
- Maintain adequate intake of dietary potassium.
- Maintain adequate intake of dietary calcium and magnesium for general health.
- Smoking cessation
- Reduce intake of dietary saturated fat and cholesterol.

Coronary Artery Disease. See Chapter 11.

Pulmonary Disorders and Diseases

Chronic Bronchitis/Chronic Obstructive Pulmonary Disease (COPD). See Chapter 10.

Asthma. See Chapter 10.

Pneumonia. See Chapter 10.

Lung Cancer. See Chapter 10.

Integumentary Disorders and Diseases

Decubitus Ulcers. See Chapter 13.

Metabolic Pathologies

Diabetes Mellitus. See Chapter 12.

ETHICAL AND LEGAL ISSUES

The Living Will (Advanced Care and Medical Directive)

Advance directives are documents signed by a competent person giving direction to health care providers about treatment choices in certain circumstances. There are two types of advance directives:

- A durable power of attorney for health care ("durable power") allows a patient to name a "patient advocate" to act on behalf of the patient and carry out his or her wishes (see Health-Care Proxy below).
- A living will that allows a patient to state his or her wishes in writing, but does not name a patient advocate.

The regulations for The Advanced Care Medical Directive (ACMD) vary state to state; however, in order to be deemed a legal document the ACMD must be signed by the principal and witnessed by two adults. There are generally two broad types of situations in which the directive may apply:

- Terminal illness, where death is expected in a relatively short time.
- Permanent disability in an intolerable situation. This is a highly individualized decision.

Many standard health care declarations instruct physicians to withhold "extraordinary care" or "life-sustaining or life-prolonging" treatments.

Refusal of Treatment/Informed Consent

Every adult (if deemed mentally competent) has the right to decide to accept or refuse any medical treatment. Informed consent is the process by which a competent and fully informed patient can participate in choices about his or her health care. It is generally accepted that complete informed consent includes a discussion of the following elements:

- The nature and purpose of the decision/procedure.
- Reasonable alternatives to the proposed intervention.
- The relevant risks, benefits, consequences, and uncertainties related to each alternative.
- The likelihood of success or failure of the intervention.
- An assessment of patient understanding. In order for the patient's consent to be valid, he or she must be considered competent to make the decision at hand and his consent must be voluntary. If the patient is not deemed competent, consent must be obtained from a legal guardian or health-care proxy.
- The acceptance of the intervention by the patient.

There are basically two broad reasons why a patient may refuse a certain treatment:

- The benefit of the treatment is not great enough to justify its risk or discomfort. This is the basis for most treatment decisions, and involves the individual attitudes each patient will bring to the decision.
- The treatment will prolong life under intolerable conditions. Even an easily tolerated treatment with minimal discomfort, such as a feeding tube, might be unacceptable if it prolongs life in the face of unwanted circumstances.

Do Not Resuscitate (DNR) Orders

These orders apply only to cardiopulmonary resuscitation (CPR) and there are specific rules concerning how they are to be written and who may authorize them.

Health-Care Proxy

A health-care proxy is an agent who makes health care decisions for the patient when he or she has been determined to be incapable of making such decisions.

COMMON FUNCTIONAL PROBLEM AREAS IN THE GERIATRIC POPULATION

Immobility-Disability

Immobility is a common pathway by which a host of diseases and problems in the elderly produce further disability. Persons who are

TABLE 14-6. PATHOPHYSIOLOGIC ALTERATIONS DUE TO IMMOBILITY

BODY SYSTEM	EFFECTS
Musculoskeletal	Decreased range of motion
	Decreased joint flexibility
	Development of contractures
	Loss of muscular strength (muscular atrophy)
	Loss of muscular endurance (deconditioning)
	Loss of bone mass
	Loss of bone strength
Integumentary	Development of pressure sores
	Skin atrophy and break down
Psychological/neurological	Depression
	Decreased perceptual ability
	Social isolation
	Learned helplessness
	Altered sleep patterns
	Anxiety, irritability, hostility
Cardiopulmonary	Decreased ventilation
	Atelectasis
	Aspiration pneumonia
	Deterioration of respiratory system
	Increased cardiac output
	Increased resting heart rate
	Orthostatic hypotension
Genitourinary	Urinary infection
	Urinary retention
	Bladder calculi
Metabolic	Negative balance
	Loss of calcium

Data from Gillette PD: Exercise in aging and disease. In: Placzek JD, Boyce DA, eds. *Orthopaedic Physical Therapy Secrets.* Philadelphia, PA: Hanley & Belfus, Inc. 2001:235-242; and Thompson LV: Iatrogenic effects. In: Kaufmann TL, ed. *Geriatric Rehabilitation Manual.* New York, NY: Churchill Livingstone. 1999:318-324.

chronically ill, aged, or disabled are particularly susceptible to the adverse effects of prolonged bed rest, immobilization, and inactivity. The effects of immobility are rarely confined to only one body system (Table 14-6). Common causes for immobility in the elderly include

- Musculoskeletal system: causes include arthritis, osteoporosis, fractures (especially hip and femur), and podiatric problems.
- Cardiopulmonary system: causes include chronic coronary heart disease, chronic obstructive lung disease, severe heart failure, and peripheral vascular disease.
- Neurologic system: causes include cerebrovascular accident, Parkinson disease, cerebellar dysfunction, neuropathies, cognitive, psychological, and sensory problems (dementia, depression, fear and anxiety), pain, impaired vision.
- Environmental causes: including forced immobilization (restraint use), inadequate aids for mobility.
- Malnutrition.
- Deconditioning.

Physical Therapy Intervention. Intervention strategies should include the following, while monitoring vital signs:

- Minimize duration of bed rest. Avoid strict bed rest unless absolutely necessary.
- Be aware of possible adverse effects of medications.
- Encourage the continuation of daily activities that the patient is able to perform as tolerated but avoiding overexertion.
- Bathroom privileges or bedside commode.
- Let patient stand 30 to 60 seconds during transfers (bed to chair).
- Encourage taking meals at a table.
- Encourage the wearing of street clothes.
- Encourage daily exercises as a basis of good care. Exercises should emphasize
  - Balance and proprioception
  - Strength and endurance
  - Coordination and equilibrium
  - Aerobic capacity
  - Posture
  - Gait
    - Cadence
    - Base of support
    - Gait deviations
- Assistive device. Design possible ways to enhance mobility through the use of assistive devices (eg, walking aids, wheelchairs) and making the home accessible.
- Ensure that a sufficient fluid intake is being maintained (1.5-2 L fluid intake per day as possible), and adequate nutritional levels.
- Encourage socialization with family, friends, or caregivers.
- If the patient is bed-bound, maintain proper body alignment and change positions every few hours. Pressure padding and heel protectors may be used to provide comfort and prevent pressure sores.
  - Skin integrity
  - Protective sensations
  - Discriminatory sensations

FALLS AND INSTABILITY

Falls can be markers of poor health and declining function, and they are often associated with significant morbidity.[48] More than 90% of hip fractures occur as a result of falls, with most of these fractures occurring in persons over 70 years of age. One-third of community-dwelling elderly persons and 60% of nursing home residents fall each year. Risk factors for falls in the elderly include increasing age, medication use (Table 14-7), cognitive impairment and sensory deficits. Common causes of falls in the elderly include[49]

- Accident, environmental hazard, fall from bed
- Gait disturbance, balance disorders or weakness, pain related to arthritis
- Vertigo
- Medications or alcohol

TABLE 14-7. DRUGS THAT MAY INCREASE THE RISK OF FALLS

Sedative-hypnotic and anxiolytic drugs (especially long-acting benzodiazepines)
Tricyclic antidepressants
Major tranquilizers (phenothiazines and butyrophenones)
Antihypertensive drugs
Cardiac medications
Corticosteroids
Nonsteroidal anti-inflammatory drugs
Anticholinergic drugs
Hypoglycemic agents
Any medication that is likely to affect balance

Reproduced, with permission, from Fuller GF: Falls in the elderly. *Am Fam Physician.* 2000;61:2159-2168, 2173-2174.

- Confusion and cognitive impairment
- Postural (orthostatic) hypotension
- Visual disorder
- Central nervous system disorder, syncope, drop attacks, epilepsy

Elderly persons who survive a fall experience significant morbidity. Hospital stays are almost twice as long in elderly patients who are hospitalized after a fall than in elderly patients who are admitted for another reason.

Evaluation of the Elderly Patient Who Falls. Elderly patients with known risk factors for falling should be questioned about falls on a periodic basis. A single fall is not always a sign of a major problem and an increased risk for subsequent falls. The fall may simply be an isolated event. However, recurrent falls, defined as more than two falls in a 6-month period, should be evaluated for treatable causes. A thorough history is essential to determine the mechanism of falling, specific risk factors for falls, impairments that contribute to falls and the appropriate diagnostic workup.

The clinician should ask about the activity the patient was engaged in just before and at the time of the fall, especially if the activity involved a positional change. The location of the fall should be ascertained. It is also important to know whether anyone witnessed the fall and whether the patient sustained any injuries. The patient and, if applicable, any witnesses or caregivers should be asked in detail about previous falls and whether the falls were the same or different in character. The clinician also needs to determine who is available to assist the patient. A mnemonic (I HATE FALLING) can be used to remind the clinician of key physical findings in patients who fall or nearly fall (Table 14-8).[50]

A home visit is invaluable for assessing modifiable risk factors and determining appropriate interventions. A home safety checklist can guide the visit and ensure a thorough evaluation (Table 14-2). It is particularly important to assess caregiver and housing arrangements, environmental hazards, alcohol use and compliance with medications. An algorithm for the evaluation of falls is presented in Figure 14-1.[48]

Balance and Gait Testing. Several simple tests have exhibited a strong correlation with a history of falling. These functional balance

TABLE 14-8. I HATE FALLING: A MNEMONIC FOR KEY PHYSICAL FINDINGS IN THE ELDERLY PATIENT WHO FALLS OR NEARLY FALLS

I	Inflammation of joints (or joint deformity)
H	Hypotension (orthostatic blood pressure changes)
A	Auditory and visual abnormalities
T	Tremor (Parkinson disease or other causes of tremor)
E	Equilibrium (balance) problem
F	Foot problems
A	Arrhythmia, heart block or valvular disease
L	Leg-length discrepancy
L	Lack of conditioning (generalized weakness)
I	Illness
N	Nutritional status (poor, weight loss)
G	Gait disturbance

Data from Sloan JP: Mobility failure. In: Sloan JP, ed. *Protocols in Primary Care Geriatrics*. New York, NY: Springer. 1997:33-38.

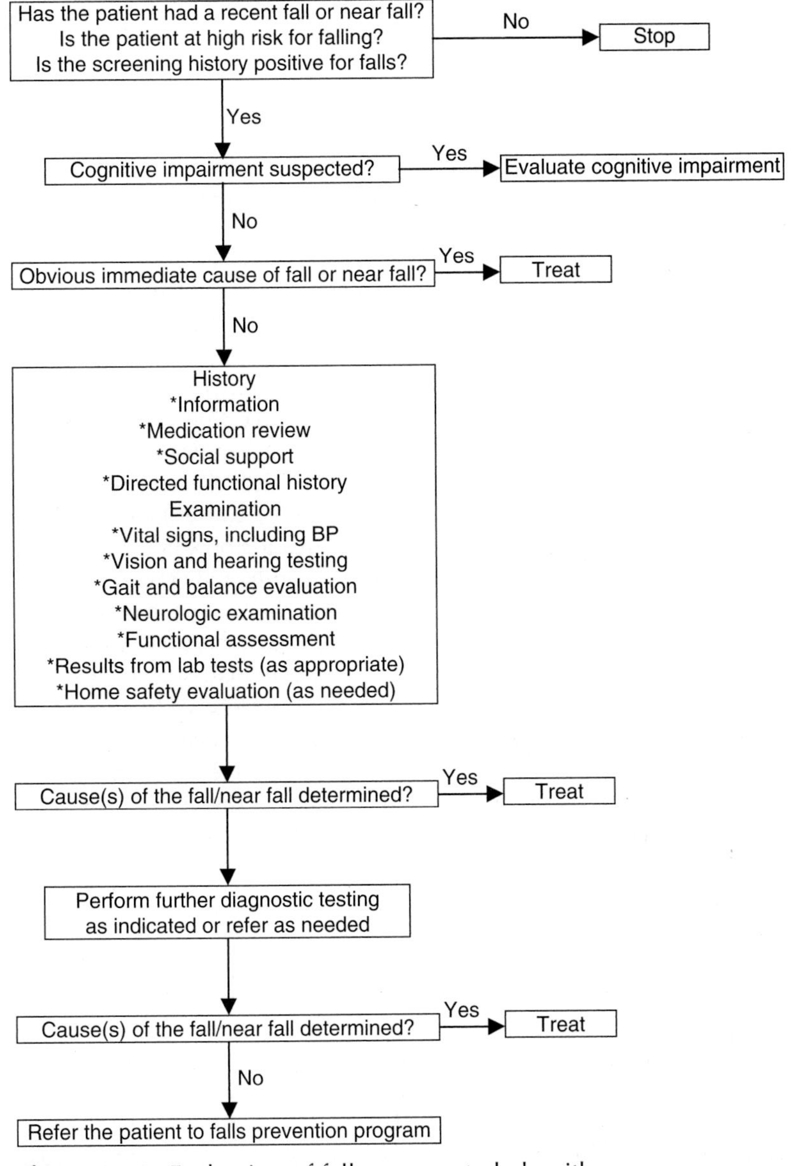

Figure 14-1. Evaluation of falls—suggested algorithm.

TABLE 14-9. TIMED "UP AND GO" TEST

Task	Get up out of a standard armchair (seat height of approximately 46 cm [18.4 in]), walk a distance of 3 m (10 ft), turn, walk back to the chair and sit down again.	
Requirement	Ambulate with or without assistive device and follow a three-step command.	
Trials	One practice trial and then three actual trials. The times from the three actual trials are averaged.	
Time	1-2 minutes	
Equipment	Armchair, stopwatch (or wristwatch with a second hand) and a measured path	
Predictive results	Seconds	Rating
	< 10	Freely mobile
	< 20	Mostly independent
	20-29	Variable mobility
	> 30	Impaired mobility

Data from Podsiadlo D, Richardson S: The timed "Up & Go": a test of basic functional mobility for frail elderly persons. *J Am Geriatr Soc.* 1991;39:142-148.

measures are quantifiable and correlate well with the ability of older adults to ambulate safely in their environment. The tests can also be used to measure changes in mobility after interventions have been applied.

- One-leg balance: tested by having the patient stand unassisted on one leg for 5 seconds. The patient chooses which leg to stand on (based on personal comfort), flexes the opposite knee to allow the foot to clear the floor and then balances on one leg for as long as possible. The clinician uses a watch to time the patient's one-leg balance.[30] This test predicts injurious falls but not all falls.
- The timed "Up & Go" test (Table 14-9) evaluates gait and balance. The patient gets up out of a standard armchair (seat height of approximately 46 cm [18.4 in]), walks a distance of 3 m (10 ft), turns, walks back to the chair and sits down again. The patient wears regular footwear and, if applicable, uses any customary walking aid (eg, cane or walker). No physical assistance is given. The clinician uses a stopwatch or a wristwatch with a second hand to time this activity. A score of 30 seconds or greater indicates that the patient has impaired mobility and requires assistance (ie, has a high risk of falling). This test has been shown to be as valid as sophisticated gait testing. A simpler alternative is the "Get-Up and Go" test. In this test, the patient is seated in an armless chair placed 3 m (10 ft) from a wall. The patient stands, walks toward the wall (using a walking aid if one is typically employed), turns without touching the wall, returns to the chair, turns and sits down. This activity does not need to be timed. Instead, the clinician observes the patient and makes note of any balance or gait problems.

Overall physical function should also be assessed. This is accomplished by evaluating the patient's ADLs and instrumental activities of daily living (IADLs).

Physical Therapy Intervention. With patients who have a history of falling, the intervention is directed at the underlying cause

TABLE 14-10. CRITICAL STEPS IN REDUCING THE RISK OF FALLS IN THE ELDERLY
Eliminate environmental hazards.
Improve home supports.
Provide opportunities for socialization and encouragement.
Modify medication.
Provide balance training.
Modify restraints.
Involve the family.
Provide follow-up.

Data from Tinetti ME, Baker DI, McAvay G, et al: A multifactorial intervention to reduce the risk of falling among elderly people living in the community. *N Engl J Med.* 1994;331:821-827.

of the fall and in preventing recurrence. Interventions that may be successful in reducing falls are listed in Tables 14-10 and 14-11. Functional training should include

- Sit to stand transitions.
- Turning.
- The provision of appropriate assistive devices/adaptive equipment.

TABLE 14-11. INTERVENTIONS BASED ON RISK FACTORS TO REDUCE THE RISK OF FALLS IN THE ELDERLY

RISK FACTORS	INTERVENTIONS
Postural hypotension: a drop in systolic blood pressure of ≥ 20 mm Hg or to < 90 mm Hg on standing	Behavioral recommendations, such as ankle pumps or hand clenching and elevation of the head of the bed. Decrease in the dosage of a medication that may contribute to hypotension; if necessary, discontinuation of the drug or substitution of another medication. Pressure stockings. If indicated, fludrocortisone (Florinef), in a dosage of 0.1 mg two or three times daily, to increase blood pressure. If indicated, midodrine (ProAmatine), in a dosage of 2.5-5 mg three times daily, to increase vascular tone and blood pressure.
Use of a benzodiazepine or other sedative-hypnotic drug	Education about appropriate use of sedative-hypnotic drugs. Nonpharmacologic treatment of sleep problems, such as sleep restriction. Tapering and discontinuation of medications.
Use of four or more prescription medications	Review of medications.
Environmental hazards for falling or tripping	Home safety assessment with appropriate changes, such as removal of hazards, selection of safer furniture (correct height, more stability) and installation of structures such as grab bars in bathrooms or handrails on stairs.
Any impairment in gait	Gait training. Use of an appropriate assistive device Balance or strengthening exercises if indicated.
Any impairment in balance or transfer skills	Balance exercises and training in transfer skills if indicated. Environmental alterations, such as installation of grab bars or raised toilet seats.
Impairment in leg or arm muscle strength or range of motion (hip, ankle, knee, shoulder, hand, or elbow)	Exercises with resistive bands and putty resistance training two or three times a week, with resistance increased when the patient is able to complete 10 repetitions through the full range of motion.

Data from Tinetti ME, Baker DI, McAvay G, et al: A multifactorial intervention to reduce the risk of falling among elderly people living in the community. *N Engl J Med.* 1994;331:821-827.

- Patient and family/caregiver education:
  - Identification of risks.
  - Safety issues.
  - Adequate lighting at home.
  - Contrasting colors.
  - Reduce clutter.
  - Minimize polypharmacy and medication errors (refer to Chapter 19).

NUTRITIONAL DEFICIENCY

Nutritional status is a "vital sign" of health. Nutrition takes on greater importance in the context of chronic illness.[51-57] With increase in age, there is an increase risk of developing nutritional deficiencies that can lead to such debilitating consequences like functional dependency, morbidity and mortality. Some older persons are at increased risk for nutritional deficiency because of multiple drug therapies, dental problems, economic hardship, and reduced social contacts. These problems arise from many varied environmental, social, and economic factors that are compounded by physiological changes of aging. A statement on nutrition screening is needed in order to

- Incorporate nutritional screening in the clinical care of older persons.
- Heighten awareness of the multiple risk factors having an impact upon nutritional status of older persons.

The Food and Nutritional Board of the Institute of Medicine no longer uses the term, Recommended Daily Allowances. Rather, they use Dietary Reference Intakes (DRI). DRIs are reference values to estimate the nutrient intakes to be used for planning and assessing diets for healthy people. Many of the DRIs for older adults are not based on large studies of older people, rather they are derived by extrapolation from data obtained for younger persons. The DRI adjustments for older adults have been made based on the reduction in physiologic function, changes in body composition and metabolic adaptation in adults over 51 years of age and then again over 71 years of age. Table 14-12 shows the most current DRIs.

Physical Therapy Role. A proper and continuous nutritional assessment of a patient's nutritional status is important to identify those patients that are at risk (Tables 14-13 and 14-14). Although not directly involved with the patient's nutritional status, the physical therapist should attempt to

- Maintain or improve the patient's physical function.
- Assist in the monitoring of the patient's nutritional intake by observing any physical or mental changes that could be nutritionally related.
- Request nutritional consults as necessary:
  - Communication with social worker for elderly food programs (Meals on Wheels, federal food stamp programs).

TABLE 14-12. RDI FOR OLDER ADULTS OVER 70

REQUIREMENTS	HEALTHY ELDERLY WOMEN	HEALTHY ELDERLY MEN	ADDITIONAL COMMENTS
Protein	1 g/kg body weight	1 g/kg body weight	Acute and chronic diseases increases protein requirements
Carbohydrate	55%-60% of total calories/day	55%-60% of total calories/day	
Fat	30% of total calories/day	30% of total calories/day	Healthy elderly in their 60s-70s but overweight, hypercholesterolemic and/or hypertensive, should reduce calories, fat and sodium under the supervision of a clinician. Aging does not alter any of the specific requirements for any essential lipids
Water	1 mL/kcal or 30 mL/kg body weight	1 mL/kcal or 30 mL/kg body weight	Dehydration and Diarrhea. The amount of fluid that is lost must be replaced, and replaced soon after the fluid loss. Patients and families must be educated to the importance of maintaining adequate fluid intake at all times, especially with acute conditions.
Calories	1900 kcal/d or 30 kcal/d	2300 kcal/d or 30 kcal/d	
Calcium	1200-1500 mg	1200-1500 mg	
Zinc	8 mg	11 mg	
Iron	8 mg	8 mg	
Selenium	55 µg	55 µg	
Vitamin C	75 mg	90 mg	
Thiamin	1.1 mg	1.2 mg	
Folate	400 µg	400 µg	
Vitamin B_{12}	2.4 µg	2.4 µg	
Vitamin D	600 IU	600 IU	If no sun exposure, 800-1600 IU/d.
Vitamin E	15 IU	15 IU	

Data from Food and Nutrition Board, the National Academies of Sciences. *Dietary Reference Intakes (DRI)*. Washington, DC: The Institute of Medicine, National Academies of Sciences. 2001.

TABLE 14-13. NUTRITIONAL ASSESSMENT IN OLDER ADULTS

Past medical history
Current symptoms
History suggestive of depression
Use of tobacco, alcohol or illicit drugs
Current medications including OTCs
Socioeconomic status
Weight loss (> 10% in 6 mo or > 5% in 1 mo)
Alteration in functional status
Comprehensive metabolic panel
Serum levels of total protein, albumin, prealbumin, total cholesterol
Thyroid function tests
Serum vitamin and mineral levels: iron, folic acid, vitamin B_{12}
Daily energy intake and recent changes
Anthropometrics
Oral/dental status
Signs of vitamin or mineral deficiency
Functional status

TABLE 14-14. THE NUTRITIONAL RISK SCREENING SCALES

Sadness	Yesavage geriatric mood assessment scale (Table 14-15) of 15 or greater out of 30.
Cholesterol	Less than 160 mg/dL
Albumin	Less than 4 g/dL
Loss of weight	5% in 1 month and/or 10% in 6 months
Eat	Problems feeding self either because of physical or cognitive problems
Shopping	Sufficient money to buy food and the ability to obtain and prepare it

Reproduced, with permission, Morley J: The nutritional risk screening SCALES. *J Am Geriatrics Soc.* 1991;39:1139-1140.

- Recommendations for home health aides:
  - Assistance in grocery shopping
  - Meal preparation

GENERAL PRINCIPLES OF GERIATRIC REHABILITATION

The following areas should be emphasized in the intervention of the elderly population:

- Safety
  - Level of cognition, vision, hearing, proprioception
  - Appropriate and safe use of assistive devices
  - Home/living environment
- Level of activity/exercise. The absolute contraindications for exercising all the adults include, but are not limited to
  - Severe coronary artery disease with unstable angina pectoris
  - Acute myocardial infarction (< 2 days after infarction)
  - Severe valvular heart disease
  - Rapid or prolonged atrial or ventricular arrhythmias/tachycardias
  - Uncontrolled hypertension
  - Profound orthostatic hypotension
  - Acute thrombophlebitis
  - Acute pulmonary embolism (< 2 days after event)
  - Known or suspected dissecting aneurysm
- Health promotion
  - Determine effects of normal aging versus disease pathologies.
  - Education on healthy lifestyle and prevention of disability.
  - Improving mood level (Table 14-15)
  - Maximize independence.
  - Enhance coping skills.
- Support systems
  - Help prevent social isolation.
  - Educate caregivers, friends and family.
  - Provide empowerment.
  - Involve patient in decision-making.
  - Be the patient's advocate for needed services.

TABLE 14-15. YESAVAGE GERIATRIC MOOD ASSESSMENT SCALE

1. Are you basically satisfied with your life?
2. Have you dropped many of your activities and interests?
3. Do you feel that your life is empty?
4. Do you often get bored?
5. Are you hopeful about the future?
6. Are you bothered by thoughts you can't get out of your head?
7. Are you in good spirits most of the time?
8. Are you afraid that something bad is going to happen to you?
9. Do you feel happy most of the time?
10. Do you often feel helpless?
11. Do you often get restless and fidgety?
12. Do you prefer to stay at home, rather than going out and doing new things?
13. Do you frequently worry about the future?
14. Do you feel you have more problems with memory than most?
15. Do you think it is wonderful to be alive now?
16. Do you often feel downhearted and blue?
17. Do you feel pretty worthless the way you are now?
18. Do you worry a lot about the past?
19. Do you find life very exciting?
20. Is it hard for you to get started on new projects?
21. Do you feel full of energy?
22. Do you feel that your situation is hopeless?
23. Do you think that most people are better off than you are?
24. Do you frequently get upset over little things?
25. Do you frequently feel like crying?
26. Do you have trouble concentrating?
27. Do you enjoy getting up in the morning?
28. Do you prefer to avoid social gatherings?
29. Is it easy for you to make decisions?
30. Is your mind as clear as it used to be?

This is the original scoring for the scale. One point for each of these ansvers. Cutoff: normal, 0-9; mild depressives, 10-19; severe depressives, 20-30.

1. no	6. yes	11. yes	16. yes	21. no	26. yes
2. yes	7. no	12. yes	17. yes	22. yes	27. no
3. yes	8. yes	13. yes	18. yes	23. yes	28. yes
4. yes	9. no	14. yes	19. no	24. yes	29. no
5. no	10. yes	15. no	20. yes	25. yes	30. no

Data from Torres RM, Miralles R, Garcia-Caselles MP, et al: Observational scale and geriatric depression scale of Yesavage to identify depressive symptoms in older patients. *Arch Gerontol Geriatr.* 2004;9:437-442.

Questions for this chapter and the entire book appear on the included CD-ROM, with additional questions at www.DuttonNPTE.com.

REFERENCES

1. Harman D: Aging: phenomena and theories. *Ann N Y Acad Sci.* 1998;854:1-7.
2. Bjorksten J: Some therapeutic implications of the crosslinkage theory of aging. *Adv Exp Med Biol.* 1977;86B:579-602.
3. Bjorksten J: The crosslinkage theory of aging: clinical implications. *Compr Ther.* 1976;2:65-74.

4. Bjorksten J: The crosslinkage theory of aging. *J Am Geriatr Soc.* 1968;16:408-427.
5. Effros RB: Roy Walford and the immunologic theory of aging. *Immun Ageing.* 2005;2:7.
6. Kent S: Can normal aging be explained by the immunologic theory. *Geriatrics.* 1977;32:111, 113, 116.
7. Walford RL: Immunologic theory of aging: current status. *Fed Proc.* 1974;33:2020-2027.
8. Walford RL: The immunologic theory of aging. *Gerontologist.* 1964;57:195-197.
9. Harman D: Free radical involvement in aging. Pathophysiology and therapeutic implications. *Drugs Aging.* 1993;3:60-80.
10. Hall C, Thein-Brody L: Impairment in muscle performance. In: Hall C, Thein-Brody L, eds. *Therapeutic Exercise: Moving toward Function.* Baltimore, MD: Lippincott Williams & Wilkins; 2005: 57-86.
11. Evans WJ: High-velocity resistance training for increasing peak muscle power in elderly women. *Clin J Sport Med.* 2003;13:66.
12. Fielding RA, LeBrasseur NK, Cuoco A, et al: High-velocity resistance training increases skeletal muscle peak power in older women. *J Am Geriatr Soc.* 2002;50:655-662.
13. Treatment of dementia and agitation: a guide for families and caregivers. *J Psychiatr Pract.* 2007;13:207-216.
14. Elble RJ: Gait and dementia: moving beyond the notion of gait apraxia. *J Neural Transm.* 2007;114:1253-1258.
15. Holthe T, Thorsen K, Josephsson S: Occupational patterns of people with dementia in residential care: an ethnographic study. *Scand J Occup Ther.* 2007;14:96-107.
16. Man-Son-Hing M, Marshall SC, Molnar FJ, et al: Systematic review of driving risk and the efficacy of compensatory strategies in persons with dementia. *J Am Geriatr Soc.* 2007;55:878-848.
17. Missotten P, Ylieff M, Di Notte D, et al: Quality of life in dementia: a 2-year follow-up study. *Int J Geriatr Psychiatry.* 2007;22: 1201-1207.
18. Mitchell SL, Kiely DK, Miller SC, et al: Hospice care for patients with dementia. *J Pain Symptom Manage.* 2007;34:7-16.
19. Newton JP: Dementia, oral health and the failing dentition. *Gerodontology.* 2007;24:65-66.
20. Pedraza O, Smith GE, Ivnik RJ, et al: Reliable change on the Dementia Rating Scale. *J Int Neuropsychol Soc.* 2007;13:1-5.
21. Solfrizzi V, D'Introno A, Colacicco AM, et al: Alcohol consumption, mild cognitive impairment, and progression to dementia. *Neurology.* 2007;68:1790-1799.
22. Buckwalter JA, Brandser EA: Stress and insufficiency fractures. *Am Fam Physician.* 1997;56:175-182.
23. Richards B, Riego de Dios R: Radius, distal fractures. Available at: http://www.emedicine.com/radio/topic822.htm, 2004.
24. Dutton M: Geriatric Physical Therapy. In: Dutton M, ed, *Physical Therapist Assistant Exam Review Guide & JB Test Prep: PTA Exam Review.* Sudbury, MA: Jones & Bartlett Learning. 2011: 407-427.
25. Afifi M: Clinical spectrum of Parkinson's disease. *Singapore Med J.* 2007;48:484-485; author reply, 486.
26. Playfer JR: Ageing and Parkinson's disease. *Pract Neurol.* 2007; 7:4-5.

27. Clarke CE, Moore AP: Parkinson's disease. *Am Fam Physician.* 2007;75:1045-1048.
28. Konczak J, Krawczewski K, Tuite P, et al: The perception of passive motion in Parkinson's disease. *J Neurol.* 2007;254:655-663.
29. Bertucci Filho D, Teive HA, Werneck LC: Early-onset Parkinson's disease and depression. *Arq Neuropsiquiatr.* 2007;65:5-10.
30. Schrag A, Dodel R, Spottke A, et al: Rate of clinical progression in Parkinson's disease. A prospective study. *Mov Disord.* 2007; 22:938–945.
31. Hermanowicz N: Drug therapy for Parkinson's disease. *Semin Neurol.* 2007;27:97-105.
32. Idiaquez J, Benarroch EE, Rosales H, et al: Autonomic and cognitive dysfunction in Parkinson's disease. *Clin Auton Res.* 2007; 17:93-98.
33. Ross OA, Farrer MJ, Wu RM: Common variants in Parkinson's disease. *Mov Disord.* 2007;22:899-900.
34. Vaugoyeau M, Viel S, Assaiante C, et al: Impaired vertical postural control and proprioceptive integration deficits in Parkinson's disease. *Neuroscience.* 2007;146:852-863.
35. Haehner A, Hummel T, Hummel C, et al: Olfactory loss may be a first sign of idiopathic Parkinson's disease. *Mov Disord.* 2007;22: 839-842.
36. Ziemssen T, Reichmann H: Non-motor dysfunction in Parkinson's disease. *Parkinsonism Relat Disord.* 2007;13:323-332.
37. Whitton PS: Inflammation as a causative factor in the aetiology of Parkinson's disease. *Br J Pharmacol.* 2007;150:963-976.
38. Hoehn MM, Yahr MD: Parkinsonism: onset, progression and mortality. *Neurology.* 1967;17:427-442.
39. Avdic S, Mujcinovic Z, Asceric M, et al: Left ventricular diastolic dysfunction in essential hypertension. *Bosn J Basic Med Sci.* 2007;7:15-20.
40. Binder A: A review of the genetics of essential hypertension. *Curr Opin Cardiol.* 2007;22:176-184.
41. Cuspidi C, Meani S, Valerio C, et al: Age and target organ damage in essential hypertension: role of the metabolic syndrome. *Am J Hypertens.* 2007;20:296-303.
42. El-Shafei SA, Bassili A, Hassanien NM, et al: Genetic determinants of essential hypertension. *J Egypt Public Health Assoc.* 2002;77:231-246.
43. Hollenberg NK, Williams GH: Nonmodulation and essential hypertension. *Curr Hypertens Rep.* 2006;8:127-131.
44. Kennedy S: Essential hypertension 2: treatment and monitoring update. *Community Pract.* 2006;79:64-66.
45. Kennedy S: Essential hypertension: recent changes in management. *Community Pract.* 2006;79:23-24.
46. Krzych LJ: Blood pressure variability in children with essential hypertension. *J Hum Hypertens.* 2007;21:494-500.
47. Parrilli G, Manguso F, Orsini L, et al: Essential hypertension and chronic viral hepatitis. *Dig Liver Dis.* 2007;39:466-472.
48. Pierdomenico SD: Blood pressure variability and cardiovascular outcome in essential hypertension. *Am J Hypertens.* 2007;20:162-163.
49. Fuller GF: Falls in the elderly. *Am Fam Physician.* 2000;61: 2159-2168, 2173-2174.
50. Rubenstein LZ: Falls. In: Yoshikawa TT, Cobbs EL, Brummel-Smith K, eds. *Ambulatory Geriatric Care.* St. Louis, MO. 1993:296-304.

51. Sloan JP: Mobility failure. In: Sloan JP, ed. *Protocols in Primary Care Geriatrics.* New York, NY: Springer. 1997:33-38.
52. Baxter J: Screening and treating those at risk of nutritional deficiency. *Community Nurse.* 2000;6:S1-S2, S5.
53. Callen BL, Wells TJ: Screening for nutritional risk in community-dwelling old-old. *Public Health Nurs.* 2005;22:138-146.
54. Corish CA, Flood P, Kennedy NP: Comparison of nutritional risk screening tools in patients on admission to hospital. *J Hum Nutr Diet.* 2004;17:133-139; quiz 141-143.
55. Hedberg AM, Garcia N, Trejus IJ, et al: Nutritional risk screening: development of a standardized protocol using dietetic technicians. *J Am Diet Assoc.* 1988;88:1553-1556.
56. Melnik TA, Helferd SJ, Firmery LA, et al: Screening elderly in the community: the relationship between dietary adequacy and nutritional risk. *J Am Diet Assoc.* 1994;94:1425-1427.
57. Reilly HM: Screening for nutritional risk. *Proc Nutr Soc.* 1996;55: 841-853.

Prosthetics, Orthotics, and Assistive Devices

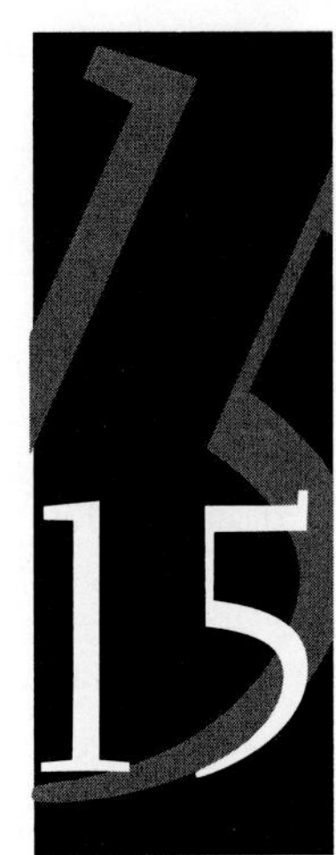

Orthotic, adaptive, protective, and assistive devices are implements and equipment used to support or protect weak or ineffective joints or muscles, and serve to enhance performance.[1] The uses of appropriate orthotic, protective, and supportive devices are outlined in this chapter.

AMPUTATION

The major rationales for amputation include disease (diabetes, peripheral vascular disease [PVD]), infection (post joint replacement, osteomyelitis), tumor, trauma, and fractures that fail to heal (non-union).

Major improvements in noninvasive diagnosis, revascularization, and wound healing techniques have lowered the overall incidence of amputations for vascular disease.[2]

Study Pearl

- Amputation refers to the cutting of a limb along the long axis of the bone.
- Disarticulation refers to cutting of a limb through the joint.

Levels of Amputation[3]

Traumatic amputations may be performed at any level (Table 15-1). Whatever the level the surgeon attempts to maintain the maximum bone length and to keep as many joints intact as possible.[2] The specific type of surgery depends on the status of the extremity at the time of amputation. Conservation of the residual limb and uncomplicated wound healing are both important.

Postoperative Period

Numerous factors influence the expected outcomes for each patient[2]:

- The individual's psychological status. One of the greatest difficulties for a person undergoing amputation surgery is overcoming the psychological stigma that society associates with loss of a limb.

TABLE 15-1. LEVELS OF AMPUTATION

LEVEL OF AMPUTATION	DESCRIPTION
Partial toe	Excision of any part of one or more toes
Toe disarticulation	Disarticulation of one or more toes at the metatarsophalangeal joint
Partial foot/ray resection	Resection of the third, fourth, fifth metatarsals and digits
Tarsometatarsal (LisFranc) disarticulation	The disarticulation of all five metatarsals and the digits
Transmetatarsal (Chopart)	Amputation through the midsection of all metatarsals leaving only the calcaneus and talus
Syme's	Ankle disarticulation which may include removal of the malleoli and distal tibial/fibular flares to create a smooth bony distal end with the attachment of the heel pad to the distal end of the tibia.
Long transtibial (below knee)	More than 50% of tibial length
Transtibial (below knee)	Between 20% and 50% of tibial length
Short transtibial (below knee)	Less than 20% of tibial length
Knee disarticulation	Amputation through the knee joint with shaping of the distal femur, squaring the condyles for an even weight-bearing surface. The knee disarticulation is most often used in children and young adults, but is nearly always avoided in the elderly and patients with ischemic disease. Several advantages of the knee disarticulation include: ▶ A large distal end covered by skin and soft tissues that is naturally suited for weight bearing ▶ A long lever arm controlled by strong muscles ▶ Increased stability of the patient's prosthesis A main disadvantage of the knee disarticulation is cosmetic—the patient's prosthetic leg will have a knee that extends far beyond his own knee in the sitting position.
Long transfemoral (above knee)	More than 60% of the femoral length
Transfemoral (above knee)	Between 35% and 60% of the femoral length
Short transfemoral (above knee)	Less than 35% of the femoral length
Hip disarticulation	An amputation through the hip joint capsule that removes the entire lower extremity, with closure of the remaining musculature over the exposed acetabulum. Hip disarticulation is generally performed as a result of failed vascular procedures following multiple lower-level amputations, or for massive trauma with crush injuries to the lower extremity.
Hemipelvectomy (HP)	Generally, the leg, hip joint and half of the pelvis are removed, and the remaining gluteal muscles are brought around and attached to the oblique abdominal muscles. The most common reason for HP is a rare form of connective tissue cancer known as sarcoma. There are various types of sarcomas such as fibrosarcoma, osteosarcoma and chondrosarcoma.
Hemicorporectomy	Involves removal of the bony pelvis below the L4-5 level, both lower limbs, the external genitalia, the bladder, rectum and anus. Necessary life functions are maintained in the upper torso. Hemicorporectomy has been performed for a variety of indications including locally invasive pelvic cancer without metastatic spread, benign spinal tumours, intractable decubitus ulcers with malignant change, paraplegia in association with intractable pelvic osteomyelitis and decubitus ulceration, and crushing trauma to the pelvis. Given the high mortality following this procedure, especially when performed for visceral malignancy, the indications for its use are very restrictive.

- ▶ The physical characteristics of the residual limb:
  - The longer the residual limb, the better potential for successful prosthetic ambulation regardless of level of amputation. One of the primary purposes of the postsurgical period is to determine an individual's suitability for prosthetic replacement. Not all people with amputations are candidates for a prosthesis, regardless of personal desire.[2]
  - A well-healed, well-shaped limb with a nonadherent scar is easier to fit than one that is poorly shaped or has redundant tissue distally or laterally.

- The vascular status of the remaining extremity.
- The physiological (not chronological) age of the patient.
- The presence of comorbidities: diabetes, cardiovascular disease, renal disease, visual impairment, limitation of joint motion, and muscle weakness can all be detrimental to the rehabilitation process.

Postoperative Dressings. The major types of postoperative dressings can be classified as soft dressings, rigid dressings, and semirigid dressings.

Soft Dressings

Elastic Wrap. During the immediate postoperative stage, an elastic compression bandage with a sterile dressing is used to provide edema control, soft tissue support, and protection of the surgical site. Following the immediate postoperative stage and removal of all surgical clips and sutures, the bandage and dressing are generally removed and reapplied a minimum of three times per day. The wrapping is applied in either a diagonal or angular pattern (not circular) and pressure is applied distally to enhance shaping. Once the wrapping is completed, there should be no signs of wrinkles in the wrapping. The elastic compression bandage is normally kept in place at all times except for reapplication, and during bathing. At the earliest opportunity, the patient is taught how to independently apply a compression wrapping or in the use of an elastic shrinker (described later). The following guidelines should be used:

- A 3 to 4 in wrap is used for transtibial amputations, while ensuring that the anchor wrap is applied above the knee.
- A 6 in wrap is useful transfemoral amputations, while ensuring the anchor wrap is applied around the pelvis.
- Following transfemoral amputations, it is important to promote full hip extension.

Rigid Dressings. A rigid dressing is sometimes used during the immediate postoperative stage in place of an elastic compression bandage with the same goals in mind.

- A rigid dressing allows early ambulation with a pylon, and earlier fitting of the permanent prosthesis, promotes circulation and healing, and stimulates proprioception.
- The disadvantages are that this dressing does not permit daily dressing changes or wound inspections as it is not removable. However, removable rigid dressings (RRD) are adjustable and may be removed as needed for wound inspection and care.

The rigid cast dressing is typically not changed until the sutures or surgical clips are to be removed.

Semirigid Dressings. The classic semirigid dressing has been the Unna paste bandage impregnated with a number of chemicals that dry to form a semirigid cast. This dressing type is typically changed once or twice weekly, depending on the amount of drainage and edema. The semirigid cast is normally only prescribed in the initial phases to help control severe edema while providing protection and soft tissue support.

Study Pearl

Individuals not fitted with a rigid dressing use elastic wrap or shrinkers to help reduce the size of the residual limb.

Elastic Shrinker. The use of an elastic shrinker, or prosthetic compression sock, is generally used once the incision line is adequately healed, and there are no areas of open drainage. Shrinkers serve to provide a degree of patient independence with those individuals who are not able to properly wrap the residual limb. Shrinkers are normally worn at all times except during bathing or use of a prosthesis for approximately the first 3 months post-amputation to maximize soft tissue edema control.

Postoperative Physical Therapy

Goals

- Relieve postoperative stump pain while promoting healing of the residual limb
- Maintain or improve strength and range of motion (ROM) of the involved limb and the uninvolved limbs
- Prevent contractures and enhance stump hygiene
- Training in the various activities of daily living (ADL)
- Preparation of the residual stump for prosthetic fitting

Examination

- Past medical history and systems review
- History of current condition
- Social history/support structure
  - Medications
  - Living environment
- Residual limb and skin assessment
  - Level of healing (scar, grafts, presence of staples, or sutures).
  - Color
  - Shape (cylindrical, conical, bulbous end, etc)
  - Pulses
  - Edema
  - Moisture
  - Temperature
  - Girth and length
  - Sensation
- Pain
  - Phantom sensation
  - Phantom pain
  - Neuroma
- ROM
- Strength and endurance
- Functional status
  - Balance
  - Bed mobility and transfer skills
  - Bathing, dressing
  - Emotional status

Postoperative Intervention

Desensitization. Post-surgical desenitization of the residual stump is routinely performed to increase the tolerance of the stump to touch and pressure. A progression of contact with soft materials such as cotton or lamb's wool, and then burlap type materials is typically used. Other techniques that assist in preparing the limb for prosthetic fitting include rubbing, tapping, and performing resistive exercises with the stump.

ROM Exercises. The goal of stretching and ROM exercises is to help prevent contractures, which can develop as a result of muscle imbalance or fascial tightness, or as a result of faulty positioning such as prolonged sitting or placing the residual limb on a pillow.[2]

Positioning. Positioning techniques are performed to help prevent contractures based on the level of the amputation:

- Above-knee patient: positions are adopted that help prevent hip flexion, abduction, and external rotation contractures. The patient is advised to avoid prolonged sitting to help prevent hip flexor contractures.
- Below-knee patient: positions are used to help prevent against those contractures associated with an above knee amputation, as well as positions to help prevent knee flexion contractures.

It is important to emphasize bed and WC positioning, proper stump wrapping, early ambulation, prone lying, and supine lying with the pelvis level and the hip maintained in extension and neutral rotation.

In those individuals who present with hip or knee flexion contractures, facilitated stretching techniques (proprioceptive neuromuscular facilitation [PNF]) are more effective than passive stretching; hold-relax and hold-relax active contraction that utilizes resistive contraction of antagonist muscles may increase ROM, particularly of the knee.[2]

Strength Training. Selected and specific strengthening exercises are prescribed to increase the strength of the residual musculature, particularly the hip extensors and abductors, and the knee extensors and flexors all of which are important for prosthetic ambulation. Strengthening exercises are initiated with isometrics, progressing to concentrics with cuff weights and simple adaptations to traditional weight machines. Again, the exercise focus is based on the level of amputation:

- Above-knee patient: emphasis is placed on hip extension, abduction, adduction, pelvic tilt exercises
- Below-knee patient: hip extension, abduction, knee extension, and knee flexion exercises are emphasized

Function. For reimbursement purposes, patients with unilateral transfemoral transtibial amputations are categorized according to the following functional levels:[4]

- Level 0: patient does not have ability or potential to transfer safely with or without assistance and a prosthesis does not enhance quality of life or mobility. This patient is not a prosthetic candidate, no prosthesis is allowed, and no components can be used.
- Level 1: the patient has the ability or potential to use a prosthesis for either transfer or ambulation on a level surface using a fixed cadence. This level describes a limited or unlimited household ambulator.
- Level 2: the patient has the ability or potential for ambulation and also has the ability to traverse lower-level environmental barriers such as curbs, stairs, or uneven surfaces. This level describes the typical limited community ambulator.

- Level 3: the patient has the ability or potential for ambulation using a variable cadence. This level describes the typical community ambulator who has the ability to traverse most environmental barriers and may require vocational, therapeutic, or exercise activities that demands prosthetic utilization beyond simple locomotion.
- Level 4: the patient has the ability or potential for prosthetic utilization that exceeds basic ambulation skills and exhibits high impact, stress, or energy levels. This level is typical of the prosthetic demands of a child, active adult, or athlete.

Ambulation and Gait Training. Early fitting with a temporary prosthesis (as soon as the wound is healed) can greatly enhance the postsurgical rehabilitation program.[2] However, individuals are not fitted with any type of prosthetic appliance until the residual limb is edema-free and much of the soft tissue has adequately shrunk, a process that can take many months of conscientious limb wrapping and exercises.[2]

An understanding of the biomechanics of gait is necessary so that most problems can be discerned by means of observation (refer to "Gait Examination and Training" later). The components of the normal gait cycle are described in Chapter 7. Patients who have undergone amputations incorporate different muscles and adaptive strategies to ensure a smooth and well-coordinated gait pattern. As a result, the gait becomes less efficient and occurs at a higher metabolic cost compared to that of healthy intact persons, who require less endurance for any given distance (Table 15-2).

Patient Education. Patient education is a critical component of the postsurgical rehabilitation program. In addition to discussing the disease process, the physiological effects of the symptoms, the benefits of exercise, and lifestyle changes to reduce risk factors, the following areas should be addressed:

- Methods of edema control.
- Hygiene and skincare: the residual limb must be kept clean and dry, and care must be taken to avoid abrasions, cuts, and other skin problems.
- Limb inspection: the residual limb must be inspected with a mirror each night to make sure there are no areas of skin breakdown, especially in those areas not readily visible, and in those patients with diminished sensation.

TABLE 15-2. ENERGY EXPENDITURE FOR AMPUTATION

AMPUTATION LEVEL	ENERGY ABOVE BASELINE, %	SPEED, m/min	OXYGEN COST, mL/kg/m
Long transtibial	10	70	0.17
Average transtibial	25	60	0.20
Short transtibial	40	50	0.20
Bilateral transtibial	41	50	0.20
Transfemoral	65	40	0.28
Wheelchair	0-8	70	0.16

Data from Wu YJ, Chen SY, Lin MC, et al: Energy expenditure of wheeling and walking during prosthetic rehabilitation in a woman with bilateral transfemoral amputations. *Arch Phys Med Rehabil.* 2001;82:265-269. Traugh GH, Corcoran PJ, Reyes RL: Energy expenditure of ambulation in patients with above-knee amputations. *Arch Phys Med Rehabil.* 1975;56:67-71.

LOWER LIMB PROSTHETIC DESIGNS

A prosthesis is a man-made device designed as a replacement for a body part. Technological advances have produced a series of comfortable and responsive prosthetic devices.

PARTIAL FOOT AMPUTATIONS

Prosthetic devices for partial foot amputations include:

- Custom molded insole with a plastic insert for the transverse arch of the foot and a heel counter for rear foot stability combined with a simple foam toe filler.
- Rigid plate: used to prevent the potential equinus deformity that can occur in the absence of the foot and the subsequent adaptive shortening of the gastrocnemius and soleus muscles.
- Slipper-type elastomer prosthesis: this is a more cosmetic approach, and involves modeling of semiflexible urethane elastomers to provide a foot-shaped prosthesis with a soft socket that conforms to the residual foot.
- Syme ankle: two major types exist.
  - Veterans Administration Prosthetic Center Syme prosthesis: consists of a media window or cutout in the distal end of the socket to provide an opening for ease of donning of the bulbous end created by the anatomical heel pad.
  - Miami Syme prosthesis: an inelastic inner liner that has an expandable wall to permit the bulbous distal end of the stump to pass down and sit snugly within the socket.

TRANSPHALANGEAL (TOE DISARTICULATION)

A simple toe filler can be placed in the shoe if one to three toes are involved, not including the first ray. In cases when the great toe is involved, a steel shank spring may be used in the sole of the shoe in addition to the toe filler (if needed), to assist in terminal stance.

TRANSTIBIAL (BELOW THE KNEE)

The lower leg is comprised of four muscle compartments: the anterior, lateral, deep posterior, and superficial posterior. The choice of which muscle compartment to use for a prosthesis is based on the amount of padding each can afford. The superficial posterior compartment—the gastrocnemius and soleus—is the most commonly used.

> **Study Pearl**
>
> The goal of any amputation is to retain as much of the useful residual nerve function as possible, while simultaneously minimizing nerve scarring and painful neuromas.

TRANSFEMORAL (ABOVE THE KNEE)

The higher the level of lower limb amputation, the greater the energy expenditure required for walking.[5,6] For example, an individual with a transfemoral amputation, requires 50% to 65% more energy for ambulation (Table 15-2). Complications associated with transfemoral amputation include:

- Balance and stability problems.
- The need for a more complicated prosthetic device.
- Difficulty rising from a seated position.
- Prosthetic comfort while sitting.

HIP DISARTICULATION

Function following a hip disarticulation with a modern prosthesis is considered acceptable—patients are ambulatory at approximately 6 months with the use of one cane.

HEMIPELVECTOMY

The energy requirements for gait following a hemipelvectomy have been reported to be as much as 200% of normal ambulation. In addition, this patient type presents a particularly challenging array of clinical issues including deconditioning, pain management, altered gait mechanics, altered sexual functioning, and edema/lymphedema management.

HEMICORPORECTOMY

Serious consideration is given before performing this procedure as the postsurgical rehabilitation is long and arduous. In addition to the physical rehabilitation, most patients require vocational training, psychological counseling, sex hormone replacement, education, and dietary advice to avoid obesity.

PROSTHETIC COMPONENTS

The following sections generically describe the components and socket designs (Table 15-3).

TABLE 15-3. IMPLICATIONS OF VARIOUS KNEE, FOOT AND ANKLE DESIGNS

COMPONENT	CHARACTERISTIC	OUTCOME
Knee joint (above-knee prosthesis)	TKA line position	The more posterior the joint to the TKA line, the more knee extension is maintained. This creates a more stable leg during stance, but is harder to initiate knee flexion for the swing phase.
	Internal rotation position	Too much internal rotation creates a lateral heel whip on heel raise.
	External rotation position	Too much external rotation creates a medial heel with heel raise.
	Friction	Less friction makes it easier to bend the knee at heel raise, but permits more terminal swing impact at heel strike,
Heel	Too soft	Forces knee into extension at heel strike (can be advantageous with an above-knee socket as it speeds knee extension up),
		Causes premature foot slap at heel strike,
	Too hard	Forces knee into flexion at heel strike (can be advantageous with below knee socket with patellar-bearing prosthesis)
Toe break	Too posterior	Creates early knee flexion in midstance.
	Too anterior	Creates delayed knee flexion in midstance.
Ankle moment	Dorsiflexed	Encourages excessive knee flexion in early stance as amputee attempts to achieve foot flat.
	Plantarflexed	Encourages excessive knee extension throughout stance.
		Creates a "hill climbing" sensation of premature heel rise at the end of stance.
	Inverted or everted	Does not affect the knee. Prosthetic foot is matched to uninvolved foot.
Foot placement	Anterior	Creates a moment which increases knee extension.
	Posterior	Creates a moment which increases knee flexion.
	Lateral	Creates a valgus moment at the knee.
	Medial	Creates a varus moment at the knee.

Shanks. Refers to the area between the knee and the foot. There are two basic structural designs:

- Exoskeletal design: the exterior of the structure provides the required support for the weight of the body. Thermosetting plastic and wood are the common materials used for fabrication.
- Endoskeletal: an internal skeleton or pylon (a narrow vertical support that connects the socket to the foot–ankle assembly) supports the load with an outer covering usually made of foam to give the shank a cosmetic shape.

Foot Socket Designs

Articulated Foot–Ankle Assemblies

Single Axis Foot. The single axis foot allows dorsiflexion (5-7 degrees) and plantarflexion (15 degrees), which are controlled by rubber bumpers or spring systems. No medial/lateral or rotary motion is permitted, which makes this design suitable for only flat and even surfaces.

Multiple Axis Foot. This type of foot allows lateral and rotary movements and is therefore more suitable for uneven terrain. However, due to the complexity of design, some of these can be bulky and require frequent maintenance and adjustments.

Endolite Multiflex Ankle. This design allows inversion, eversion, and some rotation, in addition to plantar and dorsiflexion, which makes it suitable for a wide variety of terrains.

Tru-Step Foot. A three-point weight transfer system and shock absorbing heel, which permits eight motions: plantar flexion, dorsiflexion, inversion, eversion, abduction, adduction, supination, and pronation. In addition, the three interchangeable bumpers within the system can be adjusted to provide the correct resistance for a smooth gait.

Total Concept Foot. A dynamic response system with a single carbon fiber deflector plate, and a single axis ankle that has adjustable bumpers to control plantar and dorsiflexion. The design incorporates an innovative heel height adjustment of the ankle of up to 10 degrees of dorsiflexion for ascending, or 25 degrees of plantarflexion for descending ramps or hills.

Non-Articulated Foot–Ankle Assemblies

Solid-Ankle-Cushioned-Heel (SACH) Foot/Durometer. The most commonly prescribed prosthetic foot worldwide as there are no moving parts, and thus no maintenance and no noise. The molded heel cushion, which is made of a high-density foam rubber, forms the foot and ankle into one component. At initial contact, the rubber heel wedge compresses to stimulate plantarflexion. The limitations include limited adjustment of plantar/dorsiflexion, difficulty walking up inclines due to compression of the heel, and limited motion for active people.

Stationary Attachment Flexible Endoskeletal II (SAFE II) Foot. Designed to mimic the subtalar joint by incorporating two fiber bands: the long plantar ligament band provides stability, while the plantar fascia band is designed to tighten, providing a semirigid lever for a smooth transition at terminal stance.

Seattle Foot. This foot is designed for the more active individual due to its ability to "store energy" during midstance to terminal stance and transfer that energy during the propulsive phase of terminal stance.

Carbon Copy II. The Carbon Copy II is a solid ankle design with a heel made of a polyurethane foam cushion, which provides a two-stage resistance at terminal stance depending on whether the user is walking or running.

Flex Foot. This design uses the entire distance from the socket to "store energy" within an anterior deflector plate, giving it the greatest energy return of the dynamic response feet, and making it popular with athletes.

Knee Socket Designs. There are two general classifications of sockets: the hard socket, which uses a direct contact between the socket's inner surface and stump, and the soft socket, which incorporates the use of a liner as a cushion between the socket and stump, and in some cases provides suspension.

Patella Tendon Bearing Sockets. This type of socket incorporates a total contact design by creating a totally closed system around the skin at the distal end, thereby offering a more intimate fit, and avoiding skin lesion problems that can occur when the soft tissues are not completely supported.

- The anterior wall is designed to be high enough to encompass the distal half the patella.
- The posterior wall rises slightly higher than the knee joint line thereby providing an anterior force to maintain the patella on the patella bar (a small bulge in the socket) as well as preventing excessive pressure on the hamstrings through the use of a contoured socket.
- The medial and lateral walls are slightly higher than the anterior wall, which adds stability.

There are two main variations:

- PTB-supracondylar: this design has higher medial and lateral walls to encompass both femoral condyles and thereby increase medial and lateral stability of the knee.
- PTB-supracondylar/suprapatellar: this design also has higher medial and lateral walls to encompass both femoral condyles, but also raises the anterior wall to cover all of the patella, with the suprapatellar area of the socket being contoured inward to create a "quadricep bar," which results in additional suspension and resistance to recurvatum.

Transtibial Amputee Suction Socket Designs. This design utilizes a suction suspension system, which creates a vacuum between a flexible roll on the sleeve and the skin, between the sleeve and the socket, or both, in order to hold the socket on the stump. The socket is connected to the sleeve by a pin and lock system, or a one-way valve system.

- Pin and lock system: When the sleeve-covered limb is placed completely into the socket, a locking mechanism at the distal socket receives the pin, locking the sleeve securely to the socket. A release pin located on the exterior of the socket, or the sleeve can be removed.
- Valve system: This design uses a one-way valve system to permit the expulsion of air out of the socket as the limb is inserted, while preventing air from returning back into the socket. To seal the top of the socket, an external suspension sleeve that covers the socket is rolled over the thigh.

The various benefits of the suction systems include:

- Secure suspension
- Reduced pistoning
- Reduced friction
- Reduced perspiration
- Elimination of straps, cups, or sleeves

Transtibial Amputee Suspension Systems. In many cases, more than one suspension system is necessary. For example, one is needed for suspending the socket, while a secondary system is needed to provide an added sense of security. Common suspension methods include the supracondylar cuff, thigh corset or thigh lacer, inverted Y-strap and waist belt, neoprene sleeve or latex sleeve, medial wedge, lateral wedge, suction, and removable medial brim.

Transfemoral Amputee Socket Designs

Quadrilateral Socket. This design is characterized by a series of reliefs or depressions in the socket, which reduce pressure on relatively firm tissue, tendons, muscles, and bulges. The advantages of such a socket include:

- Muscular contractions are permitted, which reduces atrophy.
- Total contact between the socket and stump is present with a wider medial-lateral than anterior–posterior dimension.
- Ability to customize different sizes and shapes caused by soft tissue and bony prominences.
- The anterior wall is 2.5 in higher than the medial wall with a prominent Scarpa's bulge, maintaining the ischial tuberosity on the ischial seat by providing counter pressure against the posterior wall.
- The socket does not press on the pubic ramus because the medial brim is the same height as the posterior brim.

Ischial Containment Socket. This socket is characterized by:

- The inclusion of the ischial tuberosity within the socket via a high posterior wall.
- Greater adduction of the femur, placing the muscles in an optimal length-tension position.
- A narrow medial-lateral dimension within the socket, which allows the pelvis and the socket to act together for greater prosthetic control.

- The pocketing of the gluteus maximus within a gluteal channel, which applies a stretch to the hamstrings.
- A lateral wall that rises superiorly over the greater trochanter during femoral adduction (10-15 degrees), which is maintained via a force applied to the greater trochanter and the length of the shaft of the femur, with a counterforce applied at the ischial ramus.

Transfemoral Amputee Suspension Systems. One significant difference between the transtibial sockets and the transfemoral systems, is that the transfemoral system allows for partial suction, where stump socks are used but there is still a close fit, but where a secondary suspension system such as a Silesian bandage or pelvic belt must be incorporated into the design.

Prosthetic Knee Units

Knee Axis. There are two classifications of knee axes:

- Single: these work like a hinge joint to maintain a single stationary axis point that allows either end to move around—the most common type of axis used.
- Polycentric: this describes any knee unit with more than one axis and is traditionally referred to as the four-bar linkage system. The advantages of this system include:
  - An instantaneous center of rotation (ICR) is created as the shank moves about the knee axis.
  - During sitting, the shank moves under the distal end of the socket, preventing the prosthetic knee from protruding too far in front of the contralateral anatomic knee.
  - During ambulation, as the shank moves posteriorly with respect to the knee's center, greater toe clearance is permitted during the swing phase.

Swing Phase Control Mechanisms. Three general classifications of swing phase control mechanisms are available:

- Mechanical constant friction: with this design, the swing resistance is generated by a friction system that creates a drag on the prosthetic shank, or controls the speed of walking. However, these units do not have the ability to vary the speed of cadence. The advantages of this system include:
  - It is the simplest of the knee units and is therefore relatively low in cost.
  - The units are typically lightweight and durable with few mechanical parts.
- Pneumatic or air-controlled: this design uses air-filled cylinders that provide a cadence response using the spring action of a compressible medium, air.
  - When the knee is flexed, the piston rod compresses the air, storing energy.
  - As the knee moves into extension during late swing, the energy is returned, assisting with extension.
  - An adjustment screw controls resistance.

The key advantage to this system is its cadence-responsive function.

- Hydraulic or fluid controlled: this design incorporates liquid filled cylinders that provide a cadence response using an essentially incompressible medium; oil.
  - When the knee flexes, a piston rod is pushed into an oil-filled cylinder, forcing the oil through one or more chambers, thus regulating the speed of movement.
  - The degree of resistance can be controlled by an adjustment screw, which varies the cross-sectional area of the chamber(s):
    - A greater cross-sectional area, which lowers the resistance, is desired if the patient has a slow weak gait.
    - A smaller cross-sectional area, which increases the resistance, is desired with a faster walking speed.

Study Pearl

The major advantages of hydraulic systems are their cadence-responsive functions and the ability to withstand greater forces than the pneumatic units. The disadvantages include cost, weight, mechanical failure, and maintenance.

Extension Bias Assists. This design of unit helps advance the limb or extend the knee during the swing phase. Two basic types are available:

- Internal: a spring provides assistance with extension once knee flexion is completed during the gait cycle. If the knee flexion is greater than 60 degrees, the knee will remain flexed as in sitting.
- External: an adjustable/nonadjustable elastic strap is attached to the socket anteriorly, descending to the anterior shank.
  - As the knee is flexed, the strap is stretched.
  - Once an extension force is initiated, the strap shortens.

Stance Phase Control Mechanisms. Stance control can be customized individually through the following five major mechanisms:

Alignment. Most knee units require that the trochanter-knee-ankle (TKA) line pass anterior to the knee axis creating an extension moment, and thus enhancing knee stability.

Locks. These are designed to prevent knee motion once engaged. Locks are available with one of two basic lock systems:

- Manually operated involving a small lever or ring and a cable system that is accessible to the patient to connect or unlock as needed.
- Spring-loaded: locks automatically when the knee is extended.

Weight-Activated Fiction Knee. This unit functions as a constant friction knee during the swing phase, whereas during the stance phase, a component with a high coefficient of friction (adjustable to the user's body weight) prevents too much knee flexion.

Hydraulic Swing-N-Stance Control Units. Increased resistance is employed from the cylinder as weight is applied when the knee is in full extension, and up to 25 degrees of flexion. The cylinder controls the rate of fluid flow, preventing the knee from buckling and allowing the user to regain balance.

Polycentric Axis Knee Unit. This design, as its name suggests, has many centers of rotation for the knee component, which provides a greater zone of stability in the stance phase.

HIP JOINTS

Hip Flexion Bias System. During midstance, a coil spring is compressed and then released during terminal stance, which thrusts the prosthetic thigh anteriorly, thereby eliminating excessive pelvic rocking.

Littig Hip Strut. This design involves an adjustable carbon composite strut that connects to the socket and knee unit, so that during the stance phase, the strut bends. Conversely, as the patient moves into the swing phase, the strut recoils, thrusting the prosthetic limb forward, minimizing the need for excessive pelvic motion.

LOWER LIMB PROSTHETIC TRAINING

The anticipated goals and expected outcomes for lower limb prosthetic training are based on the following goals:[2]

- Minimize postoperative edema while promoting healing of the residual limb.
- Minimize joint contractures, physical deconditioning, and integumentary breakdown by monitoring skin and any pressure points, especially for the beginner and those with poor circulation.[7]
- Maintain or regain strength of the involved extremity.
- Maintain or increase strength in the uninvolved extremities.
- Patient independence with a home exercise program, and proper care of the remaining extremity.
- Patient independence with ambulation using the prosthesis (including ambulation on difficult terrain), applying and removing the prosthesis, care for the prosthesis, and transfers (using the commode, etc.).

PROPRIOCEPTIVE TRAINING

This includes balance and mobility training using a variety of equipment. Parallel bars provide bilateral support, whereas a sturdy table offers unilateral support (usually on the uninvolved side). The patient must learn to balance on the involved side. A typical sequence is outlined below:

- Orientation to the center the gravity (COG) and base of support (BOS) using: proprioceptive and visual feedback. The patient must learn to shift the COG anteriorly, posteriorly, medially, and laterally. The patient is taught how to detect the available sensation within the stump/socket interface and to visualize the prosthetic foot and its relationship to the ground.
- Practices in single limb standing over the prosthetic limb while advancing the sound limb.
- Stool or block stepping in the parallel bars with the uninvolved limb in front of a 4- to 8-in stool or block (depending on level of ability). The patient is asked to slowly step onto the stool with the uninvolved limb while using the parallel bars to provide bilateral upper extremity support.

- Exercises to improve stump control to maintain balance over the prosthesis.

Gait training occurs on flat even surfaces, initially within the parallel bars, then with an assisted device, and finally independently as appropriate. Once gait is mastered on a flat surface, additional challenges are added, based on the patient's needs. These can include:

- Gait training on stairs, curbs, uneven surfaces, ramps and hills
- Falling and lowering oneself to the ground
- Floor to standing transfers
- Running skills

GAIT EXAMINATION AND TRAINING

Patients often adapt a unique way of ambulating with a prosthesis, which results in challenges in the diagnosis of any gait deviations.[8] The common gait deviations of prosthetic gait are briefly addressed. Refer also to Tables 15-4 and 15-5.

Abnormal Transtibial Gait. Stance-phase problems can occur in the gait of patients with a transtibial prosthesis. Inappropriate knee flexion can occur in the early stance phase, causing knee instability from excessive ankle dorsiflexion, socket flexion, and posterior foot placement. Knee hyperextension can also occur in the early stance phase, emanating from ankle plantarflexion or socket extension, weak knee extensors, anterior foot placement, or inadequate prosthetic foot selection.

Mediolateral knee thrust can be observed in the stance phase, which is generally derived from inadequate side-to-side placement of the foot, excessive angulation of the socket, or wide mediolateral proximal socket dimensions that result in reduced knee control. If a post-transtibial patient is noted to have a foot slap in his or her gait, it may be a result of excessive socket flexion or foot dorsiflexion, the uneven placement of the foot, or a deficient heel height for correct prosthetic alignment. Excessive forward progression of the tibia, or a drop-off gait can be caused by impaired rollover, shortening of the contralateral step length and swing time, and delayed heel raise.

External rotation can occur at two different phases of the gait cycle: initial contact or terminal stance. If external rotation occurs during initial contact, the cause could be a SACH heel that is too dense, an articulated foot plantarflexion bumper that is too hard, or incorrect placement of the suspension cuff-retention points. If external rotation appears in terminal stance, it can be caused by excessive anterior placement of the foot, excessive foot plantarflexion, or excessive hardness of the forefoot.

Early heel rise at terminal stance could result from a posterior placement of the foot, flexion contracture at the hip or the knee, or excessive softness of the forefoot. Contralateral early heel rise or vaulting is a pathologic gait that allows clearance of the prosthetic limb with decreased hip and knee flexion. Vaulting compensates for a prosthesis that is too long, inadequate suspension of the prosthesis, or an incorrectly learned gait pattern.

Fewer gait problems are involved with the swing phase than with the stance phase. When prosthetic limb clearance is poor, the gait

TABLE 15-4. GAIT DEVIATIONS ACCORDING TO PROSTHETIC CAUSES AND AMPUTEE CAUSES

DEVIATION	PROSTHETIC CAUSES	AMPUTEE CAUSES
Lateral bending of the trunk	Prosthesis may be too short Improperly shaped lateral wall High medial wall Prosthesis aligned in abduction	Poor balance Abduction contracture Improper training Short residual limb Weak hip abductors on prosthetic side Hypersensitive and painful residual limb
Abducted gait	Prosthesis may be too long High medial wall Improperly shaped lateral wall Prosthesis positioned in too much abduction Inadequate suspension Excessive knee friction	Abduction contracture Improper training Adductor roll Weak hip flexors and adductors Pain over lateral residual limb
Circumducted gait (this is different from above in that the foot returns to the proper position at heel strike)	Prosthesis may be too long Too much friction in the knee Socket is too small Excessive plantar flexion of prosthetic foot	Abduction contracture Improper training Weak hip flexors Lacks confidence to flex the knee Painful anterior distal stump Inability to initiate prosthetic knee flexion
Excessive knee flexion during stance	Socket set forward in relation to foot Foot set in excessive dorsiflexion Stiff heel Prosthesis too long	Knee flexion contracture Hip flexion contracture Pain anteriorly in residual limb Decrease in quadriceps strength Poor balance
Vaulting	Prosthesis may be too long Inadequate socket suspension Excessive alignment stability Foot in excess plantar flexion	Residual limb discomfort Improper training Fear of stubbing toe Short residual limb Painful hip/residual limb
Rotation of forefoot at heel strike (usually external rotation)	Excessive toe-out built-in Loose fitting socket Inadequate suspension Rigid SACH heel cushion	Poor muscle control Improper training Weak medial rotators Short residual limb
Forward trunk flexion	Socket too big Poor suspension Knee instability	Hip flexion contracture Weak hip extensors Pain with ischial weight-bearing Inability to initiate prosthetic knee flexion
Medial or lateral whip	Excessive rotation of the knee Tight socket fit Valgus in the prosthetic knee Improper alignment of toe break	Improper training Weak hip rotators Knee instability
Foot drag (one of the most common problems of swing phase)	Inadequate suspension of the prosthesis A prosthesis that is too long	Weakness in the hip abductors or ankle plantarflexors on the contralateral side
Uneven arm swing (characterized by the arm on the prosthetic side held close to the body during locomotion)	An improperly fitting socket may cause limb discomfort	Inadequate balance Fear and insecurity accompanied by uneven timing

becomes pathologic. Most problems occur because of poor suspension, a prosthesis that is too long, insufficient prosthetic knee flexion, or inadequate transfer of power from the residual limb to the prosthesis, resulting in decreases or delays in knee flexion. A coordinated, smooth, swing phase is facilitated by energy-efficient limb clearance, which is enabled by synchronized motions at the hip and knee joints.

Any abnormal limb rotations observed during gait are usually caused by insufficient suspension of the prosthesis, misplacement of

TABLE 15-5. GAIT ANALYSIS OF THE BELOW-KNEE AMPUTEE.

PROBLEM	CAUSE	SOLUTION
Delayed, abrupt, and limited knee flexion after initial contact	Heel wedge is too soft; the foot is too far anterior	Stiffen the heel wedge; move the foot posterior
Toe stays off floor after initial contact	Heel wedge is too stiff; the foot is too anterior; there is too much dorsiflexion	Soften heel wedge; move the foot posterior; plantarflex the foot
Extended knee throughout stance phase	There is too much plantar flexion	Dorsiflex the foot
"Hillclimbing" sensation toward end of stance phase	The foot is too far anterior; there is too much plantar flexion	Move the foot posterior; dorsiflex the foot
Knee is too forcefully and rapidly flexed after initial contact; high pressure against anterior-distal tibia at initial contact and/or prolonged discomfort at this point	Heel wedge is too stiff; the foot is too dorsiflexed	Soften the heel; move the foot anterior; plantarflex the foot
Hips level, but prosthesis appears short	The foot is too far posterior; the foot is too dorsiflexed	Move the foot anterior; plantarflex the foot
Toe off floor as patient stands or knee flexed too much	The foot is too dorsiflexed	Plantarflex the foot
Uneven heel rise	Knee joint may have insufficient friction; there may be an inadequate extension aid	Modify accordingly
The foot slaps	Plantar flexion resistance is usually too soft	Increase plantar flexion resistance

the suspension cuff-retention points, or overshooting (infringement) of the hip or knee flexors to evade foot drop.

Limited knee extension or flexion problems can always be traced back to mechanical contractures, problems with the suspension, or problems with the knee joint in relation to the thigh corset.

Abnormal Transfemoral Gait. Knee flexion in the stance phase is one of the most common problems related to gait instability with transfemoral amputations. If a patient with a transfemoral amputation is concerned about putting weight on the prosthetic leg because the knee flexion moment creates instability, an inefficient gait pattern results. For these patients, one of several unique models of prosthetic knees can be prescribed based on his or her individual needs.

Additional causes of knee flexion in stance include a hard SACH heel, excessive foot dorsiflexion, excessive socket flexion, weak hip extensors, or decreased weightbearing. Prolonged knee extension in the stance phase is another problem that can occur with transfemoral amputations. This extension can result in shortening of the contralateral step and an increase in the vertical displacement of the COG.

If lateral hip thrust is the problem, immediate attention should be given to the wide dimensions of the mediolateral proximal socket that affect the stability of the hip. If the socket fits well, the patient could have weak hip abductors, or the hip adductors might not have been reattached at the time of surgery.

The most prevalent gait abnormality with transfemoral amputations is ipsilateral trunk bending during the stance phase. Similar to the compensation for Trendelenburg gait, this abnormality could indicate weak hip abductors on the ipsilateral side or an inappropriately short prosthesis. Occasionally, a person who has undergone a transfemoral amputation can have an awkward downward movement of the upper body over the prosthesis, especially during fast walking. This is referred to as a drop-off gait in terminal stance. The foot of the prosthesis should be checked for excessive dorsiflexion whenever external rotation of the leg occurs, either during heel strike or in the late stance.

In people who have undergone transfemoral amputations, gait abnormalities in the swing phase are limited in number. Stiff-knee gait patterns can be the consequence of excessive knee stability in the joint that makes the creation of a flexion moment at the knee difficult. Circumduction, or the swing of the limb in a wide arc, usually indicates inadequate suspension or an excessive length of the prosthesis. Abnormal axis rotation at the knee that results in a whipping motion is usually due to incorrect alignment of the prosthesis at the knee.

UPPER LIMB PROSTHETIC DEVICES

Levels of Upper Limb Amputation

Classification is based on the anatomic location of the amputation. Patient acceptance of prosthetic devices varies depending on the age, activity level, and comfort level of the patient.

Terminal Devices

Hooks. The split-hook type is the most common terminal device used. This device allows the patient to grasp objects between the fingers of the hook by opening and closing the hook in a pincer-type motion.

Voluntary Opening Hooks. The patient can open the fingers of the hook by exerting a force on the control. The hook is designed to act as a spring to close the fingers and provide prehension, or a pinch force.

Voluntary Closing Hooks. This type of hook permits a more precise ability to close the device as both the opening and the closing of the device is powered by the patient using a cable control.

Voluntary Opening Hands. These are similar in operation as that of the voluntary opening hook, except the fingers form the "three-jaw-chuck" pinch with the index and middle finger joining the thumb.

Passive or Cosmetic Hands. These units have no functional mechanism and are intended purely for cosmetic effect.

Wrist Units. These are designed to attach the terminal device to the forearm and to provide the ability to pronate/supinate. Wrist units, which can be controlled by either constant-friction controlled or locking, permit easier control for midline activities such as eating, grooming, and dressing.

Transradial Sockets

Split Socket. Normally used following a very short-transradial amputation because elbow flexion is often limited.

Munster (Self-Suspending) Socket. Designed for the short-transradial amputation. It has a very narrow anterior–posterior (A-P) dimension that suspends the socket on the residual limb.

Northwestern University Supracondylar Socket. Has become the most popular self-suspending socket design. Adequately suspends the unit without any loss of ROM in the sagittal plane.

Hinges. Connect the socket to a triceps cuff or pad on the posterior upper arm, and assist with suspension and stability.

Flexible Elbow Hinges. Assist with suspension of the forearm shell and permit forearm pronation/supination.

Rigid Elbow Hinges. Used following midforearm to short-transradial amputations that have normal ROM at the elbow.

Transradial Harness and Controls. Suspends the prosthesis from the shoulder and secures the socket on the stump. Movement of the scapulothoracic region increases the pull on the control cable or creates excursion, which in turn controls the terminal device or elbow joint.

Figure 8 Harness. The most commonly used harness—the axilla loop acts as a response point for the transmission of body forces to the terminal device.

Chest Strap Harness. This type of harness is used when the patient cannot tolerate an axilla loop, or if greater suspension is required. However, the chest strap harness is not appropriate for women.

Figure 9 Harness. Typically used with the self-suspending prosthesis and consists of an axilla loop and a control attachment strap, which provides greater freedom and comfort over conventional harnesses.

Elbow Units

External. Used with an elbow disarticulation prosthesis with an outside locking hinge system.

Internal. Designed for a transhumeral patient with at least 2 in. of the distal humerus removed. It has the required space to accommodate an inside locking out unit, which allows the user to lock the elbow in 11 different positions of flexion.

USE OF THE PROSTHESIS

At the earliest opportunity, the patient must learn how to don and doff the prosthesis independently and to check the fit. Gross movements are taught initially before finer motor movements are introduced as control of the prosthesis improves. Skills to practice include:

- Drinking and eating
- Washing the face
- Dressing, including practice with buttoning, using a zipper, and managing other garment fasteners
- Writing
- Advanced activities as appropriate (driving, bicycling, playing a musical instrument)

Study Pearl

- A splint: an orthotic device intended for temporary use.
- Orthotist: a healthcare professional who designs, fabricates, and fits orthoses of the limbs and trunk.
- Pedorthist: a healthcare professional who designs, fabricates, and fits only shoes and foot orthoses.

ORTHOTICS

An orthoses is an external devive that is worn to promote control, correct load transfer, enhance stabilization, or assist with dynamic movement.[9] The term "orthotic" is an adjective, often used as a noun.

GENERAL CONCEPTS

The design of all orthoses is based on three relatively simple principles:

- Pressure: the greater the surface area of the orthoses, the less force is applied to the skin. Consideration must be given to the material selected for orthotic fabrication, the forces at the interface between the orthotic materials and the skin, and the degrees of freedom at each joint. Ideally, there should be adequate padding covering the greatest area possible for comfort.
- Equilibrium: the required force is located at a point where the desired movement is either inhibited or facilitated. Consideration must be given to the level of neuromuscular control of each segment, including strength and tone. Ideally, the total force acting on the involved segment is equal to zero, or there is equal pressure throughout the orthosis.
- Lever arm: the further the point of the force from the joint upon which it acts, the greater the moment arm and the smaller the magnitude of force required to produce a given torque at that joint. Consideration must be given to the number of joint segments involved. Ideally, the length of the orthoses is suitable to provide an adequate force to create the desired effect and to avoid increased transmission of shear forces against the anatomic tissues.

LOWER LIMB ORTHOSES: COMPONENTS/TERMINOLOGY

Shoe Components. A shoe is comprised of a number of components (Figure 15-1).

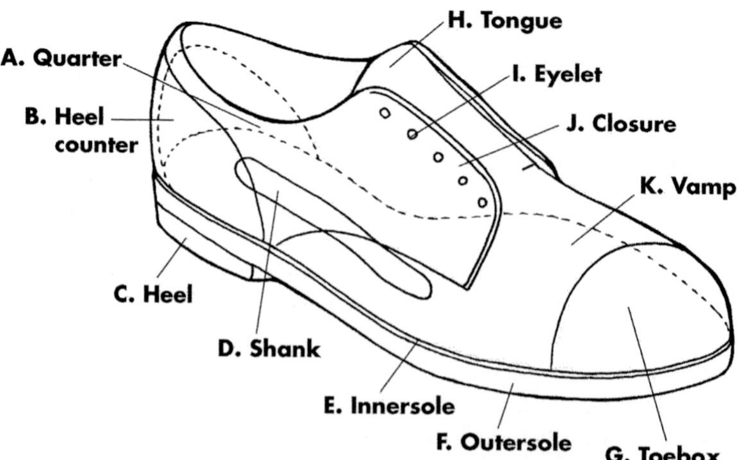

Figure 15-1. Anatomy of a shoe. (Reproduced with permission from Prentice, WE, Voight, MI: *Techniques in Musculoskeletal Rehabilitation.* McGraw-Hill. 2001:329.)

- Outersole: the hard outside layer that contacts the floor and protects the plantar surface of the foot.
- Innersole: the inner layer that interfaces with the plantar surface at the foot.
- Ball: the widest part of the sole, which is located below the metatarsal heads.
- Vamp: covers the anterior foot. The tongue is an extension of the vamp that protects the foot from the eyelet rows and laces.
- Quarters: most shoes have a medial and lateral quarter that extend posteriorly, under the malleoli in low shoes, or covers the malleoli in high shoes, and are joined at the heel.
- Closures or throat styles: the portion of the upper that influences the ease of donning and adjustability of the shoes.
- Heel: a low heel provides the greatest ability and assists in evenly distributing the weight between the rear and forefoot.
- Heel counter: a reinforcement cup that helps maintain the anatomic heel in neutral by controlling excessive movement.
- Toe box: a reinforced material used to maintain the height of the shoe to protect the toes.
- Shank: a reinforced material located between the ball and heel of the shoe.
- Last: the last determines the fit and the outward appearance of the shoe.

Study Pearl

The subtalar neutral position, used by clinicians to evaluate the amount of pronation and supination, is the position when the head of the talus is aligned with the navicular.

Foot Orthoses. A foot orthosis is primarily designed to allow the subtalar joint to function normally during the gait cycle—facilitate pronation during initial part of stance and supination during the latter part of stance. In addition, a foot orthosis can be used to alleviate symptoms by altering the mechanical function of the subtalar neutral position.

Foot orthoses can be classified into three general categories based on flexibility:

Study Pearl

Through control of one plane of motion, a well-designed foot orthosis can control all planes of motion.

- Soft: provide cushioning, improve shock absorption, decrease shear forces, and can redistribute plantar pressures.
- Semirigid: a combination of soft and rigid materials that provide some flexibility and shock absorption while simultaneously balancing or controlling the foot.
- Rigid: made of strong and durable materials to assist with transfer of weight, stabilize flexible deformities, and to control abnormal motion.

Some of the modifications available, and their purposes, include:[10]

- Arch of the orthotic shell: captures the inclination angle of the calcaneus and the architecture of the foot.
- First ray cut out: used to increase weight bearing under the second metatarsal head and to provide room for requisite plantar flexion of the first metatarsal with a patient who has a rigid plantarflexed first ray.
- Thomas heel: commonly located on the medial side of the foot under the sustentaculum tali to give added leverage for support and to stabilize motion as the foot goes from initial contact to midstance.

- Sole wedge: serves to stabilize motion but may also shift weight from one side of the shoe to the other.

Shoe Modifications. Shoe modifications can be either be internal or external.

Internal Modifications. Involve a corrective adaptation which is fixed inside the shoe. Three of the more common internal modifications include:

- Medial longitudinal arch support (scaphoid pad): often used in conjunction with a medial longitudinal counter to prevent depression of the subtalar joint.
- Metatarsal pad: a rubber or semi-soft pad that is used to relieve excessive pressure from the metatarsal heads and to support a collapsed transverse metatarsal arch.

External Modifications. External modifications include corrections to the heel or outsole:

Heel Corrections

- Medial heel wedge: used to elevate and maintain the medial margin of the shoe to decrease hyperpronation, and to shift the weight laterally.
- Lateral heel wedge: used to elevate and maintain the lateral margin of the shoe to decrease supination, and to shift the weight medially.
- Thomas heel: extends the medial aspect of heel of the shoe anteriorly by 1 in. to assist in balance, support the longitudinal arch, and assist in maintaining the subtalar joint in a neutral position. The Thomas heel is often coupled with a medial heel wedge to assist with stability.
- Reverse Thomas heel: the opposite of the Thomas heel—the lateral aspect of the heel is extended 1 in. to assist with balance, and subtalar joint alignments. Is often used in conjunction with lateral heel wedges.
- Heel flares: either a medial or lateral extension of the shoe heel designed to broaden the BOS for greater ability.

Outsole Corrections

- Medial sole wedges: used to correct forefoot eversion and promote inversion.
- Lateral sole wedge: used to correct forefoot inversion and promote eversion.
- Rocker bottom: located under and posterior to the metatarsal heads so as to redistribute the body weight over the entire plantar surface, reduce stress to the forefoot, and assist in rollover during ambulation.
- Metatarsal bar: a flat strip positioned just posterior to the metatarsal heads, designed to transfer the forces from the metatarsophalangeal joints to the metatarsal shafts.

Ankle–Foot Orthoses (AFO): designed to control the rate and direction of tibial advancement and to maintain an adequate BOS. There are several designs of AFO.

Shoe and Foot Attachments

- Stirrup (solid): a one-piece attachment with a solid metal plate riveted to the sole of the shoe, creating a U-shaped frame that forms a medial and lateral upright.
- Stirrup (split): a two-piece attachment with a metal plate riveted to the sole of the shoe that has two channels to permit donning and doffing of the removable metal uprights.
- Caliper: very similar to the split stirrup with a metal plate riveted to the sole of the shoe, except that the uprights are slightly lighter and round.
- Molded shoe insert: a plastic custom formed plate that attaches directly to the metal uprights with a calf band for proximal support.

Ankle Joints and Controls

- Plantar flexion stop: a posterior stop that restricts plantar flexion but allows full dorsiflexion.
- Dorsiflexion stop: an anterior stop that restricts dorsiflexion but allows full plantar flexion.
- Limited motion stop: an ankle joint that limits motion in all directions.
- Free motion joint: an ankle joint that provides medial and lateral stability from the uprights while permitting full plantar/dorsiflexion. Plastic AFOs use lightweight joints that permit free motion.

Assists

- Dorsiflexion assist: a posterior spring that assists with dorsiflexion by compressing the spring during the early stance phase of gait, and permits full plantar flexion.
- Dorsiflexion-plantar flexion assist (dual channel) or bi-channel adjustable ankle locks (BiCAAL): a joint with an anterior and posterior spring that assists with the plantar and dorsiflexion to varying degrees according to the settings of the springs.

Varus and Valgus Correction

- Medial T-strap: a strap that arises from the shoe that covers the medial malleolus, and buckles to the lateral upright, pushing laterally to correct a valgus deformity.
- Lateral T-strap: a strap that arises from the shoe that covers the lateral malleolus and buckles to the medial upright, pushing medially to correct a varus deformity.
- Supramalleolus orthosis (SMO): a low-profile design for subtalar joint control to limit varus or valgus. The ankle joint also assist with dorsiflexion during swing.

Knee–Ankle–Foot Orthoses. The primary purpose of most knee orthotic devices is to provide knee control in one or more planes.

- Single axis joint: designed to behave like a hinge to prevent movement in the frontal plane, and to provide medial/lateral stability, while permitting movement in the sagittal plane.

- Offset axis joint: a single axis joint designed with an axis set further posterior from the weight line than the standard single axis joint, which promotes maximal knee extension during weight bearing without having to use a mechanical lock.
- Polycentric axis joint: designed to mimic the instantaneous center of rotation present in the anatomic knee, although this two-geared mechanical joint is still confined to a uniplanar path.

Knee Locking Devices

- Drop ring locks: small rings that slide down over the proximal portion of a single axis knee joint to maintain full knee extension during standing but may be raised manually to release for sitting or free knee flexion and extension.
- Spring-loaded pull rod: a spring system that uses a control rod that can be extended to a height of convenient reach to permit easier release of the locking mechanism, which is often prescribed for clients with poor balance or dexterity issues.
- Pawl or bail locks: levers positioned posterior to the knee which provide easy release of the locking mechanism for sitting. This type of lock is typically prescribed for patients who have extreme balance disturbances or who cannot free their hands to operate another type of locking system during sitting.
- Adjustable knee lock: designed to preset and lock the knee ROM to a specific degree of flexion or extension.

Knee Orthotics

- Rigid Knee Orthotic (KO): commonly referred to as the Swedish knee cage, and typically used with patients who have knee instability. This device has a metal frame with canvas or heavy elastic thigh, and calf straps which are designed to prevent recurvatum and provide some medial and lateral support.
- Knee immobilizer: these devices are designed to comfortably restrict all motions of the knee.
- Functional knee braces: designed for patients who have returned to activity and require additional stability to protect the knee.
- Patellofemoral joint brace: designed to minimize patella compression, assist in guiding patella tracking, and to prevent excessive lateral shift of the patella.

Hip–Knee–Ankle–Foot Orthoses

Hip Joints

- Single axis: hip joints that are single axis joints permitting flexion and extension, while restricting abduction, adduction, and rotation.
- Double axis: locks two planes of motion with adjustable start to set limits as needed in each direction (flexion, extension, abduction, and adduction).

Hip Locks

- Drop locks: similar to the knee drop lock, a small ring slides down over the axis to lock the joint into extension while standing.
- Two-position hip locks: designed to lock in full extension and 90 degrees of hip flexion, used for patients with poor sitting balance.

Pelvic Bands

- Unilateral band: used when a single limb orthosis requires proximal stability—a rigid band can be incorporated that encircles the pelvis between the iliac crest and the greater trochanter, with a flexible belt that continues around the waist.
- Bilateral band: most commonly the bilateral pelvic band is used for bilateral HKAFOs where the padded metal band encompasses the pelvis around the buttock with a posterior band positioned over the sacrum.
- Double or pelvic girdle: when maximal control is required, the entire proximal pelvis is encapsulated from the iliac crest to just proximal to the greater trochanter with varying support posteriorly depending on strength and pelvis stability.
- Silesian belt: a flexible strap that attaches to a proximal portion of the orthosis and encircles the pelvis, assisting in stabilizing the orthosis and providing suspension.

Reciprocal Gait Orthosis. The reciprocal gait orthosis (RGO) is designed to permit a reciprocal gait as opposed to the traditional swing-through gait used with HKAFOs (used with spinal cord injury levels as high as C8 to T12-L1, myelodysplasia, osteogenesis imperfecta, spina bifida, paraplegia, muscular dystrophy (not the Duchenne type), and cerebral palsy). Patient requires good stability of the spine, adequate upper extremity and shoulder girdle strength and endurance, and a cardiovascular and respiratory system that is free of disease, and which provides adequate endurance. Contraindications for using this device include obesity, hip flexion contractures, and genu varum greater than 15 degrees. The reciprocal motion is facilitated by a variety of mechanisms:

- A cable system that couples the passive hip flexion and extension movements to advance the lower limbs in a reciprocal fashion.
- A bar balance system (iso-centric system) located at the lumbosacral level of the orthoses, which provides a reciprocating hip flexion action.
- A low-profile push-pull cable system (ARGO) that not only provides a reciprocating motion at the hip but also assists with standing through a hip and knee extension assist mechanism.

Standing Frame and Swivel Walker. The standing frame, designed for children, consists of broad-based, posterior non-articulated uprights that extend from a flat base to a mid torso chest band, and a posterior thoracolumbar band. The patient's shoes are strapped to the base of the frame. A similar orthosis is the Swivel Walker, which is made in both child and adult sizes. The major difference is the base, which has two distal plates that rock slightly to enable a swiveling gait.

Parapodium. The parapodium differs from the standing frame by virtue of joints that permit the wearer to sit. Parapodiums permit the wearer to stand without crutch support, freeing the hands for play or vocational activities.

Thoracic and Lumbosacral Orthoses. There are two general classifications of thoracic, lumbosacral orthoses: flexible and rigid.

Flexible

- Sacroiliac corset (binder): Encircling the waist from the iliac crest to the greater trochanter, and extending anteriorly to the symphysis pubis, these corsets function to promote stability for patients with postpartum or sacroiliac instability.
- Lumbosacral orthosis (LSO): the LSO corset is designed to encompass the torso and pelvis. The primary use is for patients with back pain.
- Thoracolumbosacral corset: relatively the same construction and function as the LSO except this one includes a shoulder strap to restrict spinal motion to the thoracic region as well as to the lumbar region.

Rigid

- Williams LSO: this orthosis incorporates a single three-point pressure system designed to limit trunk extension in the lumbar spine and to increase intra-abdominal pressure. Lordosis is decreased to limit lumbar extension while the pelvic and thoracic bands resist the medial forces that tend to limit lateral trunk motions.
- Thoracic-lumbosacral orthoses:
  - Taylor (flexion/extension control): a pelvic band connects with two posterior uprights terminating at the mid-scapular level of the thoracic region with an anterior abdominal closure and axillary straps. The orthosis is designed with two three-point pressure systems, which limit both flexion and extension of the lumbar and thoracic spine.
  - Jewett (flexion control): incorporates a three-point pressure system using two pads, one across the sternum and one at the symphysis pubis, providing the counterforce with a single pad posteriorly to promote hyperextension and thus restricting forward flexion.
  - Plastic body jacket (flexion-extension-lateral-rotary control): typically fabricated with high temperature copolymer plastics, the well-fitted body jacket will restrict motion in all planes. Body jackets are frequently used post-surgically or during an acute trauma.

Thoracic and lumbosacral orthoses offer a combination of the following therapeutic benefits:

- Intra-abdominal pressure: raises the intracavitary pressure, thereby reducing the intradiskal pressure produced with forward bending.
- Muscle relaxation: the presence of the orthosis reduces the need for the abdominal muscles to contract to support the vertebral column, thereby allowing them to relax.
- Restriction of motion: a reduction in the motion at respective intervertebral segments has been linked to a reduction in pain and spinal instability.
- Proprioceptive feedback: reinforces positive behaviors.
- Postural realignment: reduces compensatory postures related to pain.

CERVICAL ORTHOSES

- Soft collar: provides mechanical restraint for cervical flexion and extension and, to a lesser degree, side bending and rotation.
- Hard collars (Philadelphia collar): provide more rigid stabilization of the cervical spine and typically offer some type of chin and occipital support.
- Halo-cervical orthoses: provides the greatest reduction in cervical mobilization. A cranial ring is secured to the skull using four metal pins. The ring is attached by four metal bars to a plastic vest and is worn continuously.

UPPER LIMB ORTHOSES

The purpose of the majority of upper limb orthoses is to position the hand in the most functional position and/or to create usable prehension.

Hand and Wrist Orthoses

- Basic or short opponens: fabricated from low-temperature thermoplastics and designed to immobilize the first carpometacarpal (CMC) and metacarpophalangeal (MCP) joints and position the thumb in opposition and abduction to maintain the webspace and the architecture of the hand for future procedures. There is no wrist control, and therefore strong wrist flexor and extensors are required for functional use. Indications include inflammation or injury of the thumb, median nerve lesions, C6-7 spinal cord lesions, hemiplegia with loss of thumb opposition.
- Long opponens splint (anterior forearm wrist orthosis): designed to immobilize the first carpometacarpal (CMC) and metacarpophalangeal (MCP) joints and position the thumb in extension and opposition, preserving the webspace. Indications include DeQuervain's tenosynovitis, median and ulnar nerve lesions, C5-6 spinal cord lesions, wrist of thumb instability, degenerative or inflamed wrist thumb joint, scaphoid or Bennett's fracture-dislocation.
- Anterior forearm static wrist hand orthosis (resting hand splint): the object of this splint is to place the hand and wrist in a neutral, functional, or lumbrical position, with the

MCP joints flexed to 60 to 90 degrees, and the IP and PIP joints flexed to 0 to 45 degrees. The wrist is in slight extension to neutral. Indications include flaccid hand due to paralysis, burns or healing skin grafts, and post-Dupuytren's release.

- The wrist driven prehension (tenodesis) orthosis: designed specifically for patients with spinal cord injury at the C6-7 level and who have the 3−/5 to 3+/5 extensor carpi radialis muscle strength.

Elbow Orthoses

- Static orthosis: for the purpose of restricting motion and promoting tissue healing.
- Dynamic orthosis: used when there is a need to increase the resting length of the elbow.

Dynamic splints provide a low load with a prolonged stretch and are often used for patients with burns and elbow contractures.

- Shoulder–elbow–wrist (airplane) orthosis: used to protect the soft tissues of the shoulder and prevent contractures. The shoulder is abducted 70 to 90 degrees, with the majority of weight born on the iliac crest and lateral trunk.

ATHLETIC TAPING

Much controversy exists regarding the value of supported taping techniques in sport. Athletic taping is generally prescribed to:

- Support an injured body segment, or provide preventative support for a joint that is at risk.
- Limit the ROM of specific joints.
- Realign the position of a structure and thereby reduce pain (patellofemoral taping using the McConnell technique).
- Enhance proprioception.
- To secure protective devices such as felt, foam, gel or plastic padding, and to keep dressings and bandages in place.

Study Pearl

Injured ligaments should be held in a shortened position (eg, lateral inversion ankle sprains should be taped in an everted position).

Skin Preparation

The part to be taped should be properly positioned and supported. If the part to be taped has not been previously injured, it should be taped in a neutral position.

The appropriate type and width of tape is selected. Several different methods of skin preparation can be used. The most common is simply to clean and dry the skin. A layer of prewrap (a thin foam-like material) is applied to the area to be taped. In some cases it may be preferable to shave the hair from around the area and have the tape applied directly to the skin. A quick drying adherent is recommended and may be sprayed onto the skin to allow for better tape adhesion, to aid in toughening the skin, and to decrease irritation. Often, heel and lace pads (foam squares with petroleum jelly or other lubricant) are applied to areas of high friction (ie, the dorsum of the ankle and the distal Achilles tendon) to prevent blisters.

APPLICATION

When applying the tape, the clinician should avoid tape wrinkles or creases, as these can lead to blisters and discomfort. In general, tape strips should overlay each other by about one-half the width of the tape. Each area should be covered by two layers of tape. The tape should be applied with even pressure. Constriction of blood flow is possible if the tape is applied too tightly. This is especially true with circular taping.

COMPLICATIONS

- Allergic reactions to the tape, skin irritation.
- Neurologic or vascular compromise.
- The amount of restriction provided by the tape compromises the ability of the athlete/patient to perform.
- The restrictive ability of the tape typically only lasts about an hour and may therefore need to be reapplied regularly.

TRANSFER TRAINING

Prior to performing a transfer, the clinician should consider the following:

- The patient's level of cognition and mobility.
- How much assistance the patient and clinician requires. When in doubt, a second person should be utilized. It is important to communicate with the patient about the transfer details and their responsibilities during the transfer. Verbal explanation and demonstration should be used to highlight the expectations and transfer sequence. If necessary, instruct the patient in smaller segments of the transfer prior to performing the entire transfer.
- The appropriate equipment should be prepared prior to the transfer.
- Correct positioning of both the patient and the clinician. The clinician should maintain a large BOS and use proper body mechanics throughout the transfer.

Commands and counts are used to synchronize the actions of the participants involved in the transfer with the clinician giving the commands during the transfer when more than one person is involved. Manual contacts can be used with the patient to direct their participation during the transfer.

LEVELS OF PHYSICAL ASSISTANCE

The various levels of physical assistance are outlined in Table 15-6.

TABLE 15-6. LEVELS OF PHYSICAL ASSISTANCE

Independent	The patient does not require any assistance to complete the task.
Supervision	The patient requires a clinician to observe throughout completion of the task.
Contact guard	The patient requires the clinician to maintain contact with the patient to complete the task. Contact guard is usually needed to assist if there is a loss of balance.
Minimal assist	The patient requires 25% assist from the clinician to complete the task.
Moderate assist	The patient requires 50% assist from the clinician to complete the task.
Maximal assist	The patient requires 75% assist from the therapist to complete the task.
Dependent	The patient is unable to participate and the clinician must provide all of the effort to perform the task.

TYPES OF TRANSFERS

The most common types of transfers encountered by the physical therapist include:

- Pulling a patient up the bed: The clinician and an assistant stand on opposite sides of the bed. A draw-sheet is used to slide the patient up the bed. The head of the bed is lowered and the height of the bed is adjusted to the waist- or hip-level of the shorter person of the lift team. With both palms up and the elbows flexed, the two lifters grasp the draw-sheet, and point one foot in the direction the patient is to be moved. The patient is asked to bend their knees, to push down with their feet, and to pull up using a trapeze during the transfer. The lifters lean in the direction of the move using the legs and body weight, and on the count of three, the patient is lifted and pulled up the bed. This step is repeated as many times as needed.
- Out of bed to a WC: The steps of the transfer are explained to the patient. The clinician makes the determination as to whether further help is necessary based on the ability of the patient to help. A transfer belt is placed around the patient's waist to provide a firm handhold. The clinician positions and then locks the WC as close to the bed as possible and then helps the patient turn over and scoot to the edge of the bed. The clinician places their arms around the patient's chest and clasps their hands behind the patient's back. Supporting the patient's farthest leg from the WC between their legs, the clinician leans back, shifts their weight, and lifts the patient. The patient pivots toward the chair where possible, or is guided by the clinician. If the patient's legs are weak and appear to be buckling, the clinician can brace their knees against the patient's knees to lock them in extension. Once correctly positioned over the chair, the patient bends toward the clinician who bends their knees and lowers the patient into the back of the WC.
- Level surfaces (bed to gurney): The clinician and an assistant stand on opposite sides of the bed, with the clinician on the side of the direction of the transfer. A large plastic garbage bag is placed between the sheet and the draw-sheet, beneath one edge of the patient's torso, and the patient's legs are moved closer to the edge of the bed. Grasping the draw street on both sides of the bed and, on a count of three, the clinician leans backward and shifts their weight, sliding the patient toward the edge of the bed, while the assistant holds the sheet down to prevent it from slipping. The bed is raised so that it is slightly higher than the gurney, and the head of the bed is lowered. The patient's legs are moved onto the gurney, and the assistant kneels on the bed. On the count of three, the clinician and assistant grasp the drawer sheet and slide the patient onto the gurney, which may take several attempts.
- WC to toilet, tub seat: the WC is positioned as close to the destination as possible. The clinician locks the WC and fastens the transfer belt around the patient. The clinician helps the patient slide to the edge of the WC and positions the patient's

feet directly under his or her body (the patient's body). The clinician lifts the patient by grasping the back of the transfer belt, and helps the patient pivot around in front of the toilet, keeping the patient's knees between the clinician's legs. The patient grasps each of the safety rails as they are slowly and gently lowered down onto the toilet.

Dependent Transfers. See Table 15-7.

Assisted Transfers. See Table 15-8.

TABLE 15-7. DEPENDENT TRANSFERS

TYPE OF TRANSFER	DESCRIPTION
Three-person carry/lift	Used to transfer a patient from a stretcher to a bed or treatment plinth. Three clinicians carry the patient in a supine position; one clinician supports the head and upper trunk, the second clinician supports the trunk, and the third supports the lower extremities. The clinician at the head of the bed is usually the one to initiate commands. The clinicians flex their elbows and are positioned under the patient and roll the patient on their side toward them. The clinicians then lift on command and move in a line to the destination surface, lower, and position the patient properly.
Two-person lift	Used to transfer patient between two surfaces of different heights or when transferring a patient to the floor. Standing behind the patient, the first clinician should place their arms underneath the patient's axilla. The clinician should grasp the patient's left forearm with their right hand and grasp the patient's right forearm with their left hand. The second clinician places one arm under the mid to distal thighs and the other arm is used to support the lower legs. The clinician at the head usually initiates the command to lift and transfer the patient out of the chair to the destination surface.
Dependent squat pivot transfer	Used to transfer patient who cannot stand independently, but can bear some weight through the trunk and lower extremities. The clinician should position the patient at a 45° angle to the destination surface. The patient places their upper extremities on the clinician's shoulders, but should not be allowed to pull on the clinician's neck. The clinician should position the patient at the edge of the surface, hold the patient around the hips and under the buttocks, and block the patient knees in order to avoid buckling while standing. The clinician should utilize momentum, straighten his or her legs, and raise the patient or allow the patient to remain in a squatting position. The clinician should then pivot and slowly lower the patient to the destination surface.
Hydraulic or mechanical lift	A device required for dependent transfers when a patient is obese, there is only one clinician available to assist for the transfer, the patient has a weight-bearing restriction on bilateral lower extremities, or the patient is totally dependent. A body sling is required for the lift transfer. Two primary types of sling exist: full body, which covers the posterior surface of the patient from the shoulders to the back of the thighs/knees; a sling that has divided legs that cross between the patient's legs and support him or her on the posterior surface of the thighs. The hydraulic lift is locked in position before the transfer. The clinician positions the sling under the patient by rolling the patient from side to side, and then attaches the S-ring to the bars on the lift. The longer length of chain is attached at the lower end of the sling to encourage a seated position. Once all attachments are checked, the clinician should pump the handle on the device in order to elevate the patient. Once the patient is elevated, the clinician can navigate the lift with the patient to the destination surface. Once transferred, the chains should be removed, however, the webbed sling should remain in place in preparation for the return transfer.

TABLE 15-8. ASSISTED TRANSFERS

TYPE OF TRANSFER	DESCRIPTION
Sliding board	Used for a patient who has some sitting balance, some upper extremity strength, and who can adequately follow directions. The patient should be positioned at the edge of the wheelchair (WC) or bed and should lean to one side while placing one end of the sliding board sufficiently under the proximal thigh. The other end of the sliding board should be positioned on the destination surface. The patient should not hold onto the end of the sliding board in order to avoid pinching the fingers. The patient should place the lead hand 4-6 in away from the sliding board and use both arms to initiate a push-up and scoot across-the-board. The clinician should guard in front of the patient and assist as needed as the patient performs a series of push-ups across the board.
Stand pivot	Used when a patient is able to stand and bear weight through one or both of the lower extremities. The patient must possess functional balance and the ability to pivot. Patients with unilateral weight-bearing restrictions or hemiplegia may utilize this transfer and lead with the uninvolved side. The transferred may also be used therapeutically, leading with the involved side for a patient post CVA. The patient should be positioned at the edge of the WC or bed to initiate the transfer. The clinician can assist the patient to keep their feet flat on the floor while bringing the head and trunk forward. The clinician should assist the patient as needed with their feet. The clinician must guard or assist the patient through the transfer and instruct the patient to reach back for the surface before they begin to sit down. Once the stand pivot is performed, the clinician should assist as needed to insure control with lowering the patient to the destination surface.
Stand step	Used with a patient who has the necessary strength and balance to weight shift and step during the transfer. The patient requires guiding or supervision from the clinician and performs the transfer as a stand pivot transfer except that patient actually takes a step to maneuver and reposition his or her feet instead of using a pivot.
Push up (pop-over)	Used with a patient with good sitting balance who can lift buttocks clear of sitting surface (eg, a patient with a complete C7 level spinal cord injury can be independent with this transfer without a sliding board). Can be used as a progression in transfer training from using a sliding board. The patient utilizes a head-hips relationship to successfully complete the transfer—movement of the head in one direction results in movement of the hips in the opposite direction/toward the support surface being transferred to.

ASSISTIVE DEVICES

The indications for using an assistive device include:[11]

- Decreased ability to weight bear through the lower extremities (refer to "Levels of Weight Bearing")
- Muscle weakness or paralysis of the trunk or lower extremities
- Decreased balance and proprioception in the upright posture
- Joint instability and excessive skeletal loading
- Fatigue or pain

However there are a number of energy costs associated with using various assistive devices (Table 15-9).

Parallel bars can be used to provide maximum stability and security for patients during the beginning stages of ambulation or

TABLE 15-9. ENERGY COSTS ASSOCIATED WITH VARIOUS ASSISTIVE DEVICES

ASSISTIVE DEVICE	ENERGY COST
Crutches	Energy demand increased 13% to 80%, in part due to increased demands placed on arms and shoulder girdle muscles
Standard Walker	Oxygen consumption increased > 200%
Front-wheeled walker	Less impact compared with standard walker
Cain	No significant contribution

Reproduced, with permission, from Powers CM, Burnfield JM: Normal and pathologic gait. In Placzek JD, Boyce DA, eds: *Orthopaedic Physical Therapy Secrets*. Philadelphia, Hanley & Belfus, Inc. 2001:98-103.

standing. The correct height of the bar should allow for 20 to 25 degrees of elbow flexion while grasping on the bars approximately 4 to 6 in. in front of the body. The goal is to progress the patient out of the bars as quickly as possible to increase overall mobility and decrease dependence on the parallel bars.

There are three major categories of ambulatory assistive devices: canes, crutches, and walkers.

CANES

Canes are usually made out of wood, plastic, or aluminum (adjustable with a pushpin lock). The function of a cane is to widen the BOS and improve balance. However, because canes provide minimal stability and support for patients during ambulation activities, they are not intended for use with restricted weight-bearing gaits. Patients are typically instructed to hold a cane in the hand opposite the involved lower extremity. The cane and involved extremity are advanced together, followed by the uninvolved extremity.

The use of a cane in the contralateral hand helps preserve reciprocal motion and a more normal pathway for the COG.[12] Use of a cane in this fashion also helps in reducing forces created by the abductor muscles acting at the hip, as estimated by external kinematics and kinetics.[13-16] Use of a cane can transmit 20% to 25% of body weight away from the lower extremities.[17,18] Holding the cane in the hand opposite the involved extremity also allows widening the BOS and less lateral shifting of the center of mass.

In measuring cane height, the cane is placed approximately 6 in. from the lateral border of the toes.[19] Two landmarks typically are used during measurement to obtain a correct fit for a cane:[19]

- Greater trochanter: the top of the cane should come to approximately the level of the greater trochanter.
- Angle at the elbow: the elbow should be flexed 20 to 30 degrees.

An alternative method includes standing the cane at the patient's side and adjusting the handle to the level of the wrist crease at the ulnar styloid.

A variety of cane types exist:

- Standard cane: straight cane with single contact point with the ground.
- Adjustable aluminum offset (J-shaped) or offset cane: The design of this cane allows pressure to be borne over the center the cane for greater stability.
- Quad cane: four points of contact with the ground. Patients should be instructed to place all four legs of the cane on the floor simultaneously to obtain maximum stability. This type of cane provides a larger BOS than a standard cane, thereby increasing stability. However, depending on the specific design of the cane, the pressure exerted by the patient's hand may not be centered over the cane and may result in patient complaints of instability.[19]
    - Small-base quad cane is useful for stairs.
    - Wide-based quad cane provides the largest BOS but cannot be used on stairs.

Another disadvantage is that this type of cane warrants use of a slower gait pattern—faster progressions often cause the cane to rock from the rear legs to the front legs.

- Walk cane: this type of cane provides a very broad base with four points of floor contact. The legs of the cane farther from the patient's body are angled to maintain floor contact and to improve stability. Walk canes fold flat and are adjustable in height. However, this type of cane cannot be used on most stairs and requires the use of a slow forward progression.
- Rolling cane: provides a wide-wheeled base allowing uninterrupted forward progression. A pressure sensitive break is built into the handle and can be engaged using pressure from the base of the hand. This type of cane allows weight to be continuously applied as the need to lift and place the cane forward is eliminated, allowing for a faster forward progression.

CRUTCHES

Crutches (regular or standard), which are typically made from wood or aluminum, provide an increased BOS, a moderate degree of lateral stability, and can be used with all levels of weight bearing. However, crutches require a higher level of coordination than walkers, are awkward in small areas, and can cause pressure at the radial groove (spiral groove) of the humerus, creating a situation of potential damage to the radial nerve as well as to adjacent vascular structures in the axilla.[19]

The correct height for axillary crutches includes positioning the crutches 6 in. in front and 2 in. lateral to the patient with the crutch height adjusted to be no greater than three finger widths from the axilla (the handgrip is adjusted to allow for approximately 20 to 30 degrees of elbow flexion). The crutch height can be adjusted by wing nuts (pushbutton locks on the aluminum crutches) and the handgrip height is adjusted by wing nuts in both types. Alternative methods of measurement include:

- In the standing position, one can subtract 16 in. from the patient's height or measure from a point 2 in. below the axilla to a point 6 in. in front and 2 in. lateral to the foot.
- With the patient supine, measure from the axilla to a point 6 to 8 in. lateral to the heel.

Two other types of crutches are worth mentioning:

- Lofstrand (forearm): can be used at all levels of weight bearing, to provide increased ease of movement, and, because of the presence of a forearm cuff, allow the wearer to use their hands without dropping the crutches. However, this type of crutch requires the highest level of coordination for proper use. Proper fit includes 20 to 25 degrees of elbow flexion while holding the handgrip with the crutches positioned 6 in. in front and 2 in. lateral to the patient. The arm cuff should be positioned 1 to 1½ in. below the olecranon process so that it does not interfere with elbow flexion.

- Forearm platform: allow weight bearing on the forearm and are useful for patients who are unable to weight-bear through their hands. However, this type of crutch provides less lateral support owing to the absence of an axillary bar.

WALKERS

Walkers can be used with all levels of weight bearing and offer a significant BOS and good anterior and lateral stability. Attachments include fold down seats, a braking mechanism, platform attachments, wheel attachments, and carrying baskets. The correct height of the walker allows for 20 to 25 degrees of elbow flexion. The standard walker has many variations including:

- Folding (collapsible): facilitate mobility in the community, and are easier to transport in cars.
- Rolling (wheeled): available in either two wheels or four wheels, the latter of which requires a hand brake to provide added stability in stopping. The advantage of this type of walker is that it facilitates walking as a continuous movement sequence.
- Stair climbing: fitted with two posterior extensions and additional handgrips off of the rear legs for use on stairs.
- Reciprocal: fitted with hinges that allow advancement of one side of the walker at a time thereby facilitating a reciprocal gait pattern.
- Hemi: modified for use with one hand only.

Prior to initiating instruction in gait patterns using a conventional walker, several points related to the use of the walker should be emphasized to the patient:[19]

- The walker should be picked up and placed down on all four legs simultaneously to achieve maximum stability.
- The patient should be encouraged to hold their head up and to maintain good postural alignment.
- The patient should be cautioned not to step too close to the front crossbar to prevent falling.

LEVELS OF WEIGHT-BEARING

It must be remembered that most patients have difficulty replicating a prescribed weight-bearing restriction, and will need constant reinforcing.[20]

- Nonweight bearing (NWB): A patient is unable to place any weight through the involved extremity and which is not permitted to touch the ground or any surface—an assistive device is required.
- Toe touch weight bearing (TTWB): A patient is unable to place any weight through the involved extremity, however, may place the toes on the ground to assist with balance—an assistive device is required.
- Partial weight bearing (PWB): A patient is allowed to put a particular amount of weight through the involved extremity. The amount of weight bearing is expressed as allowable pounds of pressure, or as a percentage of total weight. A clinician must monitor the amount of actual weight transferred through the

involved foot during partial weight bearing (these patients often need the most reinforcing)—an assistive device is required.

- Weight bearing as tolerated (WBAT): A patient determines the proper amount of weight bearing based on comfort. The amount of weight bearing can range from minimal to full—an assistive device may or may not be required.
- Full weight bearing (FWB): A patient is able to place full weight on the involved extremity—an assistive device is not required at this level, but may be required to assist with balance.

Correct fitting for an assistive device is important for the safety of the patient, and to allow for minimal energy expenditure. Once fitted, the clinician should ensure that the correct walking technique with the device is taught to the patient.

Gait Training with Assistive Devices

The clinician must always provide adequate physical support and instruction while working with a patient using an assistive gait device. The clinician positions himself or herself on the involved side of the patient, so that they can assist the patient on the side where the patient will most likely have difficulty (the involved side).

A gait belt should be fitted around the patient's waist to enable the clinician to assist the patient. When ambulating with a patient, the clinician should be just behind the patient, standing toward the involved side, grasping the gait belt with one hand and placing the other hand on the patient's shoulder (not their arm as this will interfere).

During ambulation, the clinician's front foot should move when the patient moves, while the back leg and the assistive device should advance together.

The selection of the proper gait pattern to instruct the patient is dependent upon the patient's balance, strength, cardiovascular status, coordination, functional needs, and weight-bearing status. A number of gait patterns are recognized.

Two-Point Pattern. The two-point gait pattern, which closely approximates the normal gait pattern, requires the use of an assistive gait device (canes or crutches) on both sides of the body. This pattern requires the patient to move the assistive device and the contralateral lower extremity simultaneously.

Three-Point Gait Pattern. The three-point gait pattern involves the use of two crutches or a walker. This pattern is used when the patient is permitted to bear weight through only one lower extremity. The three-point gait pattern requires good upper body strength, good balance, and good cardiovascular endurance.

The pattern is initiated with the forward movement of one of the assistive devices. Next, the involved lower extremity is advanced. Then the patient presses down on the assistive device and advances the uninvolved lower extremity.

- If the uninvolved lower extremity is advanced to where it is parallel to the involved lower extremity, this is described as a "swing to" pattern.
- If the uninvolved lower extremity is advanced ahead of the uninvolved lower extremity, this is described as a "swing through" pattern.

Modifications of the three-point gait pattern include touchdown weight bearing (TDWB), and partial weight bearing (PWB).

This pattern is initiated with the forward movement of one of the assistive gait devices and then the involved lower extremity is advanced forward. The patient presses down on the assistive gait device and advances the uninvolved lower extremity using either a "swing to" or a "swing through" pattern.

Four-Point Pattern. The four-point gait pattern requires the use of an assistive gait device (canes or crutches) on both sides of the body. It is used when the patient requires maximum assistance with balance and stability. The pattern is initiated with the forward movement of one of the assistive devices, and then the contralateral lower extremity, the other assistive device, and finally the opposite lower extremity (eg, right crutch, then left foot; left crutch, then right foot).

Sit to Stand Transfers Using Assistive Devices. Before the patient can begin ambulation, the patient must first learn to safely transfer from a sitting position to a standing position. The wheels of the bed or WC are locked and the patient is reminded of any weight-bearing restrictions. The patient is asked to slide to the front edge of the chair or bed, and their weight-bearing foot is placed underneath the body so that their center of gravity (COG) is closer to their BOS, which makes it easier for the patient to stand.

- The patient is then instructed to lean forward and to push up with the hands from the bed or armrests.
- If the patient is being instructed on the use of walker, the patient should grasp the handgrips of the walker only after they have become upright, and should not be permitted to try to pull themselves up using the walker, as this can cause the walker to tip over, and increase the potential for falls.
- If the patient is using crutches, the patient is instructed to hold both crutches with the hand on the same side as the involved lower extremity. To stand, the patient presses down on the handgrips of the crutches, the armrest or bed, and with the uninvolved lower extremity. Once standing, the patient then moves the crutches into position and begins to ambulate.
- If the patient is using one or two canes, the patient is instructed to push up with the hands from the bed or armrests. Once standing, the patient should grasp the handgrip(s) of the cane(s) with the appropriate hand and begin to ambulate.

Stand to Sit Transfers Using Assistive Devices. The stand to sit transfer is essentially the reverse of the sit to stand transfer. In order to sit down using an assistive device, the patient must first back up against the front edge of the bed or chair. If the patient has difficulty bending the knee of the involved lower extremity, the patient is instructed to slowly advance this extremity forward. Once in position:

- the patient using a walker reaches for the bed or armrest with both hands and slowly sits down.
- the patient using crutches moves both crutches to the hand on the side of the involved lower extremity. With that hand

holding onto both handgrips of the crutches, the patient reaches back for the bed or armrest with the other hand before slowly sitting down.

- the patient using a cane(s), places the handgrip of the cane against the edge of the chair or bed. Next, the patient reaches back for the bed or armrest and slowly sits down.

Stair and Curb Negotiation

Ascending Stairs. A gait belt is recommended. To ascend steps, the patient must first move to the front edge of the step. The walker will have to be turned toward the opposite side of the handrail or wall. The clinician should remain behind the patient, usually toward the weaker side, and should place the lead foot on the same step with the patient and the other foot one step lower.

Ascending more than two to three stairs with a standard walker is not recommended. To ascend stairs using a walker, the patient is instructed to grasp the stair handrail with one hand, and to turn the walker sideways so that the two side legs of the walker are placed on the first step. When ready, the patient pushes down on the walker handgrip, and the handrail, and advances the uninvolved lower extremity on to the first step. The patient then advances the uninvolved lower extremity to the first step and then moves the legs of the walker to the next step. This process is repeated as the patient moves up the steps.

- To ascend steps or stairs with crutches, the patient should grasp the stair handrail with one hand, and grasp both crutches by the handgrips with the other hand. If the patient is unable to grasp both crutches with one hand, or if the handrail is not stable, then the patient should use both crutches only, although this is not recommended if there are more than two to three steps. When in the correct position at the front edge of the step, the patient pushes down on the crutches and handrail, if applicable, and advances the uninvolved lower extremity to the first step. The patient then advances the involved lower extremity and finally the crutches. This process is repeated for the remaining steps.
- To ascend steps or stairs with one or two canes, the patient should use the handrail and the cane. If the handrail is not stable, then the patient should use the cane(s) only. The patient pushes down on the cane or handrail, if applicable, and advances the uninvolved lower extremity to the first step. The patient then advances the involved lower extremity. This process is repeated for the remaining steps.

Descending Stairs. A gait belt is recommended. In order to descend steps, the patient must first move to the front edge of the top step. The clinician should remain in front of the patient, usually toward the weaker side, and should place the lead foot on the step the patient will step on and the other foot one step lower.

- Descending more than two to three stairs with a standard walker is not recommended. Using a walker to descend, the walker is turned sideways so that the two side legs of the walker are placed on the lower step. One hand is placed on the rear handgrip and the other hand grasps the stair handrail. When ready, the patient lowers the involved lower extremity down to the first step. Then the patient pushes down on the walker and handrail and advances the uninvolved lower extremity down the first step. This process is repeated as the patient moves down the steps.

- To descend steps or stairs with crutches, the patient should use one hand to grasp the stair handrail and the other to grasp both crutches and handrail. If the patient is unable to grasp both crutches with one hand, or if the handrail is not stable, then the patient should use both crutches only, although this is not recommended if there are more than two to three steps. When ready, the patient lowers the involved lower extremity down to the first step. Next, the patient pushes down on the crutches and handrail, if applicable, and advances the uninvolved lower extremity down to the first step. This process is repeated for the remaining steps.
- To descend steps or stairs with one or two canes, the patient should use the cane and handrail. If the handrail is not stable, then the patient should use the cane or canes only. When ready, the patient lowers the involved lower extremity down to the first step. Next, the patient pushes down on the cane(s) and handrail, if applicable, and advances the uninvolved lower extremity down to the first step. This process is repeated for the remaining steps.

Instructions. Whichever gait pattern is chosen, it is important that the patient receives verbal and illustrated instructions for use of the assistive gait device on stairs, curbs, ramps and doors, and transfers. These instructions should include any weight bearing precautions the patient may have, the appropriate gait sequence, and a contact number to reach the clinician if any questions arise.

WHEELCHAIRS

Wheelchairs are available in a variety of sizes and styles. Whenever possible, every attempt should be made to reduce the amount of resistance for wheelchair (WC) propulsion. WCs can be grouped into several classes: indoor (small wheelbase to allow maneuvering in confined spaces, but lacks the ability or power to negotiate obstacles), indoor/outdoor (provides mobility for those who stay on finished services, such as sidewalks, driveways and flooring), and active indoor/outdoor (provides the ability to travel long distances, move fast, and drive over unstructured environments such as grass, gravel and uneven terrain). WC fitting is highly individualized and requires a team effort between physiatrist, neurologist or orthopedist, occupational or physical therapists, specialists in assistive technology and driver training, and rehabilitation technology providers. When helping to choose a WC, a few patient considerations must be made:

- Physical needs
- Rental versus purchase

- Seating system
- Functional mobility
- Physical abilities
- Cognition
- Coordination
- Level of endurance
- Manual versus power

WC Measurements. To physically examine the patient for a WC, the patient should be positioned supine on a firm surface. The range of available pelvic and hip movements as they relate to spinal and pelvic alignment should be determined. The lower extremities must be well-supported by the clinician, with the knee flexed 95 to 100 degrees or as much as is needed to eliminate the influence of the hamstring muscle group.[7] ROM measurements should include hip flexion, abduction, adduction, and internal and external rotation; their effect on pelvic position and general body alignment should be noted as well. Once ROM is documented, a linear measurement of seat depth should be determined.

Once examination in the supine position is completed, the patient should be placed in a supported sitting position with the knees flexed to 100 degrees or more to eliminate the influence of the hamstring muscle group. Ideally, seated examination should be done on a simulator, a chair specifically designed for planar seated examinations. If a simulator is not available, the measurement can be done on a mat table with a thin front edge to allow 100 degrees of knee flexion (Table 15-10).

WC Components

Frame. Whereas stainless steel used to be the only frame material available, there are now choices including a variety of lightweight materials and designs. In general, the lighter the weight of the frame, the greater the ease of use, but the lesser amount of structural strength provided. The level of expected activity and environment where the WC will be used should be taken into account when deciding on frame construction.

The two most common types of frames currently available are

- Rigid frame: the frame remains in one piece and the wheels are released for storage or travel.
  - Facilitates stroke efficiency.
  - Increases distance/stroke.
- Standard cross-brace frame: enables the frame to collapse or fold for transport or storage.
  - Facilitates mobility in the community.
  - The WC is folded by first raising the footplates and then pulling up on the handles (located on either side of the seat), rather than pulling up on the middle of the upholstery, the latter of which can tear the upholstery.

Anti-Tipping Device. These are posterior extensions attached to the low-horizontal supports, which prevent the chair from tipping backward, and which limit going over curbs or over doorsills. A similar device is the Hill holder, which is a mechanical break that allows the chair to go forward, but automatically applies the brakes when the chair goes into reverse.

TABLE 15-10. STANDARD WHEELCHAIR MEASUREMENTS

DIMENSION	GUIDELINES	AVERAGE SIZE (IN)
Seat height/leg length	Measurement taken from the user's heel to the popliteal fold. 2 in are added to this measurement to allow clearance of the footrest.	Adult: 20 Narrow adult: 20 Slim adult: 20 Hemi/low seat: 17.5 Junior: 18.5 Child: 18.75 Tiny tot: 19.5
Seat depth	Measurement taken from the user's posterior buttock, along the lateral thigh to the popliteal fold. Approximately 2 in are subtracted from this measurement to avoid pressure from the edge of the seat against the popliteal space.	Adult: 16 Narrow adult: 16 Slim adult: 16. Junior: 16 Child: 11.5 Tiny tot: 11.5
Seat width	Measurement taken of the widest aspect of the user's buttocks, hips, or thighs. 2 in is added to this measurement so as to provide space for bulky clothing, orthoses, or clearance of the trochanters from the armrest side panel.	Adult: 18 Narrow adult: 16 Slim adult: 14 Junior: 16 Child: 14 Tiny tot: 12
Back height	Measurement taken from the seat of the chair to the floor of the axilla with the user's shoulder flexed to 90 degree. 4 in are subtracted from this measurement to allow the final back height to be below the inferior angles of the scapulae. NB: this measurement will be affected if a seat cushion is to be used—the person should be measured while seated on the seat cushion or the thickness of the cushion must be considered by adding that value to the actual measurement.	Adult: 16 to 16.5
Armrest height	Measurement taken from the seat of the chair to the olecranon process with the user's elbow flexed to 90°. 1 in is added to this measurement. NB: this measurement will be affected if a seat cushion is to be used—the person should be measured while seated on the seat cushion or the thickness of the cushion must be considered by adding that value to the actual measurement.	Adult: 9 in above the chair seat

Upholstery. Upholstery for WCs must withstand daily use in all kinds of weather. Many manufacturers offer a selection of materials and upholstery colors, ranging from black to neon, to allow for individual selection and differing tastes among consumers.

Seating System. Many WCs come with a fabric or sling seat. The disadvantages of a sling seat are that the hips tend to slide forward, the thighs tend to adduct and internally rotate, and the patient sits asymmetrically, which reinforces poor pelvic position. Because of these problems, and the fact that seating must be customized on an individual basis, seating surfaces are often purchased separately from the WCs themselves.

It is important when selecting a WC or a seating system to ensure that the two components are compatible.

- Insert or contour seats: these seats create a stable firm sitting surface, improved pelvic position (neutral), and reduce the tendency for the patient to slide forward or sit with a posterior pelvic tilt.
- Seat cushions: function to distribute weight bearing pressures, which assists in preventing decubitus ulcers in patients with decreased sensation, and prolongs WC sitting times.

- Pressure relieving air cushion: these lightweight cushions accommodate moderate to severe postural deformity and improve pressure distribution.
- Disadvantages: expensive, base may be unstable for some patients, require continuous maintenance.
- Pressure relieving fluid/gel or combination cushion: can be custom molded; are designed to accommodate moderate to severe postural deformity, and are easy for caregivers to reposition the patient.
- Disadvantages: require some maintenance, heavy, moderately expensive.
- Pressure relieving contoured foam cushion: uses dense, layered foam. Is designed to accommodate moderate to severe postural deformity, and is easy for caregivers to reposition patient.
- Disadvantages: may interfere with slide board transfers.
- Suspension elements: extended exposure to the vibration sustained propelling a WC in communities may lead to discomfort, chronic low back pain and disk degeneration. Suspension elements reduce the negative effects of shock and vibration.

Backrest. The standard height backrest provides support to the mid-scapula region. A number of modifications can be made to suit the user:

- A lower back height may increase functional mobility—typically seen in sports chairs—but may also increase back strain.
- Lateral trunk supports: improve trunk alignment for patients with scoliosis or poor stability.
- Insert or contour backs: improve trunk extension and overall upright alignment.
- A high back height may be necessary for patients with poor trunk stability or with extensor spasms.

Brakes. Brakes are an important safety feature. Most brakes consist of a lever system with a cam, or a ratchet. Extensions may be added to increase the ease of both locking and unlocking. When a WC has a reclining back, an additional brake is necessary. Brakes must be engaged for all transfers in and out of the chair.

Wheels/Tires. Most WCs use four wheels: two large wheels (standard spokes or spokeless) at the back (fitted with an outer rim that allows for hand grip and propulsion) and two smaller ones (casters) at the front. The tires used for the rear wheels may be narrow and hard rubber, pneumatic inflatable, semipneumatic, or radial tires. The pneumatic tires provide a smoother ride, and increased shock absorption, but require more maintenance than the solid ties. Mag wheels and off-road wheels also are options on some chairs. The standard size for the rear wheel is 24 in. Smaller and larger wheel sizes are available.

The wheels are fitted with an outer rim that enables the patient to propel himself or herself. For those patients with only one functional arm, two outer rims can be fitted on one wheel so that arm drive achieves both forward and backward propulsion. Projections (vertical, oblique, or horizontal) may be attached to the rims to facilitate with propulsion in patients with poor handgrip. However, the horizontal and oblique extensions add to the overall width of the chair and may reduce maneuverability.

Casters vary in size (ranging from six to eight inches in diameter) and composition (pneumatic, solid rubber, plastic, or a combination of these). Caster locks can be added to facilitate WC stability during transfers.

Leg Rests. Leg rests come in a variety of designs.

- Swing away: detachable leg rests that facilitate the ease in transfers, and a front approach to the WC when ambulating.
- Elevating: most frequently necessary when the patient is unable to flex the knee, for postural support, or when a dependent leg contributes to lower extremity edema. The length of the leg rest is adjustable to accommodate the full length of the patient's leg, and a padded calf support is provided. The position of the leg rest is adjusted by pushing down on a lever on the side of the chair. Elevating leg rests can be released from the WC or pivoted to one side during transfers. Elevated leg rests are contraindicated for patients with hypertonicity or adaptive shortening of the hamstrings.
- Fixed.

Footrests. A footrest is standard equipment on a WC. For rigid frame chairs, the footrests are usually incorporated into the frame of the chair as part of the design. Cross-brace folding chairs often have footrests that swivel, flip up, and/or can be removed.

Foot plates, which can be adjusted to accommodate the patient's foot, provide a resting base for the feet, so that the feet are in neutral with the knee flexed to 90 degrees.

Heel loops can be fitted to help maintain the foot position and prevent posterior sliding of the foot. Ankle and calf straps can be added to stabilize the feet onto the foot plates. Toe loops may also be used when the patient has difficulty maintaining the foot on the footplate in a forward direction.

Armrests. Armrests are available in several styles including desk length (to allow the user closer access to desks and tables) or full length, and both types may be flip-up, fixed, or detachable. The desk length design also allows the patient to remove and reverse the armrest so that the higher part is closer to the front edge in order to aid in pushing to standing. Wraparound (space saver) armrests reduce the overall width of the chair by 1½ in. The height of the armrests can also be adjustable.

Armrests can also be fitted with upper extremity support surface trays or troughs, which are helpful if the user has difficulty with upper body balance or decreased use of the upper extremities.

Many lightweight manual WCs are designed without armrests, which makes it easier for the user to roll up to a desk or table, and to perform transfers, in addition to providing a streamlined look.

Seat Belts. Seat belts can be used for safety or for positioning:

- Restraining belts are used to prevent patients from falling out of the WC.
- Seat belts can be fitted to grasp over the pelvis at a 45 degree angle to the seat to help position the pelvis. A seat belt can also be added to provide lateral or medial support at the hip

and knee to maintain alignment of the lower extremities, and/or control spasticity.

Specialized WCs

Pediatric WCs. Children with cerebral palsy, spina bifida, and osteogenesis imperfecta may be candidates for either a manual or a power WC, depending on upper extremity strength, rate of fatigue, cognitive abilities and family circumstances. Those with spinal muscular dystrophy, arthrogryposis, high-level spinal cord injuries, and those with progressively worsening Duchenne's muscular dystrophy are typically immediate candidates for powered mobility.

Seating Specifics. A pediatric WC must have approximately 4 in. of available space in the frame to accommodate growth. In addition, the seating system should be flexible enough to accommodate tonal or postural changes. Examples of flexibility in the system involve the placement of laterals, which are often attached to tracks, or the backrest can include T-nuts placed throughout the back to allow easy hardware mounting. Pediatric chairs often employ linear seating systems (to accommodate the delicate balance between providing contours in the system and accommodating growth) versus molded seats, which are more difficult to increase in size. Similarly a contoured backrest is more accommodating and provides more contact surface and thus more comfort. Caregivers should be made aware of the proper use of all accessories, including head supports and upper chest supports.

One must also always consider the aesthetic appeal of the WC and, when possible, it should reflect individuality and personality. When deciding between a manual or power WC, a number of considerations should be made:

- Power chairs are more expensive than manual chairs. Power chairs have inherent safety concerns and create issues surrounding transportation and home accessibility.
- Manual WCs are easier to transport and lift into a non-accessible home.

Reclining Wheelchairs. Reclining WCs are designed with an extended back and typically with elevating leg rests. The angle of the back is adjusted by releasing knobs on the side of the WC. A head support is required on a reclining back WC. A bar across the back of the reclining WC provides support and stability. The purpose of the reclining WC is to allow an intermittent or constant reclined positioning. Reclining WCs are indicated for patients who are unable to independently maintain an upright sitting position.

The chairs can be either manually or electrically (if the patient cannot do active push-ups or pressure relief maneuvers) controlled.

Hemi Chair. A chair that is designed to be low to the ground (seat height of approximately 17.5 inches), that allows propulsion with the noninvolved upper and/or lower extremities.

Tilt in Space. A chair that is designed to allow for a reclining position without losing the required 90 degrees of hip flexion and

90 degrees of knee flexion. This type of chair is indicated for patients with extensor spasms that may throw the patient out of the chair, or for pressure relief.

One Arm Drive. A chair that is designed with the drive mechanisms located on one wheel, usually with two outer rims (or push lever). The patient is able to propel the WC by pushing on either rim (or a lever) with one hand.

Amputee Chair. A modified WC where the drive wheels are placed posterior (approximately 2 in. backwards) to the vertical back supports, so that the BOS is lengthened and posterior stability is enhanced.

Powered Chairs. This design of chair utilizes a power source (battery) to propel the WC. Microprocessors allow the control of the WC to be adapted to various controls (joystick, head, and breath). This type of chair is usually prescribed for patients who are not capable of self-propulsion or who have very low endurance. Recent changes in the power bases have allowed for such innovations as power seat functions (power tilt, recline, elevating leg rest, seat elevator), and control interfaces (mini joysticks, head controls). Power WC bases can be classified in one of three categories, based on the drive wheel location relative to the system's COG:

- Rear-wheel drive: Drive wheels are located behind the user's COG, and the casters are located in the front, providing predictable drive characteristics and stability.
- Mid-wheel drive: Drive wheels are directly below the user's COG and generally have a set of casters or anti-tippers in the front and rear of the drive wheels. The advantage of this system is a smaller turning radius. The disadvantage is a tendency to rock or pitch forward, especially with sudden stops or fast turns.
- Front-wheel drive: Drive wheels are located in front of the user's COG. This design provides stability and a tight turning radius, and the ability to climb obstacles or curbs more easily. One of the disadvantages of this design is its rearward COG, which makes it difficult to drive in a straight line, especially on uneven surfaces.

WC Training. A number of areas need to be addressed when training a patient on how to be as functionally independent as possible with a WC.

Posture. It is important for the patient to maintain good posture in the WC. He or she should be seated well back in the chair, with the lower extremities on the footrests or leg rests. The patient should also be able to maintain a seated position when their balance is challenged.

WC Management. The various components of the WC should be reviewed with the patient, and the patient should perform all of the necessary tasks while being supervised by the clinician. WC users are susceptible to muscle imbalances. Nearly every motion and or repetitive motion is forward, working such areas as the shoulder flexors (pectoralis major and anterior deltoid) and shoulder internal rotators. These anterior muscles can become adaptively shortened, while the upper back muscles become weak and elongated. The typical posture of the WC user is rounded shoulders with mild thoracic kyphosis and a forward head. This posture can result in impingement of the soft tissue structures of the subacromial space.

WC Mobility. Depending on functional level, the patient is instructed on how to:

- Operate the wheel locks, foot supports, and armrests, and to use the mechanisms safely without tipping forward or sideways out of the chair seat.
- Transfer in and out of the chair with the least possible assistance. This may involve transfer training from the WC to the car seat.
- Propel the WC in all directions, and around corners.
- Perform a wheelie. A wheelie is performed by balancing on the rear wheels of a WC while the caster wheels are in the air. Wheelies are important for those patients who need to go up and down curbs independently when there are no curb ramps. Initially the clinician must be positioned behind the chair and move with the chair, with the hands held beneath the WC handles, ready to catch the WC if it tilts too far backwards. The patient should be taught on how to tuck their head into the chest, if they fall backward so that they do not hit the back of their head when performing the maneuver without assistance. To perform a wheelie, the patient is asked to place their hands at 11:00 on the wheels, then lean forward and arch their back. Initially the patient practices bouncing the body off the back of the chair and leaning back while holding the hands still—the front of the chair is raised by pushing backwards on the back of the chair. The patient practices until he or she can actually bounce the front end off the ground. By changing the COG (by pushing the chair forward while the body is going backwards) the patient will achieve a point of equilibrium.

Once the patient is able to bounce the front end off the ground and is able to find a point of equilibrium, they progress to reaching back and placing their hands at about 10:00 on the wheels. From this point, they lean forward, arch the back and then begin to push forward quickly while letting the body come back against the chair (when their back hits the chair, their hands should be in the 12:00 position). By continuing to lean back and while pushing the chair forward, the front end should start to leave the ground, and by the time the hands get to the 2:00 position, the front end should feel weightless, as the chair balances on the rear axle. To maintain equilibrium, the patient will need to be able to move the chair forward if the front end begins to fall down or backward if the chair begins to fall backward. This may be accomplished by sliding the hands back to about the 1:00 position, without taking the hands off the wheels. Once the chair is up and balanced, the patient will need to keep just a fraction of weight on the front end, so that if balance is lost the chair will fall forward, not backwards.

- "Pop a wheelie" and move forward and backward in the wheelie position. Once the patient is ready to try a wheelie independently, a good place to begin practicing is on carpeting, grass or sand.

Questions for this chapter and the entire book appear on the included CD-ROM, with additional questions at www.DuttonNPTE.com.

REFERENCES

1. Guide to physical therapist practice. *Phys Ther.* 2001;81:S13-S95.
2. May BJ: Amputation. In: O'Sullivan SB, Schmitz TJ, eds. *Physical Rehabilitation, 5th ed.* Philadelphia, PA: FA Davis. 2007:1031-1055.
3. Gailey RS: Considerations in treating amputees. In: Prentice WE, Voight ML, eds. *Techniques in Musculoskeletal Rehabilitation.* New York: McGraw-Hill. 2001:715-743.
4. White SC: *Health Care Financing Administration Common Procedure Coding System.* Washington, DC: US Government Printing Office. 2001.
5. Wu YJ, Chen SY, Lin MC, et al: Energy expenditure of wheeling and walking during prosthetic rehabilitation in a woman with bilateral transfemoral amputations. *Arch Phys Med Rehabil.* 2001;82:265-269.
6. Traugh GH, Corcoran PJ, Reyes RL: Energy expenditure of ambulation in patients with above-knee amputations. *Arch Phys Med Rehabil.* 1975;56:67-71.
7. Edelstein JE: Prosthetics. In: O'Sullivan SB, Schmitz TJ, eds. *Physical Rehabilitation, 5th ed.* Philadelphia, PA: FA Davis. 2007:1251-1286.
8. Ellis W, Kishner S: Gait analysis after amputation, Available at: http://www.emedicine.com/orthoped/topic633.htm, 2004.
9. Gailey RS: Orthotics in rehabilitation. In: Prentice WE, Voight ML, eds. *Techniques in Musculoskeletal Rehabilitation.* New York, McGraw-Hill. 2001:325-346.
10. Tiberio D, Hinkebein JR: Foot orthoses and shoe design. In: Placzek JD, Boyce DA, eds. *Orthopaedic Physical Therapy Secrets.* Philadelphia, Hanley & Belfus, Inc. 2001:455-462.
11. Duesterhaus MA, Duesterhaus S: *Patient Care Skills.* 2nd ed. East Norwalk, Connecticut: Appleton and Lange. 1990.
12. Baxter ML, Allington RO, Koepke GH: Weight-distribution variables in the use of crutches and canes. *Phys Ther.* 1969;49:360-365.
13. Edwards BG: Contralateral and ipsilateral cane usage by patients with total knee or hip replacement. *Arch Phys Med Rehabil.* 1986;67:734-740.
14. Oatis CA: Biomechanics of the hip. In: Echternach J ed. *Clinics in Physical Therapy: Physical Therapy of the Hip.* New York: Churchill Livingstone. 1990: 37-50.
15. Olsson EC, Smidt GL: Assistive devices. In: Smidt G, ed. *Gait in Rehabilitation.* New York: Churchill Livingstone. 1990:141-155.
16. Vargo MM, Robinson LR, Nicholas JJ: Contralateral vs. ipsilateral cane use: Effects on muscles crossing the knee joint. *Am J Phys Med Rehabil.* 1992;71:170-176.
17. Jebsen RH: Use and abuse of ambulation aids. *JAMA.* 1967;199:5-10.
18. Kumar R, Roe MC, Scremin OU: Methods for estimating the proper length of a cane. *Arch Phys Med Rehabil.* 1995;76:1173-1175.
19. Schmitz TJ: Locomotor training. In: O'Sullivan SB, Schmitz TJ, eds. *Physical Rehabilitation, 5th ed.* Philadelphia, PA: FA Davis. 2007; 523-560.
20. Li S, Armstrong CW, Cipriani D: Three-point gait crutch walking: variability in ground reaction force during weight bearing. *Am J Phys Med Rehabil.* 2001;86-92.

Pediatric Physical Therapy

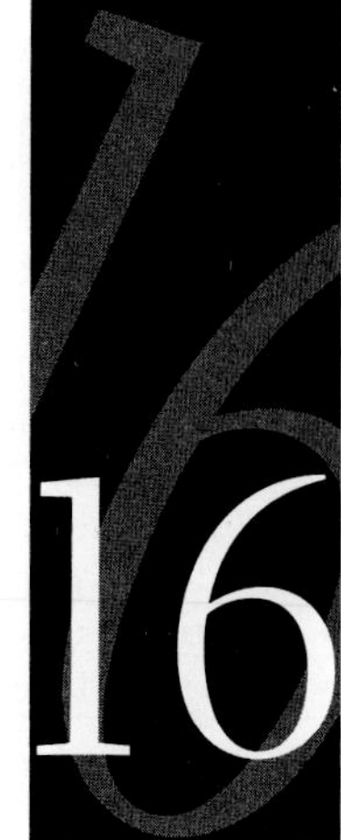

Physical therapy is a profession that focuses on the diagnosis and management of dysfunctional human movement throughout the life span. Pediatric physical therapy relates to the period (0-21 years) during which an individual ages, changes, evolves, and matures. Federal laws in the United States have been particularly supportive of pediatric practice:

- The Individuals with Disabilities Education Act (IDEA): under the requirements of this federal law, all children who have special needs must be supported in access to free and appropriate public education. This provision is based on an individualized plan. The plan for children who receive services at home (usually through age 3 years) under Part C of IDEA is called an Individual Family Service Plan (IFSP). For all children receiving services at school (usually after age 3 years to 21) under Part B of IDEA, the plan is called an Individualized Educational Plan (IEP).
  - Individual Family Service Plan (IFSP): designed to meet the needs of the family as they relate to their child's development, as well as meet the needs of the child.
  - Individual Educational Plan (IEP): identifies the student's specific learning expectations and outlines how the school will address these expectations through appropriate special education programs and services.
    - Identifies the methods by which the student's progress will be reviewed.
    - Covers all deficit areas, including communication, behavior, socialization, self-help, academics, perceptual-motor and gross-motor skills, vocational skills, and transition services, related services, and needed accommodations in both general (regular and vocational) and special education.

Study Pearl

Debates on whether changes in motor behavior result from external influences such as physical therapy, or to maturational influences remain unresolved.

Study Pearl

- A motor plan, which is made up of component motor programs, is an idea or plan for purposeful movement.[2]
- A motor program is an abstract representation that, when initiated, results in the production of a coordinated sequence of movements.[3] A motor program should be thought of as a prestructured plan in the memory that is prepared in advance of the movement, which when executed, results in a controlled contraction and relaxation of muscles causing a specific movement to occur without the involvement of feedback leading to corrections for errors in selection.

MOTOR CONTROL

The field of motor control is directed at studying the nature of movement and how the movement is controlled. Motor control refers to

TABLE 16-1. INTEGRAL ELEMENTS OF MOTOR CONTROL

The integral elements of motor control include

- The CNS functioning as a fundamentally active agent with the capacity to generate action.
- Motor patterns, which are the fundamental unit of neuromotor behavior.
- The involvement of processes of feedback and comparison of intention and result, which enable the modification of action.
  - Open loop feedback: feedback that is available to the performer but not used to control the action.
  - Closed loop feedback: a decision to move is made in the motor control center (brain). Some of the information is sent to the effector organs (muscles). The rest of the information is sent during the action and feedback monitors the effectiveness of the movement allowing for changes to be made during the movement.
- A distributed control system that delegates the control of behavior to the most appropriate subsystem.
- Memory structures such as schema that permit the transfer of skills to new situations

Data from Van Sant AF: Concepts of neural organization and movement, in Connolly BH, Montgomery PC, eds. *Therapeutic Exercise in Developmental Disabilities.* Thorofare, NJ: SLACK Inc. 2001:1-12.

processes of the brain and spinal cord that preside over the mechanisms essential to regulate or direct posture and movement using both perception and cognition.[1] Infants attain gross and fine motor control along a predetermined and sequential path. The integral elements of motor control are listed in Table 16-1.

The more common models of motor control are outlined in Table 16-2. Several factors govern movement, including the task, the environment, and the neuromotor capabilities of the individual. The multiple variables that contribute to the initiation and execution of a movement are outlined in Table 16-3.

Study Pearl

- Reflexes are evoked (involuntary, stereotyped, and graded) responses that depend on a stimulus to be initiated, such as sensory input. They have no threshold except that the stimulus must be great enough to activate the relevant input pathway.
- Fixed action patterns (sneezing, coughing), which are less graded and more complex than reflexes, are both involuntary and stereotyped. Typically these reflexes have a stimulus threshold that must be reached before they are triggered.
- Directed movements (reaching, kicking) are voluntary and complex, although generally they are neither stereotyped nor repetitive.
- Rhythmic motor patterns (walking, scratching, breathing) are complex, stereotyped, and repetitive, but they are subject to continuous voluntary control. Central pattern generators (CPGs) are neural networks that can, without rhythmic sensory or central input, produce rhythmic patterned outputs; these networks underlie the production of most rhythmic motor patterns, such as the gait cycle.[2-5]

MOTOR DEVELOPMENT

Motor development involves the processes of change in motor behavior that occur over relatively extended time periods.[1] Motor development is a complex process that has psychomotor, physiological, biochemical, biomechanical, psychosocial, and even gender considerations.[6] Motor development training is the method of producing any change in motor behavior that is related to the age of an individual, including age-related changes in posture and movement.

Motor Development Theories

Neural-Maturationist. The neural-maturation theory, pioneered by Gesell,[9,10] Shirley[11] and others, held the belief that motor patterns appear in orderly predetermined sequences, supported but not fundamentally changed by the environment. This theory is based on the existence of hierarchic maturation of neural control centers that are the main constraints for developmental progress; basic motor skills, such as standing and walking, are not learned by experience but are the result of cerebral maturation (developmental sequences and milestones of development).[12] Development follows a structural sequence:

- Superior to inferior
- Central-to-distal

Cognitive Development and Theories. Cognitive development normally occurs in a sequential manner (Table 16-4). A number of cognitive theories exist.

TABLE 16-2. THEORIES OF MOTOR CONTROL[a]

THEORY	DESCRIPTION
Maturational based	**Structure-Function Organization and Reflex-Chaining** Sensory inputs are a necessary prerequisite for efferent motor output (stimulus-evoked behavior)—movement occurs in response to a stimulus. Movement is the result of predictable anatomic changes in neural pathways and complex movement occurs as the result of a compounding of reflex movements. **Hierarchical** The nervous system is organized as a hierarchy with each successively high-level exerting control over the level below it. Separation between voluntary (higher-level) and reflexive (lower-level) movement. Reflexes work together, or in sequence to achieve a common purpose, and thus provide the building blocks of complex behavior. Forms the basis of most neurotherapeutic approaches used in physical therapy (Bobath, Brunnstrom). Useful for explaining spontaneous and volitional movement.
Learning based	**Response Chaining** More emphasis on the role of the environment—action not bound to a specific stimulus (neither spontaneous or volitional movements are dependent on external agents for their initiation). Environment is the controller of the automating process. Linkages exist between muscle groups that allow for movement combinations (synergies). A full complement of motor programs are available and used appropriately in functional contexts prior to birth.[b] Movement dysfunction may be due to motor program centers in the brain and motor program centers at lower levels. **Adams's Closed-Loop Theory**[c] In a closed loop process, sensory feedback is used for the ongoing production of skilled movement. The closed loop theory of motor learning also proposed that two distinct types of memory were important in this process: ▶ Memory trace: used in the selection and initiation of the movement. ▶ Perceptual trace: built up over a period of practice and becomes the internal reference of correctness. This theory proposes that when learning a new movement skill, an individual gradually develops a perceptual trace for the movement that serves as a guide for later movements, and that the more an individual practices the specific movement, the stronger the perceptual trace becomes. Theoretically the more time spent in practicing the movement as accurately as possible, the better the learning.
Schmidt's schema theory[d]	Schmidt's theory emphasizes open-loop control processes and the generalized motor program concept. Three constructs: general motor programs and two types of memory traces, recall schema and recognition schema. When learning a new motor program, an individual learns a general set of rules that can be applied to a variety of contexts. The generalized motor program is considered to contain the rules for creating the spatial and temporal patterns of muscle activity needed to carry out a given movement.
Dynamical-based systems[e]	Seeks to address what drives skill acquisition and how an individual moves from one developmental stage of skill to another. The system is composed of a number of identifiable variables (muscle power, body mass, arousal, neural networks, motivation, and environmental forces [gravity, friction, etc]) Movement emerges due to interaction of subsystems, which work together and which change over time. Three key hypotheses: ▶ A developing organism that is genetically endowed with spontaneously generated behaviors that make up the basic movement repertoire. ▶ A sensory system capable of detecting and recognizing movements having adaptive value. ▶ The system has the ability to select movements having adaptive value by varying synaptic strength within and between brain circuits such that successive event selections will progressively modify the movement repertoire.

(Conitnued)

TABLE 16-2. THEORIES OF MOTOR CONTROL[a] *(Conitnued)*

THEORY	DESCRIPTION
Central pattern generators (CPGs)[f-k]	These are proposed to account for the basic neural organization and function required to execute coordinated, rhythmic movements, such as locomotion, chewing, grooming (eg, scratching), and respiration. Commonly defined as inter neural networks, located in either of the spinal cord or brainstem, that can order the selection and sequencing of motor neurons independent of descending or peripheral afferent neural input. Also modulate the inputs they received, gating potentially disruptive reflex actions such as nociceptive activation of the flexor withdrawal reflex when a limb is fully loaded during the stance phase of locomotion.

[a]Bradley NS, Westcott SL: Motor control: Developmental aspects of motor control in skill acquisition. In: Campbell SK, Vander Linden DW, Palisano RJ, eds. *Physical Therapy for Children, 3rd ed.* St. Louis, MO: Saunders. 2006:77-130.
[b]Comparetti AM: The neurophysiologic and clinical implications of studies on fetal motor behavior. *Semin Perinatol.* 1981;5:183-189.
[c]Shumway-Cook A, Woollacott MH: Motor learning and recovery of function. In: Shumway-Cook A, Woollacott MH, eds. *Motor Control: Theory and Practical Applications, 2nd ed.* Philadelphia, PA: Lippincott Williams & Wilkins. 2001:26-49.
[d]Schmidt RA: Motor schema theory after 27 years: reflections and implications for a new theory. *Res Q Exerc Sport.* 2003;74:366-375.
[e]Thelen E, Corbetta D: Exploration and selection in the early acquisition of skill. *Int Rev Neurobiol.* 1994;37:75-102.
[f]Thelen E: Motor development. A new synthesis. *Am Psychol.* 1995;50:79-95.
[g]Grillner S, Wallen P: Central pattern generators for locomotion, with special reference to vertebrates. *Annu Rev Neurosci.* 1985;8:233-261.
[h]Hooper SL: Central pattern generators. *Curr Biol.* 2000;10:R176.
[i]Marder E, Bucher D: Central pattern generators and the control of rhythmic movements. *Curr Biol.* 2001;11:R986-R996.
[j]Prosiegel M, Holing R, Heintze M, et al: The localization of central pattern generators for swallowing in humans—a clinical-anatomical study on patients with unilateral paresis of the vagal nerve, Avellis' syndrome, Wallenberg's syndrome, posterior fossa tumours and cerebellar hemorrhage. *Acta Neurochir Suppl.* 2005;93:85-88.
[k]Verdaasdonk BW, Koopman HF, Helm FC: Energy efficient and robust rhythmic limb movement by central pattern generators. *Neural Netw.* 2006;19:388-400. Epub Dec 13, 2005.

Cognitive-Behavioral. Cognitive progression occurs through Pavlovian responses to previous stimulation, and by operant processes where responses are controlled by consequences.[14] Behavior is goal-oriented—actions are motivated by a desire to achieve a goal or to avoid unpleasant circumstances. Motivation has two purposes:

- To create a demand for the goal.
- To establish the actions that an individual will concentrate on.

TABLE 16-3. MOTOR CONTROL VARIABLES

VARIABLE	DESCRIPTION
Sensorimotor	Those physiologic mechanisms or processes that reside within the nervous system, eg, central pattern generators (CPGs). Movement synergies and neural mechanisms that alter or regulate them.
Mechanical	Changes in total body mass and relative distribution of mass during development are accompanied by changes in length and center of mass of the body segment, which in turn alter inertial forces due to gravity and during movement. The viscoelastic properties of musculoskeletal tissues.
Cognitive	May include variables that are dependent on conscious and subconscious processes such as reasoning, memory, or judgment to optimize performance (arousal, motivation, anticipatory or feedforward strategies, a selective use of feedback, practice, and memory).
Task requirements	May include any variable that can contribute to or in some way alter movement, including biomechanical requirements, meaningfulness, predictability, or any other variable associated with a given movement context.

Data from Bradley NS, Westcott SL: Motor control: developmental aspects of motor control in skill acquisition. In: Campbell SK, Vander Linden DW, Palisano RJ, eds. *Physical Therapy for Children, 3rd ed.* St. Louis, MO: Saunders. 2006:77-130.

TABLE 16-4. COGNITIVE DEVELOPMENT

AGE GROUP	COGNITIVE DEVELOPMENT
Preschool (3-6 years)	Can remember basic information and recall that information on demand.
	Can answer simple *who* and *what* questions.
	Tend to learn from trial and error.
	Have short attention spans (5-15 min), and poor selective attention.
	Can identify the missing parts of familiar objects.
	Can follow simple rules but need visual cues and frequent reminders.
Middle childhood (6-11 years)	See things as here and now, right or wrong, and black or white.
	Engage in magical thinking and may believe they have unique powers.
	Can understand the intent of instructions given and can follow directions.
	Can apply factual knowledge to familiar situations.
	Can recognize differences between personal performance and the performance or skill of others.

There are two main types of motivators: deprivation and incentives.

- Deprivation causes a desire to obtain the goal.
- An incentive motivates behavior based merely upon the sufficiency of the reward.

Cognitive Piagetian. Piagetian[15] theory focuses on accommodation and assimilation.

- Assimilation: the process of taking one's environment and new information and fitting it into pre-existing cognitive schemas.
- Accommodation: the process of taking one's environment and new information, and altering one's preexisting schemas in order to fit in the new information.

The four stages of development described by Piaget are

- Sensorimotor. Infants construct an understanding of the world by coordinating sensory experiences (eg, seeing and hearing) with physical or motor actions. Infants gain knowledge of the world from the physical actions they perform on it and progress from reflexive, instinctual action at birth to the beginning of symbolic thought toward the end of the stage.
- Preoperational. The child learns to use and to represent objects by images, words, and drawings.
- Concrete operational. Occurs between the ages of 7 and 11 years and is characterized by the appropriate use of logic. Important processes during this stage are outlined in Table 16-5.[15]
- Formal operational. Individuals progress beyond concrete experiences and begin to think abstractly, reason logically and draw conclusions from the information available, as well as apply all these processes to hypothetical situations.

However, as Piaget himself noted, development does not always progress in the smooth manner his theory seems to predict, and that the stage model is at best a useful approximation. Therefore, the impact of Piagetian theory on pediatric physical therapy is primarily due to the inclusion of problem-solving activities in therapeutic programs to assist in the cognitive-motivational aspects of facilitating motor development.[14]

Study Pearl

Recent motor control and development theories include[1,7,8]

- Motor control theory (Dynamical pattern theory): principles of motor coordination that include order parameters (variables that characterize coordinated behavior) and control parameters (variables that initiate change in order parameters). Some behavioral patterns are more common than others.
- Motor development theory (Dynamical action theory): movement is an evolving property based on multiple factors (eg, maturation of the neural system, muscle force, biomechanical leverages, cognitive awareness, and constraints of the task and physical environment).

Study Pearl

Pediatric physical therapy initially developed according to this theoretic model, emphasizing the assessment stages of reflex development and motor milestones as reflections of increasingly higher levels of neural maturation.[13] The intervention for children with CNS dysfunction was based around methods to inhibit the primitive reflexes and emphasize the facilitation of the righting and equilibrium reactions.[14]

TABLE 16-5. IMPORTANT PROCESSES DURING THE CONCRETE OPERATIONAL STAGE

PROCESS	DESCRIPTION
Seriation	The ability to sort objects in an order according to size, shape, or any other characteristic. For example, if given different-shaded objects they can make a color gradient.
Transitivity	The ability to recognize logical relationships among elements in a serial order (eg, if A is taller than B, and B is taller than C, then A must be taller than C).
Classification	The ability to name and identify sets of objects according to appearance, size or other characteristic, including the idea that one set of objects can include another.
Decentering	Can take into account multiple aspects of a problem to solve it. For example, will no longer perceive an exceptionally wide but short pan to contain less than a normally wide, taller pan.
Reversibility	Understands that numbers or objects can be changed, and then returned to their original state. For this reason, a child will be able to rapidly determine that if $4 + 4$ equals x, $x - 4$ will equal 4, the original quantity.
Conservation	The ability to understand that the quantity, length or number of items is unrelated to the arrangement or appearance of the object or items.

Dynamic. Thelen and colleagues[16-18] have proposed a dynamical functional perspective on motor development. This theory[18,19]

- emphasizes process rather than the finished product or hierarchically structured plans.
- places neural maturation on an equal plane with other structures and processes that interact to promote motor development.
- emphasizes that the environment is as important as the organism, and that developmental change is seen not as a series of discrete stages, but as a series of states of stability, instability, and phase shifts in which new states become stable aspects of behavior.

According to this theory, cooperating systems, including musculoskeletal components, sensory systems, central sensorimotor integrated mechanisms, and arousal and motivation, become progressively incorporated with the self organized properties of the system to gradually optimize skilled function.[19,20]

Study Pearl

- Menstrual age: the age of a fetus or newborn, in weeks, from the first day of the mother's last normal menstrual period.
- Gestational age: also known as fetal age, is the time measured from the first day of the woman's last menstrual cycle to the current date—the time inside of the uterus. A pregnancy of normal gestation is approximately 40 weeks, with a normal range of 38 to 42 weeks (Table 16-7).
- Preterm: born before 37 weeks of gestational age.[21]
- Post term: born after 42 weeks.[21]
- Conceptional age: the age of a fetus or newborn in weeks since conception.
- Chronological age: the time elapsed from date of birth to present day.
- Corrected age: based on the age the child would be if the pregnancy had actually gone to term. The corrected age, generally used for the first 2 years of life, can be calculated as the chronological age minus the number of weeks/months premature.

PRENATAL DEVELOPMENT

The prenatal period of development (Table 16-6) is also known as the gestational period.

The prenatal stage of development can be divided into three separate periods:

- Germinal: starts at the time of fertilization and last 2 weeks.
- Embryonic: starts two weeks after conception and lasts about 6 weeks.
- Fetal: starts at 7 weeks of gestation and ends at birth. All the preliminary feeding movements, including mouth opening and closing, sustained lip closure, and tongue movements, are present at 14 to 15 weeks.

TABLE 16-6. DEVELOPMENTAL CHARACTERISTICS OF THE EMBRYO ACCORDING TO GESTATIONAL AGE

GESTATIONAL AGE	DEVELOPMENTAL CHARACTERISTICS
2.5 weeks	Neural plate formation; shape and length begin to be determined.
3 weeks	Cell differentiation occurs-formation of ectoderm (nervous system, sensory systems, and many other tissues), mesoderm (muscles, skeleton, and other tissues), endoderm (respiratory system, digestive system, and other tissues).
End of 4 weeks gestation	Fetus reaches a length of 0.75-1 cm and weighs 400 mg. Spinal cord forms and fuses at the center. Lateral wings bend forward, meeting at the center and will eventually form the body. Head tilts forward and makes up about one-third of the entire structure. The rudimentary heart beats a regular rhythm. Arms and legs have the appearance of small buds. The beginnings of eyes, ears, and a nose are evident.
End of 8 weeks gestation	Embryo now a fetus. Fetus reaches a length of 1 in (2.5 cm) and weighs 20 g. The heart has a definite septum and valves. Extremities have lengthened. External genitalia are evident, but gender is not obvious.
End of 12 weeks gestation	Fetus reaches a length of 2.8-3.6 in (7-9 cm) and weighs 45 g. Some movement occurring, but usually too faint for the mother to feel. Fetal heart can be heard with a Doppler.
End of 16 weeks gestation	Fetus reaches a length of 4-7 in (10-17 cm) and weighs 55-120 g. Liver and pancreatic secretions are present. Fetus starts to make sucking motions with the mouth.
End of 20 weeks gestation	Fetus reaches a length of 10 in (25 cm) and weighs 223 g. The mother starts to feel fetal movement. Fetal heart tones can be heard with a stethoscope.
End of 24 weeks gestation	Fetus reaches a length of 11-14 in (28-36 cm) and weighs 550 g. Eyebrows and eyelashes are clearly formed. Eyelids, which fused in the 12th week, start to open. Pupils are reactive to light. Fetus could possibly be viable if born now and cared for in a neonatal intensive care unit. Surfactant, a phospholipid substance essential to lung function, is formed and excreted by cells in the alveoli.
End of 28 weeks gestation	Fetus reaches a length of 14-15 in (35-38 cm) and weighs 1200 g. Testes begin descent into the scrotal sac from the lower abdominal cavity if the fetus is male. The brain is rapidly developing.
End of 32 weeks gestation	Fetus reaches a length of 15-27 in (38-43 cm) and weighs 1600 g. Fetus hears sounds and responds with movement. Delivery presentation (vertex or breech) may be assumed. Iron stores begin to develop.
End of 36 weeks gestation	Fetus reaches a length of 17-20 in (42-49 cm) and weighs 5-6 lb (1900-2700 g). Soles of the feet have only one or two creases. The central nervous system has greater control over body functions.
End of 40 weeks gestation	Fetus reaches a length of 19-21 in (48-52 cm) and weighs 7-7.5 lb (3000 g). Fingernails have grown over the fingertips. There are creases covering at least two-thirds of the soles of the feet. Fetus kicks vigorously and may cause the mother discomfort.

Data from Forslund M, Bjerre I: Neurological assessment of preterm infants at term conceptional age in comparison with normal full-term infants. *Early Hum Dev.* 1983;8:195-208; Piper MC, Byrne PJ, Pinnell LE: Influence of gestational age on early neuromotor development in the preterm infant. *Am J Perinatol.* 1989;6:405-411; and Awoust J, Levi S: Neurological maturation of the human fetus. *Ultrasound Med Biol Suppl.* 1983;2:583-587.

DEVELOPMENTAL MILESTONES

A milestone is an important point in development or an important functional ability achieved during the developmental process. The various developmental milestones for both sensory and motor development are depicted in Tables 16-8, 16-9, and 16-10.

TABLE 16-7. ASSESSMENT OF GESTATIONAL AGE AT BIRTH

EXTERNAL CHARACTERISTIC	28 WEEKS	32 WEEKS	36 WEEKS	40 WEEKS
Ear cartilage	Pinna soft, remains folded	Pinna harder, but remains folded	Pinna harder, springs back into place when folded	Pinna firm, stands erect from head
Breast tissue	None	None	Nodule 1-2 mm in diameter	Nodule 6-7 mm in diameter
Male genitalia	Testes undescended, scrotal surface smooth	Testes in inguinal canal, a few scrotal rugae	Testes high in scrotum, more scrotal rugae	Testes descended, scrotum pendulous, covered in rugae
Female genitalia	Prominent clitoris with small, widely separated labia	Prominent clitoris; larger, well-separated labia	Clitoris less prominent, labia majora cover labia minora	Clitoris covered by labia majora
Plantar surface of foot	Smooth, no creases	1 or 2 anterior creases	2 or 3 anterior creases	Creases cover the sole

Study Pearl

- Neonatal: the period from birth until 2 weeks. The posture of the neonate is characterized by flexion.
- Infancy: the period from birth until the child is able to stand and walk. Typically infancy lasts approximately 1 year.

Approximate Ages of Epiphyseal Closures

Refer to Tables 16-11 and 16-12.

Automatic Postural Responses

Automatic postural responses (Table 16-13) permit an individual to restore or maintain body equilibrium and remain functionally oriented to space. Postural responses are dependent on correct organization of the visual, vestibular, and somatosensory systems (see Chapter 9).

MOTOR PROGRAMMING

Motor programs allow for movements to occur in the absence of sensation or in situations in which limitations in speed processing feedback negate control.[2] Two control systems coexist:

- Open-loop control system: occurs virtually without the influence of peripheral feedback or error detection processes.[2]
- Closed-loop control system: employs feedback and a reference for correctness to compute error and initiate subsequent corrections. Together with feedback, this process plays a critical role in the learning of new motor skills, and in shaping and correction of ongoing movements.[2]

TABLE 16-8. MAJOR MILESTONES

MILESTONE	APPROXIMATE AGE (IN MONTHS) ABLE TO PERFORM
Roll	3-4
Sit independently	5-6
Belly crawl	7-8
Creep (quadruped)	8-9
Pull to stand	9-10
Cruise	11
Walk	12

Data from van Blankenstein M, Welbergen UR, de Haas JH: *Le Developpement du Nourrisson: Sa Premiere Annee en 130 Photographies*. Paris, Presses Universitaires de France. 1962.

TABLE 16-9. GROSS MOTOR CHECKLIST

MONTH/YEAR	POSITION/ACTIVITY	MILESTONE
1 month	Prone	Lifts head and turns to side
2 months	Vertical	Rights head
	Prone	Recurrently lifts head to 45 degrees
	Supported sitting	Head erect and bobbing
3 months	Prone	Lifts head to 45 degrees (sustained)
		Recurrently lifts head to 90 degrees
		Supports self on forearms
		Rolls to side
4 months	Prone	Lifts head to 90 degrees (sustained)
		Rolls to supine
	Supine	Rolls to prone
		Assists with head when pulled to sit
	Supported sitting	Head steady, set forward
5 months	Prone	Supports self on extended arms
		Rolls to supine segmentally
	Supine	Lifts head when pulled to sitting
		Rolls to prone segmentally
	Supported sitting	Head erect and steady
	Standing	Takes weight on lower extremities
6 months	Prone	Can lift one arm and weight bear on the other
	Sitting	Pivots in a circle
		Erect for one minute with hands propped forward
		Protective extension sideways
7 months	Prone	Up on all fours
		Progress is forward in any manner
	Sitting	Erect without support but unsteady
		Protective extension forward
8 months	Prone	Crawls in any manner
	Sitting	Erect without support
	Standing	Pulls to stand
9 months	Prone/supine	Rotates to sitting
	Sitting	Goes to prone
		Protective extension backward
	Standing	Pulls to standing with rotation and support
10 months	Sitting	Pivots
	Locomotion	Cruises
12 months	Locomotion	Stands up without support
		Walks with high guard
15 months	Kneeling	Kneels without support
	Locomotion	Walks with medium guard
		Can stop, start, and change directions without falling
18 months	Locomotion	Walks with no guard carrying object
		Walks fast with feet flat
		Squats to play
		Goes up/down stairs on all fours
2 years	Locomotion	Walks up/down stairs one at the time holding rail
		Walks with heel-total gait
		Runs forward well
3 years	Locomotion/skills	Jumps forward on both feet
		Alternates feet going upstairs
		Walks backward easily
		Hops up to 6 times
4 years	Locomotion/skills	Walks downstairs with alternating feet, holding rail
		Skips on one foot
		Throws overhand
		Moves backward and forward with equal agility

(*Continued*)

TABLE 16-9. GROSS MOTOR CHECKLIST *(Conitnued)*

MONTH/YEAR	POSITION/ACTIVITY	MILESTONE
5 years	Locomotion/skill	Pedals and steers tricycle well Able to walk long distances on toes Gallops Hops up to nine times using 1 foot Smooth reciprocal movements in walking and running.
6 years	Skill	Throws a small ball at a target and hits the target Broad jump up to 3 ft

MOTOR LEARNING

Study Pearl

Feedback is considered one of the most powerful variables affecting motor learning.

Motor learning involves a set of processes associated with the practice or experience of new strategies for sensing as well as moving, which lead to relatively permanent changes in the capability of producing skilled action (Table 16-14). The process of motor learning leads first to attainment and later to perfection of a specific motor skill.

Feedback can be either intrinsic or extrinsic in origin:

- Intrinsic: inherent sensory information that comes from the specialized receptors in muscle, joint, tendon, and skin as well as that from visual and auditory receptors either during or following movement production.
- Extrinsic: augmented information about movement provided to the performer from an external source. Extrinsic feedback has been described as motivational as it relates to goal achievement. Two major types of extrinsic feedback are recognized:
  - Knowledge of results (KR): KR can be defined as verbal, post response, augmented feedback about the response outcome. When KR is used, subjects tend to practice longer, try harder, and stay interested in the task longer than when KR is not used.
  - Knowledge of performance (KP): in contrast to KR, KP is information about the movement pattern produced, rather than the outcome of the movement.

Study Pearl

Learning is not directly observable and can be defined as a relatively permanent change in the capability for responding that results from practice or experience. True motor learning occurs when the subject can demonstrate a performance when the extrinsic feedback is withdrawn.

In the clinical setting, KP is used more often. This is because

- The outcome (KR) is often obvious to the patient, while the movement response to cause the outcome is not so obvious and needs to be supplied by the clinician.
- There are often several components to the desired movement outcome.
- In some disease states, the intrinsic feedback is often distorted or, in severe cases absent, and must be supplemented or replaced with extrinsic feedback, usually provided by the clinician, or educated family member/caregiver.

There are four essential features related to the motor response that the performer uses when learning:

- The initial conditions before the movement
- Which parameters or motor commands were assigned to the generalized motor program

TABLE 16-10. DEVELOPMENT MILESTONES ACCORDING TO POSITION

AGE	PRONE	SUPINE	SITTING	STANDING	COMMENTS
Neonate: 0-14 days	Physiological flexor activity in the ankles, knees, hips, and elbows.		Lack of trunk muscular control—the back is round and the head flops forward.	Demonstrates the remarkable capabilities of primary standing—automatic walking when supported.	Grasp is a reflex in which the hand automatically closes on objects the baby touches due to tactile stimulation of the palm of the hand. The hands will randomly swing out wide (neonatal reaching). No organized response to postural perturbations.[2]
Newborn (0-1 month)	Arms and hands tucked in close to the body, rounded shoulders, elbows flexed, and hands are closed loosely and positioned close to the mouth.	No control of neck flexion in supine is present, so the baby cannot maintain the head in midline, but keeps it rotated to one side.	Sacral sitting if supported.		Period dominated by physiological flexion. Poor head control. Very active when awake. Random wide ranging movements primarily in supine. Soft tissue tightness holds the hips in flexion/abduction/external rotation. The baby touches and feels, and is soon sucking and learning about the hands. Vision limited to 8-9 ft. Skeletal characteristics include coxa valgus, genu varum, tibial varum and torsion, calcaneal varus, and occasionally, metatarsus adductus.
1 month	Head lifting in prone may appear to be improved. Increased cervical rotation mobility. Elbows moving forward, arms away from body.	Head to one side resulting in lateral vision becoming dominant and eye hand regard and uncontrolled swiping at toys at the baby's side is frequently observed. Wider ranges of movement. Heels hit surface.		Positive support and primary walking reflexes in supported standing.	Decreasing physiologic flexion (less "recoil"). Increasing level of arousal. Neonatal reaching. Able to visually track a moving object horizontally.
2 months	Able to hold the head steady in all positions and to raise it about 45 degrees due to increased activity of active shoulder abduction. The arms and hands begin to work to support the actions of the head and trunk. Hand movements more goal directed.	Increased asymmetry with more visual interaction.	Head lag occurs with pull to sit. Begins to develop head and trunk control and more attempts at sustained extension. Head bobs in supported sitting.	May not accept weight on lower extremities (astasia-abasia). No more neonatal stepping.	Increasing asymmetry/decreased tone Increased head and trunk control lets the baby use the arms for reaching and playing rather than for support. Holds objects placed in the hand.

(*Continued*)

TABLE 16-10. DEVELOPMENT MILESTONES ACCORDING TO POSITION *(Conitnued)*

AGE	PRONE	SUPINE	SITTING	STANDING	COMMENTS
3 months	Change occurs in the general position of the arms, from a position where the arms are tucked in close to the body with the elbows near the ribs, to one in which the elbows are almost in line with the shoulders, which allows for forearm weight-bearing. Legs abducted and externally rotated Face can be raised 45-90 degrees when prone.	Beginning of symmetry is evident—the head is in midline with chin tucking and the hands are in midline on the chest/to mouth.	Attempts pull to sit but falls forward.	Minimal weight through extended legs.	Period of controlled symmetry. The grasp becomes more controlled and voluntary and the hands can adjust to the shape of objects. Symmetry is very obvious in the lower extremities as they assume their "frog legged" position of hip abduction, external rotation and flexion and knee flexion. The feet come together and the baby is able to take some weight with toes curled in supported standing.
4 months	Able to prop up on the forearms and look around. The head and chest are lifted and maintained in midline. Prone pivots.	Can roll from prone to side and from supine to side, although these are usually accidental occurrences. Able to bring the hands together in the space above the body due to increased shoulder girdle control. Hands to knees. Active anterior and posterior pelvic tilt.	Assists in pull to sit by flexing elbows. Very minimal head bobbing—stabilized through shoulder elevation. Tends to sit in a slumped position. Protective reactions develop, first laterally, then forward, and then backward.	Because of the increased head-neck-trunk control, the baby is able to take more of his/her weight when placed in standing, and can now be held by the hands instead of at the chest. Legs are extended and the toes are clawed.	Ulnar palmar grasp develops. Able to perform bilateral reaching with the forearm pronated when the trunk is supported. Sidelying Starts hand to mouth activities. Emerging righting and equilibrium reactions. Findings of concern include poor midline orientation (persistent ATNR), imbalance between flexors and extensors, poor visual attention/tracking, persistent wide base of support in standing, and poor antigravity strength.
5 months	Equilibrium reactions begin in prone position. Can roll from prone to supine. Able to assume and maintain a position of extended arm weight bearing in prone and can weight shift from one forearm to the other and to reach out with one arm.	Chin tuck, downward gaze. Feet to mouth. Anterior and posterior pelvic tilt more active. Active roll to sideline. Manipulation and transfer of toys.	There is no head lag when the baby is pulled from supine to sit. Assists during pull to sit with chin tuck and head lift. Able to control head in supported sitting, although still leans forward from the hips.	Tends to be able to bear almost all weight.	Findings of concern include ▶ Poor antigravity flexion ▶ Poor tolerance for prone/inability to bear weight through extended arms/ poor weight shifting

6 months	Completes turning and can roll from prone to supine. Can lay prone on hands with the elbows extended and is able to weight shift on extended arms from hand to hand and to reach forward due to sufficient shoulder girdle control.	Active hip extension. Transfers toys. Flexes head independently.	Can sit independently, although initially uses the arms and hands for support.	In standing, is able to bear weight on both legs and bounce and can independently hold onto the support of a person due to sufficient trunk and hip control.	Uses rolling for locomotion. Findings of concern include: ▶ Poor tolerance for prone position. ▶ Paucity of movement patterns. ▶ Inability to sit independently. ▶ Inability to roll or rolling with neck hyperextension.
7 months	Trunk and arms free. Able to achieve and maintain the quadruped position, although prone is usually the preferred position. Can pivot on belly, often moving body in a circle.	Tends to avoid except for playing	Protective reactions more consistent. Able to perform trunk rotation in sitting. Can assume the sitting position from the quadruped position.	Can often pull to stand from the quadruped position. Able to actively flex and extend both legs simultaneously while standing and supporting independently.	Very active with large variety of movements and positions available May show fear of strangers. Findings of concern include ▶ Lack of weight shifting in prone ▶ Reliance on more primitive movement patterns as compensations in order to explore ▶ Inability to assume or maintain quadruped ▶ Poor weight-bearing in supported stance.
8 months	Minimal time spent in prone—able to creep/crawl in the quadruped position at nine months as the primary means of locomotion.		Full equilibrium reactions in sitting, and the beginning of equilibrium reactions in quadruped. Able to side-sit and is also able to go from sitting to quadruped. May also kneel	Can stand by leaning on supporting surfaces. Able to pull to stand. Early walking, cruising	Can reach out for objects and reach across the midline of the body without losing balance. The thumb can wrap around objects-now the baby can hold two small objects, such as cubes, in one hand. Findings of concern include: ▶ Poor sitting ability ▶ Unable to use hand for play ▶ Overall reliance on upper extremities
9 months			Large variety of sitting positions and movement. Pivoting/long sitting. Sitting often used as a transitional position	Uses arms, hands, and body together while pulling up to standing through half-kneel position (nine months). Immature stepping. The sequence in rising to standing is kneeling, half kneeling, weight shift forward, squat, then upright.	The index finger starts to move separately from the rest of the hand when poking at objects. This leads to the pincer grasp, with the tips of the thumb and index finer meeting in a precise pattern. The baby's ability to let go of an object smoothly has also improved. Findings of concern include: ▶ Poor standing control ▶ Poor/inadequate sitting ▶ Inability to assume quadruped

(*Continued*)

TABLE 16-10. DEVELOPMENT MILESTONES ACCORDING TO POSITION *(Conitnued)*

AGE	PRONE	SUPINE	SITTING	STANDING	COMMENTS
10 months			Arms reach above shoulders. Active side sitting. Rarely stationary	Creeping/climbing. Legs very active. "High guard" Cruising with wide base of support	
11 months			Able to play and cross midline	Mostly using legs Very symmetrical standing with a wide base of support.	
12 to 15 months				Many babies are walking unassisted.	Able to self feed. Can build a tower of two cubes.
Two years				Runs well. Goes upstairs using reciprocal pattern (reciprocal stair climbing).	

Data from van Blankenstein M, Welbergen UR, de Haas JH: *Le Developpement du Nourrisson: Sa Premiere Annee en 130 Photographies.* Paris, Presses Universitaires de France; 1962 and Prechtl HF: New perspectives in early human development. *Eur J Obstet Gynecol Reprod Biol.* 1986;21:347-355.

TABLE 16-11. APPROXIMATE AGES OF EPIPHYSEAL CLOSURES

BODY AREA	AGE
Vertebrae, sacrum, clavicle, sternum and ribs	25
Scapula	15-17
Humerus	Head fused with shaft—20
	Lateral epicondyle—16-17
	Medial epicondyle—18
Ulna	Olecranon—16
	Distal end—20
Radius	Head and shaft—18-19
	Distal end to shaft—20
Acetabulum	20-25
Femur	Greater and lesser trochanters—18
	Femoral head—18
	Distal end—20
Tibia	Proximal end—20
	Distal end—18
Fibula	Proximal end—25
	Distal end—20

Data from Pick TP, Howden R: *Gray's Anatomy.* 15th ed. New York, Barnes & Noble Books; 1995.

- The actual consequences of the movement in the form of extrinsic feedback
- The actual intrinsic sensory feedback from the response

Study Pearl

It is important to note that errors are not detrimental to learning, but rather, they can provide valuable information if extrinsic feedback is provided in the form of KR and/or KP.

MOTOR LEARNING THEORIES

Theories of motor learning (Table 16-15) describe hypotheses regarding how movement is learned. Early theories believed that learning was a process of "habit" formation.[22]

PRIMITIVE REFLEXES

Reflexes are involuntary movements or actions that help to identify normal brain and nerve activity. As a general rule, influence of the primitive reflexes is not readily observed in the healthy, normally

TABLE 16-12. APPROXIMATE CHRONOLOGICAL AGE THE EPIPHYSEAL CLOSURES

APPROXIMATE AGE	AREA
7-8	Inferior rami of pubis and ischium almost complete.
15-17	Upper extremity: scapula, lateral epicondyles of humerus, olecranon process of ulna.
18-19	Upper extremity: medial epicondyle of humerus, head and shaft of radius.
	Lower extremity: femoral head and greater and lesser trochanters, distal end of tibia.
20	Upper extremity: humeral head, distal ends of radius and ulna.
	Lower extremity: distal ends of femur and fibula, proximal end of tibia.
20-25	Lower extremity: acetabulum in pelvis.
25	Spine: vertebrae and sacrum.
	Upper extremity: clavicle.
	Lower extremity: proximal end of fibula.
	Thorax: sternum and ribs.

Data from Pick TP, Howden R: *Gray's Anatomy, 15th ed.* New York, NY: Barnes & Noble Books. 1995.

TABLE 16-13. AUTOMATIC POSTURAL RESPONSES

POSTURAL RESPONSE	DESCRIPTION
Righting	Orientation of the head in space so that the eyes and mouth are in a horizontal plane or the body parts are restored to proper alignment. Includes vertical righting (orienting head to vertical) and rotational righting (orientation following rotation of a body segment). Operates regardless of the position of the body or where the body is in the environment. Normally develops during the first 6 months of life.
Equilibrium	Complex responses to changes of posture or movement which seek to restore disturbed balance when the body's base of support is subjected to perturbation (push, pull, or tilt). Develops in a position after a child has learned to assume the position (prone, supine, sitting, quadruped, and standing) independently. Response is generally in the opposite direction of the force. ▶ Spinal column concavity on the uphill side on an unstable base of support. ▶ Spinal column concavity on the side of the pushing force on a stable base of support. ▶ Rotation of the upper trunk and head toward the midline and counter rotations of the lower trunk may occur. ▶ Abduction and extension of the extremities on the downhill side or in the direction of push.
Protective (parachute or propping)	Extension movements of the extremities generally in the same direction of the displacing force which shifts the body's center of gravity. Highly context dependent. Can be backward, forward, or laterally. Develop laterally by 6-11 months, then forwards, and finally backwards by 9-12 months.

Data from Effgen SK: Developing postural control. In: Connolly BH, Montgomery PC, eds. *Therapeutic Exercise in Developmental Disabilities.* Thorofare, NJ: SLACK Inc. 2001:111-123; Milani-Comparetti A, Gidoni EA: Routine developmental examination in normal and retarded children. *Dev Med Child Neurol.* 1967;9:631-968. Dargassies SS: Neurodevelopmental symptoms during the first year of life. I. Essential landmarks for each key-age. *Dev Med Child Neurol.* 1972;14:235-246.

developing child after six months of age (exceptions include the symmetric tonic neck reflex and the plantar grasp reflex). Some reflexes occur only in specific periods of development and are not evident later in development as they become integrated by the CNS (Table 16-16). Persistence of these reflexes can interfere with motor milestone attainment.

TABLE 16-14. THE FITS AND POSNER THREE-STAGE MODEL OF MOTOR LEARNING

STAGE	DESCRIPTION
Cognitive	An understanding of the task and general plan to accomplish it. High attentional demands (requires auditory, visual, kinesthetic, and somatosensory cues). Approach is slow and deliberate (trial and error).
Associative	Characterized by practice. Involves integration of: temporal/spatial patterns Movements develop into habit patterns. Need for external feedback decreases.
Autonomous	Tasks become automatic. Feedback begins to be replaced by feedforward. Can perform the task successfully in a variety of environments.

Data from Fitts PM, Posner MI: *Human Performance.* Belmont, CA: Brooks/Cole. 1967.

TABLE 16-15. THEORIES OF MOTOR LEARNING

Heterarchical and distributed control	Flow of information is not top-down. Decisions based on consensus of neural systems
Ecological perception-action[2]	This theory is based on the concept of search strategies—during practice there is a search for optimal strategies to solve the task, based on the task constraints. Critical to the search for optimal strategies is the exploration of the perceptual-motor workspace, which requires exploring all possible perceptual cues to identify those that are most relevant to the performance of a specific task. Perceptual information has a number of roles in motor learning: ▶ It relates to understanding the goal of the task and the movements to be learned. ▶ It serves as a method of feedback, both during the movement (knowledge of performance) and on completion of the movement (knowledge of results). ▶ It can be used to structure the search for a perceptual motor solution that is appropriate for the demands of the task.
Dynamical systems	Motor behavior emerges from the dynamic cooperation of all subsystems within the context of a specific task. Patterns of movement are flexible, adaptable, and dynamic, yet have "preferred" paths.

Data from Larin H: Motor learning: theories and strategies for the practitioner. In: Campbell SK, Vander Linden DW, Palisano RJ, eds. *Physical Therapy for Children, 3rd ed.* St. Louis, MO: Saunders. 2006:131-160; Shumway-Cook A, Woollacott MH: Motor learning and recovery of function. In: Shumway-Cook A, Woollacott MH, eds. *Motor Control: Theory and Practical Applications, 2nd ed.* Philadelphia, PA: Lippincott Williams & Wilkins. 2001:26-49.

TABLE 16-16. PRIMITIVE REFLEXES

REFLEX	DESCRIPTION
Rooting	Response to light tactile stimulation near the mouth. Infant moves head in direction of the stimulus and opens the mouth. Usually disappears around 9 months of age.
Sucking	Response to nipple or finger in mouth. Can be assessed as to whether it is sustainable and consistent.
Moro	One hand supports the infant's head in midline, the other supports the back. The infant is raised to 45 degrees and the head is allowed to fall through 10 degrees. Mature response is abduction then adduction of the limbs. Usually disappears around 3-6 months of age.
Palmar/plantar grasp	Stimulus applied to palm of hand or soles of feet. The response is a grasping of the digits. Usually disappears around 2-3 months of age.
Tonic labyrinthine	Prone position facilitates flexion. Supine position facilitates extension.
Asymmetric tonic neck reflex (ATNR)	Related to position of head turn: ▶ Extension of extremities on face side. ▶ Flexion of extremities on skull side. Usually disappears around 2-7 months of age.
Babinski	The foot twists in and the toes fan out in response to a stroke of the sole of the foot. Usually disappears around 6-9 months of age.
Symmetric tonic neck reflex (STNR)	Infant positioned in quadruped. Arm and head do the same thing, legs do the opposite, eg, head is extended, arms extend and legs flex.
Crossed extension	Pressure applied to sole of the foot produces flexion and extension of the opposite leg.
Proprioceptive placing	Pressure applied to dorsum of the foot or hand. Response is flexion, followed by extension of the extremity to bring the foot/hand on top of the stimulating surface. Usually disappears around 1 month of age.
Positive supporting	Pressure applied to sole of the foot produces extension of the extremity for weight bearing. Also known as primary standing.
Neonatal stepping	Walking motion produced as the infant is moved along a surface while being held under the arms. Also known as automatic walking.

Data from Capute AJ, Palmer FB, Shapiro BK, et al: Primitive reflex profile: a quantitation of primitive reflexes in infancy. *Dev Med Child Neurol.* 1984;26:375-383; Damasceno A, Delicio AM, Mazo DF, et al: Primitive reflexes and cognitive function. *Arq Neuropsiquiatr.* 2005;63:577-582. Epub Sep 9, 2005; Schott JM, Rossor MN: The grasp and other primitive reflexes. *J Neurol Neurosurg Psychiatry.* 2003;74:558-560; and Zafeiriou DI: Primitive reflexes and postural reactions in the neurodevelopmental examination. *Pediatr Neurol.* 2004;31:1-8.

PEDIATRIC SCREENING AND DIAGNOSTIC TOOLS

Factors to be considered when assessing a child include, but are not limited to[23]

- Current life circumstances: the child's current health, attitudes and values of the child's immediate family, and acculturation of the child.
- Health history: health and nutrition history, repeated hospitalizations etc.
- Developmental history: child's past rate of achievement of developmental milestones, events that might have had profound effects on the child either physically or psychologically.
- Extrapersonal interactions: the reaction of the child to the clinician and the conditions under which the child is observed.

Study Pearl

Developmental screening tests usually are brief, general, play-based tests of skills that do not necessarily correlate in any way with intelligence tests. Some tests use developmental ages to describe a child's physical, perceptual, social, and emotional maturity.

Study Pearl

- Norm referenced tests are those tests standardized on groups of individuals (populations) they are designed to test, and which allow the clinician to determine the exact developmental age of the child and to compare the child's performance to the performance typically expected.
- Criterion referenced test: a test that measures a child's development on particular skills in terms of absolute levels of mastery.[24] These tests have reference points which may not be dependent on a reference group—the child is competing against himself or herself, not a reference group.[24]

Infant Assessment Tools

The Brazelton Neonatal Behavioral Assessment Scale

Population. The Brazelton neonatal behavioral assessment scale (BNBAS) is a behavioral scale for infants from birth to the approximate posterm age of one month.[25]

Purpose. The BNBAS is based on the assumption that babies communicate through their behavior, and assesses the infant's use of his/her state of consciousness to maintain control of reactions to environmental and internal stimuli including

- Regulation of their autonomic nervous systems, including breathing and temperature regulation
- Control of their motor systems
- Control of their states or levels of consciousness
- Social interaction with parents and other caregivers

Content. The original BNBAS contained 26 biobehavioral items and 20 reflex items. The revised edition contains 27 biobehavioral items with increments in response to inanimate visual and auditory stimuli added to the 26 original items.[24] In addition, nine new optional supplementary items were included to address the quality of alert responsiveness, cognitive attention, examiner persistence, general irritability of the neonate, robustness and endurance, regulatory capacity, state regulation, balance of muscle tone, and reinforcement value of the infant's behavior.[24]

Administration. The BNBAS takes about 30 minutes to administer.

General Movement Assessment

Population. Requires examination of the spontaneous movements of preterm and term newborns and young infants.[26]

Purpose. An effective tool for predicting neurologic outcome at 2 years of age, in CP in particular.[27] The GMA reflects a theoretic view that maturation is not a fixed sequence of differentiation, but rather a continuous transformation of behavior. This concept acknowledges that during the development of the individual the functional repertoire of the developing neural structure must meet the requirements of the organism and its environment.

Content. Consists of an observation and classification of spontaneous movements while the infant lies in the supine position. Only movement generated while the infant is in an awake, non-crying state are analyzed and classified by movement quality. Classifications include writhing, fidgety, wiggling-oscillating, saccadic, and ballistic, and classification definitions distinguish frequency, amplitude, power, speed, flow, irregularity, and abruptness of the movements.[28]

Administration. Intertester agreement appears to be good to strong, sensitivity is strong across age groups preterm to 3 months corrected age, and specificity is strong by 3 months of age.[26]

Dubowitz Neurological Assessment of the Preterm and Full Term Infant[21]

Population. Preterm and full-term infants soon after birth and during the neonatal period.

Purpose. A screening test, based on traditional neuromaturational views of development, which is suitable for use by staff without expertise in neonatal neurology.[24] It is used to detect deviations or resolutions of neurologic problems.[21] A number of studies have shown this to be a valid tool which may be used to develop management protocols in the neonatal intensive care unit (NICU).[29,30]

Content. Consists of 32 items evaluating four areas (response decrement to repeated stimuli, movement and tone, reflexes, and behavior). Test items are drawn from the assessment tools of Saint-Anne Dargassies,[31] Prechtl,[32] Parmalee,[33] and Brazelton.[25]

Administration. Administered in a short period of time and repeated as the infant matures.[24] Scoring of the items is done on a five-point ordinal scale, although all of the items do not have to be administered with each child and no single total score is achieved. Each item is criterion-referenced and criterion-ordered according to expected changes with increasing postconceptional age.[28]

Movement Assessment of Infants

Population. For infants from birth to 1 year of age.

Purpose. To identify motor dysfunction, changes in the status of motor dysfunction, and establishment of an intervention program.[34]

Content. A criterion-referenced examination composed of 65 items selected to evaluate muscle tone (the readiness of muscles to respond to gravity), primitive reflexes (fully integrated to reflex domination of movement), automatic reactions (includes righting reaction, equilibrium reactions, and protective extension reactions), and volitional movement (includes response to visual and auditory stimuli, production of sound, and typical motor milestones, such as hands to midline, fine grasp, rolling, and walking) in the first year of life. The MAI test, when given to infants at four months and eight months of age, provides an assessment of risk for motor dysfunction.[35]

Administration. It appears that the most consistently reliable and predictive portion of the MAI is the section on volitional movement.[35]

Alberta Infant Motor Scales (AIMS)

Population. Age 0 to 12 months.

Purpose. Standardized, discriminative, evaluative, and criterion- and norm-referenced test[36] used to identify infants whose motor performance is delayed or aberrant relative to a normal group, to measure change, and to provide parents with information with regard to development.[37] The test highlights what the child can do and notes any deviations from the normal pattern of motor maturation.

Content. Dynamic systems and ecological theories evident by importance placed on the testing environment, the gravitational position of the patient, and the task in the assessment context. Maturational theory is also supported by the progression of skills achieved in a sequential, predictable manner. Observation of infant occurs in four positions (supine, prone, sit, stand) using three aspects of each (weight-bearing, posture, antigravity movements). About 58 items are scored on basis of the ability to maintain/perform certain postures, and movements.

Administration. Twenty to thirty minutes. Score is totaled and allows age equivalence to be established. Concurrent validity with the gross motor scales of the Peabody Developmental Motor Scales and the motor scales of the Bayley Scales is reported to range from 0.95 to 0.99 and 0.93 2.97, respectively.[38] High reliability (intraclass correlation coefficient [ICC] > 0.90) has been demonstrated in trained and untrained raters.[37]

Harris Infant Neuromotor Test

Population. Infants from 3 to 12 months of age.

Purpose. The Harris Infant Neuromotor Test (HINT) is designed to identify developmental delay.[39]

Content. A 22-item screening test that includes items to assess neuromotor milestones, active and passive muscle tone, head circumference, stereotypical movement patterns, behavioral interactions, and caregiver's assessment of the infant's development. Items are selected specifically because of research evidence suggesting sensitivity to delayed development.

Administration. The test takes less than 30 minutes to administer and score, is primarily observational, and can be used by a variety of health-care professionals.[14]

Comprehensive Developmental Assessment

Bayley Scales of Infant Development-II

Population. Bayley scales are applicable from birth to 15 months.

Purpose. Measures varying stages of growth at each age level, supplemented by extensive longitudinal data on groups of infants.

Content. The Bayley II, introduced in 1993,[40] is a revised and renormed version of the Bayley Scales of Infant Development (BSID),[41] necessitated by changes in infants' developmental rates since 1969.[42] As with the previous edition, the BSID-II consists of three scales used to diagnose developmental delay and plan intervention strategies:

- *Mental scale.* This part of the evaluation, which yields a score called the mental development index, evaluates several types of abilities: sensory/perceptual acuities, discriminations, and response; acquisition of object constancy; memory learning and problem solving; vocalization and the beginning of verbal communication; basis of abstract thinking; habituation; mental mapping; complex language; and mathematical concept formation.
- *Motor scale.* This part of the BSID assesses the degree of body control, large muscle coordination, finer manipulatory skills of the hands and fingers, dynamic movement, postural imitation, and the ability to recognize objects by sense of touch (stereognosis).
- *Behavior rating scale* (formerly called the Infant Behavior Record). This scale provides information that can be used to supplement information gained from the mental and motor scales. This 30-item scale rates the child's relevant behaviors and measures attention/arousal, orientation/engagement, emotional regulation, and motor quality.

Administration. The Bayley II takes about 45 to 60 minutes to administer. One strength of the test is that items have been carefully evaluated for bias based on cultural factors.[14] However, clinicians are advised to be conservative in assuming predictive capabilities of the new test until further research is available.[14]

Motor Assessments

Peabody Development Motor Scales-2 (PDMS-2)

Population. Age 0 to 6 years.

Purpose. Standardized, descriptive, and norm and criterion-referenced test used to identify children whose gross or fine motor skills are delayed or aberrant relative to a normal group. The purpose of the PDMS-2 is fivefold:

- To estimate motor competence relative to the child's peers
- To compare the gross motion motor quotient (GMQ) and fine motor quotient (FMQ) to determine if there is disparity in motor abilities
- To assess qualitative and quantitative aspects of individual skills
- To evaluate progress
- To study the nature of motor development in various populations

Content. Used to estimate a child's motor competence, aid in planning intervention, evaluate progress based on repeat testing, and conduct research on selected populations of children. Explicitly describes the level of development. Contains both gross motor and fine motor scales. Six subtests include reflexes (< 12 months age group), stationary, locomotion, object manipulation, grasping, and visual motor integration.

Administration. Takes 45 to 60 minutes to administer; 20 to 30 minutes on each composite area. Although specialized training is not required, the authors recommend that the examiner have a thorough understanding of test statistics, gross and fine motor ability, and developmental children who show deviance from normal. Criteria for "entry points" within each domain—items administered until three consecutive failures within each domain. Scoring interpretation includes a raw score, basal and ceiling, percentile, age equivalent, and standard score for each domain. Standard scores can be combined and converted into a gross motor, fine motor, and total quotient.

Bruininks Oseretsky Test of Motor Proficiency

Population. Ages 4.5 to 14.5 years of age.[43]

Purpose. The test is designed to provide educators, clinicians, and researchers with useful information to assist them in assessing the motor skills of individual students; in developing and evaluating motor training programs; and in assessing serious motor dysfunctions and developmental disabilities in children. The test may also be used as a screening device for differential diagnoses, and may be easily integrated with other types of educational and psychological measures.

Content. The test has subscales for running speed and agility, balance, bilateral coordination, strength, upper limb coordination, response speed, visual-motor control, and upper limb speed and dexterity.

Administration. Takes about 45 to 60 minutes to administer. A 15- to 20-minute short form (BOT-2) is available.

Assessments Designed for Children with Disabilities

Gross Motor Function Measure

Population. The test was specifically designed for children with CP from 6 months to 18 years of age, but can be used for any child whose motor function is below age 5 years.

Purpose. The gross motor function measure (GMFM) classification system is a clinical measure designed to evaluate change over time and with intervention in gross motor function in children with CP. Assesses motor function (what or how much a child can do) rather than the quality of movement behind motor performance. The test supports functional theory.

Content. There are two versions of the GMFM: the original 88-item measure (GMFM-88) and the more recent 66-item GMFM

(GMFM-66). Items on the GMFM-88 span the spectrum from activities in lying and rolling up to walking, running, and jumping skills. The GMFM-66 is comprised of a subset of the 88 items that has been shown to be unidimensional. The measure is widely used internationally, and is now the standard outcome assessment tool for clinical intervention in cerebral palsy (CP). The GMFM measures abilities that are usually achieved by age 5 in children without motor impairments and capability, defined as what a child can do in a standard condition.

Administration. Takes about 45 to 60 minutes to administer. The points for each of the five dimensions are totaled and a Dimension Percent Score is calculated. Intrarater and interrater reliability values for test components range from 0.87 to 0.99.[38]

Pediatric Evaluation of Disability Inventory

Population. No age limit.

Purpose. Norm-referenced when used with the appropriate age group; criterion-referenced when used with older children whose function falls in the 6-month to 7.5-year level. A descriptive and evaluative tool used to provide a comprehensive clinical assessment of key functional capabilities and performance. Focuses exclusively on what the child can accomplish and excludes information on how the child accomplishes the task. Also used for program monitoring, documentation of functional progress, and clinical decision-making. Relies on information gathered from the child's caregiver rather than on direct observation of the child.

Content. The pediatric evaluation of disability inventory (PEDI) test measures both capability and performance in three parts (functional skills—197 items, caregiver assistance—20 items, and modifications—20 items). In each part, 3 content domains are addressed (self-care, mobility, and social function).

Administration. Twenty to sixty minutes. An exact format for conducting the test is not required. Interview questionnaire and/or observational. Each item is scored, with the total scores allowing establishment of standard scores, scale scores, and frequency scores of level of modifications.

Functional Independence Measure for Children

Population. Age 6 months to 7 years.

Purpose. A minimal data set standardized functional performance measure. Evaluative, discriminative measure that uses actual performance of a child to indicate the severity of disability.

Content. Areas addressed include self-care, sphincter control, mobility, locomotion, social cognition, gross motor, fine motor, personal social and adaptive.

Administration. Easy to administer. Provides continuity with adult measures. Establishment of national database.

OTHER TESTS

School Function Assessment

Population. Kindergarten through 6th grade.

Purpose. Reflects the functional and ecological theories based on measurement of a student's performance of tasks that support participation in academic and social aspects of elementary school. Norm-referenced or criterion-referenced. Provides a seminal, comprehensive, and sophisticated method for examining a child within the contexts of the school environment.

Content. Comprehensive in three areas:

- Part I, participation: one scale appraises participation in six school settings (classroom, playground or recess, school transportation, bathroom and toileting, transitions to and from class, and meal or snack time).
- Part II, task supports: covers scales based on assistance (adult help), and adaptations (environmental or program modifications such as special equipment or adapted materials); in each two areas—physical and cognitive/behavioral.
- Part III, activity performance: covers 21 scales addressing areas such as in school travel, changing positions, using school materials, interacting with others, following school rules, and communicating needs.

Administration. The time to administer the test depends on several factors including the experience of the respondents, and the number of disciplines administering the test. Individual parts of the test may take 5 to 10 minutes, but the whole test can take 1 to 2 hours.[38] Strict administration criteria are not required. High internal consistency (0.92-0.98). Test retest reliability ranged from ICC 0.80 to 0.99. Content and construct validity are good.

Pediatric Clinical Test of Sensory Interaction for Balance

Population. Age 4 to 10 years.

Purpose. Measures standing balance when sensory input is systematically altered. The pediatric clinical test of sensory interaction for balance (PCTSIB)[44,45] assesses a child's standing stability under varying sensory conditions, including standing on stable versus foam surfaces, with and without vision, and with information from body sway relative to the surroundings occluded.

Content. Six conditions: standing on floor with eyes open, eyes closed, and with dome (eyes open, but vision stabilized); standing on foam with eyes open, eyes closed, and with dome (eyes open, but vision stabilized).[44]

Administration. The test takes 20 to 30 minutes. This test is inexpensive and requires minimal equipment.

Study Pearl

The APGAR screening test is administered to a newborn (usually by nursing) at 1, 5, 10 minutes after birth. The APGAR consists of five tests, which assess: heart rate, respiration, reflex irritability, muscle tone and color. Each test is scored 0, 1, or 2 (Table 16-17). A score of seven and above is considered good.

TABLE 16-17. DETERMINATION OF APGAR SCORE

FEATURE EVALUATED	0 POINTS	1 POINT	2 POINTS
Heart rate	Absent	Slow < 100 beats/min	> 100 beats/min
Respiratory effort	Apnea	Irregular, shallow or gasping breaths	Good, crying
Color	Pale or blue all over	Pale or blue extremities	Completely pink
Muscle tone	Absent (limp)	Weak, passive tone Some flexion of extremities	Active movement
Reflex irritability	Absent	Grimace	Active avoidance

Sum the scores for each feature. Maximum score = 10, minimum score = 0.
Data from Apgar V: The newborn (Apgar) scoring system. Reflections and advice. *Pediatr Clin North Am.* 1966;13:645-650; and Apgar V: A proposal for a new method of evaluation of the newborn infant. *Curr Res Anesth Analg.* 1953;32:260-267.

PEDIATRIC EXAMINATION AND INTERVENTIONS FOR SPECIFIC CONDITIONS

The assessment and management of infants, children, and adolescents with orthopedic, neurologic, and other disabilities requires suitably adapting the *Guide to Physical Therapist Practice.*[46] For example, in addition to the usual items of the history, the clinician asks questions related to school attendance (as appropriate) and involvement in play.

SYSTEMS REVIEW

The systems review provides additional information about the general health of the child and also provides information about communication skills, affect, cognition, language abilities, and learning style.

TESTS AND MEASURES

After analyzing the information from the history and systems review, the clinician conducts the appropriate tests and measures. With the pediatric population, this includes[38]

- Impairment-level measures such as joint motion and muscle function
- Functional limitation (activity) measures, often through standardized tests of motor or functional skills
- Disability (participation assessment through quality of life considerations)

The list of tests and measures in Table 16-18 describes those aspects relevant to pediatric physical therapy.

Following the administering of the tests and measures the clinician forms evaluation statements, a diagnosis, and a prognosis, and plans the appropriate interventions. The clinician should explain to the parent the pertinence of the examination data, discussing professional opinions about the child, diagnosis, prognosis, and preferred course of service to achieve the best outcome.[38] The main goals of physical therapy intervention in pediatric rehabilitation are to reduce barriers limiting the performance of daily routines and to facilitate the successful integration of children into the home, play, and school environments.

TABLE 16-18. TESTS AND MEASURES RELATED TO PEDIATRIC PHYSICAL THERAPY[a,b]

TEST AND MEASURE	RELEVANCE TO PEDIATRIC PHYSICAL THERAPY
Aerobic capacity/ endurance	Children with respiratory conditions such as bronchopulmonary dysplasia (see Pediatric Examination and Interventions for Specific Conditions section), or cystic fibrosis (see Pediatric Examination and Interventions for Specific Conditions), or who have ventilation assist needs should be tested in this area. In addition, those children whose movement is severely restricted by neuromotor conditions or musculoskeletal conditions such as juvenile chronic arthritis (JCA), osteogenesis imperfecta, or arthrogryposis may warrant testing in this area.
Anthropometric characteristics	Cartilage models of the long bones appear by the 6th week of gestation and primary centers of ossification appear in almost all bones of the limbs by the 12th week, and in the vertebrae by the seventh or eighth week. Children with conditions of health that affect growth directly such as pituitary gland dysfunction or bone disease such as osteogenesis imperfecta. Indirectly, cardiac or renal conditions can also retard growth. Growth can also fall below norms in children with cerebral palsy. Growth charts, with plots of height, weight, and frontal-occipital circumference are maintained by physicians and nurses. Body composition, the ratio of fat mass to fat-free mass impact performance on tests of the aerobic and muscular fitness. Obesity in American children is a growing concern and points to a community health role of the pediatric physical therapist to improve fitness in children. Baseline measurement may include girth and body fat tests.
Arousal, attention and cognition	This aspect is commonly addressed by other disciplines using tests such as the Brazelton Neonatal Assessment of Behavior Scale (BNABS), the Assessment of Preterm Infant Behavior (APIB), and the Movement Assessment of Infants (MAI).
Assistive and adaptive devices	Children with all types of conditions and varying severity of involvement can have assistive device needs ranging from temporary crutches to sophisticated power-driven wheelchairs. Adaptive devices may be needed at certain times for children who experience pain associated with JCA, or for children with spinal cord injuries, traumatic brain injuries, or severe cerebral palsy. Some standardized tests include testing with and without equipment, such as found on the Gross Motor Function Measure (GMFM), the Pediatric Evaluation of Disability Inventory (PEDI), and the School Function Assessment (SFA).
Circulation	Testing in this area is important for children with cardiac conditions, lymphatic conditions, respiratory conditions including bronchopulmonary dysplasia, diabetes, and certain genetic syndromes involving the circulatory or lymphatic systems. In addition, children with obesity should have baseline measures of at least pulse rate and blood pressure completed.
Cranial and peripheral nerve integrity	The pediatric physical therapist does not routinely examine cranial nerve integrity in children as this is often done by other disciplines with whom the physical therapist collaborates. Nonetheless, the pediatric physical therapist should be aware of the clinical signs and symptoms that may indicate cranial and peripheral nerve involvement. For example, absence or asymmetry of smiling, or other facial reactions may indicate facial nerve problems. Testing is also important for children who have severe neurological involvement following traumatic brain injury or near drowning, or in later stages of progressive disorders.
Environmental, home, and work (job/school/play) barriers	Results of these tests are often used to suggest modifications to the environment. Specific examples in pediatric physical therapy are the PEDI and the SFA.
Ergonomics and body mechanics	For children, consideration includes classroom placement for listening, attending, or functioning, as well as the height of the seat in class, and whether or not foot support is provided. This section may also include assessment of safety at school; dexterity in coordination for pointing to objects on the language board, or using hand controls on a power wheelchair; analyzing preferred postures for performance of tasks and activities; and how varied body or equipment placement improves performance or posture, or minimizes fatigue.
Gait, locomotion, and balance	Once walking has begun, clinicians will most often use observation to describe the gait pattern. The 30 Second Walk Test is an example of a quick appraisal of a child's functional performance with gait, specifically the distance the child can walk in 30 s.[c] Balance testing may be done using the original or Modified Functional Reach test, or the Pediatric Clinical Test for Sensory Interaction in Balance (PCTSIB). The Bruininks Oseretsky Test of Motor Proficiency has a subtest on balance. Similarly, the Gross Motor Scale of the Peabody Developmental Motor Scales (PDMS) has five categories, of which "balance" is one.
Integumentary integrity	The assessment of skin integrity in children is particularly important in cases of suspected abuse.

(*Continued*)

TABLE 16-18. TESTS AND MEASURES RELATED TO PEDIATRIC PHYSICAL THERAPY[a,b] *(Conitnued)*

TEST AND MEASURE	RELEVANCE TO PEDIATRIC PHYSICAL THERAPY
Joint integrity/mobility	Joint integrity measurements of children are mostly subjective. Two tests of hip joint integrity in infants under age 6 mo are used to detect hip dysplasia associated with subluxation or dislocation (see Pediatric Examination and Interventions for Specific Conditions section).
Motor function (motor control and motor learning)	Recently, the functional-ecological theories of motor control addressing function, practicality, culture, and environment seem to have attracted the greatest attention clinically. Testing of motor control may be subjective or objective, and typically focuses on a very specific aspect of motor performance. Motor learning cannot be measured directly, instead it is inferred from behavior.
Muscle performance (including strength, power, and endurance)	Muscle tone abnormalities are common in children with impaired neuromotor development and range from hypertonicity, spasticity, and rigidity to hypotonicity, hypotonia, and flaccidity. Muscle tone can be judged subjectively by observation of posture and movement as well as by hands-on examination of a muscle's response to stretch. The muscle tone section of the MAI can also be used. Methods of strength testing in children include manual muscle testing, or the appraisal of functional skills that require strength.
Neuromotor development and sensory integration	A number of standardized tests exist for the assessment of motor milestone development, most of which are based on knowledge of normal development. For example, the Alberta Infant Motor Scale (AIMS) provides motor milestone information and is extremely valuable for describing motor function in the child who is under 19 months old or who has not yet achieved walking.
Orthotic, protective, and supportive devices	Children with cerebral palsy and myelomeningocele commonly use orthotic devices. Children who incur burns may wear compression garments. Infants with congenital club foot deformity may undergo serial casting (refer to Chapter 9).
Pain	The pain-o-meter, in which children are asked to show on a scale that level of pain, has been employed with children with JCA. Visual analogue scales for pain have also been employed so children can judge the own pain levels. In pediatrics, managing pain and other sensations under one category—sensory integrity—is common for most reporting purposes.
Posture	Postural control shows a distinct, continuous developmental progression and is a critical component of skill acquisition. The development of postural control appears to follow a cephalocaudal sequence starting with the head. Delayed or abnormal development of postural control limits a child's ability to develop age-appropriate motor skills, including independent mobility and manipulation skills. Causes of poor postural control can include spasticity, insult to the motor or sensory component of the central and peripheral nervous system, Down's syndrome, cerebral palsy, abnormalities of muscle structure and function, and decreased strength. *Note:* Resting posture in recumbent, sitting, and standing positions may result in contractures. Parents can be asked about the duration of time that the child spends in postures, such as supine lying so that recommendations can be made.
Prosthetic requirements	Children with congenital amputations comprise the largest percentage of children with limb deficiencies. The examination should describe the child's level of accommodation to the prosthetic device and the time spent with or without the device.
Range of motion	Atypical neuromuscular activity during the years of musculoskeletal growth can result in modeling errors that can cause joint dysfunction and disability. Lower limb rotational deformities are also common in children with neuromuscular disorders. Range of motion may be tested passively, by moving the child's limb, or actively, by letting the child perform the movement. For example, children with JCA are often tested actively to concurrently judge the effective range of motion, whereas children with CP are often tested passively or by both means to distinguish true available motion from poor control, spasticity, or weakness.
Reflex integrity	In pediatrics, reflexes may be classified as diagnostic or developmental. Diagnostic reflexes include reflexes that might be used in a neurologic examination at any age such as muscle stretch reflexes, clonus, Babinski or variations of the Babinski reflex. Developmental reflexes tend to be more specific to neurologic examination of the developing infant and young child. This cluster of reflexes include attitudinal, righting, protection, and equilibrium reactions (see Primitive Reflexes). Rather than specifically test the primitive reflexes, many clinicians use visual appraisal of posture and movement to ascertain their persistence or influence.

(*Continued*)

TABLE 16-18. TESTS AND MEASURES RELATED TO PEDIATRIC PHYSICAL THERAPY[a,b] *(Conitnued)*

TEST AND MEASURE	RELEVANCE TO PEDIATRIC PHYSICAL THERAPY
Self-care and home management (including ADL and IADL)	A tool such as the Transdisciplinary Play-Based Assessment[d,e] can be used. In addition, two standardized functional test in pediatrics also provide information pertinent to this area: the PEDI and the SFA. Another test, the Canadian Occupational Performance Measure,[f-i] is designed to help families, children, and their parents establish goals by identifying functional limitations in daily life and rating them in importance to reducing disability in daily roles.
Sensory integrity (including proprioception and kinesthesia)	In very young children, sensation cannot be tested in the same way it is tested in adults. Rather, the examiner must look at the child's facial expression or other body reactions to judge sensory integrity. For older children more sophisticated tests of sensation and sensory perception are embedded in the Sensory Integration and Praxis Test (SIPT): This test, which requires special training and advanced clinical skills, evaluates sensory processing deficits related to learning and behavior problems, including visual, tactile, and kinesthetic perception as well as motor performance.
Ventilation and respiration (gas exchange)	The majority of clinical tests in this area produce objective data on pulmonary function such as obtained with a spirometer (measures air volume after maximal inspiration), and the oximeter (measures oxygen saturation in the blood). Infants with RDS or BPD, children with cystic fibrosis or asthma, children with cardiac conditions, and those who are ventilator dependent definitely should be examined in this area.

JCA, juvenile chronic arthritis.
[a]Data from Knutson LM: Examination, evaluation, and documentation for the pediatric client. In: Damiano D, ed. *Topics in Physical Therapy: Pediatrics.* Alexandria, VA: American Physical Therapy Association; 2001:1-36.
[b]Data from Clayton-Krasinski D, Klepper S: Impaired neuromotor development. In: Cameron MH, Monroe LG, eds. *Physical Rehabilitation: Evidence-Based Examination, Evaluation, and Intervention.* St Louis, MO: Saunders/Elsevier; 2007:333-366.
[c]Data from Campbell SK, Kolobe TH, Osten ET, et al: Construct validity of the test of infant motor performance. *Phys Ther.* 1995;75:585-596.
[d]Data from Lotan M, Manor-Binyamini I, Elefant C, et al: The Israeli Rett Syndrome Center. Evaluation and transdisciplinary play-based assessment. *Sci World J.* 2006;6:1302-1313.
[e]Data from Linder TW: *Transdisciplinary Play-Based Assessment.* Baltimore, MD: Paul H Brookes; 1996.
[f]Data from Verkerk GJ, Wolf MJ, Louwers AM, et al: The reproducibility and validity of the Canadian Occupational Performance Measure in parents of children with disabilities. *Clin Rehabil.* 2006;20:980-988.
[g]Data from Eyssen IC, Beelen A, Dedding C, et al: The reproducibility of the Canadian Occupational Performance Measure. *Clin Rehabil.* 2005;19:888-894.
[h]Data from Carswell A, McColl MA, Baptiste S, et al: The Canadian Occupational Performance Measure: a research and clinical literature review. *Can J Occup Ther.* 2004;71:210-222.
[i]Data from Law M, Baptiste S, McColl M, et al: The Canadian occupational performance measure: an outcome measure for occupational therapy. *Can J Occup Ther.* 1990;57:82-87.

PLAN OF CARE

Having identified the need for intervention, the clinician's next important decision is the plan of care. Theoretically, the goal of early intervention is the prevention or reduction of secondary impairments, such as contractures and skeletal deformities, that can develop as a result of habitual movement using compensatory patterns or over active muscles with weak antagonists or as a result of overall deficiency of movement and disuse.[19] If activity limitations persist for long periods and are not remediable or cannot be compensated for, children may fail in normal life roles, such as participation in school, play, or family activities.[19]

Study Pearl

Therapy planning should start with interdisciplinary assessment of activity and participation in natural environments when a condition that impairs developmental progress and functional capabilities is already well established.[19]

The clinician should focus on facilitating functional activity and participation, including[19]

- A determination about the constraints in subsystems that limit motor behavior, such as secondary impairments.
- The creation of an environment that supports or compensates for weaker or less mature components of the systems so as to promote activity and participation. Positioning equipment or orthoses (Chapter 15) can be prescribed to help maintain skeletal alignment, prevent or reduce secondary impairments, and

TABLE 16-19. DESIGN OPTIONS FOR PEDIATRIC ORTHOSES

DESIGN	PURPOSE
Passive deformity management	Used to reverse a flexible deformity and passively position specific joints and segments to maintain current posture and prevent further deformity.
Active deformity management	Used to reverse fixed deformity by actively stretching tissues to allow specific joints and segments to be aligned more optimally
Passive function	Used to reverse a flexible deformity and place specific joints and segments in static positions suitable for passive functional activity, such as using a standing frame or sitting in a wheelchair.
Active function	Used to enhance stability or mobility of specific joints and segments in a way that facilitates active function, such as balancing, standing or walking, or motor retraining.

to facilitate functional abilities. There are a number of design options that should be considered when prescribing an orthosis (Table 16-19).

- Awareness when setting up a therapeutic environment so that it affords opportunities to practice tasks in a meaningful and functional context.
- Utilizing activities that promote the investigation of a variety of movement patterns that might be appropriate for a task. This may necessitate addressing patient mobility in his/her environment, and/or the need for adaptive equipment (Tables 16-20 and 16-21).
- Mobility devices (eg, wheelchairs, walkers, and crutches) should provide an appropriate means of getting from one location to another efficiently. However, it is commonly agreed that positioning needs to take precedence over the issuance of a mobility device.
- The search for control parameters, such as speed of movement or force production, that can be manipulated by intervention to facilitate the attainment of therapeutic goals, especially during sensitive periods of development during which behavior is less stable.

To enhance the learning experience for the pediatric patient, the following guidelines are recommended:[47]

- Context: children learn quicker in stimulating and varied environments. Successful learning contexts are those that promote initiations by the learner, and shared control over the interaction.
- Motivation: intentional learning for improvement.

Study Pearl

It is extremely important to ensure realistic and meaningful solutions. Assistive technology, especially therapeutic positioning, can address many dimensions of impairment, particularly by helping to prevent secondary impairments due to inadequately supported body segments.

TABLE 16-20. GOALS FOR USING ADAPTIVE EQUIPMENT

Gain or reinforce normal movement.
Achieve normal postural alignment.
Prevent contractures and deformities.
Increase opportunity to participate in social or educational programs.
Provide mobility and encourage exploration.
Increase independence in activities of daily living and self-help skills.
Assist in improving physiological functions.
Increase comfort.

Data from Wilson JM: Selection and use of adaptive equipment. In: Connolly BH, Montgomery PC, eds. *Therapeutic Exercise in Developmental Disabilities.* Thorofare, NJ: SLACK Inc. 2001:167-182.

TABLE 16-21. PEDIATRIC ADAPTIVE EQUIPMENT

EQUIPMENT	TYPE	DESCRIPTION
Standers	*Supine version:* user enters the device on their backs, then they are strapped in and brought upright. Used when more support is needed posteriorly. *Prone version:* loads from the chest, and patient is strapped from behind. Used for cases when greater head and trunk control is needed.	Promotes weight-bearing and stretching, and, depending on the child's diagnosis, can help with the proper formation of the hip joint and building bone density. Promotes bone mineralization, respiratory, and bowel and bladder function. Helps teach mobility skills. Allows child to gain important emotional and social support by enabling them to interact with the rest of the world from a "normal" position.
Sidelyers		Used in cases when the patient has a tonic labyrinthine reflex (TLR), which can elicit more extensor tone in supine, and more flexor tone in prone.
Adaptive seating		Seating can be customized to meet the specific support and posture needs of the individual. As a general rule, seating systems should be customized to maintain the head in neutral position, the trunk upright, and the hips, knees, and ankles in correct alignment. For children with cerebral palsy, seating systems can be designed with a sacral pad and knee-block to correct pelvic tilt, decrease pelvic rotation and abduct/de-rotate the hip joint.
Orthoses	Various (see Orthoses section)	Orthoses are frequently required to maintain functional joint positions especially in nonambulatory or hemiplegic patients. Frequent reevaluation of orthotic devices is important as children quickly outgrow them and can undergo skin breakdown from improper use. AFOs are commonly used. Submalleolar orthosis for forefoot and midfoot malalignment.

Study Pearl

A wide variety of methods can be employed when treating the pediatric population to make the exercises more enjoyable and stimulating. These include the use of

- Balls of different sizes.
- Colored wedges.
- Swings.
- Scooter boards.
- Toys.
- Music.
- Pets. Horseback-riding therapy (hippotherapy) offers many potential cognitive, physical, and emotional benefits.[48-50]

- Creative behavior: encouraging creative behavior is a potent means of enhancing the child's learning.
- Goal setting: a major, motivational, instructional strategy.
  - Construct goals that are related to the completion of the action or to the component movements of the complete action.
  - Goals should be specific, consistent, attainable, and short in duration.
  - Standards should be high enough to foster improved performance but not so high as to provoke discouragement by repeated failure.
- Appropriate instructions: these provide a feed-forward input to convey information about the task requirements. The instructions
  - Should include a description of the task that is based on the learner's competencies as well as on the relevant environmental elements.
  - Can be verbally presented and/or demonstrated. Children tend to be more visually dependent than adults. Observational motor learning is an effective strategy for developing the perceptual skills necessary for children to selectively attend to environmental cues. Peer modeling (the use of another child to demonstrate) may also be used.
  - Assist the child to separate task relevant information from task irrelevant information.

- Purposeful tasks: these should be active, relevant, functional, voluntarily regulated, goal directed, and meaningful to the learner.
- The provision of feedback.

CONDITIONS RELATED TO THE NEONATE

Prior to the examination of the neonate, the clinician should ascertain the mother's pregnancy and birth history (prematurity, fetal distress, difficulty of labor), the mother's medical history and whether the baby was admitted to a special care unit, was incubated, on a ventilator, had surgery, and is on any medications. The clinician should observe the entire infant at the beginning of the examination, before the assessment of specific organ systems. It is important that the infant be appropriately disrobed and in a warm environment with adequate illumination.

PREMATURITY

Most of the problems associated with prematurity (preterm) occur in infants with birth weights of 1500 g (3 lb, 5 oz) or less, usually in those born at less than 32 weeks of gestational age. Causes of prematurity include, but are not limited to

- Poor prenatal care
- Multiple fetuses
- Placental abnormalities
- Preeclampsia
- Maternal age (increased age increases the risk)
- Medical condition of the mother
- Lifestyle of the mother

Characteristics associated with preterm infants include

- Global hypotonia, with the level of hypotonia related to the degree of prematurity
- Posturing of the extremities in extension and abduction, with decreased flexor patterns and midline orientation
- Absent, reduced, or inconsistent primitive reflexes
- Minimal spontaneous movement
- Dysfunction of sensory organization
- Difficulty moving between states of deep sleep, light sleep, alertness

Medical conditions associated with preterm infants include, but are not limited to

- Retinopathy of prematurity (ROP): a potentially blinding eye disorder, which is one of the most common causes of visual loss in childhood and can lead to lifelong vision impairment and blindness.
- Respiratory distress (RDS): also known as hyaline membrane disease.
- Hyperbilirubinemia.

Study Pearl

Average values of vital signs for neonates:

- Temperature 36.5 to 37.5°C
- Heart rate 120 to 160 beats/min. The infant's heart rate depends on chronological age. The heart rate averages 141 beats/min at birth, peaking to 171 beats/min at 2 months of age and gradually declining to 142 beats/min at one year of age.
- Respiratory rate: 30 to 60 per minute. The respiratory rate should be corrected for the infant's due date. In term infants, respirations, while awake, average 50 ± 19 per minute at the due date and drop to 26.5 ± 8 per minute by 12 months past the due date. Signs of increased effort of breathing, including the use of accessory muscles and abdominal breathing are as important as the respiratory rate. The respiratory rate can be up to 80 per minute if the infant is crying or stimulated.
- Systolic blood pressure 50 to 70 mm Hg. Hypertension is more common in premature infants than in term infants.

Study Pearl

Bilirubin is a tetrapyrrole created by the normal breakdown of heme. Most bilirubin is produced during the breakdown of hemoglobin and other hemoproteins. Accumulation of bilirubin (hyperbilirubinemia) or its conjugates in body tissues produces jaundice (ie, icterus), which is characterized by high plasma bilirubin levels and deposition of yellow bilirubin pigments in skin, sclerae, mucous membranes, and other less visible tissues.[51-53]

In Uterus Substance Exposure

Fetal Alcohol Syndrome. Fetal alcohol syndrome (FAS) occurs in infants whose mothers consumed more than 1 to 2 oz of alcohol a day during pregnancy.[54-56] Alcohol crosses the placenta and rapidly reaches the fetus. The likelihood of the infant developing FAS increases if the mother smokes and drinks. A diagnosis of fetal alcohol syndrome (FAS) is contingent on findings in the following three areas:

- Dysmorphology (particularly midfacial anomalies)
- Growth retardation (intrauterine growth rate and failure to experience catch-up growth)
- CNS involvement (cognitive impairment, learning disabilities, impulsiveness)

Cocaine Exposure. Among the findings in neonates associated with cocaine abuse include: low birth weight, intrauterine growth retardation, reduced head circumference, preterm birth, hemorrhagic infarctions, cystic lesions, and congenital anomalies and malformations.[57-62]

Infants born to mothers who abuse narcotics during pregnancy may show symptoms of withdrawal when they are deprived of the drug after birth. Symptoms of withdrawal increase in infants if the maternal dosage is high. The classic symptom of withdrawal in a neonate is jitteriness, which is further delineated as being stimulus-sensitive, rhythmic, and easily stopped by passive flexion of the extremities. Other common signs and symptoms include increased activity, hypotonicity, a high-pitched cry, excessive sucking behavior, and reduced sleep.

Congenital Central Hypoventilation Syndrome

Congenital central hypoventilation syndrome (CCHS), traditionally known as the Ondine curse, is traditionally defined as the failure of automatic control of breathing.[63,64] The exact pathophysiology of CCHS remains unknown.[63,64] The clinical presentation of patients with CCHS may be quite variable and is dependent on the severity of the disorder. Some infants do not breathe at birth and require assisted ventilation in the newborn nursery. Other infants may present at a later age, with cyanosis, edema, and signs of right heart failure as the first indications of CCHS.[65-67] Still others may present with unexplained apnea or an apparent life-threatening event, or some may even die and be categorized as having sudden infant death syndrome (SIDS).[65-67]

Infants with this condition may be hypotonic, display thermal lability, and have occasional and sudden hypotensive events that are unexplained by the surrounding circumstances.[65-67] The severity of respiratory dysfunction may range from relatively mild hypoventilation during quiet sleep with fairly good alveolar ventilation during wakefulness to complete apnea during sleep with severe hypoventilation during wakefulness.[65-67]

Head Trauma in Newborns

Caput Succedaneum. Caput succedaneum is a diffuse swelling of the scalp in a newborn secondary to accumulation of blood or serum above the periosteum caused by pressure from the uterus or vaginal wall during a head-first (vertex) delivery.[68] It is commonly observed after prolonged labor. Clinical features include poorly demarcated soft tissue swelling that crosses suture lines; accompanying pitting edema and overlying petechiae, ecchymoses, and purpura. The condition usually resolves within days.

Cephalhematoma. A blood cyst, tumor, or swelling of the scalp in a newborn due to an effusion of blood beneath the pericranium, often resulting from birth trauma.[68] It is less common than caput succedaneum but may occur after prolonged labor and instrumentation. Clinical features include well-demarcated, often fluctuant swelling that does not cross suture lines; no overlying skin discoloration; possibly, skull fractures; sometimes, elevated ridge of organizing tissue.[69] Complications associated with cephalhematoma include intracranial hemorrhage with resultant shock, and hyperbilirubinemia.

Treatment is not recommended for uncomplicated lesions, which usually reabsorb in 2 weeks to 3 months. However; for a suspected or detected fracture, radiographs are taken again at 4 to 6 weeks to ensure closure of linear fractures and to exclude formation of leptomeningeal cysts.[68] For depressed skull fractures, immediate neurosurgical consultation is required.

Birth Trauma

Injuries to the infant resulting from mechanical forces (ie, compression, traction) during the process of birth are categorized as birth trauma. Most birth traumas are self-limiting and have a favorable outcome. Nearly half are potentially avoidable with recognition and anticipation of obstetric risk factors. Risk factors include

- Large-for-date infants, especially larger than 4500 g
- Instrumental deliveries, especially forceps (midcavity) or vacuum
- Vaginal breech delivery
- Abnormal or excessive traction during delivery

When fetal size, presentation, or neurologic immaturity complicates the birthing event, such intrapartum forces may lead to tissue damage, edema, hemorrhage, or fracture in the neonate. The use of obstetric instrumentation may further amplify the effects of such forces or may induce injury alone.

Pulmonary System

Cyanosis. Newborns with significant cyanosis should be evaluated by the appropriate medical staff expeditiously. The numerous reasons for cyanosis in neonates and infants include pulmonary, hematologic, toxic, and cardiac causes.[70]

Diminished pulses in all extremities indicate poor cardiac output or peripheral vasoconstriction. Absent or diminished femoral pulses suggest the presence of ductal-dependent cardiac lesions (eg, coarctation of the aorta). Although hypertension is uncommon in newborns, it is rarely idiopathic.

Choanal Atresia. Choanal atresia, a congenital anomaly that results in complete nasal obstruction, is characterized by cyanosis that is relieved by crying. The condition can result in death by asphyxia. The diagnosis is usually established by the medical team due to the inability to pass a catheter through the nostril(s). Infants and children with this may present with mucus or foul-smelling secretions from the involved nares and respiratory distress associated with upper respiratory infection.

Respiratory Distress Syndrome. Originally described in adults, acute respiratory distress syndrome (ARDS), which is also known as "hyaline membrane disease," occurs in all ages. The clinical signs depend on the type, acuity, and severity of the initial insult, but include

- Dyspnea/tachypnea; over a period of hours to days, hypoxemia worsens, and the patient appears dyspneic and more tachypneic
- Flaring of the nostrils
- Use of accessory muscles
- Diffuse rales

The prognosis of infants with RDS varies with the severity of the original disease, but RDS is the leading cause of neonatal death and morbidity.[71]

Atelectasis. Atelectasis (refer to Chapter 10) is the term used to describe a collapse of part of the lung. Intrinsic airway obstruction is the most common cause of atelectasis in children, and asthma is the most common underlying disorder that predisposes patients to atelectasis.[72-83] Other causes include bronchiolitis, aspiration from swallowing disorder, endobronchial tuberculosis, aspiration from gastroesophageal reflux, airway foreign bodies, cystic fibrosis, and increased or abnormal airway secretions for other reasons. Atelectasis may occur in children with neuromuscular disease; those who have had recent thoracic or upper abdominal surgery; those on medications that decrease their minute ventilation (such as narcotics); and those with abnormally small or dysmorphic chest walls, which may be less compliant than the normal chest wall. Such children may also be predisposed to atelectasis because of poor clearance of airway secretions. An ineffective cough will allow these secretions to obstruct the airway.

Bronchopulmonary Dysplasia. Bronchopulmonary dysplasia (BPD) is a chronic lung disease of infancy, which begins with the destruction of the respiratory tract cilia followed by necrosis of the cells of the respiratory epithelium as distal as the bronchioles. The chronic lack of oxygenation often impairs neuromotor development.

Bronchiolitis. Bronchiolitis is an acute, infectious, inflammatory disease of the upper and lower respiratory tract resulting in obstruction of the small airways.[84-86] Although it may occur in all age groups, the larger airways of older children and adults better accommodate mucosal edema and severe symptoms are usually only evident in young infants. Respiratory syncytial virus (RSV) is the most commonly isolated agent. The disease is highly contagious. Viral shedding in nasal secretions continues for 6 to as long as 21 days after the development of symptoms. Hand washing and the use of disposable gloves and gowns may reduce nosocomial spread. Eighteen to twenty percent of hospitalized infants with RSV bronchiolitis develop apnea.

Diagnosis is based on the infants' age, seasonal occurrence, and physical findings. Physical examination often reveals otitis media, retractions, fine rales and diffuse, fine wheezing. The severity of the disease is directly related to post-conceptual age. Infants less than 6 months of age are the most severely affected due to smaller, more easily obstructed airways, and a decreased ability to clear secretions. First infections are usually most severe, with subsequent attacks generally milder.

Periventricular Leukomalacia (PVL)

Periventricular leukomalacia (PVL), a bilateral white matter lesion, is the most common ischemic brain injury in premature infants.[87] PVL may result from hypotension, ischemia, and coagulation necrosis at the border or watershed zones of deep penetrating arteries of the middle cerebral artery. Decreased blood flow affects the white matter at the superolateral borders of the lateral ventricles. The site of injury affects the descending corticospinal tracts, visual radiations, and acoustic radiations. Initially, most premature infants are asymptomatic. If symptoms occur, they usually are subtle. Symptoms may include the following:

- Decreased tone in lower extremities
- Increased tone in neck extensors
- Apnea and bradycardia events
- Irritability
- Pseudobulbar palsy with poor feeding
- Clinical seizures (may occur in 10%-30% of infants)

Periventricular Hemorrhage-Intraventricular Hemorrhage

Periventricular hemorrhage-intraventricular hemorrhage (PVH-IVH) remains a significant cause of both morbidity and mortality in infants who are born prematurely. PVH-IVH is thought to be caused by capillary bleeding. Two major factors that contribute to the development of PVH-IVH are (1) loss of cerebral autoregulation and (2) abrupt alterations in cerebral blood flow and pressure. Sequelae of PVH-IVH include life-long neurological deficits, such as CP, mental retardation, and seizures. PVH-IVH is diagnosed primarily through the use of brain imaging studies, usually cranial ultrasonography. As PVH-IVH can occur without clinical signs, serial examinations are necessary for the diagnosis.

Cardiovascular System

Patent Ductus Arteriosus (PDA). PDA is the fifth or sixth most common congenital cardiac defect. It involves the persistence of a normal fetal structure between the left pulmonary artery and the descending aorta beyond 10 days of life. Signs and symptoms include, but are not limited to, tachypnea, tachycardia, diaphoresis, and cyanosis.

Tetralogy of Fallot. Tetralogy of Fallot (TOF) is a complex of anatomic abnormalities arising from the maldevelopment of the right ventricular infundibulum. Cyanosis develops within the first few years of life, or at birth, which may demand surgical repair. The rare patient may remain marginally and imperceptibly cyanotic, or acyanotic and asymptomatic, into adult life.

MUSCULOSKELETAL SYSTEM

Congenital Muscular Torticollis. Congenital muscular torticollis (CMT) refers to the presentation of a neck in a twisted or bent position due to a unilateral shortening of the sternocleidomastoid (SCM) muscle.[88-95] The position adopted by the head and neck is one of

- Side bending of the neck to the same side as the contracture
- Rotation of the neck to the opposite side as the contracture
- In addition, the infant may exhibit asymmetric neck extension and forward head posture (FHP) due to upper cervical extension. There is little agreement as to the etiology of CMT. Theories include direct injury to the SCM muscle (due to birth trauma or intrauterine malpositioning), abnormal vascular patterns, rupture of the muscle, infective myositis, fibrosis of the SCM, neurogenic injury, and hereditary factors. The three subtypes of CMT are outlined in Table 16-22.
- In infants with CMT, neck range of motion is decreased for ipsilateral rotation, contralateral side flexion, and contralateral asymmetric flexion and extension. The infant is not able to maintain a midline alignment of the head with the torso in static postures or during movement because of the neck muscle imbalance and muscle contracture. Prolonged uncorrected head tilt caused by the underlying mechanism of the imbalanced muscle pull acting on the growing spinal and craniofacial skeleton may worsen any scoliosis, skull and facial asymmetry, and influence compensatory movement patterns affecting motor control development. Impaired mobility may lead to persistent asymmetry of early reflexes and reinforcement of an asymmetric postural preference. This in turn may cause neglect of the ipsilateral hand, decreased visual awareness of the ipsilateral visual field, interference of symmetric development of head and neck

Study Pearl

CMT is named for the side of the involved SCM muscle, eg, a right CMT involves the right SCM and results in sidebending of the head and neck to the right and rotation to the left.

TABLE 16-22. SUBTYPES OF CMT

SUBTYPE	DESCRIPTION
Sternomastoid tumor (Most common)	Infants often appear healthy at delivery, but over a period of 14-21 days (can be up to 3 months later), they develop a soft-tissue swelling (usually 1-3 cm in diameter and spindle shaped) over an injured sternocleidomastoid (SCM). This mass, which may be confused with a cystic hygroma or branchial cleft cyst, regresses and leaves a fibrous band in place of the SCM) muscle, causing contracture of the neck. X-rays are normal.
Muscular torticollis	There is tightness but no palpable mass within the SCM muscle and x-rays are normal.
Postural torticollis	There is no SCM muscle tightness, no palpable mass, and x-rays are normal. Causes include benign paroxysmal torticollis, congenital absence of one of several cervical muscles or of the transverse ligament, or contracture of other neck muscles.

Data from Karmel-Ross K: Congenital muscular torticollis. In: Campbell SK, Vander Linden DW, Palisano RJ, eds. *Physical Therapy for Children, 3rd ed.* St. Louis, MO: Saunders. 2006:359-380; Cheng JC, Metreweli C, Chen TM, et al: Correlation of ultrasonographic imaging of congenital muscular torticollis with clinical assessment in infants. *Ultrasound Med Biol.* 2000;26:1237-1241; and Cheng JC, Wong MW, Tang SP, et al: Clinical determinants of the outcome of manual stretching in the treatment of congenital muscular torticollis in infants. A prospective study of eight hundred and twenty-one cases. *J Bone Joint Surg Am.* 2001;83-A:679-687.

righting reactions, delayed propping and rolling over the involved side and limited vestibular, proprioceptive, and sensorimotor development. In the older child this may result in asymmetric weight-bearing in sitting, crawling, walking, and transitional movement skills as well as incomplete development of automatic postural reactions.

Physical Therapy Role. Intervention is directed toward resolving the impairments or activity limitations identified in the physical therapy examination.[93] This conservative approach typically consists of passive neck range of motion exercises (ipsilateral rotation, contralateral side flexion, and contralateral asymmetric extension from a starting point of neutral cervical spine alignment), active assistive range of motion, strengthening, and postural control exercises. Caregivers are instructed in how to carry and position the infant to promote elongation of the involved SCM, how to promote active contraction of the contralateral SCM, and in developmental exercises (Table 16-23). Assistive devices that may be used to help obtain, maintain, or restrain motion in those infants or children who are 4 months of age or older, includes a fabricated to fit, soft neck collar, or a *tubular orthosis for torticollis* (TOT).

Talipes Equinovarus (Club Foot). Clubfoot, or talipes equinovarus, is a congenital deformity consisting of hindfoot equinus, hindfoot varus, and forefoot varus. Can be classified as

- Postural or positional: not true clubfeet
- Fixed or rigid: are either flexible (ie, correctable without surgery) or resistant (ie, requires surgical release)

Treatment consists of manipulation (reducing the talonavicular joint by moving the navicular laterally and the head of the talus medially) and serial casting (refer to Chapter 9), which is most effective if started immediately after birth.

Developmental (Congenital) Dysplasia of the Hip. Developmental dysplasia of the hip involves an abnormal development of the acetabulum and the proximal femur, the labrum, capsule, and other soft tissues of the hip, which results in a failure of the femoral

TABLE 16-23. THERAPEUTIC EXERCISES FOR CONGENITAL MUSCULAR TORTICOLLIS BASED ON PATIENT POSITION (EG, LEFT CMT)

PATIENT POSITION	ACTIVITY
Supported sitting	The infant's head is prevented from tilting to the left side. Toy placement is used to promote head rotation to the left. Manual guidance is given to the left upper extremity for forward flexion, external rotation, and forearm supination during reach and grasp activities.
Supine	Toys are placed slightly to the left to promote rotation of the head to the left while the central axis alignment of head to body is maintained with sustained light traction on the occiput or base of the skull. Reaching and grasping activities allow the infant to exercise in an open kinetic chain to activate left upper extremity flexion, external rotation, elbow extension, horizontal abduction, and adduction.
Sidelying (on the left)	Soft supports are placed anterior and posterior to the infant's trunk to allow the infant to be positioned in a three quarters sidelying position.

Data from Karmel-Ross K: Congenital muscular torticollis. In: Campbell SK, Vander Linden DW, Palisano RJ, eds. *Physical Therapy for Children, 3rd ed.* St. Louis, MO: Saunders. 2006:359-380.

head to rest correctly in the acetabulum of pelvis. Although the condition may occur at any time, from conception to skeletal maturity, it occurs more frequently in early life. Two terms are used to describe this condition; the traditional term *congenital hip dysplasia (CHD)* and the current term *developmental dysplasia of the hip (DDH).* The hip may be dislocated, dislocatable, or subluxated. The following signs and symptoms may be found in the newborn:

- Asymmetric fat folds in the thigh.
- Extra skin folds on the involved side.
- Positive Ortolani test/Barlow maneuver signs. With the newborn supine, the clinician places the tips of the long and index fingers over the greater trochanter, with the thumb along the medial thigh. The infant's leg is positioned in neutral rotation with 90 degrees of hip flexion, and is gently abducted while lifting the leg anteriorly.[96] With abduction a clunk is felt as the femoral head slides over the posterior rim of the acetabulum and into the socket. This clunk, originally described by Ortolani,[97] is called the sign of entry, as the hip relocates with this maneuver. Maintaining the same position, the leg is then gently adducted while gentle pressure is directed posteriorly on the knee, and a palpable clunk is noted as the femoral head slides over the posterior rim of the acetabulum and out of the socket.[96] This clunk was originally described by Barlow,[98] and it is called the sign of exit, as the hip dislocates with this maneuver. Both tests are designed to detect motion between the femoral head and the acetabulum.[96]
- In the older child, the signs and symptoms usually include:
  - Legs that are unequal in length.
  - Positive Galeazzi sign. The patient is in supine with the hips and knees flexed. Examination should demonstrate that one leg appears shorter than the other. Although this is usually due to hip dislocation, realizing that any limb length discrepancy results in a positive Galeazzi sign is important.

The treatment of this condition depends on the child's age. From birth to 9 months the Pavlik harness has traditionally been used. The harness restricts hip extension and adduction and allows the hip to be maintained in flexion and abduction, the "protective position."[99] The position of flexion and abduction enhances normal acetabular development, and the kicking motion allowed in this position stretches the contracted hip adductors and promotes spontaneous reduction of the dislocated hip.[99] In infants older than nine months of age who are beginning to walk independently, an abduction orthosis can be used as an alternative to the Pavlik harness.[99]

Osteogenesis Imperfecta. Osteogenesis imperfecta (OI) is an inherited condition resulting from abnormality in the type I collagen (found in bones, joint capsules, fascia, cornea, sclera, tendons, meninges, and dermis), which causes the bones to be brittle. In the most severe form, the infant is born with multiple fractures sustained in utero or during the birth process. For severe cases presenting with severe osteopenia and repeated fractures, cyclic administration of intravenous aminohydroxypropylidene (ie, pamidronate) may reduce the incidence of fracture and increase bone mineral density. Surgical interventions include intramedullary rodding, surgery for basilar impression, and correction of scoliosis.

Physical Therapy Role. Typical participation restrictions for an infant with OI depend on the severity of the case. The clinician should be aware of the infant's medical history of past and present fractures and know the types of immobilizations employed before beginning the examination.[100-103] Pain is assessed using a tool such as the FLACC (face, legs, activity, cry, and consolability), which is an observational scale assessing pain behaviors quantitatively with preverbal patients. Assessing active, but not passive, range of motion is essential. Functional range of motion may prove more useful because it will assist in visualizing the whole composite of motion needed in functional abilities. Assessing muscle strength is done through observation of the infant's movements and palpation of contracting muscles rather than by using formal muscle tests. Caregiver education on proper and safe handling, positioning, and facilitation of movement is provided. Bathing, dressing, and carrying the infant are critical times when the infant is at risk for fractures.

The caregiver and clinician must be aware of the signs of a fracture which include inflammation (warmth of the site, edema, and pain), bruising, irritability, and deformity. An aquatic exercise program is an excellent therapeutic program for the child with OI. The degree of ambulation attainable varies for preschool children with OI. Gait training, which is progressed in the usual fashion (parallel bars and moving to various assistive devices), is commonly initiated when the child has achieved strength with a rating of at least 3/5 (Fair) and when range of motion has reached a plateau. In moderate to severe OI, braces and splints are usually required to begin standing activities on solid surfaces. It must be remembered that when children use walkers or crutches a large percentage of the body weight is borne through the upper extremities, necessitating precautions against bowing deformities of the radius and ulna. A walker that supports the majority of body weight through the trunk and pelvis is often used to assist in weight-bearing during initial overland ambulation. Customized mobility carts may be fabricated to encourage independent mobility when the child is immobilized, enabling the child to explore his or her environment, gain some independence, and maintain strength in the upper extremities. Children with severe types of OI often require wheelchairs for mobility. Because of the shortened extremities, these chairs are often specially ordered and may require adaptations.

> **Study Pearl**
>
> When handling the infant, it is important that forces not be put across the long bones; instead the head and trunk should be supported with the arms and legs gently draped across the supporting arm. It is also important to change the carrying position of the infant periodically because he or she develops strength by accommodating to postural changes.

Neurologic System

Hydrocephalus. Hydrocephalus is an abnormal accumulation of cerebrospinal fluid (CSF) within the ventricles inside the brain.[104-108] Intracranial pressure (ICP) rises if production of CSF exceeds absorption. This occurs if CSF is overproduced, resistance to CSF flow is increased, or venous sinus pressure is increased. Congenital hydrocephalus is thought to be caused by a complex interaction of environmental and perhaps genetic factors. Acquired hydrocephalus may result from intraventricular hemorrhage, meningitis, head trauma, tumors, and cysts. Symptoms in infants include poor feeding, irritability, reduced activity, and/or vomiting. The symptoms in children include a slowing of mental capacity, drowsiness, headaches, neck pain, visual disturbances, and gait disturbance.

> **Study Pearl**
>
> - Hydrocephalus can be characterized as either communicating or non-communicating on the basis of the location of the causative obstruction.
> - Noncommunicating hydrocephalus occurs secondary to an obstruction within the ventricular system before the exit of cerebrospinal fluid (CSF) from the forth ventricle.
> - Communicating hydrocephalus occurs when the obstruction is in the subarachnoid space. In TBI, subarachnoid obstruction is commonly caused by inflammation and impaired CSF absorption by arachnoid granulations.

Arthrogryposis. Arthrogryposis, or arthrogryposis multiplex congenita, encompasses nonprogressive neurological conditions that are characterized by multiple joint contractures and rigid joints found throughout the body at birth.[109-113] The pathogenesis of arthrogryposis has not been determined but is thought to be due to a combination of fetal abnormalities, maternal disorders (eg, infection, drugs, trauma, and other maternal illnesses) and genetic inheritance. Although joint contractures and associated clinical manifestations vary from case to case, there are several common characteristics:

- The involved extremities are fusiform or cylindrical in shape, with thin layers of subcutaneous tissue and absent skin creases.
- The deformities are usually symmetric, and the severity increases distally, with the hands and feet typically being the most deformed.
- The patient may have joint dislocations, especially the hips and, occasionally, at the knees.

Brachial Plexus Injury. Brachial plexus injury occurs most commonly in larger babies during delivery. Associated injuries include fractured clavicle, fractured humerus, subluxation of cervical spine, cervical cord injury, and facial palsy.

- Erb palsy (C5-C6) is the most common and is associated with lack of shoulder motion. The involved extremity lies adducted, prone, and internally rotated. Moro, biceps, and radial reflexes are absent on the affected side. Grasp reflex is usually present. Five percent of patients have an accompanying (ipsilateral) phrenic nerve paresis.
- Klumpke paralysis (C7-8, T1) is rare, resulting in weakness of the intrinsic muscles of the hand; grasp reflex is absent. If cervical sympathetic fibers of the first thoracic spinal nerve are involved, Horner syndrome is present.

Spina Bifida. Spina bifida includes a continuum of congenital anomalies of the spine due to insufficient closure of the neural tube and failure of the vertebral arches to fuse.[114-120] Spina bifida is classified into aperta (visible or open) and occulta (not visible or hidden). The three main types of spina bifida are listed in Table 16-24. Spina bifida aperta is often used interchangeably with myelomeningocele, which is an open spinal cord defect that usually protrudes dorsally. The neurological complications associated with spina bifida are outlined in Table 16-25. Interventions are based on clinical findings (see Chapter 9).

Prader-Willi Syndrome. Prader-Willi syndrome (PWS) is a chromosomal microdeletion/disomy disorder arising from deletion or disruption of genes in the proximal arm of chromosome 15 or maternal disomy of the proximal arm of chromosome 15 (genomic imprinting).[121-124] The condition is characterized by diminished fetal activity, respiratory and feeding difficulties in infancy, hypotonia, globally delayed motor milestones (eg, sitting at age 12 months, walking at age 24 months), strabismus, decreased skin and eye pigmentation, genital hypoplasia (eg, cryptorchidism, scrotal hypoplasia,

TABLE 16-24. TYPES OF SPINA BIFIDA

TYPE	DESCRIPTION
Spina bifida occulta	"Occulta" means hidden, thus the defect is not visible. Rarely linked with complications or symptoms. Usually discovered accidentally during an x-ray or MRI for some other reason.
Meningocele (Spina bifida aperta)	The membrane that surrounds the spinal cord may enlarge, creating a lump or "cyst." This is often invisible through the skin and causes no problems. If the spinal canal is cleft, or "bifid," the cyst may expand and come to the surface. In such cases, since the cyst does not enclose the spinal cord, the cord is not exposed. The cyst varies in size, but it can almost always be removed surgically if necessary, leaving no permanent disability.
Myelomeningocele (Spina bifida aperta)	The most complex and severe form of spina bifida. A section of the spinal cord and the nerves that stem from the cord are exposed and visible on the outside of the body; or, if there is a cyst, it encloses part of the cord and the nerves. Usually involves neurological problems that can be very serious or even fatal. This condition accounts for 94% of cases of true spina bifida. The most severe form of spina bifida cystica is myelocele, or myeloschisis, in which the open neural plate is covered secondarily by epithelium and the neural plate has spread out onto the surface.

TABLE 16-25. THE NEUROLOGICAL COMPLICATIONS ASSOCIATED WITH SPINA BIFIDA

COMPLICATION	DESCRIPTION
Syringomeningocele	The Greek word syrinx, meaning tube or plate, is combined with meninx (membrane) and kele (tumor); the term thus describes a hollow center with the spinal fluid connecting with the central canal of the cord enclosed by a membrane with very little cord substance.
Syringomyelocele	Protrusion of the membranes and spinal cord lead to increased fluid in the central canal, attenuating the cord tissue against a thin-walled sac.
Diastematomyelia	From the Greek root diastema (interval) and myelon (marrow). Is accompanied by a bony septum in some cases.
Myelodysplasia	From the Greek term myelos, meaning spinal cord, with *dys* for difficult and *plasi* for molding. This is a defective development of any part of the cord.
Arnold-Chiari deformity	Malformation of the cerebellum, with elongation of the cerebellar tonsils. The cerebellum is drawn into the fourth ventricle. The condition also is characterized by smallness of the medulla and pons and internal hydrocephalus. In fact, all patients with spina bifida cystica (failure to close caudally) have some form of Arnold-Chiari malformation (failure to close cranially). The Chiari II malformation is a complex congenital malformation of the brain, nearly always associated with myelomeningocele. This condition includes downward displacement of the medulla, fourth ventricle, and cerebellum into the cervical spinal canal, as well as elongation of the pons and fourth ventricle, probably due to a relatively small posterior fossa. Signs and symptoms include stridor, apnea, irritability, cerebellar ataxia, and hypertonia.
Craniorachischisis (total dysraphism)	A condition in which the brain and spinal cord are exposed. This often results in early spontaneous abortion, often associated with malformations of other organ systems.
Tethered cord	A longitudinal stretch of the spinal cord that occurs with growth resulting in progressive loss of sensory and motor function, long tract signs, and changes in posture and gait. Presence may be signaled by foot deformities previously braced easily, new onset of hip dislocation, or worsening of a spinal deformity, particularly scoliosis. Progressive neurologic defects in growing children may suggest a lack of extensibility of the spine or that it is tethered and low lying in the lumbar canal with the potential for progressive irreversible neurologic damage and requiring surgical release.
Hydrocephalus	Characterized by a tense, bulging fontanel and increased occipital frontal circumference. Signs and symptoms include decreased upper extremity coordination, disturbed balance, strabismus, and ocular problems. Medical intervention involves placement of a shunt between ventricle and heart/abdomen.
Neurogenic bowel and bladder	Incontinence

Data from Shaer CM, Chescheir N, Erickson K, et al: Obstetrician-gynecologists' practice and knowledge regarding spina bifida. *Am J Perinatol.* 2006;23:355-362. Epub Jul 13, 2006; Woodhouse CR: Progress in the management of children born with spina bifida. *Eur Urol.* 2006;49:777-778. Epub Feb 6, 2006; Verhoef M, Barf HA, Post MW, et al: Functional independence among young adults with spina bifida, in relation to hydrocephalus and level of lesion. *Dev Med Child Neurol.* 2006;48:114-119; Ali L, Stocks GM: Spina bifida, tethered cord and regional anaesthesia. *Anaesthesia.* 2005;60:1149-1150; Spina bifida. *Nurs Times.* 2005;101:31; Mitchell LE, Adzick NS, Melchionne J, et al: Spina bifida. *Lancet.* 2004;364:1885-1895; And Dias L: Orthopaedic care in spina bifida: past, present, and future. *Dev Med Child Neurol.* 2004;46:579.

clitoral hypoplasia), short stature, and small hands and feet. Children aged 1 to 6 years manifest symptoms of hyperphagia with progressive development of obesity.

The Role of the Physical Therapist in the Special Care Nursery

The American Physical Therapy Association, section on pediatrics has published guidelines for physical therapy practice in the NICU,[125] which provide the clinician with an algorithm for decision making, and clinical competencies based on roles, proficiencies, and knowledge areas.

The assessment of the neonate needs to focus on function (ie, skeletal alignment, range of motion, motor and sensory development, reflex development, and behavioral organization.[71] The physical therapy examination in this environment should include the following:

- Manual muscle testing: provides objective information regarding the presence of active movement and the quantity of muscle power present. As previously mentioned, conventional methods of testing are not appropriate with the neonate, so other strategies must be employed, including tickling, holding the extremities in positions such as hip and knee flexion, and holding a limb in an anti-gravity position to stimulate the infant to move or hold the limb.[71,126] Correct limb stabilization is necessary to avoid misinterpreting the origin of the movement.
- Range of motion assessment: normal neonates have physiological flexion of up to 30 degrees at the hips, 10 to 20 degrees at the knees, and ankle dorsiflexion of up to 40 or 50 degrees.[119,120]
- Sensory assessment, which is performed when the baby is in a quiet, awake state, is used to determine the level of intact sensation. Educating parents about skin care for the baby is often a shared responsibility of the nursing and therapy staff. Insensitive areas require additional protection from use and abuse.
- Reflex and behavioral testing to evaluate reflex activity such as sucking and swallowing, and the current status of the infant's organization of physiologic response to stress, state control, motor control, and social interaction.
- Pain: although it is difficult to assess pain in a neonate, physiologic manifestations of pain include increased heart rate, heart rate variability, blood pressure, and respirations, with evidence of decreased oxygenation.[71] Skin color and character when pain is present include pallor or flushing, diaphoresis, and, palmar sweating.[71] Other indicators of pain are increased muscle tone, dilated pupils, and laboratory evidence of metabolic or endocrine changes.[127,128] Several neonatal pain measures have been developed, including the Bernese Pain Scale for Neonates,[129] the Neonatal Facial Coding System,[130] and the Pain Assessment in Neonates (PAIN).[131]
- Pulmonary function: assessment of pulmonary function in the infant requires special care and includes observation, inspection, and auscultation.

- Observation and inspection: signs of respiratory distress (nasal flaring, expiratory grunting, inspiratory stridor, use of accessory respiratory muscles, and bulging of intercostal muscles during expiration), chest configuration, breathing patterns, and sneezing. Auscultation is an inexact procedure given the thin chest wall, proximity of structures, and easy transmission of sounds.

Common goals of developmental intervention in the NICU include the following[132]:

- ▶ Promote state organization. Newborns who exhibit irregular or "poorly organized" state patterns are more likely to develop conditions ranging from delayed development, aplastic anemia, and hyperactivity to SIDS.
- ▶ Promote appropriate parent-infant interaction.
- ▶ Enhance self-regulatory behavior through environmental modification.
- ▶ Promote postural alignment and more normal patterns of movement through therapeutic handling and positioning. The primary goals of therapeutic handling in premature infants are to decrease hyperextension of the neck and trunk, reduce elevation of the shoulders, decrease retraction of the scapula, and reduce extension of the lower extremities. Positioning is indicated to enhance ventilation-perfusion ratios and to drain bronchopulmonary segments. In infants aged 9 months and younger, sitting balance and support may be provided with a standard car seat, elevated 45 to 60 degrees.
- ▶ Enhance oral motor skills and assist with oral feedings. The pediatric clinician plays a crucial role in evaluating all motor skills, neurobehavioral readiness to feed, and establishment of successful feeding programs.
- ▶ Improve visual and auditory reactions.
- ▶ Prevent iatrogenic musculoskeletal abnormalities. Proper positioning reinforces the clinician's goal to enhance flexor patterns, increase midline orientation, and promote state organization. Positions are changed frequently to offer the infant various sensorimotor experiences, while protecting the respiratory capacity of the infant.
- ▶ To provide appropriate remediation of orthopedic complications and to provide consultation to team members, including the nursing staff and parents, regarding developmental intervention.
- ▶ To participate in inter-agency collaboration in order to facilitate transition to the home environment.

Outcomes include improved regulation and organization of motor behavior, interactions with caregivers and the environment, and family interaction.[133]

Developmental Interventions. Refer to Tables 16-26 and 16-27.

Discharge Planning. Discharge planning in the NICU is a multidisciplinary effort that begins with the infant's birth and admission to the unit. Important aspects include the parents' involvement in

TABLE 16-26. DEVELOPMENTAL INTERVENTIONS

INTERVENTION	RATIONALE	METHODS
Positioning	Important to promote state organization, stimulate the flexed midline positions typical of the full-term infant, and maintain range of motion. The premature infant does not have the opportunity to develop physiologic flexion and may demonstrate hypotonia. Ventilatory and infusion equipment often exaggerate extension of the neck, trunk, and extremities, which can lead to neck extensor muscle contracture. The prone position, with the heading midline and elevation of the head at 30 degrees, has the beneficial effects of decreasing intracranial pressure, gastroesophageal reflux, and aspiration and increasing stomach emptying.	Blankets, diaper rolls, sandbags, customized foam inserts, buntings, and nests can all be used to reinforce the desired posture, which includes neck flexion or chin tucking, trunk flexion, shoulder protraction, posterior pelvic tilt, and symmetric flexion of the legs. When supine positioning is used, the head is positioned in midline and blanket rolls may be placed along the infant's sides and under the shoulder girdle for support, as well as under the knees. Water mattresses and hammocks are also used in conjunction with positioning to help provide gentle vestibular and proprioceptive stimulation. Positions should be changed throughout the day.
Sensorimotor stimulation	Sensorimotor stimulation in the form of tactile, kinesthetic, visual, and auditory stimulation can have beneficial effects on weight gain, visual responsiveness, growth, development, and sensorimotor functions (behavioral organization, integration of the sensory systems). However, this form of stimulation also has the potential to be harmful necessitating careful monitoring of the infant during intervention. Avoidance responses include vomiting, sneezing, coughing, hiccupping, gagging, sighing, respiratory changes, and changes in tone.	Strategies need to be individualized—the infant who is lethargic and hypertonic needs stimulation to reach the alert state and facilitation of proximal neck and trunk musculature, whereas the infant who is irritable and hypertonic needs calming to the alert state and inhibition of increased tone. Sensory input can include the visual input of the therapist's face, physical handling, swaddling, positioning, offering visual or auditory stimuli, and social interaction.
Oral motor therapy	To help with feeding difficulties related to neurologic immaturity, abnormal muscle tone, depressed oral reflexes (tongue thrusting, sucking), or prolonged use of endotracheal tubes for mechanical ventilation.	Achieving a quiet alert state and positioning the infant in support sitting with semiflexion of the neck. Tactile stimulation of facial muscles and intraoral structure and external support to the infant's cheeks.
Family-centered care	Help the infant recognize the family as a constant in his/her life and to recognize the individual strengths and needs of each family.	Involving the parents in the decision-making process. Providing the parents with information both specific to their infant and general information about development

Data from Sweeney JK, Swanson MW: Low birthweight infants: neonatal care and follow-up. In: Umphred DA, ed. *Neurological Rehabilitation, 4th ed.* St. Louis, MO: Saunders. 2001:203-258; and Kahn-D'Angel L, Unanue-Rose RA: The special care nursery. In: Campbell SK, Vander Linden DW, Palisano RJ, eds. *Physical Therapy for Children, 3rd ed.* St. Louis, MO: Saunders. 2006:1053-1097.

their infant's care, plans for special needs such as oxygen and apnea monitoring, and teaching the parents special skills such as cardiopulmonary resuscitation. Most NICUs have no minimum weight requirement for discharge. Medical guidelines for discharge are as follows:

- Body temperature is maintained while the infant is in an open crib, usually at 34 weeks of gestational age or at 2000 g (4 lb, 6 oz) of weight.
- The infant feeds by mouth well enough to have a weight gain of 20 to 30 g/d.
- The infant is not receiving medications that require hospital management.
- No recent major changes in medications or oxygen administration have occurred.

TABLE 16-27. IDEAL PEDIATRIC POSITIONING

JOINT REGION	SITTING	PRONE	SUPINE	SIDELYING
Pelvis and hips	Pelvis in line with the trunk. Hips at 90 degrees of flexion. Neutral rotation of pelvis. Hips symmetrically abducted 10-20 degrees.	Pelvis in line with the trunk. Hips in extension. Neutral rotation of pelvis. Hips symmetrically abducted 10-20 degrees.	Pelvis in line with the trunk. Hips in 30-90 degrees of flexion. Neutral rotation of pelvis. Hips symmetrically abducted 10-20 degrees.	Pelvis in line with the trunk. Hips in flexion. Neutral rotation of pelvis. Hips symmetrically abducted 10-20 degrees.
Trunk	Straight. Shoulders over hips. Neutral rotation.	Straight. Shoulders in line with hips. Neutral rotation.	Straight. Shoulders in line with hips. Neutral rotation of trunk.	Straight. Shoulders in line with hips. Slight sidebending okay.
Head and neck	Head in neutral position. Facing forward. Head evenly on shoulders.	Head in neutral position. Facing to one side. Slight cervical flexion.	Head in neutral position. Facing forward. Slight cervical flexion.	Head in neutral position. Facing forward. Slight cervical flexion.
Shoulders and arms	Arms fully supported. Elbows in flexion. 0-45 degrees Internally rotated shoulders	Arms fully supported. Arms forward of trunk. Flexion at shoulders. Flexion at elbows.	Arms fully supported. Arms forward of trunk. Forearms rest on trunk or pillow.	Both arms supported. Lower arm forward, not lying on point of shoulders. Lower arm in neutral rotation. Upper arm may have 0-40 degrees internal rotation.
Legs and feet	Knees at 90 degrees. Ankles at 90 degrees. Feet and thighs fully supported.	Knees extended. Feet supported at 90 degrees.	Knees supported in flexion. Feet held at 90 degrees.	Knees in flexion. Feet positioned at 90 degrees. Pillow between knees.

Reproduced, with permission, from Ratliffe KT: Clinical Pediatric Physical Therapy: A Guide for the Physical Therapy Team. Philadelphia: Mosby, Inc. 1998.

PHYSICAL THERAPY ROLES FOR SPECIFIC PEDIATRIC PATHOLOGIES

ASTHMA (HYPERREACTIVE AIRWAY DISEASE)

Asthma, a chronic inflammatory disorder of the airways, is an inflammation (acute, subacute, or chronic) of the airways in susceptible individuals, that can cause intermittent airflow obstruction, and an associated increase in the existing bronchial responsiveness to a variety of stimuli.

Asthma is characterized by recurrent episodes of wheezing, breathlessness, chest tightness, and coughing. The diagnosis of asthma, which is not typically made until the child is 3 to 6 years of age, is made on the basis of history, physical examination, auscultation and palpation, and pulmonary function tests (PFTs), especially in response to a methacholine challenge.[134,135] Overt wheezing is the major presenting sign in childhood. Some children may exhibit respiratory difficulty only after exercise, at night, or in cold air. Other children may have trouble keeping up with peers or with strenuous exercise.

Study Pearl

Exercise-induced asthma (EIA) is an asthma variant in which exercise or vigorous physical activity triggers an acute bronchospasm.

The medical intervention for asthma may include pharmacologic therapy. The goals of long-term management are to[136,137]

- Prevent chronic and troublesome symptoms
- Maintain pulmonary function and activity level
- Prevent recurrent exacerbations
- Minimize the need for emergency room visits or hospitalizations
- Provide optimal pharmacotherapy
- Meet the patients and families expectations of and satisfaction with asthma care

Physical Therapy Role. Physical therapy intervention for asthma may include any or all of the following:

- Patient education on breathing exercises (specific diaphragmatic training from recumbent to upright positions, and eventually to sporting conditions), postural education, how to self monitor asthma symptoms, and to perform and record peak flow readings (as appropriate).[138,139]
- Patient instruction on relaxation techniques, endurance and strength training.[140-143]
- Manual therapy techniques including
  - Rib cage mobilization to increase chest wall and thoracic spine mobility in order to reduce respiratory workload and increased likelihood of recruiting intercostal muscles for more efficient respiration and support for the developing thorax.
  - Quadratus lumborum muscle release to promote activation of oblique and transverse abdominis muscles for lower trunk stabilization.
  - Active assisted anterior and axial glides to thoracic spine.
  - Intercostal muscle release to optimize length-tension relationship.
- Home exercise program addressing lengthening of the accessory neck muscles through active stretching, mid trunk stabilization exercises and controlled breathing techniques.

Cystic Fibrosis

Cystic fibrosis (CF), an autosomal recessive disorder involving multiple organ systems (lungs, liver, intestine, pancreas) and exocrine gland dysfunction, can result in chronic respiratory infections, pancreatic enzyme insufficiency, and associated complications in untreated patients. The root cause of CF is a malfunction of the epithelial cells' ability to conduct chloride that results in water transport abnormalities, resulting in viscous secretions occurring in the respiratory tract, pancreas, gastrointestinal tract, sweat glands, and other exocrine tissues. This increased viscosity makes the secretions difficult to clear.

The clinical characteristics of CF are listed in Table 16-28. Sweat chloride analysis is critical to distinguish CF from other causes of severe pulmonary and pancreatic insufficiencies.[144]

Physical examination of the patient includes[145]

- Inspection: can reveal postural abnormalities, modifications of breathing pattern, or signs of respiratory distress. A chronic productive cough may be apparent. Examination of the comparative dimensions of the chest in the anterior-posterior and transverse planes may reveal the barrel chest deformity common to obstructive lung diseases.[146]

TABLE 16-28. CLINICAL MANIFESTATIONS OF CYSTIC FIBROSIS

SYSTEM	SIGNS AND SYMPTOMS
Gastrointestinal tract	Intestinal, pancreatic and hepatobiliary
	Meconium ileus
	Recurrent abdominal pain and constipation
	Diabetes
	Patients may present with a history of jaundice or gastrointestinal tract bleeding.
	Minimal weight gain—failure to thrive (FTT)
Integumentary	Salty perspiration ("Kiss your Baby week" for early detection)
	Clubbing of nail beds
	Central and peripheral cyanosis
Respiratory tract	Wheezing, rales or rhonchi
	Chronic or recurrent cough, which can be dry and hacking at the beginning and can produce mucoid (early) and purulent (later) sputum
	Recurrent pneumonia, atypical asthma, pneumothorax, hemoptysis, are all complications and may be the initial manifestation.
	Dyspnea on exertion, history of chest pain, recurrent sinusitis, nasal polyps, and hemoptysis may occur.
	Pulmonary artery hypertension
	Cor pulmonale
	Bronchospasm
Urogenital tract	Males are frequently sterile because of the absence of the vas deferens.
	Undescended testicles or hydrocele may exist.

Data from Lucas SR, Platts-Mills TA: Physical activity and exercise in asthma: relevance to etiology and treatment. *J Allergy Clin Immunol.* 2005;115:928-934; Mintz M: Asthma update: part I. Diagnosis, monitoring, and prevention of disease progression. *Am Fam Physician.* 2004;70:893-898; Ram FS, Robinson SM, Black PN, et al: Physical training for asthma. *Cochrane Database Syst Rev.* 2005;CD001116; and Welsh L, Kemp JG, Roberts RG: Effects of physical conditioning on children and adolescents with asthma. *Sports Med.* 2005;35:127-141.

- Palpation: accurate evaluation of the findings of tactile fremitus, atelectasis, pneumothorax, or large airway secretions.[146]
- Percussion: examination of the resonance pattern of the chest, as demonstrated by audible changes on percussion, can provide an indication of abnormally dense areas of the lungs.[146]
- Auscultation: can contribute information on the quality of airflow and evidence of obstruction in different areas of the lungs (rales etc—see Chapter 10).

Physical Therapy Role. CF is a disorder that often requires management by a multidisciplinary team. The goals of the intervention are

- Maintenance of adequate nutritional status
- Prevention of pulmonary and other complications
- Encouragement of physical activity
- Provision of adequate psychosocial support

In the neonate, because the lungs are morphologically normal at birth, the most frequently seen symptoms are meconium ileus, malabsorption of nutrients, and failure to thrive, all of which are associated with the gastrointestinal tract. However, within a few months, some infants may develop signs of impaired respiratory function.[145]

Specific chest physical therapy techniques for the infant include, but are not limited to[145,147]

- The secretion clearance techniques of postural draining, percussion and vibrations should be performed around feeding

Study Pearl

- The quantitative pilocarpine iontophoresis test (QPIT), collects sweat and performs a chemical analysis of its chloride content.
- The sweat chloride reference value is less than 40 mEq/L, and a value of more than 60 mEq/L of chloride in the sweat is consistent with a diagnosis of CF (40-60 mEq/L are considered borderline).[144]

schedules to reduce the risk of gastroesophageal reflux. The applied force of percussion is based on the size and condition of the infant, and the infant's response to treatment.

- Ongoing family and/or caregiver education in the application of prescribed physical therapy modalities.

The physical therapy intervention for the preschool and school age period depends on the severity. The goals should address an enhancement in exercise tolerance with continued focus on secretion clearance techniques, and correction and maintenance of good postural alignment. Mechanical percussors may be used to ease the work involved with manual percussion and to provide the child with an aide to self treatment. Alternative methods for mobilizing secretions and stimulating cough have been suggested, usually involving directed breathing techniques. These include huffing, PEP (positive expiratory pressures), oscillating PEP (Flutter and Acapella), autogenic drainage, and active cycle of breathing (formerly known as FET—forced expiratory technique). Exercise has also been shown to be beneficial for secretion clearance, and for increasing peak oxygen consumption, maximal work capacity, and better expiratory flow rates.[148,149]

NURSEMAID'S ELBOW

The term nursemaid's elbow (also referred to as *pulled elbow*) refers to a subluxation of the radial head in children of preschool age, caused by a sudden longitudinal traction force on the pronated wrist and extended elbow.[150,151] These are the common causes of a pulled elbow:[152]

- The child's forearm or hand is being held firmly by a parent as the child attempts to walk away.
- The child is lifted by an adult from the ground by his hands.

The combination of patient history and limitation of motion usually make the diagnosis—a painful and dangling arm, which hangs limply with the elbow extended and the forearm pronated.[152] There is usually no obvious swelling or deformity. The common sites of pain are the forearm and wrist, the wrist alone, and the elbow alone.[153] In all cases the child resists attempted supination of the elbow.

The intervention of choice is manipulation.[152] The child's attention is diverted while the forearm is forcibly supinated with one quick motion, together with application of downward pressure on the radial head. A click in the region of the radial head (palpable and sometimes audible) is indicative of a successful reduction. Soon after the manipulation, the child usually begins to use the arm again, but sometimes there is a delay of a day or two.

TORSIONAL CONDITIONS

These include in-toeing or out-toeing, probably the most common reason for elective referral of a child to an orthopedist. Clinical examination of the child with in-toeing or out-toeing should include documentation of the foot progression angle in standing or walking, hip rotation range of motion, thigh-foot axis, and alignment of the foot:[99]

- Foot progression angle (FPA): also known as *the angle of gait*, is defined as the angle between the longitudinal axis of the foot and a straight line of progression of the body in walking.[154] While observing gait, the clinician assigns a value to the angle of both the right and left foot. In-toeing is expressed as a negative value (eg, −20 degrees), and out-toeing is expressed as a positive value (eg, +20 degrees). FPA is variable during infancy, but during childhood and adult life, it shows little change, with a mean of +10 degrees and a normal range of −3 to +20 degrees.[154]
- Hip rotation range of motion: this is measured most accurately in the prone position (or with the anxious young child being held facing the parent's chest), with the hip in a position of neutral flexion/extension. If the hip is in anteversion (anteverted), the patient will usually have more hip internal rotation than external rotation, assuming no soft tissue tightness (refer to the hip section in Chapter 8). The sum of hip internal rotation and external rotation is usually 120 degrees up to age 2 years; over age to it is 95 to 110 degrees.[155] True femoral retroversion in an infant is rare. Although many types of interventions have been tried to correct femoral anteversion, none of these has been proved effective in clinical trials.
- Thigh-foot axis: a reflection of the version of the tibia, which is assessed using the thigh-foot angle, the angular difference between the longitudinal axes of the thigh and the foot, as measured in the prone position with the knee flexed. Tibial torsion can also be described as the angle formed by a straight-line axis through the knee and the axis through the medial and lateral malleoli. By convention, internal tibial torsion is expressed as a negative value, whereas external tibial torsion is expressed as a positive value. Scoles[156] described the following approximate thigh-foot normative angles:
  - Birth: −15 degrees (normal range −30 to +20 degrees)
  - Age 3: +5 degrees (normal range −10 to +20 degrees)
  - Mid-childhood to skeletal maturity: +10 degrees (normal range −5 to +30 degrees)
- Controversy exists regarding the appropriate treatment of internal tibial torsion because the natural history of the condition is a gradual improvement in most cases. In some cases a Friedman countersplint or a Denis Browne bar may be prescribed for night wear for approximately 6 months.
- Alignment of the foot: alterations in the alignment of the foot can be divided into two categories (Table 16-29):

TABLE 16-29. DECISION MATRIX FOR FOOT DEFORMITY

	METATARSUS VARUS	CLUBFOOT	CALCANEOVALGUS
Side view (can foot dorsiflex?)	Yes	No	Yes
Foot shape (viewed from bottom)	Kidney shaped (deviated medially)	Kidney shaped	Banana shaped (deviated laterally)
Heel position	Valgus	Varus	Valgus

Data from Wenger DR, Leach J: Foot deformities in infants and children. Pediatr *Clin North Am.* 1986;33:1411-1427; And Leach J: Orthopedic conditions. In: Campbell SK, Vander Linden DW, Palisano RJ, eds. *Physical Therapy for Children, 3rd ed.* St. Louis, MO: Saunders. 2006:481-515.

- Positional (packaging): caused by a restricted intrauterine environment.
  - Metatarsus varus, also called metatarsus adductus is one of the most commonly seen positional conditions in infants. The forefoot is curved medially, the hindfoot is in the normal slight valgus position, and there is full dorsiflexion range of motion.
  - Calcaneovalgus, a common positional foot problem in newborns. The forefoot is curved out laterally, the hindfoot is in valgus, and there is full or excessive dorsiflexion.
- Manufacturing: true congenital abnormalities (talipes equinovarus)—see "Conditions Related to the Neonate" earlier.

Slipped Capital Femoral Epiphysis

Slipped capital femoral epiphysis (SCFE) is a disorder of epiphyseal growth (Table 16-30) that represents a distinctive type of instability of the proximal femoral growth plate due to a Salter-Harris type 1 fracture through the proximal femoral physis.[99,157-162] The cause of SCFE is uncertain, although it has been established that stress around the hip causes a shear force to be applied at the growth plate, which causes the epiphysis to move posteriorly and medially. In addition, the position of the proximal physis normally changes from horizontal to oblique during preadolescence and adolescence, redirecting the hip forces.

The patient usually has an antalgic limp and pain in the groin, often referred to the anteromedial aspect of the thigh and knee. The leg is usually held in external rotation, both when supine and when standing. There may be tenderness to palpation on the anterior and lateral aspect of the hip. Decreased hip motion is noted in flexion, abduction, and internal rotation. With attempts to flex the hip, the legs move into external rotation. Knowledge of SCFE and its manifestations will facilitate prompt referral by the clinician to an orthopedic surgeon. Diagnosis can be confirmed using both anteroposterior (AP) pelvis and lateral frog-leg radiographs of both hips. CT is a sensitive method of measuring the degree of tilt and detecting early disease, but it is rarely needed. MRI depicts the slippage earliest, and MRI can demonstrate early marrow edema and slippage.

Physical Therapy Role. The goals of treatment are to keep the displacement to a minimum, maintain motion, and delay or prevent premature degenerative arthritis.[99] Following surgical fixation, using one or two pins or screws, usually in situ, the clinician completes a careful and thorough examination of the motion of the hip joint and subsequent measurements should be taken after every operation and removal of the cast. Range of motion exercises for the hip should be done in all planes, with particular emphasis on hip flexion, internal rotation, and abduction.

Gait training postsurgery is initiated once lower extremity strength and range of motion is adequate for ambulation skills. The weight-bearing status can vary but is usually non-weight bearing (NWB) or touch down weight bearing (TDWB). Full weight bearing is permitted once the growth plate has fused (within approximately 3-4 months).

TABLE 16-30. EPIPHYSEAL DISORDERS: DISORDERS OF EPIPHYSEAL GROWTH

EPIPHYSEAL DISORDER	INCIDENCE	CLINICAL FEATURES AND DIAGNOSIS	INTERVENTION AND OUTCOME
Slipped capital femoral epiphysis (SCFE) (adolescent coxa vara) By far the most significant of the lower limb epiphyseal plate disorders. It is the most common hip disorder seen in adolescence.	Males (13-16 years of age) are 2-5 times more likely to be affected than females (11-14 years of age). 25%-33% bilateral, especially with boys < 12 years. More common in African Americans.	Obesity (75% of cases) Mild hip pain referred to the medial aspect of the knee. Slight limp that increases with fatigue; positive Trendelenburg sign. Posture: lower extremity unloaded into flexion, external rotation, and abduction to avoid impingement of metaphysis on the anterior lip of acetabulum. Reduced hip flexion, internal rotation, abduction. Diagnosis is confirmed with x-ray—AP and lateral views helpful, but frog view with positive Kline's line is definitive.	Prescription: prevent further slip, maintain range of motion, prevent osteoarthritis, immobilize via hip spica and non-weight-bearing status. If the slip is less than 1 cm, screwed/pin in situ, cast and weight-bearing after surgery.
Blount's disease (tibia vara) Growth suppression with premature closure of the medial portion of the upper tibial epiphyseal plate.	Girls > boys. Type in infants < 2-3 years is the most common. Juvenile type: 4-10 years. Adolescent: 11+ y. Finland and Jamaica have the highest incidence of disease.	Often seen in obese children who are early ambulators. Lateral thrust during stance. Tibial varum. Early x-ray is essential as it displays the defective ossification on the medial side of the tibia, beaked appearance of the underlying metaphysis, and obvious longitudinal growth disturbance.	Prescription: prevent progression of the varus deformity. If unilateral infantile form (< 3 y) hip, knee, ankle, foot, orthosis (HKAFO) worn 23 hr/day or night splints to correct the varus deformity. If > 4 years: splinting usually fails and osteotomy of the tibia is required. African American girls have the worst prognosis.
Madelung's deformity Localized epiphyseal dysplasia on the medial (ulnar) side of the distal radial epiphysis.	Adolescent onset. Girls > boys. Usually bilateral	Insidious onset of wrist pain. Loss of wrist/forearm range of motion (flexion and supination). Prominence of the distal end of the ulna on the dorsum of the wrist and forward displacement of the hand in relation to the forearm.	Correction of the deformity via surgical excision of the distal portion of the ulna and osteotomy of the deformed end of the radius.

Reproduced, with permission. from Hallisy KM: The adolescent population. In Boissonnault WG, ed. *Primary Care for the Physical Therapist: Examination and Triage.* St Louis, MO: Elsevier Saunders. 2005:175-237.

LEGG-CALVÉ PERTHES DISEASE

Legg-Calvé-Perthes disease (LCPD) is an idiopathic osteonecrosis of the capital femoral epiphysis of the femoral head.[163-169] LCPD has an unconfirmed etiology, but may involve

- An interruption of the blood supply to the capital femoral epiphysis—osteochondroses.
- Bone infarction, especially in the subchondral cortical bone, while articular cartilage continues to grow.

- Revascularization as new bone ossification starts. At this point, a percentage of patients develop LCPD, while other patients have normal bone growth and development.
- Changes to the epiphyseal growth plate, secondary to the subchondral fracture. When a subchondral fracture occurs, it is usually the result of normal physical activity, not direct trauma to the area.

Patients frequently have a painful limp (pain in the groin, hip, or knee), a positive Trendelenburg sign (hip abduction weakness), and limited hip range of motion, especially in hip abduction and internal rotation.[99]

Physical therapy Role. Controversy exists regarding the appropriate treatment, or whether treatment is even necessary.[99] The goal of treatment is to relieve pain, and to maintain the spherical shape of the femoral head and to prevent extrusion of the enlarged femoral head from the joint. Treatment methods include observation only, range of motion exercises in all planes of hip motion (especially internal rotation and abduction), bracing, Petrie casts (two long leg cast with a bar between, holding the hips abducted and internally rotated), and surgery.

Osgood Schlatter

Osgood-Schlatter (OS) disease is a benign, self-limiting traction apophysis at the knee, which is one of the most common causes of knee pain in the adolescent.[170] OS is manifested by pain and edema with traction apophysitis of the tibial tubercle.

During periods of rapid growth, the contraction forces of the quadriceps are transmitted through the patellar tendon onto a small portion of the tibial tuberosity that is only partially developed, which can result in a partial avulsion fracture through the ossification center. Eventually, secondary heterotopic bone formation occurs in the tendon near its insertion, producing a visible lump.

Study Pearl

The signs and symptoms of Osgood-Schlatter disease include

- A visible soft tissue edema is present over the proximal tibial tuberosity. A firm mass may be palpable.
- Patient may have tenderness to palpation over the proximal tibial tuberosity at the site of patellar insertion.
- Knee joint examination is normal; OS disease is an extra-articular disease.
- Erythema of the tibial tuberosity may be present.
- Some patients may have quadriceps atrophy.

- Approximately 25% of patients have bilateral lesions.
- Pain is the most common presenting complaint.
- May be reproduced by extending the knee against resistance, stressing the quadriceps, or squatting with the knee in full flexion.
- Running, jumping, kneeling, squatting, and ascending/descending stairs exacerbate the pain.
- Relief of symptoms occurs with rest or restriction of activities.
- Pain usually has been present intermittently for several months before the patient sees the physician.
- Approximately 50% of patients give a history of precipitating trauma.

Physical Therapy Role. The intervention for this condition is usually symptomatic, including anti-inflammatory measures. Specific procedural interventions include bracing (neoprene knee brace), quadriceps stretching exercises, including hip extension for a complete stretch of the extensor mechanism, and stretching exercises for the hamstrings. The traditional approach of activity limitations is no longer considered necessary. More persistent cases may require cast immobilization for 6 to 8 weeks. Rarely, individuals will require surgical excision of symptomatic ossicles or degenerated tendons for persistent symptoms at skeletal maturity.

Idiopathic Scoliosis

Scoliosis represents a disturbance of a series of spinal segments that produces a three-dimensional deformity of the spine including lateral curvature and vertebral rotation.[171-184] The cause of idiopathic scoliosis remains unclear, although there does appear to be a familial prevalence.

Scoliosis has three age distinctions based on the James classification system, which have prognostic significance.

- Infantile idiopathic: usually manifests shortly after birth. This type accounts for less than 1% of all cases. Although 80% to 90% of these curves spontaneously resolve, many of the remainder of cases will progress throughout childhood, resulting in severe deformity. In the most common curve pattern (right thoracic), the right shoulder is consistently rotated forward and the medial border of the right scapula protrudes posteriorly.
- Juvenile idiopathic: occurs during the ages of 3 to 9 years.
- Adolescent idiopathic: occurs at or around the onset of puberty, accounting for approximately 80% of all cases.

The following are the main factors that influence the probability of progression in the skeleton of the immature patient:

1. The younger the patient at diagnosis, the greater the risk of progression.
2. Double-curve patterns have a greater risk for progression than single-curve patterns.
3. Curves with greater magnitude are at a greater risk to progress.
4. Risk of progression in females is approximately 10 times that of males with curves of comparable magnitude.
5. Greater risk of progression is present when curves develop before menarche.

Scoliosis is described based on the location of the curve or curves, and whether the convexity of the curve points to the right or left. If there is a double curve, each curve is described and measured. As the disease progresses, the vertebrae and spinous processes in the area of the major curve rotate toward the concavity of the curve. On the concave side of the curve, the ribs are close together. On the convex side, they are widely separated. As the vertebral bodies rotate, the spinous processes deviate more and more to the concave side and the ribs follow the rotation of the vertebrae. The posterior ribs on the convex side are pushed posteriorly, causing the characteristic rib hump seen in thoracic scoliosis. The anterior ribs on the concave side are pushed anteriorly. The magnitude of a rib hump is quantified using a scoliometer (a form of inclinometer) with the forward bending test. The scoliometer is placed over the spinous process at the apex

TABLE 16-31. RISSER GRADES

GRADE	INTERPRETATION
0	Absence of ossification
1	25% ossification of the iliac apophysis
2	50% ossification of the iliac apophysis
3	75% ossification of the iliac apophysis
4	100% ossification of the iliac apophysis
5	The iliac apophysis has fused to the iliac crest after 100% ossification.

Data from Biondi J, Weiner DS, Bethem D, et al: Correlation of Risser sign and bone age determination in adolescent idiopathic scoliosis. *J Pediatr Orthop.* 1985;5:697-701; and Little DG, Sussman MD: The Risser sign: a critical analysis. *J Pediatr Orthop.* 1994;14:569-575.

of the curve to measure the angle of trunk rotation. Radiographs, which are usually only considered when a patient has a curve that might require treatment or could progress to a stage requiring treatment (usually 40-100 degrees), can be used to determine location, type, and magnitude of the curve (using the Cobb method), as well as skeletal age. Skeletal maturity is determined using the Risser sign, which is defined by the amount of calcification present in the iliac apophysis, measures the progressive ossification from anterolaterally to posteromedially (Table 16-31). Children usually progress from a Risser grade 1 to a grade 5 over a 2-year period.

Most curves can be treated nonoperatively through observation with appropriate intermittent radiographs to check for the presence or absence of curve progression. However, 60% of curvatures in rapidly growing prepubertal children will progress and may require bracing (Boston, or custom thoracolumbosacral [TLSO]) or surgery. The primary goal of scoliosis surgery is to achieve a solid bony fusion. Even in the setting of adequate correction and solid fusion, up to 38% of patients still have occasional back pain.

Study Pearl

If scoliosis is neglected, the curves may progress dramatically, creating significant physical deformity and even cardiopulmonary problems with especially severe curves.

Study Pearl

Scoliosis screening is done in schools across the United States. Generally, curvatures less than 30 degrees will not progress after the child is skeletally mature.

Physical Therapy Role. The patient's history should emphasize information relative to other family members with spinal deformity, assessment of physiologic maturity (eg, menarche), and presence or absence of pain. Observation may reveal trunk, shoulder (uneven shoulder heights and protruding scapulae), and pelvic asymmetries (waist creases). Children with such asymmetries should be referred to an orthopedic surgeon for a baseline evaluation.

During the physical examination, a determination should be made as to whether the deformity is structural (cannot be corrected with active or passive movement and there is rotation toward the convexity of the curve) or nonstructural (fully corrects clinically and radiographically on lateral bending toward the apex of the curve, and lacks vertebral rotation). Height measurements should be taken in sitting and standing. Changes in sitting height can be less than changes in standing height and give a better estimate of truncal growth rate. Trunk compensation can be assessed using a plumb-line, and a leg length measurement should also be obtained.

The intervention is based on the skeletal maturity of the child, the child's growth potential, and the magnitude of the curve. The indication for orthotic use depends on curve type, magnitude, and location. Orthoses are typically prescribed for children with idiopathic scoliosis who are skeletal immature (with a Risser sign of 0, 1, or 2) and have a curve from 25 to 45 degrees. Theoretically, curve progression is prevented by muscle contractions responding to the brace wear. Exercises to be performed while wearing a brace, such as pelvic tilts, thoracic flexion, and lateral shifts, are often taught to patients to improve the active forces, although there is little evidence to support this.

Electrical muscle stimulation, spinal manipulation, and nutritional therapies, have all been shown to be ineffective for managing the spinal deformity associated with idiopathic scoliosis. It must also be remembered that the majority of studies have indicated that exercise does not have any effect on either reducing the curve or on preventing its progression. However, a 2003 study from Germany suggested that an intensive inpatient rehabilitative exercise program (6 h/d for a minimum of 4 to 6 weeks, including both group and individual therapy) has the potential to reduce the incidence of progression in children with idiopathic scoliosis.[185] At the time of writing, the primary benefits of exercise are to help with correct alignment following the bracing program; maintain proper respiration and chest mobility; maintain muscle strength, particularly in abdominals; maintain or improve range of motion and spinal flexibility; to help reduce back pain, to improve overall posture, and to resume prebracing functional skills.

Cerebral Palsy

Cerebral palsy (CP), the neurologic condition most frequently encountered by pediatric clinicians, is generally considered to be a non-progressive defect or lesion in single or multiple locations in the immature brain.[27,48,49,186-229] CP is diagnosed when a child does not reach motor milestones while also exhibiting abnormal muscle tone or movement pattern dysfunctions such as asymmetry. Despite advances in neonatal care, CP remains a significant clinical problem. In most cases of CP the exact cause is unknown but is most likely multifactorial.

CP can be classified in a number of ways, including a diagnosis based on the area of the body exhibiting motor impairment: monoplegia (one limb), diplegia (lower limbs), hemiplegia (upper and lower limbs on one side of the body), and quadriplegia (all limbs). Another classification, which is based on the most obvious movement abnormalities, is outlined in Tables 16-32 to 16-34. CP impairments, which involve problems of the neural and musculoskeletal systems, can be either primary or secondary:

- Primary impairments of the muscular system include insufficient muscle force generation, spasticity, abnormal extensibility, and exaggerated or hyperactive reflexes.
- Primary impairments of the neuromuscular system include poor selective control of muscle activity, reduced anticipatory regulation, and a decreased ability to learn distinctive movements.
- Secondary impairments of the skeletal system include malalignment such as torsion or hip deformities.

> **Study Pearl**
>
> The clinical term *tone* is commonly used to describe the impairments of spasticity and abnormal extensibility.

Physical Therapy Role. In few conditions do physical therapists play such a central role, or have as much potential to influence the outcome of children's lives.[225] Children with CP have variable but

TABLE 16-32. CEREBRAL PALSY CLASSIFICATIONS AND MANIFESTATIONS

	SPASTIC	ATHETOID	ATAXIC	HYPOTONIC
Muscle stiffness	Excessively stiff and taut, especially during attempted movement	Low	Variable	Diminished resting muscle tone and decreased ability to generate voluntary muscle force
Posture	Abnormal postures and movements mass patterns of flexion/extension	Poor functional stability, especially in proximal joint	Low postural tone with poor balance	Variable
Visual tracking	Some deficits	Poor visual tracking	Poor visual tracking, nystagmus	Variable
Muscle tone	Increased in antigravity muscles. Imbalance of tone across joints that can cause contractures and deformities	Fluctuates, but generally decreased—floppy baby syndrome	Slightly decreased	Minimal to none
Initiating movement	Difficult	No problems	No problems	Difficult
Sustaining movement	Able to in some	Unable	No problems	Unable
Terminating movement	Unable	Variable	No problems	Uncontrolled
Muscle co-activation	Abnormal	Poorly timed	No problems	None
ROM limitations	Passive ROM, overall decreased	Hypermobile	In spine	Hypermobile

TABLE 16-33. GROSS MOTOR FUNCTION CLASSIFICATION SYSTEM

LEVEL	DESCRIPTION
I	Walks without restrictions, limitations in more advanced gross motor skills
II	Walks without assistive devices; limitations walking outdoors and in the community
III	Walks with assistive mobility devices; limitations walking outdoors and in the community
IV	Self mobility with limitations; are transported or use power motor mobility outdoors and in the community
V	Self mobility is severely limited even with the use of assistive technology

Data from Palisano R, Rosenbaum P, Walter S, et al: Development and reliability of a system to classify gross motor function in children with cerebral palsy. *Dev Med Child Neurol.* 1997;39:214-223.

TABLE 16-34. PHYSICAL ATTRIBUTES OF DIFFERENT TYPES OF CEREBRAL PALSY

TYPE	ATTRIBUTES
Spastic (ie, pyramidal)	Constitutes 75% of patients with cerebral palsy. Patients have signs of upper motor neuron involvement, including hyperreflexia, clonus, extensor Babinski response, persistent primitive reflexes, and overflow reflexes (ie, crossed adductor). Cognitive impairment is present in approximately 30% of these patients, but most patients with spastic quadriplegia have some cognitive impairment.
Dyskinesia (ie, extrapyramidal)	Characterized by extrapyramidal movement patterns, abnormal regulation of tone, abnormal postural control, and coordination deficits. Athetosis, chorea, and choreoathetoid or dystonic movements can be seen. Patients often have pseudobulbar involvement with dysarthria, swallowing difficulties, drooling, oromotor difficulties, and abnormal speech patterns. Generally, the child is hypotonic at birth with abnormal movement patterns emerging at 1-3 years. The arms are usually more involved than the legs. Abnormal movement patterns may increase with stress or purposeful activity. Muscle tone is normal during sleep. Intelligence is normal in 78% of patients with athetoid cerebral palsy. A high incidence of sensorineural hearing loss is reported.
Spastic diplegia	Patients will often have a period of hypotonia followed by extensor spasticity in the lower extremities with little or no functional limitation of the upper extremities. Patients have a delay in developing gross motor skills. Spastic muscle imbalance often causes persistence of infantile coxa valga and femoral anteversion. Scissoring gait (ie, hips flexed and adducted, knees flexed with valgus stress, equinus ankles) is observed.
Hemiplegia	Characterized by weak hip flexion and ankle dorsiflexion, overactive posterior tibialis, hip hiking/circumduction, supinated foot in stance, upper extremity posturing (eg, often held with shoulder adducted, elbow flexed, forearm pronated, wrist flexed, hand clenched in a fist with the thumb in the palm), impaired sensation, impaired 2-point discrimination, and/or impaired position sense. Some cognitive impairment is found in about 28% of these patients.

significant disruptions in the accomplishment of life habits, particularly in the categories of recreation, community roles, personal care, education, mobility, housing, and nutrition, and are most associated with locomotion capabilities. The clinician must be able to identify the abilities as well as participation restrictions, activity limitations, and impairment of body structure and function of the patient. At all ages examination of impairment involves qualitative and, when possible, quantitative assessment of single system and multisystem impairments (Table 16-18).

The physical therapy intervention for the patient with cerebral palsy is highly individualized and is usually part of a multidisciplinary team, which consists of the family, various allied health professionals, and appropriate school staff. In general, the more one practices the more one learns, therefore activities should be repeated many times in each treatment session and throughout each day.[230]

The foremost set of goals at all ages is to educate families about CP, to provide support in their acceptance of their child's problems, and to be of assistance when parents make decisions about managing both their own and their child's lives. From infancy to adulthood, physical therapy goals for patients with CP should focus on the promotion of participation by maximizing the gross motor activity allowed by the organic deficits and helping the child compensate for activity limitations when necessary.[230] This necessitates a cognizance of environmental and personal factors that could enhance activity or participation or, conversely, that could increase existing activity limitations and participation restrictions.[230] Habilitation interventions should include tasks that are purposeful, relevant, developmentally appropriate, active, voluntarily regulated, goal directed, and meaningful to the child.[230]

Infancy. Physical therapy in infancy is focused on educating the family, facilitating caregiving, and promoting optimal sensorimotor experiences and skills.[225] Abnormal postures and movements resulting from impairments can make an infant difficult to handle and position. Emphasis during this period should focus on

- Using a variety of movement and postures to promote sensory variety and to allow the emergence of motor skills such as reaching, rolling, sitting, crawling, transitional movements, standing, and prewalking skills.
- Frequently including positions that promote the full lengthening of spastic or hypoextensible muscles. This can be accomplished by carrying the child in a symmetric position that does not allow axial hyperextension and keeps the knees and hips flexed. Positioning of all playing with the upper extremities free allows the infant to see his or her hands, practice midline play, reach for his or her feet, or suck on fingers.
- Using positions that promote functional voluntary movement of the limbs. This can be accomplished by incorporating active movements such as the handling of toys that require two hands and that encourage the infant to develop flexor control and symmetry while promoting anterior, posterior, and lateral control.

Preschool. The aims of the intervention during this period include optimal postural alignment and movements of the body that are conducive to musculoskeletal development, neurophysiologic control, fitness, and function, to exercise, positioning, and equipment.[225] Age-appropriate play and adaptive toys and games based on the desired exercises are important to elicit the child's full cooperation. The clinician should encourage performance at a level of success to maintain the child's interest and cooperation. Activities such as transitional movements against gravity, ball gymnastics, treadmill use, and practice of functional skills such as ascending and descending stairs can help to improve force generation of muscles and prevent atrophy.

School Age and Adolescent. The focus of the physical therapy intervention during this period should include[225]

- Addressing impairments that could interfere with function, or lead to further secondly impairment, such as scoliosis.
- The maintenance of muscle extensibility and force generation, joint integrity, and fitness is important in preventing secondary impairments that can result from the stresses of aging.
- Casting may be necessary to increase the range of joint movement by lengthening muscles or tendons or both.
- Joint mobilizations may be used to regain joint mobility, particularly after immobilization.
- Daily range-of-motion (ROM) exercises are important to prevent or delay contractures secondary to spasticity and to maintain mobility of joints and soft tissues. Stretching exercises are performed to increase motion.
- Maintaining or improving the level of functional activity and participation while considering the stresses of growth, maturation, and increasing demand in life skills and participation in community activities. Many adapted or integrated sports activities are suitable for people with CP, including horseback riding, swimming, skiing, sailing, canoeing, camping, fishing, yoga, and tai chi.
- Involving the patient in setting goals and determining programming.

MYELODYSPLASIA

Myelodysplasia, of which spina bifida is a subclassification, refers to a defective development of any part (especially the lower segments) of the spinal cord.[231] The next most common form of myelodysplasia is a lipoma of the spinal cord. Diastematomyelia is a fibrous, cartilaginous, or bony band or spicule separating the spinal cord into hemicords, each surrounded by a dural sac. The least common of the myelodysplasias, myelocystoceles, are cysts that separate from the central canal of the spinal cord and from the subarachnoid space. The descriptions in this section refer to myelomeningocele and its associated malformations.

The broad spectrum of problems encountered, which includes spinal and lower limb deformities and joint contractures, and poor postural habits, require a multidisciplinary team approach in a comprehensive care outpatient clinic setting. The intervention strategies for the neonate and infant are described in "The Role of the Physical Therapist in the Special Care Nursery" section, earlier.

Physical Therapy Role

Function. See Table 16-35.

Positioning. Postural stability is essential to effectively perform functional tasks. Symmetric alignment is important to minimize joint stress and deforming forces and to permit muscles to function at the optimal length.[231] Typical postural problems include forward head, rounded shoulders, kyphosis, scoliosis, excessive lordosis, anterior pelvic tilt, rotational deformities of the hip or tibia, flexed hips and knees, and pronated feet. Static and dynamic balance should be observed in sitting, four-point positioning, kneeling, half-kneeling, and standing, as well as during transitions between these positions. Postural deviations and contractures that are typical for individual lesion levels are summarized in Table 16-36. Adaptive equipment is recommended based on age. For example,

- A standing frame may be used in children aged 1 to 2 years to diminish the degree of osteoporosis and to limit the contracture of the hip, knee, and ankle.
- A parapodium may be helpful for children aged 3 to 12 years, allowing patients in an erect posture greater experience standing and manipulating work with their upper extremities at a table or desk.

Bracing. The goal of bracing is to prevent contractures and to allow patients to function at the maximum level possible with their neurological lesion and their intelligence. Bracing also ensures a normal developmental progression, allowing for appropriate age-related activities, with the goal of ambulation.

Orthotics. Orthotics should aid in minimizing energy expenditure to maintain mobility levels. A knee-ankle-foot orthosis (KAFO) may be helpful in allowing ambulation. Hip-knee-ankle-foot orthoses (HKAFOs) generally are useful during therapy sessions but are not practical for long-term use.

Exercise. Passive range of motion exercises should be brief, and should be performed only two to three times each day. Passive range of motion exercises must continue throughout the child's life. Exercises, including stretching, can also be used for the correction of muscle imbalances.

Gait Training. Independent ambulation generally is a function of having an intact quadriceps muscle with good or excellent plus strength levels. Patients who do not have adequate quadriceps function may require bilateral Lofstrand crutches or may be primarily restricted to a wheelchair. Functional ambulation generally is described according to the following levels, developed by Hoffer[232]:

TABLE 16-35. IMPAIRMENT AND FUNCTION IN MYELODYSPLASIA

NEURO SEGMENTAL LEVEL	MUSCLES INNERVATED	GOALS	AMBULATION ORTHOSES	ASSISTIVE DEVICES	FUNCTIONAL PROGNOSIS	ASSOCIATED PROBLEMS
Cervical-thoracic (C1-T4)	Neck Upper limb Shoulder girdle Trunk	Maintain a straight spine, level pelvis and symmetric lower limbs	Reciprocating gait orthosis (RGO) Parapodium	Parallel bars Walker Forearm crutches Sliding boards	Wheelchair	Involvement of other CNS areas Spinal deformity Decubiti
High lumbar (L1-2)	All of the above and hip flexors, adductors and rotators	Short distance household ambulation or therapeutic ambulation	RGO KAFO	Parallel bars Walker Forearm crutches	Wheelchair (community) Standing transfers Independent living status	Hip flexion contractures
Mid lumbar (L3-4)	All of the above and knee extensors	Some potential for full time competitive employment	HKAFO/KAFO AFO (depending on quad strength)	Parallel bars Forearm crutches	Wheelchair for community, orthoses for household ambulation	Calcaneal foot deformities
Low lumbar (L5-S1)	All of the above and lateral hamstrings,hip abductors, ankle and foot dorsiflexors, evertors, inverters, toe flexors	Ambulate without orthosis Ambulate without orthosis or upper limb support (with S1 level function)	KAFO AFO	Parallel bars Walker Forearm crutches None	Household or community ambulators	Hindfoot valgus deformities Gluteal lurch with gait
Sacral (S2-3)	All of the above and ankle plantar flexors, foot intrinsic muscles	Potential for normal ambulation	AFO or none Orthoses recommended to maintain gait quality and decrease compensatory overactivity of muscles	Walker None	Community ambulators	Weak ankle muscles Foot pressure sores

Data from Kahn-D'Angel L: Pediatric physical therapy. In: O'Sullivan SB, Siegelman RP, eds. *National Physical Therapy Examination: Review and Study Guide, 9th ed.* Evanston, IL: International Educational Resources. 2006:232; Ryan K, Eman J, Ploski C: Goal attainment and habilitation of infants and children with spina bifida. APTA, National Conference. 1991; and Hinderer KA, Hinderer SR, Shurtleff DB: Myelodysplasia. In: Campbell SK, Vander Linden DW, Palisano RJ, eds. *Physical Therapy for Children, 3rd ed.* St. Louis, MO: Saunders. 2006:735-799.

TABLE 16-36. POSTURAL DEVIATIONS AND CONTRACTURES BASED ON LESION LEVELS

LESION LEVEL	POSTURAL DEVIATIONS AND CONTRACTURES
High-level (thoracic to L2)	Hip flexion, abduction, and external rotation contractures Knee flexion and ankle plantar flexion contractures Lordotic lumbar spine Crouched standing
Mid to lower lumbar (L3-L5)	Hip and knee flexion contractures Increased lumbar lordosis Genu and calcaneal valgus malalignment Pronated position of the foot when weight-bearing Crouched standing
Sacral level	Mild hip and knee flexion contractures Increased lumbar lordosis Ankle and foot can either be in varus or valgus, combined with a pronated or supinated forefoot Crouched standing

Data from Hinderer KA, Hinderer SR, Shurtleff DB: Myelodysplasia. In: Campbell SK, Vander Linden DW, Palisano RJ, eds. *Physical Therapy for Children, 3rd ed.* St. Louis, MO: Saunders. 2006:735-799.

- Community ambulator: indoors or outdoors, crutches with or without braces
- Household ambulator: only indoors, crutches with or without braces
- Nonfunctional ambulator: wheelchair, crutches and braces in therapy
- Nonambulator: wheelchair bound. Focus is on wheelchair mobility, transfers, transitions, decubiti prevention.

DOWN SYNDROME (TRISOMY 21)

The extra chromosome 21 that occurs in Down syndrome affects almost every organ system and results in a wide spectrum of phenotypic consequences. Impairments associated with this condition include hypotonia, decreased force generation of muscles, congenital heart defects, visual and hearing losses, and cognitive deficits (mental retardation).

Physical Therapy Role. The role of physical therapy varies according to the severity of the symptoms, and includes

- Minimizing gross motor delay
- Encouraging oral motor function
- Emphasis on exercise and fitness for the management of obesity
- Balance and coordination exercises
- Maximizing respiratory function
- Nutritional consult

BRAIN INJURY

Traumatic Brain Injury. There are numerous mechanisms of traumatic brain injury in the pediatric population. Traumatic brain injury is a disability category under the Individuals with Disabilities Educational Act (IDEA). The pathophysiology of TBI can be separated into primary injury and secondary injury (refer to Chapter 9):

- Primary injury: due to mechanical forces at the time of impact. This type may be grouped with respect to the role played by

Study Pearl

Shaken baby syndrome is the most common cause of death or serious neurologic injury resulting from child abuse.[233-239] Shaking is usually in response to prolonged inconsolable crying and the injuries sustained are a result of the combination of the mechanism of the shaking and the unique anatomic features of an infant: a relatively large head with weak neck muscles.

Study Pearl

The duration of loss of consciousness can be used to grade the severity of a TBI:

- 30 min or less is defined as mild TBI
- Loss of consciousness between 30 min and 6 h is moderate TBI
- Loss of consciousness of greater than 6 h is considered severe TBI.

acceleration factors, which occur when a force (translational or rotational) is applied to a movable head.

- Secondary injury occurs after the impact secondary to the body's response to primary injury and can be influenced by medical interventions. Causes include
  - Neurochemical and cellular changes
  - Hypotension
  - Hypoxia
  - Increased ICP with decreased cerebral perfusion pressure (CPP) and a risk of herniation
  - Electrolyte imbalances
  - Ischemia

Three scales are commonly used to measure severity of TBI in children[149]:

- Glasgow Coma Scale (GCS)—see Chapter 9.
- Rancho Los Amigos Scale—see Chapter 9
- The Children's Orientation and Amnesia Test (COAT).[240] Used to evaluate the level of coma in children. Test questions are based on facts commonly known by children.

Medical complications after TBI arise from the concomitant injuries, alterations in neurologic function, and the effects of prolonged immobility. Cerebral swelling and increased intracranial pressure (hydrocephalus) can be life-threatening. In addition, some of the more common complications of TBI include fever and infection, fracture, posttraumatic seizures, spasticity, heterotopic ossification, deep venous thrombosis, weakness, balance and coordination problems, and cognitive and perceptual changes.

Near-Drowning. Drowning is the fourth leading cause of fatal injuries in children between 0 and 19 years of age.[241-243] Near-drowning has been defined as an episode in which someone survives a period of underwater submersion. The most devastating outcome of new drowning is the sequelae of global hypoxic-ischemic brain injury. The magnitude of the neuronal injury that occurs is related to both the level of blood flow during the complete ischemic interval and the total duration of the ischemia.

Brain Tumors. Primary central nervous system tumors are those that originate in the brain rather than tumors that are a result of metastasis to the brain. Pediatric brain tumors may be generally classified into infratentorial (occur in the posterior fossa, which is below the tentorium cerebelli and contains the cerebellum, the brainstem, and the fourth ventricle) tumors, and supratentorial (occur in the cerebral hemispheres, the lateral ventricles, and the third ventricle) tumors (Table 16-37).

Reports or signs of any of the following should alert the clinician to the presence of a neurological disorder and should indicate a requirement for medical referral (radiographic imaging, such as CT scan and MRI [with and without contrast]):

- Altered mental status
- Cognitive impairment

TABLE 16-37. PEDIATRIC BRAIN TUMORS

CLASSIFICATION	TYPE	DESCRIPTION
Infratentorial	Astrocytomas	Neoplasms in which the predominant cell type is derived from an astrocyte. Regional effects of astrocytomas include compression, invasion, and destruction of brain parenchyma, arterial and venous hypoxia, competition for nutrients, release of metabolic end products (eg, free radicals, altered electrolytes, neurotransmitters), release and recruitment of cellular mediators (eg, cytokines) that disrupt normal parenchymal function. The type of neurological symptoms that result from astrocytoma development depends foremost on the site and extent of tumor growth in the CNS. Astrocytomas of the spinal cord or brainstem are less common and present with motor/sensory or cranial nerve deficits referable to the tumor's location. The etiology of diffuse astrocytomas has been the subject of analytic epidemiological studies that have yielded associations with various disorders and exposures.
	Ependymomas	Found in the infratentorial region about 65% of the time, and represent 10% of all childhood brain tumors. These tumors arise from ependymal cells in the ventricles and spinal column. Initial signs and symptoms relate to increased intracranial pressure in posterior fossa ependymomas.
	Medulloblastoma	Infiltrate the floor or lateral wall of the fourth ventricle and extend into the cavity. These are fast growing tumors and they may spread throughout the CNS via cerebrospinal fluid.
Supratentorial	Craniopharyngioma	Benign tumors located near the pituitary gland. Cause problems from compression rather than invasion of tissues. Progression of the tumor is related to symptoms of increasing intracranial pressure, visual complaints, and endocrine disturbances.
	Optic tract glioma	Generally slow growing astrocytomas. Visual disturbances are the predominant clinical symptom.
	Pineal	Symptoms are often related to increased intracranial pressure and include headache.

Data from Kerkering GA: Brain injuries: traumatic brain injuries, near drowning, and brain tumors. In: Campbell SK, Vander Linden DW, Palisano RJ, eds. *Physical Therapy for Children, 3rd ed.* St. Louis, MO: Saunders. 2006:709-734.

- Headaches
- Vomiting
- Visual disturbances
- Motor impairment
- Seizures
- Sensory anomalies
- Ataxia, dysmetria

Physical Therapy Role. The clinician must perform a complete and thorough neurological examination (refer to Chapter 9). The intervention will depend on the impairments and functional limitations found in the examination (Table 16-38), but in general, will involve purposeful and skillful interactions of the clinician with the child and family to produce changes that are consistent with the diagnosis and prognosis.[241] Specific goals for the intervention may include

- Maintain or improve joint range of motion using positioning, casting, and passive range of motion.
- Maximizing functional mobility by assisting the child in the achievement of the highest possible levels of independent functioning in his or her home, school, and residential community.
- Maximizing strength and postural control.
- Stimulating/arousing the level of consciousness.

TABLE 16-38. COMMON IMPAIRMENTS, ACTIVITY LIMITATIONS, AND PARTICIPATION RESTRICTIONS IN CHILDREN WITH BRAIN INJURIES

IMPAIRMENTS	ACTIVITY LIMITATIONS	PARTICIPATION RESTRICTIONS
Abnormal muscle tone	Decreased age-appropriate mobility	Dependent mobility
Postural asymmetry	Delayed gross motor skills	Dependent self-help skills
Decreased muscle strength	Poor school performances	Social isolation
Loss of range of motion	Decreased attention to environment	Limited play with peers
Ataxia		
Poor balance		
Behavior state changes		
Poor motor planning		
Poor visual perceptual skills		
Impaired cognition		

Reproduced, with permission, from Kerkering GA: Brain injuries: traumatic brain injuries, near drowning, and brain tumors. In: Campbell SK, Vander Linden DW, Palisano RJ, eds. *Physical Therapy for Children, 3rd ed.* St. Louis, MO: Saunders. 2006:709-734.

- Facilitating gross and fine motor development through appropriate positioning, postures and movements.
- Maximizing patient/caregiver competence with:
  - Therapeutic positioning and handling.
  - Home program.

SEIZURE DISORDERS

Seizures can be defined as neurologic manifestations of involuntary and excessive neuronal discharge.[244-246] The symptoms depend on the part of brain that is involved and may include an altered level of consciousness, tonic-clonic movements of some or all body parts, visual, auditory or olfactory disturbance. Differential diagnosis includes epilepsy, drugs (noncompliance with prescription, withdrawal syndrome, overdose, multiple drug abuse), hypoxia, brain tumor, infection (eg, meningitis), metabolic disturbances (eg, hypoglycemia, uremia, liver failure, electrolyte disturbance), and head injury.

Most seizures in children involve loss of consciousness and tonic-clonic movements, but auditory, visual, or olfactory disturbance, behavioral change or absences in attention may also occur. The various types of seizures are outlined in Table 16-39.

DUCHENNE MUSCULAR DYSTROPHY

The muscular dystrophies (MD) associated with defects in dystrophin range greatly from the very severe Duchenne muscular dystrophy (DMD) to the far milder Becker muscular dystrophy (BMD).[247-256] The types and subtypes of MD include those listed in Table 16-40.

Duchenne muscular dystrophy (DMD), the best-known form of muscular dystrophy, is due to a mutation in a gene on the X chromosome that prevents the production of dystrophin, a normal protein in muscle. DMD affects boys and, very rarely, girls. DMD typically manifests with weakness in the pelvis and upper limbs, resulting in frequent falling, an inability to keep up with peers while playing, and an unusual gait (waddling). Around the age of 8 years, most patients notice difficulty climbing stairs or rising from the ground. Because of this proximal lower back and extremity weakness, parents often note that the child pushes on his knees in order to stand (Gower sign). The

TABLE 16-39. SEIZURE DISORDERS

TYPE	DESCRIPTION
Generalized	Affects both hemispheres Characterized by change in level of consciousness Bilateral motor involvement
Simple partial	Affects only part of brain (focal, motor or sensory) Formerly called focal seizures May progress to generalized seizures The history is important, because the anticonvulsants used for partial seizures differ from those used for generalized seizures.
Complex partial	Partial seizure with affective or behavioral changes
Febrile	Associated with temperature > 38°C Occurs in children < 6 years old (prevalence is 2%-4% among children < 5 years old) No signs or history of underlying seizure disorder Often familial Uncomplicated and benign if seizure is of short duration (< 5 min) Involves tonic-clonic movements

Data from Camfield P, Camfield C: Advances in the diagnosis and management of pediatric seizure disorders in the twentieth century. *J Pediatr.* 2000;136:847-849; Nelson LP, Ureles SD, Holmes G: An update in pediatric seizure disorders. *Pediatr Dent.* 1991;13:128-135; Sanger MS, Perrin EC, Sandler HM: Development in children's causal theories of their seizure disorders. *J Dev Behav Pediatr.* 1993;14:88-93; and Tharp BR: An overview of pediatric seizure disorders and epileptic syndromes. *Epilepsia.* 1987;28(suppl 1):S36-S45.

posterior calf is usually enlarged as a result of fatty and connective tissue infiltration, or by compensatory hypertrophy of the calves secondary to weak tibialis anterior muscles. Respiratory muscle strength begins a slow but steady decline. The forced vital capacity gradually wanes, leading to symptoms of nocturnal hypoxemia such as lethargy and early morning headaches.

As DMD progresses, a wheelchair may be required. Most patients with Duchenne MD die in their early twenties because of muscle-based breathing and cardiac problems.

Physical Therapy Role. The role of exercise in the treatment of muscular dystrophy is controversial. One of the primary considerations in the early management program of the young school-age child is to retard the development of contractures. This can be achieved through range of motion exercises, stretching of the iliotibial band/tensor fascia latae, iliopsoas, hamstrings, and Achilles tendon, and the use of night splints. Braces, such as ankle-foot orthoses and knee-ankle-foot orthoses, are important adjuncts in prolonging the period of ambulation/mobility and delaying wheelchair dependency, which usually occurs during adolescence. However, the use of orthoses for a standing program or continuation of supported walking is not appropriate for all individuals; in fact, it should be considered a personal rather than therapeutic decision.[257] However, a standing program may help address the issue of decreased bone mineral density and subsequent increased risk of fracture.[257] Independent walking usually ceases by age 10 to 12. A power scooter should be considered as an initial power wheelchair prescription for the child who is hesitant to use a power wheelchair when walking is no longer possible.[257] If a power scooter is initially used, transition to a power wheelchair will be necessary when the adolescent is seen propping on the arm rest for trunk control.[257] Once wheelchair dependency becomes inevitable, attention should shift to prophylaxis against the deleterious consequences of immobility:

TABLE 16-40. TYPES AND SUBTYPES OF MUSCULAR DYSTROPHY

TYPE	SUBTYPE
X-linked recessive	Duchenne Becker
Autosomal recessive	Limb girdle Congenital Others
Facioscapulohumeral	Distal Ocular Charcot Marie Tooth Werdnig-Hoffman

- The chair should be customized to the patient's requirements. Eventually, a power wheelchair is necessary because upper extremity and truncal weakness will typically not tolerate use of a motorized scooter.[257]
- The fit of the wheelchair is closely monitored to maintain adequate support. Cushioning and supports can help maintain alignment of the spine and pelvis, thereby reducing the incidence of skin breakdown. The footrests should be customized to support the ankle in a neutral position. A reclining back will permit a position change while sitting in a wheelchair and will assist to deter flexion contracture formation at the hip.[257]
- Adaptive devices (wheelchair tables and ball-bearing splints) can be prescribed to maximize upper extremity mobility in muscles that cannot resist gravity.

In addition, the emphasis should shift toward an exercise program of active assistive and active exercises of the upper extremities. Key muscle groups include the shoulder depressors and triceps (strength for transfers), and the shoulder flexor and abductor and elbow flexor muscle groups (to maintain routine ADL such as self-feeding and hygiene).[257,257] Breathing exercises, postural drainage, or intermittent pressure breathing techniques should be included based on results of pulmonary evaluation.

Spinal Muscular Atrophy

The spinal muscular atrophies (SMAs) are a clinically and genetically heterogeneous group of disorders. They are characterized by primary degeneration of the anterior horn cells of the spinal cord and often of the bulbar motor nuclei without evidence of primary peripheral nerve or long-tract involvement. Classification of SMA in the pediatric population (an adult onset form of the disease exists) into three groups is based on clinical presentation and progression (Table 16-41). SMA is typically inherited as autosomal recessive.[257] No cure or treatment is currently available for SMA, but physical therapy is commonly advocated.[257]

Patients with disorders of the motor unit present with predominantly lower motor neuron signs that include hypotonia, flaccid weakness, decreased or absent deep tendon reflexes, fasciculations, and atrophy.

Physical Therapy Role. The impairments associated with SMA can be primary or secondary:[2]

- Primary: muscle weakness. Respiratory distress is present early in acute childhood SMA.

TABLE 16-41. CLASSIFICATION OF SPINAL MUSCLE ATROPHY IN PEDIATRICS

TYPE	ONSET	COURSE
Childhood-onset, type I, Werdnig-Hoffman (acute)	0-3 months	Rapidly progressive, severe hypotonia, death within first year
Childhood-onset, type II, Werdnig-Hoffman (chronic)	3 mo-4 yr	Rapid progression, then stabilizes; moderate to severe hypotonia; shortened life span
Juvenile-onset, type III, Kugelberg-Welander	5-10 yr	Slowly progressive; mild impairment

Reproduced, with permission, from Stuberg WA: Muscular dystrophy and spinal muscular atrophy. In: Campbell SK, Vander Linden DW, Palisano RJ, eds. *Physical Therapy for Children*. St. Louis, MO: Saunders. 2006:421-451.

- Secondary: postural compensations resulting from muscle weakness, contractures, and occasionally scoliosis.

The goals of physical therapy are to improve the quality of life while minimizing disability. A background knowledge of therapeutic exercise, functional use of orthoses and adaptive equipment, and strategies to minimize disabilities secondary to the impairments allow the clinician to provide a comprehensive intervention.

> **Study Pearl**
>
> Common signs and symptoms of cancer in the pediatric population can include fever, pain, a mass or swelling, bruising, pallor, headaches, neurologic changes, and visual disturbances.

Oncology

Cancer is the main cause of death by disease, and the second-leading cause of death in children ages one to 14 years.

Leukemia. Acute lymphoblastic leukemia is a malignant disease of the bone marrow, resulting in a marked decrease in the production of normal blood cells.

Neuroblastoma. Neuroblastoma is an embryonic malignancy of the sympathetic nervous system, and is the most common extracranial childhood cancer and the most common tumor occurring during infancy.[258] Most patients present with signs and symptoms related to tumor growth, although small tumors have been detected in infants on prenatal ultrasound.[258] Large abdominal tumors often result in increased abdominal girth and other local symptoms (eg, pain). Generally, symptoms include abdominal pain, emesis, weight loss, anorexia, fatigue, bone pain, and chronic diarrhea.[258] Because more than 50% of patients present with advanced-stage disease, usually to the bone and bone marrow, the most common presentation includes bone pain and a limp.[258]

Lymphomas

Hodgkin's Lymphoma. Hodgkin's lymphoma, formerly known as Hodgkin's disease, is a malignant disorder of unknown etiology that arises primarily in peripheral lymph nodes.[259-261] Signs and symptoms include

- Constitutional symptoms (eg, unexplained weight loss, fever, night sweats).
- Chest pain, cough, and/or shortness of breath (if there is a large mediastinal mass or lung involvement).
- Back or bone pain occurs rarely.
- Splenomegaly and/or hepatomegaly may be present.
- Central nervous system (CNS) symptoms or signs may be due to paraneoplastic syndromes.

Clinical staging occurs through assessment of the disease extent by clinical examination and imaging techniques. For staging classifications, the spleen is considered a lymph node area. The Ann Arbor classification is used most commonly (Table 16-42).[262,263]

The medical options for HL, which are based on the stage, include

- Radiation therapy. The involved field encompasses the involved lymph node area plus one contiguous region.
- Chemotherapy (nonleukemogenic chemotherapy [ABVD]).

TABLE 16-42. ANN ARBOR CLASSIFICATION OF HODGKIN'S LYMPHOMA

STAGE	CRITERIA
Stage I	A single lymph node area or single extranodal site
Stage II	Two or more lymph node areas on the same side of the diaphragm
Stage III	Lymph node areas on both sides of the diaphragm
Stage IV	Disseminated or multiple involvement of extranodal organs
	Involvement of the liver or the bone marrow is considered stage IV disease

These letters can be appended to some stages: A or B designations denote the presence or absence of B symptoms.
B designation: includes the presence of 1 or more of the following: (1) fever (temperature > 38°C), (2) drenching night sweats, and (3) unexplained loss of more than 10% of body weight within the preceding 6 months.
A designation: the absence of the above.
Data from Rosenberg SA: Validity of the Ann Arbor staging classification for the non-Hodgkin's lymphomas. *Cancer Treat Rep.* 1977;61:1023-1027; and Ultmann JE, Moran EM: Diagnostic evaluation and clinical staging in Hodgkin's disease: usefulness and problems of the Ann Arbor staging classification in primary staging and staging in relapse. *Natl Cancer Inst Monogr.* 1973;36:333-345.

- High-dose chemotherapy with transplantation. High-dose chemotherapy (HDC) at doses that ablate the bone marrow is feasible with reinfusion of the patient's previously collected hematopoietic stem cells (autologous transplantation) or infusion of stem cells from a donor source (allogeneic transplantation).

Non-Hodgkin Lymphoma. The non-Hodgkin lymphomas (NHLs) constitute a heterogeneous group of lymphoid system neoplasms with varying presentation and natural history.[264-268] Presentation of NHL in children is acute or subacute. The clinical manifestations are diverse and depend on the site of disease involvement.

In general, patients often appear mildly to moderately ill and occasionally have a low-grade fever. They may present with pallor, respiratory distress, pain, and discomfort. Staging of NHL is shown in Table 16-43. The intensity of current treatment regimens, particularly for advanced stages of disease, dictates inpatient administration of chemotherapy, as well as aggressive support by a team experienced in the care of immunosuppressed children.

Wilms Tumor. Wilms tumor (WT) is the fifth most common pediatric malignancy and the most common renal tumor in children.[258,269-274] The tumor may arise in three clinical settings: sporadic, association with genetic syndromes, and familial. The etiology essentially remains unknown. Most cases are not part of a genetic malformation syndrome

TABLE 16-43. STAGING FOR NON-HODGKIN LYMPHOMA

STAGE	DEFINITION
I	Single tumor (extranodal) or single anatomic area (nodal), excluding mediastinum or abdomen
II	Single tumor (extranodal) with regional node involvement, OR
	Primary gastrointestinal tumor ± associated mesenteric node involvement, with gross total resection, OR
	On same side of diaphragm: two or more nodal areas, or two single (extranodal) tumors ± regional node involvement
III	Any primary intrathoracic tumor (mediastinal, pleural, thymic), OR
	Any extensive abdominal tumor (unresectable), OR
	Any primary paraspinous or epidural tumor, regardless of other sites, OR
	On both sides of the diaphragm: two or more nodal areas, or two single (extranodal) tumors ± regional node involvement
IV	Any of the above with initial CNS or marrow (< 25%) involvement

Data from Crist WM, Mahmoud H, Pickert CB, et al: Biology and staging of childhood non-Hodgkin lymphoma. *An Esp Pediatr.* 1988;29(suppl 34):104-109.

and have no familial history; however, familial WT arises with high frequency in certain families. The mean age at diagnosis is 3.5 years. The most common feature at presentation is an abdominal mass. Abdominal pain occurs in 30% to 40% of cases. Other signs and symptoms include hypertension, fever from tumor necrosis, hematuria, and anemia.

Bone Tumors

Osteogenic Sarcoma. Any sarcoma that arises from bone is called an osteogenic sarcoma. This term includes fibrosarcoma, chondrosarcoma, and osteosarcoma, based on their cell of origin.[275-281] Osteosarcoma is the most common form of bone cancer in children, and the third most common cancer in adolescence. Although an osteosarcoma can occur in any bone, it most commonly occurs in the long bones of the extremities near metaphyseal growth plates. The most common sites are the femur (42%, with 75% of tumors in the distal femur), tibia (19%, with 80% of tumors in the proximal tibia), and humerus (10%, with 90% of tumors in the proximal humerus). Other significant locations are the skull or jaw (8%) and pelvis (8%). Symptoms may be present for weeks or months before osteosarcoma is diagnosed. The most common presenting symptom of osteosarcoma is pain, particularly with activity. Patients may complain of a sprain, arthritis, or so-called growing pains. Often, the patient has a history of trauma, though pathologic fractures are not particularly common. If in an extremity, the pain may result in a limp. Systemic symptoms, such as fever and night sweats, are rare. Tumor spread to the lungs only rarely results in respiratory symptoms, and such symptoms usually indicate extensive lung involvement. Metastases to other sites are extremely rare; therefore, other symptoms are unusual.

Ewing's Sarcoma. Ewing's sarcoma is a highly malignant primary medullary bone tumor, which is derived from red bone marrow and is most frequently observed in the bone shaft of children and adolescents aged 4 to 15 years.[282-286] The most important and earliest symptom is pain, which initially is intermittent but becomes intense. The pain may radiate to the limbs, particularly with tumors in the vertebral or pelvic region. Rarely, a patient may have a pathologic fracture. Occasionally, the clinical picture may be similar to that of acute or chronic osteomyelitis and include tenderness, remittent fever, mild anemia, leukocytosis, and an elevated sedimentation rate. After the diagnosis is made, treatment options include adjunctive chemotherapy, radiation therapy, and surgery.

Physical Therapy Role in Oncology Cases. The intervention varies according to the physical condition of the patient, the stage of cancer, and the treatment the patient is undergoing:

- Patient and family education on the expected goals, processes involved, and the expected outcomes. May also involve assisting the patient/family in coping mechanisms and through the grieving process.
- Proper positioning to prevent or correct deformities, preserve integrity, and provide comfort.
- Edema control: elevation of extremities, active range of motion, massage.
- Pain control: TENS, massage.

Study Pearl

- Systemic-onset JRA: characterized by spiking fevers. May also be accompanied by an evanescent rash affecting the trunk and extremities. Arthralgia is often present. Frank joint swelling is atypical.
- Pauciarticular disease is characterized by arthritis affecting four or fewer (typically, larger joints) joints.
- Polyarticular disease affects at least five joints. Both large and small joints can be involved.

- Preserving or correcting loss of range of motion through passive, active-assisted, active range of motion exercises, and loss of muscle mass and strength within patient tolerance, weight-bearing limits, and prescribed guidelines.
- Preserving activity tolerance and cardiovascular endurance.
- Preserving or increasing functional independence.

RHEUMATOLOGY: JUVENILE RHEUMATOID ARTHRITIS

Juvenile rheumatoid arthritis (JRA) is a group of diseases that are associated with chronic joint inflammation. JRA is a persistent arthritis, lasting at least 6 weeks, in one or more joints of a child (younger than 16 years of age), when all other causes of arthritis have been excluded.[287,288]

The exact etiology of JRA is unclear, but it is an autoimmune inflammatory disorder. General history and observation of JRA includes the following:

- Morning stiffness.
- A school history of absences and their abilities to participate in physical education classes may reflect severity of the disease.
- Gait deviations. Limping tends to occur in individuals with more severe JRA; however, the presence of limping also raises the possibility of trauma or another orthopedic problem. Very severe joint pain raises the possibility of acute rheumatic fever, acute lymphocytic leukemia, septic arthritis, or osteomyelitis. Also consider Legg-Calvé-Perthes disease; toxic synovitis of the hip; or, in an older child, slipped capital femoral epiphysis or chondrolysis of the hip.
- A preceding illness, which could indicate the possibility of infectious trigger of JRA or postinfectious arthritis.
- Acute or chronic uveitis.
- History of travel, which could indicate exposure to ticks (Lyme disease).
- Gastrointestinal symptoms raise the possibility of inflammatory bowel disease.
- Weight loss with diarrhea may be observed in persons with inflammatory bowel disease.

A detailed physical examination is a critical tool in diagnosing JRA. Physical findings are important to provide criteria for diagnosis and to detect abnormalities suggestive of other possible diagnoses. Several standardized instruments can be used to examine a child's activities. The Childhood Health Assessment Questionnaire (CHAQ), a pediatric modification of the Stanford Health Assessment Questionnaire (HAQ), has been shown to be a valid and sensitive tool in the evaluation of functional outcomes in children with chronic arthritis, and is a component of the validated JRA core set criteria used to measure improvement and flare in clinical trials (Table 16-44). The CHAQ includes 30 activities organized into eight categories. Other questionnaires designed to measure physical function include the Juvenile Arthritis Functional Assessment Index (JASI)[289] and the Juvenile Arthritis Functional Assessment Report (JAFAR) (Table 16-45).[290] Two other instruments measure both physical function and quality of life in children with JRA:

- Juvenile Arthritis Quality of Life (JAQQ).[287] The JAQQ is a recently developed disease-specific health-related quality of

TABLE 16-44. CHILDHOOD HEALTH ASSESSMENT QUESTIONNAIRE

JRA Outcome Study   Form: Haq

Childhood Health Assessment Questionnaire (CHAQ)

For all children with JRA (all ages)

Patient's Name (print) ______________________________ (First MI Last)

Patient Date of Birth: ______________________

Date of Office Visit:__________

Date this Form Completed: ____________

In this section we are interested in learning how your child's illness affects his/her ability to function in daily life. Please feel free to add any comments on the back of this page. In the following questions, please check the one response which best describes your child's usual activities (**averaged over an entire day**) **OVER THE PAST WEEK. ONLY NOTE THOSE DIFFICULTIES OR LIMITATIONS WHICH ARE DUE TO ILLNESS**. If most children at your child's age are not expected to do a certain activity, please mark it as "Not Applicable." For example, if your child has difficulty in doing a certain activity or is unable to do it because he/she is too young but NOT because he/she is RESTRICTED BY ILLNESS, please mark it as "Not Applicable."

	Due to JRA Illness Only				
	Without ANY Difficulty	**With SOME Difficulty**	**With MUCH Difficulty**	**UNABLE To Do**	**Not Applicable**
Dressing & Grooming					
Is your child able to:					
1 Dress, including tying shoelaces and doing buttons?	___	___	___	___	___
2 Shampoo his/her hair?	___	___	___	___	___
3 Remove socks?	___	___	___	___	___
4 Cut fingernails?	___	___	___	___	___
Arising					
Is your child able to:					
5 Stand up from a low chair or floor?	___	___	___	___	___
6 Get in and out of bed or stand up in crib?	___	___	___	___	___
Eating					
Is your child able to:					
7 Cut his/her own meat?	___	___	___	___	___
8 Lift a cup or glass to mouth?	___	___	___	___	___
9 Open a new cereal box?	___	___	___	___	___
Walking					
Is your child able to					
10 Walk outdoors on a flat ground?	___	___	___	___	___
11 Climb up five steps?	___	___	___	___	___

Please check any AIDS or DEVICES that your child usually uses for any of the above activities:

______ Cane	______ Devices used for dressing (button hook, zipper pull, long-handled shoe horn, etc.
______ Walker	______ Built up pencil or special utensils
______ Crutches	______ Special or Built-up chair
______ Wheelchair	______ Other Specify: ______________________

Please check any categories for which your child usually needs help from another person BECAUSE OF ILLNESS:

______ Dressing and Grooming	______ Eating
______ Arising	______ Walking

(*Continued*)

TABLE 16-44. CHILDHOOD HEALTH ASSESSMENT QUESTIONNAIRE *(Conitnued)*

	Due to JRA Illness Only				
Hygiene Is your child able to:	**Without ANY Difficulty**	**With SOME Difficulty**	**With MUCH Difficulty**	**UNABLE To Do**	**Not Applicable**
12 Wash and dry entire body?	___	___	___	___	___
13 Take a tub bath (get in & out of tub)?	___	___	___	___	___
14 Get on and off the toilet or potty chair?	___	___	___	___	___
15 Brush teeth?	___	___	___	___	___
16 Comb/Brush hair?	___	___	___	___	___
Reach Is your child able to:					
17 Reach and get down a heavy object such as a large game or books from just above his/her head?	___	___	___	___	___
18 Bend down to pick up clothing or a piece of paper from the floor?	___	___	___	___	___
19 Pull on a sweater over his/her head?	___	___	___	___	___
20 Turn neck to look over shoulder?	___	___	___	___	___
Grip Is your child able to:					
21 Write or scribble with a pen or pencil?	___	___	___	___	___
22 Open car doors?	___	___	___	___	___
23 Open jars which have been previously opened?	___	___	___	___	___
24 Turn faucets on and off?	___	___	___	___	___
25 Push open a door when he/she has to turn knob?	___	___	___	___	___
Errands, Chores, and Play Is your child able to:					
26 Run errands and shop?	___	___	___	___	___
27 Get in and out of car or toy car or school bus?	___	___	___	___	___
28 Ride bike or tricycle?	___	___	___	___	___
29 Do household chores (e.g. wash dishes, take out trash, vacuuming, yardwork, make bed, clean room)?	___	___	___	___	___
30 Run and play?	___	___	___	___	___

Please check any AIDS or DEVICES that your child usually uses for any of the above activities:

______ Raised Toilet Seat ______ Jar Opener (for jars previously opened)
______ Bathtub Seat ______ Long-Handled Appliances for Reach
______ Bathtub bar ______ Long Handled Appliances in Bathroom

Please check any categories for which your child usually needs help from another person BECAUSE OF ILLNESS:

______ Hygiene ______ Gripping and Opening things
______ Reach ______ Errands, Chores, and Play

We are also interested in learning whether or not your child has been affected by pain because of his or her illness. How much pain do you think your child has had because of his/her illness IN THE PAST WEEK?
Place mark on the line below to indicate the severity of the pain.

--	
0 No Pain	100 Very Bad Pain

Return to: Researcher Suzanne L. Bowyer, Riley Hospital For Children, Rm 5863, 1 Children's Square, Indianapolis, Indiana 46202

TABLE 16-45. JUVENILE ARTHRITIS FUNCTIONAL ASSESSMENT REPORT FOR PARENTS

Juvenile Arthritis Functional Assessment Report for Parents (JAFAR)

For children 7 and older with JRA

Patient's Name (print) ______________________ First MI Last

Date of Office Visit:______________

Patient Date of Birth: ______________________

Date this Form Completed: ______________

Part 1 Ability Scale

On this questionnaire, we are interested in learning how your child's illness affects her/her ability to function in daily life. Please feel free to add any comments on the back of this page.
Please check the one response which best describes your child's usual abilities **OVER THE PAST WEEK**.

please answer all questions **In the past week, was Patient able to:**		**All the time**	**Sometimes**	**Almost never**
1	Take shirt off hanger	___	___	___
2	Button shirt	___	___	___
3	Pull on sweater over head	___	___	___
4	Turn on water faucet	___	___	___
5	Sit on floor, then stand up	___	___	___
6	Dry back with towel	___	___	___
7	Wash face with wash cloth	___	___	___
8	Tie shoelaces	___	___	___
9	Pull on socks	___	___	___
10	Brush teeth	___	___	___
11	Stand up from chair without using arms	___	___	___
12	Get into bed	___	___	___
13	Cut food with knife and fork	___	___	___
14	Lift empty glass to mouth	___	___	___
15	Reopen previously opened food jar	___	___	___
16	Walk 50 feet without help	___	___	___
17	Walk up 5 steps	___	___	___
18	Stand on tiptoes	___	___	___
19	Reach above head	___	___	___
20	Get out of bed	___	___	___
21	Pick up something from floor from standing position	___	___	___
22	Push open door after turning knob	___	___	___
23	Turn head and look over shoulder	___	___	___

(*Continued*)

TABLE 16-45. JUVENILE ARTHRITIS FUNCTIONAL ASSESSMENT REPORT FOR PARENTS *(Conitnued)*

2 Aids or Devices

Please check any AIDS or DEVICES that your child uses for any of these activities

		Have Used	Have not used
1	Cane	_____	_____
2	Walker	_____	_____
3	Crutches	_____	_____
4	Wheelchair	_____	_____
5	Built-up pencil	_____	_____
6	Button hook	_____	_____
7	Zipper Horn	_____	_____
8	Shoe horn	_____	_____
9	Special eating utensils	_____	_____
10	Special chair	_____	_____
11	A special kind of toilet seat	_____	_____
12	Bathtub seat	_____	_____
13	Jar opener	_____	_____
14	Bathtub bar	_____	_____
15	Reacher	_____	_____

Does your child use any other kind of special tool, appliance, aid or device that helps him or her do things more easily?

IF YES: Could you describe it? ____________________________

____

3 Help from Others

Please check any categories for which your child needs HELP FROM ANOTHER PERSON.

		No Help	Some Help
1	Get dressed in the morning	_____	_____
2	Get washed in the morning	_____	_____
3	Get in and out of bed	_____	_____
4	Eat dinner	_____	_____
5	Move around the house	_____	_____
6	Get in and out of chairs	_____	_____
7	Reach and get things for you	_____	_____

4 Pain Scale

We are also interested in learning whether or not your child has been affected by pain because of his/her illness.
How much pain do you think your child has had because of his/her illness IN THE PAST WEEK?
Place a mark on the line below to indicate the severity of the pain.

0 No Pain	--	100 Very Bad Pain

Comments:____

____

____Jafar1.doc

Return to: Researcher **Suzanne L. Bowyer, Riley Hospital For Children, Rm 5863, 1 Children's Square, Indianapolis, Indiana 46202**

Data from JRA Outcome Study Form: Jafar Juvenile Arthritis Functional Assessment Report for Parents (JAFAR).

life questionnaire for children with arthritis; it consists of 74 items divided into five subclasses (gross motor function, fine motor function, psychosocial function, general symptoms and a pain assessment section).

- Pediatric Quality of Life (PedsQL™): comprised of three separate, self-administered questionnaires. The age-appropriate version (ages 5-7, 8-12, and 13-18) of the PedsQL™ questionnaire should be self-administered to all pediatric patients (≤ 18 years of age):

The Pediatric Quality of Life Inventory consists of 23 items that assess physical, emotional, social, and school functioning. A 5-point response scale is used based on a 1-month recall period. The instrument takes less than 10 minutes to complete.

- The Multidimensional Fatigue Scale consists of 18 items that assess general fatigue, sleep/rest fatigue, and cognitive fatigue. A 5-point response scale is used based on a 1-month recall period. The instrument takes less than 10 minutes to complete.
- The Pediatric Pain Questionnaire assesses present pain, worst pain intensity and disease severity using a Visual Analog Scale (VAS). The instrument takes less than 5 minutes to complete, and a ruler will be provided.

The only instrument that measures the child's actual performance is the Juvenile Arthritis Functional Assessment Scale (JAFAS).[291] The Juvenile Arthritis Functional Assessment Scale, was developed for, and validated in, patients with juvenile rheumatoid arthritis (JRA). Standards for this 10-item tool were developed using the scores of 63 normal school children as controls and comparing these results with those of 71 age-matched JRA patients (age 7-16 years). The JRA patients scored statistically significantly higher on the scale, which also demonstrated excellent internal and convergent validity and internal reliability.[291] The test is easily administered in 10 minutes by a physical or occupational therapist in a clinical or office setting.

Medical care of children with JRA must be provided in the context of a team-based approach, considering all aspects of their illness (eg, physical functioning in school, psychological adjustment to disease).

Physical Therapy Role. Physical therapists are essential members of the pediatric rheumatology team that includes the rheumatologist, nurse, occupational therapist, ophthalmologist, orthopedist, and pediatrician.[292] Other specialists, including cardiologists, dermatologists, orthotists, psychologists, and social workers provide occasional consultation as needed.

Following the comprehensive examination to identify impairments caused by the disease, a determination is made as to the relationship between the impairments and observed or reported activity restrictions. A prioritized problem list and an intervention plan is devised to reduce current impairments, maintain or improve function, prevent or minimize secondary problems, and provide education and support to the child and family. Specific interventions can include any or all of the following based on the stage of the disease (acute/subacute or chronic):

- Acute/subacute
  - Range of motion and stretching exercises: passive and active assisted to avoid joint compression
  - Strengthening: isometric exercises progressing cautiously to resistive
- Chronic
  - Range of motion and stretching exercises: active exercises
  - Strengthening: judicious use of concentrics
- Endurance exercises: fun and recreational activities, swimming
- Joint protection strategies and body mechanics education
- Mobility/assistive devices
- Rest, as needed
- Posture and positioning to maintain joint range of motion
  - Patients should spend 20 min/d in prone to stretch the hip and knee flexors
  - Assess leg length discrepancy in standing and avoid scoliosis.
- Therapeutic modalities for pain control
  - Instructions on the wearing of warm pajamas, sleeping bag, electric blanket
  - Paraffin for hands

HEMATOPOIETIC SYSTEM: HEMOPHILIA

Hemophilia is the most common inherited coagulation (blood clotting) disorder. It is inherited as a sex-linked autosomal recessive trait. Because the genes involved are located on the X-chromosome, males are affected because they have only one X-chromosome. Hemophilia, which is caused by an abnormality of plasma-clotting proteins necessary for blood coagulation,[293] is characterized by prolonged bleeding, although the blood flow is not any faster than what occurred in a normal person at the same injury. Two primary types exist

- Hemophilia A (classic hemophilia—factor VIII deficiency): 80% of all cases
- Hemophilia B (Christmas disease—factor IX deficiency)

The classification of the severity of hemophilia has been based on either clinical bleeding symptoms or on plasma procoagulant levels, which are the most widely used criteria.

The trademark characteristic of hemophilia is hemorrhage into the joints, which is painful and leads to long-term inflammation and deterioration of the joint. This, in turn, results in permanent deformities, misalignment, loss of mobility, and extremities of unequal lengths.

Various FVIII and FIX concentrates are now available to treat HA and HB.

Physical Therapy Role. Physical therapy for the child with hemophilia is aimed at maintaining ROM and strength in all joints and at preventing or diminishing disability. Specific goals include

- Prevention of contractures
- Manual traction and mobilization

Study Pearl

Kawasaki disease (KD), a febrile illness of childhood, is a self-limited acute vasculitic syndrome of unknown etiology.[294,295] KD is characterized by prolonged fever, rash, mucocutaneous involvement, extremity changes, cervical adenopathy, conjunctivitis, and the development of coronary artery aneurysms.[294-297] Outside the United States, the disease is most frequently observed in Japan.[294,296]

The medical management of KD involves the use of gamma globulin and aspirin as anti-inflammatory agents and long-term anticoagulation.[297]

- Progressive/dynamic splinting
- Serial casting (refer to Chapter 9)/drop-out casts
- Active ROM exercises (passive ROM is generally contraindicated)
- Maintaining strength: isometric strengthening exercises initially, then graded progressive exercises
- Preventing or diminishing disability
- Gait training
- Proprioceptive training
- Bracing/splints—provides stabilization and protecti

Questions for this chapter and the entire book appear on the included CD-ROM, with additional questions at www.DuttonNPTE.com.

REFERENCES

1. Van Sant AF: Concepts of neural organization and movement. In: Connolly BH, Montgomery PC, eds. *Therapeutic Exercise in Developmental Disabilities, 2nd ed.* Thorofare, NJ: SLACK, Inc. 2001:1-12.
2. O'Sullivan SB: Strategies to improve motor function. In: O'Sullivan SB, Schmitz TJ, eds. *Physical Rehabilitation, 5th ed.* Philadelphia, PA: FA Davis. 2007:471-522.
3. Schmidt R, Lee T: *Motor Control and Learning, 4th ed.* Champaign, IL, Human Kinetics. 2005.
4. Thompson S, Watson WH, III: Central pattern generator for swimming in Melibe. *J Exp Biol.* 2005;208:1347-1361.
5. Yamaguchi T: The central pattern generator for forelimb locomotion in the cat. *Prog Brain Res.* 2004;143:115-122.
6. Lewis C: Physiological response to exercise in the child: considerations for the typically and atypically developing youngster. *Proceedings from the American Physical Therapy Association combined sections meeting.* San Antonio, Texas. 2001.
7. Schöner G, Kelso JAS: Dynamic pattern generation in behavioral and neural systems. *Science.* 1988;239:1513-1520.
8. Kelso JAS: A dynamical basis for action systems. In: Gazzaniga MS, ed. *Handbook of Cognitive Neuroscience.* New York, NY: Plenum Press. 1984:321-356.
9. Gesell A: *Infancy and Human Growth.* New York, NY: MacMillan. 1928.
10. Gesell A: *The Mental Growth of the Pre-School Child: A Psychological Outline of Normal Development from Birth to the Sixth Year, Including a System of Developmental Diagnosis.* New York, NY: MacMillan. 1928.
11. Shirley MM: *The First Two Years: A Study of Twenty-Five Babies.* Vol I. *Postural and Locomotor Development.* Minneapolis, MN: University of Minnesota Press. 1931.
12. Gesell A: *The Embryology of Behavior.* New York, NY: Harper & Row. 1945.
13. Horak FB: Assumptions underlying motor control for neurologic rehabilitation. In: Lister MJ, ed. *Contemporary Management of Motor Control Problems: Proceedings of the II STEP Conference.* Alexandria, VA: Foundation for Physical Therapy. 1991:11-27.

14. Campbell SK: The child's development of functional movement. In: Campbell SK, Vander Linden DW, Palisano RJ, eds. *Physical Therapy for Children.* St. Louis, MO: Saunders. 2006:33-76.
15. Piaget J: *The Origins of Intelligence in Children.* New York, NY: International Universities Press. 1952.
16. Thelen E, Ulrich BD: Hidden skills: a dynamic systems analysis of treadmill stepping during the first year. *Monogr Soc Res Child Dev.* 1991;56:1-98.
17. Thelen E, Corbetta D: Exploration and selection in the early acquisition of skill. *Int Rev Neurobiol.* 1994;37:75-102.
18. Thelen E: Motor development. A new synthesis. *Am Psychol.* 1995;50:79-95.
19. Palisano RJ, Campbell SK, Harris SR: Evidence-based decision-making in pediatric physical therapy. In: Campbell SK, Vander Linden DW, Palisano RJ, eds. *Physical Therapy for Children.* St. Louis, MO: Saunders. 2006:3-32.
20. Shumway-Cook A, Woollacott MH: The growth of stability: postural control from a development perspective. *J Mot Behav.* 1985;17:131-147.
21. Dubowitz L, Dubowitz V: *The Neurological Examination of the Full-Term Newborn Infant.* Philadelphia, PA: JB Lippincott. 1981.
22. Larin H: Motor learning: theories and strategies for the practitioner. In: Campbell SK, Vander Linden DW, Palisano RJ, eds. *Physical Therapy for Children, 3rd ed.* St. Louis, MO: Saunders. 2006: 131-160.
23. Connolly BH, Lupinnaci NS, Bush AJ: Changes in attitudes and perceptions about research in physical therapy among professional physical therapist students and new graduates. *Phys Ther.* 2001;81:1127-1134.
24. Connolly BH: Tests and assessment. In: Connolly BH, Montgomery PC, eds. *Therapeutic Exercise in Developmental Disabilities.* Thorofare, NJ: SLACK Inc. 2001:15-33.
25. Brazelton TB: *Neonatal Behavioral Assessment Scale.* Philadelphia, PA: JB Lippincott. 1973.
26. Einspieler C, Prechtl HF, Ferrari F, et al: The qualitative assessment of general movements in preterm, term and young infants—review of the methodology. Early *Hum Dev.* 1997;50: 47-60.
27. Prechtl HF: State of the art of a new functional assessment of the young nervous system. An early predictor of cerebral palsy. *Early Hum Dev.* 1997;50:1-11.
28. Bradley NS, Westcott SL: Motor control: developmental aspects of motor control in skill acquisition. In: Campbell SK, Vander Linden DW, Palisano RJ, eds. *Physical Therapy for Children, 3rd ed.* St. Louis, MO: Saunders. 2006:77-130.
29. Campbell SK: Test-retest reliability of the Test of Infant Motor Performance. *Pediatr Phys Ther.* 1999;11:60-66.
30. Mercuri E, Guzzetta A, Laroche S, et al: Neurologic examination of preterm infants at term age: comparison with term infants. *J Pediatr.* 2003;142:647-655.
31. Saint-Anne Dargassies S: *Neurological Development in the Full Term and Premature Neonate.* London, England: Excerta Medica. 1977.
32. Prechtl HFR: *The Neurological Examination of the Full-Term Newborn Infant.* Philadelphia, PA: JB Lippincott. 1977.

33. Parmalee AH, Michaelis R: Neurological examination of the newborn. In: Hellmuth J, ed. *Exceptional Infant.* Volume 2. *Studies in Abnormalities.* London, England: Butterworths. 1971.
34. Chandler LS, Andrews MS, Swanson MW: *Movement Assessment of Infants.* Rolling Bay, WA: Chandler, Andrews, and Swanson. 1980.
35. Swanson MW, Bennett FC, Shy KK, et al: Identification of neurodevelopmental abnormality at four and eight months by the movement assessment of infants. *Dev Med Child Neurol.* 1992;34:321-337.
36. Blanchard Y, Neilan E, Busanich J, et al: Interrater reliability of early intervention providers scoring the alberta infant motor scale. *Pediatr Phys Ther.* 2004;16:13-18.
37. Piper MC, Pinnell LE, Darrah J, et al: Construction and validation of the Alberta Infant Motor Scale (AIMS). *Can J Public Health.* 1992;83(suppl 2):S46-S50.
38. Knutson LM: Examination, evaluation, and documentation for the pediatric client. In: Damiano D, ed. *Topics in Physical Therapy: Pediatrics.* Alexandria, VA: American Physical Therapy Association. 2001:1-36.
39. Harris SR, Daniels LE: Content validity of the Harris Infant Neuromotor Test. *Phys Ther.* 1996;76:727-737.
40. Bayley N: *Bayley II.* San Antonio, TX: Psychological Corporation. 1993.
41. Bayley N: *Manual for the Bayley Scales of Infant Development.* New York, NT: Psychological Corporation. 1969.
42. Campbell SK, Siegel E, Parr CA, et al: Evidence for the need to renorm the Bayley Scales of Infant Development based on the performance of a population-based sample of 12-month-old infants. *Top Early Childhood Spec Ed.* 1986;6:83-96.
43. Bruininks RH: *Bruininks Oseretsky Test of Motor Prociency: Examiner's Manual.* Circle Pines, MN: American Guidance Service. 1978.
44. Richardson PK, Atwater SW, Crowe TK, et al: Performance of preschoolers on the Pediatric Clinical Test of Sensory Interaction for Balance. *Am J Occup Ther.* 1992;46:793-800.
45. Deitz JC, Richardson PK, Westcott SL, et al: Performance of children with learning disabilities on the Clinical Test of Sensory Interaction for Balance. *Phys Occup Ther Pediatr.* 1996; 16:1-21.
46. Guide to physical therapist practice. *Phys Ther.* 2001;81:S13-S95.
47. Larin HM: Motor learning. In: Campbell SK, ed. *Physical Therapy for Children.* Philadelphia, PA: WB Saunders. 1995:157-181.
48. Sterba JA: Does horseback riding therapy or therapist-directed hippotherapy rehabilitate children with cerebral palsy? *Dev Med Child Neurol.* 2007;49:68-73.
49. Casady RL, Nichols-Larsen DS: The effect of hippotherapy on ten children with cerebral palsy. *Pediatr Phys Ther.* 2004;16:165-172.
50. Meregillano G: Hippotherapy. *Phys Med Rehabil Clin N Am.* 2004;15:843-854, vii.
51. Tiker F, Tarcan A, Kilicdag H, et al: Early onset conjugated hyperbilirubinemia in newborn infants. *Indian J Pediatr.* 2006;73:409-412.
52. Watchko JF: Neonatal hyperbilirubinemia—what are the risks? *N Engl J Med.* 2006;354:1947-1949.
53. Schwoebel A, Gennaro S: Neonatal hyperbilirubinemia. *J Perinat Neonatal Nurs.* 2006;20:103-107.

54. Merrick J, Merrick E, Morad M, et al: Fetal alcohol syndrome and its long-term effects. *Minerva Pediatr.* 2006;58:211-218.
55. O'Leary C, Bower C, Payne J, et al: Fetal alcohol syndrome. *Aust Fam Physician.* 2006;35:184.
56. Abel EL: Fetal alcohol syndrome: a cautionary note. *Curr Pharm Des.* 2006;12:1521-1529.
57. Accornero VH, Anthony JC, Morrow CE, et al: Prenatal cocaine exposure: an examination of childhood externalizing and internalizing behavior problems at age 7 years. *Epidemiol Psichiatr Soc.* 2006;15:20-29.
58. Tronick EZ, Messinger DS, Weinberg MK, et al: Cocaine exposure is associated with subtle compromises of infants' and mothers' social-emotional behavior and dyadic features of their interaction in the face-to-face still-face paradigm. *Dev Psychol.* 2005; 41:711-722.
59. Bauer CR, Langer JC, Shankaran S, et al: Acute neonatal effects of cocaine exposure during pregnancy. *Arch Pediatr Adolesc Med.* 2005;159:824-834.
60. Minnes S, Singer LT, Arendt R, et al: Effects of prenatal cocaine/polydrug use on maternal-infant feeding interactions during the first year of life. *J Dev Behav Pediatr.* 2005;26:194-200.
61. Bae S, Zhang L: Prenatal cocaine exposure increases apoptosis of neonatal rat heart and heart susceptibility to ischemia-reperfusion injury in 1-month-old rat. *Br J Pharmacol.* 2005;144:900-907.
62. Harvey JA, Romano AG, Gabriel M, et al: Effects of prenatal exposure to cocaine on the developing brain: anatomical, chemical, physiological and behavioral consequences. *Neurotox Res.* 2001;3:117-143.
63. Ley R: The Ondine curse, false suffocation alarms, trait-state suffocation fear, and dyspnea-suffocation fear in panic attacks. *Arch Gen Psychiatry.* 1997;54:677-678.
64. Rolak LA: Who was Ondine and what was his curse? *J Child Neurol.* 1996;11:461.
65. Lin Z, Chen M, Keens T, et al: Noninvasive assessment of cardiovascular autonomic control in congenital central hypoventilation syndrome. *Conf Proc IEEE Eng Med Biol Soc.* 2004;5:3870-3873.
66. Movahed MR, Jalili M, Kiciman N: Cardiovascular abnormalities and arrhythmias in patients with Ondine's curse (congenital central hypoventilation) syndrome. *Pacing Clin Electrophysiol.* 2005;28:1226-1230.
67. Kumar R, Macey PM, Woo MA, et al: Neuroanatomic deficits in congenital central hypoventilation syndrome. *J Comp Neurol.* 2005;487:361-371.
68. Parker LA: Part 1: early recognition and treatment of birth trauma: injuries to the head and face. *Adv Neonatal Care.* 2005;5:288-297; quiz 298-300.
69. Miranda P, Vila M, Alvarez-Garijo JA, et al: Birth trauma and development of growing fracture after coronal suture disruption. *Childs Nerv Syst.* 2006;5:5.
70. Grifka RG: Cyanotic congenital heart disease with increased pulmonary blood flow. *Pediatr Clin North Am.* 1999;46:405-425.
71. Kahn-D'Angel L, Unanue-Rose RA: The special care nursery. In: Campbell SK, Vander Linden DW, Palisano RJ, eds. Physical Therapy for Children. 3rd ed. St. Louis, MO: Saunders. 2006: 1053-1097.

72. McCarthy CF, DeCesare JA, Widell JK: Effect of chest physical therapy on the prevention of atelectasis in children following cardiac surgery. *Ann Surg.* 1983;198:116-117.
73. Hammon WE, Martin RJ: Chest physical therapy for acute atelectasis. A report on its effectiveness. *Phys Ther.* 1981;61: 217-220.
74. Harbord RP, Bosomworth PP: Therapy for atelectasis: chest physical and inhalation therapy combined with postural drainage and tracheobronchial suction—a preliminary study. *Anesth Analg.* 1966;45:684-695.
75. Bye MR: *Atelectasis, Pulmonary.* Available at: http://www.emedicine.com/PED/topic158.htm, 2005.
76. Bloomfield FH, Teele RL, Voss M, et al: The role of neonatal chest physiotherapy in preventing postextubation atelectasis. *J Pediatr.* 1998;133:269-271.
77. Al-Alaiyan S, Dyer D, Khan B: Chest physiotherapy and post-extubation atelectasis in infants. *Pediatr Pulmonol.* 1996;21:227-230.
78. Odita JC, Kayyali M, Ammari A: Post-extubation atelectasis in ventilated newborn infants. *Pediatr Radiol.* 1993;23:183-185.
79. Igarashi A, Amagasa S, Oda S, et al: Pulmonary atelectasis manifested after induction of anesthesia: a contribution of sinobronchial syndrome? *J Anesth.* 2007;21:66-68.
80. Duggan M, Kavanagh BP: Atelectasis in the perioperative patient. *Curr Opin Anaesthesiol.* 2007;20:37-42.
81. Wong AY, Fung LN: Pulmonary atelectasis following spinal anaesthesia for caesarean section. *Anaesth Intensive Care.* 2006;34:687-688.
82. Westerdahl E, Lindmark B, Eriksson T, et al: Deep-breathing exercises reduce atelectasis and improve pulmonary function after coronary artery bypass surgery. *Chest.* 2005;128:3482-3488.
83. Schulz-Stubner S, Rickelman J: Intermittent manual positive airway pressure for the treatment and prevention of atelectasis. *Eur J Anaesthesiol.* 2005;22:730-732.
84. Clover RD: Clinical practice guideline for bronchiolitis: key recommendations. *Am Fam Physician.* 2007;75:171.
85. Perrotta C, Ortiz Z, Roque M: Chest physiotherapy for acute bronchiolitis in paediatric patients between 0 and 24 months old. *Cochrane Database Syst Rev.* 2007;CD004873.
86. Diagnosis and management of bronchiolitis. *Pediatrics.* 2006;118:1774-1793.
87. Sugai K, Ito M, Tateishi I, et al: Neonatal periventricular leukomalacia due to severe, poorly controlled asthma in the mother. *Allergol Int.* 2006;55:207-212.
88. Britton TC: Torticollis—what is straight ahead? *Lancet.* 1998;351: 1223-1224.
89. Kiesewetter WB, Nelson PK, Pallandino VS, et al: Neonatal torticollis. *JAMA.* 1955;157:1281-1285.
90. Morrison DL, MacEwen GD: Congenital muscular torticollis: observations regarding clinical findings, associated conditions, and results of treatment. *J Pediatr Orthop.* 1982;2:500-505.
91. Anastasopoulos D, Nasios G, Psilas K, et al: What is straight ahead to a patient with torticollis? *Brain.* 1998;121:91-101.
92. Kiwak KJ: Establishing an etiology for torticollis. *Postgrad Med.* 1984;75:126-134.
93. Karmel-Ross K: Congenital muscular torticollis. In: Campbell SK, Vander Linden DW, Palisano RJ, eds. *Physical Therapy for Children.* 3rd ed. St. Louis, MO: Saunders. 2006:359-380.

94. Bredenkamp JK, Hoover LA, Berke GS, et al: Congenital muscular torticollis. A spectrum of disease. *Arch Otolaryngol Head Neck Surg.* 1990;116:212-216.
95. Whyte AM, Lufkin RB, Bredenkamp J, et al: Sternocleidomastoid fibrosis in congenital muscular torticollis: MR appearance. *J Comput Assist Tomogr.* 1989;13:163-164.
96. Aronsson DD, Goldberg MJ, Kling TF, et al: Developmental dysplasia of the hip. *Pediatrics.* 1994;94:201-208.
97. Ortolani M: Un segno poco noto e sue importanza per la diagnosi precoce di prelussazione congenita dell'anca. *Pediatria.* 1937;45:129-136.
98. Barlow TG: Early diagnosis and treatment of congenital dislocation of the hip. *J Bone Joint Surg [Br].* 1962;44:292-301.
99. Leach J: Orthopedic conditions. In: Campbell SK, Vander Linden DW, Palisano RJ, eds. *Physical Therapy for Children.* 3rd ed. St. Louis, MO: Saunders. 2006:481-515.
100. Bleakney DA, Donohoe M: Osteogenesis imperfecta. In: Campbell SK, Vander Linden DW, Palisano RJ, eds. *Physical Therapy for Children, 3rd ed.* St. Louis, MO: Saunders. 2006:401-419.
101. Binder H: Rehabilitation of infants with osteogenesis imperfecta. *Connect Tissue Res.* 1995;31:S37- S39.
102. Gerber LH, Binder H, Weintrob J, et al: Rehabilitation of children and infants with osteogenesis imperfecta. A program for ambulation. *Clin Orthop Relat Res.* 1990;251:254-262.
103. Binder H, Hawks L, Graybill G, et al: Osteogenesis imperfecta: rehabilitation approach with infants and young children. *Arch Phys Med Rehabil.* 1984;65:537-541.
104. Kinsman D: The child with hydrocephalus or myelomeningocele. II. Comprehensive physical therapy program. *Phys Ther.* 1966;46:611-615.
105. Fredrickson D: The child with hydrocephalus or melomeningocele. I. Initial and continuing physical therapy evaluation. *Phys Ther.* 1966;46:606-611.
106. Andersson S, Persson EK, Aring E, et al: Vision in children with hydrocephalus. *Dev Med Child Neurol.* 2006;48:836-841.
107. Bergsneider M, Egnor MR, Johnston M, et al: What we don't (but should) know about hydrocephalus. *J Neurosurg.* 2006;104:157-159.
108. Rizvi R, Anjum Q: Hydrocephalus in children. *J Pak Med Assoc.* 2005;55:502-507.
109. Mallia Milanes G, Napolitano R, Quaglia F, et al: Prenatal diagnosis of arthrogryposis. *Minerva Ginecol.* 2007;59:201-202.
110. Mennen U, van Heest A, Ezaki MB, et al: Arthrogryposis multiplex congenita. *J Hand Surg [Br].* 2005;30:468-474.
111. Bernstein RM: Arthrogryposis and amyoplasia. *J Am Acad Orthop Surg.* 2002;10:417-424.
112. Hardwick JC, Irvine GA: Obstetric care in arthrogryposis multiplex congenita. *BJOG.* 2002;109:1303-1304.
113. O'Flaherty P: Arthrogryposis multiplex congenita. *Neonatal Netw.* 2001;20:13-20.
114. Shaer CM, Chescheir N, Erickson K, et al: Obstetrician-gynecologists' practice and knowledge regarding spina bifida. *Am J Perinatol.* 2006;23:355-362. Epub Jul 13, 2006.
115. Woodhouse CR: Progress in the management of children born with spina bifida. *Eur Urol.* 2006;49:777-778. Epub Feb 6, 2006.

116. Verhoef M, Barf HA, Post MW, et al: Functional independence among young adults with spina bifida, in relation to hydrocephalus and level of lesion. *Dev Med Child Neurol.* 2006;48:114-119.
117. Ali L, Stocks GM: Spina bifida, tethered cord and regional anaesthesia. *Anaesthesia.* 2005;60:1149-1150.
118. Spina bifida. *Nurs Times.* 2005;101:31.
119. Mitchell LE, Adzick NS, Melchionne J, et al: Spina bifida. *Lancet.* 2004;364:1885-1895.
120. Dias L: Orthopaedic care in spina bifida: past, present, and future. *Dev Med Child Neurol.* 2004;46:579.
121. Cassidy SB, Dykens E, Williams CA: Prader-Willi and Angelman syndromes: sister imprinted disorders. *Am J Med Genet.* 2000;97:136-146.
122. Martin A, State M, Koenig K, et al: Prader-Willi syndrome. *Am J Psychiatry.* 1998;155:1265-1273.
123. Cassidy SB, Schwartz S: Prader-Willi and Angelman syndromes. Disorders of genomic imprinting. *Medicine (Baltimore).* 1998;77:140-151.
124. Cassidy SB: Prader-Willi syndrome. *J Med Genet.* 1997;34: 917-923.
125. Sweeney JK, Heriza CB, Reilly MA, et al: Practice guidelines for the physical therapist in the neonatal intensive care unit (NICU). *Pediatr Phys Ther.* 1999;11:119-132.
126. Schneider JW, Krosschell K, Gabriel KL: Congenital spinal cord injury. In: Umphred DA, ed. *Neurological Rehabilitation.* 3rd ed. St. Louis, MO: 1995:454-483.
127. Stevens BJ, Franck LS: Assessment and management of pain in neonates. *Paediatr Drugs.* 2001;3:539-558.
128. Chiswick ML: Assessment of pain in neonates. *Lancet.* 2000;355: 6-8.
129. Cignacco E, Mueller R, Hamers JP, et al: Pain assessment in the neonate using the Bernese Pain Scale for Neonates. *Early Hum Dev.* 2004;78:125-131.
130. Grunau RE, Holsti L, Whitfield MF, et al: Are twitches, startles, and body movements pain indicators in extremely low birth weight infants? *Clin J Pain.* 2000;16:37-45.
131. Hudson-Barr D, Capper-Michel B, Lambert S, et al: Validation of the Pain Assessment in Neonates (PAIN) scale with the Neonatal Infant Pain Scale (NIPS). *Neonatal Netw.* 2002;21:15-21.
132. Sheahan MS, Farmer-Brockway N: The high-risk infant. In: Tecklin JS, ed. *Pediatric Physical Therapy, 2nd ed.* Philadelphia, PA: JB Lippincott. 1994:56-88.
133. Sweeney JK, Swanson MW: Low birthweight infants: neonatal care and follow-up. In: Umphred DA, ed. *Neurological Rehabilitation.* 4th ed. St. Louis, MO: 2001:203-258.
134. Massery M, Magee CL: Asthma: multisystem implications. In: Campbell SK, Vander Linden DW, Palisano RJ, eds. *Physical Therapy for Children, 3rd ed.* St. Louis, MO: Saunders. 2006: 851-879.
135. Joseph-Bowen J, de Klerk NH, Firth MJ, et al: Lung function, bronchial responsiveness, and asthma in a community cohort of 6-year-old children. *Am J Respir Crit Care Med.* 2004;169:850-854. Epub Jan 23, 2004.
136. National Asthma Education and Prevention Program. Expert panel report: guidelines for the diagnosis and management of

asthma update on selected topics—2002. *J Allergy Clin Immunol.* 2002;110:S141-S219.

137. Fitzgerald ST: National Asthma Education Program Expert Panel report: guidelines for the diagnosis and management of asthma. *Aaohn J.* 1992;40:376-382.
138. Calfee CS, Katz PP, Yelin EH, et al: The influence of perceived control of asthma on health outcomes. *Chest.* 2006;130: 1312-1318.
139. Manning P, Greally P, Shanahan E: Asthma control and management: a patient's perspective. *Ir Med J.* 2005;98:231-232, 234-235.
140. Lucas SR, Platts-Mills TA: Physical activity and exercise in asthma: relevance to etiology and treatment. *J Allergy Clin Immunol.* 2005;115:928-934.
141. Mintz M: Asthma update: part I. Diagnosis, monitoring, and prevention of disease progression. *Am Fam Physician.* 2004;70:893-898.
142. Ram FS, Robinson SM, Black PN, et al: Physical training for asthma. *Cochrane Database Syst Rev.* 2005;CD001116.
143. Welsh L, Kemp JG, Roberts RG: Effects of physical conditioning on children and adolescents with asthma. *Sports Med.* 2005;35: 127-141.
144. Shah U, Moatter T: Screening for cystic fibrosis: the importance of using the correct tools. *J Ayub Med Coll Abbottabad.* 2006;18: 7-10.
145. Agnew JL, Ashwell JA, Renaud SL: Cystic fibrosis. In: Campbell SK, Vander Linden DW, Palisano RJ, eds. *Physical Therapy for Children, 3rd ed.* St. Louis, MO: Saunders. 2006:819-850.
146. Humberstone N: Respiratory assessment and treatment. In: Irwin S, Tecklin JS, eds. *Cardiopulmonary Physical Therapy.* St. Louis, MO: Saunders. 1990:283-322.
147. Thomas J, Cook DJ, Brooks D: Chest physical therapy management of patients with cystic fibrosis. A meta-analysis. *Am J Respir Crit Care Med.* 1995;151:846-850.
148. Zach MS, Purrer B, Oberwaldner B: Effect of swimming on forced expiration and sputum clearance in cystic fibrosis. *Lancet.* 1981;2:1201-1203.
149. Orenstein DM, Franklin BA, Doershuk CF, et al: Exercise conditioning and cardiopulmonary fitness in cystic fibrosis. The effects of a three-month supervised running program. *Chest.* 1981;80: 392-398.
150. Salter RB, Zaltz C: Anatomic investigations of the mechanism of injury and pathologic anatomy of pulled elbow in young children. *Clin Orthop.* 1971;77:134-143.
151. Dee R, Carrion W: Pulled elbow. In: *Principles of Orthopaedic Practice.* New York, NT: McGraw-Hill. 1997:579.
152. Sai N: Pulled elbow. *J R Soc Med.* 1999;92:462-464.
153. Hagroo GA, Zaki HM, Choudhary MT, et al: Pulled elbow-not the effect of hypermobility of joints. *Injury.* 1995;26:687-690.
154. Staheli LT: Rotational problems of the lower extremity. *Orthop Clin North Am.* 1987;18:503-512.
155. Engel GM, Staheli LT: The natural history of torsion and other factors influencing gait in childhood. A study of the angle of gait, tibial torsion, knee angle, hip rotation, and development of the arch in normal children. *Clin Orthop Relat Res.* 1974; 99:12-17.
156. Scoles PV: *Pediatric Orthopaedics in Clinical Practice.* 2nd ed. Chicago, IL: Year Book. 1988.

157. Kalogrianitis S, Tan CK, Kemp GJ, et al: Does unstable slipped capital femoral epiphysis require urgent stabilization? *J Pediatr Orthop B.* 2007;16:6-9.
158. Kamarulzaman MA, Abdul Halim AR, Ibrahim S: Slipped capital femoral epiphysis (SCFE): a 12-year review. *Med J Malaysia.* 2006;61(suppl A):71-78.
159. Flores M, Satish SG, Key T: Slipped capital femoral epiphysis in identical twins: is there an HLA predisposition? Report of a case and review of the literature. *Bull Hosp Jt Dis.* 2006; 63:158-160.
160. Aronsson DD, Loder RT, Breur GJ, et al: Slipped capital femoral epiphysis: current concepts. *J Am Acad Orthop Surg.* 2006;14: 666-679.
161. Umans H, Liebling MS, Moy L, et al: Slipped capital femoral epiphysis: a physeal lesion diagnosed by MRI, with radiographic and CT correlation. *Skeletal Radiol.* 1998;27:139-144.
162. Busch MT, Morrissy RT: Slipped capital femoral epiphysis. *Orthop Clin North Am.* 1987;18:637-647.
163. Herring JA, Kim HT, Browne R: Legg-Calve-Perthes disease. Part II: Prospective multicenter study of the effect of treatment on outcome. *J Bone Joint Surg Am.* 2004;86-A:2121-2134.
164. Herring JA, Kim HT, Browne R: Legg-Calve-Perthes disease. Part I: Classification of radiographs with use of the modified lateral pillar and Stulberg classifications. *J Bone Joint Surg Am.* 2004; 86-A:2103-2120.
165. Moens P, Fabry G: Legg-Calve-Perthes disease: one century later. *Acta Orthop Belg.* 2003;69:97-103.
166. Thompson GH, Price CT, Roy D, et al: Legg-Calve-Perthes disease: current concepts. *Instr Course Lect.* 2002;51:367-384.
167. Gross GW, Articolo GA, Bowen JR: Legg-Calve-Perthes disease: imaging evaluation and management. *Semin Musculoskelet Radiol.* 1999;3:379-391.
168. Roy DR: Current concepts in Legg-Calve-Perthes disease. *Pediatr Ann.* 1999;28:748-752.
169. Townsend DJ: Legg-Calve-Perthes disease. *Orthopedics.* 1999;22:381.
170. Mital MA, Matza RA: Osgood-Schlatter's disease: the painful puzzler. *Physician Sports Med.* 1977;5:60.
171. Patrick C: Spinal conditions. In: Campbell SK, Vander Linden DW, Palisano RJ, eds. *Physical Therapy for Children.* St. Louis, MO: Saunders. 2006:337-358.
172. McKenzie RA: Manual correction of sciatic scoliosis. *N Z Med J.* 1972;76:194-199.
173. Blum CL: Chiropractic and pilates therapy for the treatment of adult scoliosis. *J Manip Physiol Ther.* 2002;25:E3.
174. Miller NH: Genetics of familial idiopathic scoliosis. *Clin Orthop Rel Res.* 2002;401:60-64.
175. Kane WJ: Scoliosis prevalence: a call for a statement of terms. *Clin Orthop.* 1977;126:43–46.
176. Miller NH: Cause and natural history of adolescent idiopathic scoliosis. *Orthop Clin North Am.* 1999;30:343-352, vii.
177. Dobbs MB, Weinstein SL: Infantile and juvenile scoliosis. *Orthop Clin North Am.* 1999;30:331-341, vii.
178. Greiner KA: Adolescent idiopathic scoliosis: radiologic decision-making. *Am Fam Physician.* 2002;65:1817-1822.

179. Lonstein JE, Winter RB: Adolescent idiopathic scoliosis. Nonoperative treatment. *Orthop Clin North Am.* 1988;19:239-246.
180. Lenke LG: Lenke classification system of adolescent idiopathic scoliosis: treatment recommendations. *Instr Course Lect.* 2005;54:537-542.
181. Lenke LG, Edwards CC, II, Bridwell KH: The Lenke classification of adolescent idiopathic scoliosis: how it organizes curve patterns as a template to perform selective fusions of the spine. *Spine.* 2003;28:S199-S207.
182. Weinstein SL, Ponseti IV: Curve progression in idiopathic scoliosis. *J Bone Joint Surg Am.* 1983;65:447-455.
183. Ponseti IV, Pedrini V, Wynne-Davies R, et al: Pathogenesis of scoliosis. *Clin Orthop Relat Res.* 1976;120:268-280.
184. Ponseti IV, Friedman B: Prognosis in idiopathic scoliosis. *J Bone Joint Surg Am.* 1950;32A:381-395.
185. Weiss HR, Weiss G, Petermann F: Incidence of curvature progression in idiopathic scoliosis patients treated with scoliosis in-patient rehabilitation (SIR): an age- and sex-matched controlled study. *Pediatr Rehabil.* 2003;6:23-30.
186. Witt P, Parr C: Effectiveness of Trager psychophysical integration in promoting trunk mobility in a child with cerebral palsy, a case report. *Phys Occup Ther Pediatr.* 1988;8:75-94.
187. Gage JR, Deluca PA, Renshaw TS: Gait analysis: principles and applications with emphasis on its use with cerebral palsy. *Inst Course Lect.* 1996;45:491-507.
188. Abel MH, Damiano DL, Pannunzio M, et al: Muscle-tendon surgery in diplegic cerebral palsy: functional and mechanical changes. *J Pediatr Orthop.* 1999;19:366-375.
189. Blair E, Stanley F: Issues in the classification and epidemiology of cerebral palsy. *Mental Retard Devel Disab Res Rev.* 1997;3:184-193.
190. Davids JR, Foti T, Dabelstein J, et al: Voluntary (normal) versus obligatory (cerebral palsy) toe-walking in children: a kinematic, kinetic, and electromyographic analysis. *J Pediatr Orthop.* 1999;19:461-469.
191. Gage JR: *Gait Analysis in Cerebral Palsy.* London, MacKeith Press. 1991.
192. Mayston M: Evidence-based physical therapy for the management of children with cerebral palsy. *Dev Med Child Neurol.* 2005;47:795.
193. Harris SR, Roxborough L: Efficacy and effectiveness of physical therapy in enhancing postural control in children with cerebral palsy. *Neural Plast.* 2005;12:229-243.
194. Palisano RJ, Snider LM, Orlin MN: Recent advances in physical and occupational therapy for children with cerebral palsy. *Semin Pediatr Neurol.* 2004;11:66-77.
195. Wilton J: Casting, splinting, and physical and occupational therapy of hand deformity and dysfunction in cerebral palsy. *Hand Clin.* 2003;19:573-584.
196. Engsberg JR, Ross SA, Wagner JM, et al: Changes in hip spasticity and strength following selective dorsal rhizotomy and physical therapy for spastic cerebral palsy. *Dev Med Child Neurol.* 2002;44:220-226.
197. Engsberg JR, Ross SA, Park TS: Changes in ankle spasticity and strength following selective dorsal rhizotomy and physical therapy for spastic cerebral palsy. *J Neurosurg.* 1999;91:727-732.

198. Barry MJ: Physical therapy interventions for patients with movement disorders due to cerebral palsy. *J Child Neurol.* 1996;11(suppl 1):S51-S60.
199. Campbell SK, Gardner HG, Ramakrishnan V: Correlates of physicians' decisions to refer children with cerebral palsy for physical therapy. *Dev Med Child Neurol.* 1995;37:1062-1074.
200. Harryman SE: Lower-extremity surgery for children with cerebral palsy: physical therapy management. *Phys Ther.* 1992;72: 16-24.
201. Mayo NE: The effect of physical therapy for children with motor delay and cerebral palsy. A randomized clinical trial. *Am J Phys Med Rehabil.* 1991;70:258-267.
202. Stine SB: Therapy—physical or otherwise—in cerebral palsy. *Am J Dis Child.* 1990;144:519-520.
203. Campbell SK, Anderson JC, Gardner HG: Use of survey research methods to study clinical decision making: referral to physical therapy of children with cerebral palsy. *Phys Ther.* 1989;69: 610-615.
204. Bower E: The effects of physical therapy on cerebral palsy. *Dev Med Child Neurol.* 1989;31:266.
205. Harris SR: Commentary on "The effects of physical therapy on cerebral palsy: a controlled trial in infants with spastic diplegia." *Phys Occup Ther Pediatr.* 1989;9:1-4.
206. Horton SV, Taylor DC: The use of behavior therapy and physical therapy to promote independent ambulation in a preschooler with mental retardation and cerebral palsy. *Res Dev Disabil.* 1989;10:363-375.
207. Physical therapy for cerebral palsy. *N Engl J Med.* 1988;319: 796-797.
208. Palmer FB, Shapiro BK, Wachtel RC, et al: The effects of physical therapy on cerebral palsy. A controlled trial in infants with spastic diplegia. *N Engl J Med.* 1988;318:803-808.
209. Sommerfeld D, Fraser BA, Hensinger RN, et al: Evaluation of physical therapy service for severely mentally impaired students with cerebral palsy. *Phys Ther.* 1981;61:338-344.
210. Sussman MD, Cusick B: Preliminary report: the role of short-leg, tone-reducing casts as an adjunct to physical therapy of patients with cerebral palsy. *Johns Hopkins Med J.* 1979;145:112-114.
211. Abdel-Salam E, Maraghi S, Tawfik M: Evaluation of physical therapy techniques in the management of cerebral palsy. *J Egypt Med Assoc.* 1978;61:531-541.
212. Marx M: Integrating physical therapy into a cerebral palsy early education program. *Phys Ther.* 1973;53:512-514.
213. Mathias A: Management of cerebral palsy. Physical therapy in relation to orthopedic surgery. *Phys Ther.* 1967;47:473-482.
214. Stroumbou-Alamani S: Current concepts in the medical treatment of cerebral palsy. Physical therapy. *Arch Ital Pediatr Pueric.* 1967;25:113-120.
215. D'Wolf N, Donnelly E: Physical therapy and cerebral palsy. *Clin Pediatr (Phila).* 1966;5:351-355.
216. Footh WK, Kogan KL: Measuring the effectiveness of physical therapy in the treatment of cerebral palsy. *J Appl Toxicol.* 1963;43:867-873.
217. Paine RS: Physical therapy in the management of cerebral palsy. *Dev Med Child Neurol.* 1963;5:193.

218. Gelperin A, Payton O: Evaluation of equanil as adjunct to physical therapy for children with severe cerebral palsy. *Phys Ther Rev.* 1959;39:383-388.
219. Schwartz FF: Physical therapy for children with cerebral palsy. *J Int Coll Surg.* 1954;21:84-87.
220. Brooks W, Callahan M, Schleich-Korn J: Physical therapy and the adult with cerebral palsy; report of a conference on vocational guidance. *Phys Ther Rev.* 1953;33:426-428.
221. Bailey LA: Physical therapy in the treatment of cerebral palsy. *Phys Ther Rev.* 1950;30:230-231.
222. Grogan DP, Lundy MS, Ogden JA: A method for early postoperative mobilization of the cerebral palsy patient using a removable abduction bar. *J Pediatr Orthop.* 1987;7:338-3340.
223. Katz K, Arbel N, Apter N, et al: Early mobilization after sliding achilles tendon lengthening in children with spastic cerebral palsy. *Foot Ankle Int.* 2000;21:1011-1014.
224. Palisano R, Rosenbaum P, Walter S, et al: Development and reliability of a system to classify gross motor function in children with cerebral palsy. *Dev Med Child Neurol.* 1997;39:214-223.
225. Olney SJ, Wright MJ: Cerebral palsy. In: Campbell SK, Vander Linden DW, Palisano RJ, eds. *Physical Therapy for Children.* St. Louis, MO: Saunders. 2006:625-664.
226. Rosenbaum P: Cerebral palsy: what parents and doctors want to know. *BMJ.* 2003;326:970-974.
227. Lepage C, Noreau L, Bernard PM: Association between characteristics of locomotion and accomplishment of life habits in children with cerebral palsy. *Phys Ther.* 1998;78:458-469.
228. Westberry DE, Davids JR, Jacobs JM, et al: Effectiveness of serial stretch casting for resistant or recurrent knee flexion contractures following hamstring lengthening in children with cerebral palsy. *J Pediatr Orthop.* 2006;26:109-114.
229. Hoare B, Wasiak J, Imms C, et al: Constraint-induced movement therapy in the treatment of the upper limb in children with hemiplegic cerebral palsy. *Cochrane Database Syst Rev.* 2007;CD004149.
230. Clayton-Krasinski D, Klepper S: Impaired neuromotor development. In: Cameron MH, Monroe LG, eds. *Physical Rehabilitation: Evidence-Based Examination, Evaluation, and Intervention.* St Louis, MO: Saunders/Elsevier. 2007:333-366.
231. Hinderer KA, Hinderer SR, Shurtleff DB: Myelodysplasia. In: Campbell SK, Vander Linden DW, Palisano RJ, eds. *Physical Therapy for Children, 3rd ed.* St. Louis, MO: Saunders. 2006:735-799.
232. Hoffer MM, Feiwell E, Perry R, et al: Functional ambulation in patients with myelomeningocele. *J Bone Joint Surg Am.* 1973;55:137-148.
233. Douglas M, Archer P: Shaken baby syndrome-related traumatic brain injuries: statewide surveillance findings. *J Okla State Med Assoc.* 2004;97:487-490.
234. Clemetson CA: Shaken baby syndrome: a medicolegal problem. *N Z Med J.* 2004;117:U1160.
235. Smith J: Shaken baby syndrome. *Orthop Nurs.* 2003;22:196-203; quiz 204-205.
236. Geddes JF, Whitwell HL, Tasker RC: Shaken baby syndrome. *Br J Neurosurg.* 2003;17:18.

237. Levin AV: Shaken baby syndrome. *Br J Neurosurg.* 2003;17: 15-16.
238. Stephenson JB: Shaken baby syndrome. *J R Soc Med.* 2003;96: 102-103; author reply 103.
239. Blumenthal I: Shaken baby syndrome. *Postgrad Med J.* 2002;78:732-735.
240. Ewing-Cobbs L, Levin HS, Fletcher JM, et al: The Children's Orientation and Amnesia Test: relationship to severity of acute head injury and to recovery of memory. *Neurosurgery.* 1990;27:683-691; discussion 691.
241. Kerkering GA: Brain injuries: traumatic brain injuries, near drowning, and brain tumors. In: Campbell SK, Vander Linden DW, Palisano RJ, eds. *Physical Therapy for Children, 3rd ed.* St. Louis, MO: Saunders. 2006:709-734.
242. Hwang V, Shofer FS, Durbin DR, et al: Prevalence of traumatic injuries in drowning and near drowning in children and adolescents. *Arch Pediatr Adolesc Med.* 2003;157:50-53.
243. Fisher DH: Near-drowning. *Pediatr Rev.* 1993;14:148-151.
244. Camfield P, Camfield C: Advances in the diagnosis and management of pediatric seizure disorders in the twentieth century. *J Pediatr.* 2000;136:847-849.
245. Tharp BR: An overview of pediatric seizure disorders and epileptic syndromes. *Epilepsia.* 1987;28(suppl 1):S36-S45.
246. Nelson LP, Ureles SD, Holmes G: An update in pediatric seizure disorders. *Pediatr Dent.* 1991;13:128-135.
247. Eagle M, Bourke J, Bullock R, et al: Managing Duchenne muscular dystrophy—the additive effect of spinal surgery and home nocturnal ventilation in improving survival. *Neuromuscul Disord.* 2007;17:470-475.
248. King WM, Ruttencutter R, Nagaraja HN, et al: Orthopedic outcomes of long-term daily corticosteroid treatment in Duchenne muscular dystrophy. *Neurology.* 2007;68:1607-1613.
249. Freund AA, Scola RH, Arndt RC, et al: Duchenne and Becker muscular dystrophy: a molecular and immunohistochemical approach. *Arq Neuropsiquiatr.* 2007;65:73-76.
250. Zhang S, Xie H, Zhou G, et al: Development of therapy for Duchenne muscular dystrophy. *Zhongguo Xiu Fu Chong Jian Wai Ke Za Zhi.* 2007;21:194-203.
251. Velasco MV, Colin AA, Zurakowski D, et al: Posterior spinal fusion for scoliosis in duchenne muscular dystrophy diminishes the rate of respiratory decline. *Spine.* 2007;32:459-465.
252. Main M, Mercuri E, Haliloglu G, et al: Serial casting of the ankles in Duchenne muscular dystrophy: can it be an alternative to surgery? *Neuromuscul Disord.* 2007;17:227-230.
253. Karol LA: Scoliosis in patients with Duchenne muscular dystrophy. *J Bone Joint Surg Am.* 2007;89(suppl 1):155-162.
254. Grange RW, Call JA: Recommendations to define exercise prescription for Duchenne muscular dystrophy. *Exerc Sport Sci Rev.* 2007;35:12-17.
255. Deconinck N, Dan B: Pathophysiology of duchenne muscular dystrophy: current hypotheses. *Pediatr Neurol.* 2007;36:1-7.
256. Wagner KR, Lechtzin N, Judge DP: Current treatment of adult Duchenne muscular dystrophy. *Biochim Biophys Acta.* 2007;1772: 229-237.

257. Stuberg WA: Muscular dystrophy and spinal muscular atrophy. In: Campbell SK, Vander Linden DW, Palisano RJ, eds. *Physical Therapy for Children.* St. Louis, MO: Saunders. 2006:421-451.
258. Kim S, Chung DH: Pediatric solid malignancies: neuroblastoma and Wilms' tumor. *Surg Clin North Am.* 2006;86:469-487, xi.
259. Roman E, Ansell P, Bull D: Leukaemia and non-Hodgkin's lymphoma in children and young adults: are prenatal and neonatal factors important determinants of disease? *Br J Cancer.* 1997;76:406-415.
260. Fiorillo A, Migliorati R, Fiore M, et al: Non-Hodgkin's lymphoma in childhood presenting as thyroid enlargement. *Clin Pediatr (Phila).* 1987;26:152-154.
261. Brecher ML, Sinks LF, Thomas RR, et al: Non-Hodgkin's lymphoma in children. *Cancer.* 1978;41:1997-2001.
262. Rosenberg SA: Validity of the Ann Arbor staging classification for the non-Hodgkin's lymphomas. *Cancer Treat Rep.* 1977;61: 1023-1027.
263. Ultmann JE, Moran EM: Diagnostic evaluation and clinical staging in Hodgkin's disease: usefulness and problems of the Ann Arbor staging classification in primary staging and staging in relapse. *Natl Cancer Inst Monogr.* 1973;36:333-345.
264. Medina-Sanson A, Chico-Ponce de Leon F, Cabrera-Munoz Mde L, et al: Primary central nervous system non-Hodgkin lymphoma in childhood presenting as bilateral optic neuritis. *Childs Nerv Syst.* 2006;22:1364-1368.
265. Cairo MS, Raetz E, Lim MS, et al: Childhood and adolescent non-Hodgkin lymphoma: new insights in biology and critical challenges for the future. *Pediatr Blood Cancer.* 2005;45:753-769.
266. Sandlund JT, Santana V, Abromowitch M, et al: Large cell non-Hodgkin lymphoma of childhood: clinical characteristics and outcome. *Leukemia.* 1994;8:30-34.
267. Traggis D, Jaffe N, Vawter G, et al: Non-Hodgkin lymphoma of the head and neck in childhood. *J Pediatr.* 1975;87:933-936.
268. Crist WM, Mahmoud H, Pickert CB, et al: Biology and staging of childhood non-Hodgkin lymphoma. *An Esp Pediatr.* 1988; 29(suppl 34):104-109.
269. Nathan PC, Ness KK, Greenberg ML, et al: Health-related quality of life in adult survivors of childhood wilms tumor or neuroblastoma: a report from the childhood cancer survivor study. *Pediatr Blood Cancer.* 2006;49:704-715.
270. Kutluk T, Varan A, Buyukpamukcu N, et al: Improved survival of children with wilms tumor. *J Pediatr Hematol Oncol.* 2006;28:423-426.
271. Breslow NE, Beckwith JB, Perlman EJ, et al: Age distributions, birth weights, nephrogenic rests, and heterogeneity in the pathogenesis of Wilms tumor. *Pediatr Blood Cancer.* 2006;47:260-267.
272. Seyed-Ahadi MM, Khaleghnejad-Tabari A, Mirshemirani A, et al: Wilms' tumor: a 10 year retrospective study. *Arch Iran Med.* 2007;10:65-69.
273. Abd El-Aal HH, Habib EE, Mishrif MM: Wilms' Tumor: the experience of the pediatric unit of Kasr El-Aini Center of Radiation Oncology and Nuclear Medicine (NEMROCK). *J Egypt Natl Canc Inst.* 2005;17:308-311.
274. Cook A, Farhat W, Khoury A: Update on Wilms' tumor in children. *J Med Liban.* 2005;53:85-90.

275. Dahlin DC, Coventry MB: Osteogenic sarcoma: a study of six hundred cases. *J Bone Joint Surg Am.* 1967;49A:101–110.
276. Wilson AW, Davies HM, Edwards GA, et al: Can some physical therapy and manual techniques generate potentially osteogenic levels of strain within mammalian bone? *Phys Ther.* 1999;79: 931-938.
277. Picci P: Osteosarcoma (Osteogenic sarcoma). *Orphanet J Rare Dis.* 2007;2:6.
278. Berg EE: Osteogenic sarcoma. *Orthop Nurs.* 2006;25:348-349; quiz 350-1.
279. Lin SY, Chen WM, Wu HH, et al: Extraosseous osteogenic sarcoma. *J Chin Med Assoc.* 2005;68:542-545.
280. Wang LL: Biology of osteogenic sarcoma. *Cancer J.* 2005;11: 294-305.
281. Deitch J, Crawford AH, Choudhury S: Osteogenic sarcoma of the rib: a case presentation and literature review. *Spine.* 2003;28:E74-E77.
282. Iwamoto Y: Diagnosis and treatment of Ewing's sarcoma. *Jpn J Clin Oncol.* 2007;37:79–89.
283. Scotlandi K: Targeted therapies in Ewing's sarcoma. *Adv Exp Med Biol.* 2006;587:13-22.
284. Chun JM, Kim SY, Kim JH: Ewing's sarcoma of the rotator cuff tendon: a case report. *J Shoulder Elbow Surg.* 2006;15:e41-e43.
285. Bernstein M, Kovar H, Paulussen M, et al: Ewing's sarcoma family of tumors: current management. *Oncologist.* 2006;11: 503-519.
286. Hajdu SI: The enigma of Ewing's sarcoma. *Ann Clin Lab Sci.* 2006;36:108-110.
287. Duffy CM, Arsenault L, Duffy KN, et al: The Juvenile Arthritis Quality of Life Questionnaire—development of a new responsive index for juvenile rheumatoid arthritis and juvenile spondyloarthritides. *J Rheumatol.* 1997;24:738-746.
288. Brewer EJ, Jr, Bass J, Baum J, et al: Current proposed revision of JRA criteria. JRA Criteria Subcommittee of the Diagnostic and Therapeutic Criteria Committee of the American Rheumatism Section of The Arthritis Foundation. *Arthritis Rheum.* 1977;20: 195-199.
289. Wright FV, Law M, Crombie V, et al: Development of a self-report functional status index for juvenile rheumatoid arthritis. *J Rheumatol.* 1994;21:536-544.
290. Howe S, Levinson J, Shear E, et al: Development of a disability measurement tool for juvenile rheumatoid arthritis. The Juvenile Arthritis Functional Assessment Report for Children and their Parents. *Arthritis Rheum.* 1991;34:873-880.
291. Lovell DJ, Howe S, Shear E, et al: Development of a disability measurement tool for juvenile rheumatoid arthritis: the Juvenile Arthritis Functional Assessment Scale. *Arthritis Rheum.* 1989;32:1390-1395.
292. Klepper SE: Juvenile rheumatoid arthritis. In: Campbell SK, Vander Linden DW, Palisano RJ, eds. *Physical Therapy for Children.* St. Louis, MO: Saunders. 2006:291-323.
293. Goodman CC: The cardiovascular system. In: Goodman CC, Boissonnault WG, Fuller KS, eds. *Pathology: Implications for the Physical Therapist, 2nd ed.* Philadelphia, PA: Saunders. 2003: 367-476.

294. Coskun KO, Coskun ST, El Arousy M, et al: Pediatric patients with Kawasaki disease and a case report of Kitamura operation. *Asaio J.* 2006;52:e43-e47.
295. Pannaraj PS, Turner CL, Bastian JF, et al: Failure to diagnose Kawasaki disease at the extremes of the pediatric age range. *Pediatr Infect Dis J.* 2004;23:789-791.
296. Yanagawa H, Nakamura Y, Yashiro M, et al: Incidence of Kawasaki disease in Japan: the nationwide surveys of 1999-2002. *Pediatr Int.* 2006;48:356-361.
297. Tsai MH, Huang YC, Yen MH, et al: Clinical responses of patients with Kawasaki disease to different brands of intravenous immunoglobulin. *J Pediatr.* 2006;148:38-43.

section III

Procedural Interventions

Therapeutic Exercise

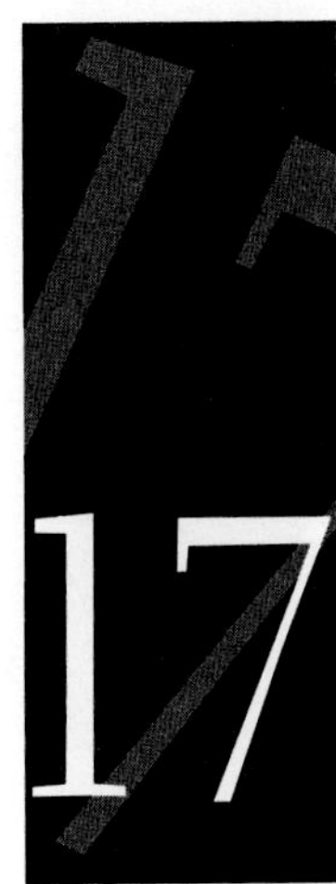

Therapeutic exercise is a fundamental component of the vast majority of physical therapy interventions. Prescribed accurately, therapeutic exercise can be used to restore, maintain, and improve a patient's functional status by increasing strength, endurance, and flexibility. When prescribing a therapeutic exercise program it is important to consider the functional loss and disability of the patient.

PHYSIOLOGY OF EXERCISE

ENERGY SYSTEMS

The creation of energy for the metabolically active muscles occurs initially from the breakdown of specific nutrients from foodstuffs. The energy is stored in a compound called adenosine triphosphate (ATP), which is produced in muscle tissue from blood glucose or glycogen, of which glycogen is the initial substrate. Two of the most important energy generating systems that function in muscle tissue include the anaerobic and aerobic metabolism, both of which produce ATP:

- Anaerobic metabolism: this process metabolizes glucose to generate small amounts of ATP energy without the need for oxygen.
- ATP-PCr system: used for ATP production during high-intensity, short-duration exercise. Phosphocreatine (PCr) decomposes and releases a large amount of energy that is used to construct ATP—it is the short-term energy system and provides energy for muscle contraction for up to 15 seconds.
- Anaerobic glycolysis (glycolytic system): a major supplier of ATP during high-intensity, short-duration activities. While unable to produce as much energy per unit time as the phosphocreatine system (ie, unable to sustain maximum sprinting speed), it lasts considerably longer before intensity must

be further reduced. This is the intermediate energy system—provides the majority of energy for a sustained performance lasting between 20 seconds and two minutes (sprinting 400 or 800 m).

- Aerobic metabolism (oxidative system): if exercise continues beyond a certain point the body can no longer rely solely on anaerobic metabolism and has to switch to this more complex form of carbohydrate and fat metabolism in order to generate ATP. This is the long-term energy system.

Ultimately, all exercise has an oxygen cost, and the faster this can be met during recovery, the better the preparation for the next high-intensity exercise bout. Delivery of oxygen to the fatigued muscles replenishes stores of PCr and lowers levels of lactic acid. This means the aerobic system must not be overlooked during rehabilitation.

In most activities, both aerobic and anaerobic systems function simultaneously with the ratio being determined by the intensity and duration of the activity. In general, high-intensity activities of short duration rely more heavily on the anaerobic system, whereas low-intensity activities of longer duration rely more on the aerobic system.

The normal and abnormal responses to exercise, and the signs and symptoms of exercise intolerance, are described in Chapter 11.

COORDINATION OF THE MUSCULAR SYSTEM

For motion to take place, the muscles producing movement must have a stable base from which to work from. Muscles perform a variety of roles depending on the required movement. These roles include

- Prime movers/agonists: a muscle that is directly responsible for producing movement.
- Synergists: performs a cooperative muscle function in relation to the agonist. Synergists can function as stabilizers, neutralizers, or rotators.
  - Stabilizers: the muscles contract statically to steady or support some part of the body against the pull of the contracting muscles, against the pull of gravity, or against the effect of momentum and recoil in certain vigorous movements.
  - Neutralizers: a muscle or muscle group that acts to prevent an undesired action of one of the movers.
  - Rotators: a combination of muscle forces that produce a desired motion, usually referred to as force couples.
- Antagonists: a muscle or muscle group that has an effect opposite to that of the agonist.

NERVE AND MUSCLE PHYSIOLOGY

Nerves and muscles are both excitable tissues. This excitability is dependent on the cell membrane, which regulates the interchange of substances between the inside of the cell and the environment outside the cell. The potential difference between electrical charges on the inside and outside of the cell membrane is known as the resting membrane potential (−60 to −90 mV for excitable cells).

RESTING MEMBRANE POTENTIAL

All cells under resting conditions have an electrical potential difference across the plasma membrane (resting membrane potential [RMP]) so that the inside of the cell is negatively charged with respect to the outside. The resting membrane potential is determined mainly by two factors:

- The differences in ion concentration of the intracellular and extracellular fluids
- The permeabilities of the plasma membrane to the different ion species

Both electrical and chemical gradients are established along in cell membrane with a greater concentration of diffusible positive ions on the outside of the membrane than on the inside. Thus,

- The cell membrane is more permeable to potassium (K^+) as compared to sodium (Na^+) and negatively charged proteins (anions).
- An electrical potential is generated across the cell membrane due to the high concentration of K^+ and anions on the inside of the cell relative to the concentration of Na^+ on the outside.
- A negative charge is produced within the cell and a positive charge develops on the outside of the cell as the positively charged K^+ diffuses from the cell.

The RMP is maintained by an active sodium-potassium pump that takes in K^+ and extrudes Na^+. To create transmission of an impulse in the nerve tissue, the RMP must be reduced below a threshold level thereby causing a change in the membrane's permeability. These changes create an action potential (AP) that will propagate the impulse along the nerve in both directions from the location of the stimulus.

ACTION POTENTIAL

An AP is a stimulus that causes the cell membrane to become more permeable to Na^+ ions.

Not all stimuli are effective in causing an AP. To be an effective agent, a stimulus must have:

- An adequate intensity and amplitude to cause the membrane potential to be lowered sufficiently to reach threshold levels. Since a single excitatory synaptic event (excitatory postsynaptic potential or EPSP) does not bring the postsynaptic membrane to its threshold level, further depolarization is necessary before the initial EPSP has died away. This further depolarization can occur at different times (temporal summation) or simultaneously from different sources (spatial summation).
- A rapid enough rise of the current peak intensity to prevent accommodation, which is the rapid adjustment of the membrane to stimuli to prevent depolarization.
- A sufficient duration to produce a depolarization of the cell membrane.

Study Pearl

The polarization is sometimes described as nonresponse in that set threshold changes do not generate an AP.

Study Pearl

Temporal summation: the process whereby a stimulus that is below threshold will elicit a reflex if the stimulus occurs repeatedly.

Spatial summation: the process whereby two or more stimuli that are individually below threshold will elicit a reflex if they occur simultaneously at different points on the body.

When the transmembrane potential reaches a critical threshold level (−55 mV), the voltage sensitive Na^+ and K^+ channels open widely.

- Na^+ permeability increases rapidly.
- K^+ permeability increases slowly.

During depolarization, the transmembrane potential might rise as high as +35 mV. The flow of ions produces a characteristic charge:

- A positive charge is generated inside the cell.
- A negative charge is produced outside of the cell.

The K^+ channels are fully open about the time the Na^+ channels are closed. Thus

- K^+ rushes rapidly out of the cell making the transmembrane potential progressively more negative (repolarization).
- The K^+ channels remain open long enough to repolarize the membrane (hyperpolarization).
- The K^+ channels close and passive diffusion of the ions rapidly returns the RMP to its initial level.

Following excitation and propagation of the impulse along the nerve fiber, there is a brief period during which an ordinary stimulus is not able to generate another impulse. This brief period is termed the *refractory period.* The refractory period consists of two phases, the absolute refractory period and the relative refractory period.

Propagation of the Action Potential. The opening of the Na^+ and K^+ channels and voltage changes that produce an AP at one segment of the membrane triggers successive depolarizations in adjacent regions of the nerve, muscle or membranes. Movement of the AP occurs along the surface of the nerve or muscle cell.

- Unmyelinated nerve: AP movement is generated by a sequential depolarization along neighboring sites in the membrane. Speed of conduction is slow due to the greater internal resistance in the small diameter fibers.
- Myelinated nerve: AP movement is generated by saltatory conduction, which occurs at discrete junctures in the myelin sheath which surrounds the nerve, called nodes of Ranvier. Myelin is an excellent insulator with a high resistance to current flow. Because myelin is absent over the nodes of Ranvier, current flows from one node to the next. The Na^+ and K^+ ion exchange and current flow is concentrated at these nodes, with the impulse jumping from node to node at speeds greater than those in the smaller unmyelinated nerve fibers.

THE TYPES OF MUSCLE CONTRACTION

Three types of contraction are commonly recognized: isometric, concentric, and eccentric:

- Isometric contraction. An isometric contraction occurs when there is tension produced in the muscle without any appreciable change in muscle length or joint movement.[1]
- Concentric contraction. A concentric contraction produces a shortening of the muscle. This occurs when the tension generated by the agonist muscle is sufficient to overcome an external resistance, and to move the body segment of one attachment toward the segment of its other attachment.[1]
- Eccentric contraction. An eccentric contraction occurs when a muscle slowly lengthens as it gives in to an external force that is greater than the contractile force it is exerting.[1] In reality, the muscle does not actually lengthen, it merely returns from its shortened position to its normal resting length. Eccentric muscle contractions, which are capable of generating greater forces than either isometric or concentric contractions,[2-4] are involved in activities that require a deceleration to occur. These include slowing to a stop when running, lowering an object, or sitting down. Because the load exceeds the bond between the actin and myosin filaments (see Chapter 5) during an eccentric contraction, some of the myosin are probably torn from the binding sites on the actin filament, whilst the remainder are completing the contraction cycle.[5] The resulting force is substantially larger for a torn cross-bridge than for one being created during a normal cycle of muscle contraction. In addition, eccentric contractions consume less oxygen and fewer energy stores than concentric contractions against similar loads. Consequently, the combined increase in force per cross-bridge and the number of active cross-bridges results in a maximum lengthening muscle tension which is greater than that which could be created during a shortening muscle action.[5]

Four other contractions are worth mentioning:

- Isotonic contraction. An isotonic contraction is a contraction in which the tension within the muscle remains constant as the muscle shortens or lengthens.[1] This state is very difficult to produce and measure. Although the term isotonic is used to describe concentric and eccentric contractions alike, its use in this context is erroneous as in most exercise forms the tension produced in muscles will vary with muscle length according to cross bridge formation and with the variation in external torque.[1]
- Isokinetic contraction. An isokinetic contraction occurs when a muscle is maximally contracting at the same speed throughout the whole range of its related lever.[1] Isokinetic contractions require the use of special equipment that produces an accommodating resistance. Both high-speed/low-resistance, and low-speed/high-resistance regimens result in excellent strength gains.[6-9] The disadvantage of this type of exercise is its expense. In addition, there is the potential for impact loading and incorrect joint axis alignment.[10] Isokinetic exercises may also have questionable functional carryover due to their performance in open kinetic chain and training a single motion/muscle group.[11]

- Econcentric contraction. This type of contraction combines both a controlled concentric and a simultaneous eccentric contraction of the same muscle over two separate joints.[12] Examples of an econcentric contraction include the standing hamstring curl and the squat. In the standing hamstring curl, the hamstrings work concentrically to flex the knee, while the hip tends to flex eccentrically, lengthening the hamstrings. When rising from a squat the hamstrings work concentrically as the hip extends and work eccentrically as the knee extends. Conversely the rectus femoris works eccentrically as the hip extends and works concentrically as the knee extends.
- Isolytic contraction. The term isolytic contraction is used in osteopathic circles to describe a type of eccentric contraction, where a greater force than the patient can overcome is used. This type of contraction is used with muscle energy techniques to stretch fibrotic tissue.

Study Pearl

According to Cyriax, pain with a contraction generally indicates an injury to the muscle or a capsular structure (see Chapter 8).[13]

RECRUITMENT OF MOTOR UNITS

The force and speed of a muscle contraction are based on the requirement of an activity and are dependent on the ability of the central nervous system (CNS) to control the recruitment of motor units.[14] Slow-twitch fiber motor units have low thresholds and are relatively more easily activated than the motor units of the fast-twitch fibers (see Chapter 5). Consequently the slow-twitch fibers are the first to be recruited, even when the resulting limb movement is rapid.[15]

Study Pearl

As the force requirement, speed requirement, and/or duration of the activity increases, motor units with higher thresholds are recruited. Type IIa are recruited before type IIb.[16]

ELECTROMECHANICAL DELAY

Following the stimulation of a muscle, a brief period elapses before the muscle begins to develop tension. This period is referred to as the *electromechanical delay* (EMD). The length of the EMD varies considerably between muscles. Fast twitch fibers have shorter periods of EMD when compared to slow twitch fibers.[17] It has been suggested that injury increases the EMD and therefore increases the susceptibility to injury.[18] One of the purposes of neuromuscular re-education is to return the EMD to a normal level.[19]

FACTORS AFFECTING MUSCLE PERFORMANCE

Muscle is the only biological tissue capable of actively generating tension (see Chapter 5). This characteristic enables human skeletal muscle to perform the important functions of maintaining upright body posture, moving body parts, and absorbing shock. Human skeletal muscle possesses four biomechanical properties: extensibility, elasticity, irritability, and the ability to develop tension.

- Extensibility. Extensibility is the ability to be stretched or to increase in length.
- Elasticity. Elasticity is the ability to return to normal resting length following a stretch.

- Irritability. Irritability is the ability to respond to a stimulus. With reference to skeletal muscle, this stimulus is provided electrochemically.
- Ability to develop tension. Skeletal muscle has the ability to contact, thereby developing tension.

The maximum tension that is generated within a fully activated muscle is not a constant, and depends on a number of factors.[14]

> **Study Pearl**
>
> Factors affecting muscle performance include[20]
> - Muscle fiber type (see Chapter 5)
> - Muscle fiber size
> - Force-length relationships
> - Force-velocity relationships
> - Muscle design (angle of insertion and angle of pennation)
> - Fatigue
> - Neural control
> - Age (refer to Chapters 14 and 16)
> - Level of cognition

MUSCLE FIBER SIZE

Sedentary men and women and young children possess 45% to 55% slow-twitch fibers.[21] Individuals who achieve high levels of sports performance have the predominance and distribution characteristic of their sport.[22]

FORCE-LENGTH RELATIONSHIP

The number of cross-bridges that can be formed is dependent on the extent of the overlap between the actin and myosin filaments.[23] Thus, the force a muscle is capable of exerting depends on its length.

If the muscle is in a shortened position, the overlap of actin and myosin reduces the number of available sites for cross-bridge formation. *Active insufficiency* of a muscle occurs when the muscle is unable to shorten to the extent required to produce full range of motion at all joints crossed simultaneously.[12,14,24,25] For example, the finger flexors cannot produce a tight fist when the wrist is fully flexed as compared to when it is in neutral.

If a muscle is in a lengthened position compared to the resting length, the actin filaments are pulled away from the myosin heads, such that they cannot create cross-bridges.[5] *Passive insufficiency* of the muscle occurs when the muscle cannot stretch to the extent required for full range of motion in the opposite direction at all joints crossed.[12,14,24,25] For example, a larger range of dorsiflexion is possible at the ankle when the knee is not fully extended.

> **Study Pearl**
>
> For each muscle cell, there is an optimum length, or range of lengths, where the contractile force is strongest. At the natural resting length of the muscle, there is near optimal overlap of actin and myosin allowing for the generation of maximum tension at this length.

THE FORCE-VELOCITY RELATIONSHIP

The rate at which a muscle shortens or lengthens significantly affects the force that a muscle can develop during contraction.

Shortening Contractions. As the speed of a muscle shortening increases, the force it is capable of producing decreases (Figure 17-1).[2,4] At very slow speeds, the force that a muscle can resist or overcome rises rapidly up to 50% greater than the maximum isometric contraction.[2,4]

> **Study Pearl**
>
> For maximal effectiveness of muscle force production, slow concentric movements should be emphasized.[2,4]

Lengthening Contractions. When a muscle contracts while lengthening, the force production differs from that of a shortening contraction:

- Rapid lengthening contractions generate more force than do slower lengthening contractions.
- During slow lengthening muscle actions, the work produced approximates that of an isometric contraction.[2,4]

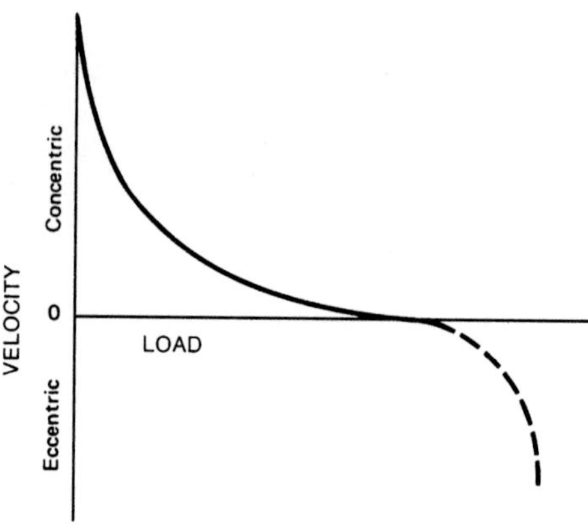

Figure 17-1. Force velocity relationship. (Reproduced, with permission, from Luttgens K, Hamilton N: *Kinesiology: Scientific Basis of Human Motion, 10th ed.* New York, NY: McGraw-Hill. 2002:56.)

ANGLE OF INSERTION

Although each muscle contains the contractile machinery to produce the forces for movement, it is the tendon that transmits these forces to the bones in order to achieve movement or stability of the body in space.[26] The interface between the muscle and tendon is called the myotendinous junction (MTJ). The angle of insertion the tendon makes with a bone determines the line of pull. The tension generated by a muscle is a function of its angle of insertion. A muscle whose line of pull is oriented at a 90-degree angle to the bone and anatomically attached as far from the joint center as possible generates the greatest amount of torque.[14] There are optimal insertion angles for each of the muscles. The angle of insertion of a muscle, and therefore its line of pull, can change during dynamic movements.[5]

ANGLE OF PENNATION

The *angle of pennation* is the angle created between the fiber direction and the line of pull (Figure 17-2). When the fibers of a muscle lie parallel to the long axis of the muscle, there is no angle of pennation. The number of fibers within a fixed volume of muscle increases with the angle of pennation.[5] Although maximum tension can be improved with pennation, the range of shortening of the muscle is reduced. Muscles that need to have large changes in length without the need for very high tension, such as the sartorius, do not have pennate muscle fibers.[5] In contrast, pennate muscle fibers are found in those muscles in which the emphasis is on a high capacity for tension generation rather than range of motion (eg, gluteus maximus).

FATIGUE

Skeletal muscle fatigue can compromise exercise tolerance and work productivity while retarding rehabilitation of diseased or damaged muscle. The development of fatigue probably involves several factors that influence force production in a manner dependent on muscle fiber type and activation pattern.[27]

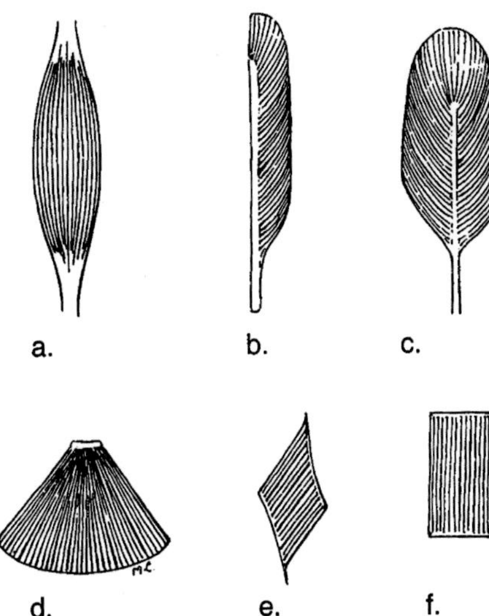

Figure 17-2. Examples of muscles of different shapes and internal structure. **A.** Fusiform or spindle. **B.** Penniform. **C.** Bipenniform. **D.** Triangular or fan shaped. **E.** Rhomboidal (quadrate). **F.** Rectangular (quadrate). (Reproduced, with permission, from Luttgens K, Hamilton N: *Kinesiology: Scientific Basis of Human Motion, 10th ed.* New York, NY: McGraw-Hill. 2002:50.)

Characteristics of muscle fatigue include reduction in muscle force production capability and shortening velocity, a reduction in the release and uptake of intracellular calcium by the sarcoplasmic reticulum, as well as prolonged relaxation of motor units between recruitment.[27,28]

Study Pearl

Skeletal muscle blood flow increases 20-fold during muscle contractions.[29] The muscle blood flow generally increases in proportion to the metabolic demands of the tissue, a relationship reflected by positive correlations between muscle blood flow and exercise.

MUSCLE PERFORMANCE

Muscle performance includes strength, endurance, and power.

- Strength. Strength is defined as the maximum force that a muscle can develop during a single contraction. Muscular strength is derived both from the amount of tension a muscle can generate and from the moment arms of contributing muscles with respect to the joint center. Both sources are affected by several factors (see "Factors Affecting Muscle Performance" earlier). Muscle strength can be measured using a number of methods:
  - Manual muscle testing (MMT)—see Chapter 5.
  - Using a dynamometer: a device that measures strength through the use of a load cell or spring-loaded gauge.
  - Isokinetic machine: measures the strength of a muscle group during a movement with constant, predetermined speed.
- Endurance. Endurance is defined as the ability of a muscle to sustain or perform repetitive muscular contractions for an extended period. The ability to perform endurance activities is based on the patient's aerobic capacity (see Chapter 5).
- Power. Power is the rate of performing work. Work is the magnitude of force acting on an object multiplied by the

TABLE 17-1. RESISTIVE EXERCISE VARIABLES

Resistance (load or weight)
Duration and volume (the total number of repetitions performed multiplied by the resistance used)
Frequency (weekly, daily)
Intensity
Point of application
Sequence (exercising large muscle groups before small; perform multi-joint before single-joint activities)
Bouts (timed sessions of exercise)
Sets and repetition
Mode (type of contraction)
Rests

distance through which the force acts. Muscular power is the product of muscular force and velocity of muscle shortening. Maximum power occurs at approximately one-third of maximum velocity.[30] Muscular power is an important contributor to activities requiring both speed and strength. Individuals with a predominance of fast twitch fibers generate more power at a given load than those with a high composition of slow twitch fibers.[31] The ratio for mean peak power production by type IIb, type IIa, and type I fibers in skeletal tissue is 10:5:1.[32]

Study Pearl

- The dosage of an exercise refers to each particular patient's exercise capability, and is determined by a number of variables (Table 17-1) and the goals of the intervention (increasing strength, endurance, or power).[34]
- Intensity and duration are inversely proportional: the higher the intensity, the fewer repetitions are performed.

Improving Muscle Performance

The promotion and progression of tissue repair while exercising involves a delicate balance between protection, and the application of controlled functional stresses to the damaged structure. The goal of the functional exercise progression is to identify the motion, or motions that the patient is able to exercise into without eliciting symptoms other than post-exercise soreness.[33] Patients must be advised to let pain be their guide and that pain-free range of motion activities must be continued to prevent loss of function.

A hierarchy for ROM (Table 17-2) and resistive exercise progression (Table 17-3) exists. This hierarchy is based on patient tolerance and response to ensure that any progress made is done in a safe and controlled fashion. A number of principles can be used to guide the clinician in the progression of therapeutic exercise:[35]

- The exercise prescription will vary according to the stage of healing and degree of irritability. Greater irritability is associated

TABLE 17-2. THE HIERARCHY FOR THE ROM EXERCISES

1. Passive ROM
2. Active assisted ROM
3. Active ROM

TABLE 17-3. THE HIERARCHY FOR THE PROGRESSION OF RESISTIVE EXERCISES

1. Single angle submaximal isometrics performed in the neutral position
2. Multiple angle submaximal isometrics performed at various angles of the range
3. Multiple angle maximal isometrics
4. Small arc submaximal isotonics
5. Full ROM submaximal isotonics
6. Functional ROM submaximal isotonics

with very acutely inflamed conditions, whereas chronic conditions usually have low irritability. The degree of movement and the speed of progression are both guided by the signs and symptoms.

- The patient should be taught initially to exercise in cardinal planes before progressing as quickly as allowed to exercising in the functional planes.
- The exercise protocol should initiate with exercises that utilize a short lever arm. These exercises serve to decrease the amount of torque at the joint. Extremity exercises can be adapted to include short levers by flexing the extremity, or by exercising with the extremity closer to the body.
- The goal should be to achieve the closed pack position at the earliest opportunity. The closed pack position of a joint is its position of maximum stability.
- The prescribed exercises should reproduce the forces and loading rates that will approach the patient's functional demands, as the rehabilitation progresses.

All exercise progressions should include[36]

- Variation. Variation to the exercises can be provided by altering
  - The plane of motion
  - The range of motion
  - The body position
  - The exercise duration
  - The exercise frequency
- A safe progression. A safe progression is ensured if the exercises are progressed from
  - Slow to fast
  - Simple to complex
  - Stable to unstable
  - Low force to high force

IMPROVING STRENGTH

To increase strength, the load or resistance must be gradually increased during the muscle contraction. Strengthening of a muscle occurs when the muscle is forced to work at a higher level than that to which it is accustomed. To most effectively increase muscle strength, a muscle must work with increasing effort against progressively increasing resistance.[3,37] If a resistance is applied to a muscle as it contracts so that the metabolic capabilities of the muscle are progressively overloaded, adaptive changes occur within the muscle, which make it stronger over time.[4,38] These adaptive changes include[2,3,39-43]

- Remodeling (hypertrophy). The muscle hypertrophies due to an increase in the number and size of the myofilaments (actin and myosin).
- An increase in the efficiency of the neuromuscular system.
- The endurance of the muscle improves.
- The power of the muscle improves.
- Improved bone mass (Wolfe's law).

- Increase in metabolism/calorie burning/weight control.
- Cardiovascular benefits, when using large muscle groups.

Conversely, a muscle can become weak or atrophied through:

- Disease
- Neurological compromise
- Immobilization
- Disuse

TYPES OF EXERCISE

Isometric Exercises

This type of exercise has an obvious role where joint movement is restricted, either by pain, or by bracing/casting. Their primary role in this regard is to prevent atrophy and prevent a decrease of ligament, bone, and muscle strength. A 6-second hold of 75% of maximal resistance is sufficient to increase strength when performed repetitively. The disadvantages of isometric exercises are

- The strength gains occur at a specific point in the range of motion and not throughout the range (unless performed at multi-angles).
- Not all of a muscle's fibers are activated—there is predominantly an activation of slow twitch (type I) fibers.
- There are no flexibility or cardiovascular fitness benefits.
- Peak effort can be detrimental to the tissues due to vasoconstriction and joint compression forces.
- There is limited functional carry over.[11]
- Considerable internal pressure can be generated, especially if the breath is held during contraction, which can result in further injury to a patient with a weakness in the abdominal wall (hernia), and/or cardiovascular impairment (increase blood pressure through the Valsalva maneuver, even if the exercise is performed correctly).

Concentric Exercises

Concentric exercises are dynamic and allow the clinician to vary the load from constant, using free weights, to variable, using an exercise machine. The speed of contraction can also be manipulated depending on the goal of the intervention.

Eccentric Exercises

Eccentric strength is important for many functional activities, and can provide a source of shock absorption during closed chain functional activities. The clinical indications for the use of eccentric exercise are numerous.[34]

Functional Exercises

Functional strength is the ability of the neuromuscular system to perform combinations of concentric and eccentric contractions involved with multijoint functional activities in an efficient manner and in a multiplanar environment, based on a patient's needs and requirements (see "Specificity of Training" later).[44,45]

Isokinetic Exercise

Isokinetic exercise produces an accommodating and variable resistance such that peak torque (the maximum force generated through the range of motion), is inversely related to angular velocity (the speed that a body segment moves through its range of motion). Thus, an increase in angular velocity decreases peak torque production. Advantages for this type of exercise include

- Both high-speed/low-resistance, and low-speed/high-resistance regimens can result in excellent strength gains.[6-9]
- Both concentric and eccentric resistance exercises can be performed on isokinetic machines.
- The machines provide maximum resistance at all point in the range of motion as a muscle contracts.
- The gravity-produced torque created by the machine adds to the force generated by the muscle when it contracts resulting in a higher torque output than is actually created by the muscle.

The disadvantages of this type of exercise include

- Expense
- The potential for impact loading and incorrect joint axis alignment[10]
- Questionable functional carryover[11]

TYPES OF RESISTANCE

Resistance can be applied to a muscle by any external force or mass, including any of the following.

Gravity

With respect to gravity, muscle actions may occur in

- The same direction of gravity (downward)
- In the opposite direction to gravity (upward)
- In a direction perpendicular to gravity (horizontal)
- In the same or opposite direction to gravity, but at an angle

Body Weight

A wide variety of exercises have been developed using no equipment and relying on the patient's body weight for the resistance (push-up).

Small Weights

Small weights are typically used to strengthen the smaller muscles or to increase the endurance of larger muscles by increasing the number of reps. Free weights also provide more versatility than exercise machines, especially for three-dimensional exercises.

SURGICAL TUBING/THERABAND

Elastic resistance offers a unique type of resistance. The amount of variable resistance offered by elastic bands or tubing is a factor of the internal tension produced by the material, which in turn is a factor of the elastic material's coefficient of elasticity, the surface area of the elastic material, and how much the elastic material is stretched.[46]

EXERCISE MACHINES

In the more advanced stages of a rehabilitation program, when the larger muscle groups require strengthening, a multitude of specific indoor exercise machines can be used. Although these machines are a more expensive alternative to dumbbell or elastic resistance, they do offer some advantages:

- Provide more sufficient resistance for large muscle groups that can be achieved with free weights/cuff weights, or manual resistance.
- Typically safer than free weights.
- Provide the clinician with the ability to quantify and measure the amount of resistance that the patient can tolerate over time.

The disadvantages of exercise machines include

- The inability to modify the exercise to be more functional or three-dimensional.
- The inability to modify the amount of resistance at particular points of the range.

MANUAL RESISTANCE

An example of manual resistance is proprioceptive neuromuscular facilitation (PNF)—refer to "Proprioceptive Neuromuscular Facilitation" later in the chapter.

The advantages of manual resistance, when applied by a skilled clinician, are[47]

- Control of the extremity position and force applied.
- More effective re-education of the muscle or extremity.
- Critical sensory input to the patient through tactile stimulation and appropriate facilitation techniques.
- Accurate accommodation and alterations in the resistance applied throughout the range.
- Ability to limit the range.

The disadvantages of manual resistance include

- The amount of resistance applied cannot be measured quantitatively.
- The amount of resistance is limited by the strength of the clinician/caregiver or family member.

Study Pearl

Water can be used as a form of resistance (see "Specialized Exercise Regimes"). Water provides resistance proportional to the relative speed of movement of the patient and the water and the cross-sectional area of the patient in contact with the water.[48]

CORRECT PROGRESSION OF EXERCISES

For exercises to be effective, the patient must be able to train without exacerbating the condition.[49] Each progression is made more challenging by altering one of the parameters of exercise (type/mode of exercise, intensity, duration, and frequency), which are modified according to patient response.

- *Intensity*: refers to how much effort is required to perform the exercise.[50]
- *Type of exercise*: relates to the specific activity being performed
- *Related perceived exertion (RPE)*: an individual's perception of effort (relative perceived exertion) is closely related to the level of physiological effort (Table 11-10).[51,52]
- *Duration:* refers to the length of the exercise session.
- *Frequency*: refers to how often the exercise is performed.

Exercise progression in the following populations is determined by a number of factors including the general health of the patient, the stage of healing and the degree of irritability of the structure, and the patient's response to exercise:

- Patients with an acute illness/fever
- Patients with an acute injury
- Postsurgical patients
- Patients with cardiac disease—edema, weight gain, unstable angina
- Patients who are obese

Delayed Onset Muscle Soreness

Muscular soreness may result from any form of exercise. Acute muscle soreness develops during or directly after strenuous and aerobic exercise performed to the point of fatigue. Theoretically, the soreness is related to the decreased blood flow and reduced oxygen that creates a temporary buildup of lactic acid and potassium. A type of post-exercise soreness that is related to eccentric exercise is delayed onset muscle soreness (DOMS).[34] DOMS occurs between 48 and 72 hours after exercise, and may last for up to 10 days. The intervention for DOMS includes aerobic submaximal exercise with no eccentric component, pain-free flexibility exercises, and high speed concentric only isokinetic training.[34,53]

EXERCISE HIERARCHY

A hierarchy exists for ROM and resistive exercises to ensure that any progression is done in a safe and controlled fashion. The hierarchy for the ROM exercises is outlined in Table 17-2. The hierarchy for the progression of resistive exercises is outlined in Table 17-3. Gentle resistance exercises can be introduced very early in the rehabilitative process. Although some soreness can be expected, sharp pain should not be provoked.

Study Pearl

Neuromuscular electrical stimulation (NMES) can be an effective component of a rehabilitation program for muscle weakness (see Chapter 18).

At regular intervals, the clinician should ensure that

- The patient is adherent with their exercise program at home.
- The patient is aware as to the rationale behind the exercise program.
- The patient is performing the exercise program correctly and at the appropriate intensity.
- The patient's exercise program is being updated appropriately based on clinical findings and patient response.

EXERCISE PRESCRIPTIONS

The greatest amount of tension the muscle can achieve is a 20% increase in fiber length measured from the resting length.[54] The clinical implications for this are that the patient can tolerate less resistance in the beginning of range, and at the end of range of a contraction, but can overcome more resistance at a point in the range 20% beyond the resting contraction.[49]

A number of precautions must be observed with patients who are performing strength training:

- Substitute motions: Muscles that are weak or fatigued rely on other muscles to produce the movement if the resistance is too high. This results in incorrect stabilization and poor form.
- Overworking of the muscles: this can occur if the exercise parameters (frequency, intensity, duration) are progressed too quickly.
- Adequate rest must be provided after each vigorous exercise. The rest period between sets can be determined by the time the breathing rate, or pulse, of the patient returns to the steady state.

Study Pearl

Progressive resistive exercises use the repetition maximum (RM) or the greatest amount of weight a muscle can move through the range of motion a specific number of times (resistance maximal).

- Repetition maximum (RM). This is based on the premise that whatever exercise progression is used to achieve an increase in the total number of repetitions while maintaining a sufficient effort, the number of sets must also be increased. This increase in sets must occur in conjunction with a reduction in the number of repetitions per set by 10% to 20%,[49] or a reduction in the resistance.
- Resistance maximal. A concept introduced by DeLorme[40] that refers to the amount of resistance a group of muscles can overcome exactly 10 times. This amount of resistance is then used for exercise.

Caution must be taken with patients diagnosed with osteoporosis whose bones are unable to withstand normal stresses and are highly susceptible to pathological fracture. Osteoporotic features may also occur as a result of prolonged immobilization, bed rest, the inability to bear weight on an extremity and as a result of nutritional or hormonal factors.

A number of programs have been designed for the progression of concentric exercise programs (Tables 17-4 to 17-6). It is important to remember, that any exercise progression should always be based on sound rationale (optimal resistance, the number of repetitions, the number of sets, and the frequency of training) and the symptomatic response.

WARM-UP AND COOL-DOWN PERIODS

Each exercise session should include a 5 to 15 minute warm-up and a 5 to 15 minute cool-down period.

The length of the warm-up and cool-down sessions may need to be longer for deconditioned or older individuals.

OVERLOAD PRINCIPLE

The principle of overload states that a greater than normal stress or load on the body is required for training adaptation to take place.

TABLE 17-4. EXERCISE PRESCRIPTIONS

	SET OF 10	AMOUNT OF WEIGHT	REPETITIONS
DeLorme program	1	50% of 10 RM	10
	2	75% of 10 RM	10
	3	100% of 10 RM	10
Oxford technique	1	50% of 10 RM	10
	2	75% of 10 RM	10
	3	100% of 10 RM	10
MacQueen technique	3 (beginning /intermediate)	100% of 10 RM	10
	4-5 (advanced)	100% of 2-3 RM	2-3
Sander program	Total of 4 sets (3 times per week)	100% of 5 RM	5
	Day 1 4 sets	100% of 5 RM	5
	Day 2 4 sets	100% of 3 RM	5
	Day 3 1 set	100% of 5 RM	5
	2 sets	100% of 3 RM	5
	2 sets	100% of 2 RM	5
Knight DAPRE program	1	50% of RM	10
	2	75% of RM	6
	3	100% of RM	Maximum
	4	Adjusted working weight	Maximum

TABLE 17-5. EXERCISE PROGRESSIONS

	SET(S) OF 10	AMOUNT OF WEIGHT	REPETITIONS
DeLorme program	1	50% of 10 RM	10
	2	75% of 10 RM	10
	3	100% of 10 RM	10
Oxford technique	1	100% of 10 RM	10
	2	75% of 10 RM	10
	3	50% of 10 RM	10
MacQueen technique	3 (beginning/intermediate)	100% of 10 RM	10
	4-5 (advanced)	100% of 2-3 RM	2-3
Sander program	Total of 4 sets (3 times per week)	100% of 5 RM	5
	Day 1: 4 sets	100% of 5 RM	5
	Day 2: 4 sets	100% of 3 RM	5
	Day 3: 1 set	100% of 5 RM	5
	2 sets	100% of 3 RM	5
	2 sets	100% of 2 RM	5
Knight DAPRE program	1	50% of RM	10
	2	75% of RM	6
	3	100% of RM	Maximum
	4	Adjusted working weight	Maximum

DAPRE, daily adjustable progressive resistive exercise; RM, repetition maximum.

TABLE 17-6. ADJUSTMENT SEQUENCE FOR DAPRE ISOTONIC PROGRAM

NUMBER OF REPS PERFORMED DURING SET	ADJUSTED WORKING WW FOR 4TH SET	NEXT EXERCISE SESSION
0-2	−5-10 lb	−5-10 lb
3-4	−0-5 lb	Same weight
5-6	Same weight	+5-10 lb
7-10	+5-10 lb	+5-15 lb
11	+10-20 lb	+10-20 lb

To increase strength, the muscle must be challenged at a greater level than it is accustomed to. High levels of tension will produce adaptations in the form of hypertrophy and recruitment of more muscle fibers.

Specificity of Training

Specificity of training is an accepted concept in rehabilitation. This concept involves the principle of the specific adaptation to imposed demand (SAID). Thus, the focus of the exercise prescription should be to improve the strength and coordination of functional or sports-specific movements with exercises that approximate the desired activity.

Resistance training performed concentrically improves concentric muscle strength and the eccentric training improves eccentric muscle strength.

The SAID principle can be applied by exercising the muscles along each extremity and within the trunk in functional patterns.[55] The exercise component of the intervention should be as specific as the manual technique used in the clinic.

Maintaining Strength

In order to maintain the benefits of training, exercise must be maintained. Based on studies of isokinetic and concentric exercise[56,57]

- Muscle strength recovery follows a steady, nonlinear, and predictable increase over time.[34]
- Reversibility: a lack of training results in decreased muscle recruitment and muscle fiber atrophy.

If an injured patient can maintain some form of strength training, even once per week, their strength can be fairly well maintained over a 3-month period.[58]

THE KINETIC CHAIN

The term *kinetic chain* is used to describe the function or activity of an extremity and/or trunk in terms of a series of linked chains, in which each of the joint segments of the body involved in a particular movement constitutes a link along one of these kinetic chains.[59]

Closed Kinetic Chain

A variety of definitions for a closed kinetic chain (CKC) activity have been proposed. Palmitier defined an activity as "closed" if both ends of the kinetic chain are connected to an immovable framework, thus preventing translation of either the proximal, or distal joint center, and creating a situation where movement at one joint produces a predictable movement at all other joints.[55]

An example of a closed kinetic chain exercise (CKCE) involving the lower extremities is the leg press. An example of a CKCE for the upper extremities is the push-up.

Open Kinetic Chain

It is generally accepted that the movement of the end segment determines the difference between open kinetic chain (OKC) and CKC activities. The traditional definition for an "open" chain activity included all activities that involved the end segment of an extremity moving freely through space, resulting in isolated movement of a joint.

Examples of an open kinetic chain activity include lifting a drinking glass, or kicking a soccer ball. Open kinetic chain exercises (OKCE) involving the lower extremity include the hamstring curl, and hip abduction using the multi-hip machine. Upper extremity examples of OKCE include the triceps curl and the upright row.

Open chain exercises have traditionally deemed to be less functional in terms of many athletic movements, primarily serving as a supportive role in strength and conditioning programs. As a result, the use of OKCE in clinical settings declined, and there has been a shift in emphasis toward the use of CKCE, although evidence supports the skillful use of both.

CONTRAINDICATIONS OF STRENGTH TRAINING

Absolute contraindications to strength training include unstable angina, uncontrolled hypertension, uncontrolled dysrhythmias, hypertrophic cardiomyopathy, and certain stages of retinopathy. Patients with congestive heart failure, myocardial ischemia, poor left ventricular function, or autonomic neuropathies must be carefully evaluated before initiating a strength-training program.

IMPROVING MUSCULAR ENDURANCE

Muscle Endurance

Muscle endurance can be enhanced by performing exercises against light resistance for many repetitions, so that the amount of energy expanded is equal to the amount of energy supplied (referred to as steady state). Although working at a level to which the muscle is accustomed does not increase its strength, exercise programs that increase strength also increase muscular endurance.

Muscular endurance programs are prescribed early in a rehabilitation program as they are more comfortable, increase the vascular supply to muscle, minimize muscle soreness and joint irritation, and reduce the risk of injury.

Aerobic Capacity and Cardiorespiratory Endurance

Cardiorespiratory endurance is the capacity to perform whole body activities such as walking and swimming for an extended period of time without undue fatigue. A number of training adaptations occur within the circulatory system in response to exercise:

- Heart rate (HR): as the oxygen demand of the muscles increases, the heart must pump more oxygenated blood to meet this increased demand.

- Stroke volume (SV): the volume of blood being pumped out with each beat increases with exercise.
- Cardiac output (CO): cardiac output increases with exercise. A training effect that occurs with regard to CO is that the SV increases while the exercise HR is reduced at a given standard exercise load.
- Blood pressure (BP): during exercise, there is a decrease in total peripheral vascular resistance. Systolic pressure increases in proportion to oxygen consumption and cardiac output, while diastolic pressure shows little or no increase (see Chapter 11).
- Hemoglobin concentration: the concentration of hemoglobin in circulating blood may actually decrease slightly.

Lung changes that occur due to exercise include:

- An increase in the diffusing capacity of the lungs.
- Oxygen consumption rises rapidly during the first minutes of exercise.
- Fitter individuals have a respiratory system that is more capable of delivering oxygen to sustain aerobic energy production at increasingly higher levels of intensity.
- In cases of severe pulmonary disease, the cost of breathing can reach 40% of the total exercise oxygen consumption, thereby decreasing the amount of oxygen available for the exercising muscles.
- A decrease in pulmonary resistance to air flow.

The maximal amount of oxygen that can be used during exercise is referred to as maximal aerobic capacity (VO_2 max)—refer to Chapter 10. A number of precautions need to be taken when exercising patients who have a compromised cardiovascular or pulmonary system.

An appropriate level of intensity must be chosen:

- Too high a level can overload the cardiorespiratory and muscular systems and potentially cause harm.
- A sufficient period of time should be allowed for warm-up and cool down to permit adequate cardiorespiratory and muscular adaptation.

Techniques for Maintaining or Improving Cardiorespiratory Endurance. Several different training factors must be considered when attempting to maintain or improve cardiorespiratory endurance:

- To see at least minimal improvement in cardiorespiratory endurance, it is necessary for the average person to engage in no less than three sessions per week.
- Recommendations regarding training intensity vary. Relative intensity for an individual is calculated as a percentage of the maximum function, using VO_2 max or maximum heart rate (HR max). To see minimal improvement in cardiorespiratory endurance, the average person must train with a heart rate elevated to at least 60% of its maximal rate.

Obese individuals should exercise at longer durations and lower intensities–able to exercise while maintaining a conversation (talk test). Two common methods of monitoring intensity are employed:

- Monitoring heart rate using one of two formulas:
  - Karvonen equation: target training HR = resting HR + (0.6 [maximum HR − Resting HR])
  - Maximum heart rate: 220 − age
- Rating of perceived exertion (RPE)—Table 11-10. A cardiorespiratory training effect can be achieved at a rating of "somewhat hard" or "hard" (13-16).

IMPROVING MUSCLE POWER

Having a muscle work dynamically against resistance within a specified timeframe increases power. Plyometric exercises, described next, are commonly used to improve the ability of the muscles to generate power, speed, and agility.[60] In the context of rehabilitation, plyometric training is the bridge between strength and power exercises.[61]

PLYOMETRICS

Movement patterns in both athletics and activities of daily living (ADL) require the ability to accelerate and decelerate.[49] Muscle power involves converting an eccentric movement into a concentric movement in the desired direction. Plyometric training decreases the amount of time required between the yielding eccentric contraction, and the initiation of the overcoming concentric contraction by improving the reactivity of various neurological receptors. Plyometric training uses muscle stretch-shortening exercises, which consist of three distinct phases:

- A setting or eccentric phase in which the muscle is eccentrically stretched and slowly loaded.[62]
- An amortization (reversal) phase in which the amount of time between undergoing the yielding eccentric contraction and the initiation of a concentric force is reduced.[62]
- A concentric response contraction in which a large amount of momentum and force is developed.

By reproducing these stretch-shortening cycles during physiologic function, plyometric activities fine-tune muscle activity patterns by exposing the neuromuscular system to increased strength loads, and improving the stretch reflex (see Chapter 9).[62]

Minimal performance criteria for initiating plyometrics include the ability to perform one repetition of a parallel squat with a load of body weight on the subject's back (for jumps over 12 inches) for the lower extremity, and a bench press with one third body weight for the upper extremity.[61]

Plyometric exercises can incorporate diagonal and multiplanar motions with tubing or isokinetic machines. These exercises may be used to mimic any of the required motions, and can be performed in the standing, sitting, or supine positions.

IMPROVING JOINT MOBILITY AND RANGE OF MOTION

Normal mobility includes osteokinematic motion, arthrokinematic motion, and neuromuscular coordination (see Chapter 8). This mobility is a factor of muscle flexibility, joint stability, and central neurophysiologic mechanisms, which are highly specific in the body.[63] A loss of motion at one joint may not prevent the performance of a functional task, although it may result in the task being performed in an abnormal manner. For example, the act of walking can still be accomplished in the presence of a knee joint that has been fused into extension by hiking the hip on the involved side, side bending the lumbar spine to the involved side, and through excessive motion of the foot.

The amount of available joint motion is based on a number of factors, including

- Integrity of the joint surfaces and the amount of joint motion.
- Mobility and pliability of the soft tissues that surround a joint.
- Degree of soft tissue approximation that occurs.
- Amount of scarring that is present.[64] Interstitial scarring or fibrosis can occur in and around the joint capsules, within the muscles, and within the ligaments as a result of previous trauma.
- Age. Joint motion tends to decrease with increasing age.
- Gender. In general, females have more joint motion than males.

The extensibility and habitual length of connective tissue is a factor of the demands placed upon it. The examination of flexibility is performed to determine if a particular structure, or group of structures, has sufficient extensibility to perform a desired activity. A decrease in the length of the soft tissue structures, or adaptive shortening is very common in postural dysfunctions. Adaptive shortening can also be produced by

- Restricted mobility.
- Tissue damage secondary to trauma.
- Prolonged immobilization.
- Disease.
- Hypertonia: the muscle will feel hard and may stand out from those around it.

Joint mobility and range of motion can be improved using a number of techniques including flexibility training and joint mobilizations (see Chapter 18).

Flexibility training has long been recognized as an essential component of any conditioning program as a means to prevent injury and improve performance. However, whether muscle flexibility, or stretching before activity, results in a decrease in muscle injuries has yet to be proven. The techniques of stretching all involve the stretch reflex (refer to Chapter 9). A reflex is a programmed unit of behavior in which a certain type of stimulus from a receptor automatically leads to the response of an effector.

The elasticity of a muscle diminishes with cooling. Optimal flexibility is based on physiologic, anatomic, and biomechanical considerations. To stretch a muscle appropriately, the stretch must be applied parallel to the muscle fibers. The orientation of the fibers can be determined by palpation. Typically, in the extremities, the muscle fibers run parallel to the bone. The viscoelastic changes are not permanent, whereas plasticity changes, which are more difficult to achieve, result in a residual or permanent change in length. Frequent stretching ensures that the lengthening is maintained before the muscle has the opportunity to recoil to its shortened state.[65]

It is important for the patient to realize that the initial session of stretching may increase symptoms in the stretched muscle.[66] However, this increase in symptoms should only be temporary, lasting for a couple of hours at most.[65,67] The stretch should be performed at the point just shy of the pain, although some discomfort may be necessary to achieve results.[68] The muscle usually requires a greater stretching force initially, possibly to break up adhesions or cross-linkages, and to allow for viscoelastic and plastic changes to occur in the collagen and elastin fibers.[68]

STATIC FLEXIBILITY

Static flexibility is defined as the passive ROM available to a joint or series of joints.[64,69] Increased static flexibility should not be confused with joint hypermobility, or laxity, which is a function of the joint capsule and ligaments. Decreased static flexibility indicates a loss of motion. The end-feel encountered may help differentiate between adaptive shortening of the muscle (muscle stretch) versus a tight joint capsule (capsular), or arthritic joint (hard). Static flexibility can be measured by a goniometer, or by a number of tests, such as the toe-touch and the sit and reach, all of which have been found to be valid and reliable.[70,71]

DYNAMIC FLEXIBILITY

Dynamic flexibility refers to the ease of movement within the obtainable ROM. Dynamic flexibility is measured actively. The important measurement in dynamic flexibility is stiffness, a mechanical term defined as the resistance of a structure to deformation.[72,73] An increase in ROM around a joint does not necessarily equate to a decrease in the passive stiffness of a muscle.[74-76] However, strength training, immobilization, and aging have been shown to increase stiffness.[77-80] The converse of stiffness is pliability. When a soft tissue demonstrates a decrease in pliability, it has usually undergone an adaptive shortening, or an increase in tone, termed *hypertonus*.

METHODS OF STRETCHING

A variety of stretching techniques can be used to increase the extensibility of the soft tissues.

Passive Stretching

The clinician or another individual partner can perform passive stretching. Because of the higher risk of injury with this type of stretching, it should only be administered after close supervision, and with the assurance that there is excellent communication between the operator and the patient.

Ideally, the passive stretch should involve a gentle, controlled, low intensity, and prolonged elongation of the tissues.

Static Stretching

Static stretching involves the application of a steady force for a sustained period.

Small loads applied for long periods of time produce greater residual lengthening than heavy loads applied for short periods.[82] Weighted traction, specific low-load braces, or pulley systems may be modified accordingly to provide this type of stretching.

Study Pearl

Applying small loads to the musculotendinous unit for 20 minutes or more in an exercise session is necessary for adequate soft tissue lengthening to occur.[81,82]

Ballistic Stretching

This technique of stretching uses bouncing movements to stretch a particular muscle. This method appears to cause more residual muscle soreness or muscle strain, than static stretching and those techniques that incorporate relaxation into the technique.[85-87]

In comparisons of the ballistic and static methods, two studies[83,84] have found that both produce similar improvements in flexibility.

Clinical Application

Restoration of normal length of the muscles may be accomplished using the following guidelines:

- The muscle activity is inhibited and in the inhibitory period, the muscle should be stretched.
- With true muscle shortness, stronger resistance is used to activate the maximum number of motor units, followed by vigorous stretching of the muscle.
- Stretching should be performed at least 3 times a week using:
  - Low force, avoiding pain
  - Prolonged duration
- Heat should be applied to increase intramuscular temperature prior to, and during, stretching.[88,89] This heat can be achieved with either through low-intensity warm-up exercise using relevant muscle groups, or through the use of thermal modalities.[89] The application of a cold pack following the stretch is used to take advantage of the thermal characteristics of connective tissue, by lowering its temperature and thereby theoretically prolonging the length changes.[90]
- Post-isometric relaxation techniques such as muscle energy are advocated.
- Rapid cooling of the muscle while it is maintained in the stretched position.

Study Pearl

Effective stretching, in the early phase, should be performed every hour, but with each session lasting only a few minutes.

Some areas of the body are difficult to stretch adequately using a lengthening technique. In these instances, techniques of localized, manual release, using varying degrees of manual pressure along the length of the muscle and myofascial tissue, may be used.[91]

NEUROMUSCULAR FACILITATION

The PNF techniques of "hold-relax," "stretch-relax," and "agonist contract-relax" can be used to actively stretch the soft tissues.

- Hold-relax (HR)—autogenic inhibition: a relaxation technique usually performed at the point of limited range of motion in the agonist pattern:
  - An isometric contraction of the range-limiting antagonist is performed against slowly increasing resistance.
  - This is followed by a voluntary relaxation by the patient and then passive movement of the extremity by the clinician into the newly gained range of the agonist pattern.
- Hold-relax-active (HRA)—reciprocal inhibition: following application of the hold-relax technique, the patient performs an active contraction into the newly gained range of the agonist pattern.
- Contract-relax (C-R): a relaxation technique usually performed at the point of limited range of motion in the agonist pattern:
  - An *isotonic* movement in rotation is performed followed by an isometric hold of the range-limiting muscles in the antagonist pattern against slowly increasing resistance, voluntary relaxation, and active movement into the new range of the agonist pattern.

A majority of studies have shown the PNF technique to be the most effective stretching technique for increasing ROM through muscle lengthening when compared to the static or slow sustained, and the ballistic or bounce techniques,[92-96]

IMPROVING BALANCE

Balance, or postural equilibrium, is the most significant factor in movement strategies involving a closed kinetic chain environment and involves synchronization between the neurologic system and the musculoskeletal system. In order for balance to be effective, an individual must be able to maintain their center of gravity (COG), which is located just above the pelvis, within the body's base of support. A wide base of support provides the best balance.

Balance training involving a change in the base of support can be performed with the patient lying, sitting, or standing, depending on the ability of the patient and the goals of the intervention. The usual progression employed involves narrowing of the base of support, raising the center of gravity (COG), and changing the weight-bearing surface from hard to soft, or from flat to uneven, while increasing the perturbation. Challenges to the patient's position can be added in a variety of ways (see Chapter 9).

> **Study Pearl**
>
> Since afferent input is altered after joint injury, the training must focus on the restoration of proprioceptive sensibility to retrain these altered afferent pathways and enhance the sensation of joint movement.[97]

IMPROVING JOINT STABILIZATION

Joint stabilization implies that a person has increased joint range of motion and the ability to stabilize and control the movement throughout the range. Stabilization exercises, which are designed to train the body to limit and control any excessive movement, include patient education, mobility exercises for hypomobile joints, strengthening exercises for hypermobile segments, and neuromuscular re-education (NMR). Neuromuscular control is administered by the CNS via the integration of information from the vestibular, vision, and proprioceptive systems (refer to Chapter 9).

NMR training enhances the correct selection of unconscious motor responses by stimulating the afferent signals and central mechanisms responsible for dynamic joint control, thereby restoring proximal stability, muscle control, and flexibility.[98] The neuromuscular mechanism that contributes to joint stability is mediated by the articular mechanoreceptors. These receptors provide information about joint position sense and kinesthesia.[106,107,109,110] The objective of NMR is to improve the ability of these control mechanisms to generate a fast and optimal muscle-firing pattern, enhance joint stability, minimize joint forces, and to relearn movement patterns and skills.[98]

The NMR progression is initiated as early as possible in the rehabilitative process with simple activities and progresses to more complex activities requiring more proprioceptive and kinesthetic awareness.[99,100]

According to Voight,[97,101] the standard progression for neuromuscular re-education involves

- Static stabilization exercises with closed chain loading and unloading (weight shifting). This phase initially employs isometric exercises around the involved joint on solid and even surfaces, before progressing to unstable surfaces. The early training involves balance training and joint repositioning exercises, and is usually initiated (in the lower extremities) by having the patient place the involved extremity on a 6- to 8-in. stool, so that the amount of weight bearing can be controlled more easily. The proprioceptive awareness of a joint can also be enhanced by using an elastic bandage, orthotic, or through taping around the involved joint.[102-107] As full weight bearing through the extremity is restored, a number of devices such as a mini-trampoline, balance board, Swiss ball, and wobble board can be introduced. Exercises on these devices are progressed from double limb support, to single leg support, to support while performing sports-specific skills.
- Transitional stabilization exercises. The exercises during this phase involve conscious control of motion without impact, and replace isometric activity with controlled concentric and eccentric exercises throughout a progressively larger range of functional motion. The physiological rationale behind the exercises in this phase is to stimulate dynamic postural responses, and to increase muscle stiffness. Muscle stiffness has a significant role in improving dynamic stabilization around the joint, by resisting and absorbing joint loads.[79]
- Dynamic stabilization exercises. These exercises involve the unconscious control and loading of the joint, and introduce both ballistic and impact exercises to the patient.

A delicate balance between stability and mobility is achieved by coordination between muscle strength, endurance, flexibility, and neuromuscular control.[108]

Initially, closed chain exercises are performed within the pain-free ranges or positions. Open chain exercises, including mild plyometric exercises, may be built upon the base of the closed chain stabilization program to allow normal control of joint mobility.

The neuromuscular emphasis during these exercises is to concentrate on functional positioning during exercise rather than isolating open and closed chain activities.[108] The activities should involve sudden alterations in joint positioning that necessitate reflex muscular stabilization coupled with an axial load.[107,108] Such activities include rhythmic stabilization performed in both a closed and open chain position,[111] and in the functional position of the joint.[108] The use of a stable, and then unstable, base during closed chain exercises encourages co-contraction of the agonists and antagonists.[111]

Weight shifting exercises are ideal for this. For example, the following weight shifting exercises may be used for the upper extremity:

- Standing and leaning against a treatment table or object.
- In the quadruped position, rocking forward and backward with the hands on the floor or on an unstable object.
- Kneeling in the three-point position. A Body Blade® can be added to this exercise to increase the difficulty.
- Kneeling in the two-point position.
- Weight shifting on a Fitter® while in a kneeling position.
- Weight shifting on a Swiss ball.
- Slide board exercises in the quadruped position moving the hands in opposite diagonals and in opposite directions.

Following treatment of any joint, retraining of the muscles must be carried out to reestablish coordination. Proprioceptive neuromuscular facilitation (PNF) techniques are especially useful in this regard (see "Specialized Exercise Regimes"). PNF techniques require motions of the extremities in all three planes.[112] PNF techniques that use combinations of spiral and diagonal patterns are designed to enhance coordination and strength.[113] The diagonal patterns 1 and 2 are appropriate with resistance being added as appropriate.

SPECIALIZED EXERCISE REGIMES

AQUATIC THERAPY

Current research shows aquatic therapy to be beneficial in the treatment of everything from orthopedic injuries to spinal cord damage, chronic pain, cerebral palsy, multiple sclerosis, and many other conditions.[114] The indications for aquatic therapy include instances when partial weight-bearing ambulation is necessary, to increase range of motion, when standing balance needs to be improved, when endurance/aerobic capacity needs improved, or when the goal is to increase muscle strength via active assisted, gravity assisted, active or resisted exercise.

Contraindications include incontinence, urinary tract infections, unprotected open wounds, heat intolerance, severe epilepsy, uncontrolled diabetes, unstable blood pressure, or severe cardiac and/or pulmonary dysfunction.

Physical Properties and Resisted Forces. There are several physical properties of water, which make exercising in water differ from that on land:

- Density: any object with a specific gravity less than that of water will float. Although the human body is mostly water, the body's density is slightly less than that of water and averages a specific gravity of 0.974, with men averaging higher density than women. The buoyant values of different body parts vary according to a number of factors:
  - Bone to muscle weight: lean body mass, which includes bone, muscle, connective tissue, and organs, has a typical density near 1.1.
  - The amount and distribution of fat: fat mass, which includes both essential body fat plus fat in excess of essential needs, has a density of about 0.9.

Consequently, the human body displaces a volume of water that weighs slightly more than the body, forcing the body upward by a force equal to the volume of the water displaced, as discovered by Archimedes.

- Hydrostatic pressure: pressure is directly proportional to both the liquid density and to the immersion depth when the fluid is incompressible. Water exerts a pressure of 22.4 mm Hg/ft of water depth, which translates to 1 mm Hg/1.36 cm (0.54 in.) of water depth. Thus a human body emerged to a depth of 48 in. is subjected to a force equal to 88.9 mm Hg, slightly greater than normal diastolic blood pressure.[115] The effects of hydrostatic pressure, which is also the force that aids resolution of edema in an injured body part, begin immediately on immersion, causing plastic deformation of the body over a short period. This results in a cranial displacement of blood, a rise in right atrial pressure, and increase in pleural surface pressure, compression of the chest wall, and a cranial displacement of the diaphragm.
- Buoyancy: as the body is gradually immersed, water is displaced, creating the force of buoyancy. A human with a specific gravity of 0.97 reaches floating equilibrium when 97% of his or her total body volume is submerged[115]:
  - With neck depth immersion, only about 15 lb of compressive force is exerted on the spine, hips, and knees.
  - With immersion up to the symphysis pubis, 40% of the body weight is effectively offloaded.
  - With immersion up to the umbilicus, 50% of the body weight is effectively offloaded.
  - With immersion up to the xiphoid, 60% or more (depending on whether the arms are overhead or beside the trunk) of the body weight is effectively offloaded.
- Viscosity: refers to the magnitude of internal friction specific to a fluid during motion. A limb moving relative to water is subjected to the resistive effects of the fluid called drag force and turbulence when present.[115]
  - Drag force: a factor of the shape of an object and its speed of movement. Objects that are more streamlined (minimizing the surface area at the front of the object) produce less drag force.

- Turbulence: under turbulent flow conditions, resistance increases as a log function of velocity.

Viscous resistance increases as more forces are exerted against it, but that resistance drops to zero almost immediately upon the cessation of force.

Thermodynamics. The heat capacity of water is 1000 times greater than the equivalent volume of air. The therapeutic utility of water depends greatly on both its ability to retain heat and its ability to transfer heat energy. Heat transfer begins immediately on immersion, and as the heat capacity of the human body is less than that of water (0.83 versus 1.00), the body equilibrates faster than the water does.

Study Pearl

Water is an efficient conductor, transferring heat 25 times faster than air. This thermal conductive property, in combination with the high specific heat of water, makes the use of water in rehabilitation very versatile because water retains heat or cold while delivering easily to the immersed body part.[115]

Design and Special Equipment. If a pool is to be used for rehabilitation purposes, it should have certain characteristics:

- It should not be smaller than 10' × 12'.
- It should have both a shallow (1.25 m/2.5 ft) and a deep (2.5 m/5 ft plus) area to allow for standing exercises and swimming or nonstanding exercise.
- The bottom of the pool should be flat and the depth gradations must be clearly marked.

Variable temperature control for the water should be available (water that is too warm can lead to fatigue or even heat exhaustion because evaporation of perspiration is not possible in water, whereas water that is too cool can cause shivering, increase muscular tension, or produce hypothermia):

- Cold plunge tanks are often used at temperatures of 10 to 15°C to produce a decrease in muscle pain and speed recovery from overuse injury.
- Most public and competitive pools operate in the range of 27 to 29°C.
- Typical therapy pools operate in the range of 33.5 to 35.5°C.
- Hot tubs are usually maintained at 37.5 to 41°C.

Rescue tubes, inner tubes, and wet vests should be purchased to assist in floatation activities. Hand paddles and pull buoys can be used for strengthening the upper extremity. Kick boards and fins are useful for strengthening the lower extremity.

Advantages

- The buoyancy of the water allows active exercise while providing support and thus allows a gradual transition from non-weight-bearing to full weight-bearing exercises by adjusting the amount the body is submerged.
- The intensity of exercise can be controlled by adjusting the body's position or through the use of exercise equipment.

Disadvantages

- Cost of building, maintenance, and staff training.
- Potential adverse effects on the cardiovascular system. Because an individual immersed in water is subjected to

external water pressure in a gradient, which within a relatively small depth exceeds venous pressure, blood is displaced upward to the venous and lymphatic systems, first into the thighs, then into the abdominal cavity vessels, and finally into the great vessels of the chest cavity and into the heart.[115] The following cardiovascular changes can occur with immersion of the body:

- An increase in central venous pressure
- An increase in pulse pressure as a result of the increased cardiac filling and decreased heart rate during thermoneutral or cool immersion
- An increase in central blood volume
- An increase in cardiac volume, cardiac output, and stroke volume
- A decrease in sympathetic vasoconstriction resulting in a reduction in both peripheral venous tone and systemic vascular resistance

PROPRIOCEPTIVE NEUROMUSCULAR FACILITATION TECHNIQUES

The concept of proprioceptive neuromuscular facilitation (also termed complex motions) was developed by Dr. Hermann Kabat, then by Sherrington, and finally by Margaret Knott and Dorothy Voss.[116] The theory behind PNF is that the human muscular system is a diagonal and spiral arrangement and that when muscles contract in proper sequence of synergistic muscle patterns, the stressed muscle group effectively overcomes the demand made on it. The naturally occurring spiral or diagonal patterns of the muscular system consist of three components:

- Flexion or extension
- Adduction or abduction
- Internal or external rotation

PNF uses the stimulation of muscle and joint receptors to improve, assist, and accelerate the reactions of the neuromuscular mechanism. Total patterns of movement and posture are important preparatory patterns for advanced functional skills, whereas evasive motions, which are uneconomical and which develop from an acute protected position taken to avoid pain, need to be eliminated.

PNF techniques can be used for a number of purposes including strengthening, increasing range of motion, and improving coordination. During the rehabilitative stage, the patient is first made to sense the tension in the muscles. Patterns of motion are then taught, first without stress, and then with stress.

Basic Principles

The position of the patient, which often uses developmental positions, allows for consistency of measurement and plays a major role in influencing postural tone. Manual contacts are used to isolate muscle groups, provides tactile clues, and to influence the strength of the contraction. The application of an appropriate resistance facilitates specific motor patterns.

PNF Terms and Techniques

Each of the following definitions include a description explaining the intent of the techniques:

- Approximation: joint compression stimulates afferent nerve endings, and encourages extensor muscles and stabilizing patterns (co-contraction), thereby inhibiting tone and enhancing stabilization of the proximal segment. This technique is commonly used with neurologically involved patients.
- Combination of isotonics (formerly referred to as agonist reversals): a slow isotonic, shortening contraction through the range followed by an eccentric, lengthening contraction using the same muscle groups. Indications include weak postural muscles, and inability to eccentrically control body weight during movement transitions, eg, sitting down.
- Stabilizing reversals (formerly referred to as alternating isometrics): isometric holding is facilitated first on one side of the joint, followed by alternate holding of the antagonist muscle groups, which can be applied in any direction (anterior-posterior, medial-lateral, diagonal). Indications include instability in weight bearing and holding, poor antigravity control, weakness, and ataxia.
- Contract-relax (C-R): a relaxation technique usually performed at a point of limited range of motion in the agonist pattern: isotonic movement in rotation is performed followed by an isometric hold of the range-limiting muscles in the antagonist pattern against slowly increasing resistance, then voluntary relaxation, and active contraction in the newly gained range of the agonist pattern. The patient is then asked to contract the muscle(s) to be stretched (agonists). The clinician resists this contraction except for the rotary component. The patient is then asked to relax and the clinician moves the joint further into the desired range. Indications include limitations in range of motion caused by muscle adaptive shortening, spasticity. Although primarily used as a stretching technique, due to the isometric contractions involved, some strengthening does occur.
- Hold-relax (H-R): a similar technique in principle to contract-relax, except that, when the patient contracts, the clinician allows no motion (including rotation) to occur. Following the isometric contraction the patient's own contraction causes the desired movement to occur. Typically used as a relaxation technique in the acutely injured patient as it tends to be less aggressive than the contract/relax technique.
- Replication (formerly referred to as hold-relax-active motion): an isometric contraction performed in the mid to shortened range followed by a voluntary relaxation and passive movement into the lengthened range, and resistance to an isotonic contraction through the range. This technique can be used with patients who have an inability to initiate movement, hypotonia, weakness, or marked imbalances between antagonists.

- Manual Contact: a deep but painless pressure is applied through the clinician's contact to stimulate muscle, tendon, and/or joint afferents.
- Maximal resistance: resistance is applied to stronger muscles to obtain overflow to weaker muscles. Indications include weakness, muscle imbalances.
- Quick stretch: a motion applied suddenly stimulates the tendon receptors resulting in a facilitation of motor recruitment and thus more force.
- Reinforcement: the coordinated use of the major muscle groups, or other body parts, to produce a desired movement pattern. This technique is often used to increase the stability of the proximal segments.
- Repeated contractions (RC): a unidirectional technique that involves repeated isotonic contractions induced by quick stretch and which is enhanced by resistance performed to the range or part of range at the point of weakness. Indications include weakness, incoordination, muscle imbalances, lack of endurance.
- Resisted progression (RP): a stretch and tracking resistance is applied in order to facilitate progression in walking, creeping, knee-walking, or movement transitions. Indications include impaired strength, timing, motor control, and endurance.
- Rhythmic initiation (RI): unidirectional or bidirectional voluntary relaxation followed by passive movement through increasing range of motion, followed by active-assisted contractions progressing to light tracking resistance to isotonic contractions. Indications include spasticity, rigidity, inability to initiate movement, motor learning deficits, communication deficits.
- Rhythmic rotation: voluntary relaxation combined with slow, passive, rhythmic rotation of the body or body part around a longitudinal axis and passive movement into the newly gained range. Active holding in the new range is then stressed. Indications include hypertonia with limitations in functional range of motion.
- Rhythmic stabilization (RS): the application of alternating isometric contractions of the agonist and antagonist muscles to stimulate movement of the agonist, develop stability, and relax the antagonist. Indications include instability in weight bearing and holding, poor antigravity control, weakness, and ataxia. May also be used to decrease limitations in range of motion caused by adaptive muscle shortening and painful muscle splinting.
- Dynamic reversals of antagonists (formerly referred to as slow reversal): uses alternating isotonic contractions of opposing muscle groups to stimulate active motion of the agonist, relaxation of the antagonist, and coordination between agonist and antagonist patterns. Indications include inability to reverse directions, muscle imbalances, weakness, incoordination, and instability.
- Slow reversal-hold: uses alternating activity of opposing muscle groups with a pause between reversals to achieve relaxation of the antagonist and to stimulate the agonist.
- Slow reversal-hold-relax: the patient is asked to actively move the involved joint to the point of limitation and then to reverse

TABLE 17-7. PNF PATTERNS FOR THE LOWER EXTREMITY

	PNF PATTERNS FOR THE LOWER EXTREMITY			
JOINT (PROXIMAL TO DISTAL)	DIAGONAL ONE (D1) FLEXION	DIAGONAL ONE (D1) EXTENSION	DIAGONAL TWO (D2) FLEXION	DIAGONAL TWO (D2) EXTENSION
Hip	External rotation, adduction, flexion	Internal rotation, abduction, extension	Internal rotation, abduction, flexion	External rotation, adduction, extension
Knee (may be kept flexed or extended)	Flexion or extension	Extension or flexion	Flexion or extension	Extension or flexion
Ankle	Dorsiflexion	Plantar flexion	Dorsiflexion	Plantar flexion
Subtalar	Inversion	Eversion	Eversion	Inversion
Toes	Extension, abduction to the tibial side	Flexion, adduction to the fibular side	Extension, abduction to the fibular side	Flexion, adduction to the tibial side

the direction of the motion, while the clinician resists. This technique is used to increase motion of the agonist.

- Timing for emphasis: the application of maximal resistance in specific parts of the range of motion to the more powerful muscle groups to obtain "overflow" to weaker muscle groups. Can be performed within a limb (ipsilateral from one muscle group to another) or using overflow from one limb to contralateral limb, or trunk to limb. Typically combined with repeated contractions to the weak components, or superimposed upon normal timing in a distal to proximal sequence. Indications include weakness, incoordination.
- Traction: the joint is distracted by use of a traction force, resulting in a decrease of muscular tone and a subsequent increase in range of motion. Indications include stimulation of a fair and nerve endings and facilitation of flexor muscles and mobilizing patterns. May also be used to help decrease spasticity.

PNF PATTERNS

See Tables 17-7 and 17-8.

TABLE 17-8. PNF PATTERNS FOR THE UPPER EXTREMITY

	PNF PATTERNS FOR THE UPPER EXTREMITY			
JOINT (PROXIMAL TO DISTAL)	DIAGONAL ONE (D1) FLEXION	DIAGONAL ONE (D1) EXTENSION	DIAGONAL TWO (D2) FLEXION	DIAGONAL TWO (D2) EXTENSION
Scapulothoracic	Rotation, abduction, anterior elevation	Rotation, adduction, posterior depression	Rotation, adduction, posterior elevation	Rotation, abduction, anterior depression
Glenohumeral	External rotation, adduction, flexion	Internal rotation, abduction, extension	External rotation, abduction, flexion	Internal rotation, adduction, extension
Elbow (may be kept flexed or extended)	Flexion	Extension	Flexion	Extension
Radio ulnar	Supination	Pronation	Supination	Pronation
Wrist	Flexion, radial deviation	Extension, ulnar deviation	Extension, radial deviation	Flexion, ulnar deviation
Fingers	Flexion, adduction to the radial side	Extension, abduction to the ulnar side	Extension, abduction to the radial side	Flexion, adduction to the ulnar side
Thumb	Flexion, abduction	Extension, abduction	Extension, adduction	Flexion, abduction

Questions for this chapter and the entire book appear on the included CD-ROM, with additional questions at www.DuttonNPTE.com.

REFERENCES

1. Luttgens K, Hamilton K: The musculoskeletal system: the musculature. In: Luttgens K, Hamilton K, eds. *Kinesiology: Scientific Basis of Human Motion.* 9th ed. Dubuque, IA: McGraw-Hill. 1997:49-75.
2. Astrand PO, Rodahl K: *The Muscle and Its Contraction: Textbook of Work Physiology.* New York, NY: McGraw-Hill. 1986.
3. Komi PV: *Strength and Power in Sport.* London: Blackwell Scientific Publications. 1992.
4. McArdle W, Katch FI, Katch VL: *Exercise Physiology: Energy, Nutrition, and Human Performance.* Philadelphia, PA: Lea and Febiger. 1991.
5. Lakomy HKA: The biomechanics of human movement. In: Maughan RJ, ed. *Basic and Applied Sciences for Sports Medicine.* Woburn, MA: Butterworth-Heinemann. 1999:124-125.
6. Worrell TW, Perrin DH, Gansneder B, et al: Comparison of isokinetic strength and flexibility measures between hamstring injured and non-injured athletes. *J Orthop Sports Phys Ther.* 1991;13:118-125.
7. Anderson MA, Gieck JH, Perrin D, et al: The relationship among isokinetic, isotonic, and isokinetic concentric and eccentric quadriceps and hamstrings force and three components of athletic performance. *J Orthop Sports Phys Ther.* 1991;14:114-120.
8. Steadman JR, Forster RS, Silfverskold JP: Rehabilitation of the knee. *Clin Sports Med.* 1989;8:605-627.
9. Montgomery JB, Steadman JR: Rehabilitation of the injured knee. *Clin Sports Med.* 1985;4:333-343.
10. Delsman PA, Losee GM: Isokinetic shear forces and their effect on the quadriceps active drawer. *Med Sci Sports Exerc.* 1984;16:151.
11. Albert MS: Principles of exercise progression. In: Greenfield B, ed. *Rehabilitation of the knee: A Problem Solving Approach.* Philadelphia, PA: FA Davis. 1993:110-136.
12. Deudsinger RH: Biomechanics in clinical practice. *Phys Ther.* 1984;64:1860-1868.
13. Cyriax J: Textbook of Orthopaedic Medicine, Diagnosis of Soft Tissue Lesions. 8th ed. London: Bailliere Tindall. 1982.
14. Hall SJ: The biomechanics of human skeletal muscle. In: Hall SJ, ed. *Basic Biomechanics.* New York, NY: McGraw-Hill. 1999:146-185.
15. Desmendt JE, Godaux E: Fast motor units are not preferentially activated in rapid voluntary contractions in man. *Nature.* 1977;267:717.
16. Gans C: Fiber architecture and muscle function. *Exerc Sport Sci Rev.* 1982;10:160.
17. Nilsson J, Tesch PA, Thorstensson A: Fatigue and EMG of repeated fast and voluntary contractions in man. *Acta Physiol Scand.* 1977;101:194.
18. Sell S, Zacher J, Lack S: Disorders of proprioception of arthrotic knee joint. *Z Rheumatol.* 1993;52:150-155.

19. Mattacola CG, Lloyd JW: Effects of a 6 week strength and proprioception training program on measures of dynamic balance: a single case design. *J Athl Training.* 1997;32:127-135.
20. Hall C, Thein-Brody L: Impairment in muscle performance. In: Hall C, Thein-Brody L, eds. *Therapeutic Exercise: Moving Toward Function.* Baltimore, MD: Lippincott Williams & Wilkins. 2005:57-86.
21. Bell RD, MacDougall JD, Billeter R, et al: Muscle fiber types and morphometric analysis of skeletal msucle in six-year-old children. *Med Sci Sports Exerc.* 1980;12:28-31.
22. Russell AP, Feilchenfeldt J, Schreiber S, et al: Endurance training in humans leads to fiber type-specific increases in levels of peroxisome proliferator-activated receptor-gamma coactivator-1 and peroxisome proliferator-activated receptor-alpha in skeletal muscle. *Diabetes.* 2003;52:2874-2881.
23. Edman KAP RC: The sarcomere length-tension relation determined in short segments of intact muscle fibres of the frog. *J Physiol.* 1987;385:729-732.
24. Boeckmann RR, Ellenbecker TS: Biomechanics. In: Ellenbecker TS, ed. *Knee Ligament Rehabilitation.* Philadelphia, PA: Churchill Livingstone. 2000:16-23.
25. Brownstein B, Noyes FR, Mangine RE, et al: Anatomy and biomechanics. In: Mangine RE, ed. *Physical Therapy of the Knee.* New York, NY: Churchill Livingstone. 1988:1-30.
26. Teitz CC, Garrett WE, Jr., Miniaci A, et al: Tendon problems in athletic individuals. *J Bone and Joint Surg.* 1997;79-A:138-152.
27. Williams JH, Klug GA: Calcium exchange hypothesis of skeletal muscle fatigue. A brief review. *Muscle & Nerve.* 1995;18:421.
28. Allen DG, Lannergren J, Westerblad H: Muscle cell function during prolonged activity: cellular mechanisms of fatigue. *Exp Physiol.* 1995;80:497.
29. Lash JM: Regulation of skeletal muscle blood flow during contractions. *Proceedings of the Society for Experimental Biology & Medicine.* 1996;211:218-235.
30. Hill AV: The heat and shortening and the dynamic constants of muscle. *Proc R Soc Lond.* 1938;B126:136-195.
31. Tihanyi J, Apor P, Fekete GY: Force-velocity—power characteristics and fiber composition in human knee extensor muscles. *Eur J Appl Physiol.* 1982;48:331-343.
32. Fitts RH, Widrick JJ: Muscle mechanics; adaptations with exercise training. *Exerc Sport Sci Rev.* 1996;24:427-473.
33. Hyman J, Liebenson C: Spinal stabilization exercise program. In: Liebenson C, ed. *Rehabilitation of the Spine: A Practitioner's Manual.* Baltimore, MD: Lippincott Williams & Wilkins. 1996: 293-317.
34. Albert M: Concepts of muscle training. In: Wadsworth C, ed. *Orthopaedic Physical Therapy: Topic—Strength and Conditioning Applications in Orthopaedics.* Home Study Course 98A. La Crosse, WI: Orthopaedic Section, APTA, Inc. 1998.
35. Litchfield R, Hawkins R, Dillman CJ, et al: Rehabilitation of the overhead athlete. *J Orthop Sports Phys Ther.* 1993;2:433-441.
36. Cook G, Voight ML: Essentials of functional exercise: a four-step clinical model for therapeutic exercise prescription. In: Prentice WE, Voight ML, eds. *Techniques in Musculoskeletal Rehabilitation.* New York, NY: McGraw-Hill. 2001:387-407.

37. Matsen FA, III., Lippitt SB, Sidles JA, et al: Strength. In: Matsen FA, III., Lippitt SB, Sidles JA, et al, eds. *Practical Evaluation and Management of the Shoulder.* Philadelphia, PA: WB Saunders Company. 1994:111-150.
38. Kisner C, Colby LA: *Therapeutic Exercise. Foundations and Techniques.* Philadelphia, PA: FA Davis. 1997.
39. Astrand PO, Rodahl K: *Physical Training: Textbook of Work Physiology.* New York, NY: McGraw-Hill. 1986.
40. DeLorme T, Watkins A: *Techniques of Progressive Resistance Exercise.* New York, NY: Appleton-Century. 1951.
41. Soest A, Bobbert M: The role of muscle properties in control of explosive movements. *Biol Cybern.* 1993;69:195-204.
42. Komi PV: The stretch-shortening cycle and human power output. In: Jones NL, McCartney N, McComas AJ, eds. *Human Muscle Power.* Champlain, IL: Human Kinetics. 1986:27-39.
43. Bandy W, Lovelace-Chandler V, Bandy B, et al: Adaptation of skeltal muscle to resistance training. *J Orthop Sports Phys Ther.* 1990;12:248-255.
44. Clark MA: *Integrated Training for the New Millenium.* Thousand Oaks, CA: National Academy of Sports Medicine; 2001.
45. Lange GW, Hintermeister RA, Schlegel T, et al: Electromyographic and kinematic analysis of graded treadmill walking and the implications for knee rehabilitation. *J Orthop Sports Phys Ther.* 1996;23:294-301.
46. Simoneau GG, Bereda SM, Sobush DC, et al: Biomechanics of elastic resistance in therapeutic exercise programs. J Orthop Sports Phys Ther. 2001;31:16-24.
47. Engle RP, Canner GC: Proprioceptive neuromuscular facilitation (PNF) and modified procedures for anterior cruciate ligament (ACL) instability. *J Orthop Sports Phys Ther.* 1989;11:230.
48. Manske RC, Reiman MP: Muscle weakness. In: Cameron MH, Monroe LG, eds. *Physical Rehabilitation: Evidence-Based Examination, Evaluation, and Intervention.* St Louis, MO: Saunders/Elsevier. 2007:64-86.
49. Grimsby O, Power B: Manual therapy approach to knee ligament rehabilitation. In: Ellenbecker TS, ed. *Knee Ligament Rehabilitation.* Philadelphia, PA: Churchill Livingstone. 2000:236-251.
50. American College of Sports Medicine: *Guidelines for Exercise Testing and Prescription, 4th ed.* Philadelphia, PA: Lea & Febiger. 1991.
51. Borg GAV: Psychophysical basis of perceived exertion. *Med Sci Sports Exerc.* 1992;14:377-381.
52. Borg GAV: Perceived exertion as an indicator of somatic stress. *Scand J Rehabil Med.* 1970;2:92-98.
53. Hasson S, Barnes W, Hunter M, et al: Therapeutic effect of high speed voluntary muscle contractions on muscle soreness and muscle performance. *J Orthop Sports Phys Ther.* 1989; 10:499.
54. Blix M: Length and tension. *Scand Arch Physiol.* 1892;27:93-94.
55. Palmitier RA, An KN, Scott SG, et al: Kinetic chain exercises in knee rehabilitation. *Sports Med.* 1991;11:402-413.
56. Grimby G, Thomee R: Principles of rehabilitation after injuries. In: Dirix A, Knuttgen HG, Tittel K, eds. *The Olympic Book of Sports Medicine.* Oxford, England: Blackwell Scientific Publications. 1984.

57. Thomee R, Renstrom P, Grimby G, et al: Slow or fast isokinetic training after surgery. *J Orthop Sports Phys Ther.* 1987;8:476.
58. Graves JE, Pollock SH, Leggett SH, et al: Effect of reduced training frequency on muscular strength. *Sports Med.* 1988;9:316-319.
59. Marino M: Current concepts of rehabilitation in sports medicine. In: Nicholas JA, Herschman EB, eds. *The Lower Extremity and Spine in Sports Medicine.* St. Louis, MO: Saunders. 1986:117-195.
60. Malone T, Nitz AJ, Kuperstein J, et al: Neuromuscular concepts. In: Ellenbecker TS, ed. *Knee Ligament Rehabilitation.* Philadelphia, PA: Churchill Livingstone. 2000:399-411.
61. Voight ML, Draovitch P, Tippett SR: Plyometrics. In Albert MS, ed. *Eccentric Muscle Training in Sports and Orthopedics.* New York, NY: Churchill Livingstone. 1995.
62. Wilk KE, Voight ML, Keirns MA, et al: Stretch-shortening drills for the upper extremities: theory and clinical application. *J Orthop Sports Phys Ther.* 1993;17:225-239.
63. Harris ML: Flexibility. *Phys Ther.* 1969;49:591-601.
64. Gleim GW, McHugh MP: Flexibility and its effects on sports injury and performance. *Sports Med.* 1997;24:289-299.
65. Kottke FJ: Therapeutic exercise to maintain mobility. In: Kottke FJ, Stillwell GK, Lehman JF, eds. *Krusen's Handbook of Physical Medicine and Rehabilitation.* Baltimore, MD: WB Saunders. 1982:389-402.
66. Travell JG, Simons DG: *Myofascial Pain and Dysfunction: The Trigger Point Manual.* Baltimore, MD: Williams & Wilkins. 1983.
67. Swezey RL: Arthrosis. In: Basmajian JV, Kirby RL, eds. *Medical Rehabilitation.* Baltimore, MD: Williams & Wilkins. 1984:216-218.
68. Joynt RL: Therapeutic exercise. In: DeLisa JA, ed. *Rehabilitation Medicine: Principles and Practice.* Philadelphia, PA: JB Lippincott. 1988:346-371.
69. The American Orthopaedic Society for Sports Medicine: *Flexibility.* Chicago, IL: The American Orthopaedic Society for Sports Medicine; 1988.
70. Kippers V, Parker AW: Toe-touch test: a measure of validity. *Phys Ther.* 1987;67:1680-1684.
71. Jackson AW, Baker AA: The relationship of the sit and reach test to criterion measures of hamstring and back flexibility in young females. *Res Q Exerc Sport.* 1986;57:183-186.
72. Litsky AS, Spector M: Biomaterials. In: Simon SR, ed. *Orthopaedic Basic Science.* Chicago, IL: The American Orthopaedic Society for Sports Medicine. 1994:447-486.
73. Johns R, Wright V: Relative importance of various tissues in joint stiffness. *J Appl Physiol.* 1962;17:824-830.
74. Toft E, Espersen GT, Kalund S, et al: Passive tension of the ankle before and after stretching. *Am J Sports Med.* 1989;17:489-494.
75. Halbertsma JPK, Goeken LNH: Stretching exercises: effect of passive extensibility and stiffness in short hamstrings of healthy subjects. *Arch Phys Med Rehab.* 1994;75:976-981.
76. Magnusson SP, Simonsen EB, Aagaard P, et al: A mechanism for altered flexibility in human skeletal muscle. *J Physiol.* 1996;497:291-298.
77. Klinge K, Magnusson SP, Simonsen EB, et al: The effect of strength and flexibility on skeletal muscle EMG activity, stiffness and viscoelastic stress relaxation response. *Am J Sports Med.* 1997;25:710-716.

78. Lapier TK, Burton HW, Almon RF: Alterations in intramuscular connective tissue after limb casting affect contraction-induced muscle injury. *J Appl Physiol.* 1995;78:1065-1069.
79. McNair PJ, Wood GA, Marshall RN: Stiffness of the hamstring muscles and its relationship to function in ACL deficient individuals. *Clin Biomech.* 1992;7:131-137.
80. McHugh MP, Magnusson SP, Gleim GW, et al: A cross-sectional study of age-related musculoskeletal and physiological changes in soccer players. *Med Exerc Nutr Health.* 1993;2:261-268.
81. Bohannon RW: Effect of repeated eight-minute muscle loading on the angle of straight-leg-raising. *Phys Ther.* 1984;64:491.
82. Yoder E: Physical therapy management of nonsurgical hip problems in adults. In: Echternach JL, ed. *Physical Therapy of the Hip.* New York, NY: Churchill Livingstone. 1990:103-137.
83. DeVries HA: Evaluation of static stretching procedures for improvement of flexibility. *Res Quart.* 1962;33:222-229.
84. Logan GA, Egstrom GH: Effects of slow and fast stretching on sacrofemoral angle. *J Assoc Phys Ment Rehabil.* 1961;15:85-89.
85. Davies CT, White MJ: Muscle weakness following eccentric work in man. *Pflugers Arch.* 1981;392:168-171.
86. Friden J, Sjostrom M, Ekblom B: A morphological study of delayed muscle soreness. *Experientia.* 1981;37:506-507.
87. Hardy L: Improving active range of hip flexion. *Res Q Exerc Sport.* 1985;56:111-114.
88. Murphy P: Warming up before stretching advised. *Phys Sports Med.* 1986;14:45.
89. Shellock F, Prentice WE: Warm-up and stretching for improved physical performance and prevention of sport-related injury. *Sports Med.* 1985;2:267-278.
90. Sapega AA, Quedenfeld T, Moyer R, et al: Biophysical factors in range of motion exercise. *Phys Sports Med.* 1981;9:57-65.
91. Sucher BM: Thoracic outlet syndrome—a myofascial variant: Part 2. Treatment. *JAOA.* 1990;90:810-823.
92. Markos PD: Ipsilateral and contralateral effects of proprioceptive neuromuscular facilitation techniques on hip motion and electromyographic activity. *Phys Ther.* 1979;59:1366.
93. Holt LE, Travis TM, Okita T: Comparative study of three stretching techniques. *Percep Motor Skills.* 1970;31:611-616.
94. Tanigawa MC: Comparison of hold-relax procedure and passive mobilization on increasing muscle length. *Phys Ther.* 1972;52:725-735.
95. Sady SP, Wortman MA, Blanke D: Flexibility training: ballistic, static or proprioceptive neuromuscular facilitation? *Arch Phys Med Rehab.* 1982;63:261-263.
96. Prentice WE: A comparison of static stretching and PNF stretching for improving hip joint flexibility. *Athl Train.* 1983;18:56-59.
97. Voight M, Blackburn T: Proprioception and balance training and testing following injury. In: Ellenbecker TS, ed. *Knee Ligament Rehabilitation.* Philadelphia, PA: Churchill Livingstone. 2000:361-385.
98. Risberg MA, Mork M, Krogstad-Jenssen H, et al: Design and implementation of a neuromuscular training program following anterior cruciate ligament reconstruction. *J Orthop Sports Phys Ther.* 2001;31:620-631.

99. Lephart SM, Borsa PA: Functional rehabilitation of knee injuries. In: Fu FH, Harner C, eds. *Knee Surgery.* Baltimore, MD: Williams & Wilkins. 1993.
100. Lephart SM, Henry TJ: Functional rehabilitation for the upper and lower extremity. *Orthop Clin North Am.* 1995;26:579-592.
101. Voight ML, Cook G: Impaired neuromuscular control: reactive neuromuscular training. In: Prentice WE, Voight ML, eds. *Techniques in Musculoskeletal Rehabilitation.* New York, NY: McGraw-Hill. 2001:93-124.
102. Jerosch J, Prymka M: Propriozeptive Fahigkeiten des gesunden Kniegelenks: Beeinflussung durch eine elastische Bandage. *Sportverletz. Sportsch.* 1995;9:72-76.
103. Jerosch J, Hoffstetter I, Bork H, et al: The influence of orthoses on the proprioception of the ankle joint. *Knee Surg Sports Traumatol Arthrosc.* 1995;3:39-46.
104. Perlau R, Frank C, Fick G: The effect of elastic bandages on human knee proprioception in the uninjured population. *Am J Sports Med.* 1995;23:251-255.
105. Robbins S, Waked E, Rappel R: Ankle taping improves proprioception before and after exercise in young men. *Br J Sports Med.* 1995;29:242-247.
106. Barrett DS: Proprioception and function after anterior cruciate ligament reconstruction. *J Bone Joint Surg.* 1991;73B:833-837.
107. Lephart SM, Pincivero DM, Giraldo JL, et al: The role of proprioception in the management and rehabilitation of athletic injuries. *Am J Sports Med.* 1997;25:130-137.
108. Borsa PA, Lephart SM, Kocher MS, et al: Functional assessment and rehabilitation of shoulder proprioception for glenohumeral instability. *J Sport Rehabil.* 1994;3:84-104.
109. Lephart SM, Warner JJP, Borsa PA, et al: Proprioception of the shoulder joint in healthy, unstable and surgically repaired shoulders. *J Shoulder Elbow Surg.* 1994;3:371-380.
110. Fremerey RW, Lobenhoffer P, Zeichen J, et al: Proprioception after rehabilitation and reconstruction in knees with deficiency of the anterior cruciate ligament: a prospective, longitudinal study. *J Bone Joint Surg [Br].* 2000;82:801-806.
111. Irrgang JJ, Whitney SL, Harner C: Nonoperative treatment of rotator cuff injuries in throwing athletes. *J Sport Rehabil.* 1992;1:197-222.
112. Voss DE, Ionta MK, Myers DJ: Proprioceptive Neuromuscular Facilitation: Patterns and Techniques, *3rd ed.* Philadelphia, PA: Harper and Row. 1985:1-342.
113. Janda DH, Loubert P: A preventative program focussing on the glenohumeral joint. *Clin Sports Med.* 1991;10:955-971.
114. Martin G: Aquatic therapy in rehabilitation. In: Prentice WE, Voight ML, eds. *Techniques in Musculoskeletal Rehabilitation.* New York, NY: McGraw-Hill. 2001:279-287.
115. Becker BE: Aquatic therapy: scientific foundations and clinical rehabilitation applications. *PM&R: the journal of injury, function, and rehabilitation.* 2009;1:859-872.
116. Kuprian W: Proprioceptive neuromuscular facilitation—PNF complex motions. In: Kuprian W, ed. *Physical Therapy for Sports, 2nd ed.* Philadelphia, PA: Saunders. 1995:99-119.

Adjunctive Interventions

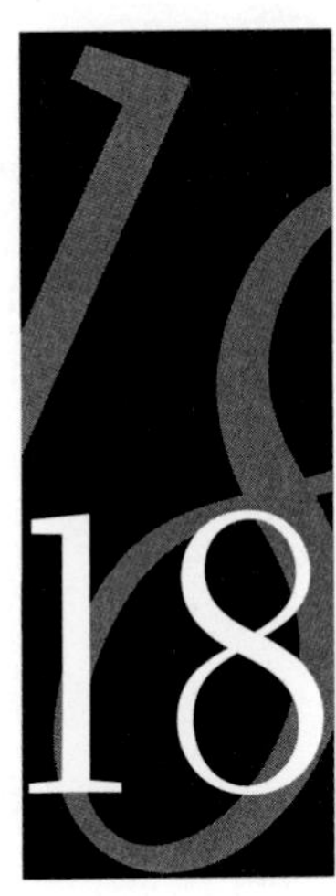

The physical therapist has a number of adjunctive interventions at his or her disposal, the use of which is determined by the goals of the intervention (Tables 18-1 and 18-2). Three categories of adjunctive interventions are recognized:

- Physical agents
- Electrotherapeutic modalities
- Mechanical modalities

Study Pearl

Temperature conversions:

- Fahrenheit = (temperature in Celsius × 9/5) + 32 or (temperature in Celsius × 1.8) + 32
- Celsius = (temperature in Fahrenheit − 32) × 5/9 or (temperature in Fahrenheit − 32) × 0.55

PHYSICAL AGENTS

Thermal modalities, of which there are four major types, involve the transfer of thermal energy (Table 18-3).

CRYOTHERAPY

Cryotherapy is the therapeutic use of cold. The physiological effects of a local cold application are principally due to vasoconstriction, reduced metabolic function,[1] and reduced motor and sensory nerve conduction velocities.[2,3] These effects include

- A rapid decrease in skin temperature. Subcutaneous temperature falls less rapidly and displays a smaller temperature change. The ideal tissue temperature to achieve the optimal physiologic effects of cryotherapy is 15 to 25°C.[4]
- A decrease in muscle and intraarticular temperature.
- Localized vasoconstriction of all smooth muscle by the central nervous system to conserve heat.[8] Maximum vasoconstriction occurs at tissue temperatures of 15°C (59°F). Localized vasoconstriction is responsible for the decrease in the tendency toward formation and accumulation of edema, probably as a result of a decrease in local hydrostatic pressure.[9] There is also a decrease in the amount of nutrients and phagocytes delivered to the area, thus reducing phagocytic activity.[9]

TABLE 18-1. INDICATIONS AND CONTRAINDICATIONS FOR THE USE OF THERAPEUTIC MODALITIES

THERAPEUTIC MODALITY	PHYSIOLOGIC RESPONSES (INDICATIONS FOR USE)	CONTRAINDICATIONS AND PRECAUTIONS
Electrical stimulating currents—high voltage	Pain modulation Muscle reeducation Muscle pumping contractions Retard atrophy Muscle strengthening Increase range of motion Fracture healing Acute injury	Pacemakers Thrombophlebitis Superficial skin lesions
Electrical stimulating currents—low voltage	Wound healing Fracture healing Iontophoresis	Malignancy Skin hypersensitivities Allergies to certain drugs
Electrical stimulating currents—interferential	Pain modulation Muscle reeducation Muscle pumping contractions Fracture healing Increase range of motion	Same as high-voltage
Electrical stimulating currents—Russian	Muscle strengthening	Pacemakers
Electrical stimulating currents—MENS	Fracture healing Wound healing	Malignancy Infections
Shortwave diathermy and microwave diathermy	Increase deep circulation Increase metabolic activity Reduce muscle guarding/spasm Reduce inflammation Facilitate wound healing Analgesia Increase tissue temperatures over a large area	Metal implants Pacemakers Malignancy Wet dressings Anesthetized areas Pregnancy Acute injury and inflammation Eyes Areas of reduce blood flow Anesthetized areas
Cryotherapy-cold packs, ice massage	Acute injury Vasoconstriction-decreased blood flow Analgesia Reduce inflammation Reduce muscle guarding/spasm	Allergy to cold Circulatory impairments Wound healing Hypertension
Thermotherapy-hot whirlpool, paraffin, hydrocollator, infrared lamps	Vasodilation-increased blood flow Analgesia Reduce muscle guarding/spasm Reduce inflammation Increase metabolic activity Facilitate tissue healing	Acute and postacute trauma Poor circulation Circulatory impairments Malignancy
Low-power laser	Pain modulation (trigger points) Facilitate wound healing	Pregnancy Eyes
Ultraviolet	Acne Aseptic wounds Folliculitis Pityriasis rosea Tinea Septic wounds Sinusitis Increase calcium metabolism	Psoriasis Eczema Herpes Diabetes Pellagra Lupus erythematosus Hyperthyroidism Renal and hepatic insufficiency Generalized dermatitis Advanced atherosclerosis

(*Continued*)

TABLE 18-1. INDICATIONS AND CONTRAINDICATIONS FOR THE USE OF THERAPEUTIC MODALITIES (*Continued*)

THERAPEUTIC MODALITY	PHYSIOLOGIC RESPONSES (INDICATIONS FOR USE)	CONTRAINDICATIONS AND PRECAUTIONS
Ultrasound	Increase connective tissue extensibility Deep heat Increased circulation Treatment of most soft tissue injuries Reduce inflammation Reduce muscle spasm	Infection Acute and postacute injury Epiphyseal areas Pregnancy Thrombophlebitis Impaired sensation Eyes
Intermittent compression	Decrease acute bleeding Decrease edema	Circulatory impairment

Reproduced, with permission, from Prentice WE: Using therapeutic modalities in rehabilitation. In: Prentice WE, Voight ML, eds. *Techniques in Musculoskeletal Rehabilitation.* New York, NY: McGraw-Hill. 2001:289-303.

TABLE 18-2. CLINICAL DECISION MAKING ON THE USE OF VARIOUS THERAPEUTIC MODALITIES DURING THE VARIOUS STAGES OF HEALING

PHASE	APPROXIMATE TIME FRAME	CLINICAL PICTURE	POSSIBLE MODALITIES USED	RATIONALE FOR USE
Initial acute	Injury—day 3	Swelling, pain to touch, pain on motion	CRYO ESC IC LPL Rest	↓ Swelling, ↓ pain ↓ Pain ↓ Swellings ↓ Pain
Inflammatory response	Days 1-6	Swelling subsides, warm to touch, discoloration, pain to touch, pain on motion	CRYO ESC IC LPL Range of motion	↓ Swelling, ↓ pain ↓ Pain ↓ Swelling ↓ Pain
Fibroblastic repair	Days 4-10	Pain to touch, pain on motion, swollen	THERMO ESC LPL IC Range of motion Strengthening	Mildly ↑ circulation ↓ Pain-muscle pumping ↓ Pain Facilitate lymphatic flow
Maturation-remodeling	Day 7—recovery	Swollen, no more pain to touch, decreasing pain on motion	ULTRA ESC LPL SWD MWD Range of Motion Strengthening Functional Activities	Deep heating to ↑ circulation ↑ Range of motion, ↑ strength ↓ Pain ↓ Pain Deep heating to ↑ circulation Deep heating to ↑ circulation

CRYO, Cryotherapy; ESC, electrical stimulating currents; IC, intermittent compression; LPL, low-power laser; MWD, microwave diathermy; SWD, short-wave diathermy; THERMO, thermotherapy; ULTRA, ultrasound; ↓ decrease; ↑ increase.
Reproduced, with permission, from Prentice WE: Using therapeutic modalities in rehabilitation. In: Prentice WE, Voight ML, eds. *Techniques in Musculoskeletal Rehabilitation.* New York, NY: McGraw-Hill. 2001:289-303.

TABLE 18-3. TYPES OF THERMAL ENERGY TRANSFER

TYPE	DESCRIPTION	EXAMPLE
Evaporation	A change in state of a liquid to a gas and a resultant cooling takes place	Vapocoolant sprays (Fluori-Methane)
Conduction	Heat is transferred from a warmer object to a cooler object through direct molecular interaction of objects in physical contact.	Cold pack, ice pack, ice massage, cold bath
Convection	Occurs when particles (air or water) move across the body, creating a temperature variation	Whirlpool
Radiation	The transfer of heat from a warmer source to a cooler source through a conducting medium, such as air	Infrared lamp

Study Pearl

The effect of skin temperature on cutaneous blood flow involves the following[5-7]:

- Normal cutaneous flow is 200 to 250 mL/min.
- At 15°C, maximal vasoconstriction is reached, with blood flow measured at 20 to 50 mL/min.
- Below 15°C, vasoconstriction is interrupted by rhythmic bursts of vasodilation occurring 3 to 5 times per hour and lasting 5 to 10 minutes. These bursts are more frequent and longer in individuals acclimated to the cold, making them less prone to frostbite injury.
- At 10°C, neurapraxia occurs, resulting in loss of cutaneous sensation.
- Below 0°C, negligible cutaneous blood flow allows the skin to freeze.
- Without circulation, skin temperature drops at a rate exceeding 0.5°C per minute.
- Smaller blood vessels (ie, microvasculature) freeze before larger blood vessels.
- The venous system freezes before the arterial system because of lower flow rates.

TABLE 18-4. STAGES OF ANALGESIA INDUCED BY CRYOTHERAPY

STAGE	RESPONSE	TIME AFTER INITIATION OF CRYOTHERAPY (MIN)
1	Cold sensation	0-3
2	Burning or aching	2-7
3	Local numbness or analgesia	5-12
4	Deep tissue vasodilation without increase in metabolism	12-15

Data from Hocutt JE, Jaffee R, Rylander R, et al: Cryotherapy in ankle sprains. *Am J Sports Med.* 1982;10:316-319.

- Local analgesia.[10,17,19-23] The stages of analgesia achieved by cryotherapy are outlined in Table 18-4. It is worth remembering that the timing of the stages depends on the depth of penetration and varying thickness of adipose tissue.[24] The patient should be advised about these various stages, especially in light of the fact that the burning/aching phase occurs before the therapeutic phases.
- Cold induced vasodilation. It has been hypothesized that when local temperature is lowered considerably for a period of about 30 minutes, intermittent periods of vasodilation occur, lasting 4 to 6 minutes.[9] This phenomenon, known as the *hunting response,* is the mechanism by which the body responds to extreme cold and is necessary to prevent local tissue injury.[9] The vasodilation is proposed to last for 4 to 6 minutes and to be followed by a vasoconstriction lasting 15 to 30 minutes. However, recent studies have not been able to demonstrate this cycle—the hunting response is more likely a measurement artifact than an actual change in blood flow in response to cold.[9,10,23,25,26]
- Decreased cell permeability and decreased cellular metabolism.[9] The decrease in cellular metabolism results in a decrease in demand for oxygen, which in turn limits further injury, particularly in the case of acute tissue damage.
- Decreased muscle spasm.[13,17,27-29] A decrease in muscle tension is produced through a raise in the threshold of activation of the muscle spindle.
- Decrease in the excitability of free nerve endings and peripheral nerve fibers, resulting in an increase in the pain threshold.[30,31]

Study Pearl

The use of ice by itself[10] or in conjunction with compression,[11-14] has been demonstrated to be effective in minimizing the amount of edema.[15-17] However, even though the immediate application of cold will help to control edema if applied immediately following injury, the gravity-dependent positions should be avoided with acute and subacute injuries because of the likelihood of additional swelling.[18]

On occasion, adverse physiological effects can occur due to hypersensitivity to cold. These include

- Cold urticaria: erythema of the skin with a wheal formation associated with severe itching due to histamine reaction.
- Facial flush, puffiness of the eyelids, respiratory problems, and in severe cases, anaphylaxis (decreased blood pressure, increased heart rate) with syncope are also related to histamine release.
- Raynaud's phenomenon: exposure to the cold triggers blood vessel spasms that result in interruption of blood flow to the fingers, toes, ears, and nose.

Goals and Indications. The therapeutic effects and indications of cryotherapy are listed in Table 18-5.

TABLE 18-5. CRYOTHERAPY EFFECTS, INDICATIONS AND CONTRAINDICATIONS

THERAPEUTIC EFFECTS	INDICATIONS	CONTRAINDICATIONS
Initial decrease in blood flow to the treated area due to vasoconstriction	Acute or chronic pain	Area of compromised circulation
Decreased temperature resulting in decreased nerve conduction velocity	Myofascial pain syndrome	Peripheral vascular disease
Increased pain threshold	Muscle spasm	Ischemic tissue
Decreased metabolism	Bursitis	Cold hypersensitivity
Decreased edema	Acute or subacute inflammation	Infection
Reduced spasticity of muscle	Musculoskeletal trauma	Raynaud's phenomenon
Analgesic effects	Reduction of spasticity	Cold urticaria
	Tendinitis	Hypertension
		Cryoglobinemia

Data from Cwynar DA, McNerney T: A primer on physical therapy. *Lippincott's Primary Care Practice.* 1999;3:451-459; and Bell GW, Prentice WE: Infrared modalities. In: Prentice WE, ed. *Therapeutic Modalities for Allied Health Professionals.* New York, NY: McGraw-Hill. 1998:201-262.

Contraindications/Precautions. The contraindications for cryotherapy are listed in Table 18-5.

Ice Massage. Ice massage, typically performed by freezing water in paper cups and applying the ice directly to the treatment area, is recommended in all of the phases of healing when any inflammation is present, but particularly in the acute phase, because of its effectiveness in reducing both pain and edema.[4,23,34-36]

Application and Patient Preparation. The patient is kept warm throughout the treatment. The ice cup is removed from the freezer and the ice is exposed. The ice is applied to an area no larger than 4" × 6" in small, circular motions at a rate of 2 in/s, using overlapping circles or overlapping longitudinal strokes, with each stroke covering one-half of the previous circle stroke. A towel is used to dab water from the treatment area. The massage is continued until anesthesia is achieved, usually for approximately 5 to 10 minutes.

Cold Packs. Cold packs, which typically contain silica gel and are available in a variety of shapes and sizes, are applied directly to appropriate area to help in decreasing pain. Cold packs are maintained in a refrigerated unit at a temperature of 0 to 10°F.[22]

Application and Patient Preparation. The patient should be kept warm throughout the treatment. A towel is dampened with warm water and the excess water wrung out. The ice pack is wrapped in the moistened towel, placed on the patient, and covered with a dry towel to retard warming. The pack is secured to the treatment area. The treatment time is typically 10 to 20 minutes.

Ice Packs. An ice pack consists of crushed ice folded in a moist towel or placed in a plastic bag covered by a moist towel. The method of application, patient preparation, and treatment time is the same as for the cold packs.

Cold Bath. A cold bath is commonly used for the immersion of the distal extremities. The temperature for a cold whirlpool used for acute conditions is in the range of 50 to 60°F (10-16°C).[9] The body part is immersed for 5 to 15 minutes, depending on the desired therapeutic effect.

Study Pearl

Depth of penetration depends on the amount of cold, the length of the treatment time, the intensity and duration of the cold application, and the circulatory response to the body segment exposed.[9]

Study Pearl

The application of cold packs and ice bags over superficial peripheral nerves (ie, the deep peroneal [fibular] nerve at the fibular head) can result in temporary or permanent injury to these nerves.[32,33]

Study Pearl

Prior to the application of cold, the area to be treated should be assessed for protective sensation to avoid skin damage.

Study Pearl

Increased heart rate and blood pressure are associated with cold application to large areas of the body.[9] Conditioned patients should not have a problem with dizziness after cold applications, but care should be taken when transferring any patient from the whirlpool area.

Vapocoolant Spray. Vapocoolant sprays, which produce superficial cooling, are often used in conjunction with passive stretching and in the treatment of muscle spasms, trigger points, and myofascial referred pain.[37]

The clinician makes two to five sweeps (at approximately 4 in/s and at a 30-degree angle to the skin) with the spray in the direction of the involved muscle fibers, keeping the spray 12 to 18 in. (30 cm to 46 cm) from the skin and applying the sweeps from the proximal to the distal aspect of the muscle attachments.[37] Stretching is initiated while applying the spray and is continued after the spray is applied using steady tension. The spray is allowed to completely evaporate each time before applying the next sweep. The length of treatment varies according to the region being treated. Precautions concerning the use of cold spray include protecting the patient's face from the fumes and spraying the skin at an acute (approximately 30 degrees) rather than at a perpendicular angle.

THERMOTHERAPY

Thermotherapy is the application of therapeutic heat involving the transfer of thermal energy. This application of heat can occur at a superficial or deeper level (Table 18-6).

Superficial Thermotherapy. Heat greatly influences the hemodynamic, neuromuscular, and metabolic processes of the body. The physiological effects of a local heat application include[25,38-41]

- Skin temperature rises rapidly and exhibits the greatest temperature change; subcutaneous tissue temperature rises less rapidly and exhibits a smaller change; muscle and joint show less temperature change, if any, depending on size and structure. The increase in heat is dissipated through selective vasodilation and shunting of blood via reflexes in the microcirculation, and regional blood flow.[42]
- Increased metabolism and perspiration.
- An increase in local nerve conduction.

TABLE 18-6. THERMOTHERAPY EFFECTS, INDICATIONS AND CONTRAINDICATIONS

THERAPEUTIC EFFECTS	INDICATIONS	CONTRAINDICATIONS
Increased temperature	Pain control	Circulatory impairment
Increased blood flow to the treated area	Chronic inflammatory conditions	Area of malignancy
Decreased nerve conduction latency	Trigger point	Acute musculoskeletal trauma
Temporarily decreased muscle strength	Tissue healing	Bleeding or hemorrhage
Increased pain threshold	Muscle spasm	Sensory impairment
Increased edema	Decreased range of motion	Thrombophlebitis
Vasodilation	Desensitization	Arterial disease
Increased nerve conduction velocity		
Increased metabolic rate		
Increased muscle elasticity		
Increased collagen extensibility		
Decreased muscle tone		

- Decreased muscle spasm, thereby facilitating stretching.[3,21,42,43] The muscle relaxation likely results from a decrease in firing rates of the efferent fibers in the muscle spindle.
- Increased capillary permeability, cell metabolism, and cellular activity, which can increase the delivery of oxygen and chemical nutrients to the area, while decreasing venous stagnation.[39,44]
- Increased analgesia through hyperstimulation of the cutaneous nerve receptors.
- An increase in tissue extensibility.[42] To be therapeutic, the amount of thermal energy transferred to the tissue must be sufficient to stimulate without causing damage to the tissue.[45] In an environment of connective tissue healing, the immature collagen bonds can be degraded by heat. This has obvious implications for the application of stretching techniques. Optimum results are obtained if the heat is applied during the stretch, and the stretch is maintained until cooling occurs after removal of the heat.[42]

Indications for Thermotherapy. The choice of superficial heating modality should be made according to the patient's diagnosis, the body part being treated, and the onset of the condition, the age of patient, and the desired goal. Typical goals include

- Modulation of pain. This effect may be due to the proposed gating of the transmission of pain signals by an activation of cutaneous thermoreceptors, or it may indirectly be a result of improved healing, decreased muscle spasm, or reduced ischemia.[9]
- Removal of metabolites and other products of the inflammatory process.[9]
- Increase in connective tissue extensibility.[9] When a soft tissue is heated prior to stretching, it maintains a greater increase in length following the stretching force; therefore less force is required to achieve the increase in length while reducing the risk of tissue damage.
- Reduction or elimination of soft tissue and joint restriction and muscle spasm.[9] Soft tissue extensibility increases and joint stiffness decreases with the application of heat.
- Preparation of the area prior to electrical stimulation (decreases skin resistance); massage; ultrasound; passive and active exercise.

Study Pearl

The choice of thermal modality depends on the goal of the treatment and the tissue to be treated. For example, if the primary treatment goal is a tissue temperature increase with a corresponding increase in blood flow to the deeper tissues, the clinician should choose a modality, such as diathermy or ultrasound, that produces energy that can penetrate the cutaneous tissues and be directly absorbed by the deep tissues.[9]

Contraindications/Precautions for Thermotherapy. It is important to assess the patient's sensitivity to temperature, pain, and circulation status prior to the use of thermotherapy. Contraindications/precautions for thermotherapy include

- Acute injury/inflammation: the applied heat will increase the tissue temperature, produce vasodilation, bleeding, and edema thus aggravating the injury and delaying recovery.[46]
- Cardiac insufficiency: the increase in heat may overload the heart.[46]
- Malignancy: may increase the growth rate or rate of metastasis of malignant tissue either by increasing the circulation to the area or by increasing the metabolic rate.[46]

- Thrombophlebitis: the vasodilation and increased rate of circulation caused by increased tissue temperature may cause a thrombus (blood clot) to become dislodged from the area being treated.[46]
- Impaired circulation: may cause burning or overheating to areas of poor circulation.[46]
- Impaired thermal regulation and/or cognitive function as the patient may not be able to report that the area is becoming too hot.[46] Elderly and very young patients can have impaired/altered circulation systems.
- Open wounds: can increase bleeding.
- Hemophilia: increased blood flow.[46]
- Edema: may increase swelling.[46]
- Pregancy: although not an absolute contraindication, care must be taken to protect the developing fetus. Fetus damage through maternal hyperthermia can occur with full body heating (Hubbard tank), or applying a hot back to the lumbar spine.[46]

Study Pearl

A decrease in diastolic blood pressure can occur during and following a heat application to a large body area.[9] Care should be taken when transferring any patient following such treatments.

Application and Patient Preparation. The area to be treated should be positioned in such a way as to be easily observed, and to prevent a dependent position of the area, or any areas of the body distal to the treatment site. All clothing and jewelry should be removed from the treatment area.

- The procedure and its rationale should be explained to the patient in addition to describing what the patient may feel during the application of the agent or modality. The modality should be positioned correctly and the patient monitored during the application.

Study Pearl

Prior to the application of heat, the area to be treated should be assessed for protective sensation to avoid burning the patient.

Heating Packs. While the human body functions optimally between 36°C and 38°C, an applied temperature of 40 and 45°C is considered effective for a heat intervention. Commercial hot packs, or electric heating pads, are a conductive type of superficial moist heat. The hot packs are made of a silica gel encased in a canvas cover, which is immersed in thermostatically controlled water that is typically between 165 to 175°F (73.92-79.4°C). The hot packs are made in various sizes and shapes designed to fit different body areas. Before applying the hot pack, layers of terry cloth toweling (approximately six to eight, depending on the length of treatment and patient comfort) are placed between the skin and the hot pack. More toweling will be needed if the patient is laying on the pack. The moist heat pack causes an increase in the local tissue temperature, reaching its highest point about 8 minutes after the application.[47] The depth of penetration for the traditional heating pads (and cold packs) is about 1 cm, and result in changes in the cutaneous blood vessels and the cutaneous nerve receptors.[48] The skin should be inspected after 5 to 7 minutes.

Treatment times vary from 10 to 15 minutes, depending on the goal. The patient should be issued with a call device to notify the clinician of any discomfort.

Study Pearl

The skin normally looks pink or red following an application of heat. A dark red, or mottled appearance indicates that too much heat has been applied and that the treatment should cease.

Study Pearl

Wet heat produces a greater rise in local tissue temperature as compared to dry heat at any given temperature.[49] However, at higher temperatures, wet heat is not tolerated as well as dry heat.

Paraffin Bath. Superficial heat to the hands and feet can be applied using liquid paraffin, which has been heated in a thermostatically controlled paraffin bath unit. Paraffin baths are a commonly used modality for stiff or painful joints, and arthritis of the hands and feet. For clinical use, the wax used is a mixture of paraffin wax and mineral oil (approximately 2 lb wax/1 gal of oil). A small amount of wintergreen is often added if the paraffin is going to be used frequently. The use of liquid paraffin is contraindicated when there is evidence of an allergic rash, open wounds, recent scars and sutures, or a skin infection.

Paraffin melts rapidly at 118 to 130°F and self-sterilizes at 175 to 200°F.[50,51]

Study Pearl

Paraffin treatments provide 6 times the amount of heat available in water because the mineral oil in the paraffin lowers the melting point of the paraffin.[9] This provides the paraffin with a lower specific heat* than water, allowing for a slower exchange of heat to the skin.

Method of Application. The patient is asked to remove all jewelry (if jewelry cannot be removed it is covered with several layers of gauze) and to wash and dry the area to be treated. The clinician inspects the area for infection and open areas. Three different procedures are commonly utilized:

- Dip-wrap (glove) method. With their fingers/toes apart, the patient is asked to dip the involved part (hand or foot) in the wax bath as far as possible and tolerable, while avoiding touching the sides or bottom of the wax bath to prevent burns. After a few seconds, the patient is asked to remove their hand/foot without moving their fingers/toes to avoid cracks forming in the wax. The layer of paraffin hardens (becomes opaque). The patient repeats the process five more times.
  - After the paraffin has solidified, the body part is then wrapped in a plastic bag or wax paper and then in a towel or insulating glove to conserve the heat, thereby slowing down the rate of cooling of the paraffin. The involved extremity is elevated and the paraffin remains on for 15 to 20 minutes, until it cools, after which the therapist peels off the paraffin replacing the paraffin in the bath or discarding it.
  - Paint. As its name implies, for this method a brush is used to paint the treatment area with 6 to 10 layers of paraffin. The area is then covered and the wax remains on for approximately 20 minutes.
- Dip and immersion. This method is similar to the dip-wrap method, except that patient's extremity remains comfortably in the bath after the final dip. Extra caution must be taken with this method compared with the other two due to the potential for greater heat exchange to occur.

Study Pearl

The risk of burn with paraffin is substantial, and the clinician should weigh heavily the considerations between a paraffin bath and warm whirlpool bath.[9]

Study Pearl

When dipping into the paraffin, the first layer of wax should be the highest on the body segment and each successive layer lower than the previous one. This is to prevent subsequent layers from getting between the first layer and the skin and burning the patient.[9]

*Specific heat is the amount of heat per unit mass required to raise the temperature by 1°C. The specific heat of water is 1 calorie/g°C = 4.186 J/g°C which is approximately 4 times higher than air.

HYDROTHERAPY

Hydrotherapy offers a number of advantages that the other thermal modalities do not, including allowing the patient to mobilize the affected part during the treatment. Most of the benefits associated with hydrotherapy are related to the physical properties of water (see also Chapter 17).[52-56]

- Water provides buoyancy: Archimedes' principle, the upward force of the water, which is equal to the weight of the water that is displaced
- Hydrostatic pressure: the circumferential water pressure exerted on an immersed body part
- Resistance: the resistance provided by water while moving through it is partially due to the cohesion of the water molecules and the force needed to separate them

Whirlpool. The therapeutic use of whirlpools involves the partial or total immersion of a body or body part, in which the water is agitated and mixed with air so that it can be directed against, or around, the involve part. The whirlpool tanks come in various sizes:

- "High-boy" (used for upper extremity)
- "Low boy" (used for lower extremity)
- "Hubbard tank" (used for full body immersion)

A height-adjustable motor turbine, secured to the side, pumps a combination of air and water. This water/air jet can be directed in the desired direction to increase stimulation, help control pain, or clean an area.[9] If the area is hypersensitive the pressure can be directed away. Because of the buoyancy and therapeutic effect of the water, patients can move the extremity more easily. A whirlpool may be utilized to clean a wound, facilitate the resorption of effusion, and to improve range of motion.[9] Various temperatures can be used depending on the desired goal (Table 18-7).

Study Pearl

Precautions when using whirlpool treatments include decreased temperature sensation, impaired cognition, recent skin graft, incontinence, confusion/disorientation, and deconditioned state.[9] Contraindications include bleeding, wound maceration, cardiac instability, and profound epilepsy.[9]

TABLE 18-7. CLINICAL APPLICATIONS OF WHIRLPOOL TREATMENT ACCORDING TO TEMPERATURE RANGES

	HYDROTHERAPY TEMPERATURES	
TEMPERATURE	DEGREES	USE
Very hot	104°F (40-43.5°C)	Used for short exposure of 7-10 min to increase superficial temperature
Hot	99-104°F (37-40°C)	Used to increase superficial temperature
Warm	96-99°F (35.5-37°C)	Used to increase superficial temperature where a prolonged exposure is wanted, such as to decrease spasticity of a muscle in conjunction with passive exercise
Neutral	92-96°F (33.5-35.5°C)	Used with patients that have an unstable core body temperature
Tepid	80-92°F (27-33.5°C)	May be used in conduction with less vigorous exercise
Cool	67-80°F (19-27°C)	May be used in conduction with vigorous exercise
Cold	55-67°F (13-19°C)	Used for longer exposure of 10-15 min to decrease superficial temperature
Very cold	32-55°F (0-13°C)	Used for short exposure of 1-5 min to decrease superficial temperature

Clinical Application. The clinician should always use universal precautions when treating a patient with an open wound or lesion, and wear gloves, waterproof gown, goggles, and a mask, particularly when working with the possibility of splashing. In addition, safety precautions must be taken with any modality that potentially exposes the patient or clinician to electrical hazard from faulty electrical connections.

The tank is filled to the desired level and appropriate temperature (Table 18-7). A whirlpool liner may be used for patients with burns, wounds, or who are infected with blood-borne pathogens. If an antimicrobial agent is to be used it should be added to water during this time.

- Sodium hypochlorite (bleach): dilution 200 parts per million (ppm)
- Povidone-iodine: dilution of 4 ppm
- Chloramine-T: dilution 100 to 200 ppm

The patient is asked to uncover the area to be treated adequately. As appropriate, any wound dressing is removed, and the skin is tested for thermal sensitivity. The checking of vital signs prior to and during immersion may also be appropriate. Patient comfort is ensured by avoiding pressure of the limb on the edge of the whirlpool, which can compromise circulation—any pressure points should be padded. Once the patient is comfortable, the force, direction, and depth of the jet are adjusted appropriately and any exercise instructions are given to the patient. The patient should be supervised throughout the treatment session and their vital signs monitored as whirlpool treatments can provide a sedative effect, and depending on the temperature of the water, can cause fluctuations in blood pressure.[57]

Once the treatment is completed, the patient is asked to remove the body part from the water, and the area is dried and inspected. If appropriate, a clean dressing is applied.

The whirlpool is then drained, cleaned, and rinsed. Cleaning procedures vary according to each clinical setting. After cleaning, draining, and rinsing the tank, the areas that were in contact with water are wiped with a clean dry towel.

Aquatic therapy. Aquatic therapy is a form of hydrotherapy (refer to Chapter 17).

Contrast Bath. Contrast baths provide an alternating cycle of warm and cold water that theoretically creates a cycle of alternating vasoconstriction and vasodilation—a kind of vascular exercise. Contrast baths are used most frequently in the management of arthritis and extremity injuries (sprains and strains) for pain modulation and edema control, or can also be used for any condition requiring stimulation of peripheral circulation such as peripheral vascular disease, or complex regional pain syndrome (see Chapter 12).[58,59] Contraindications include advanced arteriosclerosis, malignancies, hemorrhage, arterial sufficiency, loss of sensation to heat and cold, and cardiac problems.

Method of Application. The procedure is explained to the patient and the patient is appropriately draped so that the exposed area can

Study Pearl

A ground fault circuit interrupter (GFI) should be installed at the circuit breaker at the receptacle of all whirlpools and Hubbard tanks, and the unit should be checked periodically for current leakage.

Study Pearl

Contrast baths can cause fluctuations in blood pressure, requiring that the patient be monitored throughout the treatment.[57]

Study Pearl

Electrotherapy terminology:

- Accommodation: the increased threshold of excitable tissue when a slowly rising stimulus is used. Both nerve and muscle tissues are capable of accommodating to an electrical stimulus, with nerve tissue accommodating more rapidly than muscle tissue. The quicker the rise time, the less the nerve can accommodate to the impulse.
- Alternating current (biphasic): this type of current allows for the constant change in the direction of flow of the ions.
- Amplitude: refers to the magnitude of current. Amplitude controls are often labeled intensity or voltage. Lower amplitudes are used for sensory stimulation, whereas higher intensities are used for motor stimulation.
- Anode: the anode used during direct current (the flow of electrons is unidirectional and the polarity is constant) electrotherapy is the positively charged electrode that attracts negative ions.
- Biphasic: describes a pulse that moves in one direction, returns to baseline, then in the other direction and back to the baseline again within a predetermined amount of time.
- Cathode: electrically negative; usually the active electrode (not always with iontophoresis).
- Direct current (DC): unidirectional current, sometimes called galvanic. Direct current produces polar effects (Table 18-9). It is important to remember that intact skin cannot tolerate a current density of > 1 mA/cm^2.[61]

be treated. The treatment usually begins with warm water (80-100°F) or hot water (100-110°F). The body part is placed in the warm water for 4 minutes, and then transferred to cold water (55-65°F) for 1 minute. This 4:1 sequence is continued for approximately 20 minutes, ending in warm water (or cold water when treating for edema). Even though contrast baths are prescribed for edema control, the gravity-dependent positions should be avoided with acute and subacute injuries because of the likelihood of additional swelling.[18]

The extremity is removed from the bath and is dried using a towel. The clinician notes any changes and retakes girth measurements as appropriate.

ELECTROTHERAPEUTIC MODALITIES

All living cells are electrically charged or polarized; the inside of the cells being grossly negative in charge when compared with the outside of the cell.[60] This polarization is due to the unequal distribution of ions on either side of the cell membrane and can be measured as a difference in electrical potential between the inside and outside of the cell—membrane potential. A change in the membrane potential is referred to as an action potential, which is the basis for the transmission of a nerve impulse (refer to Chapter 17). The key points to remember when using electrical modalities are listed in Table 18-8.

ELECTRICAL STIMULATION

Components of Electrical Currents. All matter is composed of atoms that contain positively and negatively charged particles called ions. These charged particles possess electrical energy and therefore have the ability to move about.

- Electrons are particles of matter possessing a negative charge and a very small mass. The net movement of electrons is referred to as an electrical current.
- The unit of measurement that indicates the rate at which electrical current flows is the ampere (amp). In the case of therapeutic modalities, current flow is generally described in milliamperes (mA).
- The electromotive force, which must be applied to produce a flow of electrons is called a volt (V).

TABLE 18-8. KEY POINTS TO REMEMBER WHEN USING ELECTROTHERAPEUTIC MODALITIES

- The introduction of electricity to a patient affects the whole body.
- The physical condition of the patient must be considered before introducing an electrical current.
- The effect of the electrical current is produced in the electrically active tissue, such as muscles and nerves.
- The response of the tissue is based on the current density (current amplitude, placement of the electrodes, relative size of the electrodes).
- Electrical current affects type II muscle fibers at lower density levels than it does for type I muscle fibers, which results in an abnormal recruitment order.
- The current is sensed more by the skin, due to the local resistance and ion concentrations in the local areas around the electrodes.

TABLE 18-9. POLAR EFFECTS PRODUCED BY THE CATHODE AND THE ANODE WITH DIRECT CURRENT

NEGATIVE (CATHODE)	POSITIVE (ANODE)
Depolarizes nerve fibers	Hyperpolarizes nerve fibers
Reduces pain in chronic conditions	Reduces pain in acute conditions
Attracts bases	Repels bases
Increases the potential for hemorrhage	Prevents hemorrhage
Stimulates	Sedates
Softens tissues	Hardens tissues

Reproduced, with permission, from Pociask FD: Electrotherapy. In: Placzek JD, Boyce DA, eds. *Orthopaedic Physical Therapy Secrets*. Philadelphia, PA: Hanley & Belfus, Inc. 2001:60-74.

- ▶ Voltage is the force resulting from an accumulation of electrons at one point in an electrical circuit, usually corresponding to a deficit of electrons at another point in the circuit. Commercial current flowing from wall outlets produces an electromotive force of either 115 or 220 V.

Electrotherapeutic Currents. Electrotherapeutic devices generate three different types of current:

- ▶ Monophasic or direct (galvanic): a unidirectional flow of electrons toward the positive pole.
- ▶ Biphasic or alternating: the flow of electrons constantly changes direction or, stated differently, reverses its polarity.
- ▶ Pulsed: usually contains three or more pulses grouped together, which are interrupted for short periods of time and repeat themselves at regular intervals. Can be monophasic or biphasic.

Waveforms. Waveforms are a graphic representation of the shape, direction, amplitude (intensity), phase duration (pulse width), and frequency (pulse rate or pulses per second) of the electrical current being produced by the electrotherapeutic device (Figure 18-1).

These waveforms may take on a sine, rectangular, or triangular configuration (Figure 18-2). An individual waveform is referred to as a pulse. A pulse may contain either one or two phases, which is that portion of the pulse that rises above or below the baseline displayed on an oscilloscope.

- ▶ Monophasic: a unidirectional flow of charged particles that occurs over a finite period of time (phase), which have only a single phase in each pulse.
- ▶ Biphasic waveforms have two separate phases during each individual pulse. The waveforms may be symmetrical or asymmetrical. They may also be balanced or unbalanced.
- ▶ Pulsed: these waveforms are called polyphasic and consist of three or more phases in a single pulse.

Pulse Charge. The term pulse charge refers to the total amount of electricity being delivered to the patient during each pulse:

- ▶ Monophasic current: the phase charge and the pulse charge are the same and always greater than zero.

Study Pearl (*continued*)

- • Electrons move along a conducting medium as an electrical current.
- • Electrotherapeutic devices generate three different types of current, alternating (AC) or biphasic, direct (DC) or monophasic, or pulsed or polyphasic.
- ▶ Fasciculation: involuntary motor unit firing. May see skin move, but no joint motion
- ▶ Fibrillation: involuntary firing of a single muscle fiber; indicative of denervation
- ▶ Frequency: represents the number of cycles or pulses per second (rate of oscillation). Normally described in the unit of Hz.
- ▶ Ground fault interrupters (GFI): a safety device that automatically shuts off current flow and reduces the chances of electrical shock.
- ▶ Ohm's law expresses the relationship between current flow (I), voltage (V), and resistance (R); ($I = V/R$). The current flow is directly proportional to the voltage and inversely proportional to the resistance. Therefore:
  - • When resistance decreases, current increases
  - • When resistance increases, current decreases
  - • When voltage increases, current increases
  - • When voltage decreases, current decreases
  - • When voltage is 0, current is 0
- ▶ Volt: the electromotive force that must be applied to produce a movement of electrons—a measure of electrical power
- ▶ Watt: a measure of electrical power (watts = volts × amperes)

Study Pearl

Conductance is a term that defines the ease with which current flows along a conducting medium.

- Metals are good conductors of electricity.
- Air, wood, and glass are all considered to be poor conductors (insulators).

Study Pearl

The opposition to electron flow in a conducting material is referred to as resistance or electrical impedance and is measured in a unit known as an ohm. Factors that can typically increase skin impedance include cooler skin temperature, the presence of hair and oil, increased skin dryness, and increased skin thickness.

Study Pearl

An analogy can be used to clarify the relationship between current flow, voltage, and resistance.

- In order for water to flow, some type of pump must create a force to produce movement. With electricity, the volt is the pump that produces the electron flow.
- The resistance to water flow is dependent on the length, diameter, and smoothness of the water pipe. The resistance to electrical flow (ohm) depends on the characteristics of the conductor (pipe).
- The amount of water flowing is measured in gallons. The amount of electricity flowing is measured in amperes.
- The amount of energy produced by flowing water is determined by two factors:
    - The number of gallons flowing per unit of time.
    - The pressure created in the pipe.
- Electrical energy is a product of the voltage or electromotive force and the amount of current flowing.

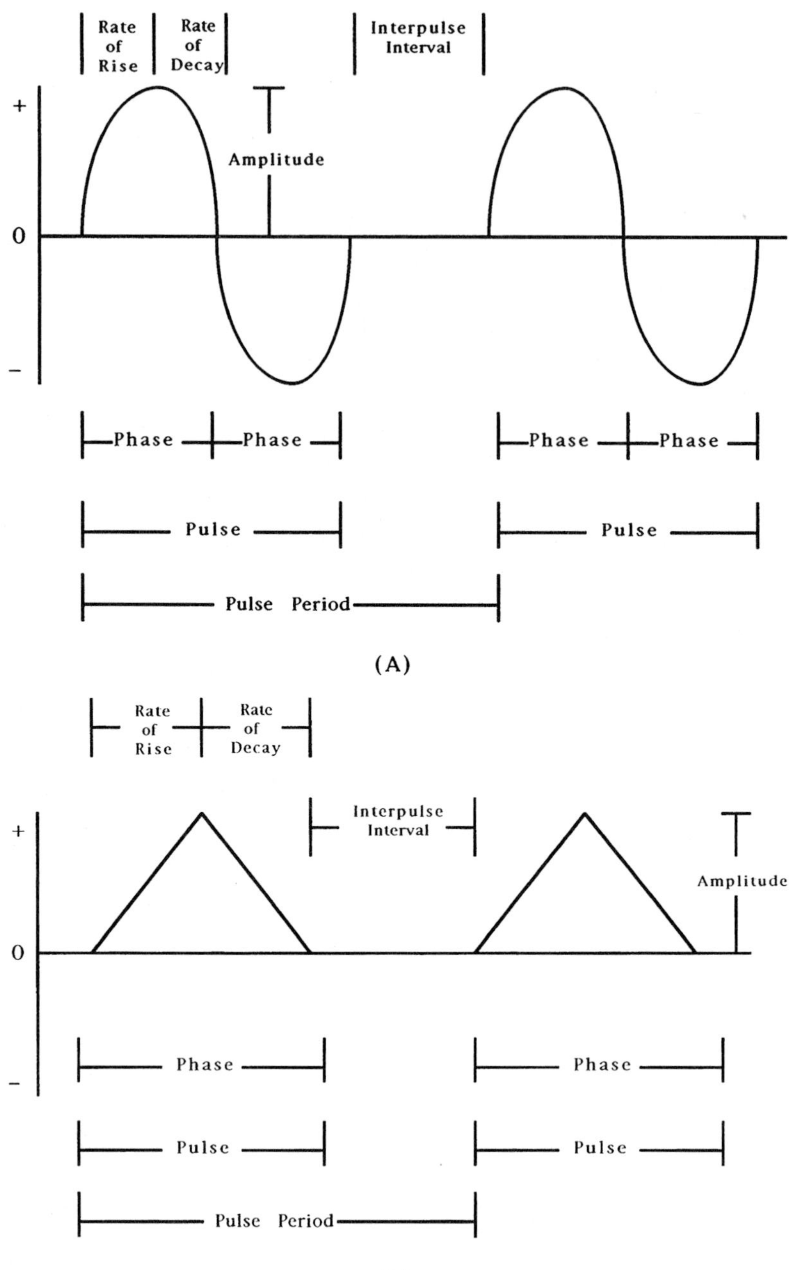

FIGURE 18-1. An individual waveform is referred to as a pulse. A pulse may contain either one or two phases, which is that portion of the pulse that rises above or below the baseline for some period of time. **A.** Biphasic pulse. **B.** Monophasis pulse. (Reproduced, with permission, from Prentice, WE: *Therapeutic Modalities for Allied Health Professionals.* New York, NY: McGraw-Hill. 1998:56.)

- Biphasic current: the pulse charge is equal to the sum of the phase charges, unless unbalanced in which case there is a net charge.

Pulse Duration. The duration of each pulse indicates the length of time current is flowing in one cycle.

- Monophasic: the phase duration is the same as the pulsed duration.

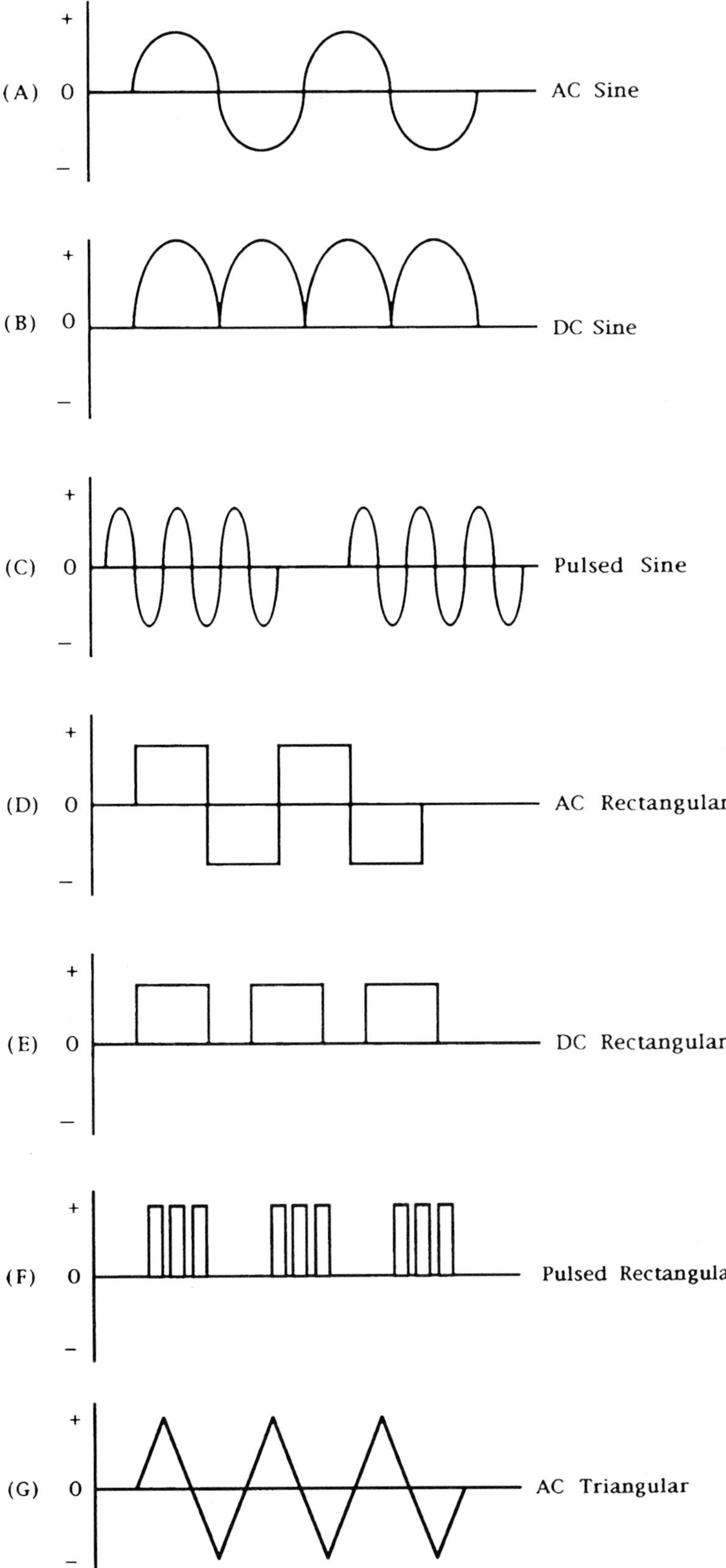

FIGURE 18-2. Waveforms of AC, DC, or pulsed current. (Reproduced, with permission, from Prentice, WE. *Therapeutic Modalities for Allied Health Professionals.* New York, NY: McGraw-Hill. 1998:57.)

Study Pearl

The phase duration contributes to the comfort of the stimulation, the amount of chemical change that occurs in the tissues, and nerve discrimination.[62] A duration of 50 to 100 μs typically is used for sensory stimulation, and 200 to 300 μs is typically used for motor stimulation.[62]

Study Pearl

- Intrapulse interval: used to increase patient comfort
- Interpulse interval: needed to ensure the absolute refractory
- Interburst interval: used with some protocols as a form of modulation
- Rise time: the time taken for the wave to go from 0 to its peak amplitude
- Fall-time: the time taken for the wave to go from its peak amplitude to 0
- Duty cycle: the relative proportion of time between the stimulation period and the rest period

Study Pearl

- Very short pulse durations with low intensities can depolarize sensory nerves.
- Longer pulse durations are required to stimulate motor nerves.
- Very long pulse durations with high intensities are needed to elicit a response from a denervated muscle.

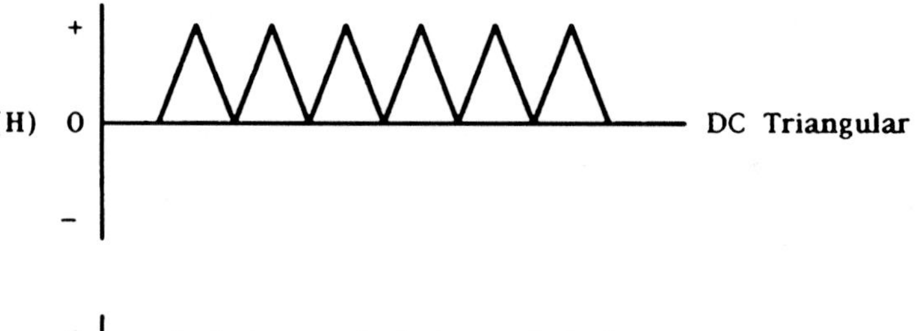

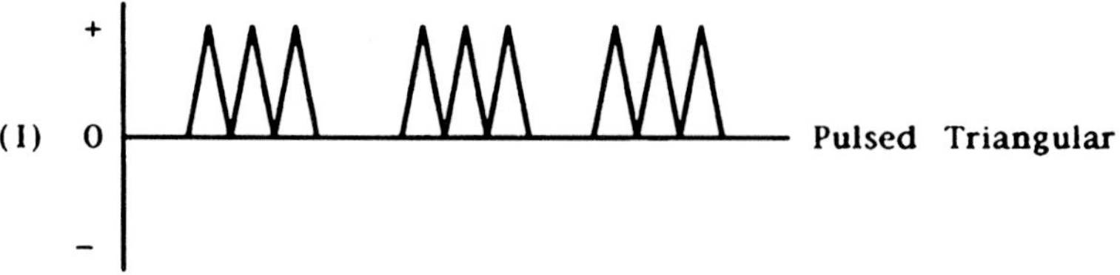

FIGURE 18-2. *(Continued)*

- Biphasic: the pulse duration is determined by the combined phase durations.

> **Study Pearl**
>
> Commercial stimulators are clinically labeled as low-, medium-, or high-frequency generators.

Pulse Frequency. Pulse frequency indicates the pulse rate or number of pulses per second (Hz). Frequency contributes to the type of contraction (Table 18-10) as well as theorized opiate-mediated effects.[62] As the frequency of any waveform is increased, the amplitude tends to increase and decrease more rapidly.

Current Modulation. Modulation refers to any alteration or any variation of the pulses of various waveforms (duration, width, frequency). For example, ramp up time is the time it takes to reach the peak amplitude. This can be used to improve the patient's tolerance to the stimulation.

Physiologic Responses to Electrical Current. Electrical current tends to choose the path of the least resistance to flow. Electricity has an effect on each cell and tissue that it passes through. The type and extent of the response are dependent on the type of tissue and its response characteristics. Typically, tissue that is highest in water content and consequently highest in ion content is the best conductor of electricity.

- Skin: offers the chief resistance to current flow and is considered an insulator. The greater the impedance of the skin, the higher the voltage of the electrical current must be to stimulate the underlying nerve and muscle.
- Blood: composed largely of water and ions and is consequently the best electrical conductor of all tissues.

TABLE 18-10. FREQUENCY AND TYPE OF CONTRACTION

FREQUENCY (HZ)	TYPE OF CONTRACTION
1-10	Twitch contraction
> 30	Tetanic contraction
30-70	Nonfatiguing tetanic contraction
100-1000	Fatiguing tetanic contraction

Reproduced, with permission, from Pociask FD: Electrotherapy. In: Placzek JD, Boyce DA, eds. *Orthopaedic Physical Therapy Secrets.* Philadelphia, PA: Hanley & Belfus, Inc. 2001:60-74.

TABLE 18-11. CHANGES IN PHYSIOLOGIC FUNCTIONING THAT OCCUR AT THE VARIOUS LEVELS OF THE BODY SYSTEM DUE TO ELECTRICITY

BODY SYSTEM LEVEL	CHANGES
Cellular level	Excitation of nerve cells
	Changes in cell membrane permeability
	Protein synthesis
	Stimulation of fibroblasts, osteoblasts
	Modification of microcirculation
Tissue level	Skeletal muscle contraction
	Smooth muscle contraction
	Tissue regeneration
Segmental level	Modification of joint mobility
	Muscle pumping action to change circulation and lymphatic activity
	An alteration of the microvascular system not associated with muscle pumping
	An increased movement of charged proteins into the lymphatic channels with subsequent oncotic force bringing increases in fluid to the lymph system
	Note: Transcutaneous electrical stimulation cannot directly stimulate lymph smooth muscle or the autonomic nervous system without also stimulating a motor nerve
Systematic effects	Analgesic effects as endogenous pain suppressors are released and act at different levels to control pain
	Analgesic effects from the stimulation of certain neurotransmitters to control neural activity in the presence of pain stimuli

- Muscle: composed of about 75% water and is therefore a relatively good conductor.
- Tendons: denser than muscle and contain relatively little water—poor conductors.
- Fat: only about 14% water—poor conductor.
- Bone: extremely dense, contains only about 5% water—the poorest biological conductor.

As electricity moves through the body, changes in physiologic functioning occur at the various levels of the system (Table 18-11).

MUSCLE AND NERVE PHYSIOLOGY RELATED TO ES

- Rheobase: the minimum intensity of current required to produce a minimum muscle contraction when applied for a maximum duration.
- Chronaxie: the length of time (pulse duration) for a current of twice the intensity of the rheobase current to produce tissue excitation.

A graphic illustration of this threshold and propagation and contraction is the strength-duration curve (Figure 18-3). The strength-duration curves for different classes of nerve and muscle tissue illustrate different thresholds of excitability of these tissues (Figure 18-4).

Motor Point. A motor point is the area of greatest excitability on the skin surface at which a small amount of electrical current generates a muscle response.

- Innervated muscle: the motor point is located at or near where the motor nerve enters the muscle, usually over the muscle belly.

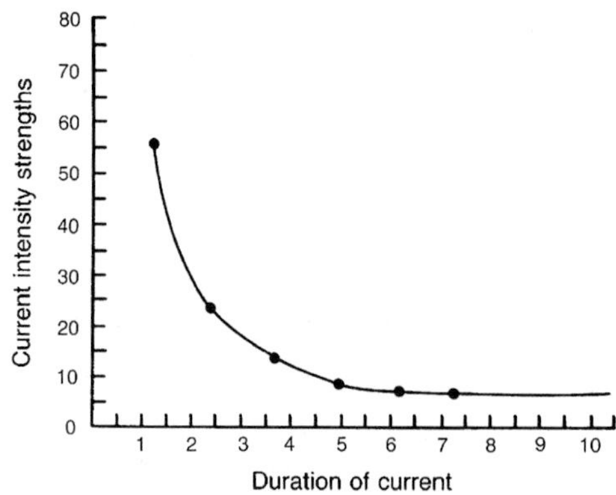

FIGURE 18-3. Strength-Duration curve. (Reproduced, with permission, from Prentice, WE. *Therapeutic Modalities for Allied Health Professionals.* New York, NY: McGraw-Hill. 1998:79.)

Study Pearl

Once a stimulus reaches a depolarizing threshold, the nerve or muscle membrane depolarizes, and propagation of the impulse or muscle contraction occurs. This reaction remains the same regardless of increases in the strength of the stimulus used—either the stimulus causes depolarization (the all) or its does not cause depolarization (the none)—there is no gradation of response.

- Denervated muscle: the area of greatest excitability is located over the muscle distally toward the insertion.

Stimulation of the motor nerves is the method used in most clinical applications of electrical muscular contractions. The all-or-none response is an important concept in applying electrical current to nerve or muscle tissue.

Manipulating the Parameters. When using electrical stimulation protocols for muscle or nerve tissue, several concepts must be understood with regard to how alterations in the available parameters can change the physiology of the body area being treated.

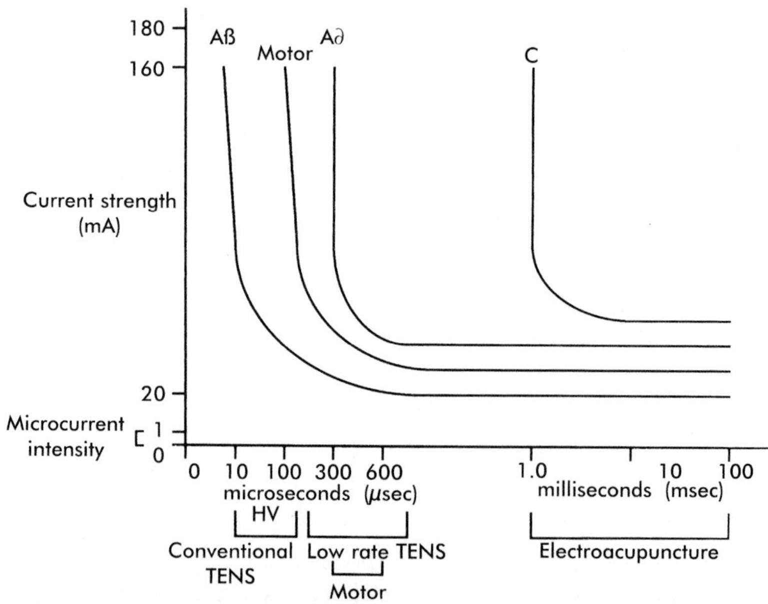

FIGURE 18-4. Strength-duration curves of the various sensory, motor and nerve fibers. (Reproduced, with permission, from Prentice, WE. *Therapeutic Modalities for Allied Health Professionals.* New York, NY: McGraw-Hill. 1998:79.)

Alternating versus Direct Current. The characteristics of direct current include

- The flow of electrons is unidirectional.
- The polarity is constant.
- The cell membrane is hyperpolarized as long as the current is on.
- The duration of current flow is > 1 second.

If continuous direct current were the only current mode available a muscle contraction would only occur when the current intensity rose to a stimulus threshold, and once the membrane depolarized, another change in the current intensity would be needed to force another depolarization and contraction. Monophasic or direct current which is most commonly used in iontophoresis, wound healing, and also for contractions of denervated muscle, has the ability to cause chemical changes. The exception is HVPC, discussed separately.

Biphasic or alternating current (AC) is characterized by sine wave modulation and has a constantly fluctuating voltage and a symmetric pattern. The characteristics of AC include

- The direction of flow reverses.
- The magnitude of flow of electrons changes.
- There are no polar effects.

AC is used in muscle retraining, spasticity, and for pain control.

Tissue Impedance. When electrical current passes through cutaneous tissues, by surface electrodes, an opposition to the flow of current is encountered. Impedance is the resistance of the tissue to the passage of electrical current. If a low-impedance tissue (nerve and muscle) is located under a large amount of high-impedance tissue (bone and fat), the current will never become high enough to cause a depolarization. Any unit that produces pulses of short durations (< 100 μs) is proficient at reducing tissue impedance.

Study Pearl

If the electrodes are spaced closely together, the area of higher current density is relatively superficial (Figure 18-5). Conversely, electrodes placed a greater distances from each other result in deeper penetration, provided that all other parameters and variables remain constant.

Current Density. Current density is the amount of current flow per cubic area. In order for a depolarization to occur the current density must be high enough. Current density is at its highest when the electrodes meet the skin and diminishes as electricity penetrates into the deep tissues.

If there is a large fat layer between the electrodes and the nerve, the electrical energy may not have a high enough density to cause depolarization (Figure 18-5).

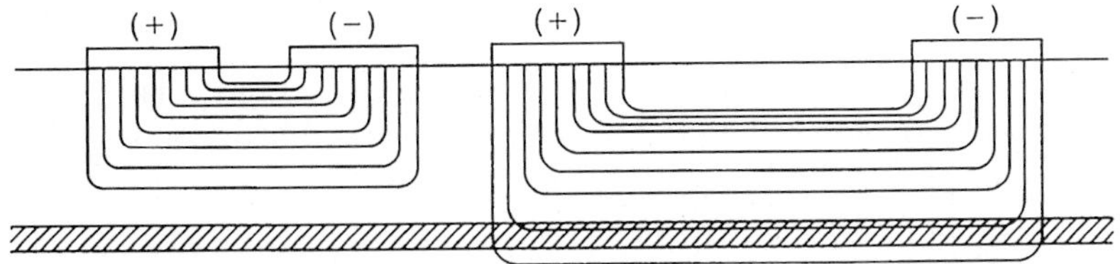

FIGURE 18-5. Electrode size and positioning. **A.** Electrodes are very close together, producing a high-density current in the superficial tissues. **B.** Increasing the distance between the electrodes increases the current density in deeper tissues. (Reproduced, with permission, from Prentice, WE. *Therapeutic Modalities for Allied Health Professionals.* New York, NY: McGraw-Hill. 1998:91.)

TABLE 18-12. THE EFFECT OF ELECTRODE SIZE ON CURRENT DENSITY, CURRENT SPREAD, SELECTIVITY, AND DISCRIMINATION

ELECTRODE SIZE	CURRENT DENSITY	CURRENT SPREAD	SELECTIVITY	DISCRIMINATION
Small	Greater	Decreased	Higher	Greater
Large	Less	Increased	Lower	Less

Data from Pociask FD: Electrotherapy. In: Placzek JD, Boyce DA, eds. *Orthopaedic Physical Therapy Secrets.* Philadelphia, PA: Hanley & Belfus, Inc. 2001:60-74.

Current density is also affected by electrode size (Table 18-12). If using two different sized electrodes, the smaller of the two electrodes should be placed as close as possible to the nerve or motor point, as the smaller electrode concentrates the current more than the larger electrode (Figure 18-5).

Frequency. The amount of frequency determines the amount of shortening of the muscle fiber and the amount of recovery allowed the muscle fiber.[63] The primary difference between an electrically induced muscle contraction and a voluntary muscle contraction is the asynchrony of firing of motor units under voluntary control versus the synchronous firing of electrically stimulated motor units.[63] Each time the electrical stimulus is applied, the same motor units respond—this may lead to greater fatigue in the electrically stimulated muscles.[63]

Intensity. Increasing the intensity of electrical stimulus causes the current to reach deeper into the tissue. The polarization of more fibers is accomplished using two methods:

- Higher threshold fibers within the range of the first stimulus are depolarized by the high-intensity stimulus.
- Fibers with the same threshold but deeper in the structure are depolarized by the deeper spread of that current.

Duration. By increasing the length of time (duration) that an adequate stimulus is available, more nerve fibers can be stimulated with the same current intensity because the current is available for a longer period of time.[63]

Polarity. The electrode that has a greater level of electrons is called the negative electrode or the cathode. The other electrode is called the positive electrode or the anode (when referring to monophasic current).

- The negative electrode attracts positive ions.
- The positive electrode attracts negative ions and electrons.

With biphasic or AC current, the electrodes change polarity with each cycle. By controlling the polarity, the clinician can control three characteristics:

- Chemical effects: the following chemical changes can occur under each electrode:
  - Changes in pH. Negative ions accumulating at the positive pole or anode produce an acidic reaction through the formation of hydrochloric acid. Positive ions that accumulate at the negative pole produce an alkaline reaction with the formation of sodium hydroxide.

- Reflex vasodilation.
- The ability to drive oppositely charged ions through the skin into the tissue (iontophoresis).

▶ Ease of excitation: the polarity of the active electrode usually should be negative when the desired result is a muscle contraction, because of the greater facility for membrane depolarization at the negative pole.[63] However, in treatment programs requiring sensory nerve stimulation, patient comfort should dictate the choice of positive or negative polarity, although usually negative polarity is found to be the most comfortable.[63]

▶ Directions of current flow: generally speaking, the negative electrode is positioned distally and the positive electrode proximally in an attempt to replicate the naturally occurring pattern of electrical flow in the body.[63] Clinically, polar effects are an important consideration in iontophoresis, stimulating motor point or peripheral nerves, and in the biostimulative effect on non-excitatory cells.[63]

Electrode Placement. The configuration of the electrodes depends on the intent of the intervention[63]:

▶ Monopolar: the stimulating or active electrode is placed over the target area (eg, motor point). A second dispersive electrode is placed at another site away from the target area. This technique is used with wounds, iontophoresis, neuromuscular electrical stimulation (NMES), and in the treatment of edema.

▶ Bipolar: two active electrodes of equal size are placed over the target area. This technique is used for muscle weakness, neuromuscular facilitation, spasms, and to increase range of motion.

▶ Quadripolar: two electrodes from two separate stimulating circuits are positioned so that the individual currents intersect with each other. This technique is utilized with interferential current.

There are several guidelines when using electrical stimulation of sensory nerves for pain suppression (transcutaneous electrical nerve stimulation or TENS). Electrodes may be placed over specific dermatomes, myotomes, or sclerotomes that correspond to the painful area.

▶ Electrodes may be placed close to the spinal cord segment that innervates a painful area.

▶ Placing electrodes over sites where the nerve becomes superficial and can be stimulated easily may stimulate peripheral nerves that innervate a painful area.

▶ Vascular structures contain neural tissue as well as ionic fluids that would transmit electrical stimulating current and may be most easily stimulated by electrode placement over superficial vascular structures.

▶ Electrodes can be placed over trigger points and acupuncture locations.

INDICATIONS FOR USE OF ELECTRICAL STIMULATION

The traditional uses of electrical stimulation are listed in Table 18-13.

TABLE 18-13. TRADITIONAL USES OF ELECTRICAL STIMULATION

USE	METHOD
Pain relief	▸ High frequency stimulation (80-120 Hz) and short duration should be used to stimulate the smallest unmyelinated nerve (C and delta) fibers in order to reduce pain (gate control theory). ▸ Low frequency (longer duration) stimulation, which stimulates the larger myelinated (alpha) fibers, should be used when producing muscle contractions is the goal. ▸ Ultra low frequencies can produce an increased endorphin production through initiation of the descending inhibition mechanisms (opiate pain control theory).
Reduce edema	▸ By producing a muscle pump action that increases the lymph and venous flow towards the heart. ▸ Increasing ion flow by attracting specific ions in a desired direction, as edema is believed to be slightly negatively charged.
Wound healing	▸ Through modification of the local inflammatory response (+ polarity produces an increase in inflammation), increasing circulation (− polarity). ▸ Pulsed currents (monophasic, biphasic, or polyphasic) with interrupted modulations can increase circulation and thus hasten metabolic waste disposal. ▸ Restoration of electrical cell charges through the use of monophasic currents (low-volt continuous modulations and high-volt-pulsed currents). May also have a bactericidal effect (cathode), by producing disruption of DNA, RNA synthesis or cell transport system of microorganisms. ▸ Low intensity continuous (nonpulsed and low volt) direct current, and high-volt-pulsed current can be applied for wound healing (by use of ionic effects).
Decrease atrophy, increase strength and endurance	▸ Using electrical stimulation to produce a depolarization of motor nerves and thus a muscle contraction. The limited studies on postsurgical or acutely injured patients seem to indicate that NMES is either as effective as, or more effective, than isometric exercises at increasing muscle strength and bulk,[a-e] in both atrophied[f] and normal muscles.[g,h] ▸ Producing a depolarization of muscle fibers due to ionic flow with direct current.
Muscle re-education	Using electrical stimulation to bring motor nerves and muscle fibers closer to threshold for depolarization. Reeducating muscles to respond appropriately using volitional effort by ▸ Providing proprioceptive feedback. ▸ Assisting with active exercise to help produce a contraction (active-assisted). ▸ Assisting in the coordination of muscle movement. Current intensity must be adequate for muscle contraction, and pulse duration should be set as close as possible to the duration needed for chronaxie of the tissue to be stimulated.[i] The pulses per second (pps) should be high enough to give a titanic contraction (20-40 pps).[i]
Improving peripheral circulation	Producing an "artificial" muscle pump through stimulation of both the agonist and antagonist muscles using alternating channels. Current intensity must be high enough to provide a strong, comfortable muscle contraction; pulse duration is preset (as close as possible to the duration needed for the chronaxie of the motor nerve to be stimulated) in most therapeutic generators, pps should be in the tetany range (20 pps).[i]
Administering medications (iontophoresis)	Directly affecting the direction of flow of specific ions within the tissues.
Stimulation of denervated muscle (monophasic current):	▸ Help minimize the extent of atrophy during the period while the nerve is regenerating. ▸ Electrically stimulated contractions of denervated muscle may limit edema and venous stasis, thus delaying muscle fiber fibrosis and degeneration.
Promotion of fracture healing	▸ Using low intensity direct current. ▸ Particularly useful in fractures prone to nonunion.

[a]Data from Delitto A, Rose SJ, McKowen JM, et al: Electrical stimulation versus voluntary exercise in strengthening thigh musculature after anterior cruciate ligament surgery. *Phys Ther.* 1988;68:660-663.
[b]Data from Goth RS, Hershkowitz S, Juris PM Electrical stimulation effect on extensor lag and length of hospital stay after total knee arthroplasty. *Arch Phys Med Rehab.* 1994;75:957.
[c]Data from Laughman RK, Youdas JW, Garrett TR, et al: Strength changes in the normal quadriceps femoris muscle as a result of electrical stimulation. *Phys Ther.* 1983;63:494-499.
[d]Data from McMiken DF, Todd-Smith M, Thompson C: Strengthening of human quadriceps muscles by cutaneous electrical stimulation. *Scand J Rehabil Med.* 1983;15:25-28.
[e]Data from Snyder-Mackler L, Delitto A, Bailey SL, et al: Strength of the quadriceps femoris muscle and functional recovery after reconstruction of the anterior cruciate ligament. A prospective, randomized clinical trial of electrical stimulation. *J Bone Joint Surg Am.* 1995;77:1166-1173.
[f]Data from Gould N, Donnermeyer BS, Pope M, et al: Transcutaneous muscle stimulation as a method to retard disuse atrophy. *Clin Orthop.* 1982;164:215-220.
[g]Data from Selkowitz DM: Improvement in isometric strength of quadriceps femoris muscle after training with electrical stimulation. *Phys Ther.* 1985;65:186-196.
[h]Data from Currier DP, Mann R: Muscular strength development by electrical stimulation in healthy individuals. *Phys Ther.* 1983;63:915-921.
[i]Data fromHooker DN: Electrical stimulating currents. In: Prentice WE, ed. *Therapeutic Modalities for Allied Health Professionals.* New York, NY: McGraw-Hill; 1998:73-133.

PRECAUTIONS WITH ELECTRICAL STIMULATION

- Allergies to tapes and gels
- Areas of absent or diminished sensation
- Electrically sensitive patients
- Placement of electrode over area of significant adipose tissue, near the stellate ganglion, over the temporal and orbital region, or over damaged skin

CONTRAINDICATIONS FOR ELECTRICAL STIMULATION

- The presence of any electronic implants (cardiac pacemaker, bladder stimulator, etc) in close proximity to the treatment area[63]
- Use over a carotid sinus (anterior transcervical area)
- Seizure disorders
- Phlebitis
- Malignancy
- Use over a pregnant uterus
- Cardiac arrhythmia
- Osteomyelitis

ELECTRICAL EQUIPMENT CARE AND MAINTENANCE

Electrical safety in the clinical setting is critical.

- The two-pronged plug has only two leads both of which carry some voltage—consequently the electrical device has no true ground (connected to the earth), and relies instead on the chassis or casing of the power source to act as a ground, which increases the potential for electrical shock.
- With three-pronged plugs, the third prong is grounded directly to the earth. Although three-pronged plugs generally work well in dry environments, they are unlikely to provide sufficient protection from electrical shock in a wet or damp area. In such instances, it is mandated that any equipment used in a wet or damp environment should be fitted with a ground fault interrupter (GFI).

> **Study Pearl**
>
> A GFI constantly compares the amount of electricity flowing from the wall outlet to the clinical unit with the amount returning to the outlet. If there is any leakage in the current flow detected, a ground fault circuit breaker will automatically interrupt current flow.

Other safety considerations include those listed in Table 18-14.

TRANSCUTANEOUS ELECTRICAL NERVE STIMULATION

Transcutaneous electrical nerve stimulation (TENS) is a safe, noninvasive, and drug-free method for treating various chronic and acute pain syndromes. TENS offers several modes of therapy depending on the

TABLE 18-14. SAFETY CONSIDERATIONS WHEN USING ELECTRICAL DEVICES

- The entire electrical system of the clinic should be designed or routinely evaluated by a qualified electrician.
- Equipment should be reevaluated on an annual basis and should conform to National Electrical Code guidelines. This includes the lead wires.
- Never assume that all three-pronged wall outlets are automatically grounded.
- Any defective equipment should be removed from the clinic immediately.
- Do not jerk plugs out of the wall by pulling on the cable.
- Extension cords or multiple adapters should never be used.

TABLE 18-15. TENS PARAMETERS AND EFFECTS

TYPE	FREQUENCY (Hz)	WIDTH (ms)	MUSCLE CONTRACTION
Conventional	> 80	~ 150	No
Low frequency (acupuncture)	< 10	> 150	Yes
Burst	< 10 (60-150 pps)	200-500	Yes
Brief intense	1-4	250+	No

parameters of electrical stimuli applied, resulting in different contributions of hyperemic, muscle-relaxing, and analgesic components of TENS (Table 18-15). TENS has been shown to be effective in providing pain relief in the early stages of healing following surgery,[64-69] and in the remodeling phase of tissue healing.[70-73]

The percentage of patients who benefit from short-term TENS pain intervention has been reported to range from 50% to 80%, with good long-term results with TENS observed in 6% to 44% of patients.[70,72,74,75] However, most of the TENS studies rely solely on subjective pain reports to establish efficacy and rarely on other outcome measures such as activity, socialization, or medication use.

TENS units typically deliver symmetrical or balanced asymmetrical biphasic waves of 100 to 500 ms pulse duration, with zero net current to minimize skin irritation,[76] and can be applied for extended periods.

Three modes of action are theorized for the efficacy of this modality:

- Spinal gating control through stimulation of the large myelinated A-alpha fibers inhibits transmission of the smaller pain transmitting unmyelinated C fibers, and myelinated A-delta fibers.[68,77] Current intensity must be adjusted to tolerance but should not cause a muscle contraction; pulse duration (width) should be 75 to 150 μs; pps should be 80 to 125.[63]
- Endogenous opiate control. When subjected to certain types of electrical stimulation of the sensory nerves, there may be a release of enkephalin from local sites within the CNS, and the release of β-endorphin from the pituitary gland into the cerebrospinal fluid.[76,78,79] Current intensity should be very high but a muscle contraction is not desirable; pulse duration (width) should be 10 ms; pps should be 80.[63]
- Central biasing. Intense electrical stimulation, approaching a noxious level, of the smaller C or pain fibers, produces a stimulation of the descending neurons. Current intensity should be high; a muscle contraction is acceptable; pulse duration should be 200 μs to 10 ms; pps should be between 1 and 5.[63] High voltage pulsed current should be used.

HIGH-VOLTAGE STIMULATION

High-volt current therapy, also referred to as high-voltage galvanic therapy or high-voltage pulsed galvanic stimulation (HVPGS), utilizes a twin peak (pair of monophasic spiked waveforms) monophasic, pulsed current. Because the waveform is fixed and small in duration,

TABLE 18-16. THE DIFFERENCES BETWEEN HIGH-VOLTAGE AND DIRECT CURRENT

HIGH-VOLTAGE	DIRECT CURRENT
Used to excite peripheral nerves	Ineffective in exciting peripheral nerves
Ineffective in exciting denervated tissues	Used to excite denervated tissues
Creates no measurable thermal reaction under the electrodes	Creates thermal and chemical reactions under the electrodes
Ineffective current for iontophoresis	Effective current for iontophoresis
Affects superficial and deep tissues	Affects only superficial tissues
Useful in discriminating between sensory, motor, and painful stimulation	Discrimination almost impossible and stimulation usually painful
Used to resolve many clinical pathologies	Restricted benefit to a limited number of clinical pathologies

Reproduced, with permission, from Pociask FD: Electrotherapy. In: Placzek JD, Boyce DA, eds. *Orthopaedic Physical Therapy Secrets.* Philadelphia, PA: Hanley & Belfus, Inc. 2001:60-74.

two peaks are required to depolarize nerve cells.[62] These units have a phase duration of 5 to 20 μs, a short pulse duration that ranges between 100 to 200 μs, and a voltage greater than 100 V to a maximum of 500 V, and a high peak current; however, the average current is only 50% of the peak current.[62] There is usually one large dispersive pad along with 1, 2, or 4 active electrodes, with the active electrode being much smaller than the dispersive electrode. A polarity switch typically is present and can be used to set the polarity of the active electrode.[62] The differences between high-voltage current therapy and direct current are listed in Table 18-16. HVPGS units are used for

- Wound management. Used as a therapy for pressure ulcers that fail to respond to conventional therapy, and for low oxygen chronic (ischemic) wounds. Has good strength of evidence rating. Electrotherapy improves oxygen perfusion by improving blood flow to damage skin areas. Electrotherapy is administered by placing two active electrodes and one return electrode in contact with the skins—one (cathode for bactericidal effect or anode if the wound is clean) in the wound bed and one on the skin a short distance away from the wound. A conductive dressing, such as wet gauze or hydrogel, is applied to the wound, and electrodes are placed over the area. After turning on the device, clinicians can increase polarity until the patient feels a tingling sensation. For large wounds, two small active electrodes are placed over the wound, with a conductive dressing between them. Electrotherapy is most effective when it is performed five days to seven days a week.[63]
- Pain management. Potential sites for electric placement used in the treatment of pain include[62]
  - At the site of pain
  - Over acupuncture points
  - Over trigger points
  - Over motor points related to the origin of pain
  - Along peripheral nerve roots
  - Paravertebral, even if the pain is only on one side
  - Contralateral to pain
  - Distal or proximal

- Soft tissue edema
- Muscle spasm
- Muscle weakness
- Specific conditions—Bell's palsy, levator ani syndrome

RUSSIAN CURRENT OR MEDIUM-FREQUENCY ALTERNATING CURRENT

Russian current is a medium-frequency polyphasic (AC) waveform. The intensity is produced in a burst mode that has a 50% duty cycle, with a pulse width range of 50 to 200 μs, and an interburst interval of 10 ms.[63] Medium-frequency currents can reduce resistance to current flow (when compared with low-frequency units that generate longer pulse durations) thus making this type of current more comfortable than some, especially if the current is delivered in bursts or if an interburst interval is used. Because medium frequency stimulation is capable and effective at stimulating deep and superficial tissues, Russian current is believed to augment muscle strengthening via polarizing both sensory and motor nerve fibers resulting in tetanic contractions that are painless and stronger than those made voluntarily by the patient.

INTERFERENTIAL CURRENT

Interferential current works by combining two high-frequency alternating waveforms that are biphasic, but that vary in relation to one another in amplitude, frequency, or both. Where these two distinct currents meet in the tissue, an electrical interference pattern is created based on the summation or the subtraction of the respective amplitudes or frequencies. Interferential current can be used for[63]

- Muscle contraction (20-50 pps) together with the overall shorter pulse widths (100-200 μs)
- Pain management: using a frequency of 50 to 120 pps and a pulse width of 50 to 150 μs
- Acustim pain relief: using a frequency of 1 pps

FUNCTIONAL ELECTRICAL STIMULATION

This form of electrical stimulation, a type of neuromuscular electrical stimulation (NMES) known as FES, is used primarily with patients who have sustained spinal cord injury or suffered a stroke. The unit, which utilizes multiple channel electrical stimulators and is controlled by a microprocessor, is used to recruit muscles in a programmed synergistic sequence that will allow the patient to accomplish a specific functional movement pattern.[63]

Electrical stimulation of the denervated muscle has been used in an attempt to maintain the muscle, however there is little documented evidence that supports this treatment option.

Typical parameters used include an interrupted or surged current with a frequency range of 20 to 40 pulses/s and an on time of 6 to 10 seconds followed by an off time of approximately 50 to 60 seconds in order to avoid immediate motor fatigue.[63] The treatment time is usually 15 to 20 minutes and can be repeated several times each day.

TRANSDERMAL IONTOPHORESIS

Transdermal iontophoresis is the administration of ionic therapeutic agents through the skin by the application of a low-level electric current. Iontophoresis has proved to be valuable in the intervention of musculoskeletal disorders. Iontophoresis causes an increased penetration of drugs and other compounds into tissues by the use of an applied current through the tissue.

Ionized medications or chemicals do not ordinarily penetrate tissues, and if they do, it is not normally at a rate rapid enough to achieve therapeutic levels.[80] This problem is overcome by providing a direct current energy source that provides penetration and transport.[80,81]

Iontophoresis has therefore been used for the controlled transdermal delivery of systemic drugs.[82] The various factors that can impact the transdermal iontophoretic transport include pH, the intensity of the current, or current density, at the active electrode, ionic strength, the concentration of the drug, molecular size and the duration of the current flow.

The proposed mechanisms by which iontophoresis increases drug penetration are[83]

- The electrical potential gradient induces changes at the cellular level.[84]
- Pore formation in the stratum corneum (SC), the outermost layer of the skin.[85]
- Hair follicles, sweat glands, and sweat ducts act as diffusion shunts for ion transport.[86]

It is important to remember the expected depth of penetration is only approximately 1 to 2 cm at best.[61]

A wide variety of chemicals can be used with iontophoresis (Table 18-17). Ideally, the clinician should shave any excessive hair and vigorously clean the skin area to be treated with isopropyl alcohol.

The positively charged ions are placed under the positive electrode, while the negatively charged ions are placed under the negative electrode so that the active electrode that contains the ions

Study Pearl

The principle behind iontophoresis is that an electrical potential difference will actively cause ions in solution to migrate according to their electrical charge.

Study Pearl

Negatively charged ions are repelled from a negative electrode (cathode) and attracted toward the positive electrode (anode). In contrast, the positive ions are repelled from the positive electrode and attracted toward the negative electrode.[80,81]

Study Pearl

Increasing the concentration of the drug does not increase the amount delivered to the target tissue. When the drug concentration becomes too high, the ions increase their attraction to one another, impeding the effect of the active electrode to push the drug across the tissue.[61]

TABLE 18-17. VARIOUS IONS USED IN IONTOPHORESIS

ION	POLARITY	SOLUTION	PURPOSE/CONDITION
Acetate	–	2%-5% acetic acid	Calcium deposits
Atropine sulfate	+	0.001%-0.01%	Hyperhidrosis
Calcium	+	2% calcium chloride	Myopathy, muscle spasm
Chlorine	–	2% sodium chloride	Scar tissue, adhesions
Copper	+	2% copper sulfate	Fungus infection
Dexamethasone	+	4 mg/mL dexamethasone Na-P	Tendonitis, bursitis
Lidocaine	+	4% lidocaine	Trigeminal neuralgia
Hyaluronidase	+	Wydase	Edema
Iodine	–	Iodex ointment	Adhesions, scar tissue
Magnesium	+	2% magnesium sulfate (Epsom salts)	Muscle relaxant, bursitis
Mecholyl	+	0.25%	Muscle relaxant
Potassium iodide	–	10%	Scar tissue
Salicylate	–	2% sodium salicylate	Myalgia, scar tissue
Tap water	+/–	—	Hyperhidrosis

+, positive; –, negative.

that are to be repelled is placed over the treatment tissue, and the depressive electrode is placed about 18 in away to encourage a greater depth of penetration.[61] Although electrons flow from negative to positive, regardless of electrode size, having a larger negative pad than the positive one will help shape the direction of flow. If the ionic source is an aqueous solution, it is recommended that a low concentration be used (2%-4%).[87]

The duration of the treatment may vary from 10 to 30 minutes. Longer durations produce a decrease in the skin impedance, thus increasing the likelihood of burns from an accumulation of ions under the electrodes.[88]

- An accumulation of negative ions under the positive electrode produces hydrochloric acid.
- An accumulation of positive ions under the negative electrode produces sodium hydroxide.

However, the causes of most burns include poor skin-electrode interface, setting the intensity too high, using the wrong polarity, or using electrodes that are too small, too dry, and with not enough of a size differential between the anode and cathode.[61]

Other complications have included prolonged erythema that resolved in 24 hours, tingling, burning, and pulling sensations that were especially apparent at the start of the current, or if the amperage was turned up too rapidly. The visible erythema demonstrates the clear increase of blood flow and the influence of the iontophoresis.

ELECTROMYOGRAPHIC BIOFEEDBACK

Electromyographic (EMG) biofeedback is a modality that uses an electromechanical device to provide visual and/or auditory feedback related to motor performance, kinesthetic performance or physiological response. Biofeedback units can be used to measure peripheral skin temperature, changes in blood volume through vasodilation, and vasoconstriction using finger phototransmission, sweat gland activity, or electrical activity during muscle contraction.[89]

Physical therapists primarily use biofeedback units for muscle reeducation:[89]

- The patient's skin is inspected and then the two active electrodes are placed parallel to the muscle fibers to be tested while being kept close to each other. The reference or ground electrode can be placed anywhere on the body.
- The sensitivity of the biofeedback unit is set at a low sensitivity setting and adjusted so that the patient can perform the repetitions at a ratio of two-thirds of the maximal muscle contraction.
- The patient is asked to perform isometric or functional contractions of the muscle. These contractions should continue for 6 to 10 seconds with relaxation in between each contraction. Treatment duration for a single muscle group is usually 5 to 10 minutes.
- As the patient improves with relaxation, the electrodes should be placed further apart, and the sensitivity setting increased.

ACOUSTIC RADIATION: ULTRASOUND

The acoustic spectrum is divided into three frequency ranges of infrasound, audible sound, and ultrasound. Ultrasound (US) is primarily used for its ability to deliver heat to deep musculoskeletal tissues such as tendon, muscle, and joint structures. The application of ultrasound requires a homogenous medium (mineral oil, water, commercial gel) for effective sound wave transmission and to act as a lubricant. US produces a high-frequency alternating current. The waves are delivered through the transducer, which has a metal face-plate with a piezoelectric crystal cemented between two electrodes. This crystal can vibrate very rapidly, converting electrical energy to acoustical (sound) energy (via the reverse piezoelectric effect) with little dispersion of energy. This energy leaves the transducer in a straight line (collimated beam). As the energy travels further from the transducer, the waves begin to diverge.

Ultrasound transducers come in a variety of sizes from 1 to 10 cm^2, although the 5 cm^2 size is the most common. The transducer size is selected relative to the size of the treat an area:

- 1 cm^2 squared = wrist; 5 cm^2 = shoulder, leg.
- The size of sound head: the recommended treatment area is only 2 to 3 times the size of the ERA.

The depth of penetration of the ultrasound depends on the absorption and scattering of the beam. Scar tissue, tendon and ligament demonstrate the highest absorption. Tissues that demonstrate poor absorption include bone, tendinous, and aponeurotic attachments of skeletal muscle, cartilaginous covering of joint surfaces and peripheral nerves lying close to bone.[92]

Clinical units typically deliver ultrasound of 85 KHz to 3 MHz, with duty cycles ranging from 20% to 100%, and intensities ranging between zero and 3 W/cm^2. The depth of penetration of the ultrasound is roughly inversely related to its frequency (Table 18-18).[93,94]

- 3 MHz is more superficial, reaching a depth of approximately 1 to 2 cm.
- 1 MHz is effective to a depth of 5 to 8 cm.[95]

Duty cycles less than 100% are usually termed pulsed ultrasound, while a 100% duty cycle is referred to as continuous ultrasound.

Study Pearl

- Beam nonuniformity ratio (BNR)[61]: the measure of the variability of the ultrasound wave intensity (W/cm^2) produced by the machine. The lower the ratio, the more uniform the machine, resulting in a more uniform treatment. Each transducer produces sound waves in response to the vibration of the crystal. This vibration has different intensities at points on the transducer head, having peaks and valleys of intensity. The greater ratio difference in the BNR, the more likely the transducer will have hot spots (areas of high intensity). A BNR of 5:1 means that the hot spots will have intensity 5 times greater than the intensity the unit is set to. High intensities have been shown to cause unstable cavitational effects (see later) and to retard tissue repair.[90,91] Moving the sound head or using pulsed ultrasound will tend to reduce the effect of the hotspot.
- Effective radiating area (ERA)[61]: the portion of the sound head that produces the sound wave is referred to as the effective radiating area (ERA). The ERA should be close to the size of the sound head or transducer. If it is smaller than the sound head, it may be misleading when treating.

TABLE 18-18. CHARACTERISTICS AND PHYSIOLOGICAL EFFECTS OF ULTRASOUND FREQUENCIES

FREQUENCY	CHARACTERISTICS	PHYSIOLOGICAL EFFECTS
1 MHz	Beam divergence Lower frequency Greater depth of penetration (5-8 cm) Less absorption of sound	Focus of ultrasound beam in the deeper tissues Can be used for phonophoresis
3 MHz	Parallel beam profile Faster frequency Less depth of penetration (1-2 cm) Greater absorption of sound	Increase in motor and sensory conduction velocities Increase in cell membrane permeability Increase in human skin fibroblasts

Both thermal and nonthermal effects are believed to be responsible for the therapeutic actions of ultrasonic energy. Continuous mode ultrasound produces a thermal effect, whereas pulsed ultrasound does not. The thermal effects of ultrasound are similar to those previously described for thermotherapy. The nonthermal or mechanical properties of US are less well defined, but are believed to involve an increase in cellular permeability and metabolism (known as cavitation and acoustic streaming), an increase in capillary density and improved blood flow, and may be important in the promotion of wound healing by increasing protein synthesis, reducing edema, pain, and muscle spasms.[90,96-98]

Intensities of 0.1 to 0.3 W/cm^2 are recommended for acute lesions, while intensities of 0.4 to 0.8 cm^2 are recommended for the chronic lesions (Table 18-19).[99] The term *spatial average intensity* is used as the measurement in documenting ultrasound treatments and is calculated by dividing the total power (watts) by the area (cm^2) of the transducer head. One study[100] demonstrated that to achieve a tissue temperature rise of 4°C in human muscle, using continuous ultrasound, the following parameters and application times are necessary:

- 1 MHz at 1.5 W/cm^2 for 13 minutes
- 3 MHz at 1.5 W/cm^2 for 4.5 minutes

Study Pearl

It must be remembered that the effects of ultrasound are predominantly empirical and are based on reported biophysical effects within tissue,[101,102] and on anecdotal experience in clinical practice.[103-105]

Treatment times for ultrasound are based on the principle of 1 minute of ultrasound per treatment head area, though account must be taken of the pulse ratio employed. Theoretically, the pulse ratio needs to be higher for the more acute lesions (1:4) and lower for the more chronic (1:1, or continuous).

Despite the paucity of documented evidence in terms of randomized control studies,[106] many benefits have been ascribed to ultrasound. These include

- The production of cellular excitation, enhancing cellular activity rather than dampening it, and enhancing the inflammatory cascade, thereby encouraging the tissues to move into their next phase.[92,107-109]
- Decreased swelling when applied in a pulsed format during the inflammatory stage of healing.[99,101,102,110-115]
- Stimulation of the active cells and a maximization of scar production activity and quality, if applied during the neurovascular phase.[115-117] During the later phase, ultrasound appears to enhance the remodeling of tissue.[91,113,116]

An alteration of the parameters of ultrasound changes the intent of the intervention (Table 18-19).[118]

TABLE 18-19. CLINICAL DOSAGES FOR ULTRASOUND

INTENSITY (W/CM^2)	PURPOSE
0.1-1.0	Wound healing
0.5-1.0	Pain and spasm relief
0.5-1.5	Hematoma resorption
1.0-1.5	Increase plasticity of scar and connective tissue

INDICATIONS

The indications for ultrasound are to modulate pain, increase connective tissue extensibility, reduce or eliminate soft tissue and joint restriction and muscle spasm.[119] Precautions include acute inflammation, breast implants, open epiphysis and healing fractures.[119]

CONTRAINDICATIONS

Contraindications include healing fractures, impaired circulation, impaired cognitive function, impaired sensation, thrombophlebitis, plastic components, over vital areas such as the brain, ear, eyes, heart, cervical ganglia, carotid sinuses, reproductive organs, spinal cord, over cardiac pacemakers or pregnant uterus.[119]

APPLICATION AND PATIENT PREPARATION

Ultrasound can be applied directly or indirectly[119]:

- Direct contact (transducer-skin interface): used on relatively flat areas. The clinician applies generous amounts of coupling medium (gel/cream) to the treatment area and then selects an appropriate sound head size (ERA should be one half the size of the treatment area). The area covered should not be greater than 2 to 3 times the size of the affecting radiating area (ERA) for 5 minutes of treatment. The transducer is placed at right angles to the skin surface, and the clinician sets the intensity to the desired level while moving the sound head slowly (approximately 1.5 in/s) in overlapping circles or longitudinal strokes while maintaining the sound head-body surface angle. Periosteal pain occurring during treatment may be due to any of the following: high intensity, momentary slowing, or cessation of the moving head. The treatment time varies according to the previously mentioned factors, but is typically 3 to 10 minutes.
- Indirect contact (water immersion): the application of ultrasound over irregular body parts. The clinician fills a plastic container (it reflects less acoustic energy than a metal one) with water high enough to cover the treatment area. The body part to be treated and transducer are immersed in the water. The transducer is kept 1/2 to 1 in from the skin surface and at right angles to the body part being treated. The clinician moves the sound head slowly while turning up the intensity to the desired level. If a stationary technique is being applied, the clinician should reduce the intensity. It may be necessary to periodically wipe off any air bubbles that may form on the sound head or body part during treatment.

PHONOPHORESIS

Phonophoresis is a specific type of US application in which pharmacological agents are driven transdermally into the subcutaneous tissues.[111,120-126] Both the thermal and mechanical properties of US have been cited as possible mechanisms for the penetration of the pharmacological agents.[111,121,122]

Study Pearl

- Ions are introduced with iontophoresis
- Molecules are introduced by phonophoresis

The efficacy of phonophoresis has not been conclusively established. The proposed indications include pain modulation, and to decrease inflammation in subacute and chronic musculoskeletal conditions. The method of application for phonophoresis is similar to that used in the direct technique method of ultrasound, except that a medicinal agent is used as, or is, part of the coupling medium, which must itself transmit the US beam. The typical treatment lasts 5 to 10 minutes and uses an intensity of 1 to 3 W/cm^2. Using lower intensities and a longer treatment time are thought to be more effective for introducing medication into the skin.

MECHANICAL MODALITIES

PROLOTHERAPY

Prolotherapy, also known as proliferation therapy, is a relatively controversial pain management technique that may be used as an intervention for degenerative or chronic injury to ligaments, tendons, fascia, and joint capsular tissue.[127-129] Although prolotherapy, is not administered by physical therapists, patients seen in the clinic may have received a course of prolotherapy from their physician and is thus included for completeness. Prolotherapy is purported to allow rapid production of new collagen and cartilage through stimulation of the immune system's healing mechanism using injections of mild chemical or natural irritants, such as dextrose sugar, manganese, and glucosamine sulfate.[130] The number of injections required per interventions are based on the type of injury.[127-129]

SPINAL TRACTION

Spinal traction involves the use of a distraction force applied to the spine to:

- Separate or attempt to separate the articular surfaces between the zygapophysial joints, and the vertebral bodies, thereby decreasing joint stiffness through a joint mobilization effect.
- Tense the ligamentous structures of the spinal segment.
- Widen the intervertebral foramen and release pressure from a spinal nerve. Adjunct treatments to be used in the lumbar spine include flexion exercises and positioning.
- Temporarily straighten the spinal curves.
- Improve nutrition to the intervertebral disk through intermittent distraction.
- Reduce disk herniation.
- Apply stretch to spinal musculature to help decrease muscle spasm.

The relative degree of flexion or extension of the spine during the applied traction force determines which of these effects are most pronounced. For example:

- Greater separation of the intervertebral foramen is achieved with the spine in a flexed position.
- Greater separation of the disk space is achieved with the spine in a neutral position.

A number of methods can be employed to apply a distraction through the spine including positional, autotraction, manual traction, and inversion/gravity assisted techniques, but this discussion will focus on the use of mechanical traction, which can be continuous or intermittent, as this is the most common method.

Some of the precautions with mechanical traction include acute inflammation aggravated by distraction, acute strains and sprains, claustrophobia, joint instability, osteoporosis, pregnancy (in lumbar traction) TMJ problems with halter use (in cervical traction). Contraindications to mechanical traction include impaired cognitive function, rheumatoid arthritis, spinal tumors, spinal infections, spondylolisthesis, vascular compromise, and very old or young patients.

Study Pearl

The VAX-D (VAX-D Medical Technologies USA, Palm Harbor, FL) and DRS (Professional Distribution Systems, Inc, Boca Raton, FL) systems are examples of relatively expensive traction devices that are marketed as decompression devices.[131] Decompression is simply unweighting due to distraction and positioning and is essentially a synonym for traction.[131]

Application and Patient Preparation for Cervical Traction

Cervical traction can be applied with the patient sitting or supine, although the supine position is generally preferred.

If using intermittent traction, a duty cycle of either 1:1 or 3:1 is used, and the treatment time varies according to condition—5 to 10 minutes are recommended for acute conditions and disk protrusion, 15 to 30 minutes are recommended for other conditions.[132-134] Weights of 25 to 40 lb appear necessary to produce vertebral separation with cervical traction.[131] Less force appears to be necessary when treatment is directed to the upper cervical area.[131]

Two methods of cervical traction can be used: the halter method, or the use of the sliding device (The Saunders Group, Inc, Chaska, MN). The halter device should not be used with patients with TMJ dysfunction or with patients who suffer from claustrophobia. The traction force used is determined by the treatment goals and by patient tolerance:

Study Pearl

Compression or narrowing of the joint space occurs with cervical traction applied in the sitting position. When the same force is applied in supine, separation is noted.[131]

Acute Phase. Approximately 10 to 15 lb or 7% to 10% of the patient's body weight is recommended to treat disk protrusions, muscle spasm, and to elongate soft tissue.[132-134]

Halter Method. The head halter is placed under the occiput and the mandible, and is then attached to the traction cord directly, or to the traction unit through a spreader bar.

The clinician removes the slack within the cord while maintaining the patient's neck in approximately 20 to 30 degrees of flexion, using a pillow if necessary.[132-134] It is possible to apply traction more specifically by varying the angle of neck flexion.[132-134]:

The clinician should ensure that the traction force is applied to the occipital region and not to the mandible, and that the patient can tolerate neck position.

Sliding Device. The clinician places the patient's head on the padded headrest, which positions the cervical spine in 20 to 30 degrees of flexion.

- The clinician adjusts the neck yoke so that it fits firmly just below the mastoid processes.
- A head strap is typically used across the forehead to secure the head in place.

- The clinician attaches the sliding device to the spreader bar.
- The clinician chooses between a continuous or intermittent mode.

The total treatment times to be used in cervical traction are only partially research-based and can range from 5 to 30 minutes. The number of traction sessions that are necessary to achieve optimum results varies. Justification to continue includes demonstration by the patient of consistent, progressive improvement. Home traction units can be prescribed for the more chronic cases to help self-manage flare-ups and increase function.

Application and Patient Preparation for Lumbar Traction

A split table is a prerequisite for effective lumbar traction so as to eliminate friction between body segments and the table surface. Additionally, a nonslip traction harness is required to transfer the traction force comfortably to the patient while stabilizing the trunk during the traction. The patient should be suitably disrobed as clothing between the harness and the skin promotes slipping.

The pelvic harness is applied with the patient standing next to the traction table so that the contact pads and upper belt are at or just above the level of the iliac crest. The contact pads are adjusted so that the harness loops provide a posteriorly directed pull, encouraging lumbar flexion. The rib belt is then applied so that the rib pads are positioned over the lower rib cage in a comfortable manner. The rib belt is then fitted snugly and the patient is asked to lie on the table:

- For disk protrusions the patient is positioned in the prone position with a normal to slightly flattened lumbar lordosis.
- For spinal stenosis, a neutral spine position allows for the largest intervertebral foramen opening.
- In the supine position, the hip position can affect vertebral separation—as hip flexion increases from 0 to 90 degrees, the traction produces a greater posterior intervertebral separation. Overall, patient positioning should be determined by patient needs and comfort.
- A call bell or cutoff switch is issued to the patient, and the patient should be closely monitored for any adverse reaction.
- The clinician chooses between a continuous or intermittent mode.

The total treatment times to be used in lumbar traction are only partially research-based and can range from 5 to 30 minutes.[135-137] The traction force necessary to cause effective vertebral separation varies (approximately 50% of the patient's body weight).[135-137] Following the treatment session, the patient is reexamined and any changes in their symptoms are noted so that the parameters for the next session can be determined, or the decision can be made to discontinue the traction if there was an adverse reaction. The number of traction sessions that are necessary to achieve optimum results varies. Justification to continue includes demonstration by the patient of consistent, progressive improvement. Home traction units can be prescribed for the more chronic cases to help self-manage flare-ups and increase function.

CONTINUOUS PASSIVE MOTION

Continuous passive motion (CPM) is a postoperative treatment method that is designed to aid recovery after joint surgery, tendon or ligament repair, or post immobilization from a fracture, by passively moving the joint within limits set by the physician. Once the patient is able to participate in physical therapy, the CPM may be no longer medically necessary, although this is not conclusive.

Indications

- Decrease soft tissue stiffness
- Increase range of motion
- Promote healing of the joint surfaces (promotes cartilage growth) and soft tissue
- Prevention of adhesions

Contraindications

- Nonstable fracture sites
- Excessive edema
- Patient intolerance

Application and Patient Preparation. The procedure is explained to the patient. Any wound area must be covered. The clinician adjusts the unit so that the patient's anatomical joint is aligned with the mechanical hinge joint of the machine. The patient's limb is secured in the machine using the safety straps. The clinician sets the beginning and end range of motion degrees, and then turns the unit on. The patient is monitored during the first few minutes to ensure correct fit and patient comfort. Treatment duration varies from 1 hour a day to 24 hours a day, depending on physician preference. Range of motion is typically progressed at 5 to 10 degrees every 24 hours, based on patient tolerance.

TILT TABLE

The tilt table is used to evaluate how a patient regulates blood pressure in response to simple stresses, including gravity. The tilt table was originally designed to evaluate patients with fainting spells (syncope), but may also be useful for patients who have symptoms of severe lightheadedness or dizziness.

- The patient is asked to lie supine on the tilt table and is secured by a series of straps or belts around the hips, knees, and trunk if needed.
- Baseline data is recorded including pulse rate, blood pressure, and subjective reports.
- The table is raised up to a 30-degrees angle so that the head is above the feet.
- The patient is maintained in this position for proximally 5 minutes.
- The patient's pulse rate, blood pressure, and subjective reports are noted. If the patient experienced no adverse effects at 30 degrees, the tilt table is raised to 60 degrees.
- The new position is maintained for about 45 minutes based on tolerance (because many of the patients that develop a

TABLE 18-20. INDICATIONS FOR MANUAL MODALITIES

- Mild pain.
- A nonirritable condition, demonstrated by pain that is provoked by motion but that disappears very quickly
- Intermittent musculoskeletal pain
- Pain reported by the patient that is relieved by rest
- Pain reported by the patient that is relieved or provoked by particular motions or positions
- Pain that is altered by postural changes

sudden drop in their blood pressure do so after 30 minutes) during which time the vital signs and subjective reports are recorded.

Over a period of time, or sessions, the tilt table is raised further while monitoring both vital signs and subjective reports.

MANUAL MODALITIES

See Tables 18-20 and 18-21.

TABLE 18-21. CONTRAINDICATIONS FOR MANUAL MODALITIES

Absolute

- Bacterial infection
- Malignancy
- Systemic localized infection
- Sutures over the area
- Recent fracture
- Cellulitis
- Febrile state
- Hematoma
- Acute circulatory condition
- An open wound at the treatment site
- Osteomyelitis
- Advanced diabetes
- Hypersensitivity of the skin
- Inappropriate end-feel (spasm, empty, bony)
- Constant, severe pain, including pain that disturbs sleep, indicating that the condition is likely to be in the acute stage of healing
- Extensive radiation of pain
- Pain unrelieved by rest
- Severe irritability (pain that is easily provoked, and that does not go away within a few hours)

Relative

- Joint effusion or inflammation
- Rheumatoid arthritis
- Presence of neurologic signs
- Osteoporosis
- Hypermobility
- Pregnancy, if technique is to be applied to the spine
- Dizziness
- Steroid or anticoagulant therapy

MASSAGE

Massage is a mechanical modality that produces physiologic effects through different types of stroking, kneading rubbing, slapping, and vibration:

- Reflexive effects: an autonomic nervous system phenomenon produced through stimulation of the sensory receptors in the skin and superficial fascia. Causes sedation, relieves tension, increases blood flow.
- Pain reduction: most likely regulated by both the gate control theory and through the release of endogenous opiates.
- Circulatory effects: increases lymphatic and blood flow.
- Metabolism: indirectly affects metabolism due to the increase in lymphatic and blood flow.
- Mechanical effects: stretching of the intramuscular connective tissue, retard muscle atrophy, increase range of motion.
- Skin: increasing skin temperature and decreased skin resistance to galvanic current.

Indications

- Increase coordination
- Decrease pain
- Decreased neuromuscular excitability
- Stimulate circulation
- Facilitate healing
- Restore joint mobility
- Remove lactic acid
- Alleviate muscle cramps
- Increase blood flow
- Increase venous return
- Breaking adhesions
- Myositis, bursitis, fibrositis, tendonitis
- Intermittent claudication

Contraindications

- Arteriosclerosis
- Thrombosis
- Embolism
- Severe varicose veins
- Acute phlebitis, cellulitis, synovitis
- Skin infections
- Malignancies
- Acute inflammatory conditions

Specific Massage Techniques

Hoffa, Classic, or Swedish. A classical massage technique that uses a variety of superficial strokes, including

- Effleurage: produces a reflexive response. Effleurage is typically performed at the beginning and at the end of a massage to allow the patient to relax. Massage is begun at the peripheral areas and moves from the extremity toward the heart. At the beginning of the massage, the pressure should be light, using flat hands with fingers slightly bent and thumbs spread apart. In the course of the massage, the pressure can be increased. The direction of the strokes should be toward the heart.

- Petrissage: described as a kneading or working stroke, which is directed primarily at the muscle system—the muscle being squeezed and rolled under the clinician's hands. Applied in a distal to proximal sequence, petrissage is used primarily for
  - Increasing the local blood supply
  - Reduction of edema.
  - Loosening of adhesions.
  - Improving lymphatic return.
  - Removal of metabolic waste.
- Rubbing (friction): used primarily in areas of local, deep lying hardening and myogelosis to produce a strong, hyperemic effect in small surface areas of the muscle. The motion applied is circular to elliptical, or transverse (transverse frictional massage).
- Tapotment/percussion: a massage technique that provides stimulation to rapid and alternating movements such as tapping, hacking, cupping, and slapping to enhance circulation and stimulate peripheral nerve endings. This type of massage is used almost exclusively for the athletic population.
- Vibration: manual vibration, which is particularly strenuous for the clinician involves a rapid shaking motion that causes vibration to the treatment area. This type of massage is used primarily for relaxation, but can also have a stimulating effect.
- Manual lymphatic drainage (MLD) according to the Vodder and/or Leduc techniques is a gentle technique that stimulates superficial lymphatics and reroutes lymph toward healthy lymphatic vessels. MLD is designed to clear the healthy quadrant (central areas), and then progress systematically down the involved extremity. The approach involves combining a number of strokes, described as stationary circles, pumping, scooping, and rotary strokes. Each stroke consists of a working (stretching) and resting phase, where the pressure is smoothly increased then decreased. Each stroke lasts at least one second and is repeated 5 to 7 times, and all strokes are applied in the direction of lymph flow. In those areas where there is congestion or obstruction caused by surgery, trauma, or radiation, strokes are applied toward the intact lymphatic pathways. MLD may be used in cases of high-protein edema, such as postsurgical swelling, wounds that do not heal because of chronic swelling, and to promote a sympathetic and parasympathetic response in those patients who experience chronic pain. Compression garments are essential between treatments. Contraindications to this form of therapy include congestive heart failure, deep vein thrombosis, and active infection.

JOINT MOBILIZATIONS

The techniques of joint mobilization are used to improve joint mobility or to decrease joint pain by restoring accessory movements to the joint and thus allow full, nonrestricted, pain-free range of motion. Additional benefits attributed to joint mobilizations include decreasing muscle guarding, lengthening the tissue around a joint, neuromuscular influences on muscle tone, and increased proprioceptive awareness.[139,140]

Consideration must be given to the stage at healing, the direction of force, and the magnitude of force. Joint mobilizations should be performed with the joint in the loose-packed or open-packed position (Table 18-22). Joint mobilizations are applied in a direction that is either parallel or perpendicular to the treatment plane to restore the physiological articular relationship within a joint, and to decrease pain (Table 18-23).[141]

To apply joint mobilizations, a number of components can be utilized, depending on the method employed:

- Direct method. An engagement is made against a barrier in several planes.
- Indirect method. Maigne[142] postulated "the concept of painless and opposite motion" where disengagement from the barrier occurs and a balance of ligamentous tension is sought.

Study Pearl

The primary indications for joint mobilizations are
- Limited passive range of motion
- Limited joint accessory motion as determined with joint mobility testing
- Tissue texture abnormality in the area of dysfunction
- Pain
- If the symptoms are aggravated by activity but relieved by rest

TABLE 18-22. SHAPE, RESTING POSITION AND TREATMENT PLANES OF THE JOINTS

JOINT	CONVEX SURFACE	CONCAVE SURFACE	RESTING POSITION	TREATMENT PLANE
Sternoclavicular	Clavicle[a]	Sternum[a]	Arm resting by side	In sternum
Acromioclavicular	Clavicle	Acromion	Arm resting by side	In acromion
Glenohumeral	Humerus	Glenoid	55 degrees of abduction, 30 degrees of horizontal adduction	In glenoid fossa in scapular plane
Humeroradial	Humerus	Radius	Elbow extended, forearm supinated	In radial head perpendicular to long axis of radius
Humeroulnar	Humerus	Ulna	70 degrees of elbow flexion, 10 degrees of forearm supination	In olecranon fossa, 45 degrees to long axis of ulna
Radioulnar (proximal)	Radius	Ulna	70 degrees of elbow flexion, 35 degrees of forearm supination	In radial notch of ulna, parallel to long axis of ulna
Radioulnar (distal)	Ulnar	Radius	Supinated 10 degrees	In radius, parallel to long axis of radius
Radiocarpal	Proximal carpal bones	Radius	Line through radius and third metacarpal	In radius, perpendicular to long axis of radius
Metacarpophalangeal	Metacarpal	Proximal phalanx	Slight flexion	In proximal phalanx
Interphalangeal	Proximal phalanx	Distal phalanx	Slight flexion	In proximal phalanx
Hip	Femur	Acetabulum	Hip flexed 30 degrees, abducted 30 degrees, slight external rotation	In acetabulum
Tibiofemoral	Femur	Tibia	Flexed 25 degrees	On surface of tibial plateau
Patellofemoral	Patella	Femur	Knee in full extension	Along femoral groove
Talocrural	Talus	Mortise	Plantarflexed 10 degrees	In the mortise in anterior/posterior direction
Subtalar	Calcaneus	Talus	Subtalar neutral between inversion/eversion	In talus, parallel to foot surface
Intertarsal	Proximal articulating surface	Distal articulating surface	Foot relaxed	In distal segment
Metatarsophalangeal	Tarsal bone	Proximal phalanx	Slight extension	In proximal phalanx
Interphalangeal	Proximal phalanx	Distal phalanx	Slight flexion	In distal phalanx

[a]In the sternoclavicular joint the clavicle surface is convex in a superior/inferior direction and concave in anterior/posterior direction.
Reproduced, with permission, from Prentice WE: Joint mobilization and traction. In: Prentice WE, ed. *Therapeutic Modalities for Allied Health Professionals*. New York, NY: McGraw-Hill. 1998:443-478.

TABLE 18-23. INDICATIONS FOR GENTLE VERSUS VIGOROUS MOBILIZATIONS

TYPE OF MOBILIZATION	INDICATIONS
Gentle (performed in the pain-free range)	From the history:
	Significant joint irritability
	Pain with most or all movements (consider immobilization)
	Pain with a specific posture
	Limb pain
	Difficulty sleeping
	Distal pain with coughing or sneezing
	Muscle spasm protecting the joint
	From the physical examination:
	Pain sufficient to produce facial distortion
	Spinal movement produces distal limb symptoms
	Pain/paresthesia that increases after testing
	Significant increase in pain with gentle testing
	Presence of a neurological deficit
Vigorous	From the history:
	Moderate pain that has been static for some time
	Symptoms that are not aggravated much by joint motion
	Symptoms do not linger following aggravation
	No difficulty sleeping
	Minimal distal pain
	No pain with coughing or sneezing
	Symptoms not aggravated by a specific posture
	No protective muscle spasm
	From the physical examination:
	Joint irritability minimal with no muscle guarding on movement
	Limited mobility testing, but does not aggravate symptoms
	No neurological deficit
	Motion limited by tissue tension rather than pain

- Combined method. Disengagement is followed by direct retracement of the motion.

Rationale for Joint Mobilizations

1. Need to restore motion and strength to the connective tissues that have been altered by injury, inflammation, and/or immobilization.
2. Motion and strength must be restored without reinjuring the connective tissues since this will result in further information.
3. The force used must be controlled with the intention of
   - Stimulating cellular activity—collagen and proteoglycan
   - Producing extracellular change—realignment of old fibers, increase in length of fibers, increase of interfiber distance and lubrication, proper orientation of new fibers
4. Restoration of flexibility.

TABLE 18-24. APPROPRIATE TECHNIQUE BASED ON BARRIER TO MOTION AND END-FEEL

BARRIER	END-FEEL	TECHNIQUE
Pain	Empty	None
Pain	Spasm	None
Pain	Capsular	Oscillations
Joint adhesions	Early capsular	Passive articular motion stretch
Muscle adhesions	Early elastic	Passive physiologic motion stretch
Hypertonicity	Facilitation	Hold-relax
Bone	Bony	None

Grades of Mobilization. See Table 18-24.

Kaltenborn. Kaltenborn's techniques use a combination of traction and mobilization to reduce pain and mobilize hypomobile joints. Three grades of traction are defined:

- Grade I—Piccolo (loosen). This involves a distraction force that neutralizes pressure in the joint without producing any actual separation of the joint surfaces. This grade of distraction is used to reduce the compressive forces on the articular surfaces, and is used both in the initial intervention session, and with all of the mobilization grades. Grade I techniques are used in the inflammatory stage of healing.
- Grade II (take up the slack). This grade of distraction separates the articulating surfaces and eliminates the play in the joint capsule.
- Grade III (stretch). This grade of distraction actually stretches the joint capsule and the soft tissues surrounding the joint to increase mobility. Grade III traction is used in conjunction with mobilization glides according the convex-concave rules to treat joint hypomobility.[143] These techniques are typically used during the remodeling stage of healing.

Study Pearl

Kaltenborn's Piccolo and Slack movements are generally used in the treatment of joint problems in which the predominant feature is pain, while Stretch is used to improve range of motion in a joint condition whose predominant feature is stiffness.

Maitland. Maitland described five grades of joint mobilization/oscillations, each of which falls within the available range of motion that exists at the joint—a point somewhere between the beginning point and the anatomic limit. Although the relationship that exists between the five grades in terms of their positions within the range of motion is always constant, the point of limitation shifts further to the left as the severity of the motion limitation increases.

- Grade I: a small amplitude movement at the beginning of the range of movement.
- Grade II: a large amplitude movement within the mid range of movement.
- Grade III: a large amplitude movement up to the physiological limit in the range of movement.
- Grade IV: a small amplitude movement at the very end of the range of movement.
- Grade V: small amplitude, quick thrust delivered at the end of the range of movement, usually accompanied by a popping sound, which is called a manipulation.

Maitland's grades I and II are used solely for pain relief and have no direct mechanical effect on the restricting barrier but do have a hydrodynamic effect. Grade I and II joint mobilizations are theoretically effective in pain reduction by improving joint lubrication and circulation in tissues related to the joint.[144,145] Rhythmic joint oscillations also possibly activate articular and skin mechanoreceptors that play a role in pain reduction.[146,147]

Maitland's grades III and IV (or at least III+ and IV+) do stretch the barrier and have a mechanical, as well as a neurophysiological effect. Grade III and IV joint distractions and stretching mobilizations may, in addition to the above-stated effects, activate inhibitory joint and muscle spindle receptors, which aid in reducing restriction to movement.[144-147]

Whichever technique or grade is employed, a number of further considerations help guide the clinician.

- The patient is placed in the position of maximum comfort and should be relaxed.
- The position of the joint to be treated must be appropriate for the stage of healing and the skill of the operator:
  - The resting position is used for the acute stage and/or inexperienced operator
  - Other starting positions may be employed by a skilled operator in the nonacute stages.
- The operator must be in a position that employs good body mechanics and utilizes gravity as an assist to the mobilization whenever possible.
- One half of the joint should be stabilized while the other half is mobilized. Both the stabilizing and mobilizing hands should be placed as close as possible to the joint line. The other parts of the clinician involved in the mobilization should make maximum contact with the patient's body to spread the forces over a larger area and reduce pain from contact of bony prominences. The maximum contact also results in more stability and increased confidence from the patient. An alternative technique, which produces the desired results, must be sought if the contact between opposite sexes is uncomfortable to either the patient or the clinician.
- The direction of the mobilization is almost always parallel or perpendicular to a tangent across adjoining joint surfaces, and is appropriate for the arthrokinematics of the joint being treated.
- The mobilization should not move into or through the point of pain throughout the duration of the technique.
- The velocity and amplitude of movement is carefully considered and is based on the goal of the intervention, to restore the joint motion or to alleviate the pain, or both.
- Slow stretches are used for large capsular restrictions.
- Fast oscillations are used for minor restrictions.
- One movement is performed at a time, at one joint at a time.
- The patient is reassessed after a few movements if the joint is in the acute stage of healing, less frequently for other stages of healing.
  - The intervention should be discontinued for the day when a large improvement has been obtained or when the improvement ceases.

Muscle re-education is essential after mobilization or manipulation and often produces a noticeable reduction in posttreatment soreness. While the joint is maintained in the new range, five to six gentle isometric contractions are asked for from the agonists and antagonists of the motion mobilized.[148]

Questions for this chapter and the entire book appear on the included CD-ROM, with additional questions at www.DuttonNPTE.com.

REFERENCES

1. Clarke R, Mellon R, Lind A: Vascular reactions of the human forearm to cold. *Clin Sci.* 1958;17:165-179.
2. Fox RH: Local cooling in man. *Br Med Bull.* 1961;17:14-18.
3. Kalenak A, Medlar CE, Fleagle SB, et al: Athletic injuries: heat vs cold. *Am Fam Phys.* 1975;12:131-134.
4. Zemke JE, Andersen JC, Guion WK, et al: Intramuscular temperature responses in the human leg to two forms of cryotherapy: ice massage and ice bag. *J Orthop Sports Phys Ther.* 1998; 27:301-307.
5. Mack GW: Assessment of cutaneous blood flow by using topographical perfusion mapping techniques. *J Appl Physiol.* 1998;85:353-359.
6. Scotto G, Miniaci MC, Silipo F, et al: Reduction of cutaneous blood flow in cold fingers. *Boll Soc Ital Biol Sper.* 1998;74:35-41.
7. Vayssairat M, Chabbert-Buffet N, Gaitz JP, et al: Measurement of the cutaneous blood flow reserve in normal humans by laser-Doppler flowmetry. *Int Angiol.* 2004;23:255-258.
8. Olson JE, Stravino VD: A review of cryotherapy. *Phys Ther.* 1972;52:840-853.
9. Bell GW, Prentice WE: Infrared modalities. In: Prentice WE, ed. *Therapeutic Modalities for Allied Health Professionals.* New York, NY: McGraw-Hill. 1998:201-262.
10. Knight KL: *Cryotherapy: Theory, Technique, and Physiology.* Chattanooga, TN: Chattanooga Corp. 1985.
11. Hocutt JE, Jaffee R, Rylander R, et al: Cryotherapy in ankle sprains. *Am J Sports Med.* 1982;10:316-319.
12. Quillen WS, Rouillier LH: Initial management of acute ankle sprains with rapid pulsed pneumatic compression and cold. *J Orthop Sports Phys Ther.* 1981;4:39-43.
13. Starkey JA: Treatment of ankle sprains by simultaneous use of intermittent compression and ice packs. *Am J Sports Med.* 1976;4:142-143.
14. Wilkerson GB: Treatment of ankle sprains with external compression and early mobilization. *Phys Sports Med.* 1985;13:83-90.
15. Lamboni P, Harris B: The use of ice, air splints, and high voltage galvanic stimulation in effusion reduction. *Athl Training.* 1983; 18:23-25.
16. McMaster WC: Cryotherapy. *Phys Sports Med.* 1982;10:112-119.
17. McMaster WC, Liddle S, Waugh TR: Laboratory evaluation of various cold therapy modalities. *Am J Sports Med.* 1978;6:291-294.

18. Cote DJ, Prentice WE, Jr., Hooker DN, et al: Comparison of three treatment procedures for minimizing ankle sprain swelling. *Phys Ther.* 1988;68:1072-1076.
19. Daniel DM, Stone ML, Arendt DL: The effect of cold therapy on pain, swelling, and range of motion after anterior cruciate ligament reconstructive surgery. *Arthroscopy.* 1994;10:530-533.
20. Konrath GA, Lock T, Goitz HT, et al: The use of cold therapy after anterior cruciate ligament reconstruction. A prospective randomized study and literature review. *Am J Sports Med.* 1996;24:629-633.
21. Michlovitz SL: The use of heat and cold in the management of rheumatic diseases. In: Michlovitz SL, ed. *Thermal Agents in Rehabilitation.* Philadelphia, PA: FA Davis. 1990:158-174.
22. Speer KP, Warren RF, Horowitz L: The efficacy of cryotherapy in the postoperative shoulder. *J Shoulder Elbow Surg.* 1996;5:62-68.
23. Knight KL: *Cryotherapy in Sports Injury Management.* Champaign, IL: Human Kinetics. 1995.
24. Kellett J: Acute soft tissue injuries: a review of the literature. *Med Sci Sports Exerc.* 1986;18:5.
25. Knight KL, Aquino J, Johannes SM, et al: A re-examination of Lewis' cold induced vasodilation in the finger and ankle. *Athl Training.* 1980;15:248-250.
26. Knight KL, Londeree BR: Comparison of blood flow in the ankle of uninjured subjects during therapeutic applications of heat, cold, and exercise. *Med Sci Sports Exerc.* 1980;12:76-80.
27. McMaster WC: A literary review on ice therapy in injuries. *Am J Sports Med.* 1977;5:124-126.
28. Hartviksen K: Ice therapy in spasticity. *Acta Neurol Scand.* 1962;3(suppl):79-84.
29. Basset SW, Lake BM: Use of cold applications in the management of spasticity. *Phys Ther Rev.* 1958;38:333-334.
30. Knutsson E: Topical cryotherapy in spasticity. *Scand J Rehabil Med.* 1970;2:159-163.
31. Waylonis GW: The physiological effects of ice massage. *Arch Phys Med Rehabil.* 1967;48:42-47.
32. Nehme AE, Warfield CA: Cryoanalgesia: freezing of peripheral nerves. *Hosp Pract (Off Ed).* 1987;22:71-72, 77.
33. Marsland AR, Ramamurthy S, Barnes J: Cryogenic damage to peripheral nerves and blood vessels in the rat. *Br J Anaesth.* 1983;55:555-558.
34. Doucette SA, Goble EM: The effect of exercise on patellar tracking in lateral patellar compression syndrome. *Am J Sports Med.* 1992;20:434-440.
35. Fisher RL: Conservative treatment of patellofemoral pain. *Orthop Clin North Am.* 1986;17:269-272.
36. Meeusen R, Lievens P: The use of cryotherapy in sports injuries. *Sports Med.* 1986;3:398-414.
37. Travell JG, Simons DG: *Myofascial Pain and Dysfunction: The Trigger Point Manual.* Baltimore, MD: Williams & Wilkins. 1983.
38. Clark D, Stelmach G: Muscle fatigue and recovery curve parameters at various temperatures. *Res Q.* 1966;37:468-479.
39. Baker R, Bell G: The effect of therapeutic modalities on blood flow in the human calf. *J Orthop Sports Phys Ther.* 1991;13:23.
40. Zankel H: Effect of physical agents on motor conduction velocity of the ulnar nerve. *Arch Phys Med Rehabil.* 1994;47:197-199.

41. Abramson DI, Bell B, Tuck S: Changes in blood flow, oxygen uptake and tissue temperatures produced by therapeutic physical agents: effect of indirect or reflex vasodilation. *Am J Phys Med.* 1961;40:5-13.
42. Frizzell LA, Dunn F: Biophysics of ultrasound. In: Lehman JF, ed. *Therapeutic Heat and Cold, 3rd ed.* Baltimore, MD: Williams & Wilkin. 1982:353-385.
43. Lehman JF, Masock AJ, Warren CG, et al: Effect of therapeutic temperatures on tendon extensibility. *Arch Phys Med Rehabil.* 1970;51:481-487.
44. Barcroft H, Edholm OS: The effect of temperature on blood flow and deep temperature in the human forearm. *J Physiol.* 1943;102:5-20.
45. Griffin JG: Physiological effects of ultrasonic energy as it is used clinically. *J Am Phys Ther Assoc.* 1966;46:18.
46. Cwynar DA, McNerney T: A primer on physical therapy. *Lippincott's Primary Care Practice.* 1999;3:451-459.
47. Lehmann JF, Silverman DR, Baum BA, et al: Temperature distributions in the human thigh produced by infrared, hot pack and microwave applications. *Arch Phys Med Rehabil.* 1966;47:291.
48. Oosterveld FGJ, Rasker JJ, Jacobs JWG, et al: The effect of local heat and cold therapy on the intraarticular and skin surface temperature of the knee. *Arthritis Rheum.* 1992;35:146-151.
49. Abramson DI, Tuck S, Lee SW, et al: Comparison of wet and dry heat in raising temperature of tissues. *Arch Phys Med Rehabil.* 1967;48:654.
50. Sandqvist G, Akesson A, Eklund M: Evaluation of paraffin bath treatment in patients with systemic sclerosis. *Disabil Rehabil.* 2004;26:981-987.
51. Stimson CW, Rose GB, Nelson PA: Paraffin bath as thermotherapy: an evaluation. *Arch Phys Med Rehabil.* 1958;39:219-227.
52. Epps H, Ginnelly L, Utley M, et al: Is hydrotherapy cost-effective? A randomised controlled trial of combined hydrotherapy programmes compared with physiotherapy land techniques in children with juvenile idiopathic arthritis. *Health Technol Assess.* 2005;9:iii-iv, ix-x, 1-59.
53. Bender T, Karagulle Z, Balint GP, et al: Hydrotherapy, balneotherapy, and spa treatment in pain management. *Rheumatol Int.* 2004;25:220-224. Epub Jul 15, 2005.
54. McCulloch J: Physical modalities in wound management: ultrasound, vasopneumatic devices and hydrotherapy. *Ostomy Wound Manage.* 1995;41:30-32, 34, 36-37.
55. Goldby LJ, Scott DL: The way forward for hydrotherapy. *Br J Rheumatol.* 1993;32:771-773.
56. O'Byrne J: Hydrotherapy: the healing waters. *Nurs Stand.* 1990;4:22.
57. Downey JA: Physiological effects of heat and cold. *Phys Ther.* 1964;44:713-717.
58. Cox JS: The diagnosis and management of ankle ligament injuries in the athlete. *Athl Training.* 1982;18:192-196.
59. Marino M: Principles of therapeutic modalities: implications for sports medicine. In: Nicholas JA, Hershman EB, eds. *The Lower Extremity and Spine in Sports Medicine.* St. Louis, MO: C. V. Mosby. 1986:195-244.
60. Prentice WE: Using therapeutic modalities in rehabilitation. In: Prentice WE, Voight ML, eds. *Techniques in Musculoskeletal Rehabilitation.* New York, NY: McGraw-Hill. 2001:289-303.

61. Pociask FD, Kahn J, Galloway K: Iontophoresis, ultrasound, and phonophoresis. In: Placzek JD, Boyce DA, eds. *Orthopaedic Physical Therapy Secrets.* Philadelphia, PA: Hanley & Belfus, Inc. 2001:74-80.
62. Pociask FD: Electrotherapy. In: Placzek JD, Boyce DA, eds. *Orthopaedic Physical Therapy Secrets.* Philadelphia, PA: Hanley & Belfus, Inc. 2001:60-74.
63. Hooker DN: Electrical stimulating currents. In: Prentice WE, ed. *Therapeutic Modalities for Allied Health Professionals.* New York, NY: McGraw-Hill. 1998:73-133.
64. Smith MJ: Electrical stimulation for the relief of musculoskeletal pain. *Phys Sports Med.* 1983;11:47-55.
65. Gotlin RS, Hershkowitz S, Juris PM, et al: Electrical stimulation effect on extensor lag and length of hospital stay after total knee arthroplasty. *Arch Phys Med Rehabil.* 1994;75:957.
66. Magora F, Aladjemoff L, Tannenbaum J, et al: Treatment of pain by transcutaneous electrical stimulation. *Acta Anaesthesiol Scand.* 1978;22:589-592.
67. Mannheimer JS, Lampe GN: *Clinical Transcutaneous Electrical Nerve Stimulation.* Philadelphia, PA: FA Davis. 1984:440-445.
68. Woolf CF: Segmental afferent fiber-induced analgesia: transcutaneous electrical nerve stimulation (TENS) and vibration. In: Wall PD, Melzack R, eds. *Textbook of Pain.* New York, NY: Churchill Livingstone; 1989:884-896.
69. Smith MJ, Hutchins RC, Hehenberger D: Transcutaneous neural stimulation use in post-operative knee rehabilitation. *Am J Sports Med.* 1983;11:75-82.
70. Long DM: Fifteen years of transcutaneous electrical stimulation for pain control. *Stereotact Funct Neurosurg.* 1991;56:2-19.
71. Fried T, Johnson R, McCracken W: Transcutaneous electrical nerve stimulation: its role in the control of chronic pain. *Arch Phys Med Rehabil.* 1984;65:228-231.
72. Eriksson MBE, Sjölund BH, Nielzen S: Long-term results of peripheral conditioning stimulation as an analgesic measure in chronic pain. *Pain.* 1979;6:335-347.
73. Fishbain DA, Chabal C, Abbott A, et al: Transcutaneous electrical nerve stimulation (TENS) treatment outcome in long term users. *Clin J Pain.* 1996;12:201-214.
74. Ishimaru K, Kawakita K, Sakita M: Analgesic effects induced by TENS and electroacupuncture with different types of stimulating electrodes on deep tissues in human subjects. *Pain.* 1995; 63:181-187.
75. Eriksson MBE, Sjölund BH, Sundbärg G: Pain relief from peripheral conditioning stimulation in patients with chronic facial pain. *J Neurosurg.* 1984;61:149-155.
76. Murphy GJ: Utilization of transcutaneous electrical nerve stimulation in managing craniofacial pain. *Clin J Pain.* 1990;6:64-69.
77. Melzack R: The gate theory revisited. In: LeRoy PL, ed. *Current Concepts in the Management of Chronic Pain.* Miami, FL: Symposia Specialists. 1977.
78. Salar G: Effect of transcutaneous electrotherapy on CSF B-endorphin content in patients without pain problems. *Pain.* 1981; 10:169-172.
79. Clement-Jones V: Increased B endorphin but not metenkephalin levels in human cerebrospinal fluid after acupuncture for recurrent pain. *Lancet.* 1980;8:946-948.

80. Gangarosa LP: *Iontophoresis in Dental Practice.* Chicago, IL: Quintessence Publishing. 1982.
81. Coy RE: *Anthology of Craniomandibular Orthopedics.* Seattle, WA: International College Of Craniomandibular Orthopedics. 1993.
82. Burnette RR: Iontophoresis. In: Hadgraft J, Guy RH, eds. *Transdermal Drug Delivery: Developmental Issues and Research Initiatives.* New York, NY: Marcel Dekker. 1989:247-291.
83. Prentice WE: Iontophoresis. In: Prentice WE, ed. *Therapeutic Modalities for Allied Health Professionals.* New York, NY: McGraw-Hill. 1998:134-148.
84. Chien YW, Siddiqui O, Shi M, et al: Direct current iontophoretic transdermal delivery of peptide and protein drugs. *J Pharm Sci.* 1989;78:376-384.
85. Grimnes S: Pathways of ionic flow through human skin in vivo. *Acta Dermatol Venereol.* 1984;64:93-98.
86. Lee RD, White HS, Scott ER: Visualization of iontophoretic transport paths in cultured and animal skin models. *J Pharm Sci.* 1996;85:1186-1190.
87. O'Malley E, Oester Y: Influence of some physical chemical factors on iontophoresis using radioisotopes. *Arch Phys Med Rehabil.* 1955;36:310-313.
88. Zeltzer L, Regalado M, Nichter LS, et al: Iontophoresis versus subcutaneous injection: a comparison of two methods of local anesthesia delivery in children. *Pain.* 1991;44:73-78.
89. Prentice WE: Biofeedback. In: Prentice WE, ed. *Therapeutic Modalities for Allied Health Professionals.* New York, NY: McGraw-Hill. 1998:149-166.
90. Dyson M, Pond JB: The effect of pulsed ultrasound on tissue regeneration. *Physiotherapy.* 1970;56:136.
91. Dyson M, Suckling J: Stimulation of tissue repair by therapeutic ultrasound: A survey of the mechanisms involved. *Physiotherapy.* 1978;64:105-108.
92. Dyson M: Mechanisms involved in therapeutic ultrasound. *Physiotherapy.* 1987;73:116-120.
93. Lehman JF, deLateur BJ, Stonebridge JB, et al: Therapeutic temperature distribution produced by ultrasound as modified by dosage and volume of tissue exposed. *Arch Phys Med Rehabil.* 1967;48:662-666.
94. Lehman JF, deLateur BJ, Warren CG, et al: Heating of joint structures by ultrasound. *Arch Phys Med Rehabil.* 1968;49:28-30.
95. Goldman DE, Heuter TF: Tabulator data on velocity and absorption of high frequency sound in mammalian tissues. *J Acoust Soc Am.* 1956;28:35.
96. Dyson M: Non-thermal cellular effects of ultrasound. *Br J Cancer.* 1982;45:165-171.
97. Paaske WP, Hovind H, Sejrsen P: Influence of therapeutic ultrasound irradiation on blood flow in human cutaneous, subcutaneous and muscular tissue. *Scand J Clin Invest.* 1973;31:388.
98. Warren CG, Koblanski JN, Sigelmann RA: Ultrasound coupling media: their relative transmissivity. *Arch Phys Med Rehabil.* 1976; 57:218-222.
99. Binder A, Hodge G, Greenwood AM, et al: Is therapeutic ultrasound effective in treating soft tissue lesions? *BMJ.* 1985; 290:512-514.
100. Draper DO, Castel JC, Castel D: Rate of temperature increase in human muscle during 1-MHz and 3-MHz continuous ultrasound. *J Orthop Sports Phys Ther.* 1995;22:142-150.

101. Dyson M, Pond JB, Joseph J, et al: The stimulation of tissue regeneration by means of ultrasound. *Clin Sci.* 1968;35: 273-285.
102. Dyson M, Suckling J: Stimulation of tissue repair by ultrasound: a survey of the mechanisms involved. *Physiotherapy.* 1978; 64:105-108.
103. Ebenbichler GR, Resch KL, Graninger WB: Resolution of calcium deposits after therapeutic ultrasound of the shoulder. *J Rheumatol.* 1997;24:235-236.
104. Aldes JH, Klaras T: Use of ultrasonic radiation in the treatment of subdeltoid bursitis with and without calcareous deposits. *West J Surg.* 1954;62:369-376.
105. Flax HJ: Ultrasound treatment for peritendinitis calcarea of the shoulder. *Am J Phys Med Rehabil.* 1964;43:117-124.
106. Robertson VJ, Baker KG: A review of therapeutic ultrasound: effectiveness studies. *Phys Ther.* 2001;81:1339-1350.
107. Nussbaum EL, Biemann I, Mustard B: Comparison of ultrasound, ultraviolet C and laser for treatment of pressure ulcers in patients with spinal cord injury. *Phys Ther.* 1994;74:812-823.
108. Dyson M, Luke DA: Induction of mast cell degranulation in skin by ultrasound. *IEEE Trans Ultrasonics. Ferroelectrics and Frequency Control UFFC.* 1986;33:194-201.
109. Nussbaum EL: Ultrasound: to heat or not to heat—that is the question. *Phys Ther Rev.* 1997;2:59-72.
110. Makulolowe RTB, Mouzos GL: Ultrasound in the treatment of sprained ankles. *Practitioner.* 1977;218:586-588.
111. Dinno MA, Crum LA, Wu J: The effect of therapeutic ultrasound on the electrophysiologic parameters of frog skin. *Med. Biol.* 1989;25:461-470.
112. Falconer J, Hayes KW, Chang RW: Therapeutic ultrasound in the treatment of musculoskeletal conditions. *Arthritis Care Res.* 1990;3:85-91.
113. Maxwell L: Therapeutic ultrasound. Its effects on the cellular & mollecular mechanisms of inflammation and repair. *Physiotherapy.* 1992;78:421-426.
114. Ter Haar GR, Stratford IJ: Evidence for a non-thermal effect of ultrasound. *Br J Cancer.* 1982;45:172-175.
115. Young SR, Dyson M: The effect of therapeutic ultrasound on angiogenesis. *Ultrasound Med Biol.* 1990;16:261-269.
116. Dyson M, Niinikoski J: Stimulation of tissue repair by therapeutic ultrasound. *Infect Surg.* 1982;26:37-44.
117. Young SR, Dyson M: Effect of therapeutic ultrasound on the healing of full-thickness excised skin lesions. *Ultrasonics.* 1990; 28:175-180.
118. Watson T: The role of electrotherapy in contemporary physiotherapy practice. *Manual Ther.* 2000;5:132-141.
119. Draper DO, Prentice WE: Therapeutic ultrasound. In: Prentice WE, ed. *Therapeutic Modalities for Allied Health Professionals.* New York, NY: McGraw-Hill. 1998:263-309.
120. Antich TJ: Phonophoresis: the principles of the ultrasonic driving force and efficacy in treatment of common orthopedic diagnoses. *J Orthop Sports Phys Ther.* 1982;4:99-102.
121. Bommannan D, Menon GK, Okuyama H, et al: Sonophoresis II: examination of the mechanism(s) of ultrasound-enhanced transdermal drug delivery. *Pharm Res.* 1992;9:1043-1047.

122. Bommannan D, Okuyama H, Stauffer P, et al: Sonophoresis. I: the use of high-frequency ultrasound to enhance transdermal drug delivery. *Pharm Res.* 1992;9:559-564.
123. Byl NN: The use of ultrasound as an enhancer for transcutaneous drug delivery: phonophoresis. *Phys Ther.* 1995;75:539-553.
124. Byl NN, Mckenzie A, Haliday B, et al: The effects of phonophoresis with corticosteroids: a controlled pilot study. *J Orthop Sports Phys Ther.* 1993;18:590-600.
125. Ciccone CD, Leggin BG, Callamaro JJ: Effects of ultrasound and trolamine salicylate phonophoresis on delayedonset muscle soreness. *Phys Ther.* 1991;71:39-51.
126. Davick JP, Martin RK, Albright JP: Distribution and deposition of tritiated cortisol using phonophoresis. *Phys Ther.* 1988; 68:1672-1675.
127. Hakala RV: Prolotherapy (proliferation therapy) in the treatment of TMD. *Cranio.* 2005;23:283-288.
128. Kim SR, Stitik TP, Foye PM, et al: Critical review of prolotherapy for osteoarthritis, low back pain, and other musculoskeletal conditions: a physiatric perspective. *Am J Phys Med Rehabil.* 2004;83:379-389.
129. Britton KR: Is prolotherapy safe and effective for back pain? *Postgrad Med.* 2000;108:37-38.
130. Reeves KD, Hassanein K: Randomized prospective double-blind placebo-controlled study of dextrose prolotherapy for knee osteoarthritis with or without ACL laxity. *Alt Ther Health Med.* 2000;6:68-74, 77-80.
131. Saunders HD, Ryan RS: Spinal traction. In: Placzek JD, Boyce DA, eds. *Orthopaedic Physical Therapy Secrets.* Philadelphia, PA: Hanley & Belfus, Inc. 2001:93-98.
132. Colachis SC, Strohm BR: Cervical traction: relationship of traction time to varied tractive force with constant angle of pull. *Arch Phys Med Rehabil.* 1965;46:815-819.
133. Deets D, Hands KL, Hopp SS: Cervical traction: a comparison of sitting and supine positions. *Phys Ther.* 1977;57:255-261.
134. Harris PR: Cervical traction: review of literature and treatment guidelines. *Phys Ther.* 1977;57:910-914.
135. Austin R: Lumbar traction a valid option. *Aust J Physiother.* 1998;44:280.
136. Lee RY, Evans JH: Loads in the lumbar spine during traction therapy. *Aust J Physiother.* 2001;47:102-108.
137. Pellecchia GL: Lumbar traction: a review of the literature. *J Orthop Sports Phys Ther.* 1994;20:262-267.
138. Hooker DN: Intermittent compression devices. In: Prentice WE, ed. *Therapeutic Modalities for Allied Health Professionals.* New York, NY: McGraw-Hill. 1998:392-407.
139. Tanigawa MC: Comparison of hold-relax procedure and passive mobilization on increasing muscle length. *Phys Ther.* 1972; 52:725-735.
140. Barak T, Rosen E, Sofer R: Mobility: passive orthopedic manual therapy. In: Gould J, Davies G, eds. *Orthopedic and Sports Physical Therapy.* St Louis, MO: CV Mosby. 1990.
141. Mennel J: *Joint pain and diagnosis using manipulative techniques.* New York, NY: Little, Brown. 1964.
142. Maigne R: *Orthopedic Medicine.* Springfield, IL: Charles C Thomas. 1972.

143. Kaltenborn FM: *Manual Mobilization of the Extremity Joints: Basic Examination and Treatment Techniques, 4th ed.* Oslo, Norway: Olaf Norlis Bokhandel, Universitetsgaten. 1989.
144. Grieve GP: Manual mobilizing techniques in degenerative arthrosis of the hip. *Bull Orthop Section APTA.* 1977;2:7.
145. Yoder E: Physical therapy management of nonsurgical hip problems in adults. In: Echternach JL, ed. *Physical Therapy of the Hip.* New York, NY: Churchill Livingstone. 1990:103-137.
146. Wyke BD: The neurology of joints. *Ann R Coll Surg Engl.* 1967;41:25-50.
147. Freeman MAR, Wyke BD: An experimental study of articular neurology. *J Bone Joint Surg.* 1967;49B:185.
148. Meadows JTS: The principles of the Canadian approach to the lumbar dysfunction patient, Management of Lumbar Spine Dysfunction—Independent Home Study Course. La Crosse, WI: APTA, Orthopaedic Section. 1999.

Pharmacology for the Physical Therapist

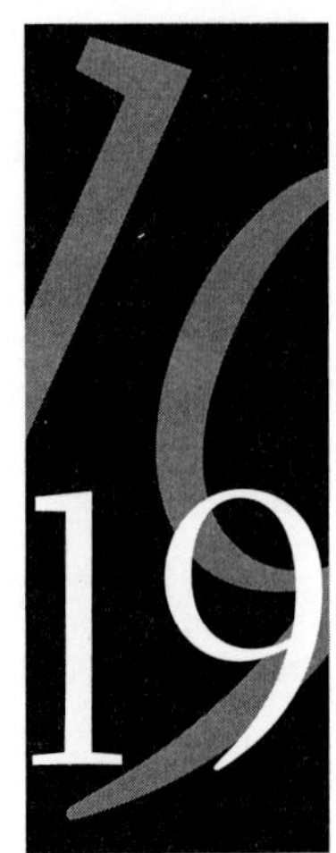

Pharmacology is the branch of medicine concerned with the study of how a drug's actions affect living tissue (Table 19-1). It is important for the physical therapist to have a working knowledge of pharmacology because of the number of drugs currently on the market and the number of physical therapy patients that are likely to have been prescribed medications.

> **Study Pearl**
>
> Some of the beneficial effects of drugs may be enhanced by physical therapy interventions, but in other cases the interventions may have negative consequences.

DRUG DEVELOPMENT AND REGULATION

The Food and Drug Administration (FDA):

- Directs the drug development process
- Gives approval for marketing a new drug
- Approves a new use for an older drug

Drug regulation is essential to ensure a safe and effective product. The purposes of drug regulation include

- Balancing the need of the pharmaceutical companies to show a profit with the need for patients to have easy access to effective medications
- To ensure safety and efficacy of the drugs and review product labeling
- To regulate the manufacturing process to ensure stability in the product
- To control public access to drugs that have the potential for abuse

Controlled Substances

Controlled substances are drugs classified according to their potential for abuse. These drugs are regulated under the Controlled Substances Act, which classifies these compounds into schedules from I to V.

TABLE 19-1. PHARMACOLOGY TERMS AND DEFINITIONS

TERM	DEFINITION
Drug	Any substance that can be used to modify a chemical process or processes in the body, for example to treat an illness, relieve a symptom, enhance a performance or ability, or to alter states of mind The word "drug" is etymologically derived from the Dutch/Low German word "droog," which means "dry," since in the past, most drugs were dried plant parts.
Pharmacology	The science of studying both the mechanisms and the actions of drugs, usually in animal models of disease, to evaluate their potential therapeutic value
Pharmacy	The mixing and dispensing of drugs The monitoring of drug prescriptions for appropriateness and the monitoring of patients for adverse drug interactions
Pharmacotherapeutics	The use of chemical agents to prevent, diagnose, and cure disease
Pharmacokinetics	The study of how the body absorbs, distributes, metabolizes and eliminates a drug
Pharmacodynamics	The study of the biochemical and physiologic effects of drugs and their mechanisms of action at the cellular or organ level
Pharmacotherapy	The treatment of a disease or condition with drugs
Pharmacogenetics	The study of how variation in human genes leads to variations in our response to drugs and helps direct therapeutics according to a person's genotype
Toxicology	A study of the negative effects of chemicals on living things, including cells, plants, animals, and humans

- Schedule I: these drugs are available only for research. They have a high abuse potential, leading to dependence without any acceptable medical indication. Examples include heroine, LSD, marijuana.
- Schedule II: these drugs also have a high abuse potential but have accepted medical uses. Examples include amphetamines, morphine, and oxycodone.
- Schedule III: although these drugs have a lower abuse potential and dosing schedule than I or II, they may also be abused and can result in some physical and psychological dependence. Examples include mild to moderately strong opioids, barbiturates, and steroids.
- Schedule IV: these drugs have less of an abuse potential. No more than five refills within 6 months are allowed per prescription. Examples include opioids, benzodiazepines, and some stimulants.
- Schedule V: these drugs have the lowest abuse potential and are often available without prescription. Examples include various cold and cough medicines containing codeine.

DRUG NOMENCLATURE

Typically, drugs have three names:

- Chemical: based on the specific structure of the compound
- Generic: considered the official name of the compound, and the name listed in the United States Pharmacopeia
- Trade/brand: the name given to the drug by the pharmaceutical company that copyrights the name

DRUG CLASSIFICATION

Drugs may be classified in one of four ways:

- Specific categories that provide an explanation of the overall pharmacological action on a specific disease process. Examples include antivirals, antibiotics, and antihypertensives.
- Their pharmacological action. Examples include arterial vasodilators and anesthetics.
- Their molecular action. Examples include calcium channel blockers.
- Their chemical makeup or the source of the drug. Examples include atropine and penicillin.

PHARMACODYNAMICS

Pharmacodynamics refers to the affect the drug has on the body. For the physical therapist, the study of pharmacodynamics includes four important areas[1]:

- The drug's mode of action:
  - Potency: the dose of the drug required to produce a given effect relative to a standard. It is important to relate response to drug concentrations at the active site (eg, plasma) to truly classify the potency of a given drug.
  - Efficacy: the capacity to stimulate or produce an effect for a given occupied receptor (the maximum response to a drug). Drugs in which a small difference exists between the effective and toxic concentrations are defined as having a narrow therapeutic index. These medications need to be monitored closely because the interindividual variability that exists in pharmacokinetics and pharmacodynamics.
  - Tolerance: the sensitivity of the receptor. Tolerance to a drug occurs when increasing amounts of the drug are required to produce the same effect or when the same dose on repeated occasions produces lower responses. Narcotic analgesics are a class of drugs that exhibit tolerance.
- Indications for use of the drug: refers to the use of that drug for treating a particular disease. A drug often has more than one indication, which means that it can be used to treat more than one disease. Indications for drugs can be classified as FDA-approved (labeled indications) and non-FDA approved (off-label indications).
- The drug's safety profile: the evolving safety profile of a drug both during its development in clinical trials, and after its FDA approval for availability to the general public to ensure that the benefits of taking the drug outweigh any safety concerns.
- The site of action: for a drug to have an effective action it must have a target. Sites of drug action may include receptors, ion channels, transport molecules, and enzymes. The binding of drugs to receptors has a certain specificity and selectivity.

RECEPTORS

Most receptors are transmembrane receptors in that they contain receptors responding to ligands (an extracellular substance that binds to receptors) outside the cell that contains structural proteins that link this region to the intracellular domain.[2-6] A number of receptors are recognized:

- Ion channels: transmembrane proteins arranged around a central aqueous channel which open in response to a voltage change in the membrane, allowing a selective transfer of ions from a greater concentration to a lesser concentration.
- Ligand-gated channels: protein subunits surrounding a central pole, where opening of the port depends on binding of the neurotransmitters to one of the peptide subunits.
- G-protein-linked receptors: consists of a transmembrane receptor coupled to an intracellular system by a guanosine-binding protein (G-protein), which then activates other effectors such as ion channels and enzymes.
- DNA-coupled receptors: intracellular receptors that stimulate gene transcription, leading to the synthesis of proteins and enzymes.
- Kinase-linked receptor: consists of a single transmembrane helical region with a large extracellular domain for ligand binding.
- Kidney tubules: many diuretics bind to sodium transporters in the renal tubules to block reabsorption of sodium.
- Enzymes.

PHARMACOKINETICS

Pharmacokinetics is the study of how the body absorbs, distributes, metabolizes, and eliminates a drug.

ABSORPTION

Absorption is the process by which a drug is made available to the body fluids that distribute the drug to the organ systems. A prerequisite to absorption is drug dissolution. Solid drug products (eg, tablets) disintegrate and deaggregate, but absorption can occur only after drugs enter solution. The physicochemical properties of drugs (bioavailability), their formulations, and routes of administration determine the level of drug absorption. When given by most routes (excluding intravenously), a drug must traverse several semipermeable cell membranes before reaching the systemic circulation.[7-14] These membranes are biologic barriers that selectively inhibit the passage of drug molecules and are composed primarily of a bimolecular lipid matrix, containing mostly cholesterol and phospholipids. The lipids provide stability to the membrane and determine its permeability characteristics. Globular proteins of various sizes and composition are embedded in the matrix; they are involved in transport and function as receptors for cellular regulation. Drugs may cross a biologic barrier by diffusion through the water filled channels or specialized ion channels, passive diffusion through the lipid membrane, carrier-mediated processes that include a facilitated diffusion or active transport, or pinocytosis.

- Diffusion: most drugs are weak organic acids or bases, existing in un-ionized and ionized forms in an aqueous environment. The un-ionized form is usually lipid soluble and diffuses readily across cell membranes. The ionized form cannot penetrate the cell membrane easily because of its low lipid solubility and high electrical resistance, resulting from its charge and the charged groups on the cell membrane surface. Thus, drug penetration may be attributed mostly to the un-ionized form. However, whether a drug is acidic or basic, most of its absorption occurs in the small intestine.
- Passive diffusion: in this process, transport across a cell membrane depends on the concentration gradient of the solute. Most drug molecules are transported across a membrane by simple diffusion from a region of high concentration (eg, GI fluids) to one of low concentration (eg, blood). Because drug molecules are rapidly removed by the systemic circulation and distributed into a large volume of body fluids and tissues, drug concentration in blood is initially low compared with that at the administration site, producing a large gradient. The diffusion rate is directly proportional to the gradient but also depends on the molecule's lipid solubility, degree of ionization, size, and on the area of the absorptive surface. Because the cell membrane is lipoid, lipid-soluble drugs diffuse more rapidly than relatively lipid-insoluble drugs. Small molecules tend to penetrate membranes more rapidly than large ones.
- Facilitated passive diffusion: for certain molecules (eg, glucose), the rate of membrane penetration is greater than expected from their low lipid solubility. One theory is that a carrier component combines reversibly with the substrate molecule at the cell membrane exterior, and the carrier-substrate complex diffuses rapidly across the membrane, releasing the substrate at the interior surface. Carrier-mediated diffusion is characterized by selectivity and saturability. The carrier transports only substrates with a relatively specific molecular configuration, and the process is limited by the availability of carriers. The process does not require energy expenditure, and transport against a concentration gradient does not occur.
- Active transport: this process is characterized by selectivity and saturability and requires energy expenditure by the cell. Substrates may accumulate intracellularly against a concentration gradient. Active transport appears to be limited to drugs structurally similar to endogenous substances. These drugs are usually absorbed from sites in the small intestine. Active transport processes have been identified for various ions, vitamins, sugars, and amino acids.
- Pinocytosis: a cell engulfs a fluid or particles. The cell membrane invaginates, encloses the fluid or particles, then fuses again, forming a vesicle that later detaches and moves to the cell interior. This mechanism requires energy expenditure. Pinocytosis probably plays a minor role in drug transport, except for protein drugs.

TABLE 19-2. METHODS FOR DRUG ADMINISTRATION

METHOD	DESCRIPTION
Parenteral/intravenous	Direct placement of a drug into the bloodstream
Oral	Chewed, sucked, or swallowed
Sublingual	Placed under the tongue
Intramuscular	Injected into the muscle
Subcutaneous	Beneath or under the skin
Inhalational	Breathed in
Topical	Placed on the skin

DRUG ROUTES OF ADMINISTRATION

When a drug is administered to a patient, a certain response will occur. The response is a factor of the route of administration and the dosage formulation. The primary routes of administration include oral (enteral) including, buccal, sublingual, and rectal, and parenteral (intravenous, intramuscular, subcutaneous, and intra-articular). Other routes of administration include topical, transdermal, and inhalational (Table 19-2). As the target cells become exposed to increasing concentrations of the drug, increasing numbers of receptors become activated, and the magnitude of the response increases until there is a maximal response. This phenomenon is illustrated by graphing a dose-response curve (Figure 19-1).

> **Study Pearl**
>
> Absorption after oral administration is confounded by differences in luminal pH along the GI tract, surface area per luminal volume, blood perfusion, the presence of bile and mucus, and the nature of epithelial membranes.

Oral Administration. For oral administration, the most common route used, absorption refers to the transport of drugs across membranes of the epithelial cells in the GI tract. The oral mucosa has a thin epithelium and a rich vascularity that favors absorption, but contact is usually too brief, even for drugs in solution, for appreciable absorption to occur. A drug placed between the gums and cheek (buccal administration) or under the tongue (sublingual administration) is retained longer so that absorption is more complete.

Stomach Absorption. The stomach has a relatively large epithelial surface, but because it has a thick mucous layer and the time that the

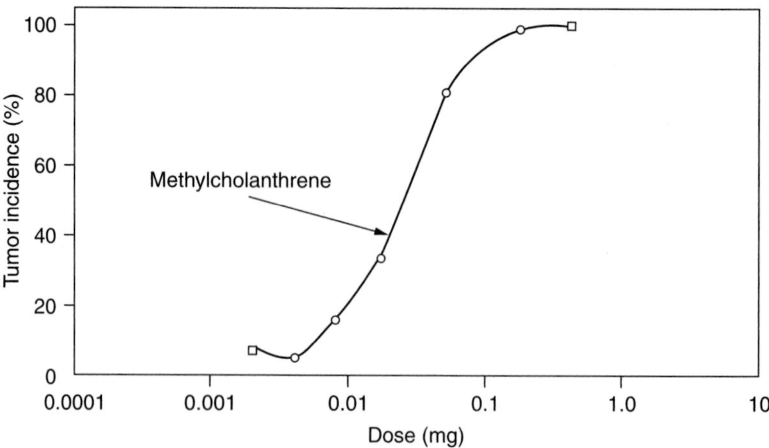

Figure 19-1. Example of a dose-response curve. (Data from Eaton DL, and Klaassen CD: Principles of Toxicology. In *Casarett & Doulls' Toxicology: The Basic Science of Poisons, 5th ed.* New York: McGraw-Hill. 1996.)

drug remains there is usually relatively short, absorption is limited. Therefore, gastric emptying is the rate-limiting step. Food, especially fatty foods, slows gastric emptying (and the rate of drug absorption), explaining why some drugs should be taken on an empty stomach when a rapid onset of action is desired. Food may enhance the extent of absorption for poorly soluble drugs, reduce it for drugs degraded in the stomach (eg, penicillin G), or have little or no effect. Drugs that affect gastric emptying (eg, parasympatholytic drugs) affect the absorption rate of other drugs.

Small Intestine Absorption. Absorption of virtually all drugs is faster from the small intestine than from the stomach due to the larger surface area and greater permeability of the membranes in the small intestine. The intraluminal pH is 4 to 5 in the duodenum but becomes progressively more alkaline, approaching 8 in the lower ileum.[15,16] GI microflora may inactivate certain drugs, reducing their absorption. Decreased blood flow (eg, in shock) may lower the concentration gradient across the intestinal mucosa and decrease absorption by passive diffusion. Decreased peripheral blood flow also alters drug distribution and metabolism.

Intestinal transit time can influence drug absorption, particularly for drugs that are absorbed by active transport (eg, B vitamins), that dissolve slowly, or that are too polar (ie, poorly lipid-soluble) to cross membranes readily (eg, many antibiotics).[15,16] For such drugs, transit may be too rapid for absorption to be complete.

Liver Absorption. For any drug to be effective after oral administration, it must be absorbed through the intestinal epithelium and enter the blood vessels of the intestinal tract.[1] The drug is then carried directly to the liver by the hepatic portal system before it reaches the systemic circulation. Thus, if a drug has properties that allow the liver to rapidly metabolize it, then little if any will actually enter the systemic circulation. The liver extraction is called the "first-pass effect" and may render an orally administered drug ineffective.

Large Intestine Absorption. For controlled-release dosage forms, absorption may occur primarily in the large intestine, particularly when the drug release continues for > 6 hours, the time for transit to the large intestine.

Absorption from Solution. A drug given orally in solution is subjected to numerous GI secretions and, to be absorbed, must survive encounters with low pH and potentially degrading enzymes. Usually, even if a drug is stable in the enteral environment, little of it remains to pass into the large intestine. Drugs with low lipophilicity (ie, low membrane permeability), such as aminoglycosides, are absorbed slowly from solution in the stomach and small intestine; for such drugs, absorption in the large intestine is expected to be even slower because the surface area is smaller.[17-19] Consequently, these drugs are not candidates for controlled release.

Absorption from Solid Forms. Most drugs are given orally as tablets or capsules primarily for convenience, economy, stability, and patient acceptance. These products must disintegrate and dissolve before absorption can occur. Disintegration greatly increases the drug's surface area in contact with GI fluids, thereby promoting drug dissolution and absorption. Disintegrants and other excipients (eg, diluents, lubricants, surfactants, binders, dispersants) are often added during manufacture to facilitate these processes.[20-22] Surfactants increase the dissolution rate by increasing the wetability, solubility, and dispersibility of the drug.[20-22] Disintegration of solid forms may be retarded by excessive pressure applied during the tableting procedure or by special coatings applied to protect the tablet from the digestive processes of the gut. Hydrophobic lubricants (eg, magnesium stearate) may bind to the active drug and reduce its bioavailability.

Dissolution rate determines the availability of the drug for absorption. When slower than absorption, dissolution becomes the rate-limiting step.[20-22] Dissolution rate is affected by whether the drug is in salt, crystal, or hydrate form.

Manipulating the Absorption Rate. Manipulating the formulation can significantly change absorption properties.

- Reducing the particle size increases the drug's surface area, thus increasing the rate and extent of GI absorption of a drug whose absorption is normally limited by slow dissolution.
- Timed-release or sustained-release formulations are designed to produce slow, uniform dissolution of the drug and thus allow more of the drug to reach the systemic circulation.
- Enteric-coated (delayed release) formulations may be used with orally administered medications to alter absorption. This method is particularly useful if a medication is prone to acidic degradation in the stomach.

Parenteral Administration. Direct placement of a drug into the bloodstream (usually by IV) ensures delivery of the dose to the systemic circulation. However, delivery of the entire dose is not ensured if a route requires movement through one or more biologic membranes to reach the systemic circulation (intramuscular [IM] or subcutaneous [SC] injection).[23,24]

Because capillaries tend to be highly porous, perfusion (blood flow/gram of tissue) greatly affects the absorption rate of small molecules.[23,24] Thus, the injection site can markedly influence a drug's absorption rate.

Study Pearl

Oral controlled–release forms are often designed to maintain therapeutic drug concentrations for ≥ 12 hours. The absorption rate can be controlled by coating drug particles with wax or other water-insoluble material, by embedding the drug in a matrix from which it is released slowly during transit through the GI tract, or by complexing the drug with ion-exchange resins.

Controlled-Release Forms. Controlled-release dosage forms are designed to reduce dosing frequency and to reduce fluctuation in plasma drug concentration, providing a more uniform therapeutic effect. Less frequent dosing is more convenient and may improve patient compliance. These dosage forms are suitable for drugs that otherwise require frequent dosing because their elimination half-life and duration of effect are short.

Transdermal controlled-release forms are designed to provide drug release for extended periods; eg, clonidine diffusion through a membrane provides controlled drug delivery for 1 week, and nitroglycerin-impregnated polymer bonded to an adhesive bandage provides controlled drug delivery for 24 hours.

THE EFFECTS OF EXERCISE ON PHARMACOKINETICS

According to the limited information available, exercise has no substantial effect on the absorption of orally given drugs.[25-30] However, it appears to enhance absorption from intramuscular, subcutaneous, transdermal and inhalation sites. The effects of exercise on drug distribution are complex. Exercise increases muscular blood flow resulting, for example, in the increased binding of digoxin in working skeletal muscle. On the other hand, exercise may sequester some drugs such as propranolol in muscle and reduce the availability of the drug for elimination.[31,32] In addition, exercise decreases the clearance of highly extracted drugs and increases their plasma concentration. It may also increase the clearance of drugs by increasing biliary excretion. Since exercise reduces renal blood flow, the plasma concentrations of those drugs that are primarily eliminated by the kidneys may increase. In conclusion, if maintaining the plasma concentration of a drug at a certain level is important, consideration should be given to alternative drugs if the patient is on intermittent or irregular exercise.

DISTRIBUTION OF DRUGS

The distribution of a drug refers to the process by which drugs leave the systemic circulation and are transported to the extravascular spaces of the body. The rate at which this distribution occurs depends on a variety of factors including[1]

- The rate of organ blood flow.
- The degree of drug ionization in different compartments.
- The binding of a percentage of the drug molecules to serum protein. The primary protein that binds drug molecules is serum albumin. Binding prevents the drug from exerting any pharmacologic action. The unbound molecules are the portions of the drug that can penetrate capillary walls to reach the site of action.
- The number of competing drugs within the system. Some drugs compete for the same binding sites. This competition may result in higher levels of the unbound drug acting on the body.
- Molecular weight of the drug.
- Blood–brain barrier. Many drugs that easily penetrate other body organs do not appreciable enter the brain because of the sieve-like action of the blood–brain barrier.
- Lipid solubility of the drug:
  - Lipid soluble drugs are more likely to penetrate the blood–brain barrier than other drugs because they pass through the cell membrane.
  - Lipid soluble drugs may be stored in adipose tissue, which acts as a drug repository.
- Any local metabolism that occurs at any tissue other than the target organ.

METABOLISM OF DRUGS

Metabolism refers to the process of transforming a drug into more water-soluble compounds so that the kidneys can excrete them. Metabolism occurs primarily in the liver with the goal of decreasing the drugs pharmacological activity and lipid solubility. Drug metabolism involves two processes or phases:

- Phase I: these reactions are catabolic and involve oxidation, reduction, full hydrolysis reactions, with oxidation occurring most frequently.
- Phase II: during this phase the drug undergoes conjugation reactions.

DRUG ELIMINATION

Drug elimination refers to the irreversible removal of a drug from the body by all routes of elimination. This process typically is broken into two major physiological components: metabolism (biotransformation) and excretion.

- Metabolism: the major metabolizing organ in the body is the liver.
- Elimination: drugs are eliminated from the body by a variety of routes including elimination in fluids (urine, breast milk, saliva, tears, and sweat), through the GI tract in the feces, expelled in exhaled air through the lungs, and through the kidneys. Excretion of a drug by the kidneys occurs by two processes[1]:
  - Glomerular filtration: the process in which drugs are filtered through the glomerulus and then carried through the tubule into the urine.
  - Active secretion of the drug by the tubule into the urine.

DRUG HALF-LIFE

The rate at which a drug disappears from the body, through metabolism, excretion, or a combination, is called the half-life. It is the amount of time required for half of the drug that is in the body to be eliminated. Two terms are used to describe half-life:

- Elimination half-life:
  - The time in which the concentration of the drug in the plasma falls to one-half of its original amount.
  - A drug's rate of disappearance from the body, whether by metabolism, excretion or a combination of both.
- Biological half-life:
  - The time in which the duration of action falls to one half of its original duration.
  - The time of the drug's response rather than its plasma concentration.

Study Pearl

Knowing the half-life of a drug is critical in determining how often and in what dosage a drug must be administered to achieve and maintain therapeutic levels of concentration.

The dosage interval (time between administrations of the drug) is equal to the half-life of a particular drug. The shorter the half-life, the more often the patient must take the medication. Theoretically a steady state will be reached when the amount of the drug taken equals the amount that is excreted. A steady state is usually reached after five half lives of the drug have occurred. Thus, drugs with long half-lives may take several days to weeks to reach a steady state.

Study Pearl

Clearance describes the efficiency of irreversible elimination (by biotransformation and/or excretion) from the body. From a physiological sense, clearance is the volume of blood cleared of a drug per unit time. Clearance is the parameter that determines the maintenance dose required to achieve an average plasma concentration of a drug.

DRUG ALLERGY AND DRUG-INDUCED ILLNESSES

Drug allergies, or hypersensitivities, range from mild presentations to very severe life-threatening events. For a drug to produce a reaction, it must have antigenic effects and stimulate antibody formation or the formation of sensitized T-lymphocytes, which is immune-related. Drug allergies are generally classified into four types:

- Type I (anaphylactic reactions): anaphylaxis is the most severe allergic reaction and involves the skin and pulmonary and cardiovascular systems, producing cardiovascular and respiratory collapse. The signs and symptoms associated with anaphylactic shock, which usually occur within minutes after antigen exposure but may still occur up to one out later, include
  - Neurological: dizziness, weakness, and seizures
  - Ocular: pruritis, lacrimation, edema around the eyes
  - Respiratory: nasal congestion, hoarseness, stridor, cough, dyspnea, tachypnea, bronchospasm, and respiratory arrest
  - Cardiac: tachycardia, hypotension, arrhythmias, myocardial infarction
  - Integumentary: flushing, erythema, urticaria
  - Gastrointestinal: nausea, vomiting, and diarrhea
- Type II (cytotoxic reaction): the antigens adhere to the target cell and begin to destroy the target tissue. The clinical manifestations include
  - Fever
  - Arthralgia
  - Rash
  - Splenomegaly
  - Lymph node enlargement
- Type III (autoimmune reaction): a complex mediated hypersensitivity reaction in which the body has difficulty eliminating antigen-antibody complexes. Manifestations include serum sickness, glomerulonephritis, vasculitis, and pulmonary disorders.
- Type IV (cell-mediated hypersensitivity): this type of reaction is mediated through T-lymphocytes as opposed to antibodies. Manifestations include local or tissue reaction.

PHARMACOTHERAPY

Although physical therapists are not permitted by law to prescribe or dispense prescription drugs, an understanding of the potential effects of certain types of drugs commonly encountered during the rehabilitation process is essential.[33]

MUSCULOSKELETAL PHARMACOLOGY

Drugs are widely used in the management of both acute and chronic pain and inflammation. The following discussion emphasizes those drugs that are prescribed to control pain and/or inflammation. In the absence of data supporting a therapeutic benefit for a drug, toxicity associated with the drug can still occur. It is critical, therefore, for physicians to continually assess the balance between therapeutic benefit and safety.

Opioid Analgesics. Most of the narcotics used in medicine are referred to as opioids, as they are derived directly from opium or are synthetic opiates. Examples of these opioids include codeine, Darvon (propoxyphene hydrochloride), morphine, and Demerol (meperidine). Refer to "Narcotic Analgesics" later in the chapter.

Non-Opioid Analgesics. Non-opioid analgesics comprise a heterogeneous class of drugs including the salicyclates (eg, aspirin), para-aminophenol derivatives (primarily acetaminophen), and the NSAIDs. Despite their diverse structures, non-opioid analgesics have similar therapeutic effects, oral efficacy, and similar side effect profiles. Non-opioid analgesics are better tolerated than opioids by ambulatory patients, have less sedative effects, and are much less likely to produce tolerance or dependence. Conversely, the hazards of long-term administration of these drugs are recognized.

NSAIDs have antipyretic, analgesic, and anti-inflammatory effects. The analgesic and anti-inflammatory activity of NSAIDs is primarily due to the inhibition of arachidonic acid metabolism.[34] NSAIDs also seem to promote the inhibition of the release of cyclooxygenase-1 (Cox-1) and cyclooxygenase-2 (Cox-2) and the synthesis of prostaglandins at an injury site.[34] Inhibition of COX-1 can also produce gastrointestinal toxicity including inflammation, ulceration, and bleeding, and can lead to perforation.[35] Suppression of prostaglandins is not limited to the site of injury and may result in alteration of normal function in the gastrointestinal mucosa and kidney blood flow. NSAIDs may also alter kidney blood flow by interfering with the synthesis of prostaglandins in the kidney involved in the autoregulation of blood flow and glomerular filtration.[36]

Cox-2 inhibitors do not produce the same gastrointestinal effects as Cox-1 inhibitors; therefore, they are safer to use in patients who are predisposed to gastric or kidney malfunctions. Cox-2 drugs only block the Cox-2 enzyme, which is responsible for triggering pain and inflammation.[34] Because Cox-1 is not affected, the patient's stomach lining is protected and bleeding tendencies are avoided.[34]

Corticosteroids. Corticosteroids are natural anti-inflammatory hormones produced by the adrenal glands under the control of the hypothalamus. Synthetic corticosteroids (cortisone, dexamethasone) are commonly used to treat a range of immunological and inflammatory musculoskeletal conditions. Corticosteroids exert their anti-inflammatory effects by binding to a high-affinity intracellular cytoplasmic receptor present in all human cells.[37] As a result, these agents are capable of producing undesirable and sometimes severe systemic adverse effects that may offset clinical gains in many patients. The side effects from corticosteroids emulate from exogenous hypercortisolism, which is similar to the clinical syndrome of Cushing's disease. These side effects include:[38]

- Cutaneous manifestations. Cutaneous manifestations of hypercortisolism include delayed wound healing, acanthosis nigricans (a velvety, thickened, hyperpigmented plaque that usually occurs on the neck or in the axillary region), acne, ecchymoses after minor trauma, hyperpigmentation, hirsutism, petechia, and striae.
- Hypokalemia. Hypokalemia is a well-recognized side effect of corticosteroid therapy and is probably related to the mineralocorticoid effect of hydrocortisone, prednisone, and prednisolone. Dexamethasone has no mineralocorticoid effect.
- Myopathy. There are two recognized forms of corticosteroid-induced myopathy: acute and chronic. Acute myopathy may in part be caused by hypokalemia, although corticosteroids (especially massive dosages) may have a direct affect on skeletal muscle. Both proximal and distal muscle weakness occur acutely, usually with an associated and significant elevation in serum creatinine phosphokinase, which is indicative of focal and diffuse muscle necrosis. In the more chronic form of myopathy, weakness is more insidious in onset and primarily involves proximal muscle groups.
- Hyperglycemia. Although the mechanism behind this is not clear, hyperglycemia, especially when combined with the immunosuppressive effect of corticosteroids, may significantly increase the risk for infection.
- Neurological impairments. These can include vertigo, headache, convulsions and benign intracranial hypertension.
- Osteoporosis. Corticosteroids inhibit bone formation directly via inhibition of osteoblast differentiation and type I collagen synthesis, and indirectly by inhibition of calcium absorption and enhancement of urinary calcium excretion.
- Ophthalmologic side effects. Corticosteroids increase the risk of glaucoma by increasing intraocular pressure, regardless of whether administered intranasally, topically, periocularly, or systemically.
- Growth suppression. Corticosteroids interfere with bone formation, nitrogen retention, and collagen formation, all of which are necessary for anabolism and growth.

Muscle Relaxants. Muscle relaxants, such as Robaxin and Soma, are thought to decrease muscle tone without impairment in motor function by acting centrally to depress polysynaptic reflexes. There presently exists a discrepancy between the common clinical use of skeletal muscle relaxants and the results of controlled clinical trials evaluating their efficacy in comparison with placebo. Supporting evidence does not exist for their efficacy in pain of myogenic origin, nor is it clear if they provide an additive effect with exercises aimed at muscle relaxation.

Neurologic System Pharmacology

Antianxiety Medications

Selective Serotonin Reuptake Inhibitors. Selective serotonin reuptake inhibitors (SSRIs) are prescribed as psychotherapeutic agents. The most serious drug-related adverse effect of SSRIs is serotonin syndrome (SS). Serotonin is a neurotransmitter synthesized from the amino acid L-tryptophan. Synthesis is necessary in both the central and peripheral nervous systems because serotonin cannot cross the blood–brain barrier. Once synthesized, serotonin is either stored in neuronal vesicles or metabolized by monamine oxidase (MAO) to 5-hydroxyindoleacetic acid. SS, characterized by mental status changes, neuromuscular dysfunction, and autonomic instability. Symptoms attributed to serotonin excess may include restlessness, hallucinations, shivering, diaphoresis, headache, and nausea.

Monoamine Oxidase Inhibitors. Monoamines generally function as neurotransmitters. When neurotransmitters are released into the synaptic space, they are either reabsorbed into the proximal nerve or destroyed by monoamine oxidase (MAO) within the synaptic cleft. The two types of MAO are MAO-A and MAO-B. MAO-A is found primarily in the liver and gastrointestinal tract with some found in the monoaminergic neurons. MAO-A present in the liver is involved in the elimination of ingested monoamines such as dietary tyramine. Circulating monoamines such as epinephrine, norepinephrine, and dopamine, are inactivated when they pass through a liver rich in MAO-A. MAO-B, on the other hand, is found primarily in the brain and in platelets.

Monoamine Oxidase Inhibitors (MAOIs) indirectly degrade the monamines and inhibit breakdown of norepinephrine, serotonin, and dopamine, thereby increasing the available monamines available within the CNS. This can result in hypertension, tachycardia, tremors, seizures, and hyperthermia.

Benzodiazepines. Benzodiazepines (BZDs) are used for a variety of situations that include seizure control, anxiety, alcohol withdrawal, and insomnia. They also are combined frequently with other medications for conscious sedation before procedures or interventions.

Gamma-aminobutyric acid (GABA) is the major inhibitory neurotransmitter in the CNS. BZDs exert their action by potentiating the activity of GABA. They bind to a specific receptor on the GABA-A receptor complex, which facilitates the binding of GABA to its specific receptor site. BZD binding causes increased frequency of opening of the chloride channel complexes with the GABA-A receptor. Chloride channel opening results in membrane hyperpolarization, which inhibits cellular excitation.

Enhanced GABA neurotransmission results in sedation, striated muscle relaxation, and anticonvulsant effects. Stimulation of peripheral nervous system (PNS) GABA receptors may cause decreased cardiac contractility, vasodilation, and enhanced perfusion.

Beta Blockers. Beta-blockers (eg, propranolol) have been used to block the autonomic response in persons with social phobia.

Sedatives/Hypnotics. Benzodiazepines (see above) and barbiturates are the most commonly used sedative-hypnotics in this class. Other agents include the nonbarbiturate nonbenzodiazepine sedative-hypnotics, such as buspirone, zolpidem, ethchlorvynol, glutethimide, chloral hydrate, meprobamate, methaqualone, methyprylon, carisoprodol, and gamma-butyrolactone (GBL). Most sedative-hypnotics stimulate the activity of GABA, the principal inhibitory neurotransmitter in the CNS.

Mild toxicity resembles ethanol intoxication; moderate poisoning leads to respiratory depression and hyporeflexia; severe poisoning leads to flaccid areflexic coma, apnea, and hypotension.

Narcotic Analgesics. In current practice, narcotic refers to any of the many opioids or opioid derivatives.

Activation of the opiate receptors results in the inhibition of synaptic neurotransmission in the central nervous system (CNS) and peripheral nervous system (PNS). Opioids bind to and enhance neurotransmission at opiate receptors. The opiate antagonists (eg, naloxone, nalmefene, naltrexone) antagonize the effects at all opiate receptors.

Opioids decrease the perception of pain, by inducing slight euphoria rather than by eliminating or reducing the painful stimulus. The GI tract and the respiratory mucosa provide easy absorption for most opioids. Following therapeutic doses, most absorption occurs in the small intestine. Toxic doses may have delayed absorption because of delayed gastric emptying and slowed gut motility. Certain opiates (eg, propoxyphene, fentanyl, and buprenorphine) are more lipid soluble and can be stored in the fatty tissues of the body.

Opiate metabolites are excreted in the urine, making urine toxicology useful. Renal failure also leads to toxic effects from accumulated drug or active metabolites (eg, normeperidine).

Opioid toxicity characteristically presents with a depressed level of consciousness, and should be suspected when the clinical triad of CNS depression, respiratory depression, and pupillary miosis are present. Other important presenting signs are euphoria, ventricular arrhythmias, acute mental status changes, and seizures.

Study Pearl

All opioids have a prolonged duration of action in patients with liver disease (eg, cirrhosis) because of impaired hepatic metabolism. This may lead to drug accumulation and opioid toxicity.

Antidepressants

Tricyclic Antidepressants. Tricyclic antidepressants (TCAs), as their name suggests, are used in the treatment of depression, as well as in the treatment of chronic pain, and enuresis (involuntary discharge of urine).

TCAs affect the CNS and the cardiovascular, pulmonary, and GI systems. The toxic effects on the myocardium are related to the blocking of fast sodium channels, which involves the same mechanism as type IA antiarrhythmics (eg, quinidine). The result is a slowing myocardium depolarization that leads to arrhythmia, myocardial depression, and hypotension. Hypotension also results from peripheral alpha-adrenergic blockade, which causes vascular dilatation. Inhibition of norepinephrine reuptake and subsequent depletion causes further hypotension.

CNS toxicity results from the anticholinergic effects and direct inhibition of biogenic amine reuptake. An excitation syndrome is the initial result and manifests as confusion, hallucinations, ataxia, seizures, and coma.

The adverse effects on the pulmonary system include pulmonary edema, adult respiratory distress syndrome (ARDS), and aspiration pneumonitis. The etiologies of the first two remain unclear, but the third, aspiration pneumonitis, is secondary to an altered mental status.

The anticholinergic effects of TCAs cause a slowing of the gastrointestinal (GI) system, which results in delayed gastric emptying, decreased motility, and prolonged transit time.

Parkinson Disease and Parkinsonian Syndrome. The basal ganglia motor circuit modulates cortical output necessary for normal movement. Levodopa, coupled with a peripheral decarboxylase inhibitor (PDI), remains the criterion standard of symptomatic treatment for PD.[40-46] It provides the greatest antiparkinsonian benefit with the fewest adverse effects. Dopamine agonists provide symptomatic benefit comparable to levodopa/PDI in early disease but lack sufficient efficacy to control signs and symptoms by themselves in later disease.

Medications for Parkinson's usually provide good symptomatic control for 4 to 6 years. Whether levodopa has a toxic or protective effect in the brain with PD is unknown. As PD progresses, fewer dopamine neurons are available to store and release levodopa-derived dopamine. The patient's clinical status begins to fluctuate more and more closely in concert with plasma levodopa levels. Fluctuating levodopa-derived dopamine concentrations in association with advancing disease therefore may be responsible for development of motor fluctuations and dyskinesia.

In contrast to levodopa, the long-acting dopamine agonists (ie, bromocriptine, pergolide, pramipexole, ropinirole, cabergoline) provide relatively smooth and sustained receptor stimulation.

The selection of medication depends in part on the nature and cause of the disability.

If disability is due solely to tremor, a tremor-specific medication, such as an anticholinergic agent, can be used. Anticholinergic medications provide good tremor relief in approximately 50% of patients but do not improve bradykinesia or rigidity. Because tremor may respond to one anticholinergic medication and not another, a second anticholinergic usually is tried if the first is not successful. Adverse cognitive effects are relatively common, especially in the elderly.

Most patients require symptomatic dopaminergic therapy to ameliorate bradykinesia and rigidity within 1 to 2 years after diagnosis.

For patients who are demented or those older than 70 years, who may be prone to adverse effects from dopamine agonists, and for those likely to require treatment for only a few years, physicians may elect not to use a dopamine agonist and depend on levodopa/PDI as primary symptomatic therapy.[47]

For patients aged 65 to 70 years, a judgment is made based on general health and cognitive status.

Study Pearl

Anticonvulsants in mood disorders have four major effects:

- Increasing of the seizure threshold
- Decreasing the seizure duration
- Decreasing the neurometabolic response to an episode
- Decreasing the phenomena of amygdaloid kindling

Essentially, they make it more difficult for the postsynaptic neuron to reach its excitation threshold either electrically or neurochemically, and once it has been reached, decreases the widespread effects.

Antiepileptic Drugs. Antiepileptic drugs (AEDs) are designed to modify the processes behind a seizure to favor inhibition over excitation in order to stop or prevent seizure activity. AEDs can be grouped according to their main mechanism of action, although many of them have several actions and others have unknown mechanisms of action.

Side Effects and Toxicity. AEDs can produce dose-related adverse effects, which include dizziness, diplopia, nausea, ataxia, and blurred vision. Hydantoins may not be suitable for persons with a history of thyroid, liver, or kidney disease, depressed renal function, diabetes mellitus, porphyria, lupus, mental illness, high blood presure, angina (chest pain), or irregular heartbeats and other heart problems.

GABA Receptor Agonists. GABA has two types of receptors.

- GABA-A: GABA-A receptor is stimulated, chloride channels open to allow the influx of negative ions (ie, chloride) into the neuron and cause hyperpolarization, moving the membrane potential further from the cell-firing threshold. The GABA-A receptors have multiple binding sites for benzodiazepines, barbiturates, and others substances such as picrotoxins, bicuculline, and neurosteroids.
- GABA-B: The GABA-B receptor is linked to a potassium channel.

Direct binding to GABA-A receptors, can enhance the GABA system by blocking presynaptic GABA uptake, by inhibiting the metabolism of GABA by GABA transaminase, and by increasing the synthesis of GABA. The benzodiazepines most commonly used for treatment of epilepsy are lorazepam, diazepam, clonazepam, and clobazam. The two barbiturates mostly commonly used in the treatment of epilepsy are phenobarbital and primidone.

Side Effects and Toxicity. The most common effect is sedation. Other adverse effects include dizziness, ataxia, blurred vision, diplopia, irritability, depression, muscle fatigue, and weakness. Idiosyncratic reactions are very rare and no fatal reactions have been reported so far.

GABA Reuptake Inhibitors. At least four specific GABA-transporting compounds help in the reuptake of GABA; these carry GABA from the synaptic space into neurons and glial cells, where it is metabolized. Nipecotic acid and tiagabine (TGB) are inhibitors of these transporters; this inhibition makes increased amounts of GABA available in the synaptic cleft. GABA prolongs inhibitory postsynaptic potentials (IPSPs).

Side Effects and Toxicity. The most common adverse effects include dizziness, asthenia, nervousness, tremor, depressed mood, and emotional lability. Diarrhea also was significantly more frequent among TGB-treated patients than placebo-treated patients. Other adverse effects included somnolence, headaches, abnormal thinking, abdominal pain, pharyngitis, ataxia, confusion, psychosis, and skin rash. No changes in biochemical or hematological parameters were reported. Serious idiosyncratic adverse effects were recorded as commonly in patients on placebo as in those on TGB.

GABA Transaminase Inhibitor. GABA is metabolized by transamination in the extracellular compartment by GABA-transaminase (GABA-T). Inhibition of this enzymatic process leads to an increase in the extracellular concentration of GABA. Vigabatrin (VGB) inhibits the enzyme GABA-T.

Side Effects and Toxicity. The most common adverse effect is drowsiness. Other important adverse effects include neuropsychiatric symptoms, such as depression, agitation, confusion and, rarely, psychosis. Minor adverse effects, usually at the onset of therapy, include fatigue, headache, dizziness, increase in weight, tremor, double vision, and abnormal vision.

Glutamate Blockers. Glutamate and aspartate are the most two important excitatory neurotransmitters in the brain. The glutamate system is a complex system with macromolecular receptors with different binding sites (ie, AMPA, kainate, NMDA, glycine, metabotropic site). The AMPA and the kainate sites open a channel through the receptor, allowing sodium and small amounts of calcium to enter. The NMDA site opens a channel that allows large amounts of calcium to enter along with the sodium ions. This channel is blocked by magnesium in the resting state.

The glycine site facilitates the opening of the NMDA receptor channel. The metabotropic site is regulated by complex reactions and second messengers mediate its response. NMDA antagonists have a limited use because they produce psychosis and hallucinations. In addition to these adverse effects, blocking these receptors may impair learning and memory, because NMDA receptors are associated with learning processes and long-term potentiation. Examples of glutamate blockers include topiramate and felbamate.

Side Effects and Toxicity. Common adverse effects include insomnia, weight loss, nausea, decreased appetite, dizziness, fatigue, ataxia, and lethargy. Polytherapy is associated with increases in adverse effects.

Neuroleptics (Antipsychotics). Neuroleptics are antipsychotic drugs that reduce confusion, delusions, hallucinations, and psychomotor agitation in patients with psychoses. The adverse effects of neuroleptics are not confined to psychiatric patients. Neuroleptics also are used as sedatives, for their antiemetic properties, to control hiccups, to treat migraine headaches, as antidotes for drug-induced psychosis, and in conjunction with opioid analgesia. Neuroleptics are also utilized in conjunction with antidepressants, or mood stabilizers when psychotic symptoms are present, or to enhance the effect of other medications when attempting to control mania.

Although all antipsychotic preparations share some toxic characteristics, the relative intensity of these effects varies greatly, depending on the individual drug. Generally, all neuroleptic medications are capable of causing the following symptoms:

- Hypotension.
- Anticholinergic effects such as tachycardia, hyperthermia, urinary retention, and toxic psychosis.
- Extrapyramidal symptoms such as dystonia, torticollis, acute parkinsonism, and other movement disorders.
- Neuroleptic malignant syndrome which is a life-threatening derangement that affects multiple organ systems and results in significant mortality.
- Seizures.
- Hypothermia.
- Cardiac effects.
- Respiratory depression.

SPASTICITY

Although the use of oral medications for the treatment of spasticity may be very effective,[48] at high dosages they can cause unwanted adverse effects that include sedation as well as changes in mood and cognition.

Cardiovascular System Pharmacology

Alpha-Adrenergic Blocking Drugs (Alpha Blockers). These drugs work through the autonomic nervous system (ANS) by blocking nerve receptors that are called alpha-receptors. Alpha-receptors normally promote constriction of the arterioles. Blocking constriction promotes dilation of the vessels and lowers blood pressure as well as reducing the work of the heart in some situations. Alpha-blocking drugs also inhibit the actions of one of the adrenal hormones, norepinephrine, that raises blood pressure as part of the fight-or-flight response. Alpha-blockers are usually prescribed along with other blood-pressure-lowering drugs, such as a beta blocking drug and/or a diuretic. In general, alpha-blockers are not as effective for initial therapy as some of the other blood-pressure-lowering medications. There are now several medications available that combine the effects of blocking both the beta and alpha-receptors (labetolol [Normodyne, Trandate]).

Possible Adverse Side Effects. Nausea and indigestion; these usually subside with long-term use. Less frequent effects are cold hands and feet, temporary impotence, and nightmares. Dizziness may occur initially or as dosage is increased.

Angiotensin-Converting Enzyme Inhibitors. These drugs act to prevent production of a hormone, angiotensin II, which constricts blood vessels. They belong to the class of drugs called vasodilators—drugs that dilate blood vessels, an effective way to lower blood pressure and increase the supply of blood and oxygen to the heart and various other organs. In addition to dilating blood vessels, angiotensin-converting enzyme (ACE)-inhibiting medications may produce some beneficial effects indirectly by preventing the abnormal rise in hormones associated with heart disease, such as aldosterone. ACE inhibitors are widely used to treat high blood pressure, or hypertension, a major risk factor for cardiovascular disease. Used alone or in combination with other drugs, ACE inhibitors have also proved effective in the treatment of congestive heart failure.

Possible Adverse Side Effects. Common side effects are dizziness or weakness, loss of appetite, a rash, itching, a hacking, unpredictable cough, and swelling.

Anti-Arrhythmic Drugs. These drugs correct an irregular heartbeat and slow a heart that is beating too fast. Regardless of the type of antiarrhythmic drug, patients should never take more than prescribed. Conversely, because the effectiveness of these drugs depends on maintaining the optimum level of medication in the blood, the patient should be sure to take them according to the physician's instructions. Although the vast majority of patients benefit from antiarrhythmic drugs, heart arrhythmias may paradoxically worsen in 5% to 10% of patients.

Possible Side Effects. Most significant common side effects are weakening of heart contractions, worsening of some arrhythmias, weight loss, nausea, and tremors. Other less common effects are fever, rash, dry mouth, depressed white blood cell count, liver inflammation, confusion, loss of concentration, dizziness, and disturbances in vision.

Study Pearl

Any patient who has had a heart valve replaced with a mechanical valve requires lifelong oral anticoagulants in order to prevent clots from forming on the valve.

Anticoagulants, Antiplatelets, and Thrombolytics. These drugs are sometimes referred to as "blood thinners," but this term is not truly accurate. They inhibit the ability of the blood to clot—preventing clots from forming in blood vessels and from getting bigger. Under a number of different circumstances, it becomes necessary to stop clotting. Anticoagulants, antiplatelet agents, and thrombolytics each have specific indications and uses.

Patients who develop atrial fibrillation may require anticoagulants; clot formation in the left atrium is a potential hazard of this rhythmic disturbance. Oral anticoagulants are prescribed for patients who develop thrombophlebitis, an inflammation of the veins in the legs or pelvis. One of the dangers of this condition is the development of blood clots that may travel to the lungs and cause pulmonary emboli. Lastly, some patients who have a serious heart attack involving the front surface of the heart are prescribed an anticoagulant to prevent clots from forming on the inner lining of the scar.

Heparin is an anticoagulant that is administered intravenously when rapid anticoagulation is necessary. Aspirin is not an anticoagulant but has a profound effect on platelets. Because of aspirin's ability to inhibit the clotting action of platelets, it is designated as an antiplatelet and is frequently prescribed in patients who have recovered from a heart attack, in order to prevent clots from forming in the veins used for coronary bypass surgery.

Thrombolytic drugs are given intravenously to help prevent clotting of the coronary arteries, and prevent permanent, debilitating damage. The three most commonly used thrombolytics are t-PA, streptokinase, and APSAC.

Possible Side Effects. Adverse effects are rare, but may include nausea, headache, flushing, dizziness or faintness, or rash.

Beta-Adrenergic Blockers. These drugs probably reduce blood pressure by reducing the output of blood from the heart (or perhaps by blocking the production of angiotensin). Beta-blockers are also used to treat high blood pressure. Specifically, they block responses from the beta nerve receptors. This serves to slow down the heart rate and to lower blood pressure. Beta-blockers also block the effects of some of the hormones that regulate blood pressure. During exercise or emotional stress, adrenaline and norepinephrine are released and normally stimulate the beta-receptors—sensors that transmit messages to the heart to speed up and pump harder. By blocking the receptors, beta-blockers act to reduce heart muscle oxygen demands during physical activity or excitement, thus reducing the possibility of angina caused by oxygen deprivation. Beta-blockers also dampen heart rate increases caused by stress, exercise, or anxiety.

Possible Side Effects. Lethargy and cold hands and feet because of reduced circulation may occur. Also may cause nausea, nightmares or vivid dreams, and impotence. May also precipitate asthmatic attack.

Calcium Channel Blockers. Calcium plays a central role in the electrical stimulation of cardiac cells and in the mechanical contraction of smooth muscle cells in the wails of arteries. Calcium channel blockers are relatively new synthetic drugs that work by blocking the passage of calcium into the muscle cells that control the size of blood vessels, thereby preventing the muscles of the arteries from constricting.

Possible Side Effects. Excessively slow heart rate, low blood pressure, headache, swelling of ankle/feet, constipation, nausea, tiredness, dizziness, redness of face and neck, palpitations, and rash.

Digitalis Drugs. Like many drugs, digitalis was originally derived from a plant, in this case the foxglove. Digitalis has the primary effect of strengthening the force of contractions in weakened hearts, but it is not a cardiac vitamin that can make a strong heart stronger. It is also used in the control of atrial fibrillation. The most commonly used digitalis products are digoxin and digitoxin. The drug penetrates all body tissues and reaches a high concentration in the muscle of the heart. Its molecules bind with cell receptors that regulate the concentration of sodium and potassium in the spaces between tissue cells and in the bloodstream. Digitalis preparations act by increasing the amount of calcium supplied to the heart muscle and thus enhancing its contractions. By increasing the force of heart contractions, there is an increase in the amount of blood pumped with each beat. Digitalis drugs also affect electrical activity in cardiac tissues. They control the rate at which electric impulses are released and the speed of their conduction through the chamber wails. These two actions determine the two major uses of digitalis drugs in heart disease—treatment of heart failure and control of abnormal heart rhythms. Digitalis preparations are a major class of drugs used in the treatment of heart failure. The improved pumping capacity offsets the mechanisms that lead to the enlargement of the failing heart.

Possible Side Effects. Some side effects include tiredness, nausea, loss of appetite, and disturbances in vision.

Diuretics. Diuretics, commonly referred to as water pills, lower blood pressure by increasing the kidney's excretion of sodium and water, which in turn reduces the volume of blood. There are several types of diuretics, which are classified according to their site of action in the kidney.

Possible Side Effects. Although uncommon, lethargy, cramps, rash, or impotence may occur. Some of these effects may be caused by loss of potassium and may be avoided by including a potassium supplement or potassium-sparing agent in the regimen.

Nitrates. The oldest and most frequently used coronary artery medications are the nitrates. Nitrates are potent vein and artery dilators, causing blood to pool in the veins and the arteries to open up, thus reducing the amount of blood returning to the heart. This has the effect of decreasing the work of the left ventricle and lowering the blood pressure. Nitrates may also increase the supply of oxygenated blood by causing the coronary arteries to open more fully, thus improving coronary blood flow. Nitrates effectively relieve coronary artery spasm. They do not, however, appear to affect the heart's contractions.

Possible Side Effects. Headaches, flushing, and dizziness may occur.

Pulmonary System Pharmacology

Direct drug delivery to the lungs allows a medication to interact directly with the diseased tissue and reduces the risk of adverse effects, while allowing for the reduction of dose compared to oral administration. Most of these inhaled drugs are administered through a pressurized metered-dose inhaler. The other main drug delivery system for pulmonary problems is the nebulizer, a device that dispenses liquid medications as a mist of extremely fine particles in oxygen or room air so that is inhaled.

Bronchodilator Agents. Bronchodilator agents are a group of medications that produce an expansion of the lumina of the airway passages of the lungs. Bronchodilator agents are central to the symptomatic management of chronic obstructive pulmonary disease (COPD), and asthma.

- $Beta_2$ agonists: mimic the activity of the sympathetic nervous system (sympathomimetics) thereby producing relaxation of airway smooth muscle, bronchodilation. In addition, these medications inhibit inflammatory mediator release from mast cells, and enhance mucociliary clearance. They are the most commonly prescribed drugs for the treatment of asthma. $Beta_2$ agonists can be categorized into short acting (rescue drugs) and longer acting agents. Examples of the short acting types, which are used primarily for immediate release of breakthrough symptoms of chest tightness, wheezing and shortness of breath, include Ventolin, Alupent, Maxair, albuterol, salbutamol, and terbutaline. Salmeterol, Serevent, and formoterol are examples of the longer acting agents. Side effects of $Beta_2$ agonists include tremor, tachycardia, hypokalemia, and hyperglycemia.
- Anticholinergic agents: these drugs are primarily used in the treatment of COPD and asthma. The muscarinic receptor antagonists cause bronchodilation by blocking the action of acetylcholine on airway smooth muscle (inhibit the parasympathetic nervous system). Although these medications do not prevent all types of bronchospasm, they are effective against asthma produced by irritant stimuli. In general, dry mouth and pharyngeal irritation are the major side effects, but tachycardia may occur with excessive dosing.
- Theophylline: a methylxanthine, a substance found in coffee, tea, and chocolate, which acts as a phosphodiesterase inhibitor, which in turn increases intracellular cyclic adenosine monophosphate, resulting in relaxation of smooth muscle. The drug is used for patients who do not respond to the standard asthma agents, and is occasionally used in the treatment of spinal cord injury. Adverse side effects of this drug include nausea, increased blood pressure, arrhythmias, tachycardia, nervousness, headaches, and seizures.

Anti-inflammatory Agents.

- Corticosteroids: steroids block the release of arachidonic acid from airway epithelial cells, which in turn blocks production of prostaglandins and leukotrienes. These drugs can be administered systemically or topically (MDI). Inhaled steroids have been the drugs of choice for reducing the number of asthmatic attacks in patients who have mild to moderate persistent asthma and for those who require Beta$_2$ inhalers more than once a day. Examples of inhaled steroids include beclomethasone, budesonide, and fluticasone. The side effects of systemic administration are increased blood pressure, glaucoma, sodium retention, muscle wasting, osteoporosis, dyphonia. The main side effect of inhaled steroids is oral candidiasis, although the use of the spacer device and diligent rinsing of the mouth after the inhalation can decrease the effects. Examples of these medications include Vanceril (MDI), and Azmacort (MDI).
- Leukotriene receptor antagonists: act by blocking the actions of leukotrienes that are released in an allergic reaction, decreasing the migration of eosinophils, production of mucus, and bronchoconstriction. Examples of these drugs include Montelukast and zafirlukast. Leukotriene receptor antagonists have demonstrated few adverse drug reactions.
- Cromolyn and nedocromil: act by inhibiting mast cell degranulation (ie, histamine) after exposure with allergens, thereby blocking the release of inflammatory mediators and thus decreasing airway hyperresponsiveness. These drugs are used prophylactically to prevent exercise-induced bronchospasm and severe bronchial asthma via oral inhalation. A benefit of these drugs is that they have relatively few side effects with the exception of a bitter taste. Frequent inhalation can result in hoarseness, cough, dry mouth and bronchial irritation.

Antitussives. Antitussives are drugs that suppress coughing by decreasing the activity of the afferent nerves or decreasing the sensitivity of the cough center. The stimulus to cough is relayed to the cough center in the medulla and then to the respiratory muscles via the phrenic nerve.

Antibiotics. Cultures and sensitivity results are used to describe the most effective antibiotic—refer to next section.

Metabolic and Endocrine System

Diabetes. Because patients with type II diabetes have both insulin resistance and beta-cell dysfunction, oral medication to increase insulin sensitivity (eg, metformin, a thiazolidinedione [TZD]) is often given with an intermediate-acting insulin (eg, neutral protamine Hagedorn[49]) at bedtime or a long-acting insulin (eg, glargine [Lantus] insulin, insulin detemir [Levemir]) given in the morning or evening. Medications for diabetes are typically prescribed based on their mode of action. Examples include

- Exenatide (Byetta): incretin mimetic agent that mimics glucose-dependent insulin secretion and several other antihyperglycemic actions of incretins.

- Chlorpropamide (Diabinese): may increase insulin secretion from pancreatic beta cells.
- Tolbutamide (Orinase): increases insulin secretion from pancreatic beta cells.
- Tolazamide (Tolinase): increases insulin secretion from pancreatic beta cells.
- Acetohexamide (Dymelor): increases insulin secretion from pancreatic beta cells.
- Glyburide (DiaBeta, Micronase, PresTab, Glynase): increases insulin secretion from pancreatic beta cells.
- Glipizide (Glucotrol, Glucotrol XL): second-generation sulfonylurea; stimulates insulin release from pancreatic beta cells.
- Repaglinide (Prandin): stimulates insulin release from pancreatic beta cells.
- Metformin (Glucophage): monotherapy or with sulfonylurea, TZD, or insulin. Taken with food to reduce adverse GI effects.
- Acarbose (Precose): delays hydrolysis of ingested complex carbohydrates and disaccharides and absorption of glucose. Inhibits metabolism of sucrose to glucose and fructose.
- Miglitol (Glyset): delays glucose absorption in small intestine; lowers after-dinner hyperglycemia.
- Pioglitazone (Actos): improves target cell response to insulin without increasing insulin secretion from pancreas.
- Rosiglitazone (Avandia): insulin sensitizer; major effect in stimulating glucose uptake in skeletal muscle and adipose tissue.
- Pramlintide acetate (Symlin): synthetic analogue of human amylin, hormone made in beta cells. Slows gastric emptying, suppresses after-dinner glucagon secretion, and regulates food intake.

POLYPHARMACY AND MEDICATION ERRORS

Polypharmacy is defined here as the long-term use of two or more medications. Many medications are absorbed, distributed, metabolized, and excreted differently in the elderly. The presence of multiple diagnoses in the elderly leads to multiple drug and nutrient interactions and complex medical management, with the resulting side effects of progressive loss of functional reserve and physiological homeostasis.[50]

The National Coordinating Council for Medication Error Reporting and Prevention (NCC MERP) defines a medication error as "any preventable event that may cause or lead to inappropriate medication use or patient harm while the medication is in the control of the health care professional, patient, or consumer. Such events may be related to professional practice, health care products, procedures, and systems, including prescribing; order communication; product labeling, packaging, and nomenclature; compounding; dispensing; distribution; administration; education; monitoring; and use."

The American Hospital Association lists the following as some common types of medication errors:

- Incomplete patient information (not knowing about patients' allergies, other medicines they are taking, previous diagnoses, and laboratory results, for example).

- Unavailable drug information (such as lack of up-to-date warnings).
- Miscommunication of drug orders, which can involve poor handwriting, confusion between drugs with similar names, misuse of zeroes and decimal points, confusion of metric and other dosing units, and inappropriate abbreviations. Multiple providers often are unaware of one another's new prescriptions or medication changes, especially after hospitalization.
- Lack of appropriate labeling as a drug is prepared and repackaged into smaller units; and environmental factors, such as lighting, heat, noise, and interruptions, that can distract health professionals from their medical tasks.
- Drug name confusion. Examples of drug name confusion reported to the FDA include
  - Serzone (nefazodone) for depression and Seroquel (quetiapine) for schizophrenia
  - Lamictal (lamotrigine) for epilepsy, Lamisil (terbinafine) for nail infections, Ludiomil (maprotiline) for depression, and Lomotil (diphenoxylate) for diarrhea
  - Taxotere (docetaxel) and Taxol (paclitaxel), both for chemotherapy
  - Zantac (ranitidine) for heartburn, Zyrtec (cetirizine) for allergies, and Zyprexa (olanzapine) for mental conditions, Celebrex (celecoxib) for arthritis and Celexa (citalopram) for depression
- Older patients often have visual or cognitive impairment (or both) that leads to errors in self administration.
- Older patients are often on fixed incomes and may cut doses down to save money.
- Cultural diversity can affect the perspective about the value of taking a certain medication when some natural alternative has been used for centuries in a culture to treat the same condition.
- Many older patients self-prescribe.

PHYSICAL THERAPY ROLE

Assist in adequate monitoring of drug therapy through:

- Scheduling physical therapy to coincide with drug schedule to maximize the effects of the drug.
- Recognition of drug-related side effects/adverse reactions. This includes the interaction effects of modalities certain medications (the use of heat with patients on vasodilators).
- Being aware of potential drug interactions in the elderly.
- Monitoring of patients responses to medications relative to exercise and activity.

Patient and family education/compliance:

- Encourage centralization of medications through one pharmacy.
- Safe administration of drugs.
- Medication schedule, daily pillbox.
- Appropriate dosage and frequency.

AMPHETAMINES

The phenylethylamine structure of amphetamines is similar to catecholaminergic, dopaminergic, and serotonergic agonists (biogenic amines), which may explain their actions, which are similar to those of cocaine; however, while the effects of cocaine last for 10 to 20 minutes, duration of amphetamine action is much longer, lasting as long as 10 to 12 hours. The routes of amphetamine administration may be oral (ingestion), inhalation (smoke), or injection (IV).

Patients with amphetamine intoxication often are identified by a change of mental status alone or associated with another injury and/or illness.

Questions for this chapter and the entire book appear on the included CD-ROM, with additional questions at www.DuttonNPTE.com.

REFERENCES

1. Brookfield WP: Pharmacologic considerations for the physical therapist. In: Boissonnault WG, ed. *Primary Care for the Physical Therapist: Examination and Triage.* St Louis, MO: Elsevier Saunders. 2005:309-322.
2. Brodie BB: Displacement of one drug by another from carrier or receptor sites. *Proc R Soc Med.* 1965;58:946-955.
3. Donne-Op den Kelder GM: Distance geometry analysis of ligand binding to drug receptor sites. *J Comput Aided Mol Des.* 1987;1:257-264.
4. Glossmann H, Striessnig J, Hymel L, et al: Purification and reconstitution of calcium channel drug-receptor sites. *Ann N Y Acad Sci.* 1988;522:150-161.
5. Schou JS: Drug interactions at (pharmacodynamically active) receptor sites. *Pharmacol Ther.* 1982;17:199-210.
6. Watson PJ: Drug receptor sites in the isolated superior cervical ganglion of the rat. *Eur J Pharmacol.* 1970;12:183-193.
7. Ayrton A, Morgan P: Role of transport proteins in drug absorption, distribution and excretion. *Xenobiotica.* 2001;31:469-497.
8. Davis SS, Wilding IR: Oral drug absorption studies: the best model for man is man! *Drug Discov Today.* 2001;6:127-130.
9. Fu XC, Liang WQ, Yu QS: Correlation of drug absorption with molecular charge distribution. *Pharmazie.* 2001;56:267-268.
10. Idkaidek NM, Abdel-Jabbar N: A novel approach to increase oral drug absorption. *Pharm Dev Technol.* 2001;6:167-171.
11. Jackson K, Young D, Pant S: Drug-excipient interactions and their affect on absorption. *Pharm Sci Technolo Today.* 2000;3:336-345.
12. Kimura T, Higaki K: Gastrointestinal transit and drug absorption. *Biol Pharm Bull.* 2002;25:149-164.
13. Lin J, Sahakian DC, de Morais SM, et al: The role of absorption, distribution, metabolism, excretion and toxicity in drug discovery. *Curr Top Med Chem.* 2003;3:1125-1154.

14. Stenberg P, Bergstrom CA, Luthman K, et al: Theoretical predictions of drug absorption in drug discovery and development. *Clin Pharmacokinet.* 2002;41:877-899.
15. Kennedy JM, van Rij AM: Drug absorption from the small intestine in immediate postoperative patients. *Br J Anaesth.* 2006; 97:171-180.
16. Taki Y, Sakane T, Nadai T, et al: Gastrointestinal absorption of peptide drug: quantitative evaluation of the degradation and the permeation of metkephamid in rat small intestine. *J Pharmacol Exp Ther.* 1995;274:373-377.
17. Bartal C, Danon A, Schlaeffer F, et al: Pharmacokinetic dosing of aminoglycosides: a controlled trial. *Am J Med.* 2003;114:194-198.
18. Davies JE: Aminoglycosides: ancient and modern. *J Antibiot (Tokyo).* 2006;59:529-532.
19. Turnidge J: Pharmacodynamics and dosing of aminoglycosides. *Infect Dis Clin North Am.* 2003;17:503-528, v.
20. Gouda MW, Khalafalah N, Khalil SA: Effect of surfactants on absorption through membranes V: concentration-dependent effect of a bile salt (sodium deoxycholate) on absorption of a poorly absorbable drug, phenolsulfonphthalein, in humans. *J Pharm Sci.* 1977;66:727-728.
21. Riegelman S: The effect of surfactants on drug stability. *I J Am Pharm Assoc Am Pharm Assoc.* 1960;49:339-343.
22. Utsumi I, Kono K, Takeuchi Y: Effect of surfactants on drug absorption. IV. Mechanism of the action of sodium glycocholate on the absorption of benzoylthiamine disulfide in the presence of sodium laurylsulfate and polysorbate 80. *Chem Pharm Bull (Tokyo).* 1973;21:2161-2167.
23. Adams JF: The effect of some drugs and of differing routes of administration on the urinary excretion of parenteral vitamin B_{12}. *Clin Sci.* 1963;24:431-435.
24. Benini A, Bertazzoni Minelli E: Parenteral administration of antimicrobial drugs can affect the intestinal microflora of rat. *Pharmacol Res.* 1992;25(suppl 1):75-76.
25. Collomp K, Anselme F, Audran M, et al: Effects of moderate exercise on the pharmacokinetics of caffeine. *Eur J Clin Pharmacol.* 1991;40:279-282.
26. Jessup JV, Lowenthal DT, Pollock ML, et al: The effects of exercise training on the pharmacokinetics of digoxin. *J Cardiopulm Rehabil.* 2000;20:89-95.
27. Khazaeinia T, Ramsey AA, Tam YK: The effects of exercise on the pharmacokinetics of drugs. *J Pharm Pharm Sci.* 2000;3:292-302.
28. Kim HJ, Lee AK, Kim YG, et al: Influence of 4-week and 8-week exercise training on the pharmacokinetics and pharmacodynamics of intravenous and oral azosemide in rats. *Life Sci.* 2002;70: 2299-2319.
29. Persky AM, Eddington ND, Derendorf H: A review of the effects of chronic exercise and physical fitness level on resting pharmacokinetics. *Int J Clin Pharmacol Ther.* 2003;41:504-516.
30. Ylitalo P: Effect of exercise on pharmacokinetics. *Ann Med.* 1991;23:289-294.
31. Frank S, Somani SM, Kohnle M: Effect of exercise on propranolol pharmacokinetics. *Eur J Clin Pharmacol.* 1990;39:391-394.

32. van Baak MA: Influence of exercise on the pharmacokinetics of drugs. *Clin Pharmacokinet.* 1990;19:32-43.
33. Dionne RA: Pharmacologic treatments for temporomandibular disorders. *Surg Oral Med Pathol Radiol Endodont.* 1997;83: 134-142.
34. Sperling RL: NSAIDs. *Home Healthcare Nurse.* 2001;19:687-689.
35. Holvoet J, Terriere L, Van Hee W, et al: Relation of upper gastro-intestinal bleeding to non-steroidal anti-inflammatory drugs and aspirin: a case-control study. *Gut.* 1991;32:730-734.
36. Clive DM, Stoff JS: Renal syndromes associated with nonsteroidal antiinflammatory drugs. *N Engl J Med.* 1984;310:563-572.
37. Brattsand R, Linden M: Cytokine modulation by glucocorticoids: mechanisms and actions in cellular studies. *Aliment Pharmacol Ther.* 1996;10(suppl 2):81-90; discussion 1-2.
38. Buchman AL: Side effects of corticosteroid therapy. *J Clin Gastroenterol.* 2001;33:289-294.
39. Elenbaas JK: Centrally acting oral skeletal muscle relaxants. *Am J Hosp Pharm.* 1980;37:1313-1323.
40. Charles PD, Davis TL: Drug therapy for Parkinson's disease. *South Med J.* 1996;89:851-856.
41. Hagan JJ, Middlemiss DN, Sharpe PC, et al: Parkinson's disease: prospects for improved drug therapy. *Trends Pharmacol Sci.* 1997;18:156-163.
42. Hermanowicz N: Drug therapy for Parkinson's disease. *Semin Neurol.* 2007;27:97-105.
43. Mizuno Y: Drug therapy of Parkinson's disease. An overview. *Eur Neurol.* 1992;32 (suppl 1):3-8.
44. Oertel WH, Quinn NP: Parkinson's disease: drug therapy. *Baillieres Clin Neurol.* 1997;6:89-108.
45. Robertson DR, George CF: Drug therapy for Parkinson's disease in the elderly. *Br Med Bull.* 1990;46:124-146.
46. Stevenson T: Drug therapy in the management of Parkinson's disease. *Br J Nurs.* 1997;6:144-148, 150.
47. Caird FI: Non-drug therapy of Parkinson's disease. *Scott Med J.* 1986;31:129-132.
48. Vanek ZF, Menkes JH: *Spasticity.* Available at: http://www.emedicine.com/neuro/topic706.htm, 2005.
49. Spitzer G, Adkins D, Mathews M, et al: Randomized comparison of G-CSF + GM-CSF vs G-CSF alone for mobilization of peripheral blood stem cells: effects on hematopoietic recovery after high-dose chemotherapy. *Bone Marrow Transplant.* 1997;20:921-930.
50. Bottomley JM: The geriatric population. In: Boissonnault WG, ed. *Primary Care for the Physical Therapist: Examination and Triage.* St Louis, MO: Elsevier Saunders. 2005:288-306.

section IV

Examination Prepration

Examination Preparation

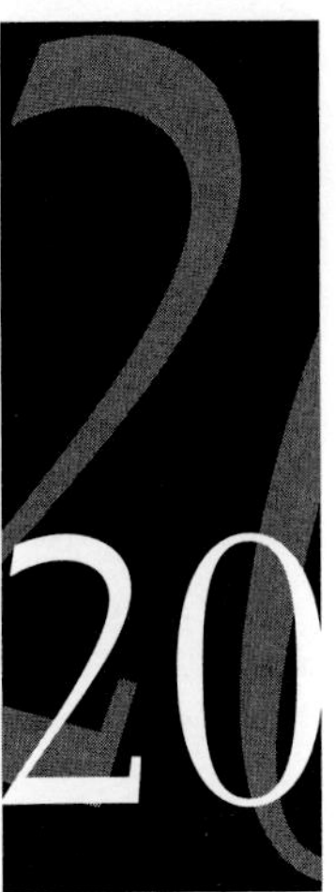

Since the examination is multiple choice and computerized, candidates should make sure they are comfortable taking multiple-choice, computerized examinations.

What are the steps for taking the examination?

- Obtain registration materials from the licensing authority of the jurisdiction in which you are seeking licensure. Some jurisdictions allow online registration for the examination at http://www.fsbpt.org.
- If you have a documented disability, you may request special accommodations to take the examination. Contact the licensing authority in the jurisdiction in which you are seeking licensure for details. You must request special accommodations at the time you register.
- Return completed registration materials, along with payment, to the appropriate organization as identified on the instructions you received from the licensing authority. If either the scannable payment form or registration is incomplete, it will be returned to you. If you register online, you will not need to complete the scannable registration form or payment form.
- The jurisdiction licensing authority will approve your eligibility and notify FSBPT.
- FSBPT will send you an "Authorization to Test" letter containing instructions on how to schedule an appointment with Prometric. Questions regarding registration processing may be directed to examregis-tration@fsbpt.org.
- Schedule an appointment for the examination with Prometric. You may schedule your appointment with Prometric by calling the number given in your "Authorization to Test" letter or you may schedule online at www.prometric.com.

- Sit for the examination at your chosen Prometric testing site. You must sit for the examination within your 60-day eligibility period as indicated on the "Authorization-to-Test" letter provided by FSBPT. If you do not sit for the examination, or withdraw your registration, within these 60 days, you will be removed from the eligibility list and will be required to begin the registration process again.

Physical Therapist Examination Content Outline
With Content Category Specifications
Federation of State Boards of Physical Therapy

	Specs	#
1000 Examination	*26.0%*	*52*
History and Systems Review	**7.5%**	**15**
1100 History Included are critical knowledge and skills related to obtaining past and current patient history information from medical records, and interviews with patients and others. Information includes demographics, general health status, chief complaint, medications, medical/surgical and social history, functional status/activity level, social/health habits, living environment, employment, and growth and development.		
1200 Systems Review. Included are critical knowledge and skills related to: 1210 Conducting a systems review of the cardiovascular/pulmonary system 1211 Conducting a systems review of the integumentary system 1212 Conducting a systems review of the musculoskeletal system 1213 Conducting a systems review of the neuromuscular system 1300 Tests and Measures. Included are critical knowledge and skills related to:		
Tests and Measures Group I: A. Strength, ROM, Posture, Body Structures, Prosthetic & Orthotic Devices B. Cognition, Nerve, Reflex and Sensory Integrity, Neurodevelopment	**11.0%**	**22**
1310 Tests and Measures A: Strength, ROM, Posture, Body Structures, Prosthetic, and Orthotic Devices 1311 Anthropometric characteristics 1312 Joint integrity and mobility 1313 Posture 1314 Prosthetic devices 1315 Range of Motion/muscle length 1316 Muscle performance 1317 Orthotic, protective and supportive devices 1320 Tests and Measures B: Cognition, Nerve, Reflex and Sensory Integrity, Neurodevelopment 1321 Arousal, attention and cognition 1322 Cranial and peripheral nerve integrity (motor and sensory) 1323 Motor function 1324 Neurodevelopment and sensory integration 1325 Reflex integrity 1326 Sensory integrity		

(*Continued*)

Physical Therapist Examination Content Outline
With Content Category Specifications
Federation of State Boards of Physical Therapy

Tests and Measures Group II: C. Cardiovascular/pulmonary System D. Integumentary System E. Functional Status/Community Integration	**7.5%**	**15**
1330 Tests and Measures C: Cardiovascular/pulmonary System 1331 Aerobic capacity/endurance 1332 Circulation (arterial, venous, lymphatic) 1333 Ventilation and respiration/gas exchange 1340 Tests and Measures D: Integumentary System 1341 Integumentary integrity 1350 Tests and Measures E: Functional Status and Community Integration 1351 Self-care and home management, including activities of daily living and instrumental activities of daily living 1352 Work (job/school/play), community and leisure integration or reintegration, including instrumental activities of daily living 1353 Assistive and adaptive devices 1354 Gait, locomotion, and balance 1355 Pain 1356 Ergonomics and body mechanics		
2000 Evaluation, Diagnosis, Prognosis, and Outcomes - Included are critical knowledge and skills related to integration of results of history, systems review, tests and measurements with the client's reported goals in order to identify relationships between pathology, impairment, functional limitation, and/or disability.	*22.5%*	*45*
Evaluation and Diagnosis	**11.5%**	**23**
2100 Identifying and prioritizing Impairments 2200 Determining the dysfunction toward which the intervention will be directed		
Prognosis and Outcomes	**11.0%**	**22**
2300 Determining the predicted optimal level of improvement in function and the amount of time needed to reach that level 2400 Determining the prognosis with consideration of modifying factors, eg, age, medications, co-morbidities, cognitive status, nutrition, social support 2500 Planning and sequencing patient interventions and progressing treatment based upon outcome 2600 Determining outcomes 2610 Collecting outcome data 2620 Determining discharge criteria based upon patient goals and functional status 2630 Differentiating between discharge of patient, discontinuation of service and transfer of care and re-evaluation 2640 Modifying tests/measures and interventions when necessary 2650 Recognizing effectiveness of PT interventions		
3000 Intervention - Include are critical knowledge and skills related to:	*41.5%*	*83*
Non - procedural Intervention	**7.0%**	**14**
3100 Coordination of Care, ie, knowledge of resources and coordination with team members (PTA, RN, OT, SLHP, SW, Psychology, etc), including appropriate referral or direction and supervision, as indicated **3200 Communication** 3210 Educating members of other healthcare disciplines regarding safe, effective patient handling techniques 3220 Conferring with members of other healthcare disciplines about the physical therapy plan of care 3230 Conferring with the patient/client and family regarding plan of care, interventions, and outcomes		

(*Continued*)

Physical Therapist Examination Content Outline
With Content Category Specifications
Federation of State Boards of Physical Therapy

3300 Documentation
3310 Documentation of objective, patient-centered, functional outcomes (goal statements)
3320 Objective documentation of examination, evaluation, diagnosis, prognosis, interventions, and outcomes
3400 Patient/Family/Client-related Instructions
3410 Utilizing teaching strategies, theories and techniques to achieve desired goals including consideration of variables that may require adjusting educational methods, eg, learning styles, communication deficits, cultural/language style, motor learning principles
3420 Educating the client/family about client's current condition/examination findings, plan of care and expected outcomes, utilizing their feedback to modify the plan as needed
3430 Providing and modifying same according to the client/family's needs

3500 Procedural Intervention - Included are critical knowledge and skills related to understanding and implementing the application of interventions. This includes the indications, contraindications, precautions and interactions related to the diagnosis for physical therapy and /or related to the intended activity	*34.5%*	*69*
Procedural Intervention Group I: Exercise and Manual Therapy	**13.5%**	**27**

3510 Exercise
3511 Aerobic capacity training/cardiovascular training
3512 Strengthening/muscular endurance
3513 Stretching/range of motion
3514 Neuromuscular re-education (including perceptual training)
3515 Balance/coordination
3516 Breathing
3517 Aquatic
3518 Postural
3519 Developmental
3540 Manual therapy
3541 Techniques, including spinal and peripheral mobilization, manual traction
3542 Techniques of soft tissue mobilization

Procedural Intervention Group II: Transfer and functional activities, gait training, assistive and adaptive devices and modification of the environment	**10.0%**	**20**

3520 Transfer activities and functional activities, including safety related to transfers
3521 Performing transfers
3522 Performing functional activities
3560 Gait training and use of gait assistive devices (normal/abnormal weightbearing status, common deviations, balance deficits, components of gait cycle)
3561 Performing gait-training techniques, including pre-gait activities
3562 Ensuring/facilitating proper weight bearing status
3570 Prescription, application and, as appropriate, fabrication of devices and equipment and environmental modification
3571 Adaptive devices
3572 Assistive devices
3573 Orthotic devices
3574 Prosthetic devices
3575 Protective devices
3576 Supportive devices
3577 Ensuring/facilitating proper weight bearing status
3578 Modification of environment for home/work/leisure activities

(*Continued*)

Physical Therapist Examination Content Outline With Content Category Specifications Federation of State Boards of Physical Therapy		
Procedural Intervention Group III: Physical agents and modalities, airway clearance techniques, wound care, promoting health and wellness (includes some components of non-procedural intervention)	**11.0%**	**22**
3530 Physical agents and modalities 3531 Intermittent compression 3532 Superficial thermotherapy, eg, hot packs, paraffin, and cryotherapy 3533 Ultrasound including phonophoresis 3534 Electrical stimulation including iontophoresis 3535 Biofeedback 3536 Mechanical modalities: traction, tilt table/standing frames, continuous passive motion 3537 Whirlpool/Hubbard tank 3550 Airway clearance techniques 3551 Breathing strategies, eg, coughing, huffing, and pacing 3552 Manual/mechanical techniques, eg, percussion, vibration, suctioning 3553 Positioning 3580 Wound care and skin integrity 3581 Skin status monitoring 3582 Patient positioning and use of adaptive/protective equipment for pressure relief 3583 Dressing application and removal 3584 Topical agent application 3585 Debridement technique 3586 Oxygen therapy 3600 Promoting health and wellness and prevention, including instructions and intervention		
4000 Standards of Care - Included are critical knowledge and skills related to:	**10.0%**	**20**
4100 Maintaining patient autonomy and obtaining consent for physical therapy evaluation and intervention 4200 Maintaining patient confidentiality 4300 Recognizing scope of physical therapy practice, including limitations of the PT role that necessitate referral to other disciplines 4400 Recognizing implications of research on PT practice and modifying practice accordingly 4500 Utilizing body mechanics/Positioning 4510 Body mechanics (utilize, teach, reinforce, observe) 4520 Positioning, draping, and stabilization of patient 4600 Considering the patient's cultural background, social history, home situation, and geographic barriers, etc 4700 Safety, CPR, Emergency Care, First Aid 4710 Ensuring patient safety and safe application of patient care 4720 Performing first aid 4730 Performing emergency procedures 4740 Performing CPR 4800 Standard precautions 4810 Sterile procedures 4820 Demonstrating appropriate sequencing of events related to universal precautions 4830 Demonstrating aseptic techniques 4840 Properly discarding soiled items 4850 Determining equipment to be used and assembling all materials, sterile, and non-sterile		

Questions for this chapter and the entire book appear on the included CD-ROM, with additional questions at www.DuttonNPTE.com.

Appendix

LABORATORY TESTS AND VALUES

Laboratory tests, which provide the clinician with insight into the physiological status of an individual, are tools helpful in determining a diagnosis when used as an adjunct to the patient history and physical examination. Laboratory tests can be used for screening, diagnosing, and monitoring patient health and disease.

The Centers for Medicare and Medicaid Services (CMS) of the Department of Health and Human Services regulate or laboratory testing (except research) performed on human beings in United States through the Clinical Laboratory Improvement Amendments (CLIA).[1]

The interpretation of a laboratory test result is made using a reference range for the age and sex of the patient which is the interval between and including below and up a reference limits. The interval is determined statistically by the assay of the analyte of interest in a selected population.[1] The range reflects the selected population only. The traditional reference range for quantitative test is the range of values of the central 95% of the healthy population.[1] Reference ranges are reported in the same units as the test result and depend on the method used.

The tables (Tables 1 to 6) that follow are intended for guidance only.

APPENDIX TABLE 1. INTERVENTION CATEGORIES

Therapeutic exercise may include performing:

A. Aerobic capacity/endurance conditioning or reconditioning:
   (1) Gait and locomotor training
   (2) Increased workload over time (modify workload progression)
   (3) Movement efficiency and energy conservation training
   (4) Walking and wheelchair propulsion programs
   (5) Cardiovascular conditioning programs
B. Balance, coordination, and agility training:
   (1) Developmental activities training
   (2) Motor function (motor control and motor learning) training or retraining
   (3) Neuromuscular education or reeducation
   (4) Perceptual training
   (5) Posture awareness training
   (6) Sensory training or retraining
   (7) Standardized, programmatic approaches
   (8) Task-specific performance training
C. Body mechanics and postural stabilization:
   (1) Body mechanics training
   (2) Postural control training
   (3) Postural stabilization activities
   (4) Posture awareness training
D. Flexibility exercises:
   (1) Muscle lengthening
   (2) Range of motion
   (3) Stretching
E. Gait and locomotion training:
   (1) Developmental activities training
   (2) Gait training
   (3) Device training
   (4) Perceptual training
   (5) Basic wheelchair training
F. Neuromotor development training:
   (1) Developmental activities training
   (2) Motor training
   (3) Movement pattern training
   (4) Neuromuscular education or reeducation
G. Relaxation:
   (1) Breathing strategies
   (2) Movement strategies
   (3) Relaxation techniques
H. Strength, power, and endurance training for head, neck, limb, and trunk:
   (1) Active assistive, active, and resistive exercises (including concentric, dynamic/isotonic, eccentric, isokinetic, isometric, and plyometric exercises)
   (2) Aquatic programs
   (3) Task-specific performance training
I. Strength, power, and endurance training for pelvic floor:
   (1) Active (Kegel)
J. Strength, power, and endurance training for ventilatory muscles:
   (1) Active and resistive

Functional training in self-care and home management may include

A. Activities of daily living (ADL) training:
   (1) Bed mobility and transfer training
   (2) Age appropriate functional skills
B. Barrier accommodations or modifications

(*Continued*)

APPENDIX TABLE 1. INTERVENTION CATEGORIES (*Continued*)

C. Device and equipment use and training:
  (1) Assistive and adaptive device or equipment training during ADL (specifically for bed mobility and transfer training, gait and locomotion, and dressing)
  (2) Orthotic, protective, or supportive device or equipment training during self-care and home management
  (3) Prosthetic device or equipment training during ADL (specifically for bed mobility and transfer training, gait and locomotion, and dressing)
D. Functional training programs:
  (1) Simulated environments and tasks
  (2) Task adaptation
E. Injury prevention or reduction:
  (1) Safety awareness training during self-care and home management
  (2) Injury prevention education during self-care and home management
  (3) Injury prevention or reduction with use of devices and equipment

Functional training in work (job/school/play), community, and leisure integration or reintegration may include

A. Barrier accommodations or modifications
B. Device and equipment use and training:
  (1) Assistive and adaptive device or equipment training during instrumental activities of daily living (IADL)
  (2) Orthotic, protective, or supportive device or equipment training during IADL for work
  (3) Prosthetic device or equipment training during IADL
C. Functional training programs:
  (1) Simulated environments and tasks
  (2) Task adaptation
  (3) Task training
D. Injury prevention or reduction:
  (1) Injury prevention education during work (job/school/play), community, and leisure integration or reintegration
  (2) Injury prevention education with use of devices and equipment
  (3) Safety awareness training during work (job/school/play), community, and leisure integration or reintegration
  (4) Training for leisure and play activities

Manual therapy techniques may include

A. Passive range of motion
B. Massage:
  (1) Connective tissue massage
  (2) Therapeutic massage
C. Manual traction
D. Mobilization/manipulation:
  (1) Soft tissue (thrust and nonthrust)
  (2) Spinal and peripheral joints (thrust and nonthrust)

Prescription, application, and, as appropriate, fabrication of devices and equipment may include

A. Adaptive devices:
  (1) Hospital beds
  (2) Raised toilet seats
  (3) Seating systems—prefabricated
B. Assistive devices:
  (1) Canes
  (2) Crutches
  (3) Long-handled reachers
  (4) Static and dynamic splints—prefabricated
  (5) Walkers
  (6) Wheelchairs
C. Orthotic devices:
  (1) Prefabricated braces
  (2) Prefabricated shoe inserts
  (3) Prefabricated splints

(*Continued*)

APPENDIX TABLE 1. INTERVENTION CATEGORIES (*Continued*)

D. Prosthetic devices (lower-extremity)
E. Protective devices:
(1) Braces
(2) Cushions
(3) Helmets
(4) Protective taping
F. Supportive devices:
(1) Prefabricated compression garments
(2) Corsets
(3) Elastic wraps
(4) Neck collars
(5) Slings
(6) Supplemental oxygen—apply and adjust
(7) Supportive taping

Airway clearance techniques may include
A. Breathing strategies:
(1) Active cycle of breathing or forced expiratory techniques
(2) Assisted cough/huff techniques
(3) Paced breathing
(4) Pursed lip breathing
(5) Techniques to maximize ventilation (eg, maximum inspiratory hold, stair case breathing, manual hyperinflation)
B. Manual/mechanical techniques:
(1) Assistive devices
C. Positioning:
(1) Positioning to alter work of breathing
(2) Positioning to maximize ventilation and perfusion

Integumentary repair and protection techniques may include
A. Debridement—nonselective:
(1) Enzymatic debridement
(2) Wet dressings
(3) Wet-to-dry dressings
(4) Wet-to-moist dressings
B. Dressings:
(1) Hydrogels
(2) Wound coverings
C. Topical agents:
(1) Cleansers
(2) Creams
(3) Moisturizers
(4) Ointments
(5) Sealants

Electrotherapeutic modalities may include
A. Biofeedback
B. Electrotherapeutic delivery of medications (eg, iontophoresis)
C. Electrical stimulation:
(1) Electrical muscle stimulation (EMS)
(2) Functional electrical stimulation (FES)
(3) High voltage pulsed current (HVPC)
(4) Neuromuscular electrical stimulation (NMES)
(5) Transcutaneous electrical nerve stimulation (TENS)

Physical agents and mechanical modalities may include
Physical agents:
A. Cryotherapy:
(1) Cold packs
(2) Ice massage
(3) Vapocoolant spray

(*Continued*)

APPENDIX TABLE 1. INTERVENTION CATEGORIES (*Continued*)

B. Hydrotherapy:
  (1) Pools
  (2) Whirlpool tanks
C. Sound agents:
  (1) Phonophoresis
  (2) Ultrasound
D. Thermotherapy:
  (1) Dry heat
  (2) Hot packs
  (3) Paraffin baths

Mechanical modalities:

A. Compression therapies (prefabricated)
  (1) Compression garments
  (2) Vasopneumatic compression devices
  (3) Taping
  (4) Compression bandaging (excluding lymphedema)
B. Gravity-assisted compression devices:
  (1) Standing frame
  (2) Tilt table
C. Mechanical motion devices:
  (1) Continuous passive motion (CPM)
D. Traction devices:
  (1) Intermittent
  (2) Positional
  (3) Sustained

APPENDIX TABLE 2. GUIDE FOR CONDUCT OF THE PHYSICAL THERAPIST ASSISTANT

A. Purpose.

1. This *Guide for Conduct of the Physical Therapist Assistant (Guide)* is intended to serve physical therapist assistant in interpreting The *Standards of Ethical Conduct for a Physical Therapist Assistant (Standards)* of the American Physical Therapy Association (APTA). The *Guide* provides guidelines by which physical therapist assistants may determine the propriety of their conduct. It is also intended to guide the development of physical therapist assistant students. The *Standards* and *Guide* apply to all physical therapist assistants. These guides are subject to change as the dynamics of the profession change and as new patterns of health-care delivery are developed and accepted by the professional community and the public. This *Guide* is subject to monitoring and timely revision by the Ethics and Judicial Committee of the Association.

B. Interpreting standards.

1. The interpretations expressed in this *Guide* reflect the opinions, decisions, and advice of the Ethics and Judicial Committee. These interpretations are intended to guide a physical therapist assistant in applying general ethical principles to specific situations. They should not be considered inclusive of all situations at a physical therapist assistant may encounter.

Standard 1

1. A physical therapist assistant shall respect the rights and dignity of all individuals and shall provide compassionate care.
   a. Attitude of a physical therapist assistant.
      1) A physical therapist assistant shall recognize, respect and respond to individual and cultural difference with compassion and sensitivity.
      2) A physical therapist assistant shall be guided at all times by concern for the physical and psychological welfare of patients/clients.
      3) A physical therapist assistant shall not harass, abuse, or discriminate against others.

Standard 2

1. A physical therapist assistant shall act in a trustworthy manner toward patients/clients.
   a. Trustworthiness.
      1) A physical therapist assistant shall always place to patient's/client's interest(s) above those of the physical therapist assistant. Working in the patients/client's best interests requires sensitivity to the patient's/client's and vulnerability and an effective working relationship between a physical therapist and a physical therapist assistant.
      2) A physical therapist assistant shall not exploit any aspect of the physical therapist assistant—patient/client relationship.
      3) A physical therapist assistant shall clearly identify him/herself as a physical therapist assistant to patients/clients.
      4) A physical therapist assistant shall conduct him/herself in a manner that supports the physical therapist—patient/client relationship.
      5) A physical therapist assistant shall not engage in any sexual relationship or activity, whether consensual or nonconsensual, with any patient/client entrusted to his/her care.
      6) A physical therapist assistant shall not invite, accept, or offer gifts or other considerations that affect or give an appearance of affecting his/her provision of physical therapy interventions.
   b. Exploitation of patients.
      1) A physical therapist assistant shall not participate in any arrangements in which patients/clients are exploited. Such arrangements include situations where referring sources in hand that personal incomes by referring to or recommending physical therapy services.
   c. Truthfulness.
      1) A physical therapist assistant shall not make statements that he/she knows or should know are false, deceptive, fraudulent, or misleading.
      2) Although it cannot be considered unethical for a physical therapist assistant to own or have a financial interest in the production, sale, or distribution of products/services, he/she must act in accordance with law and make full disclosure of his/her interest to patients/clients.
   d. Confidential information.
      1) Information relating to the patient/client is confidential and shall not be communicated to a third-party not involved in that patient's/client's care without the prior consent of the patient/client, subject to applicable law.
      2) A physical therapist assistant shall refer all requests for release of confidential information to the supervising physical therapist.

Standard 3

1. A physical therapist assistant shall provide selected physical therapy interventions only under the supervision and direction of a physical therapist.
   a. Supervisory relationship.
      1) A physical therapist assistant shall provide interventions only under the supervision and direction of a physical therapist.
      2) A physical therapist assistant shall provide only those interventions that have been selected by the physical therapist.
      3) A physical therapist assistant shall not provide any interventions that are outside his/her education, training, experience, or skill, and shall notify the responsible physical therapist of his/her inability to carry out the intervention.

(*Continued*)

APPENDIX TABLE 2. GUIDE FOR CONDUCT OF THE PHYSICAL THERAPIST ASSISTANT (*Continued*)

4) A physical therapist assistant may modify specific interventions within the plan of care established by the physical therapist in response to changes in the patient's/client's status.

5) A physical therapist assistant shall not perform examinations and evaluations, determine diagnoses and prognoses, or establish or change a plan of care.

6) Consistent with a physical therapist assistant education, training, knowledge, and experience, he/she may respond to the patient's/client's inquiries regarding interventions that are within the established plan of care.

7) A physical therapist assistant shall have regular and ongoing communication with a physical therapist regarding the patient's/client's status.

Standards 4

1. A physical therapist assistant shall comply with laws and regulations governing physical therapy.
   a. Supervision.
      1) A physical therapist assistant shall know and comply with applicable law. Regardless of the content of any law, a physical therapist assistant shall provide services only under the supervision and direction of a physical therapist.
   b. Representation.
      1) A physical therapist assistant shall not hold him/herself out as a physical therapist.

Standard 5

1. A physical therapist assistant shall achieve and maintain competence in the provision of selected physical therapy interventions.
   a. Competence.
      1) A physical therapist assistant shall provide interventions consistent with his/her level of education, training, experience, and skill.
   b. Self-assessment.
      1) A physical therapist assistant shall engage in self-assessment in order to maintain competence.
   c. Development.
      1) A physical therapist assistant shall participate in educational activities that enhance his/her basic knowledge and skills.

Standard 6

1. A physical therapist assistant shall make judgments that are commensurate with their educational and legal qualifications as a physical therapist assistant.
   a. Patient safety.
      1) A physical therapist assistant shall discontinue immediately any intervention(s) that, in his/her judgment, may be harmful to the patient/client and shall discuss his/her concerns with the physical therapist.
      2) A physical therapist assistant shall not provide any interventions that are outside his/her education, training, experience, or skill and shall notify the responsible physical therapist of his/her inability to carry out the intervention.
      3) A physical therapist assistant shall not perform interventions while his/her ability to do so safely is impaired.
   b. Judgments of patients/client status.
      1) If in a judgment of the physical therapist assistant, there is a change in the patient/client status he/she shall report this to the responsible physical therapist
   c. Gifts and other considerations.
      1) A physical therapist assistant shall not invite, except, or offer gifts, monetary incentives or other consideration that affect or give an appearance of affecting his/her provision of physical therapy interventions.

Standard 7

1. A physical therapist assistant shall protect the public and the confession from unethical, incompetent, and illegal acts.
   a. Consumer protection.
      1) A physical therapist assistant shall report any conduct that appears to be unethical or illegal.
   b. Organizational employment.
      1) A physical therapist assistant shall inform his/her employer(s) and/or appropriate physical therapist of any employer practice that causes him or her to be in conflict with the *Standards of Ethical Conduct of the Physical Therapist Assistant.*
      2) A physical therapist assistant shall not engage in any activity that puts him or her in conflict with the *Standards of Ethical Conduct for the Physical Therapist Assistant,* regardless of directives from a physical therapist or employer.

Data from Guide to physical therapist practice. *Phys Ther.* 2001;81:S13-S95.

APPENDIX TABLE 3. ACID-BASED STATUS TESTS

TEST	RELATED PHYSIOLOGY	REFERENCE RANGE EXAMPLE
Arterial Po_2	Reflects the dissolved oxygen level based on the pressure it exerts on the bloodstream	80-100 mm Hg
Arterial Pco_2	Reflect the dissolved carbon dioxide level based on the pressure it exerts on the bloodstream	36-44 mm Hg
Arterial pH	Reflects the free hydrogen on and concentration; collectively this test and the arterial Po_2 and arterial Pco_2 tests help reveal the acid-based status and how well oxygen is being delivered to the body	7.35-7.45
Oxygen saturation	Usually a bedside technique (pulse oximetry) to indicate the level of oxygen transport	95%-100%

Reproduced, with permission, from Wall LJ: Laboratory tests and values. In: Boissonnault WG, ed. *Primary Care for the Physical Therapist: Examination and Triage*. St Louis, MO: Elsevier Saunders. 2005:348-367.

APPENDIX TABLE 4. TROPONIN LAB VALUES

Normal	Troponin I (TnI): Less than 0.3 μg/L Troponin T (TnT): Less than 0.1 μg/L
Abnormal	Elevated troponin may be present with an injury to the myocardium. Blood levels of troponin typically rise within 4-6 hours after a heart attack, reach their highest levels within 10-24 hours, and fall to normal levels within 10 days.

APPENDIX TABLE 5. TOTAL **CREATINE PHOSPHOKINASE** (CPK)

Normal	Men:	55-170 IU/L
	Women:	30-135 IU/L
Abnormal	CPK levels generally rise within 4-8 hours after a myocardial infarction, peak within 12-24 hours, then return to normal within 3-4 days.	

APPENDIX TABLE 6. CPK-MB LAB VALUES

Normal	Less than 3.0 ng/mL (0% of total CPK)
Abnormal	CPK-MB is found in large amounts in the myocardium. A CPK-MB greater than 3.0 ng/mL may be present with muscle damage as a result of a myocardial infarction. Blood levels of CPK-MB typically rise within 2-6 hours after a heart attack, reach their highest levels within 12-24 hours, and fall to normal levels within 3 days. An ongoing high level of CPK-MB levels after 3 days may mean that a heart attack is progressing and more heart muscle is being damaged.

Questions for this chapter and the entire book appear on the included CD-ROM, with additional questions at www.DuttonNPTE.com.

REFERENCE

1. Wall LJ: Laboratory tests and values. In: Boissonnault WG, ed. *Primary Care for the Physical Therapist: Examination and Triage*. St Louis, MO: Elsevier Saunders. 2005:348-367.

Index

H

U

V